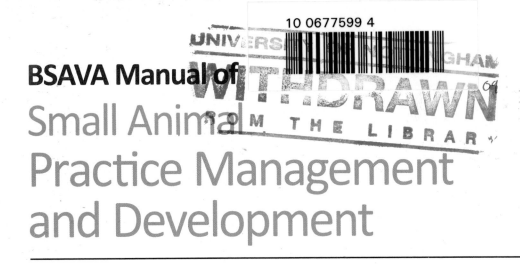

BSAVA Manual of Small Animal Practice Management and Development

Editors:

Carole J. Clarke
MA VetMB CVPM MRCVS
Mill House Veterinary Surgery and Hospital,
20 Tennyson Avenue, King's Lynn, Norfolk PE30 2QG

Marion Chapman
Elands Veterinary Clinic, St John's Church, London Road,
Dunton Green, Sevenoaks, Kent TN13 2TE

Published by:

British Small Animal Veterinary Association
Woodrow House, 1 Telford Way,
Waterwells Business Park, Quedgeley,
Gloucester GL2 2AB

A Company Limited by Guarantee in England
Registered Company No. 2837793
Registered as a Charity

Figures 16.6, 25.5 and 26.4 were drawn by S.J. Elmhurst BA Hons (www.livingart.org.uk) and are printed with her permission.

A catalogue record for this book is available from the British Library.

ISBN 978 1 905319 40 4

While the publishers, editors and contributors have used best endeavours to ensure that the information in this publication is correct at the time of publication, please note: (a) the information is general and educational in nature and is not intended to constitute a definitive or complete statement of the law on any subject, nor is any part of it intended to constitute legal advice for any specific situation; (b) the information may contain inadvertent inaccuracies and may over the course of time become incorrect or out of date; and (c) the publishers, editors and contributors cannot accept any responsibility for action taken as a result of information provided in this publication. You should take specific advice when dealing with specific situations. In addition, the publishers, editors and contributors cannot take responsibility for information provided on dosages and methods of application of drugs mentioned or referred to in this publication. Details of this kind must be verified in each case by individual users from up to date literature published by the manufacturers or suppliers of those drugs. Veterinary surgeons are reminded that in each case they must follow all appropriate national legislation and regulations (for example, in the United Kingdom, the prescribing cascade) from time to time in force.

Printed in India by Imprint Digital
Printed on ECF paper made from sustainable forests

Other titles in the BSAVA Manuals series:

Manual of Canine & Feline Abdominal Imaging
Manual of Canine & Feline Abdominal Surgery
Manual of Canine & Feline Advanced Veterinary Nursing
Manual of Canine & Feline Anaesthesia and Analgesia
Manual of Canine & Feline Behavioural Medicine
Manual of Canine & Feline Cardiorespiratory Medicine
Manual of Canine & Feline Clinical Pathology
Manual of Canine & Feline Dentistry
Manual of Canine & Feline Dermatology
Manual of Canine & Feline Emergency and Critical Care
Manual of Canine & Feline Endocrinology
Manual of Canine & Feline Endoscopy and Endosurgery
Manual of Canine & Feline Gastroenterology
Manual of Canine & Feline Haematology and Transfusion Medicine
Manual of Canine & Feline Head, Neck and Thoracic Surgery
Manual of Canine & Feline Infectious Diseases
Manual of Canine & Feline Musculoskeletal Disorders
Manual of Canine & Feline Musculoskeletal Imaging
Manual of Canine & Feline Nephrology and Urology
Manual of Canine & Feline Neurology
Manual of Canine & Feline Oncology
Manual of Canine & Feline Rehabilitation, Supportive and Palliative Care: Case Studies in Patient Management
Manual of Canine & Feline Reproduction and Neonatology
Manual of Canine & Feline Surgical Principles: A Foundation Manual
Manual of Canine & Feline Thoracic Imaging
Manual of Canine & Feline Wound Management and Reconstruction
Manual of Canine & Feline Ultrasonography
Manual of Exotic Pets
Manual of Ornamental Fish
Manual of Practical Animal Care
Manual of Practical Veterinary Nursing
Manual of Psittacine Birds
Manual of Rabbit Medicine and Surgery
Manual of Raptors, Pigeons and Passerine Birds
Manual of Reptiles
Manual of Rodents and Ferrets
Manual of Small Animal Fracture Repair and Management
Manual of Small Animal Ophthalmology
Manual of Wildlife Casualties

For further information on these and all BSAVA publications, please visit our website: www.bsava.com

Contents

Contributors

Caroline Jevring-Bäck BVetMed MRCVS
Kulladals Gård, Vellinge, Sweden

Chris Beesley FCCA
http://ChrisAndSusanBeesley.com

Susan Beesley
http://ChrisAndSusanBeesley.com

Amy Bowcott DipAVN(Surgical) RVN
Assistant Nurse Manager (Surgical), Willows Referral Service, Highlands Road, Shirley, Solihull B90 4NH

Marion Chapman
Elands Veterinary Clinic, St John's Church, London Road, Dunton Green, Sevenoaks, Kent TN13 2TE

Alison Clark CertEd TechIOSH HonMemBVNA RVN
Salus QP Health & Safety Services Manager, Salus House, 97a Main Street, Beeford, East Yorkshire YO25 8AY

Carole J. Clarke MA VetMB CVPM MRCVS
Mill House Veterinary Surgery and Hospital, 20 Tennyson Avenue, King's Lynn, Norfolk PE30 2QG

Stephen Collins BVetMed CertVC MRCVS
Southern Counties Veterinary Specialists (Cardiology), Forest Corner Farm, Hangersley, Ringwood, Hampshire BH24 3JW

Rita Dingwall MCMI CVPM
Group Practice Manager, Cinque Ports Veterinary Associates/Milbourn Equine Ltd

Mark Enright
Head of Salus QP Health & Safety (a division of Vets Now Ltd), Salus House, 97a Main Street, Beeford, East Yorkshire YO25 8AY

Peter Hundepool
Rotterdam, The Netherlands

Victoria S. Johnson BVSc DVR DipECVDI MRCVS
RCVS and European Specialist in Veterinary Diagnostic Imaging
Vet CT Specialists, St John's Innovation Centre, Cowley Road, Cambridge CB4 0WS

Margaret Keane MCIPD
HR Dept, Barclays House, Gatehouse Way, Aylesbury, Buckinghamshire HP19 8DB

Helen Kington CVPM DMS Cert(B&PS)
Practice Manager, Coach House Vets, Burlyns Ball Hill, East Woodhay, Newbury, Berkshire RG20 0NU

Alison Lambert BVSc MMRS MRCVS
Onswitch Ltd, Ground floor, South Suite, The Keep, The Old Barracks, Sandon Lane, Grantham, Lincolnshire NG31 9AS

Philip Lhermette BSc(Hons) CBiol MSB BVetMed MRCVS
Elands Veterinary Clinic, St John's Church, London Road, Dunton Green, Sevenoaks, Kent TN13 2TE

Geoff Little MVB MRCVS
The Veterinary Defence Society Ltd, 4 Haig Court, Parkgate Estate, Knutsford, Cheshire WA16 8XZ

Christine Magrath BVMS(Hons) FRCVS
The Veterinary Defence Society Ltd, 4 Haig Court, Parkgate Estate, Knutsford, Cheshire WA16 8XZ

Andy Moore FCCA
Moore Scarrott, Calyx House, South Road, Taunton, Somerset TA1 3DU

Bob Moore BVM&S DVM&S(hc) CVPM MRCVS
Somerset

Pam Mosedale BVetMed MRCVS
Chapel-en-le-Frith, Derbyshire

Roger Powell MA VetMB DipRCPath DipACVP FRCPath MRCVS
PTDS, Unit 2a, Manor Farm Business Park, Higham Gobion, Hertfordshire SG5 3HR

Pippa Reffold FCIPD, Diploma in Company Direction (IOD)
Pips1 Ltd, Business and Human Resources Consultancy (www.Pips1.com)

Deborah Roberts DipAVN(Surgical) RVN
Patient Care Supervisor, Davies Veterinary Specialists, Manor Farm Business Park,
Higham Gobion, Hertfordshire SG5 3HR

Maggie Shilcock BSc CMS
Anmer, Norfolk

Wayne Smith-Gillard BSc RVN
Chimera Consulting, 223 Alnwick Road, London SE12 9BU

Bradley Viner BVetMed MSc(VetGP) DProf MRCVS
The Blythwood Veterinary Group, Waterlane House, Sandy Lane, Northwood, Middlesex HA6 3HA

Jim Wishart DipM MCIM AssocCIPD FInstSMM
James M Wishart and Associates, Veterinary Management Consultants, PO Box 43, North Muskham,
Newark, Nottinghamshire NG23 6EJ

Foreword

This is not the first management manual from BSAVA: the first *Manual of Practice Improvement*, edited by Ian Hughes, was published in 1972; and a second edition was published in 1981, edited by my former employer Peter Fry. To pick that book up now and compare it with this new Manual exemplifies the changes that have occurred in the veterinary profession over the last 30 years but also demonstrates great insights into how practice would develop. The last book was 140 pages long, whereas this new BSAVA Manual is over 500 pages. The 1980s edition came at a time of great change when companion animal practice had emerged as a separate entity from large animal and mixed practice. Many of the topics from the original manuals remain instantly recognizable – 'Computers', 'Communications', 'Practice Finance' and 'The Pharmacy, Stock Control and Controlled Drugs' – but there is also much that is new.

The brief given to the editors was to produce a BSAVA Manual that supported practice owners and managers in improving the clinical standards of their practice through better design and management. This was no easy task. Rather than dealing with business and administration alone, the book shows how maintaining high standards of client and pet care within a framework of responsible management is the best route to sustainable and profitable practice and to team motivation and wellbeing. Carole Clarke and Marion Chapman have achieved a great deal and this Manual fulfils BSAVA's aims of improving practice 'through science and education'. I commend them for their hard work and dedication in producing this Manual.

I would also like to congratulate the authors for their practical approach to practice management, combined with a significant academic content. Reading the content I am confident that it has been written by experienced managers that have designed and built their own surgeries, managed veterinary staff, bought and used the equipment, and 'cleaned the floors'. The editors have scoured the profession for the best of both worlds – the practical and the academic. They have identified authors who have learned from their experiences, and translated this journey into a knowledge resource that will prove invaluable to anyone considering starting their own practice, becoming involved in management, or purely enquiring 'Why do they do it like that?'. The authors have carefully avoided the pitfalls of offering prescriptive advice – veterinary practices come in all shapes and sizes and this Manual has something to offer to each.

It strikes me that one thing hasn't changed through this technological revolution: in veterinary practice we remain at heart a caring profession and what we do is primarily motivated by doing the best for our patients and their owners. I am confident that this *Manual of Small Animal Practice Management and Development* will be on the practice bookshelf for many years.

Andrew Ash BVetMed CertSAM MBA MRCVS
BSAVA President 2011–12

Preface

In the area of veterinary practice, there is never just one way of doing things – in fact, get a group of vets and managers together and there will be as many opinions as there are people! This has become particularly evident as we have planned and edited this long-awaited new addition to the BSAVA Manual series.

This is not just a management book. Our 28 authors bring practical expertise from a variety of veterinary practices and businesses, and our intention has been to bring together ideas and guidelines that will be useful in improving and running your small animal veterinary business, whether you are working in an established practice, moving into a new role or just starting out.

As well as being a guide to setting up and improving practice premises, the first part of the book discusses each clinical area of the practice in turn – its design, equipment and maintenance, and the organization and management of the clinical and support teams. The second part covers communication and people management issues, including leadership skills and self-management, together with the ethical and legal framework within which we work. Thirdly, the business aspects of veterinary practice are explored, including planning, finance, marketing, the client experience and clinical governance.

This Manual is intended to be a daily source of information for veterinary surgeons and managers in companion animal practice, as an aid for all aspects of organization and delivery of clinical veterinary care. It will also be a useful resource for current and aspiring practice owners, practice managers (particularly if new to the industry), veterinary nurses, and vet and VN students; and will help support studies for the VPMA's VPAC and CVPM and the RCVS CertAVP. The Manual is expected to be the first port of call for practices preparing for RCVS Practice Standards Scheme (PSS) and VMD inspections, and will be of benefit to all practitioners wanting to improve their quality of service, premises and facilities, and the management of their clinical and support teams.

The book is intended for quick reference, with examples of forms, protocols and standard operating procedures (SOPs) which practices can adapt to their own situations and according to their specific requirements. As management information and legislation changes regularly (e.g. medicines, employment laws, health and safety regulations), readers are directed to external primary sources of information, particularly websites. Professional advice is strongly recommended in these areas.

We are very grateful to: all those who have provided images or allowed us to use images from their practice; the BSAVA Publications Committee and publishing team for their patience and enthusiasm for the project; and to family, friends and colleagues who have supported us over the past year, in particular our partners, David and Gordon, and Carole's sons Chris, Will and Nick, who have all been a great source of encouragement.

The first BSAVA *Manual of Practice Improvement* was published in 1972, with a revised edition published in 1982. Thirty years on, we hope that this completely new Manual will inspire and support a new generation of veterinary surgeons in their careers in small animal practice.

Carole Clarke
Marion Chapman
April 2012

Managing the planning and construction process

Jim Wishart

It would be difficult to overstate the potential value of well located, well presented and accessible premises to the image and promotion of a veterinary business. The premises should be seen as a major marketing tool, presenting the desired image in terms of professionalism, approachability, capability and value. The importance of creating a good first impression of the image of the practice is covered in detail in Chapter 27.

In this rapidly changing world people make decisions based on perceptions and impressions, as well as on personal recommendations. If veterinary premises are in a prominent location and well presented, this projects a positive image into the community. Easy and logical access, along with good off-street parking, adds convenience. The site and building are beginning to fulfil a number of the classic marketing requirements.

Most decision makers in veterinary practice will begin with an existing premises and site. Whether this location is owned or leased can depend on many factors. Where owned, the premises will almost always be the biggest investment involved in a veterinary business. Even with a leased building, the rent will be a major outgoing, at least equivalent to a mortgage on the property. As with any major outlay, the business should ensure maximum value for the investment. The premises are a vital component in the financial balance of the practice and any compromise could affect the whole business.

To allow the widest scope to consider the factors that impact on a location, the plot of land, and the planned premises, this chapter will focus primarily on developing a new site. This could be:

- A branch practice, where the security of continued trading at an established location remains
- A site on which to relocate an existing facility, with the original site continuing until the moving date
- A totally new start-up.

The chapter will also flag up implications for extending existing premises where the veterinary business is to continue during the construction phase. Such projects carry a whole new challenge in terms of coordination, communication, continuity and temperament. Whether a new build or a conversion, thorough planning is essential.

Development *versus* new premises

An existing location comes with some 'baggage', particularly if it is a long-term location for a long-established practice. The fact that the practice has been there for many years and '*everyone* in the town knows where it is' does not mean that it is well situated, that access is easy, or that everyone in the town really does know where it is. Often, a long-term location has seen piecemeal development over the decades, all slowly eating up the on-site parking, just when it has become a major client demand, and leaving awkward corners and spaces in the building. Eventually, the time comes when the realization dawns that the current site is no longer fit for purpose and the pull to stay must be resisted.

The traditional partnership-based model tends to go through phases, depending on the lifestages of the partners. If all the senior members are looking more towards retirement than expansion, younger members can become frustrated by the lack of drive in their colleagues. At the same time, the younger colleagues may have very limited investment resources, with large loans from when they bought into the practice and a big mortgage at home. Whatever the stage, however, it is well worth having a frank view of the existing site so that it can be judged within the overall business. Often, carefully planned reviews can make the partnership realize that change is overdue.

In Chapter 23 the process of SWOT analysis is discussed. This looks at the internal strengths and weaknesses of a situation – the aspects which can be altered – against the external opportunities and threats, which one may try to influence but cannot control. Undertaking SWOT analyses of the location, site, building, etc., can be a very useful tool to help arrive at priorities. SWOT analysis can also be used to determine facilities that are needed, such as the number of consulting rooms, internal facilities, and the RCVS Standards category it is planned to achieve, both now and in the future. This specification of requirements will be vital in the assessment of any potential new site.

Figure 1.1 sets out some of the more obvious reasons for development and alternative options.

Proposal	Reasoning	Alternative
Relocation	Existing building too small	Redevelop existing building
	Existing site too small	A relatively close branch to take some pressure
	Lease expiring	Renegotiate lease
	No parking	
Branch	Expand geographical coverage	Attract clients from further away to the existing facility
	Lower pressure on main base	
	Lease expiring	Renegotiate lease
	Develop new interest area (e.g. cats-only clinic)	

1.1 Reasons and options for development.

Each situation, however, has its own priorities and alternatives, and deciding on a goal can help maintain focus.

Professional support

Throughout any project veterinary surgeons are likely to require support from a variety of professions, from property agents to chartered engineers.

The building industry has a host of professional advisors, some with clearly recognized titles, such as architects, chartered surveyors and chartered engineers. In addition, there are many other professionals and advisors with less familiar job titles. As with *Veterinary Surgeon,* the terms *Architect, Chartered Surveyor* and *Chartered Engineer* are protected by law. However, architects work with architectural technologists and CAD (computer-aided design) technicians, who are often the ones who do the main design work. In consequence, there are 'architectural' firms that may be highly competent but do not employ actual architects but rather architectural technologists who, incidentally, have their own chartered institute. Likewise, the term 'surveyor' is only protected when it is 'Chartered Surveyor' but it does not necessarily mean that a surveyor without 'Chartered' is incompetent. This can cause confusion.

Other specialists may work on particular aspects, such as those specializing in veterinary design, or mechanical and electrical (M&E) consultants. Figure 1.2 gives a guide to the various professions that may be involved but, by the very nature of the subject, this list cannot be definitive.

Finding a site

Choosing an area

It would be very unusual to find a site exactly where one would like, so there is value in having some set-down priorities with clearly drawn boundaries of acceptance.

One of the best approaches is to buy a good street map of the area, preferably one which can be opened out flat to see the whole area as one. This will be a working document for scribbling notes on and for highlighting areas of interest. The map can be used to grade different parts of the area, highlighting zones

Development stage	Professions, job titles and roles	Aspects of role
Entire project	Project manager	Coordinates all aspects of a development project so that solicitors, agents, designers and other advisors are kept informed and to time
Site finding	Chartered surveyor/Estate agent Commercial property agent	Selling agent; search agent
Site assessment	Architectural consultant with veterinary design knowledge	To assess suitability for purpose. To review against LPA planning policies
Site valuation	Chartered surveyor (with local commercial knowledge)	Pre-offer condition survey. Valuation (possibly surveyor nominated by loan funder)
Legal searches	Solicitor	Legal conveyance
Initial ground investigations	Local authority building control officers	Good first step to assess likely ground conditions
Full site investigation (if required)	Chartered structural engineer	Ground stability; special foundations; dealing with problems
Premises design	Veterinary design consultant	Veterinary layout; room links; finish; installations
Structural design	Chartered structural engineer	Required calculations and design for large spans, some roof structures, support where walls removed, etc.
Heating, ventilation and electrical design	Mechanical and electrical (M&E) consultants	More complex ventilation and heating design; sometimes linked with electrical circuitry
Cost assessments	Quantity surveyors	Pre-contract cost estimates. (Often on larger projects.) Work stage valuation. Contractor estimators
Building control	Approved inspectors Building control officers (LPA)	Ensuring structure is built to comply with current Building Regulations

1.2 Some of the support professionals that may be involved in a veterinary development project, and their roles. (continues)

Development stage	Professions, job titles and roles	Aspects of role
Construction	Contract administrator	The professional who manages the construction contract on behalf of the employer
	Clerk of works	- A site manager, normally independently employed by the employer, to organize all the different trades, i.e. as opposed to the employer organizing everything themselves - On very large projects, the employer may use a clerk of works to monitor all activities on site, even where there is a main contractor in place - Another name for the contractor's site manager
	Site manager Site foreman (often promoted tradesman such as joiner or bricklayer)	Managing work on site for the contractor
	Contract manager	Contractor's employee that manages various sites and to whom the site manager/foreman reports

1.2 (continued) Some of the support professionals that may be involved in a veterinary development project, and their roles.

that match well with the practice's aspirations and ethos, which could be the preferred areas. Almost more important is to highlight the 'no-go' areas: those parts of the district it is proposed to avoid.

If the proposal is relocation, a pictorial view can help prioritize areas. If, on the other hand, the plan is to take pressure off an existing location by opening a branch, the client scatter will give some idea of areas where there is a minor nucleus who might move to a more convenient location.

A study of the practice database will be helpful to determine where clients reside. In city areas this can be done by analysing the postcodes of clients, using the first five characters, such as LS17 6. This will show the scatter of clients across the trading area. In rural areas, plotting the addresses more precisely is better, as the first five letters of a postcode may cover a very large area (e.g. NG23 6 is some 6 miles long and 2 miles wide).

A research tool often used is known as an 'S' survey. It happens that in most alphabetical listings surnames beginning with 'S' make up around 10% of the total. Plotting the location of, say, 2 in 10 of the 'S' surnames in a database therefore gives a representative sample of client locations. Plotting these on a map gives a useful pictorial image of a trading area. Some computer programs may be able to do this type of analysis, but the pictorial image on a street map makes it very real.

Agents and other options

When it comes to commercial sites and property there are commercial agents. Some agents will actually do some of the searching for the client, charging a finder's fee if they buy. These agents should know the local market, and the movers and shakers in that market. There may be companies or people who own land in the area which is not actively being promoted.

Many local authorities have some form of economic development department, separate from their Planning Department (see later), which holds lists of existing commercial land and sites within their area. Some also have a system for mailing updates to enquirers on a regular basis. In addition, there may be local or regional bodies linked to commercial development.

The Internet adds to the options, both for viewing properties on the books of agents and for searching for potential locations using one of the aerial mapping sites. In mature built-up areas, aerial searching is particularly useful.

It is also helpful to make a point of travelling every route looking for signboards, vacant plots, odd spaces, developers, developments and anything else of potential. Getting to know a locality well, and the characters in the market, may give rise to some surprising discoveries.

Whilst the dream may be a brand new building, it may be that untouched 'greenfield' sites do not exist. Even previously developed but cleared sites, known as 'brownfield', may be difficult to find. The only option may be to look at converting the existing building, or demolishing it to rebuild. The latter option would of course destroy part of the asset being bought and would need careful assessment. Conversions can work very well, though careful design is required to avoid or minimize any compromises that may need to be made regarding use of existing floor space, and costs can be high.

Site review

Armed with a specification of what is required, any potential locations that seem to meet the criteria can be reviewed.

Usable size

The size of a site is generally fixed and there is little that can be done to change that unless there is an option to take over an adjoining plot. If the site is too small there is little point in trying to compromise.

KEY POINT

The physical size of a plot of land and the usable size are two very different things.

Sites are advertised and sold in terms of their overall size; this may be in acres, hectares or square metres. Whilst this may determine the boundaries, it does not define the usable area.

- The access to the site may demand visibility 'splays' (Figure 1.3) at the entrance. Splays are tapering strips of land that allow a driver leaving the site a good view along the road and allow those on the road a chance to see any vehicle poised to leave the site. The size and length of a splay will be determined by the type of road, speed limit, and curvature. In some cases, there may not be sufficient site frontage to form the required splay. Vision splays can eat up a fair amount of land.
- There might be an area that cannot be developed because it would restrict visibility on the highway or position the building out of line with neighbouring properties.
- There may be a planning demand for landscaping to screen the building from public view – the last thing wanted – or to protect trees, hedgerows, etc. All affect the *real* size of the site in terms of development potential.

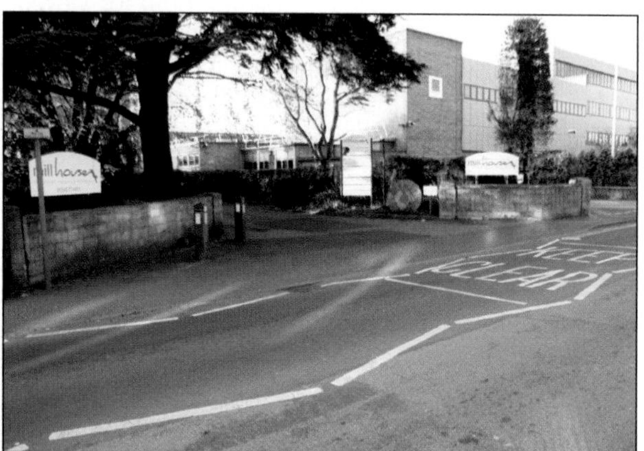

1.3 Although longstanding, these vision splays offer a view along the road for people leaving the practice, and a good view of the entrance when turning in. The bollards help protect pedestrians and the wall, and stop people thinking this is a parking bay.

Early review of the Local Plan is essential (see below), as is a visit to the local planning department to talk to the Duty Planners and then the Planning Officer, or team, dealing with the area around the site.

It may sound harsh but, if the building needed will not fit the site, taking into account the required number of parking spaces and other space, that is it. Trying to justify any shortfalls will only fool the justifier. Patience and persistence is the key.

Topography

Somewhat linked to size is the question of physical topography. This is the *lie of the land* in terms of slopes, contours, shapes and tapers. RCVS Practice Standards states that *premises must be accessible*. Just as important, so do the Building Regulations. *'Access for all'* is an often-used phrase, but it does create design challenges.

Sloping sites can be a real problem for ramps, which have a strictly controlled maximum gradient. Short ramps can be around 1:15 gradient but longer slopes may have to be gentler, with refuges (level resting places) after specified distances, which may be quite impractical.

Levelling the site could be an option, but at what cost? Earth moving, particularly if some volume of material has to leave the site, can be very costly, as can strongly engineered retaining walls.

Ground conditions and substructure

The very ground making up a site can have a host of natural factors which make for interesting construction. First, there is the soil structure and whether or not it is stable for simple strip foundations or whether it needs some engineering (see Figure 1.2). This is linked to the underlying geology and any potential for thin layers of soil before hitting rock. In addition, coal or old coal workings can be a problem.

A good source of early information can be the local building control department (see later), who may know the area well and should be able to flag up certain factors before contracts are signed. Ground conditions may add complexity to building costs by requiring a different approach to foundations. This would be advised by a consultant chartered structural engineer (see Figure 1.2).

Initial searches should reveal whether any of the utility companies have pipes, cables or pylons that cannot be moved. A gas main across the middle of a site can render it close to useless, whereas one along one side may be of little real consequence or even useful if it is the supply to the site.

Drainage

Of all the utility issues, the drainage question is both varied and vital. Ideally, there would be a main sewer to which the proposed premises can be connected, using gravity to carry waste to the drain. This is not always possible, however, and alternatives may have to be found. Most of these require an eventual ability for treated effluent to soak into the ground, or for effluent to be sufficiently treated that it is acceptable to join a watercourse. If the site is at the bottom of a hill, in a patch of clay, major problems may be encountered.

- Where mains drains are not available, a septic tank may be allowed. This is a chambered vessel where bacterial action helps neutralize the worst of the material and the liquid element is permitted to soak into the ground, in a soak-away or herringbone filter-drain. Some ground conditions are not suitable, or the authorities will not permit such limited treatment. The use of a septic tank alone is often difficult with current regulations, although some are still permitted.
- One step up would be some form of minor sewage treatment plant. This would have mechanical parts, and would need power, but gives a more effective treatment. The effluent can run into soak-aways or into a watercourse.
- On some sites, it may be possible to have a septic tank with the outfall passing through a reed bed, to purify the outfall further before it enters a watercourse (Figure 1.4). In such a situation, the reed bed could be turned into a feature, or at least add to the green credentials of the practice.
- If neither a septic tank nor minor treatment plant is acceptable, a cesspool is required. This is a large underground tank which collects the effluent which needs pumping out for disposal at regular intervals, possibly monthly.

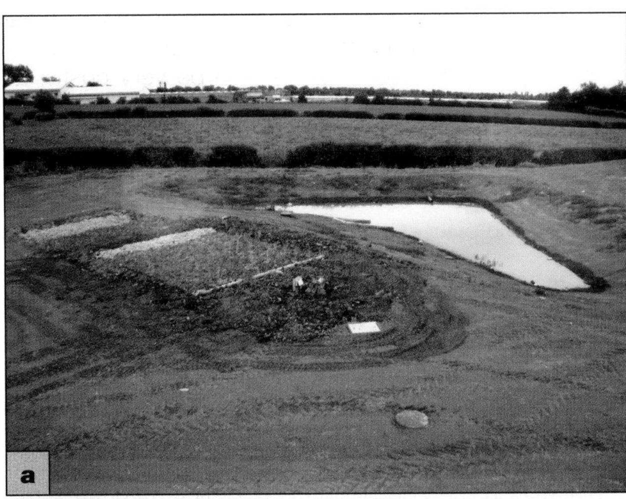

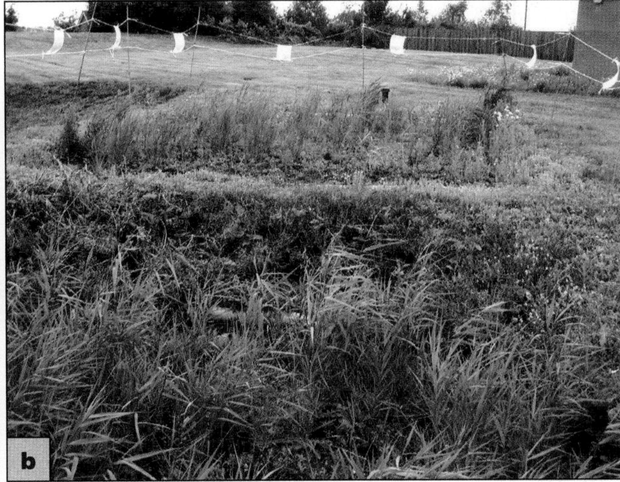

1.4 **(a)** This photograph, taken during the construction phase, offers a plan of the drainage system. The foul outflow from the practice drains into a septic tank (below the inspection chamber cover), with the outfall from that passing through a rectangular reed bed for further treatment. The treated water then drains into a balancing pond before discharge into a watercourse. **(b)** The reed bed a few months after planting.

Utilities

Water, gas and electricity are the other key utilities (see also Chapter 2). Checking out the cost of connecting these services to the site must not be overlooked. Sometimes the connection charges seem eye-wateringly large, particularly if the nearest main is a long distance away.

- Mains water can be an issue in terms of both availability and pressure. There may be an option of a borehole or other sources of potable water, which may be a cost-effective solution. Where mains water is provided, and water rates paid, some degree of rainwater recycling may be well worth considering.
- In many rural areas mains gas is not available and it is then necessary to opt for oil heating, liquid petroleum gas or some form of solid fuel.
- Electricity is often less of an issue to connect as it can be supplied on overhead lines. It is not, however, a low-cost power source, particularly for heating.

Archaeology

There can be few plots of land where anyone could really claim to be the first to dig into the ground. In known historic areas, planners may add a condition to any Consent that some degree of archaeological project is undertaken prior to construction. This can have huge costs, depending on the situation, and should be carefully checked at an early stage.

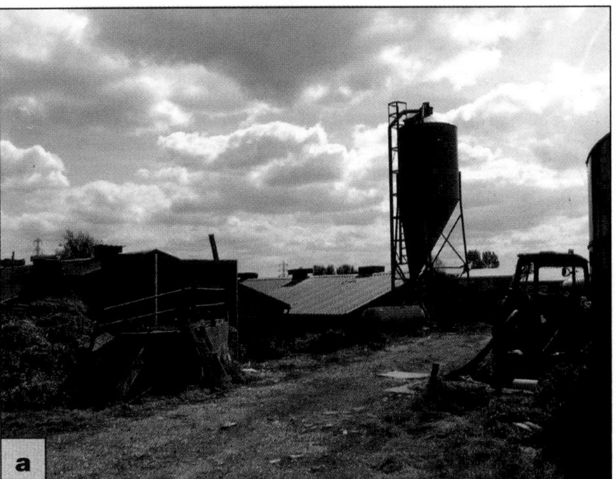

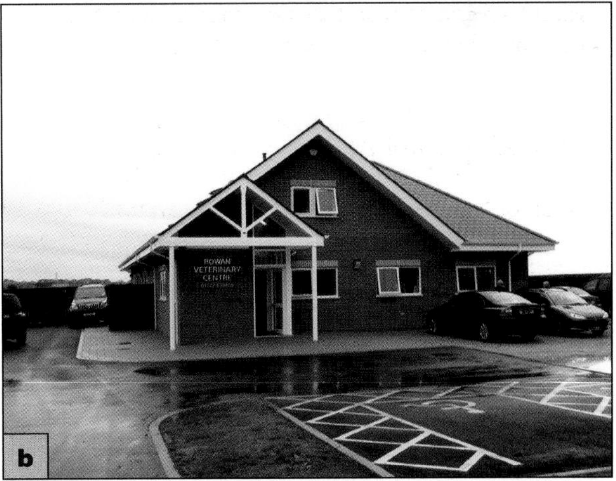

1.5 **(a)** A run-down pig and poultry farm that was purchased, demolished and decontaminated. **(b)** The finished relocation site.

Previous use

Sites that have been previously developed, whether they are formally termed 'brownfield' or not, can range from building in a garden to old industrial sites. An old factory site that is being regenerated may have been through a process of refurbishment to deal with any contamination. Other such sites may be left to the purchaser to clean up (Figure 1.5).

Fuel depots, gas works, tanneries, dye works, scrap yards and some garages can leave significant contamination, as can many sites that carried out chemical or industrial processes. Clean-up costs can be very high, sometimes more than the value of the land, so care must be taken when such risks emerge. Some sites would not be worth the investment in terms of environmental clean-up liability, whatever the purchase price. Frequently, contaminated sites can appear quite innocuous, until chemical analyses are undertaken.

Client perception

The idea of considering a site for likely client perception may seem odd – almost ephemeral – but it is hugely important. Many communities have areas that are considered less desirable, or a little bit scary at night. A building that looks like a Wild West jail, with bars at every window, communicates to visitors either 'this is a rough area, watch your back' or 'these vets don't trust us locals, look at their barricades'. Security is always better by design.

There is, of course, the opposite extreme, where the site is in an opulent area and, once built, the premises look over-palatial and vastly expensive. Images and perceptions are strange things, but need just as much consideration as everything else.

Planning Consent

It is essential to be aware of planning requirements at the very start of any development process. For the individual, there are two stages:

1. Planning Consent.
2. Building Regulations.

This process is set within some form of Local Plan produced by the Local Planning Authority (LPA) which, in turn, is written to fit within a national Government framework. As Governments change, so can the national planning framework.

The Local Plan

The LPA is required to prepare an overall plan of how it sees its area developing. The Local Plan gives details of agreed local *planning policies,* which are resolutions agreed by elected members regarding the development, or otherwise, of a local area.

This plan will designate areas as residential, industrial, food retail, non-food retail, etc. (see below). Some areas may be *Conservation areas,* where there is an aim to retain and restore the streetscape and character of that part of town. The Local Plan can be useful when deciding on the area of town in which to develop a new practice premises but, as veterinary businesses are the type of business acceptable in a residential area, the plan may also help gain some insight into the thinking of the local councillors and point to potential growth areas.

In addition to the Local Plan, the LPA may have *supplementary planning guidance (SPG)* information about how it expects certain developments to be progressed. This may include details of the approach taken in terms of design, materials, conservation areas, etc.

These plans can normally be found on the LPA's website or, for a small fee, a full copy can be purchased, with all the plans of the area. It is a useful easy document when planning veterinary premises within the jurisdiction of the LPA.

Land use classification

Within the Local Plan and planning law there is a shorthand system for classifying land use (Figure 1.6). This is designed to speed the planning process in that different uses within the same classification can change without a new planning consent. For example, shops within the A1 classification do not need to apply for *Change of Use* if a newsagents is taken over as a dress shop.

Not all businesses fall into neat classifications and 'Veterinary practice' is one such example. This is quite logical, as there is a very substantial difference

Class	Use/Description	Permitted changes
A1	Shops/Retail (broad general retail)	No permitted change outside classification
A2	Financial and professional services	A1 (with ground floor display window)
A3	Restaurants, Cafés	A1 or A2
A4	Drinking establishments (e.g. pubs, wine bars)	A1, A2 or A3
A5	Hot food takeaways	A1, A2 or A3
B1	Business (other than A2), R&D, Laboratories, Studios, Light industry	B8 (with size limit)
B2	General industry	B1 or B8 (size limit)
B8	Storage and distribution	B1 (size limit)
C1	Hotels, Guest houses (not care homes)	No permitted change
C2	Residential institution (e.g. hospitals, nursing homes, training centres)	No permitted change
C2A	Secure residential institutions (e.g. young offenders centres, secure hospitals, prisons)	No permitted change
C3	Dwelling houses	No permitted change
D1	Non-residential institutions (e.g. medical and healthcare, museums, libraries, training centres, places of worship)	No permitted change
D2	Assembly and leisure (e.g. cinemas, dance and concert halls, sports, outdoor leisure)	No permitted change
Sui Generis	Proposals not fitting into other classes (e.g. amusement arcades, motor vehicle sales, theatres, car/van hire, bingo and casinos, gymnasia)	No permitted change

1.6 Land use classification (England).

between a practice dealing exclusively with domestic pets and one with equine handling and surgical capability. All veterinary applications should fall within the catch-all class of Sui Generis, and the application taken on its individual merits. Planners, however, often seem to place companion animal practices into D1, the same as a medical GP premises. If looking to develop premises on land designated to another class, the Sui Generis card can be a very useful tool as it forces the LPA to treat the application on merit. The downside is that it may be unwise to sign up to buy a site with a designated use classification until a Change of Use Consent has been achieved. In some cases, the seller may be reluctant to wait until such consent is forthcoming without some contractual arrangement.

Planning application

This is the formal system whereby the LPA considers a proposal against planning legislation, the Local Plan, and various other parameters. This is to judge the impact on the community, the appearance, and the overall desirability in that location.

Outline Consent

In some situations, Outline Consent can be applied for. This carries a lower fee but only takes into account the concept, leaving many details to be dealt with at a further application stage. Outline Consent is sometimes appropriate where a large unit is planned and there is uncertainty about the chances of success of the proposal. However, it is not always appropriate and may leave planners, local Councillors and potential neighbours with little to see and a lot to imagine. With good prior communications with the Planning Officers, a full application is often more successful. *Outline Consent is not permitted for Change of Use applications.*

Planning Application pack

A copy of the Planning Application form, and guidance notes, can be downloaded from the website of the local LPA. In addition, it is now possible to do everything online, using the planning portal (www.planningportal.gov.uk). In the first instance, a copy and notes from the LPA site is probably the logical start for reviewing the requirements. A list of fees should also be downloaded to help with budgeting for this stage. Fees are based on a standard national system, which begins with a basic element but has additions related to the floor area being created.

The application form is set out for all developments, above the simplest domestic project. There are, therefore, sections that do not apply directly to a veterinary application. Those relating to traffic movements, employment and waste management do. There is also a range of standard questions on access, flood risk, the natural world, environmental factors, and such like. The practice may find itself involved with tree preservation orders (Figure 1.7), or may be required to conduct an ecological survey to determine the presence and status of rare, protected or endangered species such as owls, bats, nesting birds and great crested newts that may be on a potential project site.

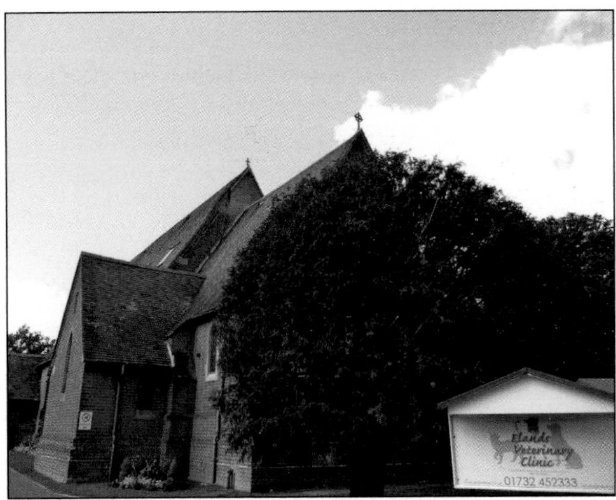

1.7 A tree with a preservation order (TPO) can block development and also needs consent for pruning, trimming or lopping.

In addition to the application form there are various supporting documents. Within the application pack there are certificates to sign such as declarations of ownership, or notice to owners, and one confirming whether or not the application site is an Agricultural Holding. The application must include:

- Site location plan, showing where the site is
- Site plan, showing the layout
- Block plan, showing parking, buildings, etc.
- All the floor plans, elevations and sections through the building, showing room heights, etc. (see Chapter 3).

Design and Access Statement (DAS)

One more recent addition is the *Design and Access Statement* (*DAS*). This is one of the *supplementary planning documents* (*SPDs*) now required, along with various other SPDs that may be specified in the planning guidance notes. The DAS is becoming increasingly complex but was originally intended as a 'talk-through' of what is planned, how it would fit within the local context, the approach to the design and covering access for all. CABE (Commission for Architecture and the Built Environment) have put out a guidance document on the subject of writing, reading and interpreting a DAS and this approach has been adopted by many LPAs. As well as the guide by CABE, the LPA often has an outline of what it expects in a Design and Access Statement. The key topics are shown in Figure 1.8.

In some ways, the DAS is the applicant doing much of the work the Planning Officers used to do. It does, however, involve working through the proposal and justifying it against the Local Plan. With veterinary projects, it also provides the opportunity to sell the project and overcome fears about noise, traffic and smells. As the DAS may be read by a wide range of people, from planners and elected Councillors, to potential neighbours who would like to find an excuse for the application to be turned down, the writing should be simple and positive.

Section	Topics for inclusion
Introduction	Always begin with a positive, but subtle, introduction about the proposal and how it will mark an advance in access to animal care and veterinary science
Context	How your proposals fit within the plan developed by the LPA. Note any relevant planning policies Note any relevant supplementary guidance notes
Design	How the size of the project fits within its setting How the scale of the 'built mass' has been managed The siting within the landscape, the layout and appearance The planned sympathy, or statement, within the community
Access	Note the factors relating to access (for all), covering public transport, cars, vans, lorries, bicycles – all within their context Practical aspects for all (ages, disability, ethnicity, or social groups)
Other	Outline any pre-planning consultations with the LPA, Highways Agency, the historic environment groups (Listed Buildings, etc.), Environment Agency, Parish Council, etc. The concept of local liaison and consultations can be very important, though commercial confidentiality may over-ride this! Particularly note factors such as trees, bats, great crested newts, nesting birds

1.8 Design and Access Statement topics.

Application validation

Once dispatched to the LPA, a Planning Application is *validated* to check that the correct fee has been sent and that all the right documents are included. Once validated, the clock begins to tick away. At times, validation is delayed due to the most minor issue. Classically, it is when one of the standard items is irrelevant, for example no overall site plan submitted because it is a rented shop with no outside ground.

Once the application has been validated, the applicant, or their agent, will be notified as to the Officer dealing with the application.

LPA consultations

The LPA has to send the application out for consultation to Parish Councils, Civil Trusts, the Highways Agency, and the like, as well as assessing the application against the Local Plan. It is a good idea to communicate with the Officer dealing with the application and to attend local Parish Council meetings dealing with the application. Whilst there is no legal right to speak at such meetings, the Parish Council Chairman may suspend the formal meeting and allow the applicant to speak, or respond to any concerns.

Contact with the Planning Officer will allow the progress of the application to be monitored. Where local objections have arisen, the applicant may be able to supply further information to overcome the concerns or to counter them if they are misguided or ill-founded. Attending LPA planning meetings can be very time-consuming and stressful. It is probably good advice to see how the contact with the Planning Officer goes.

If there are legitimate objections the application will go to a meeting of the Planning Committee of the LPA. The planners, however, must give a response within 8 weeks or they lose out in government sanctions.

With prior consultation with the LPA, study of the Local Plan and policies, along with any other guidance the hope is that the application submitted has been well thought out and is half-way to gaining consent. With the clock ticking away over the 8 weeks, and the first 4 weeks taken up by the LPA contacting other bodies, time is getting tight to counter problems, and it is wise to avoid a rejection and any 'black mark' on the file.

If, despite all the work-up, there is a fundamental factor which will cause the application to be refused, the best approach may well be to withdraw the application before it can be turned down. Hopefully, the applicant can redesign, reposition, or get positive information prepared and resubmit an adjusted application that the Planning Officer will back. There is no new fee for the re-application, as long as it is made within a set timeframe.

Decision Notice

Hopefully, if the application is good, the research thorough, and potential points of objection well covered, Planning Consent will be granted using powers delegated to the Officers of the Planning Department.

A positive decision will have conditions attached. A standard condition is that the project must begin within 3 years of the decision date. Another common condition relates to the fact that the building must be as presented on the drawings (giving their reference numbers) and the materials must be agreed with the Officer.

There may be other conditions relating to business hours, landscaping, car park bay marking out (Figure 1.9), etc. Some conditions may be very difficult such as 'no animals kept in overnight'. Planning departments often receive complaints about dogs barking at boarding kennels and it may be important to stress

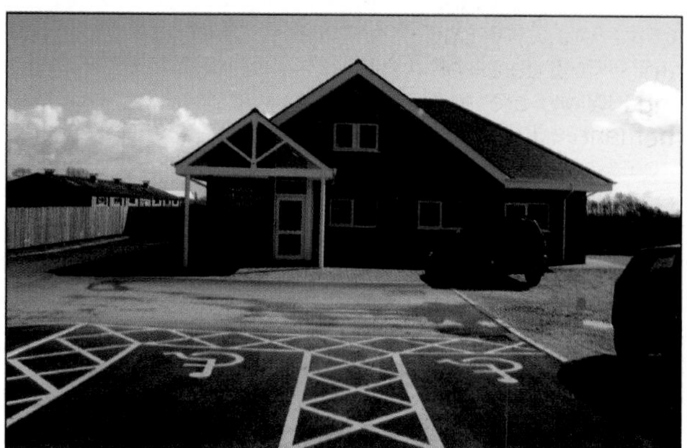

1.9 Car park bay marking, including of bays designated for disabled clients, may be a requirement of Planning Consent.

the difference between hospitalization and boarding, explaining that sick animals are usually quiet but that there may be night-time emergencies which need admitting. There is a world of difference between 'no animals housed overnight' and 'no animals housed overnight, except in an emergency'.

Building Regulations (Building Warrant in Scotland)

Entirely separate from Planning Consent is the matter of Building Regulations. This is when the design of the construction is judged against the *Building Regulations* (Building Standards in Scotland, leading to a *Building Warrant*). Like the Veterinary Medicines Regulations, the Building Regulations are covered by Parliamentary Statutory Instrument. This is where the detail of the design, the stair treads and rises, the doorways, the access, the structural components, insulation, energy efficiency, and all such technical things, are judged against the laid down requirements.

This is a major part of the project work-up and, if there is any level of doubt about gaining Planning Consent, it may be worth waiting until that is secured before investing in this area. If, however, there are *good signals* from the LPA, moving forward with these details will save some 8 weeks.

A veterinary development, or any commercial project, is quite different from domestic development. With a development at home, the home owner can instruct a builder as soon as they have planning consent. The home owner, or more often their builder, will serve notice to the Building Control Department of the LPA saying when they will start, and inspections will be carried out at key stages. The Building Control Officer will want to see the foundation footings, the foundations, and all the stages of development to ensure they meet the law. With commercial development, this route is not open. A Full Plans application has to be lodged for Building Regulations approval, which covers all the construction detail, any special foundations, and a host of other detail, like fire safety and the position of exit signs. Much of this is on the plan drawings but there may be separate calculations from structural engineers and reports from other investigations.

Whilst the planning application looked at pictures of the property, and talked of concepts, building control is the detail of the construction. With new buildings, there are a variety of other design and quality demands. Two, in particular, stand out.

- Within the design stage is the theoretical calculation relating to the **energy efficiency** of the building, rather as electrical appliances and heating boilers are rated. This is known as the Simplified Building Energy Model (SBEM – pronounced 'ess-bem'). The process involves the consideration of insulation, and other energy-saving factors, balanced against power used in heating, lighting, ventilation, etc.
- The **pressure test**. This comes right at the end of the build when the building should be close to hand-over. With all windows and doors closed, a special panel is placed to seal a doorframe and this has a fan which pressurizes the building. There follows a process of monitoring the loss of pressure due to air leakage from the building.

Traditionally, the Building Regulations application was submitted to the LPA, which had a building control department. This is still possible but this part of the market has become more competitive. Local authorities compete with each other to undertake building control inspections and, in addition, there are independent *Approved Inspectors* who may offer a more competitive service or better fit individual requirements.

Legal requirements regarding building structure

The partners or directors need to be in no doubt about legal responsibility. As the owners, or 'instigators', the law places huge responsibility on the owners or senior managers of any business, referred to as the Employer.

Asbestos

Asbestos can be found in many buildings and it is up to the owner to manage the risk (see Chapter 22). All types of asbestos were banned by 1999. This means that asbestos should not be found in buildings constructed after, say, 2000. In 2006 the various pieces of legislation were combined in the 'Control of Asbestos Regulations 2006' (see www.hse.gov.uk/asbestos) and certain terminology changed in 2010.

- There were many uses of asbestos apart from the corrugated asbestos–cement roofing sheets familiar on farm and factory roofs. Similar products were flat asbestos–cement sheeting, used for some prefabricated structures, along with a variety of flue pipes, fire boards and ceiling linings.
- Asbestos was also contained in some more surprising products, such as the thermoplastic floor tiles frequently laid in buildings with concrete floors and highly fashionable in the 1970s.
- Just as surprisingly, some textured ceiling finishes contained asbestos, as may old roofing bitumen.
- Far more worrying, however, is the asbestos found in lagging, fire-stopping materials and some packing. These were *fluffy* products, where the lethal fibres are sometimes clearly visible and can gain easy access to air. Similar material may be found in electrical components, switch gear and circuit boards.

The risk is in disturbing the asbestos. This could happen when drilling a hole to put up a cupboard, or during decorating. If identified, asbestos can be labelled so that people know to avoid it. At times it may be encapsulated behind some other cover. The important thing is to manage the substance; if buying or selling a commercial building, there must be an asbestos report available for the purchaser.

KEY POINT

Those managing buildings that could contain asbestos (the 'Duty holder') must ensure compliance with the law. The law places all responsibility on the building owner, or tenant, who needs to select the type of management required.

The simplest approach is to commission an independent asbestos surveyor to carry out a survey and undertake any sampling work. Unless about to undertake alteration work, this survey is a fairly modest one-off cost. This helps the practice comply with the law and gives the peace of mind that a specialist, who can recognize asbestos-containing products, has checked the place out, and the work is backed by the insurance policy of the surveyor. Until 2010 there were three tiers of survey but this has now been reduced to two (Figure 1.10).

Survey type	Survey outline and actions required	Pre-2010 name
Asbestos management survey	This is a first stage to see whether there is any asbestos in the premises. The survey undertakes to discover any asbestos-containing materials (ACMs). If an ACM is suspected, sampling is likely to ensure the type and management required. If there is no plan to alter the building, identified material can be noted and warning labels affixed	Types 1 and 2
Refurbishment and demolition survey	Full access, sampling and identification must be undertaken prior to disturbance. The results of this type of survey must be handed to any contractor undertaking refurbishment work on (or demolition of) the building. If asbestos is found, a specialist contractor will be required to remove it, and a clear air test proven, before the redevelopment work can commence	Type 3

1.10 Asbestos surveys.

As noted above, if a site is being considered that has existing structures, the seller, or their agent, should provide a current appropriate asbestos survey. If there is asbestos there, which has to be removed, a specialist contractor will need to be involved. They will have to serve notice on the Health and Safety Executive (HSE) when removal work is to begin so an officer can visit and check compliance with the strict removal methodology.

Construction (Design and Management) Regulations 2007

The Construction (Design and Management) Regulations (CDM) have been around for some time; 2007 is the current version. Their aim is to improve safety in the construction industry. Building sites are all different: the ground can be uneven; people can be working overhead, and drop things; and the place is under constant change. Health and safety is a constant concern, and systems have to be tight.

KEY POINTS

- When employing a firm to undertake construction work on your behalf, you are responsible for health and safety, as the employer.
- A notice (form *F10*) has to be sent to the HSE *before construction work begins*. This is normally dealt with by the CDM coordinator (see below).

Within the legislation, there is a requirement to have a named CDM coordinator on all but fairly short-term projects. That should be someone experienced in the role and, ideally, not employed by the contractor. Often, the appointment of the CDM coordinator can be discussed with the designer, as the regulations need to be considered at the drawing board stage.

The CDM Regulations are designed to apply to all types of project, including massive buildings with huge risks. Within that safety gamut are some really useful elements, such as making the designer, project manager, and contractor concentrate on safety. For many, the most useful tool of the CDM Regulations is the *handbook* which is put together at the end. This has all the plans, as built, along with instructions and leaflets for equipment installed, rather like the owner's manual for a car.

The construction phase

The construction phase (Figure 1.11) is the period when large sums of money begin to be spent. It is a time when changes of mind about the design, minor extras, and a lack of control can cause costs to run away. Options are detailed in Figure 1.12. In most cases a full specification by a designer with specialist veterinary knowledge should help avoid excesses. The full specification allows the project to go for some form of *fixed price* building contract, probably by tender.

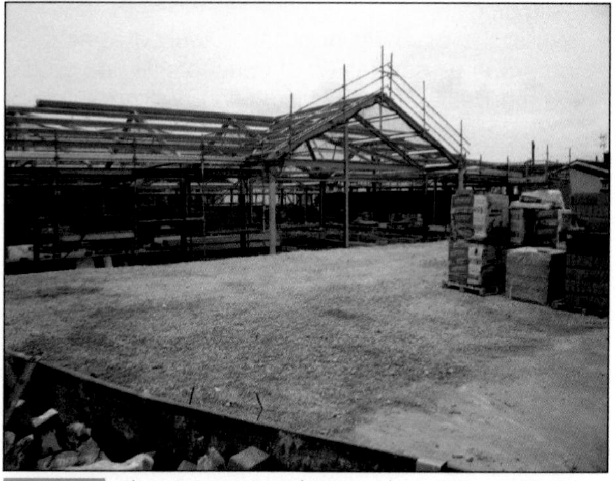

1.11 The construction phase is when costs can start to mount if changes are made to the original plans.

Options	Process	Comments
Organize the project oneself (act as Clerk of Works)	Working directly with all the various trades	Saves a 'contractor's margin' but time away from being a vet or practice manager likely to 'cost' far more. Difficult to judge quotes and estimates. Trades' coordination difficult: each trade will blame each other for hold-ups. Likely cost over-run. Almost certainly time over-run
Ask a favourite builder	Delegates sorting out the different trades. Known good and reliable firm can be asked for a fixed price quote	Could be a good option for small additions and alterations. Big risk of extra costs and disputes. No competitive pricing, so difficult to judge overall value. Design brief likely to be less exacting, so could have 'extras'
Design and build	Hand a lot of work to contractor, possibly with some loss of design control	Design and build firms not experienced in veterinary design. Difficult to know costs and value. Design rolled into construction costs and difficult to isolate. Logical to bring in an independent specialist to guide the contractor, even if adding to cost
Full specification and competitive tender	Get full design and specification developed before approaching contractors. Go out for tender to several firms to gain a competitive fixed price, all to the exact same specification	All stages costed independently. Full control of specification and compromises. Options to review price breakdowns to check quotes. Fixed price (with contingency). Overall project may seem to take slightly longer but more likely to offer better value and known completion date. Security in the competitive tender process (if well managed)
Developer	This is where a firm owns the land and builds the building; often linked to 'design and build' but with them also providing the site	May be the only way to develop preferred site (i.e. the developer will not sell the land separately). All the issues listed for design and build (above) will apply. Higher element of unknown value. Potentially difficult

1.12 The options that a veterinary practice has when facing a development project. These range from taking total responsibility, and risk, through various stages of delegation.

Construction contract

When it comes to major projects, it is vital to have some form of written agreement with the contractor. This will normally be dealt with by the Project Manager, whether architect, surveyor or specialist design firm. Within the UK there is a system known as JCT Contract. JCT stands for *Joint Contract Tribunal*, which was established in 1931. This provides a range of different contract structures for different types of construction projects. The most likely contract to be used is either the *JCT Minor Works, or Intermediate Works, Building Contract.*

Acknowledgements

The author and editors gratefully acknowledge the following practice, images of which appear in this chapter: Rowan Veterinary Centre.

References and further reading

HSE (2010) Asbestos: *The Survey Book*. (HSG264) Available from www.hse.gov.uk

Wishart J (2003) *Premises for Vets (Designing the Veterinary Habitat)*. Threshold Press, Newbury

Plant, utilities and systems

2

Jim Wishart

The bricks and mortar (or steel and concrete) are the cheaper part of any new building, and may account for much less than half the total cost. It is inside where budgets can run out of control if not carefully managed. Large costs are associated with installations (mechanical and electrical, M&E), including heating, cooling, ventilation and plumbing.

Beyond what might be called 'commodity installations' (gas, electricity, water), there are others associated with the veterinary business, in particular those linked to the data systems (telephone, computer) and peripherals (e.g. diagnostics, anaesthetic gas scavenging, fire detection and intruder alarms). In general these installations are considered separately from those of the plant room.

Whether planning a new building or retrofitting an existing practice, information technology should be considered early on in the project, as it has a key role to play in any modern business. This is especially true for veterinary practices, due to the huge range of data that must be handled and transmitted, from images (e.g. photographs, radiographs, MRI/CT studies) and video files (e.g. surgical procedures, endoscopy), to e-mail, Internet traffic, voice traffic (telephones) and possibly television. Data will also be generated by the practice management system. IT and telecommunications systems are considered in Chapter 4.

'Future proofing'

Whilst the overall structure seems fairly static, all installations have a degree of dynamism. Whether gas, oil, water or electrical, the installations all have a finite life. Upgrades and renewals are a constant factor in practice life and it can be useful if installations are accessible. In a factory, all these installations would be surface-mounted to make maintenance and uprating more cost-effective. Whilst this may not be completely acceptable in veterinary premises, and could make hygiene maintenance a problem, there is a level of compromise, and carefully planned design could help make upgrading simpler and help 'future-proof' the building.

Regulations

Along with this dynamism comes an element of risk, and there are a host of regulations covering virtually all installations. The supply of anaesthetic gases and radiological protection (see Chapter 13) are clear examples of where risks need to be accounted for. Additional problems come with aspects such as radioactive iodine suites, MRI scanners, and some other technologies. There can be many dangers, or latent dangers, in the variety of installations around any commercial premises. The law requires specifically qualified persons to undertake certain installations.

KEY POINTS

- All work to gas systems has to be undertaken by qualified engineers on the Gas Safe Register (has replaced CORGI).
- Electricians, must be 'Part P-Registered', part P being the Building Regulations section (England & Wales) dealing with electrical installations. Issues such as *PAT testing,* the inspection requirement for all portable electrical appliances, must also be considered as adding costs to the business.

Plant rooms

The complexity of installations can range from somewhere around that of a domestic property of similar size, to something resembling a 'pocket battleship' (Figure 2.1). Somewhere along the line, there can seem a big step from the domestic type of arrangement to that of a significant commercial enterprise. This step is the move from a utility area, with the heating boiler mounted on the wall, to a specialist 'plant room' to house the installations and the main controls (Figure 2.2). The advantage of a separate plant room is that all the main services and controls are in a dedicated area, which can be accessed away from clinical areas. Indeed, it is often useful to have access to the plant room from outside the building, with some form of wide doorway. This can be advantageous

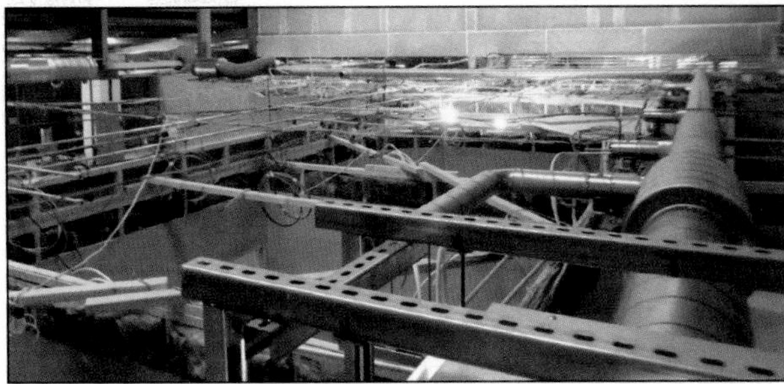

2.1 View of a mechanical installation.

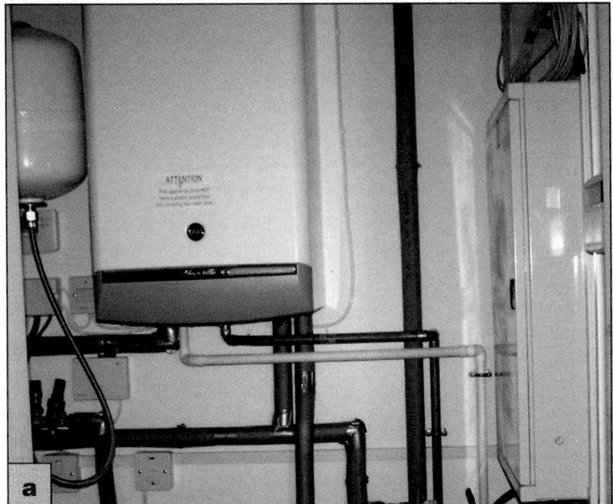

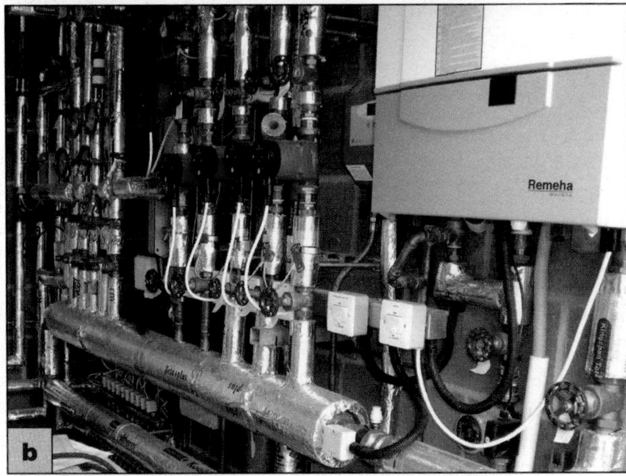

2.2 **(a)** A wall-mounted gas boiler in a small plant room. **(b)** A large plant room, showing the pipework for underfloor heating.

when large or heavy equipment, such as boilers or heat pumps, needs installation, or replacement. External access means that maintenance staff, or even breakdown engineers, cause minimum disruption to the workings within the practice. In addition, with limited access, unauthorized staff cannot access the controls.

> **KEY POINT**
>
> The vital factor is that the installations are fit for purpose and appropriate for the building, and that those managing the systems have the training and knowledge to be able to work all the controls correctly.

Energy efficiency and technological changes

The rise in energy costs over recent decades has concentrated minds within the heating and ventilation industries, leading to a constant stream of innovations. In addition, it has increased demand for insulation and energy efficiency within the Building Regulations. New ideas and concepts are coming to market which seemed out of reach not long ago.

Whatever is written here is expected to date rapidly. For this reason, it will concentrate on basic principles and the more traditional approaches. Innovative concepts will be covered in broad terms but, as the technology is in constant change, there is a need to undertake research at every stage. Most of the 'new' technologies are not all that new, as the basic processes have been known about for years. Economics, demand for alternatives, and governmental encouragement have brought these to the fore. The constant rise in energy costs is, without doubt, the main driving factor.

Although these new approaches to energy savings offer interesting options, it would be difficult to overstate the likely higher return from improving simple factors such as insulation. Heat rises; so loft insulation should be considered first, then cavity wall, followed by double glazing. Improving floor insulation is very difficult to achieve in an extant building and is normally a factor included during the build process unless major floor work, such as replacing a wood suspension floor, needs to be undertaken.

Energy costs are rising. As much energy in the UK is imported, the topic has become a major issue, with tighter controls on insulation and the efficiency of heating appliances. With new commercial buildings, there is the need to pass through the Simplified Building Energy Model (SBEM) assessment (see Chapter 1). This is a computer calculation relating to the energy consumption of a building and can get down to the level of balancing one light fitting with another to save a few Watts.

Energy sources

Energy options have remained similar for years, although some of the sources have broadened. The main options are:

- Mains gas
- Solid fuel
- LPG (liquid propane gas)
- Oil
- Electricity.

Solar power may be an option for pre-heating water, and for some electrical generation. In recent years, there have been many new sources of solid fuel, from twists on traditional coal-based sources to wood pellets and various other biofuels. There has been an even larger array of sources of electrical energy.

Mains gas

Mains gas tends to remain the most cost-effective energy source for space heating, at least in terms of the traditional sources. Most urban areas are linked to a mains gas supply, which offers low-cost installation and probably the most competitive range of boilers that can link to whichever internal heating system is desired. The management process with gas is close to automatic, in that the consumer does not have to worry about priming, fuelling and holding stocks. A very significant advantage, linked to the supply process, is that the gas is paid for after use, rather than buying up front as with oil, LPG and solid fuels.

Safety

Gas is explosive and needs qualified installation, careful management, and regular maintenance. There is an onus on owners of rented and commercial buildings to ensure that the gas system is safe for employees, tenants and other users. The Gas (Safety Installation and Use) Regulations 1998 deal with the requirements in residential and shorter-term leased commercial premises. Where employees are in practice accommodation, the residential elements will apply but, wherever staff are employed, there is a responsibility and liability to ensure gas safety. This will usually mean an annual inspection and safety check (see Chapter 22).

Solid fuel

Whilst there are many types of solid fuel, there is a common element of storage and higher management involvement which must be considered. Fuel needs to be stock-piled and the boiler may require more regular maintenance, even if there is some degree of automatic feed. In general, this leads to a larger plant area, housing fuel stocks and boilers, and more staff involvement. This is the type of fuel which, in many cases, would only be considered where mains gas is not available unless there is some exception, such as a ready supply of low-cost fuel.

LPG and oil

- Both LPG and oil have specialized containers located outside the premises: LPG has the option of exchangeable cylinders or a static tank, whereas oil has only the static tank option.
- LPG-powered boilers are similar to those used with mains gas, with some adjustments or modifications.
- Oil uses a far more expensive boiler which, where a veterinary application is considered, is less likely to be a small wall-mounted unit.

The balance, therefore, is between future fuel costs and initial installation costs. As both are petrochemicals, the expectation would be that prices would change roughly in parallel, although oil prices have proved to be more volatile. For years, running costs of oil have been lower but there is no guessing how this will pan out in the future.

New oil tank installations may need to be bunded (i.e. have internal storage capacity for the oil if the main tank fails) and must now comply with a complex range of regulations; there are several Internet resources to help with these. Dependent upon location, either the Control of Pollution (Oil Storage) (England) Regulations 2001 or the Water Environment (Oil Storage) (Scotland) Regulations 2006 will apply. Wales and Northern Ireland are exempt from these, but other legislation may apply. Security must also be considered as oil theft is not uncommon.

Electricity

The term *power* is taken to mean electrical power – the essential ingredient for light and communications in the modern world. Having a mains electrical supply to a veterinary site would seem essential, although there are probably some working with self-generation or local supply. In addition, there are probably many vets who would warm to the concept of being totally self-sufficient on all utility matters.

When considering power in veterinary practices it is advisable to install more 13 amp socket outlets than the projected power use would imply. Because many sockets are positioned for convenient access but are not constantly in use, and because much equipment carries a relatively low power rating, overloading a circuit is unlikely. All modern wiring systems have circuit breakers in them, but older installations may need upgrading where portable appliances are frequently used in a clinical setting.

In work areas it is important to consider proposed use and position of sockets. In wards, for example, power may be needed for individual patient care equipment, and also for heating and cleaning machinery. Sockets can be at a suitable height for purpose. Trailing leads can be avoided by locating sockets higher up, e.g. over cages, with wiring boxed in and wired to a fused spur or additional circuit breaker. Any trailing leads that are present must be kept out of patients' reach, and hooked up where applicable to ensure that socket wiring does not carry any weight.

KEY POINT

Sockets for cleaning appliances should be separate, and/or clearly labelled, so there is no risk of someone unplugging a vital piece of life-support equipment to plug in a floor scrubber.

The electrical power supply for domestic use is usually 'single phase'; a 'three-phase' supply may be needed for heavy motors and high-powered equipment. At the time of development or conversion of the premises, an assessment is needed to check that the power supply will be adequate. Some care is useful to communicate the likely loading on individual sockets around the building; electrical comfort cooling or air conditioning, certain diagnostic equipment (e.g. large X-ray generators), or a complex ventilation system may increase the power demand. It may be that a three-phase supply enters the building but the wiring uses only two of the phases to cover the power requirements.

Self-generation

Veterinary hospitals must be able to continue to function in the event of a power cut or other power failure, and most use some form of generator in such events.

Power sockets that link to the generator are indicated by colour (Figure 2.3). For years, self-generation meant a diesel-powered generator chugging away in an outhouse. Some were semi-automatic, starting up when switches were thrown and when power was required. This was the story for almost all areas away from a National Grid supply. Such a system would not be considered as attracting the *sustainable* tag but may still be found in certain locations.

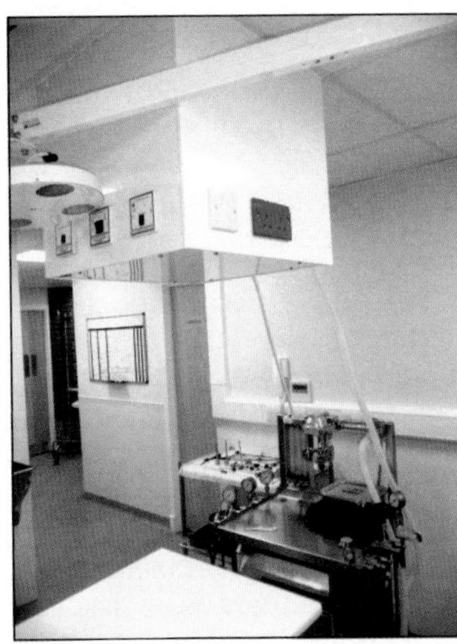

2.3 Red power sockets indicate the connection to generator power.

Today, the Government is committed to move towards a greater percentage of sustainable power generation as part of the International Climate Change and Carbon Control initiatives. These have, in effect, created a false market for power generated from sustainable sources, paying premiums to all those generating from sustainable sources. These premiums, known as Feed-in tariffs (FITs), vary depending on the sustainable power source. As more and more smaller users take advantage of the incentives, and lock themselves into premium payments, the levels of premiums are beginning to be reduced. There was a very high premium for electricity generated by photovoltaic panel (see below) but this is reducing. There is also a premium for generation through wind. The rather strange fact is that self-generators receive payment for every Watt they produce but gain most if they also use the power themselves. Hydroelectricity could be a really consistent sustainable source of electrical power, with a constant flow of sufficient water, but few veterinary practices will be in a position to exploit this type of option.

Wind power

Smaller units are receiving more attention from designers and may be a useful adjunct, although inland wind speed may not be sufficient or steady enough to make them effective. As well as the familiar unit, with aeroplane-style propeller blades, vertical axis models are being developed. These take up less room and may offer a more acceptable unit in many locations. Battery technology still needs to improve, however, and good independent advice is essential.

Solar energy

Originally, solar energy was limited to heating domestic hot water but solar power is changing rapidly. Panels can be of three types, one of which generates electricity.

Photovoltaic (PV) panels: To work efficiently, these need a south-facing position, with no risk of shadow, with an ideal backward slope of 30 degrees (Figure 2.4). The technology is developing rapidly and the feed-in tariff (FIT) is currently the highest of the self-generation options. Without an FIT premium, the technology would not be cost-effective, although it is hoped that encouraging usage and development will reduce costs over time. In the author's opinion, this technology is far more suited to south-facing sites in southern Europe, and good insulation and the management of power usage will prove far more cost-effective in the long run

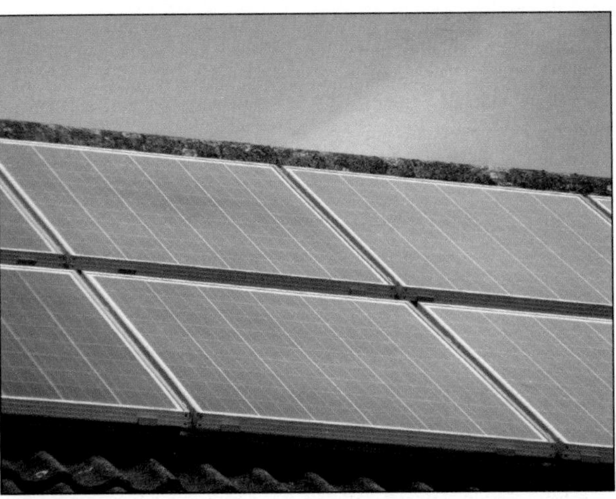

2.4 Photovoltaic panels can be used to generate some electricity.

Water heating: There are two options in solar water-heating panels; both absorb heat from the sun into water (or antifreeze) held within the pipework, and this is then pumped through a coil in a standard type of hot-water cylinder, pre-warming the water within. This reduces the cost of heating the water. One option is the flat-panel, a fairly sophisticated design of pipework within a specifically designed housing with a glass or plastic front face and a highly insulated backing; this is the modern incarnation of the original black panels, which were a little like central-heating radiators fixed to the roof. A more advanced system is the 'evacuated tube' system (Figure 2.5): within the housing are glass tubes with a vacuum inside. The process is the same, but the evacuated tubes are more efficient at absorbing energy. Again, this system links to the hot water system to transfer heat.

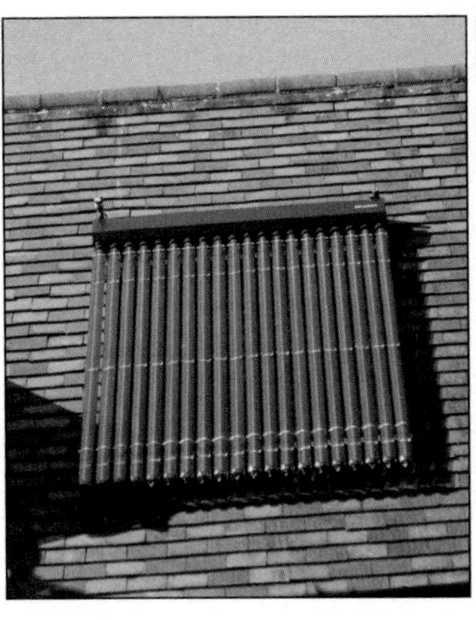

2.5 Evacuated tube solar panels used for water heating.

Water

Water is an obvious essential, and gaining a mains supply can be a very substantial cost factor if the location is some way from the nearest suitable point. As well as the actual supply, there are the issues of quantity and pressure. A normal domestic-type supply may not meet the needs of a larger veterinary building with many water outlets. An early assessment should be made. It may be impossible, or impractical to get a water main to a particular location, which could rule it out as a development site. There may, however, be the option of a borehole, natural spring, or other form of private water supply to overcome the problem.

In the UK, along with most developed countries, the water coming out of the mains supply is 'potable', i.e. fit to drink, even though only a tiny fraction of usage is for drinking or food preparation. Recycled water will be considered separately below; this is often termed 'grey water' but that is a rather too broad and generalized a term.

Water meters are generally fitted to any new build, so water-sparing appliances should always be considered to minimize costs.

Water regulations

These are designed to maintain the quality of supply and to avoid contamination. In the wider sense, water regulations extend to the countryside, with rules on muck spreading, activities near watercourses, above aquifers, and so on. This is to maintain the quality, or stop the contamination, of run-off and groundwater, which may end up in the mains supply.

As regards the mains water supply, the property owner does not need to concern themselves too much until the supply pipe leaves the water meter, often in the public footpath just outside the site, and crosses on to private land. Beyond that point responsibility is clearly with the owner or tenant. This includes leakage which, with a metered supply, is charged. The first that may be known about a leak could be a very large bill.

Private water supply

With a private supply from a well, borehole or spring or via a shared private distribution system, new regulations came into force in January 2010 (The Private Water Supply Regulations 2009). These regulations fall mostly on the local authority and are based on knowledge, risk assessment and recording. There is a 5-year introductory process and a key element would appear to be to record where private supplies exist, what they are supplying, and how they are being managed.

Water supply (water fittings) regulations

As potable water arrives in the premises, these regulations are designed to stop the installations within a building contaminating the public main through any backflow of contaminated fluids. There are a range of similar regulations in England and Wales, Scotland, and Northern Ireland. The basic theory is that, if there were to be some catastrophic failure in the water main, it could create a potential vacuum. This could suck water from end users' properties back into the main water supply. If water had become contaminated, once delivered to the premises, there is a risk that the contamination could be drawn back into the main supply to later contaminate other end users. In this risk-based world, various potential contaminated water situations are grouped together and classified into five categories: as the contaminated water is not potable, these are termed 'fluid categories' (Figure 2.6).

KEY POINT

In veterinary situations, washing machines, some X-ray developers, tub tables or shower areas with a shower head and certain hose-based systems will need to comply with Fluid Category 5.

Most fluid categories can be dealt with using a 'back flow' preventer in the water feed. These devices, however, are not considered secure enough for Fluid Category 5, when a type AA (Figure 2.7) or AB water

Category	Description	Examples
1	Wholesome water supplied by a water undertaker (water company)	Water supplied direct from the supply pipe (main)
2	Water which would be in Category 1 but for its aesthetic quality being impaired owing to a change in temperature, taste, some odour, or appearance	Hot water supply
3	Fluid which represents a slight health hazard because of the concentration of substances of low toxicity, including any fluid that contains: ethylene glycol, copper sulphate or similar chemical additive, or sodium hypochlorite (e.g. common disinfectants)	Water in primary circuits and heating systems (with or without additives) in domestic premises, e.g. fluid in central heating systems
4	Fluids which represent a significant hazard due to the concentration of toxic substances, including any fluid that contains: chemical, carcinogenic substances or pesticides or environmental organisms of potential health significance	Commercial clothes-washing machines (excluding those used for laundry contaminated with animal or human fluids or waste)
5	Fluids representing a serious health hazard because of the concentration of pathogenic organisms, radioactive or very toxic substances, including fluid which contains faecal material or other human waste, butchery or other animal waste or pathogens from any other source	'Grey water' recycling cisterns; medical equipment with submerged inlets; a cistern which also receives recycled process water; a hose union tap used in an abattoir or mortuary

2.6 Water regulations: fluid categories.

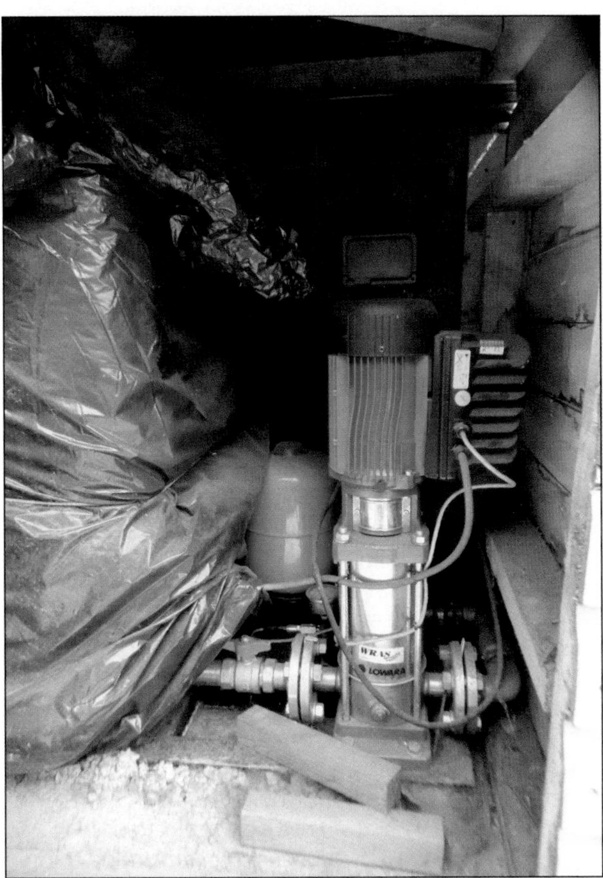

2.7 A type AA water gap system for a ground floor. Mains water enters the lagged tank (left) through a ball valve, providing the air gap. The pump then feeds water to the building at a similar pressure as would be expected from the main.

gap is required. This, in essence, requires a separate water tank to feed these items. Water from the main must flow into the tank, with the inlet discharging far enough above the water level in the tank for there to be no risk of siphoning. The overflow, which is referred to as the warning pipe, has to be large enough to take the full-flow volume of the inlet pipe.

The tank can be situated on the first floor or in the attic. Where, however, the veterinary facility is all on one floor, relying on gravity, with a simple header tank, is not an option. The only approach is to have a ground floor cistern with a pumped feed to the installations. Pump noise must be considered if close to working areas. Where type AA or AB air gaps are required, it is not that difficult, in two-storey buildings, to fit a separate water cistern, with the appropriate gap, somewhere on the first floor, to feed specific equipment on the ground floor.

Alternatively, many commercial washing machines have a built-in AB water gap, as do some more expensive domestic-style models; the technical information should be checked before purchase. Other approaches can be to keep hose fittings to a length that cannot leave the end in contaminated water. This includes tub tables with shower heads where the plug can be removed. Mains-fed X-ray developers can be replaced by models that are manually filled with water, and not connected to the mains.

Water authority inspections are routine in many areas, and non-compliant practices will be served improvement notices.

Water softeners

Hard water leads to limescale, which reduces both the efficiency and life of all systems/equipment using water, from kettles to heating boilers. The solution will depend on local conditions, and advice.

Traditional water softeners remove the calcium and magnesium that causes the limescale. They are expensive installations and require regular filling with salt. This means that the water system has to be split, with untreated outlets for drinking water, and the rest for cleaning, laundry, etc. Salt-using systems can be used in particular problem areas if that is the advice for a system. There are now, however, electronic systems; these fit around the rising main and set up a magnetic field that, although not removing the elements which cause limescale, seem to retain them in suspension within the water, at least for a time, which appears to stop limescale forming. Independent advice is recommended from an experienced plumber or water engineer.

Water safety

Whilst there is a tendency to take for granted the fact that the water arriving in the mains is safe, what is then done with it can have a range of health and safety implications. These risks link to a host of government regulations and statutory instruments. Most issues, however, can be overcome by the initial design of the water systems within the property.

Legionellosis

Legionnaires' disease, a potentially fatal disease, is just one of a range of conditions caused by various *Legionella* species. Whilst often associated with larger hotels, offices and institutions, it is not exclusively a problem of size but of systems and temperatures. Although they can survive in low temperatures, *Legionella* bacteria thrive in a water temperature range of 20–45°C, particularly if there are suitable nutrients such as scale, rust, sludge and algae. The problem is often linked to water tanks, little-used pipe runs, showers and sprays, since the bacteria are spread via inhalation of contaminated water droplets. In general, most veterinary buildings can be designed to avoid conditions where *Legionella* would thrive; for example, direct water systems with no storage tank; stored hot water kept above critical temperatures (60°C). Mechanical and electrical designers, and plumbers, are well versed in the risks and prevention of legionellosis.

KEY POINTS

- Stored hot water should be kept at a temperature higher than that at which *Legionella* can thrive.
- All shower heads and outlets should be clean and free of limescale.

Recycling water

As with alternative energy sources, the options for recycling water are advancing all the time. Interestingly, at least in country areas, this is a return to old systems. Houses fed by a well, in hard-water areas, often had 'soft water tanks' feeding a hand pump in the house; these were rainwater recycling tanks gaining their supply from the roof. There is a simple economic balance between the cost of commercial water rates and the payback on investment for rainwater recycling. Many installations use 'harvested' rainwater for flushing toilets, laundry, and similar uses. As most veterinary practices are likely to find the largest water consumption to be laundry, this alone may well give a valuable payback. As with soft-water tanks, the rain collects in an underground storage tank and is then pumped into the building. This may be to a header tank for a gravity feed, or through a pumped system. Most modern installations have a water main adjunct, which will supply the tank to a minimal level if there is no rainfall for a period.

Space heating

There are various options when it comes to heating a veterinary building, some are familiar and easy to manage, and others can be technically more involved and, therefore, need more consistent management.

Except in the most unusual of circumstances, the direct use of mains electricity is likely to be the most expensive source of energy for space heating. However, in relatively small premises, where mains gas is not an easy option, electrical heating may be a very useful solution. This could be night-storage systems or, more probably, one of the modern flat panel or convector systems. The lower cost of installation may well prove useful, particularly where short-term leases are involved, or where there is need for greater flexibility on heat control. It is interesting to note that most of the modern budget hotels use wall-mounted convector heaters, linked to room thermostats. As a heat source, however, electricity has been involved in some of the newest areas of technology such as heat pumps (see below).

Even in the depths of winter, most people will have experienced the power of winter sun creating a warm spot, either in a sheltered 'sun trap' or with heat through a windows. Sunshine, through glazing, on to a solid structure like concrete or masonry, can create a heat storage unit; a kind of 'day storage unit'. With new design, depending on the site, it may be possible to harness some of this thermal energy to directly heat the fabric of the building.

Central heating

Although sometimes misused, the term 'central heating' refers to systems where there is a single source of heat for a whole building, with the created heat being transferred around – either as warm liquid (normally water) or warmed air. With some buildings, it is suggested that having two heat sources can offer security and flexibility. This may mean having two smaller boilers, linked together, which gives some security should one fail. An alternative is to have one boiler for space heating and a separate boiler for hot water. The advantage may be that the space heating can be off most of the summer, and the building just runs with the hot-water boiler. There could, of course, be some blend of these two options. In general, however, in terms of installation cost, a single boiler is likely to offer better value.

Heat pumps

Both ground-source and air-source heat pumps work by transferring, and boosting, heat from one area to another. This is the reverse of the way in which a refrigerator works: that extracts heat from inside the unit and releases it into the room via the built-in heat pump and fins at the back. With space heating, the heat pump takes heat from the ground, or outside air, boosts it, and releases it to provide warmth inside.

Air-source heat pumps are very like an air-conditioning (comfort cooling) system working in reverse. The external unit, which appears reasonably similar to that for an air-conditioning unit, extracts heat from the outside air. The system seems quite miraculous, as it can extract heat from sub-zero temperatures, which seems to defy logic. There are, however, limitations when the external temperature crashes, such as in the winter of 2010/11, as many systems were found wanting at around –10°C.

Ground-source heat gathers warmth from the earth. It is said that 2 metres down the temperature is constantly 10°C. This is not quite true but it is a general guide, and it is certainly below the frost level. To gain the heat, the system uses underground pipes, either in a coil spread out in trenches running over a large area, or by using a borehole or piles. The latter is good where space is limited. Where the ground conditions are suitable, the former option is probably less costly if there is a large area, such as a car park, where the coil trenches can be left undisturbed. Liquid (often an antifreeze solution) is pumped through the underground pipework to pick up the background 'heat'. It continues through the heat pump, which boosts the temperature to a usable level. This has the potential of being a useful system if there is a consistent underground temperature, particularly when linked to a low-temperature heating system, such as underfloor heating (see later).

In general, both heat pump systems can be considered as new forms of electric central heating, using the ground, or outside air, as a type of storage system. Both systems are dependent on electrical power and require careful costings.

Water-filled radiators

The most common space-heating system in domestic and medium-sized commercial buildings uses the familiar water-filled radiators. The water is heated by a boiler and is then pumped around the pipes and radiators to warm the premises. Particularly where mains gas is available, this can be a highly efficient system. Other heat sources, including air-source heat, oil, solid fuel and LPG all end up working in similar ways.

One disadvantage of water-filled radiators is the radiators themselves. They take up space where it may be needed for positioning something or where people may wish to sit or stand, and they can be onerous or difficult to keep clean. Although this can be overcome with careful planning, and some localized alternatives, there will still be rooms where the heating system can be restrictive. The great advantage is that water-filled radiators do the job, are of relatively low cost, and prove highly reliable.

Underfloor heating

Run as central heating, with a central boiler and underfloor water-filled pipework, the system works at a much lower temperature than radiator heating. Keeping in mind the facts that the system provides even heat over the whole floor and uses the building fabric as a heat store, and then adding the simple science that heat rises, this system has distinct advantages whilst retaining the benefits of the single heat source.

In terms of installation costs, the underfloor pipework makes it only really practical for new buildings or for very major refurbishments when the floor is replaced. The pipe network will confirm the requirement of a dedicated plant room (see Figure 2.2b). Where budgets allow, the advantages are likely to outweigh the installation costs. Space will be gained as wall surfaces become available. As a low-temperature system, underfloor heating is the ideal if ground-source heat is to be considered.

Underfloor heating can also be run on electricity. Whilst there may be some efficiency advantage against other electrical systems, the fact that electricity is a costly power source probably makes this option unattractive.

Blown air

This was a popular system in domestic and office premises some years ago. Whilst as a *raw* system it has fallen out of favour, it has evolved into the full air-conditioning system found in major buildings and shopping malls. The challenge, when moving air around, is to avoid drying the atmosphere and to maintain a pleasant working environment. One problem can be fan noise, which needs to be kept to a minimum. In addition, there is always the challenge of removing pathogens from the air.

Localized heating

The advantage of localized heating systems is that the heating can be applied only where required. There is a huge range of localized heating options that may be suitable in veterinary premises. Many of these are electric but there are gas-fired and oil-based systems which may be used in some situations.

Whilst there may be systems which are technically more efficient, many practices find it fits their requirements to have an overall central heating system, working on a timed basis, plus some localized heating to target warmth out of hours. A good example is an isolation ward, where out-of-hours heating is only needed if there is an out-of-hours incumbent.

When designing or upgrading a central heating system, it is necessary to consider how the building will be used, and to install separate controls for inpatient areas where heating may need to be kept on overnight, and for areas where temperatures may need to be kept higher than in reception or outpatient areas. In traditional radiator or underfloor water-based systems, area heating can be controlled by thermostats and timers on different circuits, and also by individual radiator thermostatic valves for maximum efficiency.

In addition, there may be places where heating is only needed occasionally. A plant room may not normally need heating but there may be logic in having a supplementary heater, linked to a frost-stat, to ensure there are no winter freeze-ups. A practice with some mixed work may have somewhere which is only really used, say, at lambing time. Here, instant infra-red heaters may be superb when that late-night caesarean comes in during frosty weather. A similar situation could exist where a small animal practice has an unheated area where they carry out post-mortem examinations. Apart from some electrical panel or convector heaters, wall-mounted fan heaters and infra-red strips might be considered.

Where possible, some level of integrated heating system should be more efficient, in terms of energy usage. This, however, must be balanced against the initial cost and payback period.

Ventilation, air movements and cooling

Natural ventilation

In terms of inpatient safety, the options of opening a window for ventilation may not exist in many rooms within clinical areas. It can be possible, however, if windows are fitted with mesh screens, similar to the flyscreens found overseas. Many, if not most, double glazing systems can be fitted with such screens, often sliding sideways. In a move to a 'greener world', this may become a much preferred option, and there is something special about a slight natural breeze rather than a fan-forced input. However, many practices may not want even this level of risk.

There are now a number of firms developing natural ventilation systems with sophisticated design approaches. Heat rises, and if low-level inputs allow air in, to be pulled through by warm air extracted at a higher level, the basis of a good natural system may be found. A great deal of development is being undertaken regarding natural ventilation and design to create the right airflow through a building. This tends to be a specialist design area and may carry a slight premium but is worthy of consideration at the very start of a project. If the payback is a building that does not need to expend money on electrical power used by air conditioning, comfort cooling or powered fans, it could well be a wise investment.

Air movement systems

In many veterinary premises that have evolved with time, the issues created by warm humid summers may not create a need for air conditioning, more for a greater supply of fresh air. However, there are likely to be inner rooms with no natural ventilation, so the option of a simple extractor in the wall does not exist. Moreover, if air is 'dragged' from a room, using an extractor, how is the lost air replaced? It may be logical to draw the air from adjoining corridors but there will still be a need to deliver fresh air and remove stale air.

One area where drawing air through from adjoining areas proves useful is in consulting rooms. Using in-line extraction, where the electrical fan is some distance away, and incoming air is drawn from a shared supply passage, good ventilation can be achieved whilst still being able to hear a weak heartbeat.

There are various approaches to achieving this, including fairly simple systems where air is pulled through, using ducted extractors to remove stale air whilst vents in doors allow a flow of air from other areas. This does rely, however, on an adequate air supply coming in.

As the ventilation system develops, there can be a move to fully integrated systems with air-handling units which pre-heat incoming air, possibly using the warmth from the air being extracted. Heat exchangers may be used in the system and the whole process can become very sophisticated and quite complex. Whilst some of the most complex systems offer high levels of efficiency, their installation costs can make them less attractive. There is then a balance in terms of investment and payback. What is proposed may have superb energy savings, at least on paper, but the payback may take 25 years or more and the maintenance costs are difficult to judge. With very large projects, the use of mechanical and electrical consultants may be well worthwhile.

Having logical air changes is the basis of good ventilation (Figure 2.8). Whether this is managed by some electromechanical system, or by natural means, does not matter to the effectiveness of the system.

Biosecurity considerations

As with any medical building, not all the air can be recycled or re-used, due to the unwanted risk of pathogens being drawn through the building.

- For isolation and recovery areas, air can be drawn in from other parts of the practice, such as corridors, but the air inside should be extracted directly to the exterior of the building. A slight negative air pressure is required within these areas, so that air is unlikely to be drawn into the rest of the building when a door is opened.
- To a large extent, this approach should be considered for all wards, as surgical cases could well be admitted with latent infectious conditions, and levels of expired anaesthetic gases may be significant.
- Areas such as dental suites also need negative air pressure to protect colleagues from inhaling airborne particulates blasted into the air space.
- In contrast, operating theatres, particularly the main sterile space, should have positive air pressure in them, so that any air flows out from the theatre.

Creating positive and negative pressures does not have to be a drama. Good extraction from a preparation area, with air inlets in the theatres, will create this airflow. The trick with simple systems is to have some external filtration on air inlets. If the prep area has

Area	Ventilation rate	Comments
Waiting area	10 litres per second per person	General area with no specific demands
Consulting rooms	12 litres per second per person	Normally based on three people. Need quiet extraction, probably with ducted system with distant fan. If individual (through-the-wall) fan, recommend some form of manual override to switch off to listen to weak heart, etc.
Supply passage, shared dispensary	6 air changes per hour	General area, no specific issues
General wards	6 air changes per hour	Slight negative pressure ideal with extraction to outside air, though can be ducted system drawing off other areas. Not linked to lights so it can be kept on overnight if patients hospitalized
Isolation ward	6 air changes per hour	Negative pressure with dedicated dirty extract straight to outside air. Not linked to lights so it can be kept on overnight if patients hospitalized
Dental theatre/area	10 air changes per hour	Negative pressure with dirty extract direct to outside air. Useful if extractor can be close to main descaling point
Operating theatres	10 air changes per hour	Positive pressure. Filtered (ideally pre-heated) air drawn in from outside
Preparation area	8–10 air changes per hour	Good general extraction but could be ducted drawing from several areas
Laboratories	6–15 air changes per hour	Depends on activities. Most veterinary premises probably at the 6–8 level
Toilets	6 air changes per hour	Dirty extract, direct to outside air
Other examination and diagnostic rooms	8–10 air changes per hour	Good general extraction but could be ducted drawing from several areas
Dog washing/high moisture	15 air changes per hour	Good general extraction but could be ducted drawing from several areas
Office	10 litres per second per person or 6–8 air changes per hour	Whichever is the greater
Staff rest room	8–10 air changes per hour	Good general extraction but could be ducted drawing from several areas
Staff bedrooms	2–4 air changes per hour	Ideally opt for natural ventilation unless an inner room

2.8 Ventilation requirements for different areas of the practice. These figures are presented as a general guide. Advice from ventilation engineers is helpful where comfort cooling or air conditioning is included.

good extraction, this may be sufficient to create the right pull-through from theatre and avoid more costly solutions. The alternative is to have some form of air-handling unit (AHU) drawing in clean air and pre-heating it before it is passed into the theatres. The pre-heating can come from the central heating heat source, or can be a separate arrangement.

Cooling

If the only air available from outside is already rather warm, some form of 'comfort cooling' may be desirable. Consulting rooms, dispensary/pharmacy areas and offices with computing equipment all benefit from air conditioning to keep the area comfortable.

KEY POINT

Cooling may be more of a challenge than heating in areas where equipment, dogs and people generate significant heat.

Maintenance

Regular maintenance and cleaning of air grilles and fan units is essential. Routine attention with a vacuum cleaner, to remove surface dust, is useful; filters, grime and fan blades should be deep-cleaned to the manufacturer's recommendations by a competent person.

Lighting

There are two very important aspects linking to decisions on lighting.

- Lighting, temperature and ventilation are closely linked ingredients in overall comfort. This is not just for staff, but visitors and patients as well.
- Adequate general background lighting is essential, as the variation in patients and potential problems with restraint mean that localized task lighting will not always be in the right place at the right time.

Light levels

Compared with most artificial light, daylight is massively brighter. Somehow, however, as darkness falls, people are able to accept a far lower level of light than during the day. When interior light levels are discussed, the light level is measured when there is no daylight to enhance the artificial light being measured.

Light levels are measured in lux (though 'candle-power' is sometimes used). The lux scale ranges from shades of darkness, at around zero, to direct sunlight at around 100,000 lux. At night, a lit suburban street is unlikely to break 10 lux, while a large theatre light, at one metre from the source, could be matching daylight.

The basic need in veterinary practice is the light level itself, measured at working height. The type of light, however, is also important, both the tonal element, and the degree of focus. Although the essential light level is set at examination table height, the table position may need to be moved to accommodate large pets and family, so general light levels must be good for the entire room. 'Daylight' tubes are now much more cost-effective and can improve both the feel of the environment and the accuracy of colour rendering. It is usually possible to change the tubes in a standard fluorescent fitting for daylight ones.

Dimmable lighting

One item that has become available in the last decade or so is the dimmable fluorescent fitting. The ability to dim lights in imaging areas is vital, and these fittings allow good control within a low-energy unit. It is also useful to be able to dim the lights of patient wards at night, but retain enough light for visual supervision through a viewing panel in the door. Veterinary surgeons and nurses doing their rounds can observe, but not disturb unless there is concern. In the past, night-lights, in the form of bulk-head fittings with low-wattage bulbs, were fitted as a secondary system. This did work well but added to the wiring and installation costs. Dimmable fluorescents, whether strip lights or compact units, cover both uses with a single light unit. For existing installations, fitting an additional dimmable circuit can be an option.

Lighting for specific areas

Lighting requirements for a range of areas within the practice are shown in Figure 2.9; see also chapters on specific areas.

Surgical areas

In the surgical situation, the theatre needs to be generally bright and shadow-free. A level of around 1000 lux offers good light to flood the room. The critical area is that of the operating table, so light should be calculated at around 900 mm above floor level, and fairly centrally in the room. Focused surgical lighting can supplement this with directed cold light of around 15,000 lux, for some procedures, and closer to 100,000 lux for others. To gain good basic shadow-free light, one simple approach is to use an open square of fluorescent lights (Figure 2.10); whether 1200 mm or 1500 mm singles or doubles will depend on various factors. An electrical contractor, or the supplier, can calculate the lighting requirements from the light levels set.

Examination areas

The four-square approach can be useful wherever bright shadow-free light is required. In the consulting rooms, illumination of around 1000 lux should be concentrated over the examination table, with good light at floor level; this may be achieved by two parallel fluorescent units.

All areas where animals are to be examined in any detail need a high level of light and this may rule some locations out as good for examinations. However, most clinical work areas need to be bright, and lux levels of 500–1000 may be useful in many areas of the practice. Some electricians may advise that this seems high (and it is), but they are not undertaking the examinations, so it is important to insist on sufficient lighting.

Area	Light level (lux)	Comments
Waiting area	300	Warm white
Consulting rooms	500–1000	1000 at examination level
Supply passage, shared dispensary	500	
General wards	300	Dimmed for night to 100 or less
Isolation ward	300	Dimmed for night to 100 or less
Dental theatre/area	500–1000	1000 at dental table level
Examination light	15,000	At 1 metre from examination point
Operating theatres	1000	Four-square fluorescent layout for shadow-free lighting
Theatre light	<100,000	At 1 metre from incision
Preparation area	500–750	Possible additional examination lighting
Laboratories	500+	<1000 for colour inspection – daylight white
Other examination and diagnostic rooms	500	General
	1000	Examination level
Radiography and scanning	500	Dimmable
Toilets	300	
Office	300–500	
Staff rest room	300	
Staff bedrooms	100	General
	300	For reading

2.9 A general guide to lighting requirements for different areas of the practice.

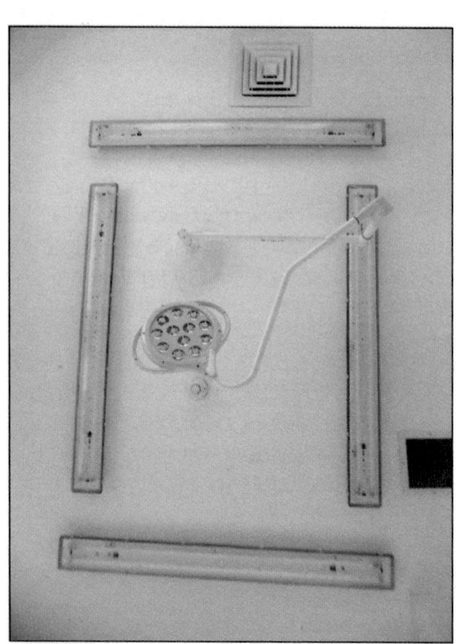

2.10 Theatre ceiling lighting: four fluorescent strip lights set in an open rectangle with a surgical light (LED 100,000 lux) mounted in the centre.

Waiting areas

There are conflicting demands for lighting within the client waiting area. Beginning outside, there is little worse than approaching a building, looking inside, and not being sure if the place is open or not. Inside, focused lights may be desirable over the reception counter, without glare on screens. Further focused lighting may be wanted on displays, noticeboards and sales items, but a warmer and more comforting light could be kinder where clients sit and wait (Figure 2.11). Whilst fluorescent tubes offer good light elsewhere, they may prove somewhat harsh in the waiting room, unless shielded in some way.

Low-energy lighting has come a long way in recent years and there is a vast range of options now available. Wall-mounted uplighters offer a softer lighting option in seating areas and flood the wall with light.

In the same way that LED (light-emitting diode) technology has produced excellent surgical and examination lights, the technology has advanced into downlights and other units. Although still quite costly,

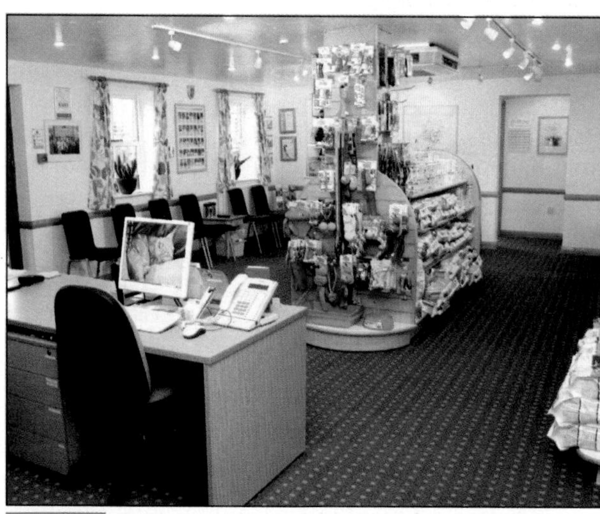

2.11 In this reception area low-energy downlighters over the seating areas are combined with directable halogen spotlights to create a warm feel, with focused lighting on the pictures and stock displays.

there is no need to put up with those little downlights where at least one bulb seems to blow every week. The latest range of LEDs offers good light, low power use, and a life to last towards a decade. The unfortunate thing about LED lighting is that there is a very broad range working upwards from the lowest bargain basement units, which are quite poor, to some really excellent products.

Emergency lighting

Building Regulations stipulate required emergency lighting to enable safe evacuation of the premises. This will not be adequate for continuing to work in the event of a power cut, as the light level from emergency lights is low and the locations will be to facilitate exit, rather than be over specific work areas. Some light fittings have emergency lighting built in, being backed up by an internal battery. Installing sufficient of these in working areas is very useful for completing procedures in the event of a power cut.

KEY POINT

Supplementary emergency lighting (by uninterruptible power supply, generator or by use of battery-powered headlamps or loupes) will still be needed for surgical procedures and is mandatory for veterinary hospitals under the RCVS Practice Standards Scheme.

Medical gases and gas scavenging

Medical gases, and the control of waste anaesthetic gases, are key factors in any premises with a surgical capability (see also Chapter 8).

Medical gases

There are a number of gases, and associated products, which come under this banner.

- In most veterinary premises the gases used are normally restricted to oxygen and nitrous oxide.
- Practices with particular orthopaedic interests may use air-driven tools, and install medical (compressed) air. A few practices that undertake long procedures may have vacuum systems.
- Carbon dioxide may be used for insufflations in endoscopic procedures.

KEY POINT

It is critical that cylinders are safely stored, that any pipework is correctly installed, and that the system is maintained and managed. In simplistic terms, the safety principle is 'What happens if...?'.

The gases are under pressure and there is, therefore, a potential risk should there be a failure. What seemed a fairly benign, if rather heavy, metal cylinder can suddenly become a 'rocket', with hugely destructive force. If such a failure happened inside an enclosed working environment, there could be very real risk to life and limb, let alone the property. The storage principle, therefore, is to house cylinders *outside the working environment*, ideally in some form of external unit. If the storage unit is fixed to the external wall of the building, as is the norm, the other sides should be weaker than the building wall and thus any failure would cause the store to blow outwards, rather than into the building. In simplistic terms, all that would be needed is a rack to keep the cylinders upright and a canopy to protect the regulators. In general, however, there is some level of security required to avoid the cylinders being stolen, either for their content or their scrap value.

Where small volumes of gases are used, there is little value in considering costly installations. However, in volumetric terms, small cylinders are very much more costly to rent and refill than are large cylinders, giving a rapid payback period for the installation costs of a pipeline if usage is fairly high.

Oxygen

Oxygen is the primary gas used in veterinary installations. Indeed, with recent changes in anaesthetic agents and approaches, many practices opt for oxygen as their only piped gas. Whilst technically not flammable, oxygen is a fire accelerant and, as such, needs managing with caution. Where the installation is seen as having any potential risk, a flashback arrestor (FBA) is fitted in the system to reduce the risk of flame travelling back up the supply pipework. In the case of excess heat a shut-off valve closes to protect the system. Storing gas cylinders outside the building (Figure 2.12) adds to this safety approach.

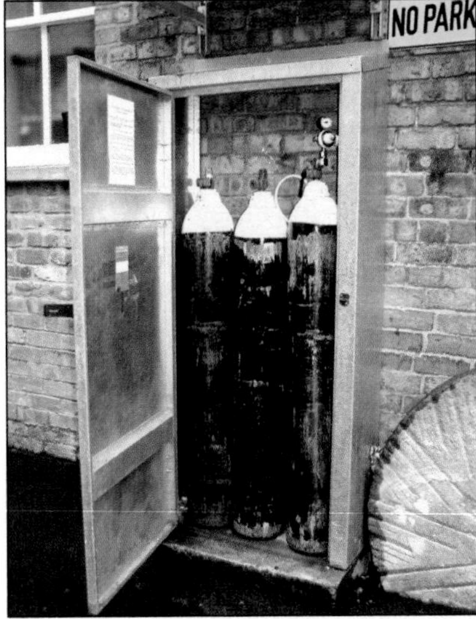

2.12 A small external storage unit housing oxygen cylinders.

Oxygen concentrators (oxygen pumps or generators) are increasingly used in small animal practice. This technology is changing rapidly but, in general, there are two options. For solo-vet practices, or some branch premises, it is possible to purchase a portable oxygen concentrator, which was originally designed to supply a single anaesthetic machine (Figure 2.13). In reality, this concept is changing, as there are already small concentrators which can supply two machines. There are also concentrators fitted to a trolley, some with an anaesthetic machine linked to the unit. Where

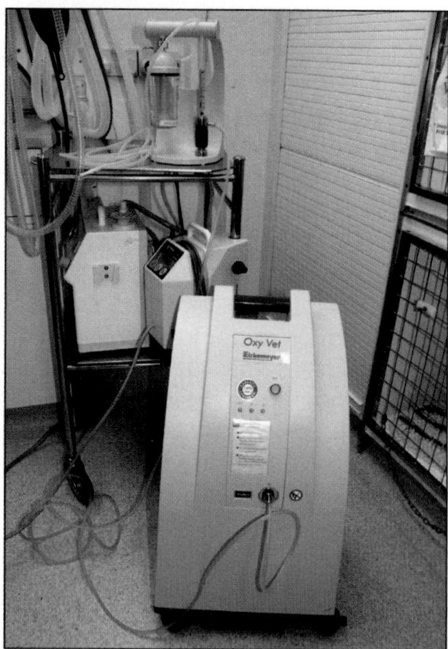

2.13 Single-user oxygen concentrators can be linked to an anaesthetic machine for surgery, or moved to wherever needed for oxygen therapy.

these concentrators are located within a working area, thought should be given to the oxygen being extracted from the air. Whilst this is not a big issue with small units, an adequate supply of fresh air is important. For larger premises, there can be a static concentrator supplying the pipeline in place of refillable oxygen cylinders; these would normally be located in the external gas store, which may need to be slightly larger. Where pressurized units are used, the Pressure Systems Safety Regulations 2000 apply.

The oxygen concentrator option can have significant long-term financial savings but, at present, there can be one very major problem: if the electrical power goes off, so does the supply of oxygen. However, with either type, there can be the addition of a traditional compressed oxygen cylinder for emergency switch over. Where a back-up supply is linked to a portable concentrator, this does make the trolley a little heavier, but it is not normally a problem, particularly if the unit is not moved very much. Most practices will maintain an emergency oxygen cylinder for power failure situations. Oxygen concentrators can be useful for maintaining oxygen flow to intensive care patients and offer similar flexibility to individual small cylinders but without the risk of depleting oxygen stocks.

Nitrous oxide

Nitrous oxide is supplied as a liquid at room temperature in blue cylinders, under 52 bar (750 psi, 50 atm). Unlike oxygen cylinders, where it is very easy to tell the volume remaining by the pressure gauge reading, the pressure gauge on a nitrous oxide cylinder will read full as long as there is any liquid nitrous oxide remaining in the cylinder. The pressure gauge will only start to drop when all the liquid has turned to gas, indicating the amount of vapour left within the cylinder. Cylinder content can be assessed by weight, deducting the empty cylinder weight (tare weight) from the current weight to give the weight of nitrous oxide remaining. The tare weight of a nitrous oxide E sized cylinder is approximately 5800–6400 g.

Compressed air

Compressed air may be required to operate surgical instruments, and also possibly patient ventilators. Pneumatic drills and saws require compressed air at 7.2 bar (105 psi) and anaesthetic patient ventilators at 4.1 bar (60 psi). It is important that medical-grade compressed air is used to operate these pieces of equipment rather than industrial compressed air. Medical-grade air should be free from toxic products, flammable or toxic vapours and odours. Medical air is not classed as sterile, but it is clean and at a standard temperature and pressure it should contain:

- No more than 0.5 mg particulate oil mist per m^3 of air
- No more than 5.5 mg carbon monoxide per m^3 of air
- No more than 900 mg carbon dioxide per m^3 of air
- No moisture
- No bacterial contamination.

Larger practices may find it more economical to install a compressor system that supplies its own compressed air rather than having cylinders. These systems consist of various parts, including air inlet, compressors, reservoirs, dryers or desiccators, coolers, filters, conduits and pipelines. They are expensive to install and maintain but prevent the need to transport medical air cylinders. Compressed air systems are covered by the Pressure Systems Safety Regulations 2000 (see www.hse.gov.uk). Compressed air systems should be maintained according to the manufacturer's recommendations and often benefit from being covered by a service contract.

Piped gases

In terms of the pipework, the installation process is largely the same for all gases. There is the source, normally the compressed gas cylinder. From this, the gas passes into the pipework through a pressure regulator, which checks the pressure in the pipework. At the end of the pipework are the outlet terminals (Figure 2.14), normally with self-sealing valves, referred to as Schrader valves. Around the Schrader outlet is a coloured ring, indicating the supply from that outlet (Figure 2.15).

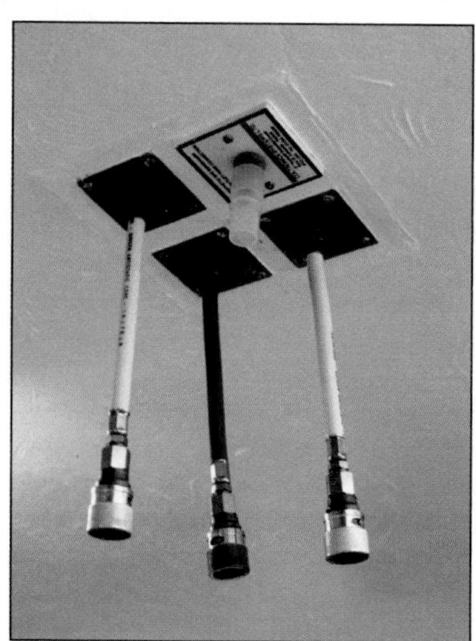

2.14 Ceiling outlets for piped oxygen (white) and nitrous oxide (blue). An active gas scavenging point is also present.

Colour code	Interpretation
White	Oxygen
Blue	Nitrous oxide
Black	Medical air
Yellow	Vacuum/Suction

2.15 Colour coding of piped gas outlets.

With any system, there is a need to provide a way for replacing a depleted cylinder with a full one. The options range from a single cylinder connection, where there is some manual handling at change over, to a fully automated system. In general, the fully automated systems are only required in large hospital systems, normally a good deal larger than veterinary premises. For most veterinary premises, there will be two cylinders of each gas, linked to a manifold. If the pressure begins to drop, an alarm sounds, giving plenty of time for someone to go to the store and turn the lever that closes the old cylinder and opens the new one. This is a good, simple, logical option with no added complexities, no requirement for reliance on a functional electrical supply, and a real safeguard for any mishaps at changeover.

KEY POINT

Where electrical switches are used to change supply from one cylinder to another, a foolproof system must be in place to ensure that change-over can be achieved during a power failure, and that the empty cylinder is replaced.

Within the veterinary premises, there are decisions to be made relating to the location of outlets. Nitrous oxide, for example, may only be needed in certain surgical areas, and medical air where air-driven tools are to be used. Oxygen, however, may have a much more extensive network. Oxygen can be piped into the wards or small cylinder trolley units can be used, the choice influenced by costs and space requirements. A full anaesthetic trolley may not be needed. The requirements for dedicated intensive care units, dedicated high-observation cages or fixed locations of cages with oxygen fronts should be taken into consideration when locating piping and outlets. The use of piped gases may be balanced against the higher degree of flexibility of a mobile oxygen cylinder, or generator. These options are explored further in Chapter 7.

Pipework installation

There are a number of options when it comes to considering the installation of the pipework for gases. Whilst there is nothing particularly difficult in plumbing terms, there is a need for degreased pipework, testing, and correctly fitting outlets. Best practice would suggest the use of a recognized installer with veterinary understanding. Such firms will design the installation to minimize pipe runs and offer a logical system for a particular premises.

For many veterinary premises it is probably wisest to opt for surface-fixed pipework (Figure 2.16a). This allows simple access if, say, there is a need to alter the pipe runs and outlets or to add another supply line at any future time. Where it is unlikely that gas lines will ever be altered, concealed pipework may be considered, possibly with some blanked-off pipework where later extensions could be made if ever needed. Whilst surface-mounted pipework may require some neat boxing in, normally in wipe-clean plastic trunking, the accessibility is useful. A popular approach has trunking which carries both gases and active scavenging (Figure 2.16b).

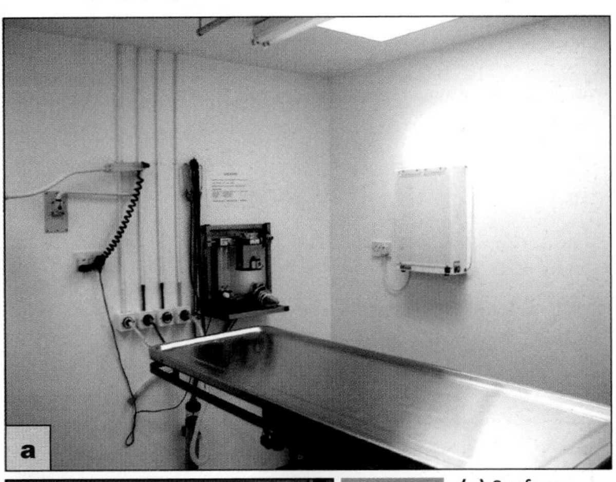

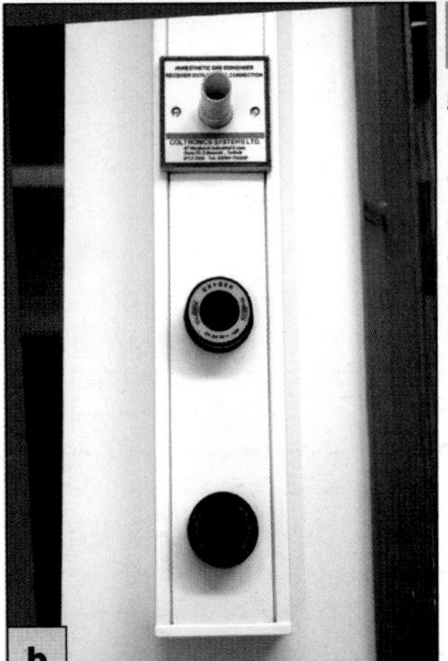

2.16 **(a)** Surface-mounted piped gases are accessible but can represent a hygiene challenge. **(b)** Piping within smooth plastic trunking offers a good compromise between accessibility and cleanability.

Waste gas scavenging

Waste anaesthetic gases are a potential problem, both in areas where anaesthesia is induced and maintained, and where recovering animals are exhaling. Some practices use consumable absorbers to deal with the waste gas. Absorbers are available from most veterinary wholesalers and should be weighed daily and disposed of correctly when exhausted. This can be quite costly in the longer term, however, and some form of scavenging is usually considered preferable.

Scavenging systems carry the waste gas directly from the anaesthetic machine to mix with the air outside the building. This may be achieved by simple outlet pipes linked to the anaesthetic machine (passive scavenging) or by using suction (active scavenging).

Passive scavenging

Passive scavenging is a low-cost system that is perfectly effective where there is easy access to outside air. All that is involved is a pipe, quite low on the wall, with a diameter large enough to take the outlet from the anaesthetic machine/patient. The passive scavenging pipe on the wall has a 90-degree elbow and passes horizontally through the external wall to a similar elbow which turns the final outlet downwards. To improve this, the outlet could terminate with a 'T' piece which will help airflow, and some form of small mesh cover to protect the pipe and stop ingress of small native species. Although some manufacturers supply passive scavenging kits, standard plastic sink wastepipe is all that is needed to create a system just as good (Figure 2.17).

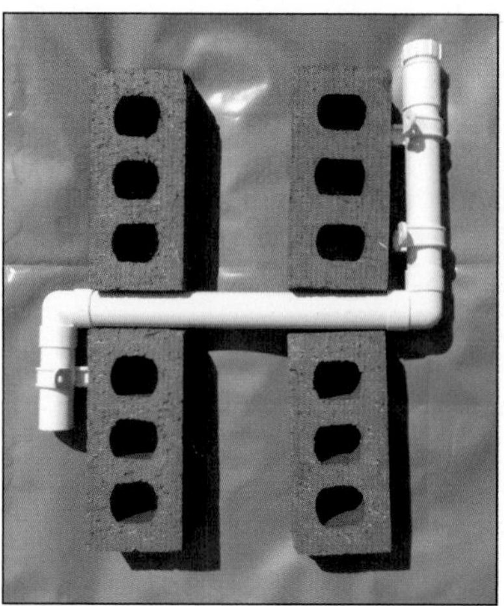

2.17 A passive scavenging system can be constructed using standard plastic sink wastepipe.

Active scavenging

Active scavenging is at its most useful where anaesthesia is to be induced or maintained in rooms with no external wall. In addition, because it is mechanically controlled, and can be checked, it is likely to find favour with the safety legislation surrounding such systems.

The concept centres on an extraction unit (Figure 2.18a) that draws the waste gases to outside air, where it is dispersed in line with passive scavenging. There is one small complication. If the waste gas output from the anaesthetic machine is connected directly to an extractor, there is a risk that anaesthetic could be drawn out of the breathing system, compromising patient safety. To avoid this occurring, a unit called an air break receiver (ABR) or Barnsley unit (Figure 2.18b) is fixed between the waste gas pipe from each anaesthetic machine and the extraction pipework. What begins as a simple network of extraction pipes becomes somewhat more complex and, with an ABR for each anaesthetic machine, quite costly. Whilst it would be very possible to fit active scavenging systems on a DIY basis, it is important to use a matched suite of components. Different systems use differing pressures, or vacuums, as some are designed specifically for the veterinary market whilst others are adaptations of systems for large NHS hospitals.

KEY POINTS

- Regular servicing is recommended for all types of scavenging, normally annually.
- Inspection of the pipework should also be undertaken regularly to ensure that it is functioning correctly.
- The pipework should be kept clean and without debris build-up where it bends.
- Negative pressure at the active scavenging port should be checked before each anaesthetic session.

Recovery scavenging

KEY POINT

Removing waste gas from recovery areas is rarely considered outside the normal ventilation processes. It should be monitored and, where large dogs recover in relatively small areas, an effective extraction system should be in place and regular anaesthetic pollution monitoring carried out.

As waste gas collects at low levels, a very simple process is to have some extraction from just above floor level. Whilst this sounds simple, normal ventilation relies on fresh air entering at a low level to be pulled

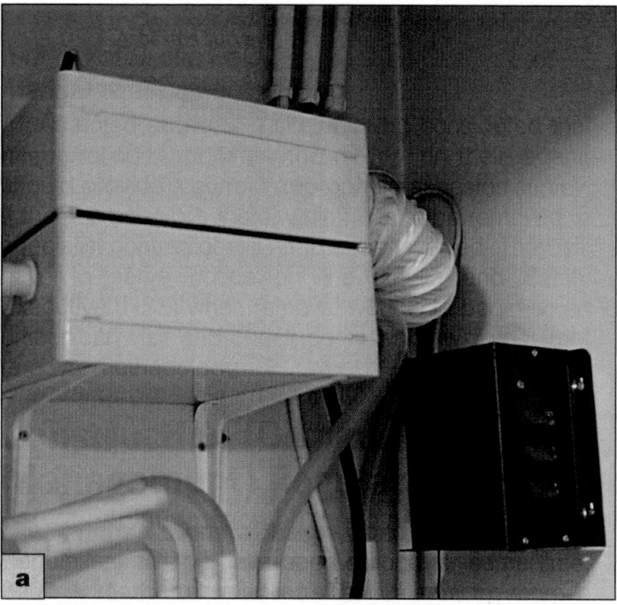

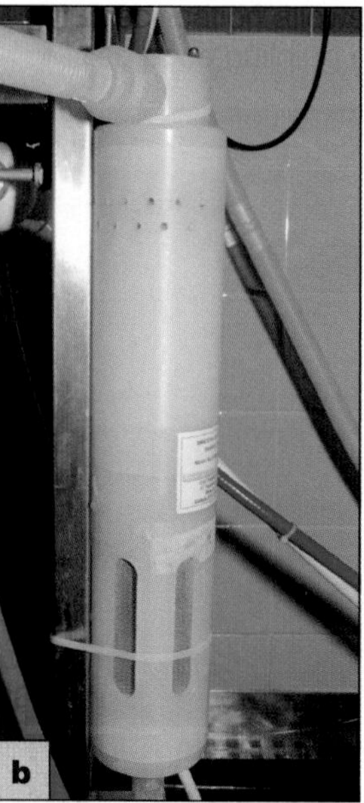

2.18 Active scavenging. **(a)** This central fan unit scavenges from several different locations. It is vital to keep pipework and tubing clean and free from condensation, and to check the functioning of the unit regularly. **(b)** An air break receiver (ABR; sometimes referred to as a Barnsley unit) which is situated between the positive scavenging system and the anaesthetic machine.

through the air space by foul air, which is warmer, being drawn out at high level. Thus, any low-level waste gas extraction must be planned so it does not interfere with the normal venting of the space.

Recovery area scavenging can be provided by a fairly low-output fan in a suitable high location, with ducting running right down the wall and an inlet grille at the bottom. This extractor can have manual controls and be used only during the postoperative recovery period.

Security and alarm systems

There are many aspects that link to the security of a veterinary premises, and some compromises have to be made. Externally, the layout and landscaping can make it difficult for a potential intruder to conceal themselves whilst breaking in, and this can be helped with lighting during the hours of darkness (Figure 2.19). Strategically placed prickly barriers, such as holly bushes or artificial barriers, are useful for protecting vulnerable fencing and climbable boundaries.

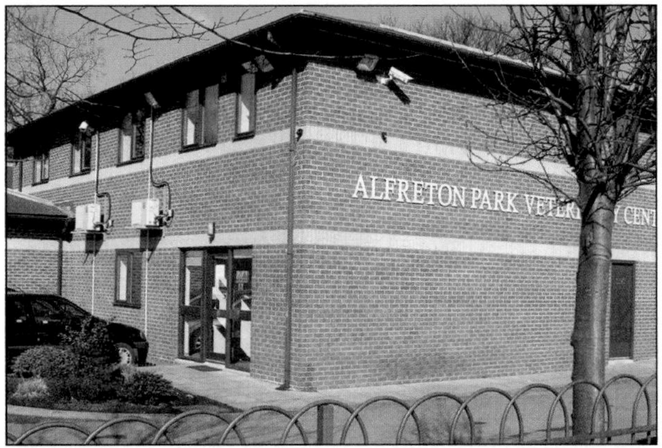

2.19 Low-wattage sodium lights mounted high on the building flood the pathways and access points without causing dazzle. CCTV cameras cover entrances and the parking areas.

Internally, vulnerable areas include unprotected staircases accessible from the outpatient area, drug storage areas and external doors used for ward access or staff entrances. Closed-circuit television and digital or card-operated security locks may help reduce unauthorized access in busy areas. Physical systems and installations, such as locks, alarms, panic buttons and security devices, may need to be considered.

It is helpful to have a protocol to ensure that the premises are secured overnight; a checklist can ensure that all doors and windows are closed securely (Figure 2.20).

External shell and doors

Locks and keys

Insurers will insist that external doors have locks compliant with BS3621. These will be deadlocks, where the bolt cannot be slid back into the casing without the key. The lock will have a minimum of five levers, and a bolt which has a throw of at least 14 mm. These locks may be of the traditional type, with a classic key which could be inserted from either side, or Euro style, with a smaller key similar to that found on many modern padlocks. Whilst the first often seems more robust, there is the disadvantage of the keyhole, right through the door, and the bulk of the key in a pocket or on a key ring. In addition, the barrel of the Euro lock can be changed without the need for a whole new lock being fitted. This could be useful if the key is lost or stolen.

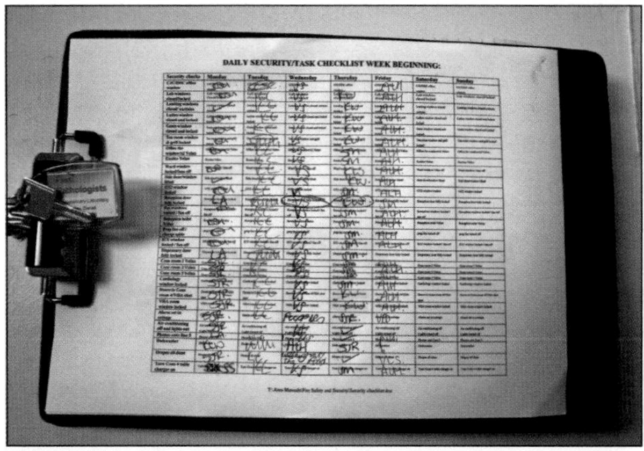

2.20 An example of a daily security checklist for staff to complete before leaving for the day. Days are across the top and items to confirm secure or completed are on the left-hand side. The list includes: locking wall and ceiling windows; locking doors; switching phones to emergency lines; setting alarms; and confirming completion of daily tasks. Such a checklist is also useful during handover to any duty staff, and could form part of the lone worker protocol.

Door strengthening

The five-lever deadlock has been the norm for a long time and few self-respecting felons would attempt to pick it. Rather, vulnerability is likely to be from the door being kicked in, smashed, cut, or ram-raided. Where there is such a worry, ram-raiding can be blocked by a secure bollard in the ground and the integral strength of the door can be increased by multiple locking anti-jemmy frames, and general strengthening (Figure 2.21). In areas of high vulnerability,

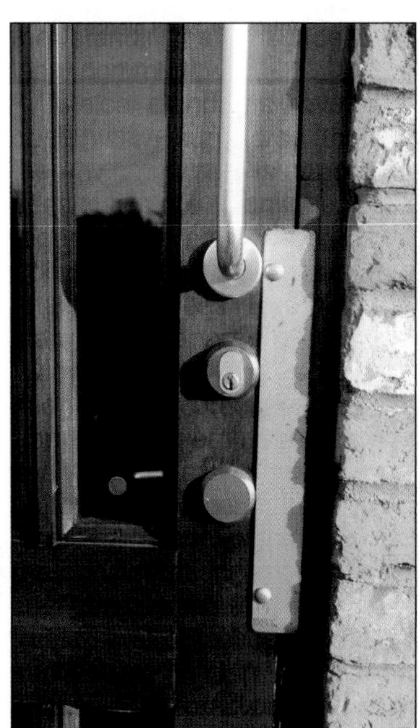

2.21 Security locks on a timber door that has also been fitted with an anti-tamper plate following an attempt to prise it open using a steel bar. The central lock is the Euro style.

external or internal roller shutters can be used, subject to Planning Consent. Where an external shutter is used, it is unwise to install a letterbox through the shutter as a steel bar, attached to a chain, can be inserted, the chain attached to a vehicle, and the shutter pulled off the wall.

In most situations, however, major visible doors can be adequately secure without the added physical barriers. Vulnerable fire doors that have push-bar or panic-pad opening can be steel or steel-faced, with no external ironmongery for a would-be thief to gain a grip (Figure 2.22).

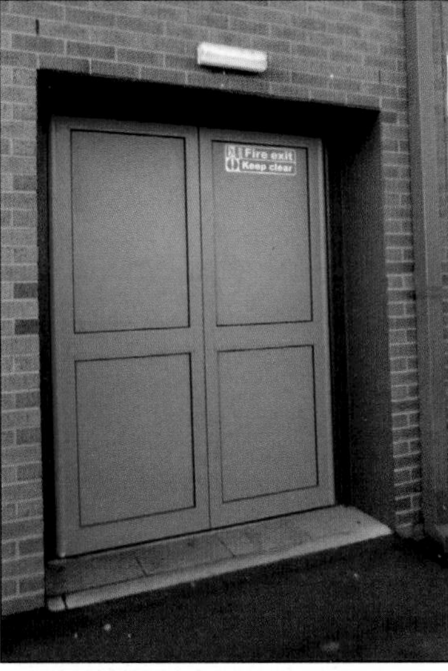

Fire exit
Keep clear

2.22 The most secure fire doors have a smooth finish with no external door furniture for anyone to try to force open. This one has double doors for easy access for large equipment.

Windows

In most areas, strong windows with window locks and double glazing will deter most would-be entrants. Where there is a risk of break-in or vandalism, roller shutters are probably the most effective option, as they protect against both criminal damage and forced entry. Where possible, the use of permanent bars should be avoided, particularly on visible external windows, as they portray a negative image of the premises and area. External roller shutters or internal foldable shutters (Figure 2.23) can be closed at night and opened up during the day.

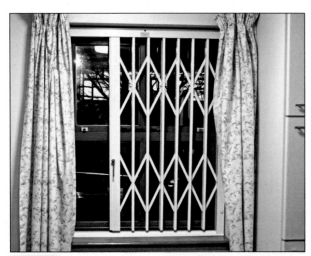

2.23 Bars at windows can look off-putting but folding shutters such as these can be drawn to one side during the day and locked in place at night.

Flat roofing and skylights

An assessment should also be made regarding areas of flat roof, which may offer access to first-floor windows, and any skylights. Any access considered vulnerable should be given special attention to avoid easy entry to thieves.

Sadly, there have been break-ins where entrance has been gained by removing roof tiles, but such entry should be picked up by an intruder alarm (see below).

Closed-circuit television

As with many technologies, costs for CCTV have reduced significantly. Coupled with adequate lighting, some strategically placed CCTV cameras (Figures 2.19 and 2.24) can deter criminals but also record any attempted entry. Sadly, modern felons tend to be careful to wear hoods and avoid looking at cameras, but many can be identified by other clothing, gait, or criminal habits. As well as out-of-hours criminal detection, CCTV can offer visual supervision of the external area, such as car parks and service yards. Internally placed systems can also be used to monitor where help might be required, e.g. Reception, and to keep a remote eye on inpatients. Where CCTV images are intended to be used for formal evidence, professional systems with date stamping and high-quality images are required and effective secure back-up is essential.

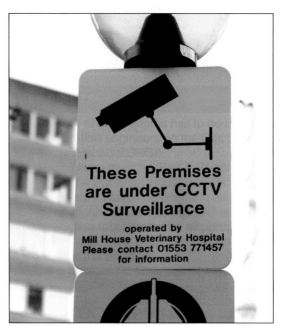

These Premises
are under CCTV
Surveillance
operated by
Mill House Veterinary Hospital
Please contact 01553 771457
for information

2.24 Where CCTV cameras are installed, clear signage with contact details should be placed to inform people of their use.

Intruder alarms

Whilst the sound of a wailing intruder alarm seems to be ignored by all and sundry, such installations seem ubiquitous. The alarm itself is not the important aspect; it is how it reports. Where a building is staffed 24 hours a day, all that is probably needed is for the alarm to sound. If there are periods where the premises are unoccupied, a link to a listening centre, referred to as red-care, and/or a dial up to a staff member's telephone, is more valuable.

Passive infra-red (PIR) sensors pick up movement by detecting body heat and can protect an entire room, and its windows and corridors. Whilst many systems also use an electromagnetic detector on doors, PIR sensors can cover corridors and central hubs, protecting each area of the practice. PIR devices have hugely reduced the cost of intruder alarms and made them far less intrusive. Gone are those silvery strips around windows or internal window bars with wires running through them. A few strategically placed PIR sensors (Figure 2.25) can cover the inside of the outer shell, to activate if the external barriers are breached.

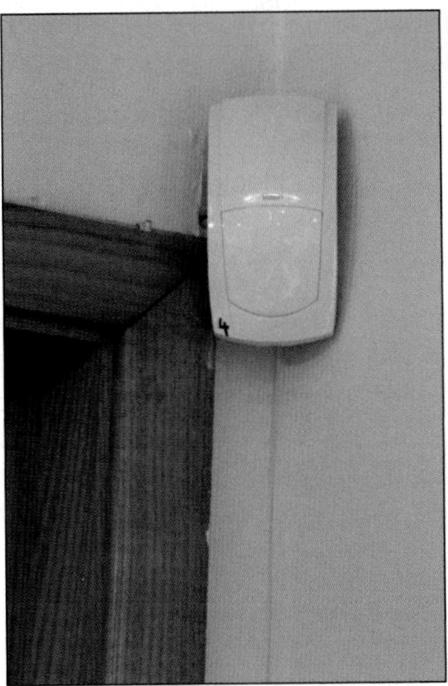

2.25 A passive infra-red (PIR) sensor mounted in a corner to pick up movement across a wide area.

Barriers and remote access

Apart from securing the building, most practice premises have car parks. If these are more than a few pull-in spaces, they could be vulnerable to misuse out of hours. In addition, they may be abused by neighbours during the day, taking up valuable client parking space.

Some form of remotely operated barrier could be useful, particularly when clients may visit for out-of-hours emergencies. During the day the barrier can raise on entry, but on exit a token or code available from reception staff is needed. At night, the barrier could be inactive, so basically locked down, unless released by staff from within the premises.

Remote access systems, such as reception-activated door locks and intercoms, can also be used for night-time client entry, particularly if there is a lockable inner lobby. Unless there were very exceptional circumstances, however, such a system could be seen as negative during normal hours.

Fire safety

Over the centuries, fire has been one of the major driving forces for building regulations. As well as structural and material considerations, within the Building Regulations (Building Standards) the means of escape from buildings has become a critical issue. This is coupled with a demand on the owners or managers of commercial buildings to undertake a regular fire risk assessment.

Rather like the legislation surrounding veterinary medicines, by the beginning of this century there was a welter of pieces of legislation dealing with fire safety. In the same way that the Veterinary Medicines Directorate coordinated all the different strands of law covering veterinary medicines into a single new piece of law, The Regulatory Reform (Fire Safety Order) 2005 did the same for fire safety.

KEY POINTS

- Known as the Fire Safety Order (FSO), the law now requires the nomination of a Responsible Person, usually referred to as a Fire Officer or Fire Marshal, for commercial buildings, and it is their responsibility to ensure legal compliance.
- Compliance requires: a risk assessment, followed by the implementation of appropriate measures to minimize the risk to life and property from fire; and keeping the assessment up to date.

Fire risk

Whilst there is plenty of guidance on government websites (www.communities.gov.uk/fire), Responsible Persons often do not feel competent at undertaking this assessment and there is an army of consultants who will undertake the process. These will protect themselves by covering every potential risk, which may lead to expensive and complicated requirements. The law does not insist on this, but pragmatism is not easy when lives could be at risk.

Fortunately, veterinary premises tend to have hard surfaces and few soft furnishings to catch fire so the risk of fire should be relatively low. There are, however, various items that will burn or act as fire accelerants, so there is no room for complacency.

Fire escape

Veterinary premises are divided into a number of relatively small rooms, making fire escape rules quite a challenge. With a few exceptions, the rule is that anyone inside should be able to escape from the room they are in, either direct to outside air or along a fire-protected corridor to outside air. This corridor will have a specific fire rating for the structure, and any doors off it will have to be fire doors.

KEY POINT

Every escape route must be protected with closed doors offering 30 minutes of fire protection.

If fire doors and patient security doors can coincide, inconvenience can be minimized. Where it is preferred that there is not a closed door, devices can be used to hold doors open; these have electromagnets in them, which release if the fire alarm is activated (Figure 2.26). These can be very useful on trolley routes.

Building interiors will be compartmentalized, each as a fire containment area. Where many larger commercial buildings can have relatively few external escape doors, because the internal rooms are larger, veterinary premises may end up with proportionately more.

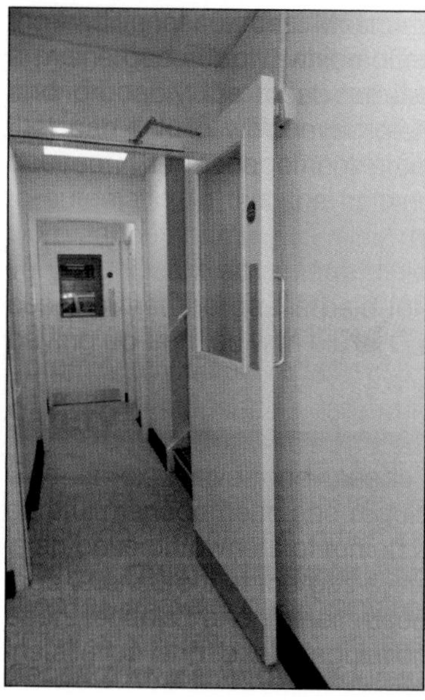

2.26 This fire door on a trolleying route is held open with an electromagnetic catch which releases if the fire alarm sounds. In this area, vision panels are only fitted to upper parts of doors, to avoid risk to glass when a trolley is pushed through.

Many practice premises can be considered in two zones. Around the waiting and reception area there could be a number of people, many of whom will be unfamiliar with the layout. Here, fire escapes need to be well marked, though there is the advantage that staff should be on hand to guide escape. Elsewhere in the premises, there may be fewer people and they will be familiar with the layout and escape routes. However, should a fire start in an unattended area, it may have a chance of gaining a strong hold before it is noticed. This means that fire detection systems are vital for all but the smallest of premises.

Fire alarms

There are two elements involved:

- Detection of fire, picking up the early signs of smoke or heat so occupants can be warned in time to escape
- Warning the occupants that a fire exists.

With small buildings, such as a lock-up branch, there may be no logical need for any system, other than a shout of 'FIRE!', but such an approach only works if people are there to raise that alarm. Should a fire arise when the building is unoccupied, there would be neither detection nor alarm. This unoccupied risk may not be considered acceptable by insurers.

The decision about the installation of a fire alarm, and the type installed, may be determined by insurers, advice from a local Fire Officer consulted by the Building Control Department of the Local Planning Authority (LPA), or the risk assessment arranged by the Responsible Person.

- **Conventional alarms** have detectors and call points wired back to a control panel, often in zones.
- One stage on are **addressable alarms** which can identify the actual sensor that detected the problem, rather than zones.
- **Analogue alarms** detect whether there is a fire, a fault, or whether a detector needs cleaning, and they can take many more interface devices.
- Today it is also possible to have reliable **wireless alarms**, which can be fully addressable.

Of more importance is the decision of what the alarm protects, addressed in BS5839 Part 1 and establishing either life or property protection (Figure 2.27).

Decisions also need to be made on the locations of sensors, and whether smoke or heat detectors are fitted. Where smoke or steam may be generated during clinical procedures or cooking, heat detectors are more practical. Modern fittings can often be set for either detection, which is very useful.

Code	Purpose
L systems have automatic detection with the aim of protecting life	
L1	Covering the entire building to give the longest possible time for escape
L2	Covering all escape routes, adjacent rooms, plus any high-risk areas
L3	Covering escape routes, with alarm sounders to warn all occupants
L4	Covering escape routes only (corridors, stairways and circulation areas)
L5	A custom system where detectors are located at specific risk areas, not covered by the above
P systems have automatic detection with the aim of protecting property	
P1	Covering the whole building to gain early detection of fire
P2	Covering specific areas of high risk
M systems are manual	
M	Manually operated alarm (smash glass), hand-bell, shout, etc.

2.27 Fire alarm classification.

Fire extinguishers

A range of fire extinguishers is available, suitable for use on different sorts of fire. The UK recognizes six fire classes:

- Class A fires involve organic solids such as paper and wood
- Class B fires involve flammable or combustible liquids. Petrol, grease and oil fires are included in this class
- Class C fires involve flammable gases
- Class D fires involve combustible metals
- Class E fires involving electrical appliances (no longer used as when the power supply is turned off an electrical fire can fall into any category)
- Class F fires involve cooking fat and oil.

According to the standard BS EN 3, fire extinguishers in the United Kingdom, as throughout the EU, are red. A circle of a second colour, covering between 5 and 10% of the surface area of the extinguisher, indicates the contents (Figures 2.28 and 2.29). Before 1997, the entire body of the fire extinguisher was colour-coded according to the type of extinguishing agent.

Fire extinguishers should be positioned to support escape as well as to deal with small incidents where there is no risk to the operator. Staff should be trained

Type	Old code	BS EN 3 colour code	Suitable for use on fire classes (brackets denote sometimes applicable)					
Water	Signal red	Signal red	A					
Foam	Cream	Red with a cream panel above the operating instructions	A	B				
Dry powder	French blue	Red with a blue panel above the operating instructions	(A)	B	C		E	
Carbon dioxide CO_2	Black	Red with a black panel above the operating instructions (see Figure 2.32)		B			E	
Wet chemical	Not yet in use	Red with a canary yellow panel above the operating instructions	A	(B)				F
Class D powder	French blue	Red with a blue panel above the operating instructions				D		
Halon 1211/BCF	Emerald green	No longer in general use	A	B			E	

2.28 UK fire extinguisher classification and colour coding.

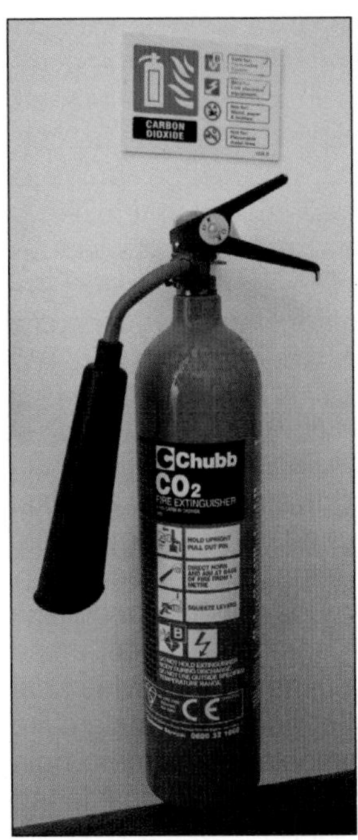

2.29 A carbon dioxide extinguisher suitable for electrical fires.

regularly in their use; a number of training packages are available, including DVDs and Internet-based programmes. Service engineers will often offer the opportunity to use an extinguisher when it is due to be recharged or is being replaced, and this is useful experience.

Testing and drills

- Fire alarm and emergency lighting systems must be tested regularly and a log kept.
- Fire extinguishers in appropriate locations should be regularly inspected and serviced according to manufacturer's recommendations.
- Fire drills should also be carried out on a regular basis to ensure that evacuation procedures are effective and that everyone knows what to do in the event of a fire.

Acknowledgements

The author and editors gratefully acknowledge the following practices, images of which appear in this chapter: Avenue Veterinary Centre; Crossings Veterinary Centre; Marshlands Veterinary Centre; Rowan Veterinary Centre; Wildbore Vetstop.

Further reading

As systems information is changing all the time, Internet searching is very useful, as is discussion with professional advisors. A useful review point is the Energy Saving Trust: www.energysavingtrust.org.uk. Fire Safety Law and Fire Guidance Documents for business are available at www.communities.gov.uk/fire.

Floor plans, design and maintenance

3

Jim Wishart

Practice managers should decide some overall objective, possibly longer term, regarding the type of practice building they wish to develop and the RCVS standard they plan to achieve on a particular site. If the designer is briefed accordingly, a design can be developed to achieve this objective, even if it has to be undertaken in planned stages over time. It is important to incorporate future plans in any current building design to avoid expensive reworking later.

Floor plans and layout

Good layout design is the critical factor in designing a building which is easy to work in, a pleasure to visit, and generates a perception of being right – without being 'over the top'. There are some very simple logical principles that, all too often, are overlooked:

- Male dogs may cock their legs on any available upright or corner
- Dogs come on leads with an owner at the end
- Opposites, in terms of species, can attract, and not always pleasantly
- Clients expect privacy in consultations
- Euthanasia requires subtlety in management
- Inpatients, outpatients and staff pets are separate issues
- Clients perceive, and their perceptions are communicated
- However good it looks, it must be kept clean
- Design to avoid expensive re-fits and close downs in the future.

One of the hardest things to grasp, in terms of practice design, is client perception. Veterinary surgeons are often good at designing around specific workstations, but that is the internal mechanics. Sadly, the client is not too aware of the inner workings, and may not want to know. It is their perception that brings them back again and again.

Walk into any *clinical environment* (dental surgery, GP practice, hospital clinic) or *hygiene environment* (from restaurant to transport café, butchers to sandwich bar) and the senses become acutely tuned to cleanliness and hygienic procedures. For the client, that sense is just as heightened when they enter a veterinary premises. Designing in easy maintenance, cleanability, longevity and simple approaches can, with a good cleansing regime, ensure the image of *clean*. So, too, can a clean smell, but the visual sense has a much longer impact and retention. As well as the visual impact of the level of cleanliness, clients are also very aware of the implications for disease control of a well maintained and clean facility.

This section will concentrate on client and animal handling areas which, hopefully, will all be on one level. Areas such as staff rooms, offices, changing rooms and overnight accommodation can be on a different floor, and their linkages are not quite so critical – though they do need careful thought, particularly within the scope of logical access and fire escape (see Chapters 2 and 16).

RCVS Practice Standards

When it comes to designing layout, a very early reference volume should be the *RCVS Practice Standards Manual.* This is true, even if a practice is not planning to join the Practice Standards Scheme (PSS) as it offers a useful checklist of factors aiming towards best practice. An early move should be to check the RCVS website (www.rcvs.org.uk) and download the current standards, probably printing them out so that there is a copy that can be referred to as a working document and on which notes can be made.

Client arrival

When travelling to any new place, the senses are heightened in expectation of what might be found. Impressions begin before arrival, possibly while following signs, and they continue well beyond arrival. The design of the approach, arrival, parking and entrance is one of the most critical parts of the overall design. Some immediate questions need to be addressed:

- Is the practice easy to find?
- Is the car park well set out, and is it easy to park?
- Is the entrance to the building obvious and well signed?
- Is pedestrian access fit for all?

- Is there sufficient privacy for the current transaction?
- Do the surroundings present a professional image?
- Do the surroundings present a caring image?
- Does the place look tidy and well maintained?
- Is it laid out with the client and patient in mind?
- Is the style within the client's comfort zone?

The car park and outside areas

Lines and signage

Clear use of lines and signage (Figure 3.1) in the car park is essential to help clients park sensibly and to maximize use of available space. Disabled parking spaces also need to be delineated (Figure 3.2). Thermoplastic lining is neatest and most durable, and should be laid by experienced contractors. Bicycle parking is a requirement of planning law and may be appreciated by some clients (Figure 3.3). Staff cycles are best parked in a secure area, if possible.

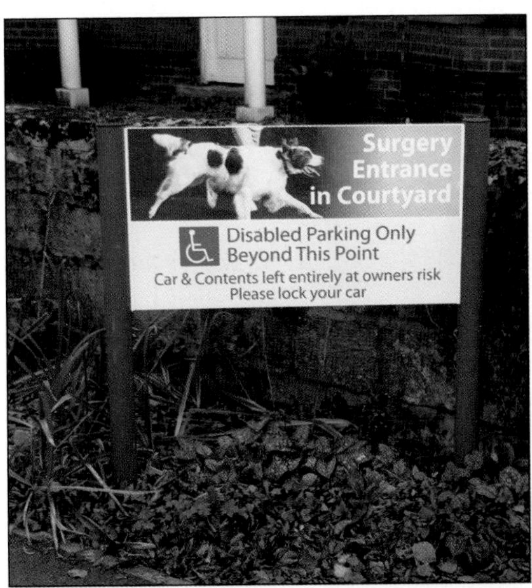
Surgery
Entrance
in Courtyard
Disabled Parking Only
Beyond This Point
Car & Contents left entirely at owners risk
Please lock your car

3.1 Clear and well branded signage helps guide clients and visitors, as well as prompting a coordinated professional image.

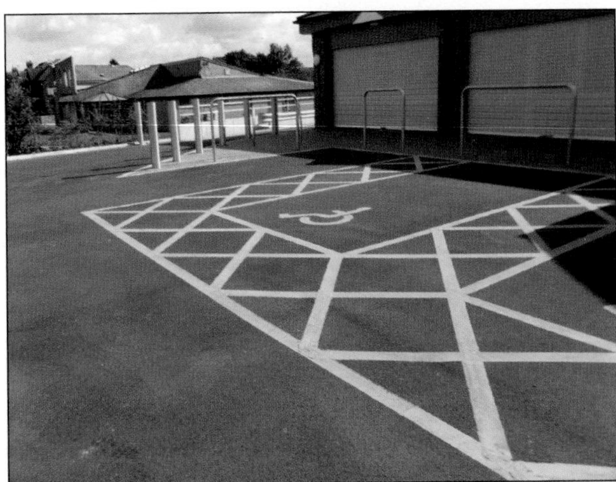

3.2 Wheelchair parking bays provide space for the disabled to get out of their cars and unload their wheelchairs. Clearly lined disabled parking bays should comply with Building Regulations and the DDA.

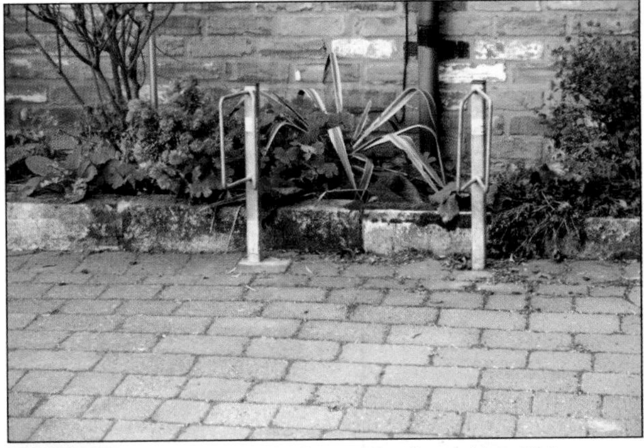

3.3 Planners now insist on bicycle parking. This demand is not onerous and may encourage some clients to use their bicycle when collecting prescriptions, etc.

Planting

Outside garden or planting areas should be designed for ease of maintenance and year-round interest, and a grassed area is handy for walking inpatients or for clients to walk their dogs on before admission. Regular litter picking and clearly labelled dog waste bins (Figure 3.4) are essential, with a supply of bags or a shovel for picking up faeces.

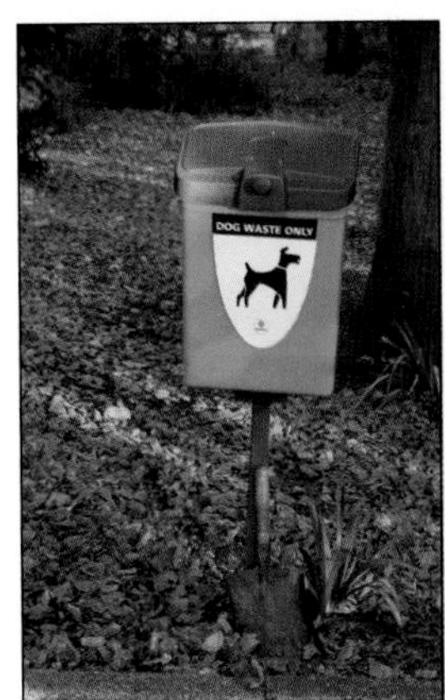
DOG WASTE ONLY

3.4 A suitable area where clients can let their dogs spend a few moments before entering the premises will allow dogs to urinate and defecate, reducing soiling around the entrance and in reception. A clearly visible bin for dog waste is essential.

Lighting

Night-time lighting should be designed to illuminate the entrance, car park, footpaths and also shady corners. The choice of light will depend on the area being lit, personal preference, and the demands of the Local Planning Authority. Car park lights should be positioned so they do not dazzle drivers: they either need to be fairly high and shining downwards, like a street lamp (Figure 3.5), or even higher on a building or pole with an angled flood light, shining across the area. Sodium lights are low energy, so good for floodlighting. An alternative to flooding the area with light can be the use of curb lights and low-energy bulkheads. These are useful where there is a risk of causing a nuisance to neighbours.

Pedestrian access points need good lighting, with no worrying shadows. Low-energy lights are ideal to light the way during business hours. These can be linked to a photocell and an over-riding 7-day timer (Figure 3.6). The lights will then come on automatically when light levels fall, but only when the practice is open. Some practices find that low-energy lighting is useful security during all hours of darkness, so a simple photocell link will do.

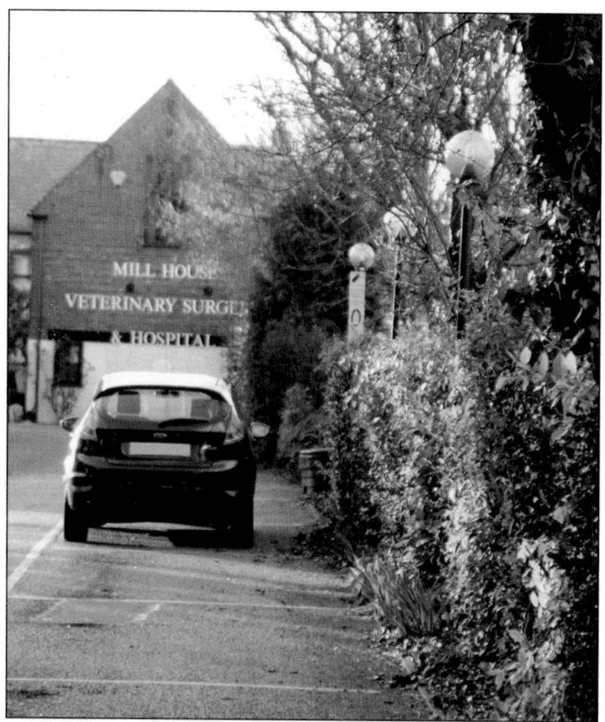

3.5 An attractive tall lamp standard gives a pleasant approach to drive and car park lighting.

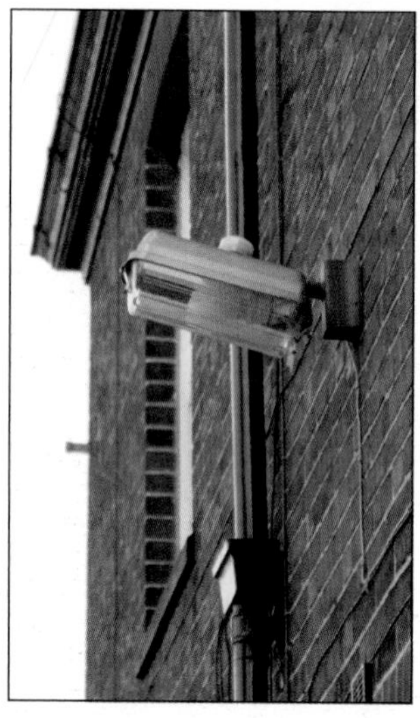

3.6 Wall mounted floodlight ideal for unobtrusive lighting. This model is fitted with an individual photocell.

Halogen lights activated by a passive infra-red (PIR) movement sensor can be useful deterrents, and will flood an area with light. Often the bulbs are 500 watts, so are expensive to run, even if of low cost to buy; lower wattage versions have recently come on to the market and may prove a useful alternative.

Entrance to the reception/waiting area

Whilst the entrance may be well signed from the car park and work well for pedestrians, it must also work for the patients.

The front door is a challenge and dilemma for veterinary premises. Most practice staff are rightly very concerned about the risk of animals escaping from the premises. Current legislation is often misunderstood, and designers can be misled into insisting on automatically opening doors. This is not required. Access must be planned, and the access of the infirm managed, but this does not mean putting animal patients at risk by having a door that opens for them just because they go near it when their owner is not competent at control. Automatic doors can be one of the most risky fitments on any veterinary building and should be resisted with logical argument. Security requirements for external doors are considered in Chapter 2.

Within the Design and Access Statement for planning, or the Access Statement at the Building Control (Building Warrant) stage (see Chapter 1), an alternative management system can be outlined, possibly with an 'assistance bell' and/or good visual supervision of the entrance by reception, and a standard operating procedure (SOP) to assist anyone who needs it. That person requiring assistance might be able-bodied – with two cat baskets, a small child and a pushchair.

The veterinary practice doorway carries a great chance of animal conflict – mostly dog to dog. Thought and design can avoid this, particularly with good visibility.

- On new designs it is useful to have an entrance with two doors, almost side by side, with the left approach in-only and the right door out-only (Figure 3.7a).
- If there is a single entrance and exit doorway, however, a fully glazed door will allow both owners and pets to see what is on the other side and avoid conflict (Figure 3.7b).

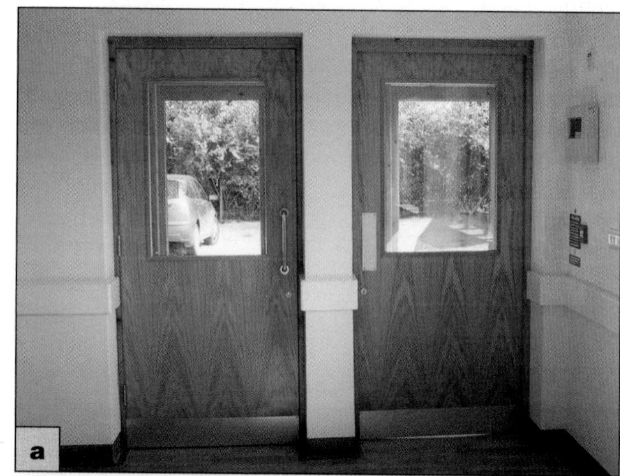

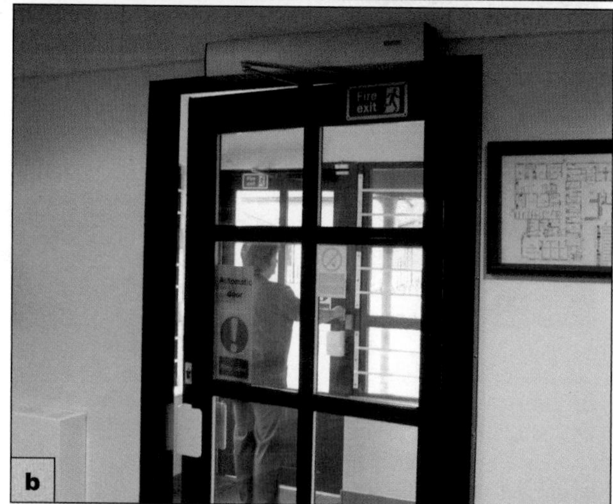

3.7 **(a)** Designated side-by-side entrance and exit doors can reduce the risk of conflict in the doorway. **(b)** Fully glazed entrance doors allow clients and pets to see what is on the other side, reducing unexpected conflicts.

There is then the issue of space beyond the entrance. Poor planning can create a bottleneck between the entrance and the reception counter, for example if the designer forgot that dogs come with leads and that owners are sometimes not that good at controlling their charge on a short 'rein'. Space must be planned so that one large dog does not block the entire ingress and egress of the practice.

Some years ago there was a design trend for completely separate entrances and exits, with a virtual one-way system for outpatients. This seemed like a great idea until it was realized that clients are individuals who do not necessarily conform to the grand plan. Sometimes, a family turned up with their pet, but only one or two went into the consulting room. If the one-way system brought them out in a different place, they then had to do a 'lap of honour' to pick up the rest of the family! This could be even more difficult if members of the family came with both a dog and a cat, and the practice had strictly segregated waiting areas.

Disabled access

We live in a world of ageing populations, both client and patient. That access ramp demanded by the planners (Figure 3.8) is a boon for 'doddery' dogs which the veterinary surgeon's skills keep going. There is more, however, to disabled access than wheelchairs and ramps, even though mobility issues affect the physical structure of the design more than other aspects. Someone in a wheelchair has a lower plane of vision and restricted reach, which must be considered as well as the requirements of Building Regulations (Building Standards). Additionally, not everyone with access difficulties sits in a wheelchair or is old. The Disability Discrimination Act (DDA) is a wide ranging piece of legislation and covers almost every possibility.

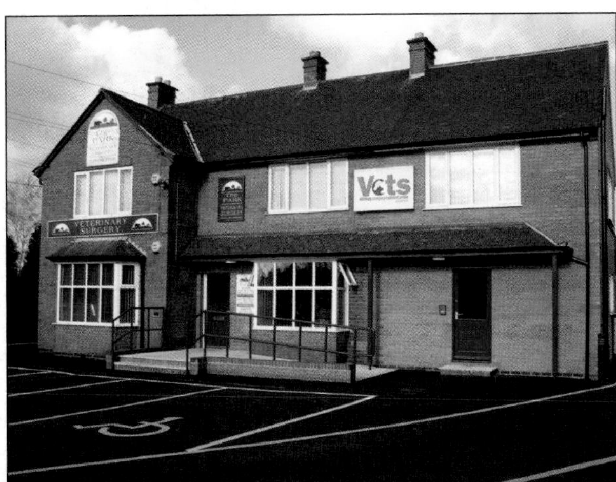

3.8 This wheelchair access ramp was added to cater for an entrance which had two steps to floor level.

Two areas of disability that add little to the building or design costs relate to the partially sighted and those with hearing impairment.

- The **partially sighted** can be helped enormously by having strong colour contrasts between the door and handle, the riser and tread on stairs, stair nosings, handrails and surroundings, etc. A little bit of thought in planning can make a huge difference.
- **Hearing aid users** can be helped with the availability of induction loop technology. These systems could be described as a personal public address system, which picks up the sounds of speech and plays them direct into the earpiece of the hearing aid. Such systems can either be wired into an area or can be portable. The latter option, in most cases, is probably the most practical in veterinary premises, as the portable loop can be stationed at the reception counter but moved into other areas as required.

Client reception

More than ever before the veterinary receptionist is 'tied' to a fixed position by the requirement for access to a computer terminal and keyboard. This means that the reception counter design must, with some degree of subtlety, bring the client to that position. In addition, to use the keyboard efficiently, the receptionist is far better seated. The design, therefore, needs to create a 'cockpit' with all the necessary ingredients readily to hand – the till drawer, credit card machine, printer, etc. (Figure 3.9).

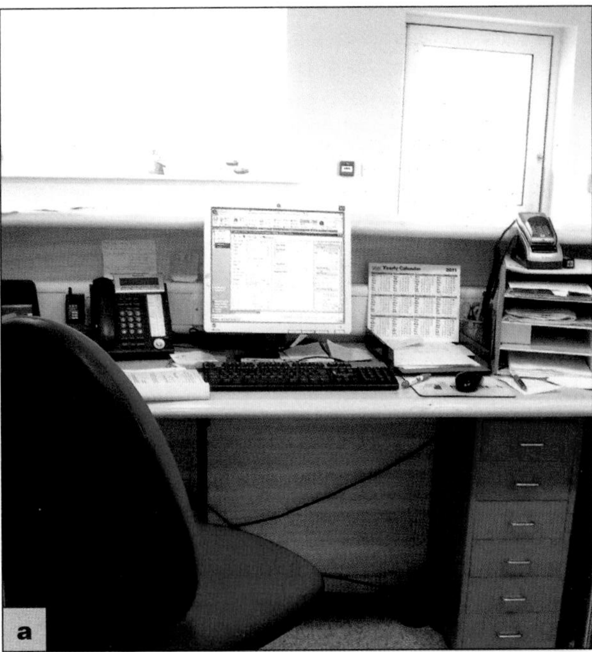

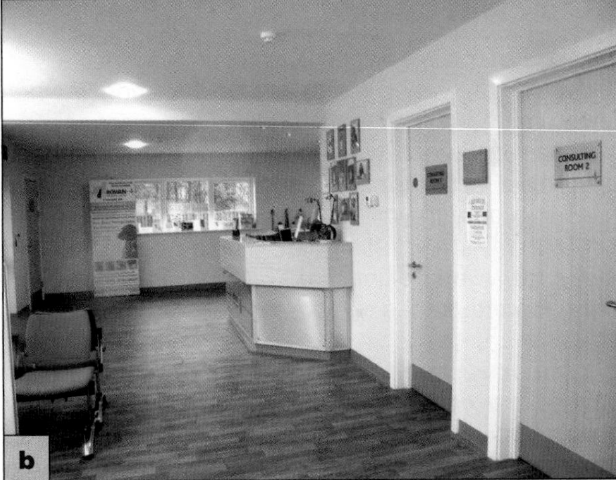

3.9 **(a)** The receptionist has everything to hand and a commanding view of the entrance, ready to greet clients. **(b)** This reception desk allows the receptionist to monitor the whole waiting area.

If the desk is high, there must be a point for serving clients in wheelchairs and others who find higher counters difficult. To give wheelchair users both time and dignity, this service point should be obvious but, if possible, out of the main thoroughfare. As usage is likely to be low, the point can double as a hinged top, where reception staff can gain access to the waiting area to help clients with animals or purchases. This is all covered within BS8300 which is combined into much of the Building Regulations (see Chapter 1).

The receptionist is in a vulnerable position, out front and exposed. Risk includes exposure to disturbed and aggressive clients and, more concerning, to attempted robbery. This adds a security dimension which should be managed, in part, by the design of the counter. Island units are particularly insecure, as receptionists would need to cross the waiting area to escape. It is far better to have the desk linking back to somewhere where there are colleagues around and where the receptionist can just back out of the way. For added security, some form of panic alarm or other device may be installed. Whilst offering security for the receptionist, the reception desk must also offer service access to all clients. The receptionist will also need a direct route into the waiting area, to interact with patients, demonstrate displayed items for sale and maintain the area between busy spells. That takes careful design and planning.

There are times when a receptionist or reception nurse may need to interact face to face with the clinical team. Direct access from reception to the 'prep' or linked dispensary area will bring the team together, permit easier interaction and ultimately improve communication and efficiency within the team. Having to access clinical areas via a consulting room is not ideal.

If the reception point is also the place where dispensed medicines are handed over, there needs to be a logical link to the dispensary area where the medications are prepared for handover. NFA-VPS, POM-VPS and POM-V medicines (see Chapter 15) must not be available for self-selection by the client and should be out of reach and secure. There is, however, no legal restriction about these being in view.

Reception and client waiting areas are discussed in more detail in Chapter 5.

Outpatient waiting

Having been dealt with efficiently and courteously at reception, the client needs a good experience when attending the outpatient services of the practice. This begins with a relatively short waiting period before being seen at the allotted appointment time.

Being able to wait for an appointment in comfort and with minimal stress is key. Single-species waiting areas may work for many, but there are clients who bring more than one species or whose dog seems to attract the unwelcome attention of another animal of the same species. Whilst it is certainly a good idea to have a 'cat only' waiting zone, it is also valuable to have different seating bays so clients can segregate themselves as they desire. It may also be handy to have an out-of-the-way area, the veterinary equivalent to the 'naughty step', for clients with decidedly unsocial or noisy dogs; a covered area outside is also helpful.

As well as the species segregation, there is the subtle management of the client who comes with particular circumstances. For example, the client who has come to the conclusion that it is time to say farewell to their cherished companion may not want to sit amongst the general hubbub for their last few moments with their beloved pet. Here, a mix of case management and design can come into play.

Consulting rooms

Ultimately, the client is paying for a private consultation with the veterinary surgeon. That privacy should be maintained by good design and careful management:

- The management comes from not disturbing the consultation with obtuse enquiries and issues
- On the design side, it is to do with the management of sound travel and having a layout that has been well planned so virtually everything needed is to hand.

The idea of a supply passage, running behind the consulting rooms, is far from new. It allows all consulting supplies to be stored in one place, and reduces the overall stock-holding requirement dramatically. Equally important, however, is having a design that allows the practice to admit and discharge animals without their crossing the waiting room, and to have a discrete exit route for cadavers and for distressed clients. An example of a floor plan for a consulting room is shown in Figure 3.10. Consulting rooms are discussed in more detail in Chapter 6.

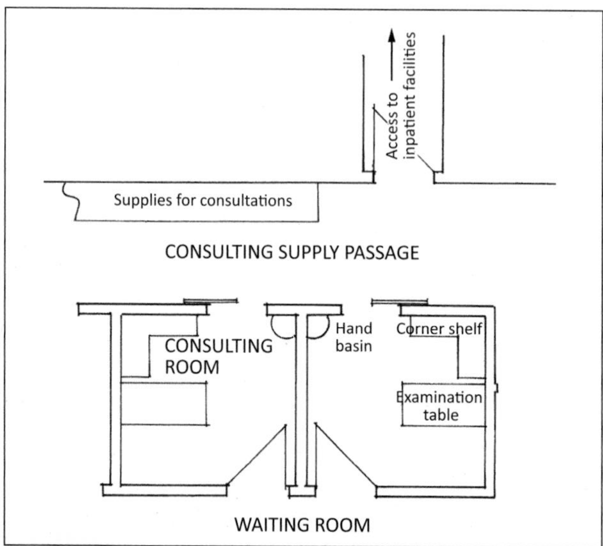

3.10 An example of a floor plan for a consulting room.

Adequate washing and disinfection facilities are essential. Best Practice is, logically, to have a handbasin in each consulting room, positioned so that the consulting vet or nurse, or the client, can wash their hands without doing an awkward dance around each other.

KEY POINT

Hand-washing and disinfection facilities are essential in every area where animals are handled or examined. Hands must be clean before touching any door.

Non-surgical areas

This term covers all inpatient handling areas other than operating theatres. In the same way as outpatient areas must flow correctly, so too must inpatient areas. Ergonomics really come into play, thinking through the various movements (Figure 3.11).

Getting the practice linkages right can be one of the most challenging parts of the design project. It is also one of the most important, as decisions made will have a permanent impact on the day-to-day workings of the clinical team, and the costs of the construction.

Corridors and movement areas

Corridors cost money and should be kept to the practical minimum. They are, however, necessary and provide a hygiene and noise barrier which can be very important.

Wards

The number of inpatients housed will vary according to the caseload and the out-of-hours policy of the practice. Facilities are needed for day cases, overnight stays, and longer hospitalization. This may well place a design challenge on ward space for patients, nursing staff, visitors and team rounds, as well as accommodation for overnight supervisory staff.

Many owners wish to visit their pets. A ward off the preparation area may therefore not be a good idea, as it restricts the time of client access. Ideally, for visits to the ward, or a quiet space, animal housing should be placed between the consulting area and the inpatient treatment areas. This means that clients can be taken beyond the consulting zone, to visit their pet, without disrupting diagnostic and surgical procedures.

Whilst many wards are 'off-square' converted rooms, a better design can be to have longer narrower wards with no animals facing each other. Whilst this is an aim, it is not always possible to achieve due to various design constraints. Figure 3.12 shows a useful layout of wards with the links to laundry, food preparation and the nursing station. Avoiding animals facing each other has been achieved, apart from the dog walk-in cages. Inpatient wards are discussed in more detail in Chapter 7.

There must be hand-washing facilities in each ward area so that there is no need for staff to open a door to access a sink. Adequate sinks for washing equipment should also be provided.

To ensure maximum cleanability of the ward it is helpful to place cages on a pre-made plinth, which has the floor coving fixed to the upright.

- For dog cages, a plinth 100 mm high allows the coving to reach the top of the plinth and to be trimmed flush, with the small front lip of the cage bank overlapping and forming a neat and clean finish (Figure 3.13).
- With cat cages, to avoid having to crouch down to drag a reluctant cat from the back of a floor-level tier, a slightly higher plinth for the floor coving, then a storage area for cat carriers, with the first tier of cages at around 635 mm above the finished floor level seems ideal (Figure 3.14).

Two tiers of cages works well. With careful planning, there is scope above cages for storage of bedding,

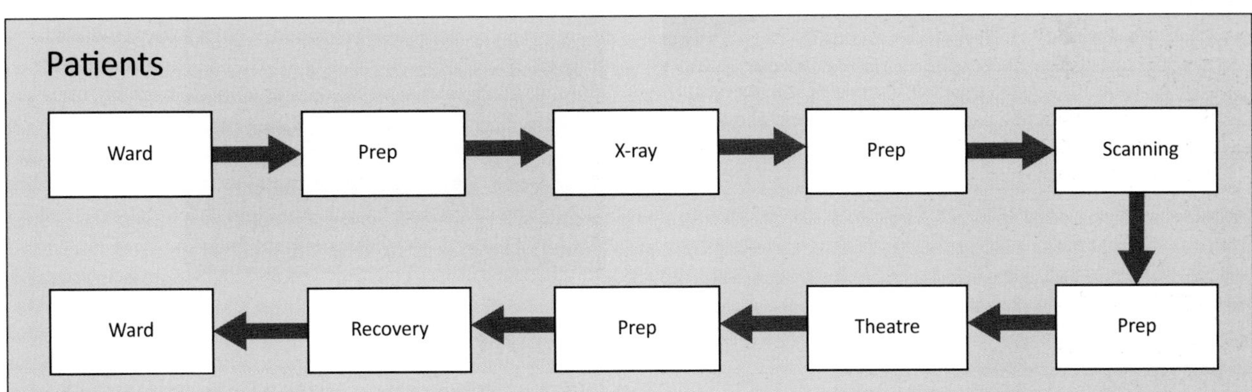

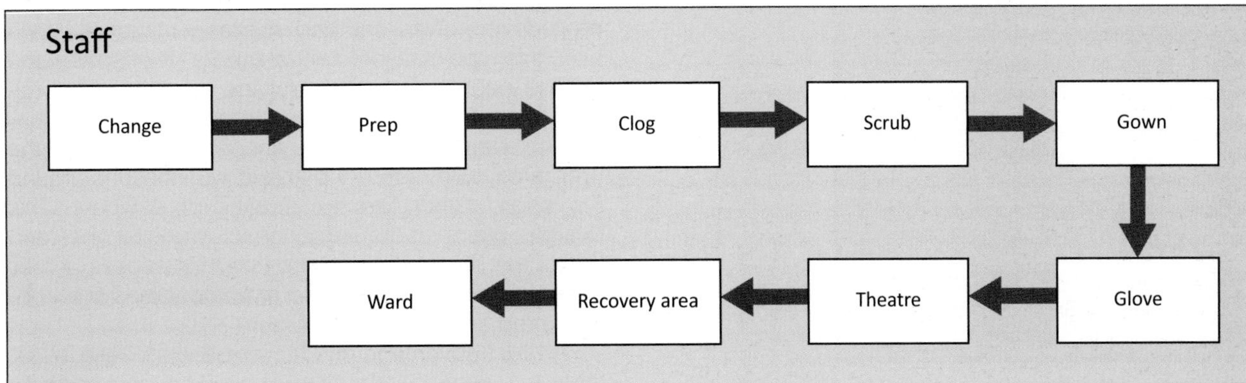

3.11 Traffic flow for patients and for staff must be carefully considered when designing how areas are linked up.

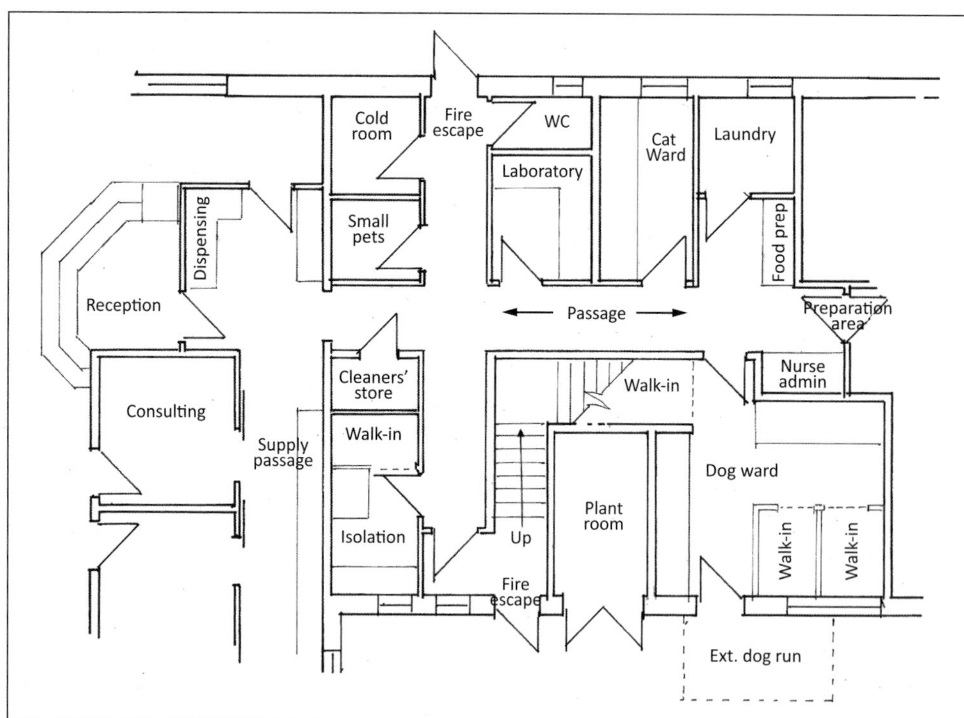

3.12 An example of a floor plan for inpatient wards and related areas.

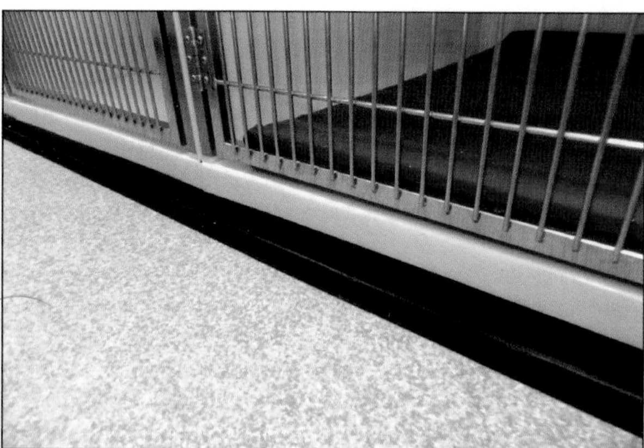

3.13 Mounting cages on a plinth makes cleaning easier, raises patients away from draughts and allows for easier replacement of cages should this be necessary.

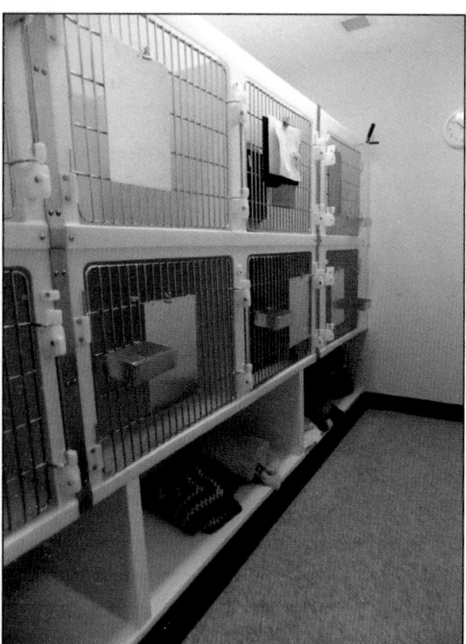

3.14 Under-cage storage can be useful for heavier items, and smaller cages are always best raised above floor level for ease of access.

and other related items, and room for some form of 'pelmet' carrying electrical sockets for heat pads, monitors, pumps, etc. (Figure 3.15). Oxygen pipelines can terminate in these pelmets or be ceiling-mounted (see Chapter 2).

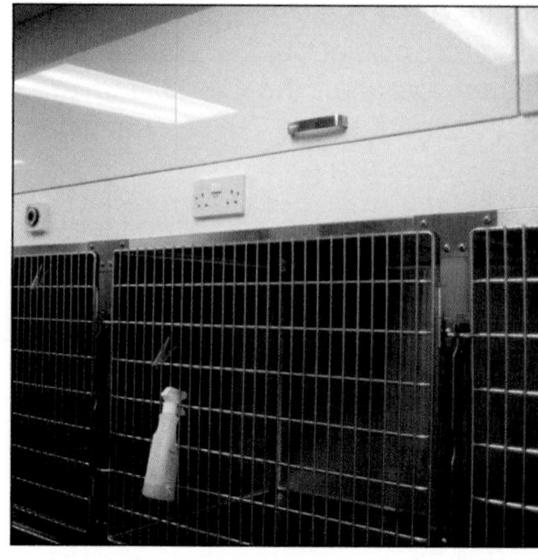

3.15 Above the kennel bank is the ideal place to design in electrical sockets, oxygen outlets and storage for bedding, etc.

Preparation area

Often, a dream is for a large preparation ('prep') area with workstations in the centre of the room and clever drop-down power, gas and scavenging points. However, this type of layout can take up a lot of space and lead to people walking round the edges of the prep area to get to where they need to go.

The alternative is to have a clear central hub to the prep area, with carefully planned workstations around the edge, rather like the spokes of a wheel. This design offers more ergonomic workstations and keeps the centre of the room clear for access across and to all parts. An example of a floor plan for a hub-type prep area is shown in Figure 3.16.

A great advantage of specialized work bays is that there is a natural separation of hygiene roles such as scrubbing up, instrument preparation, hand hygiene, and other sink use. The prep area is the centre of the

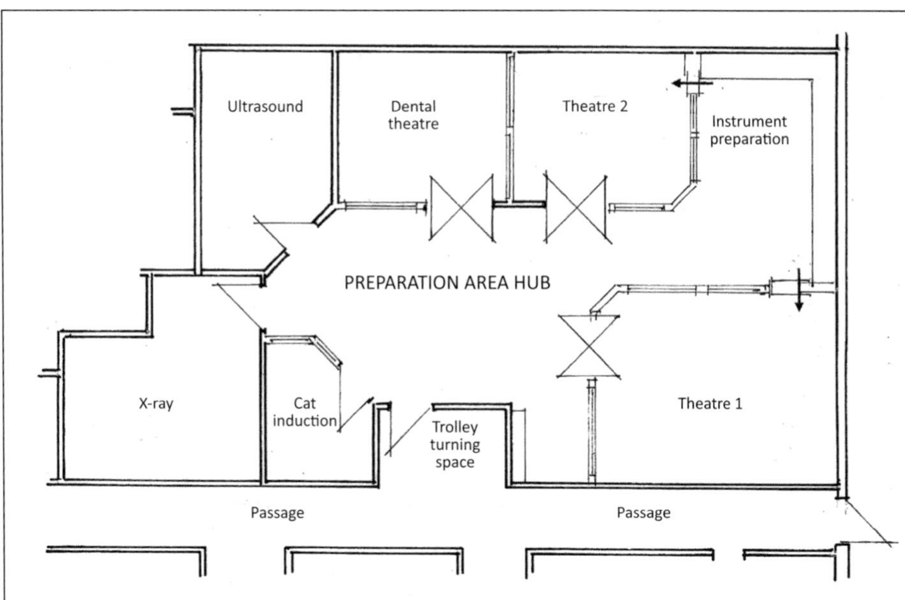

3.16 An example of a floor plan for a hub-type preparation area within a building conversion project. Note the use of angled doors into the ultrasonography and cat induction rooms, avoiding corners in the prep area. The arrows mark the positions of sterile pass-through cabinets for instruments.

diagnostic and treatment zone, and hygiene should be separate from inpatient area cleaning. With such a design, it can be useful to have enclosed spaces where the movement of the patient is limited, should they wriggle free. Such spaces can be used for induction of anaesthesia in cats, or restricted spaces for noisy patients. Off the hub are the anaesthesia induction station(s), scrub area, instrument preparation area, and the like. From the prep hub a pair of two-way-swing doors lead into the operating theatres, so trolleys can be pushed through and scrubbed staff can back out. Radiography and other diagnostic rooms surround the empty hub, and the prep area workstations are in bays.

More space can be gained in the preparation hub, and easier trolleying can be achieved, if the dedicated rooms to the side have angled doors (Figure 3.17). In essence, an unused corner of the theatre, radiography room, etc., is stolen and added to the hub area. This is often only workable in new-build projects or in conversions where there are large clear roof spans. Preparation areas are discussed in more detail in Chapter 8.

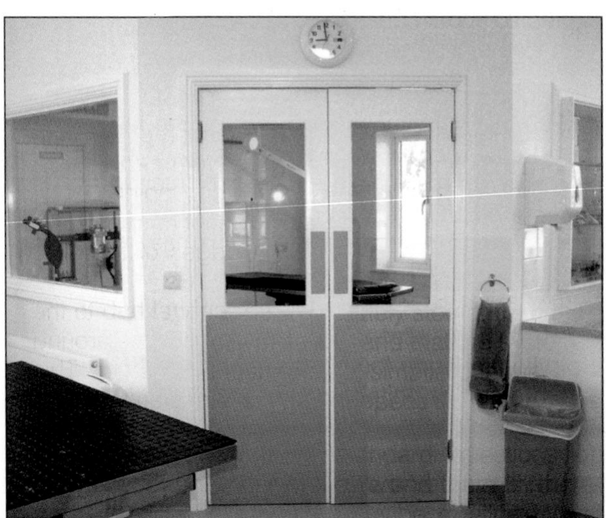

3.17 An angled theatre door can be very useful. It avoids turning trolleys 90 degrees and adds space in the prep area.

Operating theatres

Further details can be found in Chapter 8 and in the *BSAVA Manual of Surgical Principles.*

Space

Theatre layouts are fairly simple rectangles, in general. Different veterinary surgeons seem to require varying amounts of space; this seems as much to do with what they have grown used to in other environments as to the procedures being undertaken. Some procedures where large equipment is used, however, do dictate larger theatre spaces. Examples are laser surgery, orthopaedics where fluoroscopy is used, endoscopy, and procedures using an operating microscope. One way to gain space around a theatre table is to place it diagonally in the room. This gives more working space at each side and end. This is a particularly useful layout if the corner of the theatre has been angled (see above).

Hygiene and safety

Operating theatres, whether for sterile, non-sterile or dental procedures, should all be rooms that are *'no through roads'*. This is one of the key elements of best practice which helps keep them clean. Another is to have the minimum of items retained in the theatre. If, at the start and end of each day, there is just the operating table on the floor, the room will be much easier to clean. More detail about cleanable surfaces and options are discussed later in this chapter.

The concept of a sterile cabinet, or pass-through cabinet, *between* the instrument preparation area and theatres, also saves space and clutter (Figure 3.18). Sterile items can enter the theatre through the cabinet and be placed on a suitable instrument trolley during use. At the end of the procedure, they can be wheeled out of the theatre, back to the instrument preparation area for cleaning and sterilization.

Wall-mounted anaesthetic machines avoid the use of trolleys, and ceiling and wall lights keep the floor clear of trip-hazard stands.

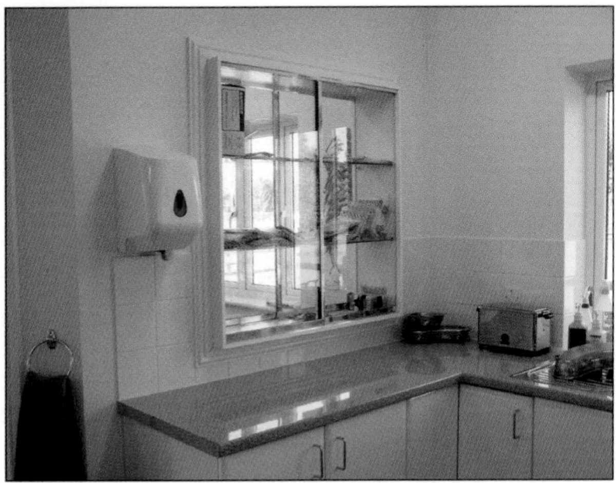

3.18 The double glazed sides of the pass-through (sterile) cabinet allow sterile kits to be stored ready for use, and improve light transfer and visual communication.

Service areas

These are discussed in more detail in Chapter 7.

Laundry

Laundry is often a difficult issue, with high volumes of water usage and the need to dry items within a moderate timescale. Where space and budget allows, the separation of human apparel, theatre laundry and animal bedding into separate laundry areas offers some useful benefits.

- A laundry for patient bedding is best located next to the wards and near to, but separate from, food preparation areas.
- The staff scrubs and uniforms laundry should be close to the changing area, so could be upstairs.
- The theatre laundry could be close to the 'prep' room and the instrument preparation area (Figure 3.19). Increasing use of disposable drapes and gowns may make this type of laundry redundant.

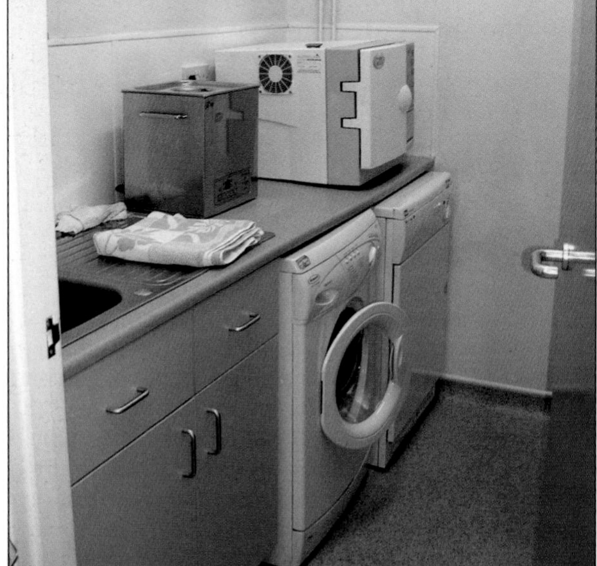

3.19 For smaller practices, a combined food prep and uniforms laundry, close to the wards, becomes an *ad hoc* nursing station.

However well intentioned, the practicality of relying on natural drying is not viable and some form of assisted drying will be required. Where possible some external drying area is useful but tumble driers, either electrical or gas-powered, are likely to be the mainstay and, ideally, should be situated against an external wall so the drier can vent to the outside. Should the external wall option be impossible, there are condensing driers that do not require direct venting, but ventilation is still essential. Another drying option could be a warm room but space costs and ventilation needs tend to make this less attractive.

Cleaning cupboard

A cleaners' cupboard (Figure 3.20) may be set aside for central use or for an out-of-hours or contract cleaner to use, but cleaning equipment must be accessible to all areas of the practice throughout the day. It is helpful to keep separate colour-coded mops and buckets to hand for each area (see Figure 3.40).

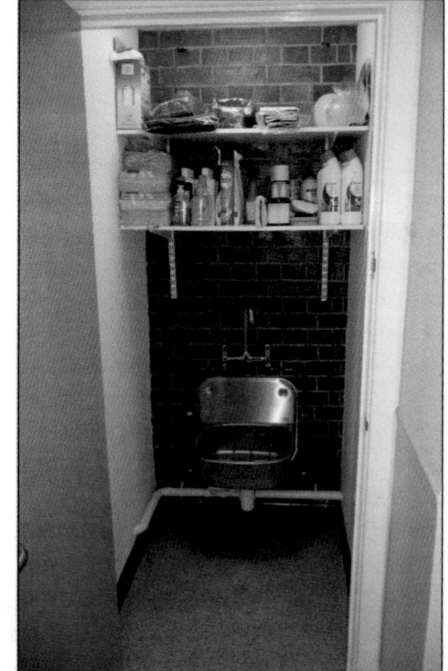

3.20 A cleaners' cupboard with a low sink for bucket filling and emptying creates a dirty sluice. It also keeps cleaning chemicals away from clinical areas.

Laboratory

The practice laboratory (see Chapter 14) can be located in a number of areas. The best position will depend on the type and range of work undertaken, as well as the equipment used. Where the laboratory is used for procedures needing peace and quiet, siting the facility away from the main hub, maybe upstairs, would seem ideal: it can give the required element of peace; and upper floor space is normally at less of a premium. However, a first-floor location will cause staff to leave their main duty area to undertake diagnostic testing.

Samples are taken in the consulting room and in the inpatient treatment area, and probably in the preparation room and theatres. A laboratory positioned between these areas, for example off the supply passage behind the consulting rooms and close to the preparation area, would be ideal. In some situations it is possible to have a hatch between the laboratory and preparation areas, so samples can be passed through for diagnostic processes.

Mortuary

The vast majority of UK practices use some variety of freezer for the storage of cadavers, after bagging and labelling. These have the benefits of being cheap and compact. However, domestic chest freezers are designed to freeze down modest quantities of garden produce, not the volume of many of the cadavers handled in veterinary practice, particularly ones not yet cold. In addition, there is the health and safety aspect of lifting the cadaver in, and the contractor's employee lifting out the frozen mass. Best Practice would therefore be to avoid these units.

Logical alternatives such as a cold room should be considered where space permits. This is simply an insulated room, kept at a temperature of around 5°C. The walls can have racking against them so that cadavers, brought in by trolley, can be slid on to the shelves, avoiding lifting. Apart from all the issues of cadaver dignity, and health and safety of staff and contractors, there is the practical aspect of maintaining a chilled corpse for a short while, just in case the client decides they wish to bury their late pet at home. Presenting and explaining a frozen block is not the easiest public relations exercise when dealing with a bereaved client. Cold rooms can be constructed, or purchased, from local refrigeration companies, some as stand-alone units, possibly reconditioned; or an existing space can be insulated and a refrigeration unit installed through an external wall. Bagged Hazardous waste and Offensive waste can also be kept in this environment, avoiding risks of odours.

Discreet removal of cadavers is important; this may be very difficult on a corner site, with views of all sides.

Dog run

External dog exercise runs are very useful, as many dogs will only defecate on grass. However, this adds both a facility and a hygiene challenge, and taking a dog outside does add an escape risk. An enclosed lawned area can be useful for walking patients, but it may not be possible or practical to have such an area.

The best approach for an outside run is to link this directly to the dog ward as the only access point. The unit should have a cage top, or a covered top but cage sides. A good cleanable surface with a drainage gulley and hose point will aid cleaning. To reduce the risk of complaints about barking dogs, the run should be screened to reduce stimuli. All runs must be totally secure in terms of being both escape-proof and theft-proof, and will require some form of double-door entrance and exit.

Support facilities

Areas are also needed for administration, staff refreshments, overnight accommodation, and the like (see Chapter 16). These facilities can often be located upstairs, one floor away from the client and patient areas. For many general practices, and some hospitals, all these facilities can be accommodated in approximately half the floor space required on the ground floor, giving the option of a partial first floor, or the use of a dormer-style roof with offices and rest rooms built into the roof space (Figure 3.21). Factors to be considered are listed in Figure 3.22. Ease of access from any overnight duty accommodation to the inpatient areas is important, as are privacy and security of duty staff.

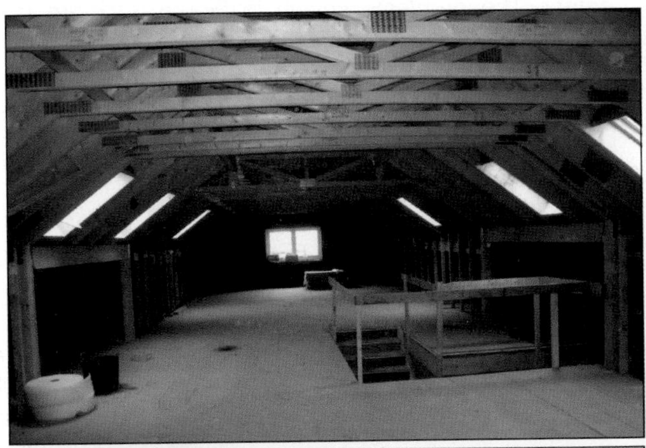
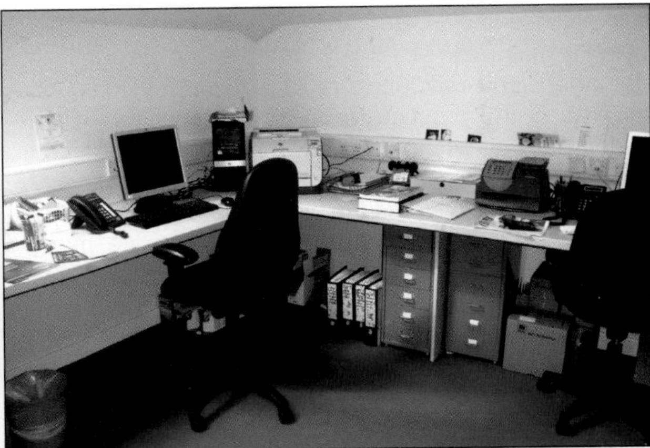
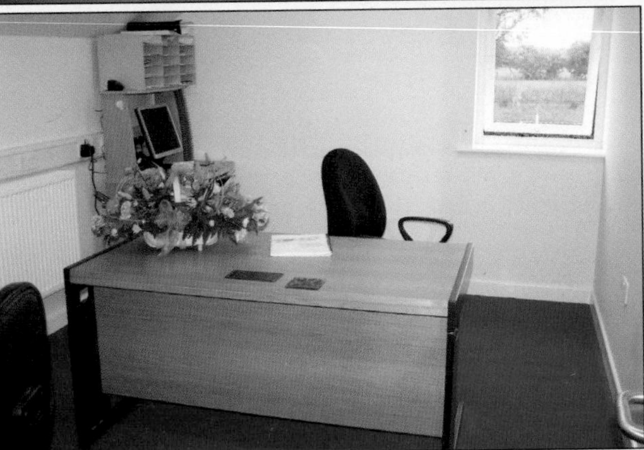
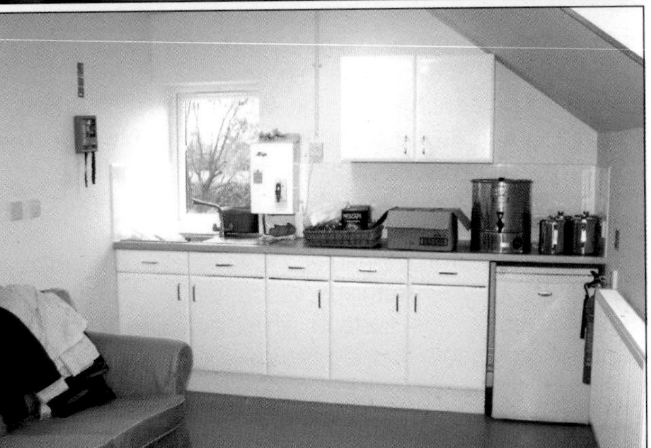

3.21 The space within a dormer-style roof can be ideal for fitting out with a residential flat, administrative office, duty rest room or staff facilities.

Administration
■ What space is required? ■ How many staff spaces? ■ Is there need for private space (cash counting, interviews)? ■ Do proprietors need individual office space? ■ Assistants/Nurses space for study? ■ Where do staff go to telephone clients? ■ What about study and training? ■ Where is the main server and telephone system?
Staff facilities
■ Coffee, breaks, lunch, and rest? ■ Safe locker storage for personal apparel and possessions? ■ Changing and showering facilities? ■ Overnight accommodation for duty staff? ■ Assistant, nurse or security person's flat? ■ Staff pets?
Other factors
■ First-floor practice facilities (laboratory, laundry, etc.)? ■ Archive storage? ■ Communications room? ■ Meeting room? ■ Library, lecture/training facilities?

3.22 Some of the facilities that can be sited on a non-clinical floor, with some of the questions that may be useful to determine requirements.

Surface finishes and materials

One of the most taxing aspects of veterinary design is to balance cost, longevity, maintenance, repair and refit disruption when it comes to the treatments of walls, floors and fitments. Some of the currently attractive finishes may date rapidly as fashions change, whilst some may be highly durable but unsightly if damaged, and difficult to replace without closing off an area of the practice for a fairly extensive refit. All sheet material, whether flooring, wall boards, or tiling, comes with joints. It is often these joints that are the vulnerable areas and cause the greatest let-down.

There is no perfect solution but there are many options. Sometimes, simple solutions can offer the most practical result and the best value.

Flooring

The RCVS Practice Standards make various references to flooring, cleanliness and safety. Of particular note is the reference to impervious walls and floors with a curved finish at the join, to aid cleaning. This coving must continue up the wall at least 75 mm. Although the Practice Standards currently only *require* this type of surface in veterinary hospitals, and only in their inpatient areas, having this finish for all inpatient areas is logical. Best practice should dictate this, as some of the greatest hygiene challenges are seen elsewhere in the premises, such as in consulting rooms. Gaining this surface whilst avoiding slipping dangers on smooth flooring is a design challenge.

Slip-resistant finishes

Smooth floor surfaces can become treacherous in the event of liquid spillages or where barrier matting is insufficient and water is brought in on shoes and paws. This creates a challenge in waiting areas, with the odd puddle, and elsewhere with other spillages. In addition, and equally important, is the fact that many dogs will not stand easily on smooth floors. These factors indicate the need for slip-resistant flooring.

- Slip-resistant flooring is not slip-proof; it just helps reduce the risk of slipping because the floor surface grips the feet.
- The downside is that what grips feet will also grip dirt.
- Whilst some older-style slip-resistant flooring is difficult to keep clean, the more modern slip-resistant vinyl products have much more cleanable surfaces. These floors, however, do need a special cleaning regime and specialist products.

The traditional way of laying coved vinyl floors involves placing a 'former' at the joint between the floor and the wall, and bending the floor covering up the wall for the required distance. Joins are welded, using a hot gun and colour-matched rods. This was quite serviceable in the days of smooth vinyl and the finish is still used in low-risk human medical situations such as hospital corridors and health centres.

With slip-resistant materials, bending them up the wall creates an area around the room that will attract dust and grip dirt; all those little gripping flecks have been squashed together, multiplying their dirt-gripping effect. What is more, mechanical scrubbers, both rotor and rotary, do not clean well on the coved area and cannot get into corners. In addition, in many situations, the top of the coving needs a special capping running around the room, adding a 5 mm shelf for dust to gather. The problems shown in Figure 3.23 are far from uncommon. The situation arises in areas of particular stress but, in doing so, ruins the entire project.

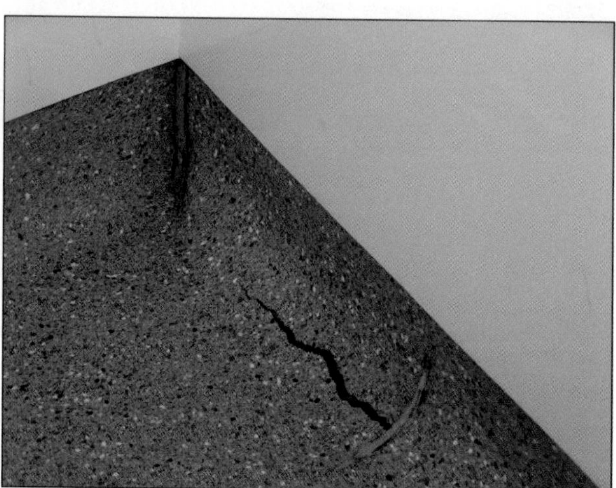

3.23 Slip-resistant flooring, coved up the wall, can split in time. This floor is only 8 years old.

The solution is to fit a smooth-surfaced coving around the room. This pre-formed coving comes in long rolls, so there is no need for difficult joins at intervals along the wall length, just neat mitres in the corners (Figure 3.24). The slip-resistant vinyl is then laid flat on the floor, with all joints hot welded as before. By not stressing the flooring by bending it up the wall, longevity seems far superior. The inset, or set-in,

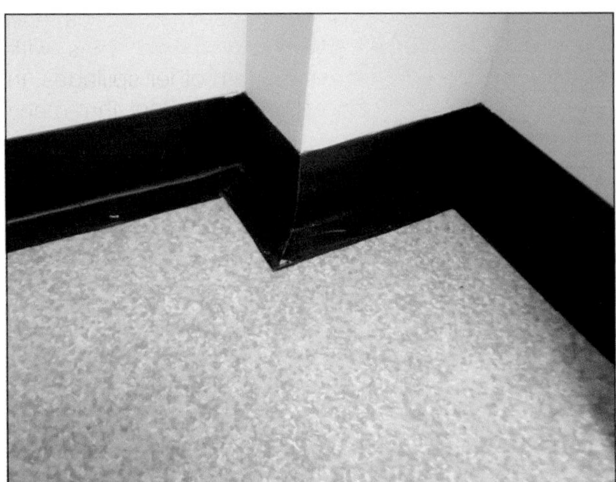

3.24 Using a smooth coving with a slip-resistant floor avoids the dirt trap that is created when vinyl is coved up a wall. It provides an easy-clean curve and, normally, a much extended life.

coving approach leaves a neat level joint between floor and cove, unlike 'sit-on' coving, which is not acceptable under RCVS standards. The set-in coving is now being used in NHS clinical areas, though with smooth flooring. See Figure 7.2 for an illustration of colour-coordinated set-in coving in a ward area.

Whilst flooring contractors may try persuasion towards the traditional approach, they do not have to clean the floor or close down for a refit ten years hence.

> **KEY POINT**
>
> Always use a contractor on the flooring manufacturers recommended list that is a member of the Contract Flooring Association (CFA).

Other floor surfaces

One of the most attractive smooth floor surfaces is traditional linoleum. This material tends to be somewhat thicker than vinyl, adding some comfort and flex, and is very hard-wearing. There are pre-formed inset coving units, and slip-resistant surfaces, so it can be fully compliant.

There are some wet-laid floor surfaces, such as epoxy and other painted or poured on surfaces. These can have slip-resistant particles added. Whilst often not as attractive, and liable to cracking should there be any substructure movement, they can offer a lower-cost alternative for utility and other areas. Such a slip-resistant finish to an external dog run, with good drain points and hosing, can help considerably with cleaning.

Foot cleaning

Where people enter with wet or dirty feet, the aim is to have a wiping and foot-cleaning area, normally a minimum of two strides. The traditional coir (coconut) door mats have given way to newer mechanisms. Many of these still face cleaning challenges in the veterinary situation, particularly in an enclosed lobby.

One excellent approach, working well with slip-resistant vinyl, is the lay-flat mat. This is a rubber-backed and -edged fabric mat, which is just laid on the floor inside the door. These mats are normally provided as part of a cleaning contract, and are collected and replaced regularly to keep them hygienic. They can have wording or logos on them and make a pleasant welcome for clients (Figure 3.25).

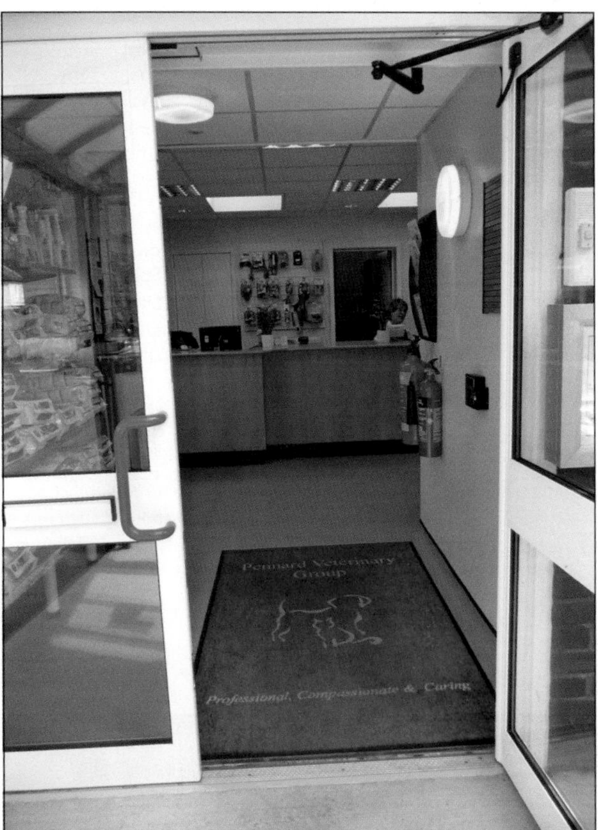

3.25 A modern lay-flat doormat, which takes two strides to cross, helps clean wet shoes and protects the floor. Most types can be laundered by commercial suppliers.

Walls

There are a vast range of options for wall finishes, from fair-faced concrete block, through a range of wall boards and laminates, and paint-on finishes, to ceramic tiles (Figure 3.26). There is, as always, a balance between costs, repair, longevity, fashion, and visual appeal.

On a cost–benefit basis, paint-on surfaces have two clear points in their favour:

- They are mostly of relatively low expense
- They give a homogeneous finish, with no joints. This has to be balanced against cleanability and longevity. Today, there are low-odour paints that can be scrubbed clean if required. They are a little more costly than normal emulsions, but demand real consideration in many hygiene areas.

Veterinary walls, like those in many situations, take more punishment on their lower half than on the upper half. Traditionally, institutional walls were painted using gloss paint at the bottom and emulsion – or colour wash – at the top. There are economic benefits of dividing some walls, top and bottom, with different finishes, or, perhaps, some physical barrier such as a plain dado strip of some kind (Figure 3.27).

Wall type	Surface finish	Comments
High hygiene (operating theatres, etc.)	Ceramic tiling and waterproof grout	Very tough: colours and styles must be chosen carefully as the surface will last decades Cleanable and non-staining Danger from impact – carry spares Concerns about the grout – probably not well founded when considering sterilization options Quite costly unless simple white 150 mm square selected
	Wall coverings (vinyl sheet/ laminate panels)	Tough, semi-homogeneous Easily cleaned Can have difficult joins; some raised and not well sealed Often poor appearance as fashions change but well within the design life
	Painted finish	Completely homogeneous Some tough options, including scrubbable vinyl Gloss – looks institutional; eggshell – OK Epoxy resin – very tough, does stain, poor appearance Sprayed/flecked – tough but easily pulled off with tape, sticky putty, etc. and then unsightly and uneven Difficult to patch
Medium hygiene	Painted finish	Completely homogeneous Some tough options, including scrubbable vinyl and eggshell Fill and repaint if damaged
Modest hygiene	Painted finish	Completely homogeneous Some tough options, including scrubbable vinyl and eggshell Fill and repaint if damaged
	Wallpaper, etc.	Can be used to good effect on upper walls in waiting and consulting rooms; depends on practice style and pattern

3.26 Wall finishes.

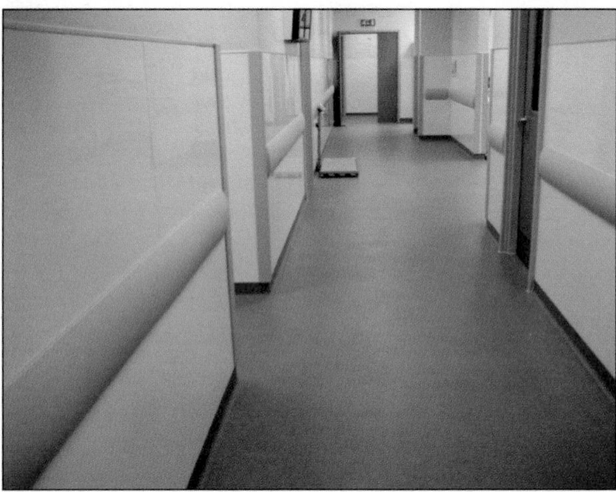

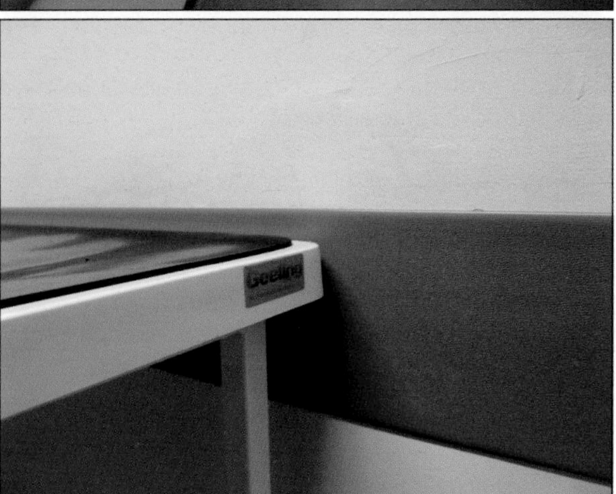

3.27 Wall protectors, set at trolley rubbing height, avoid damage to the wall surfaces and keep the place looking good for years. The same sort of approach can be used for chair rubbing, or to divide upper and lower walls for a less bland approach, or for decorative purposes.

- Where chairs will rub, some form of broad strip around the room offers protection and the opportunity to use different finishes above and below.
- In consulting rooms, the lower half gets grubby faster, with the coats of damp and dirty dogs brushing against the walls. Here, some division can, again, be useful. In this situation, some form of dado banding can avoid a room looking too plain and can give the opportunity to soften the décor above the line but maintain tough serviceability on the higher stress lower level.

Ceilings

The great thing about plaster ceilings is that they can be washed down and repainted as required. In addition, they are a sealed surface, so very useful in high-hygiene areas. However, that same sealing can be a disadvantage, in that access above is difficult without damage. In construction terms, they may be more expensive than other options.

Suspended ceilings

These consist of square or rectangular panels held within a grid. That grid is suspended from fixed points, which can be several metres above in large open spaces. The great advantage is that services can run above the ceiling, with easy access by removing the odd panel. They are also relatively cheap (less than the cost of paint, plaster skim, plasterboard and a structure to carry it).

The insert panels are normally made of mineral fibre, which is adequate for reception, waiting and consulting areas, along with internal corridors, etc. In addition, the manufacturers do make panels with tough, smooth, cleanable surfaces; however these are a major task to clean. While these ceilings are not a particularly good finish for wards and inpatient treatment areas, they do have some advantage where the area has a flat roof. Witho ut suspended ceilings, all the wiring, plumbing, and other services running above the ceiling would become inaccessible.

Ceiling heights

Many modern ceilings are installed at a height of 2400 mm. This has more to do with domestic building costs than with pleasant spaces. Where possible, such as new building projects, designing ceilings at 2500–2600 mm can make a huge difference to the working environment. As veterinary spaces tend to be quite small, however, over-high ceilings can look odd and make rooms appear out of proportion.

Doors and doorways

In terms of materials, the choice is between veneered timber, paint and inset laminate finishes (Figure 3.28).

Hinges

Door hinges should be of high quality. Three hinges on each door (often referred to as 'a pair and a half') should be used for all doors. With two-way swing doors, in clinical areas, there are two hinging options. Side-mounted hinges are like normal hinges but swing both ways. These are sometimes thought inferior compared to floor-mounted units, where the doors are hinged with metal fittings in the floor and ceiling. However, side-mounted hinges do the job very well and do not add the sort of dirt trap created by floor-mounted units.

Door furniture

This term is used to cover handles, locks, knobs, finger-plates, kick-plates, and signage (Figure 3.29). Veterinary practice doors are subject to high usage and a good deal of abuse. The handles and fitments must be tough enough to take the loading. Within the Disability Discrimination Act (DDA) there is a requirement to plan for visual impairment; a good contrast between the door finish and handles is a help. Aluminium, steel or brass against timber, or some well linked coloured handles against timber or paint, can satisfy the DDA and look really good. Finger-plates, kick-plates and protection from trolleys all need careful thought and positioning. There are now colour-coordinated push-plates and other protection that can be ordered to size and affixed to the door. They can add spark and colour to liven up any area and are an alternative to stainless steel.

Where doors have closers, such as fire doors (see Chapter 2), strong ball-catches may be considered instead of handles to turn. One side would then have a

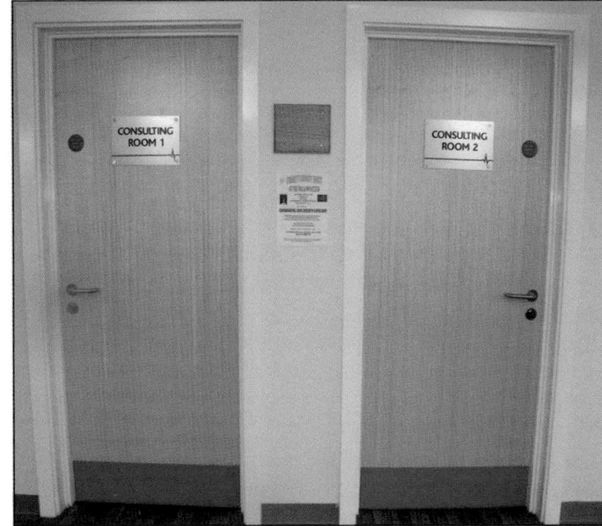

3.29 Taking the trouble to ensure that the door finish reflects other design and colour approaches in the practice adds that little extra. It should be noted that the DDA requires a good contrast between the door finish and handle for the partially sighted.

Finish	Advantages	Disadvantages	Comments
Doors			
Varnished timber	Attractive. Cleanable. Rarely need re-coating	Fixed colour. Need to replace if damaged (finish not easy to repair)	Useful in client areas (e.g. consulting room front doors, entrances, offices)
Laminate	Attractive. Colour-coordinated. Very low maintenance. Cleanable	Fixed colour. Impossible to repair if scratched	Very expensive. Need protection if exposed to rougher handling
Paint	Colour options. Readily repairable (fill scratches, sand, repaint). Cleanable (gloss)	Regular redecoration required. Silk, sheen, matt paints less cleanable	Useful in non-client areas
Doorframes			
Varnished timber	Cleanable	Can match with doors. Very expensive, as bespoke	Probably avoid
Gloss paint	Can add contrast. Tough. Cleanable. Low cost	Standard door casings: usually softwood, so easily damaged, leading to chipped paint. Maintenance required	Useful for almost all doorways
Matt/silk paint	Softer appearance. Fairly cleanable	Standard door casings: usually softwood, so easily damaged, leading to chipped paint. Higher maintenance as less easy to wipe clean	Client areas, if avoiding gloss

3.28 Door and doorframe finishes.

push-plate, the other a 'D' handle to pull. This approach makes passage quicker and uses less costly fittings, though the door closers must be set correctly.

Locks and keys

Locks are expensive items and door 'schedules', containing details of all ironmongery and locking systems for each door, should be carefully planned so that locks are only fitted to doors which will need to be locked. Main security doors will need locks compliant with insurance company demands (see Chapter 2); others may not. Often, a simple thumb-turn lock, the modern equivalent of a bolt, will be all that is needed, say, to lock the front consulting room door when not in use.

All types of key can be 'suited': this is where one key may open various doors but not others; and there can be a master key that opens all doors. Careful decisions on suiting can save people carrying and fumbling masses of keys. The door schedule should be planned so that security-critical keys are only held by staff members who need them. This reduces costs should a key be lost and locks need to be changed.

Where doors that are used frequently need to be locked, keys can become a real problem. Here, coded door locks, or card-operated systems, are preferable. Such doors are best kept to a minimum and, where possible, the swipe-card approach is the fastest, though most costly. Most practices find a button keypad system (Figure 3.30) the most practical.

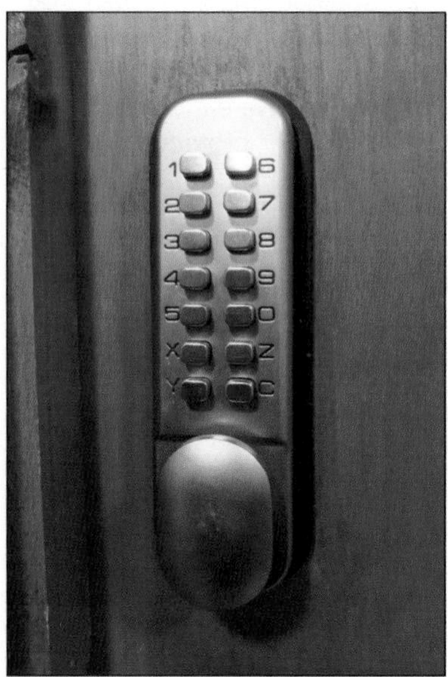

3.30 Simple coded door locks can be very useful for restricting access to certain areas.

Fitments

Further detail on storage units, etc., can be found in the chapters dealing with specific practice areas.

Fitments may be:

- Ceiling-mounted, e.g. theatre lights. These will need some form of ceiling strengthening to take their weight and forces at full stretch. This may require structural calculations to design adequate support
- Wall-mounted.

Cabinet base units

Materials

Whether from a retail DIY store, a trade supplier or a specialist medical furniture supplier, base units will appear remarkably similar. Costs, however, range enormously.

The models designed for medical use tend to be considerably more expensive for the few extras they offer (e.g. locks on doors, slightly heavier construction). There is also the option to consider units made from alternative materials, such as stainless steel. Stainless steel is a very tough material, though cost often makes it rather thin and sometimes noisy for base units. Whilst, clinically, some would claim advantages, aesthetically it is rather harsh.

Units constructed from slightly higher than normal specification timber/particle board are likely to be more attractive, of much lower cost, and often more practical. There is, however, some vulnerability to constant wetting, depending on the finish. Those with simple lines and high-gloss finish do seem capable of taking the punishment found in veterinary practice. All units, however, need regular cleaning and maintenance to retain their integrity and appearance.

Placement

If the floor is laid correctly, evidence suggests that a lifespan of 20+ years is possible. It would be a very superior base unit that would survive veterinary practice punishment for that long. There is, therefore, a need to be able to replace the units before the flooring has reached its design-life end. If the floor surface has coving to the units, which it should have in hospitals, there is a longer-term potential problem. The solution is to have a separate plinth, set in the position of the units. The floor coving can be fixed to the plinth and the units fixed on top. When units need replacing, it is a relatively simple job to take them off the plinth and install new units. This is helped by the fact that most kitchen units sit on adjustable legs and the plinths just clip on to the legs; if both legs and plinths are removed, the units can sit on the pre-fixed plinth instead (Figure 3.31).

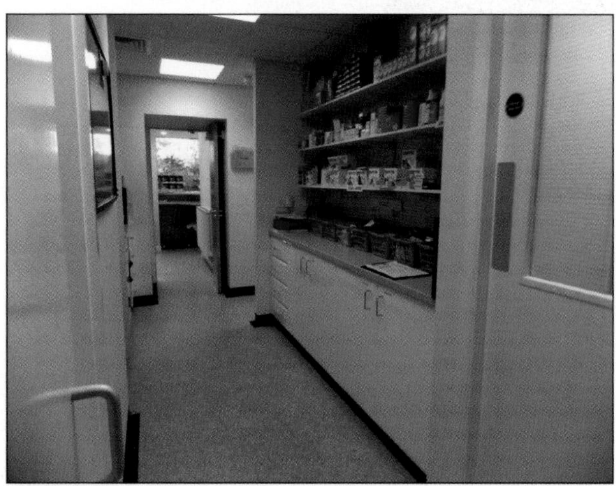

3.31 The base cupboards of this dispensing area are mounted on a pre-formed plinth which spans an alcove. The cupboards could, therefore, be replaced or altered without damage to the floor.

Most base units have a rear void of 60–100 mm. This is to leave space for plumbing runs, although some of the modern pipe support systems, and wrap-around insulation, are deeper than 100 mm. One answer is to note all pipe drops and runs, and ask the contractor to avoid using anything which takes up more than the void. If they cannot, the unit maker will need to be instructed to adjust accordingly, with bigger voids where required, but compensate with smaller voids elsewhere.

Design

Units should be chosen with care, considering planned storage and contents. In base units, deep drawers can be much easier to access than cupboards, and reduce the need to bend down and block workspace to access items at the back. Modern drawer runner mechanisms seem to be more robust and can cope with higher-capacity drawers. A mix of drawers and cupboards is ideal. Planners often fail to provide enough space for the various waste bins required. These should be positioned out of the way so that they do not cause clutter or a tripping hazard. They should be able to be opened without using the hands. This normally means some form of pedal bin or foot-operated cupboard doors concealing bins (Figure 3.32).

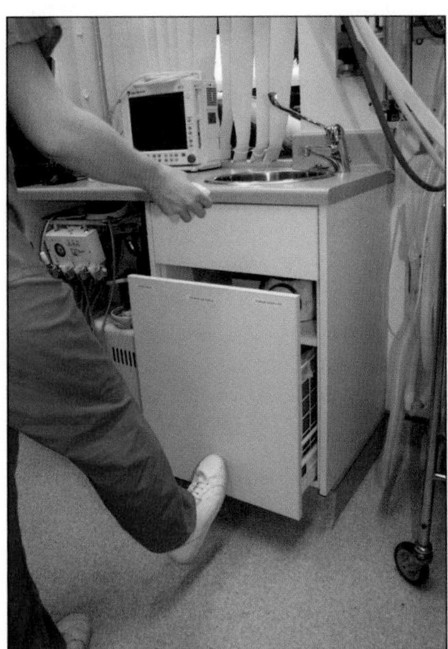

3.32 Access to bins should be hands-free where possible. A push to open, push to close foot-operated drawer, like this one in dental cabinetry, is neat, easy to use and can contain more than one receptacle to allow segregation of waste.

Worktops

Modern laminated worktops are tough and should last for years if correctly fitted and sealed. It is advisable to opt for a smooth finish, or even high gloss. Both are highly cleanable. In addition, modern router and clamping technology allows corners to be created with almost invisible joins.

Modern worktops come in lengths of up to 4.1 metres. Where possible, plan maximum runs of, say, 4 metres, ideally running wall-to-wall to avoid exposed ends. Where exposed ends are unavoidable, correct fitting and adhesion of the laminate end-strip must be ensured. This should have no edge to catch and chip.

Where the worktop meets the wall there is the choice of some form of splash-back or the use of matching upstands to give a neat finish (Figure 3.33).

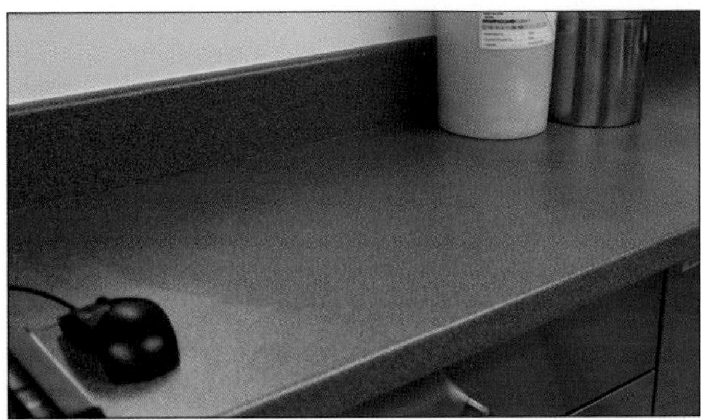

3.33 A worktop with a rear upstand can provide a neat and sealed finish and, in many areas, avoid the need for any form of 'splash-back'.

Sinks, basins and taps

Sinks with drainers

Most modern stainless steel sinks are designed to fit into a hole cut into the worktop. They are termed *inset sinks*. These are designed for domestic use and are not fully fit-for-purpose in the veterinary situation. This is because, just behind the sink, next to the wall, there is a strip of worktop which tends to gather water. In addition, the seal between the sink and worktop leaves an edge, all the way round, which, over time, can become grubby.

The better option, where a sink and draining board is required, is to go for the rectangular *sit-on* sink, which has square corners and a slight upstand against the wall (Figure 3.34). On either side they can be sealed to the adjoining worktop, using a suitable silicon-based sealer, to give a tough, cleanable sink. With some modern base units, however, there may be a need for additional support across the front, as there is no run of worktop across that space.

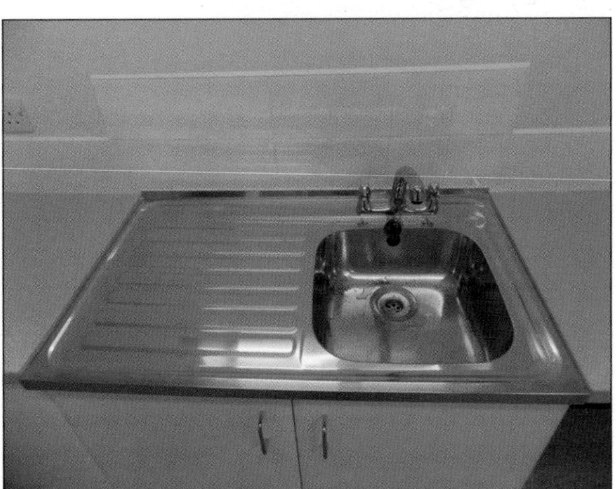

3.34 Sit-on sinks offer the best hygiene option. There is an upstand at the back, no area for water to collect behind the sink, and the sides can be sealed at the worktop joint. (Many base units will need additional struts to carry the sink firmly.)

Other sinks

There may be other locations where some form of sink is required, but without a drainer. Options include the traditional 'Belfast sink' and a variety of stainless steel sinks, which are useful in utility areas. Sinks can be low mounted for filling buckets, or situated in a laundry for soaking particularly soiled bedding.

There will be a need to have a sink in the laboratory and in the dispensary. These are usually for minor use, plus hand washing. Whilst the use of small inset sinks in the worktop might be considered, one issue can be the risk of splashes and spray dampening the surrounding worktop. Where the use is primarily hand-washing, a separate handbasin can be used, as long as it is correctly fitted and logically sited.

> **KEY POINT**
>
> Whilst the 'tub table' is, in essence, a large sink, it should be treated as a piece of fixed equipment and not used for general cleaning purposes nor relied upon for hand-washing. Other sinks and basins should be provided for such purposes.

Taps

Modern plumbing systems are often at mains pressure and have pumped hot water circulation. This means that hot taps run hot quickly, without wasting water.

Ideally, where hands are washed, taps should be capable of being used without the operator touching them with his/her hands.

- Where practical, single lever-operated mixer taps, often called 'monobloc' have some advantage. This is because they are lifted up to let water flow and pushed down to stop it, and tend to get left in a position where the water emerges at around the correct temperature. Care should be taken to ensure that water pressure is controlled to stop taps splashing water around. For hand-washing, monobloc taps are excellent. There are temperature-controlled taps, but these are very expensive and limit the range somewhat.
- There are also taps with built-in sensors which begin to flow automatically. These are particularly good for scrub sinks, as an alternative to knee operation. Whilst similar systems are available for many tap types, all with built-in temperature control, there is an added cost and maintenance factor, and the water run-on tends to make them rather wasteful.

Where a sink is used to fill bowls, taps with a higher outfall are necessary to give the clearance. Mixer taps with an inverted J-shaped outlet pipe are often the most practical (see Figure 3.20).

Signage

External signs

Some external signage requires Planning Consent (see Chapter 1); local planning authorities (LPAs) have specific leaflets and application forms for these requirements. In order to present a strong image, signage should be well designed and coordinated, with a clear and professional message. Once the practice image is agreed, it should be used to coordinate the entire look.

Permission for light-box signs or spotlit signs will depend on the LPA, the style, and the location; light-box signs tend to be frowned upon in residential areas, so a timer may be required.

Sadly, external signs may be vulnerable to vandalism. Problems are best avoided by careful positioning, possibly above spray-can range, or set back a little from the frontage. Positioning is critical and should be considered very carefully, with all viewable angles taken into the decision.

Internal signs

Having certain doors named, such as 'Consulting Room 1' or 'WC' is helpful to the client (see Figures 3.29 and 3.35). Whether the consulting room door should also name the consulting nurse or vet is a practice decision, and another management requirement. It is useful for clients but the holders must be robust enough to take frequent changes of names between consultation periods. Where doors and routes are signed, these should be coordinated with the door furniture and other fitments to add to the professional appearance.

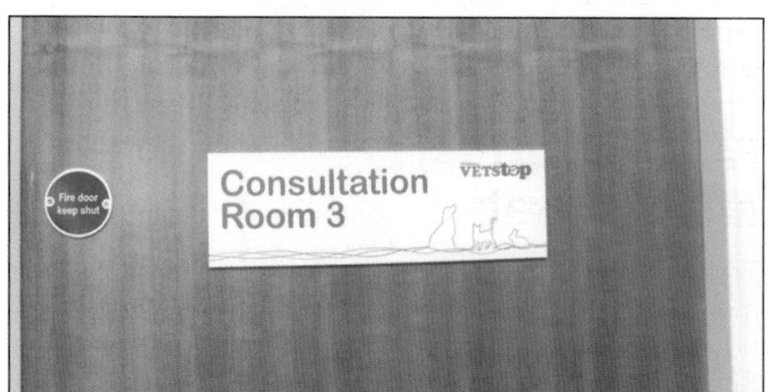

3.35 Door labelling produced to match the practice style and image can add an extra touch.

Safety signs

There are a range of safety signs and notices that are required around the building. Examples include fire exit *'running man'* signs (Figure 3.36) and X-ray warning signs (see Chapter 13). Both have levels of legislative control in terms of size, colour and style.

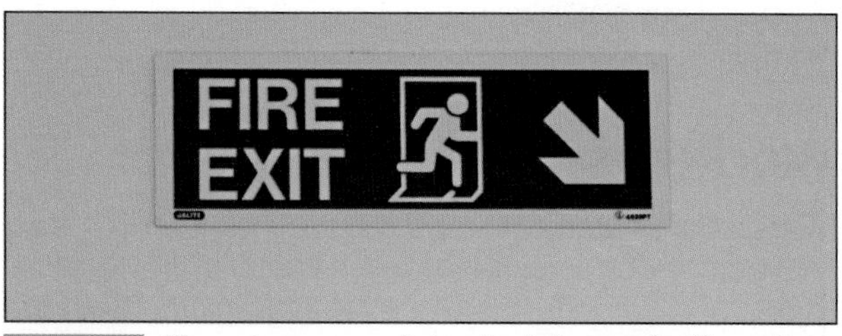

3.36 There is a range of standard signage for fire exits. All are required to have a green background and white letters. The most common sign is the 'running man'. In most areas, low-cost self-adhesive signs can be used. Illuminated signs may be required on final escape doors and exits.

In public areas, signage should guide clients out of danger in an unfamiliar environment. Away from the public areas, the staff present will be familiar with the layout. Whilst signs are needed in both areas, the need for expensive illuminated signs is restricted to client areas. Most of the remainder of the building can use the standard formats, with the possible exception of final exit doors.

Notices

Many practices have the ability to design, produce and encapsulate their own signs. These can be very helpful to clients but there is some need for caution. Language, spelling, terminology, and 'aggression' should be carefully considered. Colleagues should be asked to check out the style, wording and understanding before use. To a large extent, client notices should be kept to a minimum or they soon become just part of the environment (see Chapter 5).

Maintenance

Attractive premises, with an ergonomic design and good surface finishes can soon look dowdy or unkempt if there is no protocol for keeping them up to standard in terms of cleanliness. Clients will always notice when cleanliness is lacking, and a rigorous cleaning regime is also essential for biosecurity. Safe and efficient removal of waste is an integral part of premises maintenance, and planning segregation and storage areas for waste is an important consideration.

Fault reporting, maintenance and decorating

Practices should have a system in place whereby a manager routinely walks round the premises and notes any decorative or maintenance shortcomings. Simple jobs can be dealt with at the time, but external contractors will usually be brought in for redecoration and large or more complex repairs. Clear lines of responsibility should be in place. This system should be supplemented by a reporting system for equipment, cleaning or decorative failures, to alert the relevant manager to a problem and facilitate its resolution. Reports can be made verbally or, preferably, on a list (Figure 3.37) or on report sheets held in a central and accessible location (Figure 3.38) . The action taken and progress of the problem can be posted on a noticeboard, to keep staff aware and to prompt follow-up where issues have not been dealt with satisfactorily.

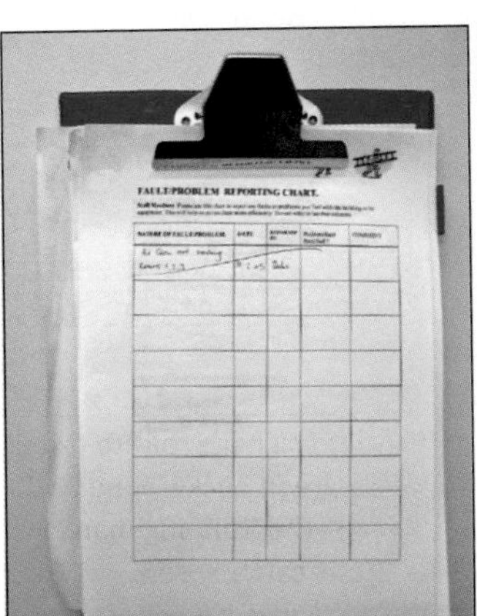

3.37 A handy reporting chart for faults and deficiencies can be hung in a central place. Details of the problem can be noted, and follow-up action recorded so everyone is aware of progress.

FAULT REPORT	
Name of person reporting fault	
Date:	Time:
Equipment description Item and location:	
Nature of fault/damage	
Reported to:	
Moved to:	
Any action already taken (e.g. sent for repair)	
Now pass this to	
Final result	

3.38 An example of a format for a fault-reporting form. These can be available in convenient places in the practice, where they can be used to record failure of any equipment or item and to note decorative deficiencies. The completed slips can be given to the relevant manager for action, or used as report forms if faults are remedied immediately. Where repairs are in progress, slips can be pinned on a noticeboard for information. Filing the completed slips with equipment manuals will provide a maintenance and fault timeline, which is useful in decision-making on replacement.

A rolling programme of area redecoration may be a preferred option but, particularly in clinical areas, decoration will usually be necessary as and when needed according to the wear and tear experienced in each area. It is worth remembering that staff members soon become used to poorly maintained areas and cease to worry about the appearance and cleanliness of a practice if they are not supported by an attentive management.

Cleanliness standards

Whilst there is an inherent thought that everyone knows what the word 'clean' means, without writing down some standards there can be different interpretations. Whilst it may be seen as a bit bureaucratic, or difficult, getting something down on paper provides a way to judge results. For example, if the protocol says that windows and walls are to be washed every 2 weeks but they look grubby after 10 days, the protocol will need to be revised to weekly. Chapters 6 and 7 contain guidance on cleaning schedules and protocols for specific areas.

Inspection and auditing

Standards and protocols only work if they are monitored. One risk area is a client lavatory not usually shared by practice staff. Here, there is an isolated unit with, potentially, no management control. Regular timed inspections should be carried out. This does not need to be onerous, just a quick check, by the reception staff, at set times during the day. Again, that inspection should be against a checklist (Figure 3.39).

Day					Date		
Time Due	**Rota**	**Time Checked**	**Initials**	**Routine Check/Task**	**Extra**	**Problem**	**Reported To**
08.15				Cleanliness, Odour, Disinfect Seat, Floor, Paper, Soap, Bin	Cleaner Check		
09.30				Cleanliness, Odour, Disinfect Seat, Floor, Paper, Soap, Bin			
10.30				Cleanliness, Odour, Disinfect Seat, Floor, Paper, Soap, Bin			
11.30				Cleanliness, Odour, Disinfect Seat, Floor, Paper, Soap, Bin			
12.30				Cleanliness, Odour, Disinfect Seat, Floor, Paper, Soap, Bin			
13.30				Cleanliness, Odour, Disinfect Seat, Floor, Paper, Soap, Bin			
14.30				Cleanliness, Odour, Disinfect Seat, Floor, Paper, Soap, Bin			
15.30				Cleanliness, Odour, Disinfect Seat, Floor, Paper, Soap, Bin			
16.30				Cleanliness, Odour, Disinfect Seat, Floor, Paper, Soap, Bin			
17.30				Cleanliness, Odour, Disinfect Seat, Floor, Paper, Soap, Bin			
18.00				Cleanliness, Odour, Disinfect Seat, Floor, Paper, Soap, Bin			
18.45					Window Locks		

3.39 An example of a checklist for a client lavatory. Whilst the rota receptionist can check before and after consultation times, it should be the role of a different rota member during the day, or the reception may be left unmanned. First check should be to make sure the out-of-hours cleaners have done a good job. The use of electric hand driers may help reduce littering in the client WC.

Cleaners

A very important factor in the cleanliness equation is: Who does the cleaning? Many practices rely on animal care staff, whether qualified nurses or otherwise, to do the entire cleaning but is this the best solution? Whoever is given responsibility for cleaning an area must have the necessary training, motivation, equipment (Figure 3.40) and time to carry this out to the required standard at all times.

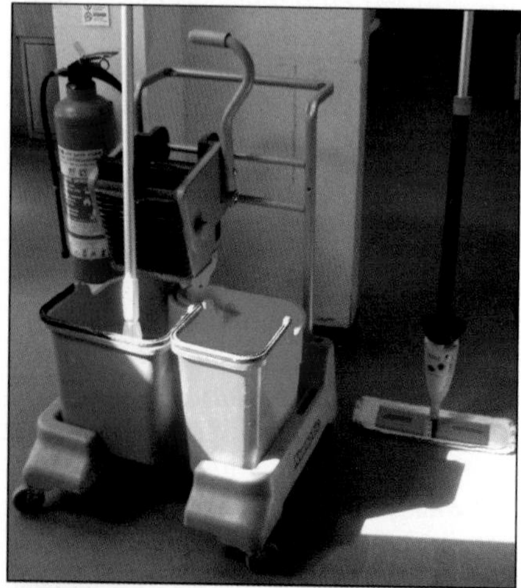

3.40 The right equipment can make cleaning easier and more effective – this cart has separate buckets for clean and contaminated areas. A wall mop is pictured to the right.

There are logical splits between routine cleaning and maintenance cleaning, and between clinical and non-clinical and outpatient areas.

- Nurses and care staff should certainly be responsible for dealing with hand-touch area cleaning (Figure 3.41), daytime accidents and spillages, and with the sterilization of theatres and other procedural areas.

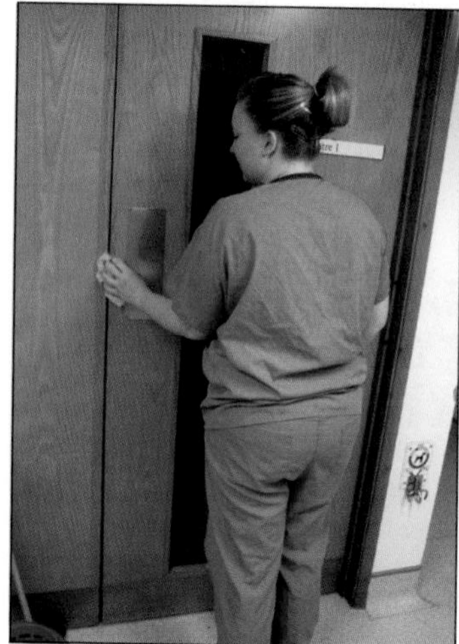

3.41 Careful attention should be paid to cleaning areas frequently soiled, such as finger-plates and door-gripping areas.

- It is probably better, however, to use other cleaners for daily floor washing, routine window cleaning, overall cleanliness and the public and administrative areas. This could be an out-of-hours cleaner employed by the practice or a contract cleaner from an independent firm. One advantage of the latter is that they would have to provide holiday cover. The disadvantage may be some aspects of security.

Duty roles

Assuming the practice employs separate people to do the routine cleaning, many practices have rotas for nursing staff to add variety to their roles. This may rotate duties between different staff, say, theatre nurse, preparation area nurse, ward duty, and such like.

Each duty should have protocols and standards for that role, to include the hygiene aspects required. These are a useful reference for performance evaluation. It is appropriate for the nursing managers to carry out regular cleaning audits (Figure 3.42) to assess the

	Date audit issued	Date audit returned	Outstanding issues	Manager's signature
CR1				
CR2				
Nurses CR				
Reception				
Dispensary				
Clinical Waste				
X-ray				
ICU				
Prep Room				
Theatre 1				
Theatre 2				
Ward 1				
Ward 2				
Exotics				
Laboratory				
Domestic Areas				

3.42 Example of a control sheet for ensuring audits are carried out.

effectiveness of the cleaning arrangements, and these should be recorded and any shortcomings acted upon and discussed should changes in procedure and responsibility be needed. Whilst, on first sight, this sounds a little cumbersome, in practice it works well and provides standards for job evaluation. Administrative staff should also have clear responsibility for maintaining the cleanliness of touch points such as phones and keyboards in between routine cleaning by dedicated cleaning staff.

An example of a checklist-style audit for monitoring the effectiveness of current cleaning protocols and schedules is given at the end of the chapter. Deficiencies should be noted and appropriate action and any necessary further training undertaken. Figure 3.42 is an example of a control sheet for ensuring that audits are carried out.

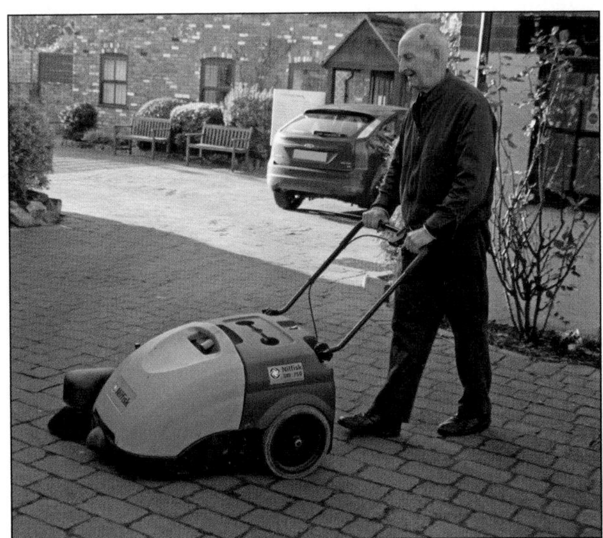

3.43 Car park maintenance. Rechargeable sweepers can be useful for larger flat surfaces where hand sweeping can be time-consuming and hard work. Alternatively, sub-contractors with compact road or path sweeping vehicles can be used to keep large areas clear.

Grounds maintenance

Grounds maintenance should not be forgotten, and can be time-consuming if grounds and car parks are extensive. Motorized aids can be useful (Figure 3.43).

Winter is always a dilemma for businesses, with worries about visitors falling on icy surfaces. Although snow and ice are infrequent in many areas of the UK, suitable clearing and grit/salt spreading equipment may be a worthwhile investment for practices with large car park areas and many metres of path in areas where snow and ice occur more regularly. Many ride-on mowers, quad bikes, and mini-tractors can have angled blades for shifting snow. Otherwise, it might be a case of keeping the odd snow shovel in a cupboard and calling 'all hands on deck' if snow arrives.

With ice, clearing and salting entrances, paths and car parks is the logical approach. Rather than reacting only when winter arrives, trying to buy bags of rock salt along with everyone else, a little forward planning is preferred. Installing a grit bin (Figure 3.44) or bunker, which is filled up out of season, is the best solution.

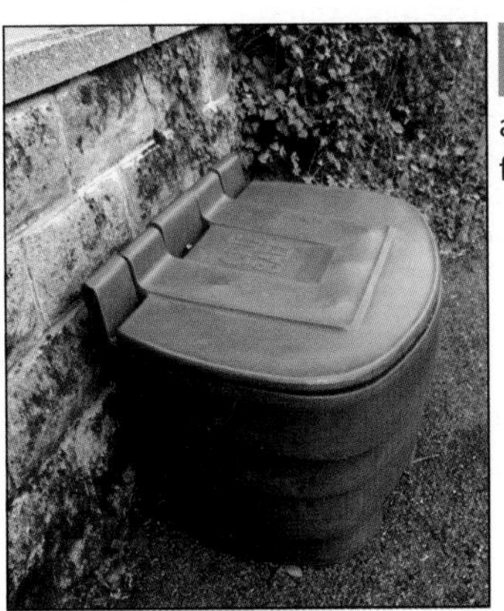

3.44 Permanent bin for rock salt and grit, ready to treat frosty paths in winter.

As important as preparation is the question about who will clear the snow and grit the ice. If the practice employs maintenance staff, they may be prepared for early starts on wintry days. Often, however, it may end up as an early start for the partners, though encouraging a team approach is advised, particularly to be prepared for when the partners may take a day off.

Waste management

Regulations

Over the last few decades there has been a gradual tightening of waste regulations. Various human health concerns have driven tightening of the controls on biological waste, particularly anything with a link to human blood or bodily waste. At the same time, concerns about drug abuse began to tighten controls on pharmaceutical waste, with the two aspects linked regarding the topic of 'sharps'. Adding to this, fears of pollution, toxic spillages and concerns about volatile organic compounds (VOCs), such as methane and oil-based substances, have heightened awareness about the environment, just as sites for landfill are becoming harder for planners to find.

Veterinary healthcare waste is governed by a diverse group of regulations that are progressively being brought under one directive. Current regulation is an amalgam of:

- The Special Waste Regulations 1996
- European Waste Catalogue (EWC) 2002
- The Landfill (England and Wales) (Amendment) Regulations 2005 or The Landfill Allowances Scheme (Scotland) Regulations 2005
- *Safe Management of Healthcare Waste* (version 2011) from the Department of Health.

Written protocol

A veterinary practice must have a written protocol for the disposal of healthcare waste. This must include details of:

- What wastes will be produced
- How they will be segregated and stored
- How they will be disposed of and to whom
- Where the contractor will take the waste and how.

Copies of all relevant licences and permits should be obtained.

This detailed assessment will include how the practice will perform a risk assessment of its wastes and, particularly, determine what is or is not hazardous waste. Details of the paperwork should be held in this document. This paperwork will fulfil the Veterinary Practices Duty of Care requirement and also serve as the legally required Pre-Collection Audit.

Specific paperwork is needed at each disposal event:

- Non-hazardous waste must be documented and recorded on a w
- Waste Transfer Note
- Hazardous waste must be logged and documented on a Consignment Note.

Types of waste

Waste is broadly divided into Hazardous and Non-hazardous waste. A poster summarizing regulations can be found at the end of this chapter. Wider and more detailed guidance should be consulted, such as BVA guidance and the *BSAVA Guide to the Use of Medicines,* available on their respective websites.

Hazardous waste

Veterinary surgeons should carry out a risk assessment to decide in each case whether waste should be deemed hazardous or not.

Infectious waste

Infectious waste is anything that has been contaminated with an infectious agent or toxin of that infection, where the infection or toxin may cause a risk to humans or animals that come into contact with it. In practice, this may be all waste from the isolation unit – bedding, contaminated disposable protective clothing, etc.

Infectious hazardous waste is collected into:

- Yellow bags (for incineration)
- Orange bags (for pre-treatment, e.g. autoclaving).

Cytotoxic and cytostatic pharmaceuticals

These include:

- Cancer chemotherapy agents
- Immunotherapy agents, e.g. interferon, ciclosporin
- Hormones, e.g. prostaglandins, androgens
- Others, e.g. chloramphenicol.

Whole medicines or anything contaminated with such products (e.g. needles, syringes, empty injection vials) must be segregated and disposed of in a purple-topped container (Figure 3.45). In practice, it is often best to have a single collection bin. This could be a purple-topped 'sharps' bin; any other waste contaminated by such products (e.g. soiled gloves or gowns, giving sets, animal bedding) can then be disposed of in the same bin.

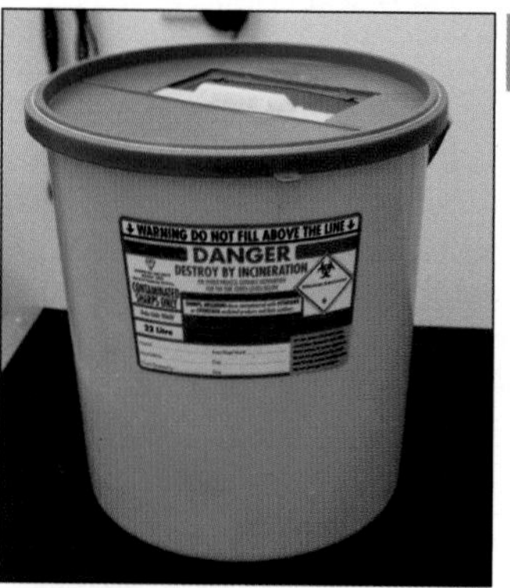

3.45 Purple-lidded cytotoxic waste bin.

Contaminated sharps

All contaminated 'sharps' (includes hypodermic needles, cannulae, microscope slides, scalpel blades and any other sharp objects) must be disposed of as Hazardous waste. Those contaminated with cytotoxic/cytostatic drugs must be separated from others (see above).

Sharps are placed in purple- or yellow-lidded sharps bins and disposed of via incineration.

It is possible to segregate out non-blood and non-pharmaceutical contaminated sharps into orange-lidded sharps bins, but in practice this is unlikely to be practical.

Heavy metals

Photographic chemicals: Both fixer and developer solutions are toxic and should be salvaged and stored in separate leak-proof containers in a well ventilated area awaiting collection. There is an option to remove the heavy metal hazard (silver trap) provided permission from the local water authority has been obtained. The full silver trap is then consigned as Hazardous waste and the chemicals (post-trap) are disposed of via the drain to the foul sewer.

Batteries: Mercury or lithium makes these Hazardous waste. It is illegal for a veterinary practice, as a commercial premises, to dispose of such items via domestic (home) sites or in Domestic waste. Batteries must be segregated as Hazardous waste and consigned to the waste contractor. This may be the Local Authority, the main waste contractor or a specialist waste contractor.

Fluorescent strips and low-energy bulbs: These also contain mercury and so should be consigned as Hazardous waste, as for batteries (see above). Specific collection boxes are available to store sufficient tubes to warrant collection cost.

Electrical wastes: Used electrical equipment is covered by separate legislation (WEEE – Waste Electrical and Electronic Equipment Directive). The heavy metals in circuit boards or solder mean that all electronic items must be disposed of as Hazardous waste. It may be possible to recycle computer items to charities, but the rest must be consigned to a specific contractor.

Non-hazardous waste

General waste

This includes staff room and office waste, and non-contaminated packaging. Where possible, this should be recycled (Figure 3.46) or composted. Availability of recycling collections will vary geographically but they are now more widely available, particularly for cardboard and paper. Ink and toner cartridges can often be recycled via the manufacturer or through schemes operated by several charities. Composting of waste non-meat food and shredded paper should be considered. These items can be removed from site for recycling.

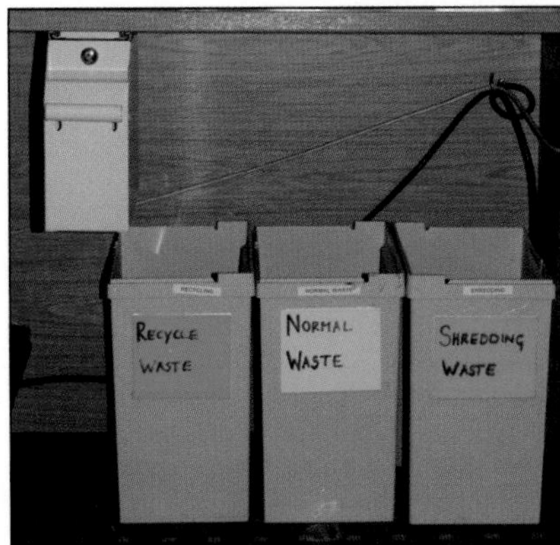

3.46 Waste should be segregated at the point of production. In reception, waste is separated into recycling for paper, general waste (mostly packaging) and confidential shredding (for patient and client records).

Pharmaceuticals (not cytotoxic or cytostatic)

Other than cytotoxic/cytostatic medicines (see above), pharmaceuticals must be segregated and disposed of in a separate leak-proof bin. It is recommended that this is a blue-lidded container.

- Whole pharmaceuticals:
  - Out-of-date medicines
  - Damaged medicines
  - Returned medicines
  - Should be placed in a Pharmaceutical waste bin and details of amount and type recorded and listed
- Residual pharmaceuticals:
  - Used syringes
  - Empty injection vials
  - Contaminated pill pots
  - Should be placed in a Pharmaceutical waste bin but volumes and details are not needed.

Controlled Drugs are disposed of as pharmaceuticals once they have been denatured (see Chapter 15).

Offensive waste

This generally accounts for all remaining waste that is judged to be free of specific hazard following risk assessment by the practice. Offensive waste will include:

- Ward bedding, including that contaminated with faeces, urine or other bodily fluids
- Blood-contaminated items, e.g. bedding, swabs drapes, and theatre waste
- Faeces from dog runs and kennels
- Sanitary towels and personal waste from washrooms.

Yellow bags with a black stripe ('tiger' bags; Figure 3.47) are used for Offensive waste, which generally goes to landfill. Hazardous waste and body parts must not be disposed of via this route.

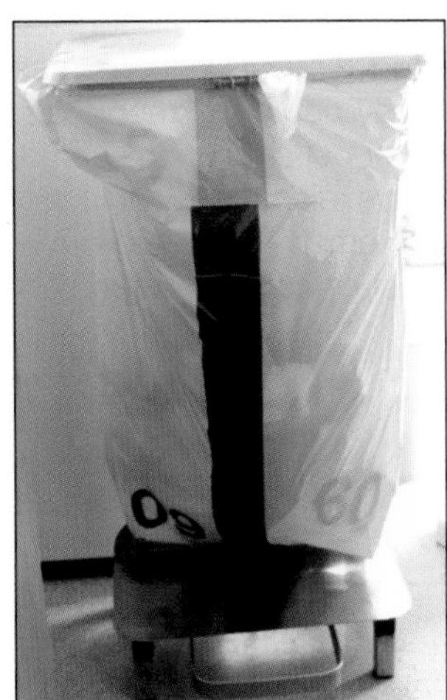

3.47 Offensive waste bin, with striped 'tiger' bag.

Cadavers and body parts

Tissue parts and amputated limbs, etc., must be segregated into a bin called a Limb bin. This must be a leak-proof container that cannot be pierced. The advice is to keep this in the freezer and send with cadavers for incineration when full.

Pet cadavers are now transferred and disposed of under animal by-product controls, except where the cadaver is suspected of harbouring a notifiable disease, in which case collection and disposal will be arranged by Defra.

Waste segregation and storage

These regulatory demands for dealing with all the differing wastes create a need for space for segregation and storage. Whatever the waste, there are two vital elements which add together to create best practice:

- The veterinary business carries out its duty of care to dispose of waste in accordance with the waste regulations
- Storage and disposal is undertaken subtly, out of public gaze, and the storage space is considered and managed effectively.

Service yard

There is a now such a wide range of waste items that some form of dedicated waste area is helpful. Although much of the waste is in relatively small volumes, some is quite bulky and commercial removal contractors will supply large wheelie bins to manoeuvre. Some form of service yard offers a good approach for keeping this necessary function out of sight of clients and onlookers, and secure from interference. In commercial terms, such a yard allows investment in storage space to be suitable for the requirements, rather than using part of a high-specification veterinary building.

Careful planning, so that the interior of the yard cannot be seen from the outside, can provide an adaptable space for: waste; anaesthetic gas storage; a main delivery and disposal point; and, possibly, secure overnight staff duty parking. The exact format of such an area may depend on location. A 2000-mm high close-boarded fence may suffice, or the location may demand something more resistant to intruders.

Cadavers

As cadavers are categorized as 'waste' there is legislation to be adhered to regarding disposal options (see earlier). Whilst some owners may opt for home burials, most practices use some form of pet cremation service that offers a range of alternative disposals to the pet owner, including communal cremations or individual cremations. Between euthanasia and departure from the practice, cadavers must be handled and stored safely, hygienically and sensitively.

Choosing a waste contractor

Most practices use one main contractor for collection and disposal of cadavers and most healthcare waste. Selecting this contractor will involve considering all aspects of the service offered, with the handling and disposal of cadavers as an important factor. Sensitivity is important, particularly where clients may want ashes returned in a particular way, or may wish to be present at the time of cremation.

Practices are advised to obtain service proposals from several companies and compare not just costs, but other factors such as convenience, collection times and the handling and confirmed destination of each waste category. A visit to the premises of the disposal company is advised, and it is often useful for practice staff to visit the cremation facility too, so they feel comfortable discussing the issues and options with clients. It is important to communicate accurately to clients what happens to their pet after it has been left at the practice, and the timescale of cremation and return of ashes, choice of casket, etc.

The destination and handling of all categories of waste should be clear and supported by the correct and current paperwork and licences.

Trade waste and recycling contracts are usually renewed annually and should be renegotiated regularly to keep costs as low as possible consistent with the desired service level.

Acknowledgements

The author and editors gratefully acknowledge the following practices, images of which appear in this chapter: Alfreton Park; Crossings Veterinary Centre; Dovecote Veterinary Hospital; Elands Veterinary Clinic; Mill House Veterinary Surgery and Hospital; Park Veterinary Group; Pennard Veterinary Group; Rowan Veterinary Centre; Wildbore Vetstop; Willows Veterinary Centre and Referral Service. The author and editors would also like to thank Mike Jessop for his advice on the waste management section.

Further reading

Wishart J (2003) *Premises for Vets (Designing the Veterinary Habitat).* Threshold Press, Newbury

The British Veterinary Hospital Association (BVHA) produces design guides and also articles on specific design issues.

Cleaning audit and waste poster 

Cleaning audit

Audit performed by .... Date: ....

This audit to be carried out at least quarterly to check that cleaning schedules are being followed effectively. Once complete and any action taken, please pass to partners. All schedules and audits are scanned to electronic archive.

Item/area Checked	**Satisfactory?**		**Action required**	**Completed by (Initial/ date)**
	Y	**N**		
Dispensary / Consult rooms				
Bin, cupboards, splashes/cleanliness/hair				
Underneath/behind computers				
Scale/sink/taps				
Under fridge/fridge clean, check temperature records				
Tile grout/handles etc.				
Window sills/models/in-use items				
Check walls for splashes				
Dust check – door frames/clocks/radiators/skirting boards/ air con units				
Drug shelves				
Books tidy/relevant/stocks of client packs/books/vaccine records/insurance and info packs				
Check business cards/practice labels/Sharps pots				
Drawer contents Drawer 1 – auriscope heads, curved and suture scissors, nail clippers, micropore, cotton buds, pens, cheque stamp Drawer 2 – PDSA treatment receipts, disposable gloves, money detector pen.				
Syringes/needles/tablet pots/dispensing packaging topped up				
Reception				
Dust check tins of food/products for sale				
Clutter check on reception				
Light bulbs				
Grille of air conditioning unit				
Bags/bins tidy in clinical waste				
Children's toys clean, good condition				
Extra food/orders current and tidy				
Skirting boards/behind chairs				
Dangling wires under reception desk				
X-ray				
Bin, cupboards, splashes/cleanliness/hair				
Behind and under X-ray table and fluoroscopy				
Scale/sink/taps				
Sand bags/foam wedges				
Ties clean and drawer in order				
Cradles clean				
Check walls for splashes esp. in darkroom				
Dust check – door frames/clocks/radiators/skirting boards				
Darkroom clean and bench dust-free				
Books tidy/relevant				
Extractor fan grilles clean				

An example of a cleaning audit form.

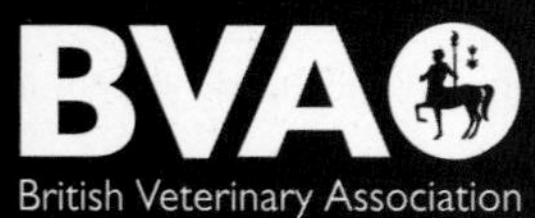

Good practice guide to handling veterinary waste in England and Wales

Introduction to handling veterinary waste

This is a practical guide to assist the veterinary profession to comply with waste regulations in England and Wales. The Environment Agency supports this guide.

Further detailed information is available at www.bva.co.uk and www.environment-agency.gov.uk

The BVA also encourages practices to discuss this further with their waste contractor.

Duty of care

All businesses have to ensure that

- All waste is stored and disposed of responsibly
- Waste is only handled or dealt with by those authorised to do so
- Appropriate records are kept of all waste that is transferred or received.

The BVA recommends that veterinary practices secure an assurance in writing that the person collecting the waste is authorised to do so.

Hazardous waste

Hazardous wastes are those that are harmful to people, the environment or animals, either immediately or over an extended period of time.

Key veterinary hazardous wastes include:

- Cytotoxic and cytostatic pharmaceuticals
- Infectious waste — any veterinary waste containing viable micro-organisms or their toxins which are known or reliably believed to cause disease in man or other living organisms
- Sharps contaminated with animal blood or pharmaceuticals that are deemed to present a risk of infection
- Photographic chemicals such as fixer or developer solutions.

All veterinary facilities that produce more than 500 kg of hazardous waste per annum need to register their premises because of the Hazardous Waste Regulations. This can be done on the Environment Agency website or by phoning or writing to them.

All people who move or receive hazardous waste need to record this and maintain a register of each waste involved for their records. Before any hazardous waste leaves the premises a consignment note needs to be completed. Sufficient copies of the note must be prepared to allow the producer, the consignor (if different), all carriers and the consignee to each have a copy. Consignment notes may be supplied by your waste contractor. They are also available from the Environment Agency in hardcopy for £1.00 or can be electronically downloaded from its website. These records must be kept for at least three years.

Non-hazardous waste

Key veterinary non-hazardous wastes include:

- Any pharmaceuticals other than cytotoxic or cytostatic pharmaceuticals.
- Offensive waste—waste that is not hazardous but which is unpleasant and may cause offence to the senses. For all waste placed in this stream the veterinary surgeon must be able to demonstrate that they implemented procedures that meet the requirements set out in the accompanying web guidance (see www.bva.co.uk).
- Domestic rubbish.

When non-hazardous waste is transferred from one party to another, the person handing it on must complete a transfer note, which both parties must sign and keep a copy. An annual transfer note may be used to cover all the movements of a regular transfer of the same non-hazardous waste between the same parties. These records must be kept for at least three years.

British Veterinary Association
7 Mansfield Street, London W1G 9NQ

Tel: 020 7636 6541
Email: bvahq@bva.co.uk
Web: www.bva.co.uk

BVA — Your Association, Your Future

Waste streams in veterinary practice. The information in this figure (available as a poster from BVA) applies to England and Wales; there are differences (mainly in terminology) in Scotland and Northern Ireland. The information is correct at the time of going to press but regulations are subject to change. (© BVA 2011 and reproduced with their permission) (continues) ▶

BVA Good practice guide to handling veterinary waste in England and Wales

British Veterinary Association

Veterinary assessment

All general waste must be subject to a veterinary risk assessment which must ask:

- Does the material arise from an animal that has any disease caused by a micro-organism, such that the material is contaminated with that micro-organism?
- Is there any other potential risk of infection?
- If the answer to either is **'yes'**, the waste is infectious, clinical waste ▼

Hazardous waste

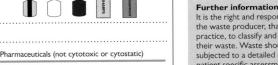

Register your premises, keep a Waste Register, use Consignment Notes, keep all records for at least three years.

Cytotoxic and cytostatic pharmaceuticals

Waste contaminated with cytotoxic and cytostatic pharmaceuticals, which are medicinal products that are toxic, carcinogenic, toxic for reproduction or mutagenic.

This includes:
- Glass bottles and vials
- Clinical items (for example, swabs, masks and gloves)
- Syringes and sharps
- Animal bedding.

DISPOSAL
- Segregate into appropriate purple and yellow containers—sharps, glass bottles and vials into purple-lidded sharps containers—for high-temperature incineration only
- EWC=18 02 07*.

Contaminated sharps

Sharps must be subject to a risk assessment. Sharps contaminated with material (other than cytotoxic or cytostatic) that is deemed to present a risk of infection to any animal or person that may come into contact with it may include:

- Partially and fully discharged sharps, hypodermic needles and other sharp instruments and objects.

DISPOSAL
- EWC=18 02 02* and 18 02 08
- Segregate into yellow sharps containers for high-temperature incineration only.

FOR BEST PRACTICE
- EWC=18 02 02*
- Non-pharmaceutically contaminated sharps can be further segregated into orange-lidded bins for suitable alternative treatment (for example, autoclaving).

Infectious, clinical waste

Infectious, clinical waste is:

Waste containing viable micro-organisms or their toxins which are known or reliably believed to cause disease in humans or other living organisms; or waste which, following a veterinary assessment, is deemed to present a risk of infection to any animal or person that may come into contact with it.

This may include:
- Items used in treatment (for example, swabs, masks and gloves, which may include blood-contaminated items
- Animal bedding
- Blood and body parts.

DISPOSAL
- Segregate into appropriate yellow containers for high-temperature incineration only
- EWC=18 02 02*.

FOR BEST PRACTICE
- Infectious waste, other than body parts and cadavers, can be further segregated into orange containers for suitable alternative treatment (for example, autoclaving) as best practice
- EWC=18 02 02*.

Photographic chemicals

This may include:
- Waste fixer and developer solutions.

DISPOSAL
- Segregate into separate fixer and developer leak-proof containers for treatment at an appropriately permitted facility
- There is no standard packaging so specific requirements should be discussed with your waste contractor
- EWC=09 01 01* (developer) and 09 01 04* (fixer).

Non-hazardous waste

Use transfer notes and keep all records for three years.

Offensive waste

Offensive waste is veterinary waste other than sharps that is not hazardous or clinical but which is unpleasant and may cause offence to the senses.

This waste must have been subjected to a detailed item and patient-specific assessment that clearly demonstrates it does not present a risk of infection or other potential hazard to any animal or person that may come into contact with it, even if mismanaged.

This is particularly important in the case of material contaminated with body fluids (for example, blood), where a veterinary surgeon must be able to demonstrate that they implemented procedures that meet the requirements set out in the accompanying web guidance (see www.bva.co.uk).

As a result of this assessment the veterinary surgeon is declaring that the waste is not hazardous, and is not clinical waste that requires incineration or other treatment prior to landfill.

Offensive waste may include:
- Items used in treatment (for example swabs, masks and gloves, which may include blood-contaminated items)
- Animal bedding
- Animal faeces

These **must not** contain body parts or body tissues.

DISPOSAL
- Landfill or other suitable permitted facility
- EWC=18 02 03.

Sharps

Sharps must be subject to a risk assessment that demonstrates they do not present a risk of infection to any animal or person that may come into contact with them.

This may include:
- An unused sharp that has been dropped on the floor prior to use.

If there is deemed to be a risk, however small, the sharp should be assumed to be hazardous and handled accordingly (see Contaminated sharps).

DISPOSAL
- EWC=18 02 01
- If the sharps are classified as 18 02 01 the vet is indicating that they are not clinical waste and do not need to be rendered safe. In such circumstances disposal outlets may be more limited and less predictable, potentially including landfill without treatment. It is unlikely that a veterinary practice would produce a sharps waste stream which could be coded 18 02 01.

Pharmaceuticals (not cytotoxic or cytostatic)

Waste contaminated with pharmaceuticals (not cytotoxic or cytostatic).

This may include:
- Denatured controlled drugs
- Prescription-only medicines
- Out-of-date drugs
- Contaminated bottles, syringe bodies and packaging.

DISPOSAL OF CONTROLLED DRUGS
- All controlled drugs must be denatured or made not readily recoverable and then be disposed of with other pharmaceuticals (not cytotoxic or cytostatic)
- For Schedule 2 controlled drugs this should be done in the presence of an authorised person (for example, a veterinary surgeon from another practice).

DISPOSAL OF OTHER PHARMACEUTICALS
- Segregate into blue leak-proof containers
- Avoid mixing
- Incineration at an appropriately permitted facility
- EWC=18 02 08.

Pet cadavers

Pet cadavers are now transferred and disposed of under animal by-product controls, except where the cadaver is suspected of harbouring a notifiable disease, in which case collection and disposal will be arranged by Defra.

DISPOSAL
- Burial at home
- Burial in a pet cemetery
- Cremation.

Domestic waste

Waste that only contains domestic rubbish. This includes separate recyclable and mixed non-recyclable materials. Batteries and hazardous items should not be placed in the mixed municipal waste.

Recyclables may include:
- Paper, card, unsoiled newspapers and magazines
- Plastic food containers
- Drink cans
- Batteries.

DISPOSAL
- Recycling or disposal at a suitably permitted or licensed site
- EWC=20 03 01 (mixed).

Further information
It is the right and responsibility of the waste producer, that is, the practice, to classify and segregate their waste. Waste should be subjected to a detailed item and patient specific assessment to determine if it presents a risk of infection or other potential hazard to any animal or person that may come into contact with it.

All businesses have a duty of care to ensure that:

- All waste is stored and disposed of responsibly
- Waste is only handled or dealt with by those authorised to do so
- Appropriate records are kept of all waste that is transferred or received

This is a practical good practice guide to assist veterinary surgeons to comply with waste regulations in England and Wales

Supported by the
ENVIRONMENT AGENCY

The **Environment Agency** supports this *Good practice guide to handling veterinary waste in England and Wales* written and published by the British Veterinary Association

Further information on handling veterinary waste is available at **www.bva.co.uk** and **www.environment-agency.gov.uk**

BVA—Your Association, Your Future

(continued) Waste streams in veterinary practice. The information in this figure (available as a poster from BVA) applies to England and Wales; there are differences (mainly in terminology) in Scotland and Northern Ireland. The information is correct at the time of going to press but regulations are subject to change. (© BVA 2011 and reproduced with their permission)

IT and telecommunications

4

Wayne Smith-Gillard and Chris Beesley

Components of the practice computer system

When planning a computerized system, the goal should be to enable staff to access as much data and functionality as possible without the need to refer to paper copies of documents. Instant access to e-mail, online resources (e.g. RCVS, VPMA, NOAH, BSAVA, BVA websites) and even radiographs and laboratory reports will streamline activities on a day-to-day basis, and should ideally be available from every terminal on the network.

The platform and operating system

The computer platform is the foundation upon which all operations and functions of the computer system are based, and is comprised of a combination of the computer hardware and the operating system.

The operating system is a computer's most crucial program, as its role is to run other programs, along with the general management of all software and many hardware components. A number of operating systems exist, including Microsoft Windows (upon which programs like Outlook and Office run), SCO Unix and MacOSX. Apple also make their own hardware.

Some programs are operating system-specific, and this must be borne in mind when deciding upon which operating system to use in the practice. The choice of operating system will affect compatibility with other programs and hardware.

Many modern systems operate via 'cloud computing', where programs and information are stored remotely on the Internet and can be accessed from almost anywhere. There are now a host of providers of 'cloud computing' solutions, some of which are freeware (programs that do not cost anything to download and use) and can be obtained via the Internet. 'Freeware' can range from spreadsheet and word processing programs to full operating systems. Google offers 'cloud computing' solutions for e-mail, calendar, spreadsheets, word processing, presentations and more. A free restricted-user licence is available, which may be suitable for small businesses; alternatively, larger businesses can pay a small monthly fee per user in return for greater functionality, more storage and a higher number of user licences.

The network

There are currently two ways in which data can be transmitted around buildings: wired and wireless networks.

Wired networks

Wired networks have several advantages over wireless networks, including greater security and a more reliable, faster service.

The cable

Installation: Cabling is the key component of a wired network; the type of cable, the length of the run, the route taken and the siting of connection ports must all be considered. As with electrical sockets, it is worth installing up to 50% more outlets/ports than the currently estimated requirement to allow for future expansion. Electrical sockets should be sited wherever a workstation might be needed at the outset, to avoid future problems. Data cables should only be installed by competent professionals, as they can be damaged by incorrect handling during installation.

Cables can be run through hidden conduits with other service cables, but they must be shielded to protect them from the electromagnetic interference of adjacent power cables. Ready-shielded cables (Figure 4.1) can be purchased easily. Shielded connectors are also necessary at cable junctions to ensure complete protection.

KEY POINT

Burying cables within walls is not advisable unless using a free-running channel; despite the desired neatness, it can cause major disruption if cables need to be replaced or moved in the future. If retrofitting a building, surface-mounted conduit can be chosen, hiding as much cable as possible within false walls, dropped ceilings or other hidden trunking.

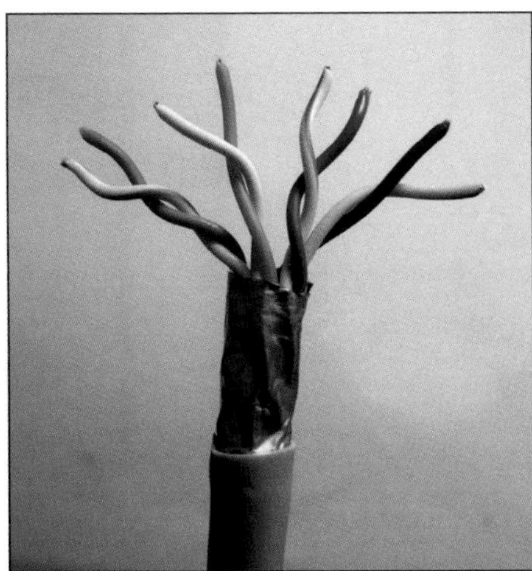

4.1 Category 5E shielded cable, showing outer sheath, foil shielding and four twisted 'pairs' of wires.

Termination: Typically, cables are run around the building and terminate in an area (preferably a dedicated room) in which the computer server, broadband line connection, telephone exchange server and other similar equipment are situated and can be kept within a pre-defined operating temperature range through the use of air conditioning. Servers and computer hardware generate a lot of heat and, if left uncontrolled, these higher temperatures will cause fluctuations in performance and will shorten the working life of the equipment. The impact of temperature must be considered when positioning servers and computer hardware close to where people will be working.

Data cables terminate in what is known as a patch panel: each connection is numbered and a corresponding number exists at the port on the other end of that cable in the different rooms of the building. The patch panel is then connected to the router via a hub, which is itself connected to the server and broadband line (Figure 4.2).

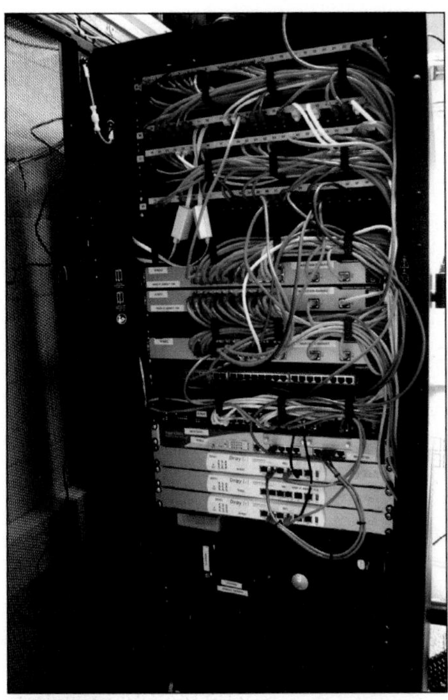

4.2 Patch panel, server and hub.

Speed

Wired networks should provide much more consistent speeds than wireless networks (usually 100 Mbps), and are able to handle a much greater amount of data. Additionally, gigabit (1000 Mbps) networks can be created easily at little extra cost.

The most common cabling standards used are Cat5 and Cat5E (enhanced; see Figure 4.1), followed by Cat6, Cat7 and fibreoptic, each bringing increased speed and quality but at higher costs. Typically, 'Cat' rated cables transmit good quality signals up to distances of 100 metres from the router, although slightly shorter cable runs are usually advised to allow for the connections at either end that go to the PC and from the patch panel to the server. For longer runs, fibreoptic cable is currently the only option.

KEY POINT

Speeds achieved on a wired network will depend upon the rating of the lowest component. Therefore, in order to maintain a gigabit network, all components (e.g. connectors, junctions, end ports, router) must be gigabit-rated.

Wireless networks

Wireless networking has improved greatly in the last few years, with increases in speed, quality and security. It also saves cabling costs and creates little disruption during installation. In spite of these benefits, wireless networking still has drawbacks over its wired counterpart.

Security

The security of a wireless network is inherently weaker than that of a wired network. With the right credentials, or some determination, the remote signal broadcast by a wireless network can be broken. Security will depend on the type chosen and its set-up.

There are three main types of wireless security:

- **WEP** (wired equivalent privacy)
- The more secure **WPA** (Wi-Fi protected access), of which there are two types: standard WPA and the more advanced WPA2. WPA or WPA2 used alone is referred to as WPA-Personal or WPA2-Personal
- **802.1 x authentication**, which can be used alongside WPA to increase security (referred to as WPA-Enterprise or WPA2-Enterprise).

Reception and speed

Wireless signals are broadcast via routers and wireless access points. Reception can vary greatly depending on:

- The location and quality of the router or access point
- The material of which walls and floors are constructed
- The distance to the connecting equipment.

Even the best routers have a maximum range of around 70 metres and speed of 300 Mbps (megabits per second), although in reality much lower speeds and range are typically achieved due to signal loss and distance from the router. It is also the case that the more equipment connected (and therefore data transmitted) concurrently, the slower the speeds. Wireless local area networks (WLANs) are represented as 802.11*x*, where *x* is either a, b, g or n. WLAN 802.11b has a theoretical speed of up to 11 Mbps, b and g up to 54 Mbps, and n up to 300 Mbps.

Mobile devices

Wireless network access is particularly useful for portable PCs, tablet PCs, smart phones and other mobile devices. By connecting to the practice's wireless network, data such as e-mails will be received via the practice broadband connection and save costly data use on the remote device's cellular plan. Transmission and receipt of files are also likely to be faster, the battery life longer, and a user will be able to move around unhindered. It is possible to view images such as radiographs on some mobile devices or to access the practice management system for billing and case history updating (Figure 4.3). However, it is questionable at this stage as to whether wireless networking is adequate for all network traffic generated by a small to medium-sized business.

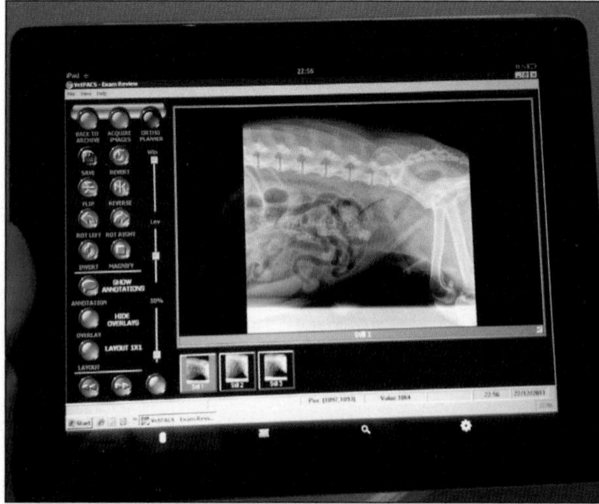

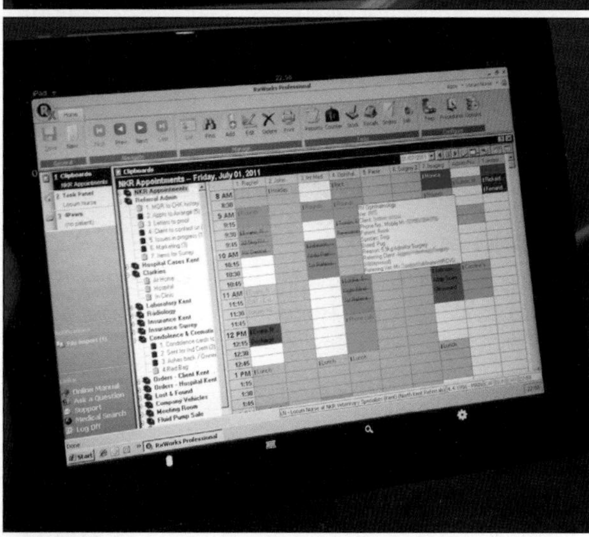

4.3 Some mobile devices allow radiographs to be viewed and/or access to the practice management system.

Broadband

All major broadband suppliers offer a domestic and business service.

- A domestic service is normally cheaper, is provided for *ad hoc* use, and will have a high 'contention ratio' (normally 50:1). This means that one line can be used by up to 50 people simultaneously; in simple terms, the speed will be reduced as more people share the line. The support and service response guarantee will be days rather than hours, as it is not critical to a domestic household if the broadband connection is down for a few days.
- A business broadband service is a specific service for businesses and is more expensive than domestic. It provides lower contention ratios, normally from 20:1 down to 1:1. The lower the ratio, the higher the cost but the better the speed and service. The support and service response guarantee will be hours, which means the business will not be without its broadband for extended periods.

The practice management system

The practice management system (PMS) is the software program used by the practice to handle everyday operations and to collect and process data in order to aid the management of the business. If used to its fullest, the PMS will be responsible for storing all clinical records, laboratory reports, transaction data, faxes, e-mails and images, including radiographs. From these data it will be possible to:

- Glean valuable performance information
- Market the practice to clients and assist them with patient care
- Manage stock control.

Some practice management systems will also handle other business functions, such as personnel records, rotas and aspects of the financial accounts. A PMS will ultimately improve the business; however, the installation of a new PMS will cause upheaval and the PMS will prove a significant ongoing investment.

Planning the installation of a new PMS

There are a number of PMS suppliers in the veterinary marketplace. For the busy veterinary surgeon, it is very easy to take the path of least resistance and upgrade to the existing supplier's latest version; for a first-time installation, it is tempting simply to ask contacts at other practices for their opinion regarding the system they currently use and whether they would recommend it. However, when investing in a business tool that will be at the heart of the practice and will be used by all members of staff, it is vital that time and resources are committed to making the project a success right from the beginning. A lack of planning and time commitment may result in a poor decision that must be lived with for years to come.

When planning the installation of a new PMS, the practice resources and skills, and the time available to dedicate to the project, should be reviewed. A target completion date is useful at this stage, and this can be confirmed or changed as the project progresses.

KEY POINT

It is important to gain the full support and input of practice staff and management – including client input – from the very start, as everybody will be affected by the project.

Identifying what the practice requires from its PMS

A clear idea of what the practice wants to get out of its new PMS, including its communication requirements, will make the job of selecting the right PMS much easier.

What is a PMS capable of?

At the basic level, all practice management systems carry out similar functions. These include:

- Storage of client and patient details
- Storage of clinical records
- An appointment and procedures diary
- The ability to charge and take money
- Stock control
- Simple reporting.

Advanced functionality will vary between systems; some examples are given in Figure 4.4. This is not an exhaustive list and there will be other advanced requirements specific to the practice that will need to be considered.

- Detailed and flexible reporting, e.g. of sales and purchases analysis
- Marketing capability, e.g. selection of clients or pets that meet certain criteria for marketing purposes
- Client communication, which may include communicating with clients via SMS (text) and e-mail
- Integration with external online systems such as those of insurance companies (for claims) or external laboratories (for results)
- Client classification and grouping, for reporting, communication and marketing
- Pricing of products and services, and the ease of updating prices and setting pricing structures
- A rota and diary system that is interlinked with client records
- Accounting and integration with the accounting system (see Chapter 24)
- Security, including the flexibility of the system to allow for different security levels and passwords to get into different parts of the program, and for editing
- Medicines management, stock control, labelling and re-ordering systems
- Accurate recording and data handling for auditing and reconciliation purposes
- Batch numbers, including compatibility with supplier systems to allow the practice to easily comply with any batch number recording requirements and legislation

4.4 Examples of advanced functionality that may be found in a PMS.

Reviewing and documenting general requirements

The chosen PMS should complement, or improve, the way in which the practice currently operates. A list of the processes that take place in the practice should be created, with the involvement of staff from the different work groups within the practice, including veterinary surgeons, veterinary nurses, receptionists, administrators and accountants. This is important, as different staff will have different requirements from the system. Examples of processes that take place in the practice are shown in Figure 4.5. Once a list has been created, each process should be documented in detail, preferably by a member of staff who carries out the procedure on a regular basis as part of their routine duties. For a start-up practice, this is the ideal time at which to document how the practice should work. This list can then be used to consider the role that can be played by the PMS in each of the processes that take place in the practice.

- Making client appointments
- The consultation process, from client arrival at the surgery, through examination and treatment of the pet by the veterinary surgeon, to the client returning to the reception area to pay
- Admitting and discharging patients
- Treatment and management of inpatients
- Dispensing and stock control
- Accounting and debt collection
- Dealing with insurance claims
- Referrals
- Laboratory tests and results
- Dealing with patients out of hours
- Dealing with supplier payments
- Preparing and targeting marketing communications

4.5 Examples of processes that take place in the practice and that need consideration when selecting a PMS.

Communication requirements

Practice communication requirements, both current and future, should be defined, considering both internal and external networks. Also, the operational requirements of multi-site practices should be considered. Questions that will help with this assessment are shown in Figure 4.6.

- Are sites completely autonomous in operation?
- Does the practice operate a central location or hospital with other sites feeding in?
- Do clients visit more than one branch?
- Do staff work 'in the field'?
- Do key staff require access from home?
- How easy is it to add a new site to the system?
- What would happen if primary communication links failed?
- Is a communication back-up required and if so how would it work?
- What internal networks are currently in place, and will they work with the new system or will they need to be upgraded?
- What Internet access does the practice need?
- What sort of broadband requirements are needed (quality and speed)?

4.6 Questions that should be asked in assessing the communication requirements of a PMS.

Identifying what the new PMS will require from the practice

As well as identifying what the practice requires from a PMS, it is also important to realize that a PMS will also require certain things from the practice.

Hardware requirements

In order to check that a PMS is compatible with the current hardware at the practice, all existing hardware should be reviewed and a list created to include the model, specification and age of each item. This will enable potential suppliers to advise the practice as to whether current hardware is suitable for use with their system. A list of hardware requirements can then be made. The practice should take into consideration that more computers and printers may be needed in the future.

Different PMS systems will have different server requirements:

- Some require a **central server**: a powerful computer that holds all of the data and manages the system for one or more locations
- Some may require **distributed servers**: computers that hold data and manage the system at each location
- Some systems are held **'in the cloud'** or **'Internet based'**: all of the data are held on professionally managed servers connected via the Internet. In this scenario, a less powerful server is needed in house to manage the network and e-mail system.

This knowledge will give the practice a place to commence discussions with potential suppliers. All suppliers will advise on the hardware requirements for their system and some will offer to supply it. This is a good stage at which to obtain an initial costing. There are a variety of ways to finance computer hardware, and financial advice should be sought (see Chapter 24).

Support requirements

All aspects of the new system will require ongoing support, and consideration should be given to the level of support the practice will need. This will be influenced by the level of computer system and network skills within the practice. For most practices this will be limited and a full support package will therefore be required. A major contributor to the cost of support is the response time following a failure. The operational and financial effects on the practice can be significant if part or all of the system is down for a period of time.

The need for external expertise

External expertise to assist with the project should be considered early on. Many PMS suppliers offer a 'turnkey' package. This means that they will offer to supply the PMS software, the hardware, the communications and a full installation and support package. This will suit many practices. Depending on the size of the practice, it may be the case that the PMS supplier has sufficient expertise and the system supplied has sufficient functions to meet the needs of the practice. Larger or more complex practices may have more specific requirements and therefore may need to consider using external expertise for specific areas of the business. Alternative systems for specific business functions may also need to be considered, e.g. using an industry-wide recognized human resources management system. It should be borne in mind, however, that this may sometimes cause problems when trying to resolve problems where it is unclear who is primarily responsible.

Selecting the right PMS for the practice

Figure 4.7 depicts the major steps that a practice needs to take in order to select and install a new practice management system.

Choosing a system

PMS suppliers should use current programming technology and their systems should function on the latest operating systems; although as technology advances at an ever-increasing pace, and with hardware now becoming more of a 'consumable' item, even a system using the most up-to-date technology should not expect an active life of more than 3 years.

Where incompatibilities are found between the practice's current system and the PMS, a decision should be made as to which method would be most effective. Many practice systems will have to be adapted to work with the new PMS, but this should not be a backward step. If reliance is placed on a promise to adapt the PMS, this should be in place before installation is agreed.

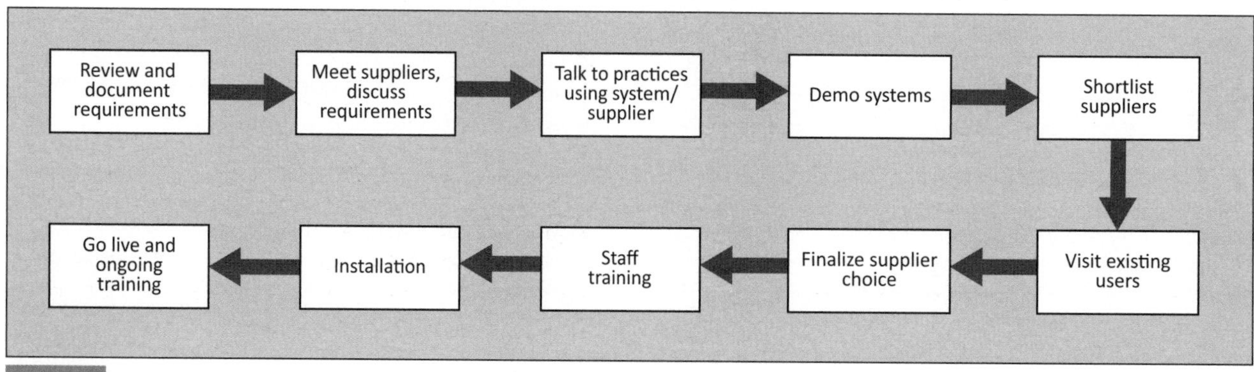

4.7 Overview of selecting and installing a PMS.

References should be contacted and views sought on the following issues:

- How the system deals with key requirements
- Installation and training
- Support service and upgrading
- Communications
- The relationship with the supplier.

In order to review available systems fully, suppliers should be contacted, the agreed requirements outlined, and an initial meeting arranged. Some suppliers may not be able to meet the practice requirements, and time should not be wasted on meeting them. One way of shortcutting the process of whittling down the list of potential suppliers is to attend a veterinary exhibition, where initial face-to-face discussions can take place with all suppliers, and details of reference sites for the systems can be obtained and followed up.

KEY POINT

Demonstrations should be arranged with shortlisted suppliers, and these should preferably take place at the practice. Plenty of time should be allowed for demonstrations, as the detail will be very important.

The ability and extent to which the provider can supply the services required by the practice should be discussed. This will most likely include the following:

- Form production, including:
  - Consent forms
  - Laboratory request forms
  - Unauthorized medicines consent
  - Referral and discharge notes
  - Out-of-hours work reports
- Storage of client and patient details, including such things as extra addresses, multiple telephone numbers, e-mail addresses and social media contacts
- Incorporation of a workable diary/rota system
- Classification/grouping of clients, e.g. referral, first opinion, bad debtors and staff
- Recording of patient insurance details (e.g. company, policy number, type, limits)
- Handling of insurance claim administration, direct claims, part payments, etc.
- Syndication (where multiple owners of an animal exist and each shares a percentage of the bill) – this can be very useful in some instances
- Entering of information during a consultation (e.g. warnings, drug reactions, important notes)
- Lists of inpatients/hospitalized patients
- Appointment scheduling
- Scheduling procedures with specific staff members
- Management of client loyalty schemes
- Marketing: ability to search for clients and/or patients using a range of criteria and then to be able to produce the information in a usable format
- Multi-branch functions such as booking appointments and stock control
- Financial reporting: the range of standard reports and the range of configurable reports
- Stock management, batch numbering, ordering and stock rotation; variable drug pricing
- Reminder generation and the ability to update and communicate with clients in a variety of ways (e.g. SMS and e-mail).

The following aspects of the system must also be discussed:

- **Data conversion**. If the practice has an existing system, the new system should be able to convert all of the essential data. If computerizing for the first time, some data entry will be necessary prior to going live. Transferring client and patient records may not be essential, as an old card or computer system can be continued in parallel for looking up historical data and clinical records. The disadvantages of this are space and risk to the data through failure of old hardware and lack of ongoing support for the old system
- **Staff training** pre- and post-installation
- Whether the PMS meets the practice's particular **communication requirements**. The supplier should have already tried and tested communication systems in the field and they should also have been seen in action. There is quite often a difference between the 'promise' and the reality, particularly in relation to speed and reliability
- How the new PMS integrates with the **Internet** to allow additional services, such as the facility for clients to order repeat prescriptions and book appointments, should be investigated. This may involve links between the PMS and the practice website
- **Security and back-up**
- All aspects of **support,** including the willingness of the supplier to take individual practice ideas on board
- The **age of the current version** (technology moves on very quickly) and the way in which upgrades are planned, applied, installed and charged
- The **pricing model** and financing options. The value of the total package agreed upon is important and can include set-up and installation, training, ongoing proactive support, ongoing software development, and free upgrades.

Staff from all disciplines should be asked to attend the demonstration. The supplier should be asked to give an overview and go through the whole system, discussing the above points. The areas that are of key importance to the practice should be demonstrated in detail, in relation to the current documented processes. Areas of concern must be highlighted and discussed with the supplier, and the process from demonstration to going live, including timescales, should be set out.

A list of existing users of similar practices should be requested so that visits to these practices can be arranged. It is useful for a demo system to be left at the practice, where staff can use it 'hands on'. This will give the practice useful feedback and ensure staff involvement.

Once a supplier has been selected, the price should be agreed, dates and timescales set and the order placed.

Staff training

The more 'hands on' staff training that can take place before installation the better. A training schedule that suits the practice should be agreed. The supplier should provide sufficient trainers to fit the training timescales. The training should be done at the practice, if possible, and ideally a training system left for the staff to practise on.

KEY POINT

It is a good idea to have one or more members of practice staff fully trained in order to support other staff.

Installation and 'go live'

The installation will have three components:

- PMS software and support
- Computer hardware and support
- Communications – internal and external networks.

KEY POINT

Installation must be planned and agreed with the supplier in meticulous detail, including estimated timings. Once these have been agreed, all staff must be fully aware of the timescales and plans.

Ideally, installation should be planned for when the practice is closed. However, for practices providing a 24-hour operation, or if the time requirements are longer than closure times, downtime will need to be planned along with any alternative working and recording arrangements required during this time. Time must also be allocated for inputting data into the new system once it goes live.

It is best to ensure that the supplier has both engineers and trainers on site immediately after the system goes live. All locations must be covered in a multi-site practice.

IT policies

Policies for the use of IT within the practice should incorporate the following:

- Compliance with relevant laws and ensuring security of data, so that the practice is not brought into disrepute and facilities are not abused
- Security protocols: including use and misuse of passwords, access to restricted areas
- Appropriate use: e-mail etiquette, use of distribution lists, disclaimers
- Data storage and the use of removable hardware, which may introduce viruses
- Personal use policy: what is and is not acceptable
- Care of the equipment
- Privacy and the rights of the practice to inspect e-mail accounts/files
- User responsibilities
- Training.

For more detail see Chapter 16.

Basic IT and data security principles

New security threats occur all the time, but some basic principles should be adhered to so that practice IT equipment and data are as safe as possible (Figure 4.8; see also chapter 16.).

- Ensure that administrator full-access log-ins and system passwords are known only by key staff. Users should have limited access, i.e. only to those programs needed for everyday work. Owners and managers are advised to have two accounts: one for day-to-day work; and a super-user account for troubleshooting, maintenance and accessing sensitive data. Time-limited log-ins and good discipline to log out of the system will prevent unauthorized access and misallocation of notes and charged work. Passwords should be changed regularly, and redundant users removed from the system
- Ensure limited access with users being able to use only those parts of the program they need for their day-to-day work
- Ensure operating systems and essential software are upgraded regularly to reduce vulnerabilities
- Use hardware and software firewalls to protect the local network from the Internet. Wireless networks should be protected by secure encryption
- Ensure antivirus software is up to date and effective, and do not permit staff to download personal e-mail attachments or programs on to the system
- Use an up-to-date browser with adequate security settings
- Surge protectors and battery back-up supplies allowing controlled shutdown are recommended
- Keep mobile computers and devices secure and password-protected. Do not allow sensitive data to be taken offsite unless absolutely necessary (e.g. for back-up)
- Use effective onsite and offsite data back-up, which is regularly verified and held securely
- Do not allow the use of personal devices on the network unless satisfied that security will not be breached

4.8 Data security principles.

IT for marketing

It is essential to take advantage of technology in order to market the practice to existing and potential clients (see also Chapter 25). The PMS can play a large part in a practice's marketing strategy, particularly in relation to e-mail and text communication, and consideration of the client 'touch points' in Figure 4.9 is recommended. Well designed and presented documents, websites, e-mails and client information require not just design expertise but also appropriate word- and image-handling software and reproduction equipment, if they are to be produced in house.

It is also important to consider the growing popularity of social media sites. Clients are spending increasingly significant amounts of time on these sites, and so veterinary practices that make use of social media are undoubtedly going to benefit.

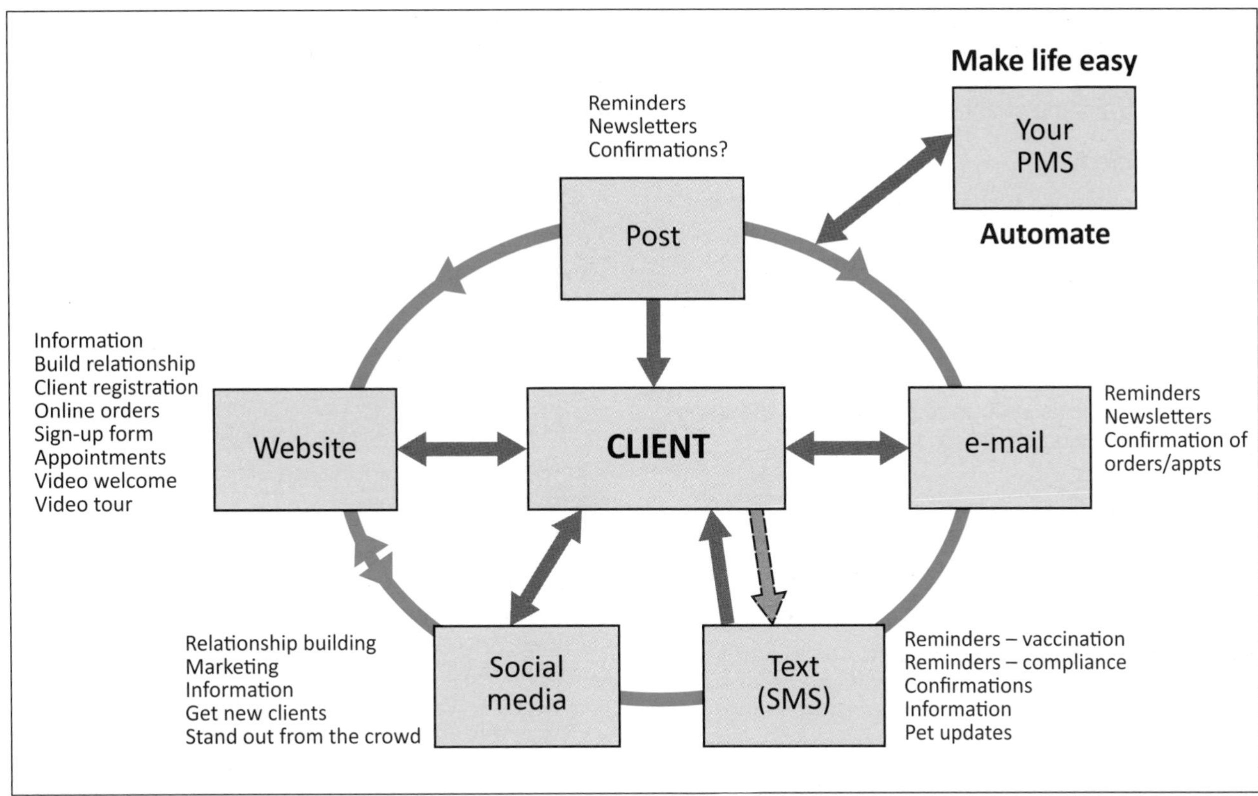

4.9 Client touch points. The practice should use multiple methods of communication with each client, and the PMS should enable them to do that with as little additional work as possible. In this diagram, grey arrows indicate communication with the client. The red lines indicate the need for electronic links. For example, any social media presence should contain links back to the practice website and *vice versa*; and any letters posted should refer the reader to the website for more information, e.g. to encourage clients to sign up for the newsletter. The link between post and e-mail is there to encourage clients to consider e-mail delivery instead of, or as well as, physical letters for things such as reminders and appointment confirmations.

Accepting payments electronically

Methods of payment

Payments can be processed in one of three ways:

- Through a standalone terminal connected to a phone line or the Internet
- Via the computer through a specific program (sometimes through the PMS)
- Through a website.

Accepting payment using a standalone terminal

Merchant services

The most common method of card payment uses a merchant service; this is the method many high street shops employ. The client's card is inserted into a PDQ ('process data quickly') machine, which is separate from the till. The PDQ machine is connected to a merchant service (acquiring bank), which has provided the seller with a unique identifier (merchant ID) via a dedicated telephone line. After the client has confirmed the card is theirs, by entry of a pin code, the merchant service receives the merchant ID plus a few key details, which are enough to be able to authorize or decline a transaction. PDQ machines can also be used in 'customer not present' mode, where the details and transaction are manually entered by staff. This introduces a potentially higher risk of fraud, as card security numbers replace entry of a pin code in order to try and ensure the remote client has authorization to use that card. All PDQ machines are tethered to a phone line or network. Because the telephone line is separate and secure, the cost of processing cards is lower using this method.

Bluetooth terminals

Portable Bluetooth terminals are a flexible option for accepting payment, although occasionally there are reliability problems. Portable Bluetooth terminals are useful where clients are not in reception, and can be helpful if reception is congested.

GPRS terminals

Mobile terminals are available that use GPRS (general practice radio service) connectivity; this can be very useful for veterinary surgeons on ambulatory visits. The terminals must be kept fully charged, as problems can be encountered if the terminal battery is allowed to run down.

Accepting payment through a website

Payment service provider and Internet merchant service

When accepting online payments, the payment service provider (PSP) and the Internet merchant service (IMS) are the online equivalents of the PDQ machine and the merchant service. The PSP provides the software to replicate the process of acquiring card details. The IMS has separate rules from those governing the use of merchant services.

Payment bureau

A payment bureau is a cost-effective solution for businesses that are just starting to accept online payments; these organizations eliminate the requirement for a PSP or an IMS as they process transactions through their own acquirer. However, their charges tend to be higher and they routinely hold on to payments for 30–60 days during the period of early trading (the period during which most fraud is recognized) to reduce the exposure of the acquiring service to fraud.

Person-to-person

Person-to-person (P2P) is a method of payment that relies on individuals setting up what is effectively an online mini bank account. This can be charged using credit, debit or direct bank transfer by the individual after paying appropriate associated costs. Once this money is in the individual's account it can be used for several purposes, including paying other individuals or paying online retailers using the same P2P service. This is a common method of payment on online auction sites and advantages include a low set-up cost and low transaction rates, with no requirement for a PSP or IMS.

The cost of processing card payments

All of the routes for accepting card payments come with additional set-up costs. The bank that provides the merchant service (the acquiring bank) need not be the practice's main banking partner and the rates for hire of PDQs and card processing costs are all negotiable, with preferential rates offered in conjunction with buying groups and professional associations. For more details on negotiating rates and managing card payments see Chapter 16.

Payment card industry data security

The Payment Card Industry Data Security Standards (PCIDSS) are a set of standards created to ensure security of payment card data and include the prevention, detection and response to security threats. The standards include 12 requirements (Figure 4.10) for any business that stores, processes or transmits payment cardholder data.

The principle is a self-assessment of the flow of cardholder data through the organization, to look for vulnerabilities and then remedy them, before attesting compliance with the standards. It is an ongoing process and requires regular review (usually each year or when significant changes to the process have occurred).

Currently, if the practice is using a standalone card terminal from a well known merchant connected to its own telephone line (not to the computer network), and as long as payment card data such as card numbers, expiry dates or card PINs are not stored, there is very little risk and a shorter self-assessment can be used. Where the card reader is attached to the computer system and/or the data are processed via a third party or payment service provider, things are more complex. Most card merchants and acquirers provide a process to assist businesses with self-assessment.

- Install and maintain a firewall configuration to protect cardholder data
- Do not use vendor-supplied defaults for system passwords and other security parameters
- Protect stored cardholder data
- Encrypt transmission of cardholder data across open, public networks
- Use and regularly update antivirus software
- Develop and maintain secure systems and applications
- Restrict access to cardholder data by business 'need to know'
- Assign a unique ID to each person with computer access
- Restrict physical access to cardholder data
- Track and monitor all access to network resources and cardholder data
- Regularly test security systems and processes
- Maintain a policy that addresses information security

4.10 Payment Card Industry Data Security Standards requirements.

There are four categories within the PCIDSS, A to D, depending on how card transactions are processed and if any of the data are stored. The Sensitive Authentication Data include the full track contents of the magnetic strip or chip, card verification codes and values, and PINs and PIN blocks. These data should *never* be stored but occasionally the equipment does this without users being aware. Most reputable merchants now supply terminals that do not do this; the merchant service should be able to advise.

If any permitted card data such as the personal account number (PAN), expiration date, cardholder name and service code are stored, the practice should consider whether this is entirely necessary and delete what is not required. All card data should then be isolated from other systems on the network and the network security itself reviewed. Doing so will allow the PCIDSS to be focused only upon the areas that matter, and will simplify the process and reduce the cost of compliance. More information can be found at www.pcisecuritystandards.org.

Telecommunication in the practice

The nature of telecommunication is constantly evolving. The change from analogue to digital signals has greatly improved call quality and enables data transmission concurrently with computer traffic. Today's fibreoptic cables are able to carry greater amounts of data with much less interference than hitherto.

Lines for transmission of data

There are three different types of line available for the transmission of data:

- The basic **analogue** line, which is of limited business use
- **ISDN** (integrated services digital network)
- **ADSL** (asymmetric digital subscriber line).

ISDN splits an analogue line into three channels: two can carry 64 kbps; the third is a control channel and can carry either 16 or 64 kbps. ISDN is flexible in that both non-control channels can be combined to give an Internet connection at 128 kbps, dropping the Internet speed if a call comes in that uses one of the channels. ISDN can therefore replace two analogue lines, which is a cost benefit.

ADSL allows concurrent transmission of voice and data, by using a different frequency for the data. (A 'splitter' or 'DSL filter' allows an analogue line to be used for both voice calls and data simultaneously.) ADSL is usually faster than ISDN and provides an 'always on' Internet connection. ADSL is affected by distance from the exchange and quality of the copper telephone cables among other things, and so the line quality may vary. There are also upstream (from user to exchange) and downstream (from exchange to user) speeds. Downstream speeds are usually faster. This is not normally a problem, as most traffic is into the business; however, upstream speeds will be important when, for instance, data from the main practice are being sent to branches that have a linked PMS.

Whether ISDN or ADSL is chosen will depend upon the distance from the exchange and the likely ADSL line quality/speed *versus* usage patterns. ISDN is better value if multiple voice lines are in use, as there are potentially two per connection (along with Internet and fax), whereas ADSL only carries one.

Telephone systems

The choice of telephone system will depend on the number of extensions and the functionality required from the internal handsets (Figure 4.11).

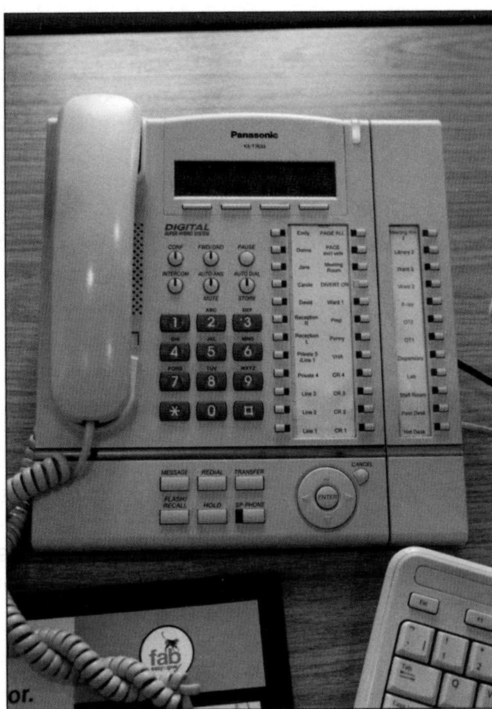

4.11 An advanced telephone handset which shows extension activity via an LED light on the unit. This can be useful for locating staff, for direct dialling of extensions and for monitoring call volume in real time. The display at the top can indicate caller identification or location and can carry system messages, call time duration, etc. This model also has a speaker for paging and hands-free use.

The simplest internal telephone system is similar to extensions in a domestic setting, with one line and several handsets (extensions). There is very little flexibility with such a system and, although some phones may be able to 'page' or talk to other handsets within the system, it does not allow easy transfer of calls or provide much useful business functionality.

- Smaller practices may manage with one incoming line and one outgoing line, which could be shared with the fax.
- Larger practices will usually have several incoming lines or a flexible number of multi-use lines using ISDN, and may allocate different numbers for functions such as accounts, appointments and enquiries.
- The number of lines used should be decided by looking at the normal call traffic and number of engaged calls, so that most calls get through to ring, as long as sufficient staff members are available to answer the calls. Call traffic reports can usually be obtained from the practice telecommunications provider (see later).
- Unlike most call centres, veterinary practices must always be ready for emergency calls, so long periods or messages on hold before answering need to be avoided.

PABX

A small piece of hardware referred to as a PBX or PABX (private (automatic) branch exchange; Figure 4.12) enables telephone extensions to be connected internally with the public telephone network. The features and cost of a PABX vary considerably

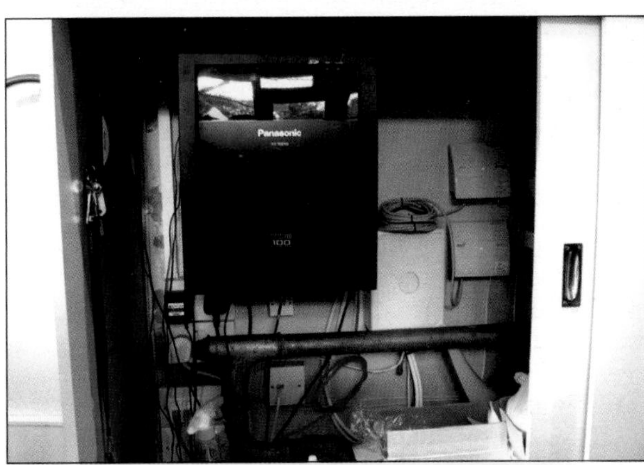

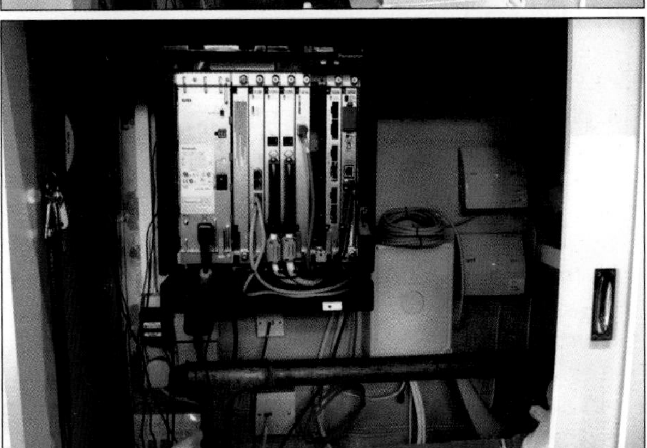

4.12 A PABX with a central control unit provides enhanced functionality to internal telephone systems. Battery back-up for power failure is essential.

depending on the functions and number of extensions needed, although it should be possible to source a PABX that is suitable for a small business for only a few hundred pounds. The PABX normally handles multiple incoming lines and offers internal calls, call forwarding, music on hold, voicemail, public address/ paging and many other features.

KEY POINT

The PABX is powered by electricity. In the event of a power cut, it will therefore cease to function and a back-up plan will be necessary, such as diversion of the practice line to a mobile number.

Automatic call answering

A PABX has the ability to enable automatic call answering, which may or may not be desired depending on practice ethos. It can be useful in larger practices, as it enables the caller to choose, and be automatically routed to, the department they require (e.g. wards, reception, accounts). It is also a useful tool out of hours and can replace a traditional answering machine by announcing a pre-recorded message that gives the caller several options and then diverts the filtered call (if the client still considers this an emergency) to the on-call staff member or elsewhere. If there are multiple incoming lines, the automated answering facility can ensure that calls are not missed by increasingly involving more extensions if a call is not answered within a certain timeframe, finally reverting to a voicemail facility as a last resort. Choice of menu options and the order in which they are offered, together with the tone of the recorded voice, will all affect how frustrated the busy or worried caller will feel. The 'emergency help' option should always come early in the list.

Communicating with mobile staff

In most practices, many staff are mobile – moving about the building constantly. There should be a method of easily reaching mobile staff so that they can be informed of relevant information, alerted to client calls and summoned should help be required. An effective system will reduce the length of time clients wait on hold, and will increase efficiency within the practice.

Perhaps the easiest method is a public address (PA) system, which can either be included as part of the phone set-up or be independent from it. Most modern phones can be set to 'speaker' mode, which allows the user to talk whilst the handset is still in place. This speaker can usually be used as a PA system (but only when that unit is not in use on another call); therefore in a busy practice it may be necessary to have several phones, which all have this feature switched on, in areas where handsets are in high demand – otherwise messages may be missed.

In an independent system there will usually be one speaker per room that will broadcast whether people are using the phone system or not. The cost implications of set-up and hardware for either system can be weighed up once the location of speakers has been decided. The practice needs to consider whether it is necessary to install PA systems in staff rest areas and in other areas, such as external buildings.

The disadvantages of PA systems must also be considered. A constant stream of messages, which are only relevant to the minority, can interfere with staff's ability to work and disturb patients. Pagers provide a less intrusive method of mobile alert (see later).

Performance monitoring

As with all aspects of the business, gathering and reviewing performance data will enable better planning and greater efficiency. Monitoring the call rates at different times, the proportion of answered and unanswered calls, those receiving an engaged tone and the pattern of incoming and outgoing calls throughout the day will help managers to adapt staffing and call management to best effect. Time-to-answer measurements are also helpful for indicating staff performance. Such services are available through most reputable telecoms providers.

Call content can also be recorded, for use in training, to improve processes, and to give evidence of transactions. However, there are certain requirements to be aware of: callers must be told the calls may be recorded (both inbound and outgoing); employees must also be informed (usually in contracts or company handbooks) and the benefits of doing so clearly explained. Any card details given verbally cannot be recorded due to payment card industry data security standards (see above), which state that this information must not be stored.

Voice over Internet protocol

Voice over Internet protocol (VoIP) is the transfer of packets of voice data over the Internet, and is now commonplace. As this is classified as digital traffic, it is often included in a data allowance and so when used with ISDN or broadband will allow for much cheaper calls. Multi-site practices can also have extensions within their branches that behave as though they were within the main practice telephone system and do not require a separate number or an external call to reach colleagues.

Skype is an example of a program that makes use of VoIP; users load the small program on to a computer, where it will then use the hardware of that terminal (microphone and video if installed, or alternatively a plug-in headset) to allow users registered with Skype to talk to each other via the Internet. The basic service is free, and enables talking, video conferences and the sending of files. Added functionality can be gained by paying a subscription. Whether this solution works for a practice will depend upon the acceptance by the staff, as it is quite a shift from using a standard telephone handset and users need to become familiar with the concept.

VoIP call quality can be variable and will depend not only upon the practice's broadband connection but also the client's connection. If using such a system it is recommended to source a broadband line with a low 'contention ratio' (see above). A telecoms provider will be able to discuss this further.

Fax

Perhaps surprisingly, facsimile (fax) remains widely used. Fax is still better than unencrypted Internet technologies as a secure method for sending documents between sites. Standalone machines can be purchased cost-effectively, and so are a good choice for small businesses. During transmission the caller pays the cost of a telephone call and the line is 'tied up' during the process. If only one line exists then the fax call prevents other calls (clients) from reaching the practice. Hence most companies pay for an extra line, which is an extra expense.

The output of a fax machine is usually thermal or plain paper. Faxes printed on thermal paper do not provide a permanent copy, so must be photocopied.

The modern alternative to the automatic printing of faxes is a fax server (computer), which receives the faxes electronically and then either securely distributes them within the organization or places them in an easily accessible digital folder for printing, electronic storage or forwarding. With a fax server installed, it is also possible to 'print' any document to a virtual fax, which then electronically transmits the file to the required destination (a scanner is required to load documents that have been signed or handwritten). If it is enabled, this facility may be accessible from any terminal on the network.

When siting a standalone fax machine, consideration should be given to who is going to use it most and whether it will be possible to check for received faxes regularly. The noise created by a fax machine must also be considered when deciding its position in the practice.

Paging

Traditionally, this was the form of communication used to alert on-call staff to an emergency. Paging signals are delivered via satellite technology. This means that pagers are more reliable than mobile phones where the cellular network coverage is poor (e.g. hospitals), in remote areas or when cellular networks may fail; this reliability is the main reason pagers are still used. However, functionality is poor compared with mobile phones: most pagers only transmit a simple one-way numeric or alphanumeric message, although two-way pagers have been developed for use by the emergency services.

'Smart' phones

Smart phones use operating systems that allow other third-party applications (or 'apps') to be loaded, and many offer integration with a corporate network. Some of these applications are useful and many are free; some practices are even setting up their own apps.

Smart phones accomplish a wide variety of tasks, from calendar scheduling to quick calculations, reference books, etc. They are perhaps most useful where they can connect to the clinic server and allow users to access business e-mails, calendar and contact functions without the need to be onsite or in possession of a computer; as the technology advances it may soon be possible to gain access to the appointment diary, billing or other functions of the PMS. Functionality of smart phones sometimes requires a server to be running specific software. Smart phones are also limited by the quality/availability of the cellular network.

Reception and client waiting areas

5

Alison Lambert and Peter Hundepool

Getting the reception and client areas right is such a fundamental part of a practice's success, yet one that many practices do not fully appreciate. There simply is no second chance to make a first impression, so it is essential to make sure that the reception and client areas are saying exactly what they should be about the practice and about the team who work there.

If the first thing a client sees when they come through the door is a bright and airy waiting area that smells pleasant, and they are greeted by name, by a receptionist in uniform, wearing a name badge and an expectant smile, that client is much more likely to think, 'I like it here. This is a modern, friendly and professional practice where my pet and I will be treated with respect.' A client who is impressed with both the look of the practice and the level of service is more likely to become a loyal client who recommends the practice to others.

If premises are a little run down and waiting areas look rather tired, this can convey the impression to clients that maybe the service is also not up to a high standard. If staff appear stressed and harassed, clients may end up wondering whether their pets are perhaps receiving second-class care from overworked employees.

These elements go hand in hand:

- A practice can look fantastic but be let down by rude or indifferent staff
- If the reception and client areas need redecorating and this has not been authorized, an excellent team may feel let down, as the look of the practice does not do them and their good work justice.

Whether a client's overall experience of a practice is good or bad is hugely dependent on how they are treated by front-of-house staff whilst waiting with their pet.

The receptionist is the first *and last* point of contact with the practice, and therefore needs to be friendly, professional, efficient, courteous, helpful and unflustered at all times with everyone who visits the practice.

Design considerations

The reception area can be used as a tool to differentiate the practice from its competitors. It is very important to get the look, feel and style of the reception and client areas right. The style should match and be incorporated into the style of the whole practice. While modern finishes and materials allow practices to maintain hygienic premises without looking too 'clinical', some simple changes to existing areas can make big improvements in both the look of the practice and the way that it operates.

The traditional reception area

Rather than being carefully planned and thought through, the reception area in many practices has evolved, which often means that compromises have had to be made. In particular, practices in older buildings may be working with logistical challenges and physical constraints. In the past it was not uncommon for the reception area to be housed in a room where only a small window looked out into the waiting area. Through this limited opening, staff were expected to carry out the current wide range of tasks (Figure 5.1).

- Arranging appointments
- Keeping an eye on waiting pets
- Giving information and advice
- Calling patients in for their appointments
- Handing out prescriptions
- Discussing confidential information
- Accepting deliveries

5.1 Key tasks that are performed in the reception/waiting area.

There was often a sliding window that was opened to allow brief face-to-face contact with clients and was then hastily closed again. Such barriers alienate practice visitors by impeding communication and interaction between client, patient and staff. The physical act of removing the walls around the reception area, to integrate it into the waiting room by making the desk more open and staff accessible, will go a long way towards making clients feel welcome.

KEY POINT

If the reception area *looks* accessible, clients will *feel* that the practice is also open, welcoming and friendly.

The modern reception and waiting area

Making the most of the reception area (Figure 5.2) is one of the key elements needed to make a practice welcoming and successful. When a reception area looks tired and worn out, this is the impression clients will form about the whole practice.

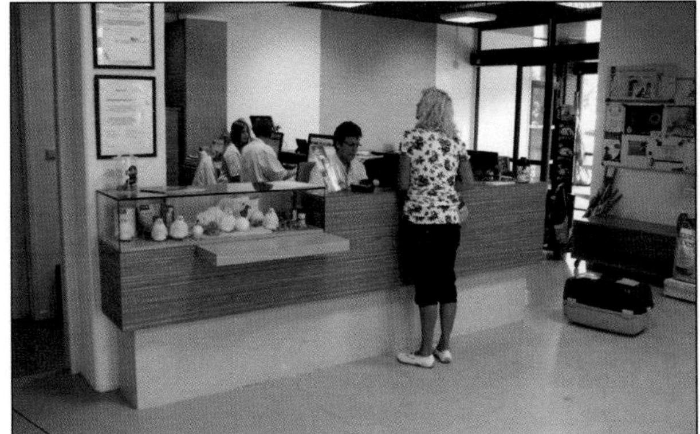

5.2 The modern reception area should be well maintained, clean and bright with good lighting and the counter should be at a user-friendly height.

The front desk

The front desk should not only look good from the front but should also be well designed at the back (Figure 5.3). When Reception is well organized and staff can find everything easily, the whole customer experience runs smoothly.

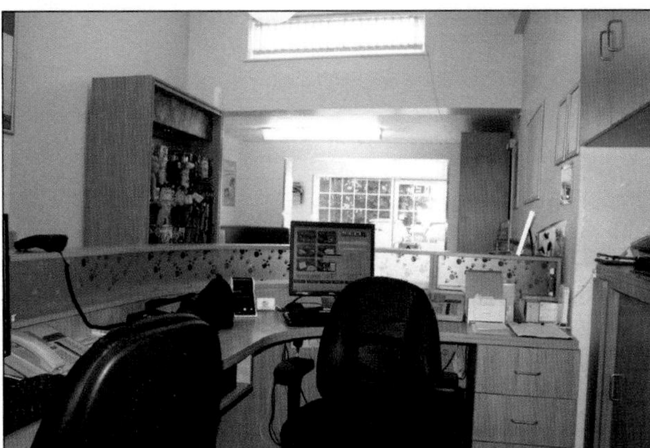

5.3 The front desk should also be well designed at the back, with enough space available to house essential items such as computers, keyboards and phones. The area should be kept neat and tidy, with cupboards and drawers provided for storage. It is important for the wellbeing of staff that chairs are comfortable and set at the right height.

Some recommended good practice points to bear in mind when designing or changing the front desk area are as follows.

- American studies have shown that the reception area should ideally fill a space of 3 m x 4 m.
- Raising the floor level behind the desk by 15–20 cm will add a subtle air of authority, and therefore improve the interaction between staff and clients.
- Raised and lowered desk areas offer defined places to write, and also spaces on which to place a small purchased item or a handbag (Figure 5.4a). A safe dog lead hook is also useful if the desk is fixed (Figure 5.4b)
- The desk should not be so high that the reception staff cannot see pets at floor level, nor maintain eye contact with clients whilst they are sitting down.
- Facilities for disabled visitors need to be taken into consideration, such as desk height for wheelchair users (Figure 5.5) and a hearing loop system for the deaf.
- Adequate leg room under the desk must be ensured at all staff seating stations.
- Temperature and ventilation should feel pleasant.
- The practice will always need at least one computer more than the number of staff working at the front desk.
- If not already computerized, there should be a prominent place for the appointment book.
- Headsets may be better for staff who spend most of their day on the phone.
- Telephone handsets must be available for summoning additional help and for communicating with staff in the rest of the practice without leaving reception.
- Practice leaflets and handouts should be easily accessible, and filed so it is quick and simple to find the information needed to give to clients.
- Shelves and cubby holes behind and/or built into the front desk must be of the correct height and width to accommodate files, storage boxes, etc.
- Space needs to be allocated for practical items, such as fire extinguishers.

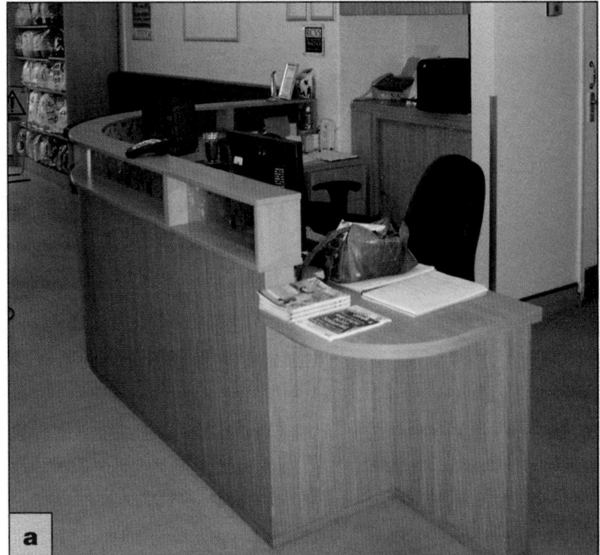

a

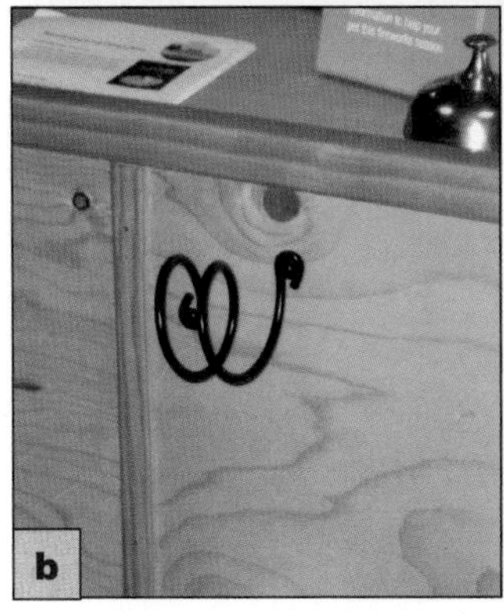

b

5.4 **(a)** Raised and lowered areas on a desk provide areas for clients to write and to place personal objects such as handbags. **(b)** A hook is useful for clients to secure a dog lead while their hands are otherwise occupied.

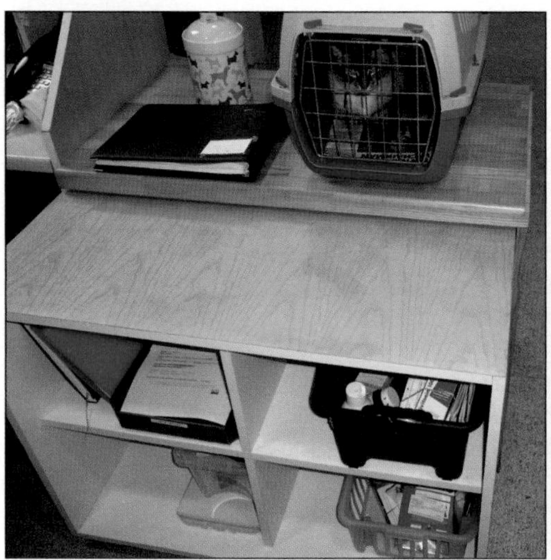

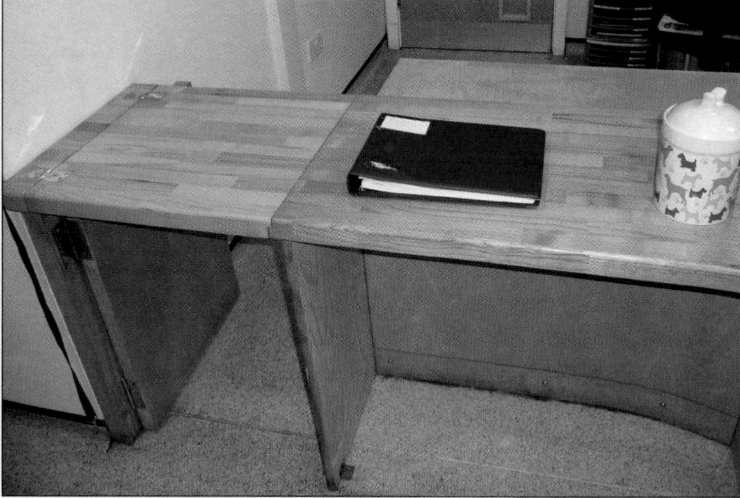

5.5 This desk has a built-in mobile drawer unit on castors. This section of the counter can be pulled back, creating a space/recess in the client area to allow knee room for a wheelchair user.

- Cleaning materials, including a spillage kit, should be kept close at hand (but out of reach of clients) for dealing with any problems quickly and efficiently.
- A set of scales for weighing pets at the front desk saves time in the consultation room (Figure 5.6). Scales flush to the floor are more aesthetically pleasing and easier for patients to use, but careful forethought is required, as once sunk into the floor their location is permanent. For cleaning purposes, particularly in the event of a dog urinating on them, the scales need to be easy to remove without staff trapping fingers in the process.
- A secure area, out of sight of any members of the public, must be available for cashing up and for emptying cash drawers and tills. A counter cache behind the desk can be used as a temporary safe store for banknotes (Figure 5.7).
- Installation of a panic button provides security for staff, who are then able to call for help quickly and discreetly if required.
- As well as improving security, CCTV systems that cover the interior and exterior of the building allow any problems, such as a queue at the front desk, to be spotted straight away.

When designing a practice, thought needs to be given to the location of the reception area in relation to other areas of the practice (see Chapter 3).

> **KEY POINT**
>
> Make the space work for staff as well as clients.

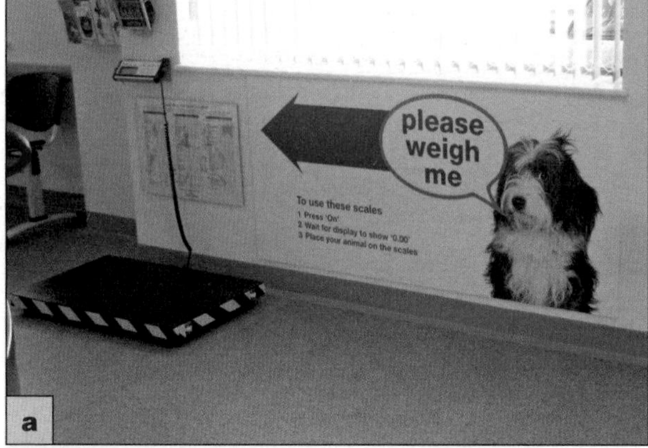

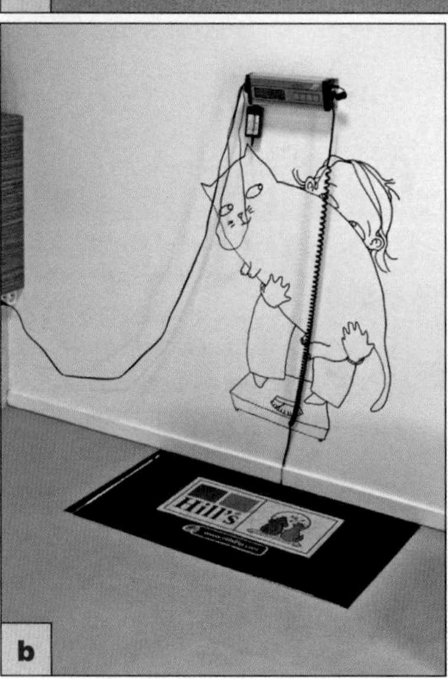

5.6 **(a)** Inviting clients to use scales to weigh their animals will encourage footfall. **(b)** Scales set into the floor can be aesthetically pleasing.

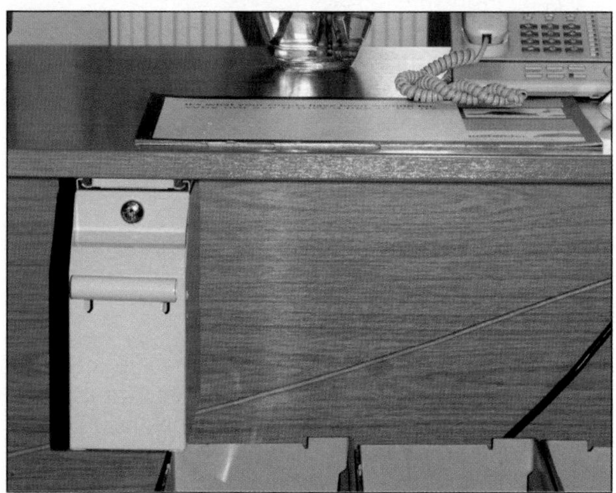

5.7 A small cache behind the desk can be used as a temporary safe store for any banknotes received.

The client waiting area

The waiting area needs to be clean and welcoming, but workable. Many practices do not use the term 'waiting room' but opt instead for 'client reception area', which has a more welcoming ring to it.

KEY POINTS

- Screens, reception layout and seating arrangements can all be used to separate nervous patients and owners from others, and to segregate species where necessary.
- A spare consulting room can often be put to use as a private waiting area, and this can be useful, for example, for euthanasia appointments.

When designing or looking to make changes, the following should be considered.

- Is the door easy to open and close?
- Is there enough room to get a pushchair or wheelchair *and* a cat basket or large dog through?
- Are there enough seats to cover the busiest times? Bench seats provide more capacity and possibly storage, but individual seating may be more flexible and give owners more personal space (Figure 5.8).
- Can nervous pets or owners wait without being too close to excited or noisy dogs? Is there flexibility for a quiet area for cats, rabbits or birds if space allows?
- Are the seats clean, matching and in a good state of repair? Padded upholstery gives a better impression than hard seating but cloth upholstery will need to be maintained with regular vacuuming and wet cleaning, whereas wipeable surfaces are easier to keep clean.
- Does the practice smell? People will forgive a whiff of wet dog on a rainy day, but if puddles left by nervous patients are not cleaned up, or there is a distinct tomcat smell in the air, there will soon be complaints. Ideally there should be a post or corner outside the front door for patients to mark before they enter the building; this will reduce the tendency to mark inside.
- Is there space to leave shopping, umbrellas, pushchairs, etc.?
- Is it too warm? Too cold? Too stuffy?
- Is the reception area bright and well lit?
- Are toilets available? If so, are they clean (Figure 5.9) and fully stocked with toilet roll, soap and towels? Toilets should not be used for storage and any cleaning materials should be removed. It is ideal to have a toilet accessible for clients and their children that is also accessible to disabled clients, and this will be a requirement for new builds and extensive practice upgrades.

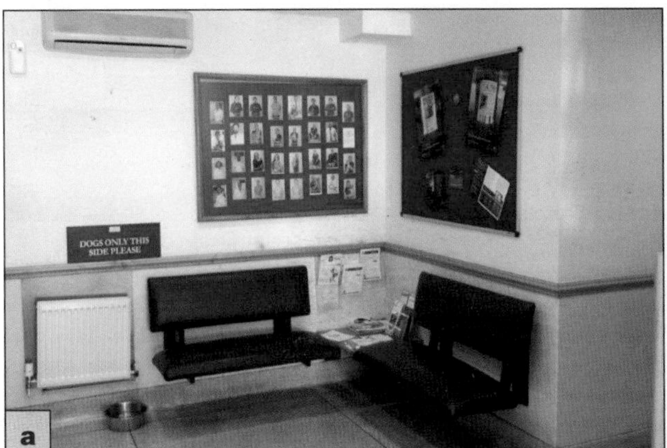
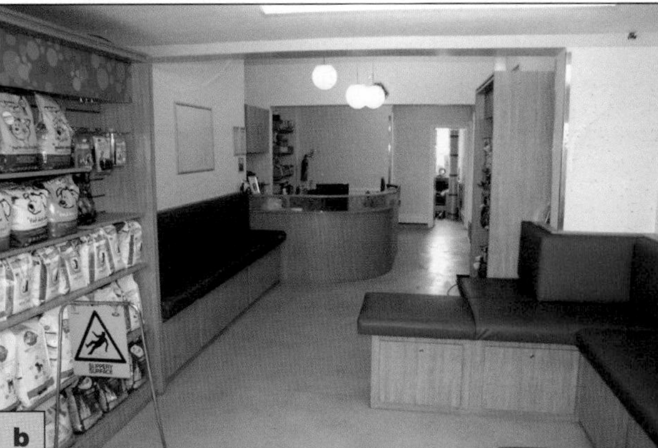
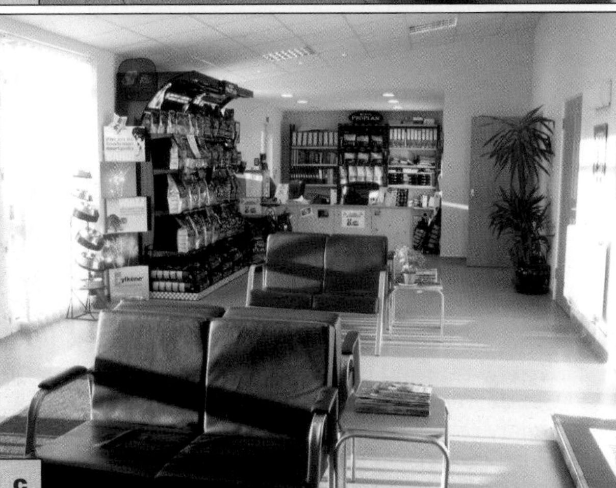
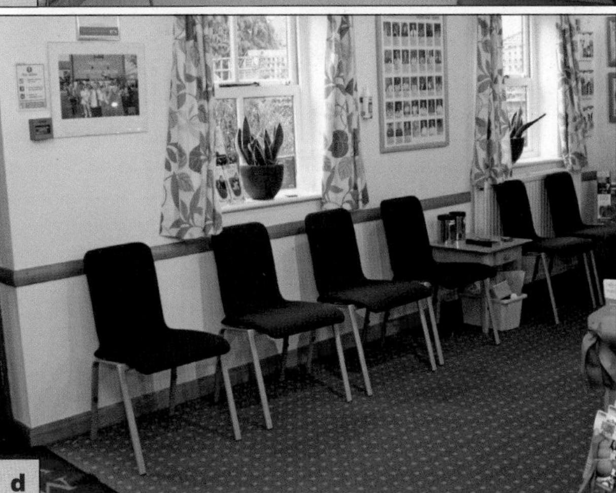

5.8 Seating. **(a)** This bench seating in the dog waiting area is easy to clean underneath and encourages dogs to stay out of the circulation area. **(b)** Bench seating can also provide underseat storage. **(c)** Long client reception areas can present a challenge for seating layout. This example, which has a welcoming appearance, uses comfortable easy-clean seating and allows some separation of waiting pets. **(d)** These individual seats have hardwearing and cleanable fabric covers with special backcare foam for improved comfort.

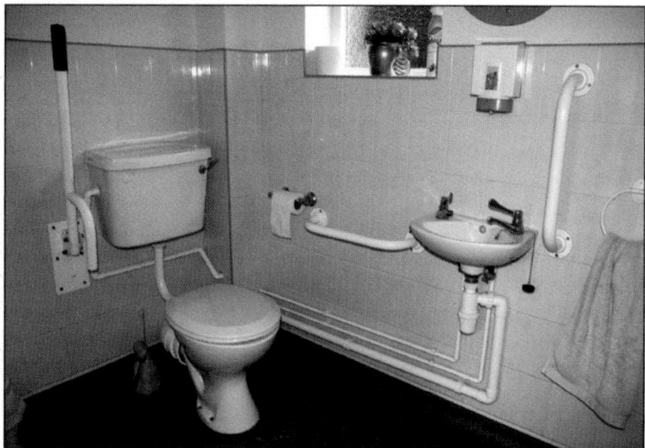

5.9 Toilet facilities must be pleasant, clean and tidy. They should be suitable for disabled users; appropriate bars and supports can be retrofitted to existing facilities.

Even where building design or lack of funds necessitates a practical and realistic approach, much can still be made of what currently exists.

- Keep fresh flowers on display.
- Create space high up to place cat baskets. (This not only reduces stress for the animals, but also allows staff to admire the inhabitants.)
- Ensure any newspapers or magazines put out are not out of date or tatty.
- Use appropriate colour schemes. Pastels and neutrals are more calming (Figure 5.10), but it is important to ensure that the colour palette is also practical (easy to clean, hides scuffs, etc.).

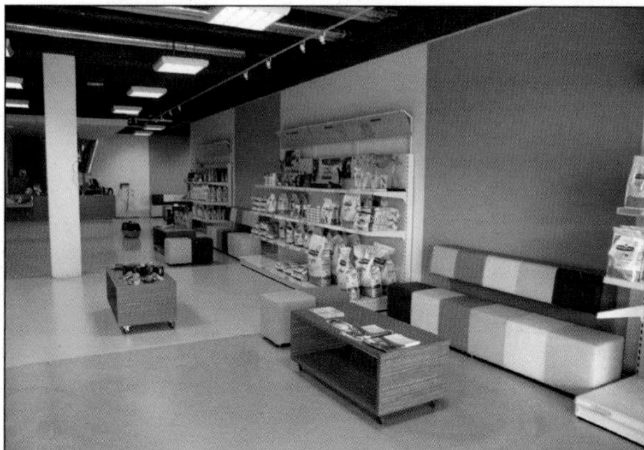

5.10 Colour schemes should be chosen carefully, both for ambience and for ease of cleaning.

- Flooring choices should be practical, hygienic, non-slip and easy to clean and maintain, especially at the edges (see also Chapter 3):
  - Carpet can quickly become smelly and is difficult to keep clean
  - Stark plain vinyl or lino can feel very hospital-like, so care should be taken with the choice of colour (Figure 5.11)
  - Most practices tend to opt for high-grade waterproof vinyl 'safety' flooring, with cove-to-wall joints and containing non-slip grains (Figure 5.12) The grains can create some cleaning problems, necessitating regular use of a professional hard floor scrubber/dryer (Figure 5.13a) but overall this choice is a stylish yet practical one and allows colour patterns (Figure 5.11) and zoning of areas
  - Waterproof and washable textile flocked floor coverings that have been treated to offer antibacterial protection have the benefit of being non-slip and very hard-wearing. Regular cleaning with a professional machine (Figure 5.13b) and minimal detergent is essential to maintain cleanliness and avoid the risk of an underlying and continuous unpleasant odour
  - Durable resin flooring is an also an option.
- Entrance mats look welcoming and help to keep the main waiting room floor cleaner, particularly on wet days when muddy paws can be a problem. A variety of mats are available and can be decorated with logos, pawprint patterns, etc (see Chapter 3). They will all need cleaning on a regular basis (Figure 5.13c), be it professionally or in house, so more than one mat may be required. Coir matting is often used but is not recommended as it is impossible to clean adequately. Mats can be sunk into the ground to avoid becoming a trip hazard.

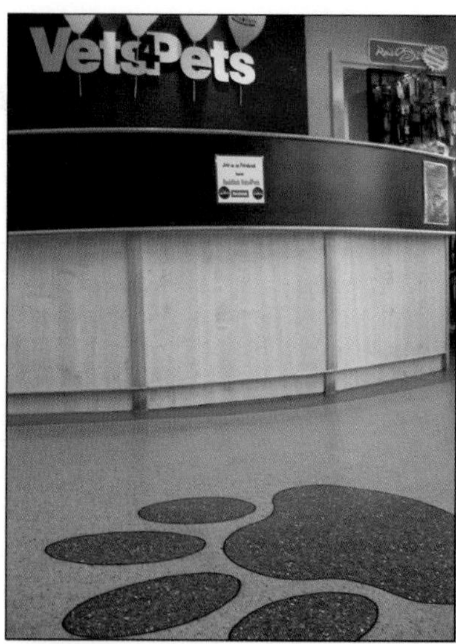

5.11 Vinyl flooring, both smooth and safety non-slip types, can be laid creatively to include patterns or images in different colours. (© Vets4Pets Ltd)

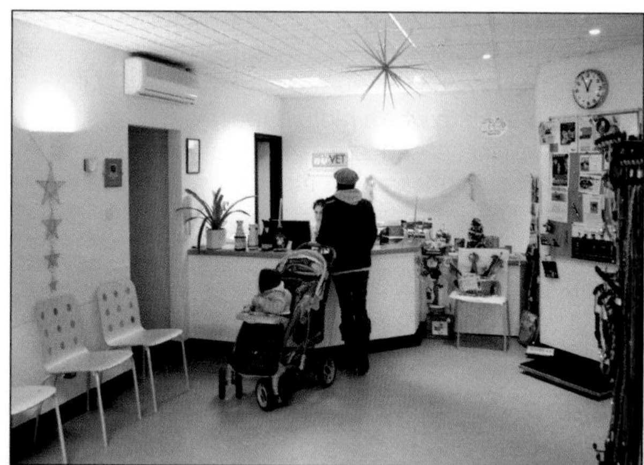

5.12 This reception area uses neutral-coloured vinyl 'safety' flooring, which is non-slip and quiet. (Courtesy of Nuvet and Veterinary Business Journal. © Veterinary Business Development)

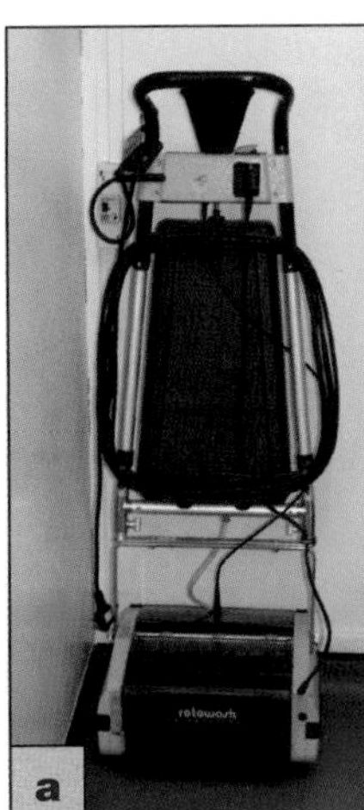

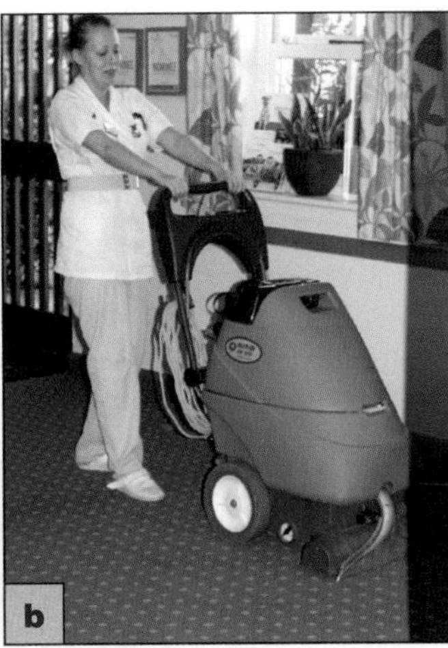

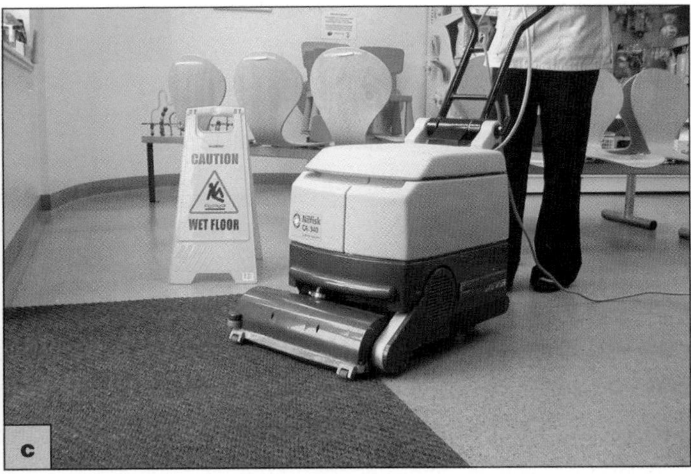

5.13 **(a)** A hard-floor scrubber/dryer is usually necessary to keep vinyl 'safety' flooring looking clean. **(b)** Flocked textile floors can be scrubbed and cleaned like vinyl, but take longer to dry. A professional carpet scrubber/dryer and minimal use of detergent are essential to keep the floor clean and looking good. **(c)** Barrier matting is essential in reception areas where people are walking in from the outside. Here the matting is inset (recessed) into the floor. Regular deep cleaning is essential; a scrubber such as the one pictured is effective on both the matting and the safety flooring. (b, © Vets4Pets Ltd)

- Walls can be hung with tasteful artwork rather than an onslaught of product posters. Anything on the walls should be in a frame or laminated; nothing looks worse than dog-eared posters stuck up on a wall. A 'who is who' staff introduction (Figure 5.14) is worth considering, but must be regularly updated. Hardwearing matt finish acrylic paints are readily available to give a professional feel, and will look less harsh than an eggshell or gloss finish. Painted surfaces should be touched up or repainted regularly, as required.
- Automatic doors greatly improve accessibility for everyone struggling with combinations of shopping, children and pet carriers. However, to minimize the risk of escape or the chance of boisterous dogs rushing out and pulling owners over, it is necessary to have two sets of doors that open independently or use a manual control (Figure 5.15).

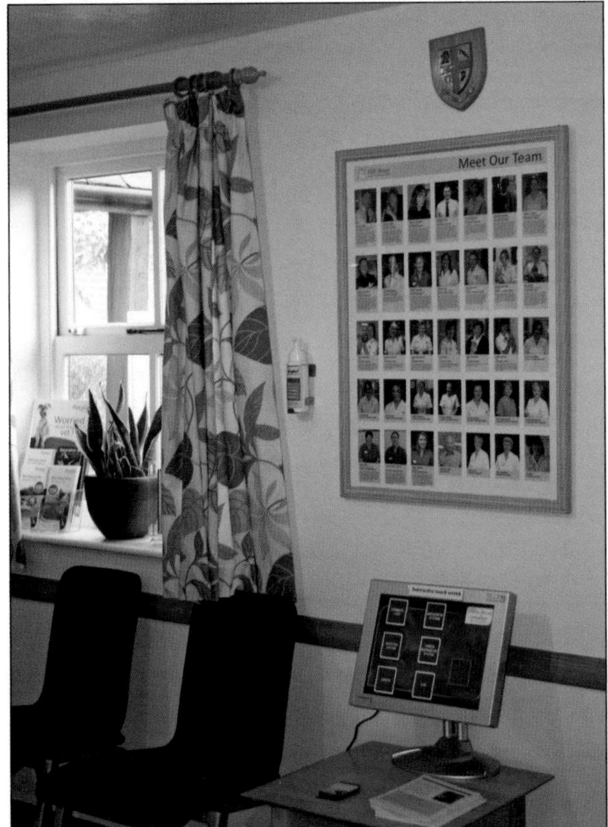

5.14 A 'who is who' board is useful for introducing the team. It must be well presented with current photographs and can be a collage of separate pictures, or a professionally printed poster prepared with photo editing software as in this example. Also shown is an interactive touch screen unit giving pet health care information, which is particularly popular with children.

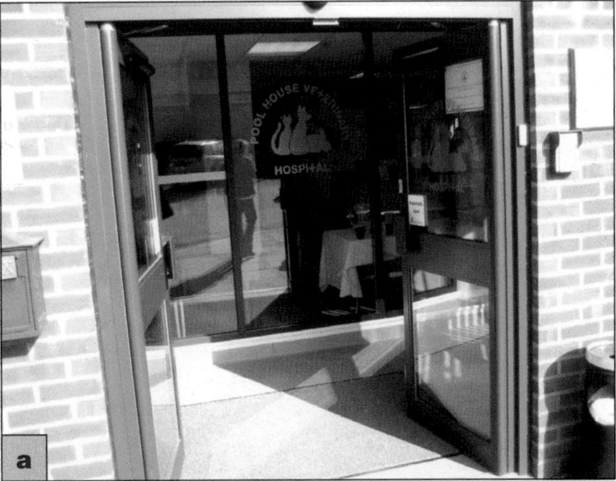

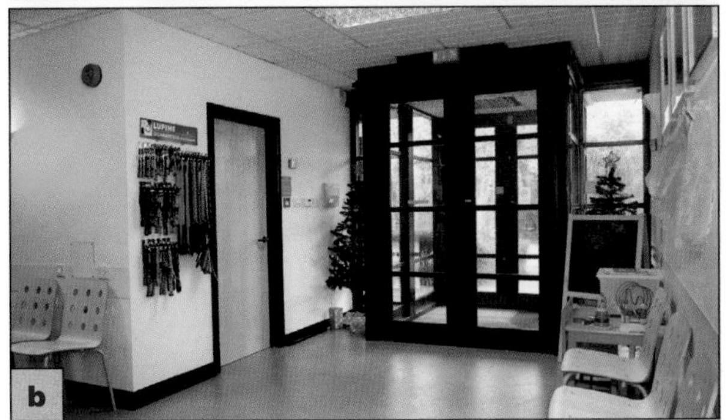

5.15 **(a)** This automatic door opens into a lobby holding area, with a second, manual, door into reception. **(b)** Manually operated double doors may be less accessible but are more secure. (b, courtesy of Nuvet and Veterinary Business Journal. © Veterinary Business Development)

KEY POINT

Making the most of the reception area does not have to be expensive, difficult or time-consuming. Do not overlook the details; it is the small things that can make the biggest impact.

Advanced design

Larger practices have the luxury of being able to opt for a practice design that allows the client to walk in one door and leave by another. This enables staff to deal with clients more efficiently, but it does mean that two teams are needed at two desks – a front desk for checking patients in, and a second area for payment and checking patients out. Such an arrangement can be awkward where some family members have been left to wait in the reception area during the consultation. However, this design does have the enormous benefit of allowing clients to exit the practice quickly after their consultation; hence, by avoiding delays at this stage of the visit, the client is not frustrated and leaves the practice on a positive note.

Where feasible, open-plan spaces throughout the reception area are always more effective:

- Lack of walls and doors bring staff and clients together, and make the practice feel more welcoming
- Communication is easier
- Watching the general goings-on around the reception area keeps clients occupied and can reduce any frustration during waiting
- Clients can see other owners buying things and booking services, thereby encouraging them to do the same (Figure 5.16).

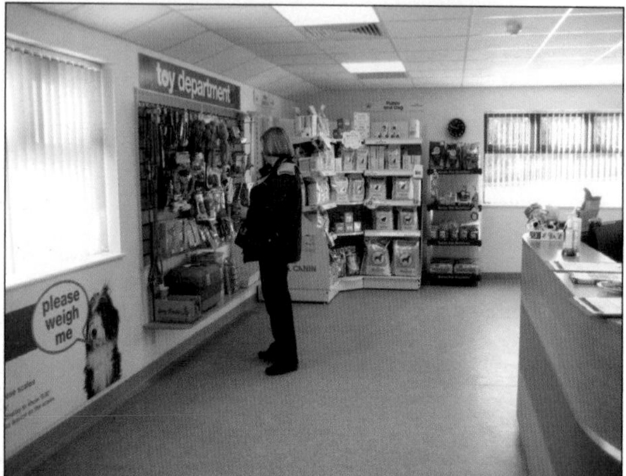

5.16 Open spaces in reception allow browsing.

The role of the receptionist

A key aspect of the receptionist's role is to welcome clients on arrival and to look after and attend to any clients in the waiting areas. The reception team is expected to handle several different tasks at once, whilst dealing pleasantly, effectively and professionally with a wide range of human emotions and personalities. The receptionist is hardly ever able to initiate tasks, being required instead to respond to the many and varied requests and demands of clients and colleagues, often at the same time.

There are two key areas where receptionists interact with clients: on the telephone; and face-to-face. Each requires mastery of different skills and techniques. Excellent telephone skills are vital (Figure 5.17); these are covered in more detail in Chapter 27. Dealing with financial transactions and asking for payment are covered in Chapter 16.

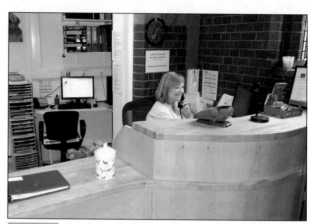

5.17 Excellent telephone skills are essential for a receptionist.

Face-to-face client interaction

This is made slightly easier than telephone interaction by the fact that, when face to face, the receptionist can read the client's body language. The essential skills needed in this area are covered in Chapter 17.

Many client frustrations arise from lack of information or from misunderstandings, so a good receptionist will address any issues head on. If possible, Reception should never be left unattended. This means having the full support of the rest of the team, and having systems in place so that everything is to hand, with other members of staff available as and when support and back-up is required.

Clients have choices; if they feel that staff are vague, evasive, unhelpful, rushed or just plain rude, they will take their pets elsewhere. Clients should always be made to feel welcome and valued:

- Always greet clients by name if known, and use the pet's name throughout the conversation
- Use positive body language (make eye contact, nod and smile, and do *not* do other things whilst they are talking) (Figure 5.18)
- Be generous with your time and advice (if it is not a good time, say so, and explain when will be, or ask a colleague to help)
- Ask lots of questions about the pet and the client's routine, so that you can personalize the advice given
- Always offer to make an appointment, where appropriate.

KEY POINT

Deliver the kind of friendly, helpful service that you would like to receive yourself.

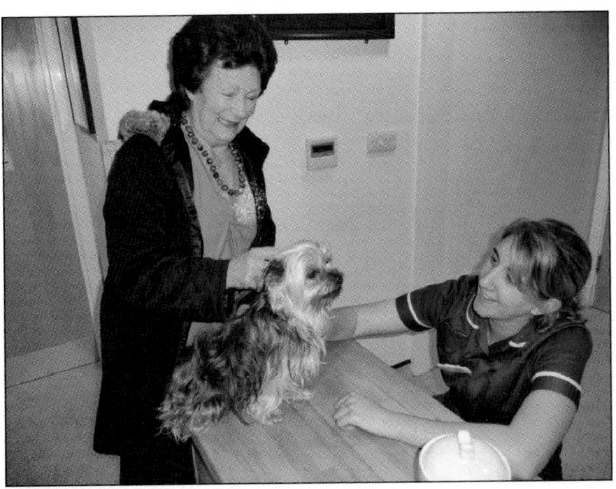

5.18 Taking an interest in clients and their pets will show that the practice cares.

Protocols for dealing with enquiries and information requests

Reception staff at a busy practice will receive hundreds of requests for information or advice in a 'typical' week. Whilst many of these will come from existing clients, others will be from potential new clients, meaning that staff can take these opportunities to promote the practice and register new patients. All members of staff dealing with the public:

- Must have had a thorough induction
- Must be fully trained
- Must be familiar with practice policies and protocols.

Induction

A comprehensive induction in this area for all the team (not just those on the reception desk who answer the telephone) must be in place; this will vary between, and be specific to, individual practices. Examples of areas to cover at induction are listed in Figure 5.19.

Training

This should include thorough training on how to handle enquiries and telephone calls. When a request for information is made, staff must be friendly and polite first and foremost. Staff should also be well informed, and take every opportunity to give out plenty of practice information (opening hours, nurse clinics, website details) and always try to close the enquiry with an appointment where appropriate.

KEY POINT

All staff that use the telephone, particularly for interacting with clients, will need to develop a good telephone manner (see Chapter 27). This includes vets, nurses and office staff, who should also therefore receive training in telephone skills.

Protocols

RCVS Practice Standards requirements include written protocols for dealing with the public (Figure 5.20). These can be filed in a reference manual that is kept in the reception desk and also by key phone points, to help ensure that enquiries are handled correctly, quickly and efficiently.

Tasks	Trainer's initials and date training given	Student is confident: signed by student
General computer training		
Computer terminals – logging on and off		
How to find a client – using search criteria		
Entering a new client		
How to make, transfer or cancel an appointment		
How to book in a procedure		
Current waiting room list options: change, move (keep clients in correct time order), insert, remove		
How to edit client records and pet details		
Telephone skills		
Speed of telephone answering		
How to answer correctly; importance of telephone manner – smile!		
How to take messages correctly		
What to say if someone is unavailable (don't just say 'busy')		
How to handle phone shoppers: engage owner; ask questions; always send out a pack/ info sheets; offer an appointment		
How to use phone features: paging system, loudspeaker, voicemail and hold (ask first!)		
How to switch phone lines over to night service		

5.19 Areas to cover during induction of reception area staff. (continues)

Tasks	Trainer's initials and date training given	Student is confident: signed by student
Client arrivals		
Greeting clients – make eye contact, smile		
Importance of making sure that everyone in reception is accounted for and keeping clients informed of progress		
How to put an emergency at the top of the list		
'No shows' – call owner		
Practice policy on case handling – always see the same vet (unless impossible), consult clinical records		
Cash and fee collection		
How to inform clients of the bill and ask for payment		
How to take cash and card payments: always give a receipt; never give the till key to anyone; count change back to client		
What to do if people cannot pay – call accounts administrator or practice manager. No products should be dispensed/given		
Petty cash: claiming, need for receipts		
How to deal with refund queries: what can/can't be refunded. How to refund to a credit card		
Insurance		
What to do with insurance claim forms: client to complete forms correctly		
Direct claims policy		
General reception duties		
Dealing with complaints		
How to deal with upset/angry clients		
Confidentiality		
How to handle clients after euthanasia/death of pet		
New starter packs, practice handouts and leaflets		
Keeping reception clean and tidy, leaflet racks full and merchandising displays looking good		
Practice protocol on leaflets and notices in reception		
Lost and found. How to deal with wildlife		
Practice protocols and giving information		
Accepting urine samples		
NEVER LEAVE RECEPTION UNATTENDED		

5.19 (continued) Areas to cover during induction of reception area staff.

The inspector will ask to see guidelines, where appropriate, for such things as:

- Staff induction procedure
- Client confidentiality
- Answering the telephone/greeting clients
- Appointment procedures and recognition of emergencies
- Practice policy for home visits
- Complaints procedure
- Practice arrangements for out-of-hours cover, referrals and second opinions
- Practice arrangements for acceptance of incoming referrals
- Vaccination, parasite control and neutering policies (where applicable)
- Prescribing/dispensing policy
- PETS passports

5.20 Written protocols required by RCVS Practice Standards for staff dealing with members of the public.

The client waiting experience

Prolonged waiting is a common cause of complaint from clients. Most people accept that there may be a short wait; they understand that vets are dealing with emergencies and that sometimes things over-run. However, after 10 or 15 minutes, the majority of clients will begin to get irritated; after all, they may have other appointments elsewhere, or children to collect from school. Inner-city practices may find that their clients are less tolerant than those in rural areas where the pace of life is generally slower.

Managing waiting time

Starting on time

It is important that consultations start on time at the beginning of each session. Any initial delays tend to have a knock-on effect, resulting in what the clients will ultimately perceive as a poor service. Whilst not many clients will complain direct to the veterinary surgeon if kept waiting, they will complain to the receptionist.

> **KEY POINT**
>
> Starting consultations on time should be seen as a professional obligation to colleagues as well as the client.

Appointments

Reception staff may opt to allocate appointments evenly throughout each session, rather than filling the diary from the beginning of the session onwards. This avoids the potential for a rush followed by an empty hour in the diary which, in reality, is then used to catch up and see disgruntled clients who have been kept waiting due to previous appointments that have overrun. Alternatively, and depending on the workload and/or preference of the veterinary surgeon on duty, staff may be requested to book back-to-back appointments to avoid any potentially time-wasting gaps, particularly if there is a busy surgery schedule which needs to start promptly. Flexible appointment scheduling can be used, with different appointment durations for different problems, but this requires good staff training and can still be thrown out by the unpredictability of many consultations and clients.

Emergencies

If delays are routinely caused by emergency admissions, setting up a triage system where nurses can assess and prioritize cases as they come in should be considered.

Communication here is vital, as clients will quickly become annoyed if they have waited 15 minutes already, only to see another animal come straight in and be taken through to see the vet immediately. Informing owners that the practice has the best interests of every pet at heart, and assuring them that should their pet ever need urgent attention, it would be immediately forthcoming, will help quell the frustration of most clients at occasionally having to wait a little longer. Informed owners will be more tolerant, so where there is a reason for the delay, clients should be told. This can be through a general announcement to the waiting area or through talking to clients individually, giving enough detail to explain the delay (rather than just a short general apology). Owners who are just left to fume quietly in the waiting area will magnify the delay and length of time that they have been kept waiting.

Alternative arrangements should also be offered, such as seeing a different vet or making another appointment.

After the consultation

Owners are less likely to accept having to wait *after* they have seen the vet. In their eyes they simply have a prescription to pick up, a bill to settle and another appointment to make, and then they need to leave. Clients do not understand why the reception team may not have their information to hand immediately in order to facilitate this. Rapid computerized transfer of information allows the administration team to see immediately what the client needs; otherwise the member of staff who has just attended to the client should walk the client through to the desk and hand over all the necessary information (which also gives the client a further opportunity to understand and discuss any next steps). It is certainly worth considering booking in surgery or follow-up appointments during the consultation. With many computer systems this takes little time, and allows direct negotiation with the clinician on alternative dates if there are problems.

One further source of irritation during waiting is when clients are asked to return for pets who have undergone procedures as day cases 'any time after 5 pm'. A much improved service can be provided when time is allocated and appointments booked, thereby reducing the risk of a logjam of owners all queuing at the desk at 5.30 and getting increasingly fractious at the end of an already busy and stressful day.

> **KEY POINT**
>
> To avoid a queue, and the risk of any confusion on behalf of the client as to what happens next and whom they need to see, surgery or follow-up appointments can be booked during the consultation.

An alternative system

Some consultation systems have been designed to maximize the time a veterinary surgeon spends with each client while examining and diagnosing their pet. Each consulting vet has access to two consulting rooms, with a nurse in each. The nurse runs the appointment, carrying out any initial work including taking the history. The vet's time can then be used more efficiently, carrying out the examination and making a diagnosis. The nurse can spend time completing the end part of the consultation, allowing the vet to see the next client in a neighbouring room.

Such a system requires a standardized approach, true teamwork and trust between staff, as it involves several members of the team. However, each member is better placed to carry out the tasks they have been trained to do to their full ability. Waiting times for clients tend to be reduced, as is the stress of the leaving client who is allowed the opportunity to raise any other issues that they may feel too small to 'bother' a busy vet with. For such a system to work, appointment times need to be much longer and have to be carefully coordinated. This model therefore may not be suitable for practices in cities and towns where clients are busy and do not have much time or in those that are restricted due to a lack of space. The model can work well for specific cases, such as bandage changes or initial puppy or kitten appointments.

Monitoring waiting times

By walking through the front door and sitting in the waiting room as if a client, staff can try to feel what clients are experiencing and will be in a better position to suggest changes and to visualize improvements.

The practice should regularly monitor individual and average waiting times (many practice management systems can do this automatically). If the average is consistently more than 15 minutes, process improvements should be implemented, such as changes to the booking system, changing staff allocation and identifying time-consuming processes during consultations that could be delegated to veterinary nurses (e.g. blood sampling). Longer appointment times may be a consideration if appointments consistently run over; however, the impact of this on profitability must be carefully assessed and prices may need to be increased where longer consultation times are required. Longer appointment times will also reduce the number of slots available per session, and consequently the number of clients seen. A practice management system that clearly shows in real time how long each client has been waiting will facilitate good management and appropriate action when clients are not seen at the expected time.

KEY POINT

Written guidelines for staff regarding the number of appointment slots to allocate when booking an appointment for certain longer procedures (e.g. second opinions, bandage changes) will help prevent delays.

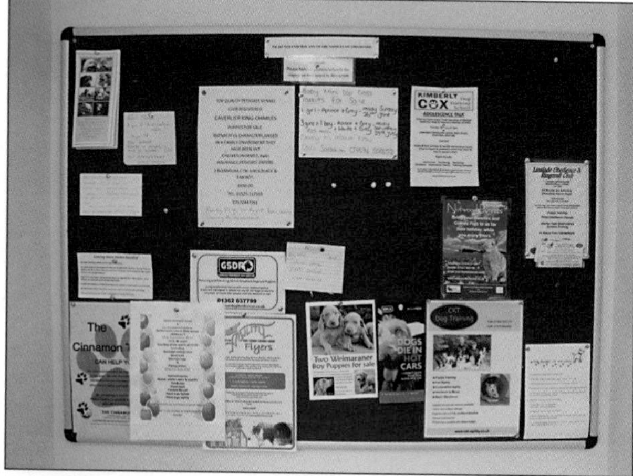

5.21 Pinboards can be used to provide useful information and to increase awareness of practice promotions.

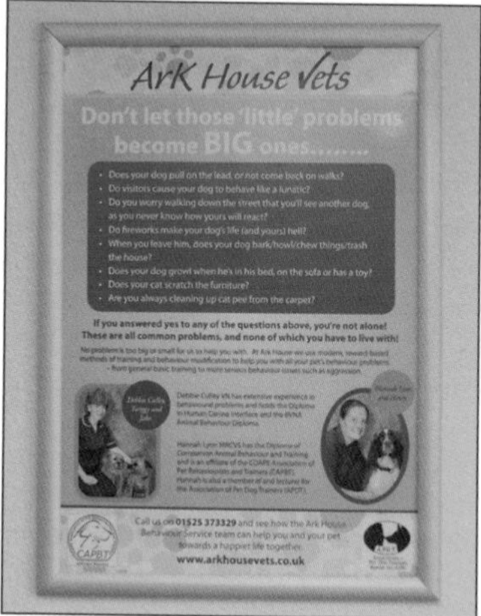

5.22 Posters should be laminated or framed, and changed regularly to tie in with marketing activity.

Information and merchandising

A potentially dull wait can be turned into something more productive.

- Offering clients information about practice goods and services will help boost income and encourage repeat business.
- Providing something to read or watch whilst clients wait will keep them occupied and so reduce any potential complaints about waiting times. Ideally, such reading material will give information about the practice or be of educational value by offering advice about pet care.
- Any other reading matter should be topical and up to date.

  Information can be provided in a number of ways.

- **Noticeboards.** A large and prominent pinboard (Figure 5.21) can contain details of practice opening hours, promotions, prices, staff members, local pet care services, additional clinics and so on. It must be kept tidy and up to date and be regularly maintained. If displaying details of local pet care services, a disclaimer should be put up to say that the noticeboard is for client information only and does not necessarily mean that the practice recommends these services; clients should take all the necessary steps before using them.
- **Posters**. These should be laminated or framed (Figure 5.22) and changed regularly to tie in with any marketing activities and promotions.
- **Leaflets**. A careful balance is required between providing enough information to give an informed choice, and giving so much that it causes confusion. Leaflet stands should be kept topped up with information covering a select few products and subjects, and staff can always direct owners to the practice website for more information. Information printed by the practice can be more specific than leaflets provided by third parties. It is important to remember that leaflets are there to be given away, as opposed to being tidied up. If leaflets are not taken, they should either be actively given to clients, or discarded as recycling waste.
- **Newsletters**. Copies should be left out so that clients can read the latest practice news whilst they wait. (For more on newsletters see Chapter 25.)
- **Television screens**. As well as helping to keep clients occupied while waiting, television screens provide the practice with an opportunity to market the services on offer and the products for sale. Displaying relevant information will help to educate and update clients on pet care issues.

TV and video displays

Equipment

One of the major expenditures is the cost of a digital flat screen. Commercial-quality screens cost more but will deteriorate less over time and will need replacing less frequently than domestic-quality display screens. Siting of the screen is important (Figure 5.23), and wiring and connections should be tidy and

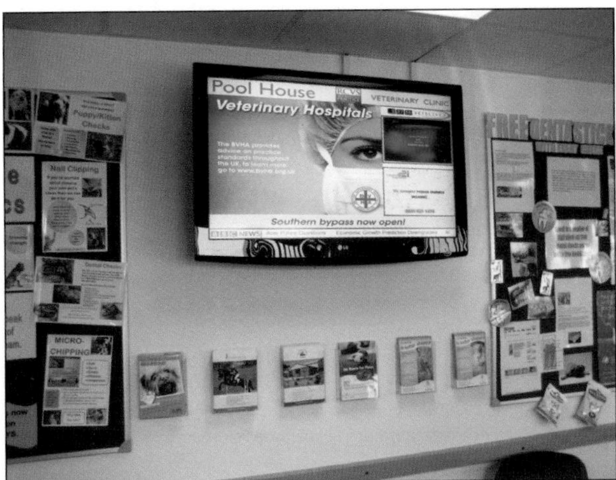

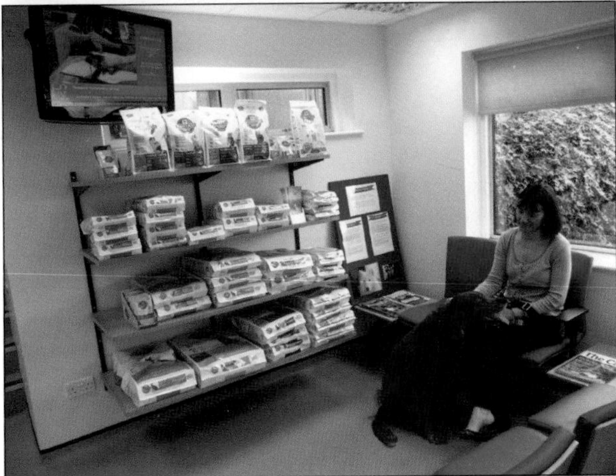

5.23 Wall space is needed for siting a TV display. Care should be taken to avoid reflections, and blinds may be needed.

safe. It is not advisable to place the screen behind the reception desk, as this distracts clients from the receptionist and can be frustrating for staff.

There are companies who will supply, fit the cabling, install, update, maintain, manage and repair such a system, providing graphic designers to put together the content. However, practices should read the small print carefully before being tied into regular ongoing costs and subscriptions. Live in-house veterinary TV channels require broadband connection. Update discs, if required, can be expensive and the practice may not have total control over content.

Videos, discs and presentation DVDs can be produced in house but there can sometimes be quality problems when presenting powerpoint displays on such screens. If converting powerpoint presentations to DVD, appropriate software must be used to ensure good slide transitions and smooth presentation. For smaller screens a built-in DVD player enables playback; for larger screens a separate DVD player or computer may be required.

A wireless adapter connected to the screen allows the DVD player to be sited elsewhere, but this set-up is not always reliable. Some screens allow playback from a portable flashdrive.

Costs can be covered by on-screen advertising from other businesses but care should be taken as, should their reputation become tarnished, this could indirectly reflect badly on the practice. Electronic displays or digital signage that can overlay live television broadcasts with practice advertising and information offer more than static images, but practices should consider whether the sound would cause a disturbance for clients and staff.

Content

Marketing and communication via screens is much more effective if the content is interesting, relevant and punchy, and it has the added benefit of reducing apparent waiting times. Clips should be kept short (no longer then 5 minutes) and content should be changed on a regular basis. The in-house responsibility for maintaining and updating the system should be clear and sufficient time allocated to the staff member(s) involved.

If the practice uses the system to watch terrestrial broadcasts a TV licence will be required. If music is played there may be copyright issues, and the practice will need to determine whether licences will need to be obtained.

KEY POINT

Waiting is almost always inevitable – the time can be used to provide information and education for clients.

Merchandising

Research by the author's company has shown that 91% of UK practices have retail displays of some kind on their premises but that there is considerable room for improvement:

- Just under half of practices were rated as 'average' or lower for ease of finding an item
- Over half of practices were rated as 'average' or lower for clarity of pricing on their displays (Figure 5.24)
- Finally, a third of practices were judged by 'mystery shoppers' not to be well stocked (scoring 'average' or lower).

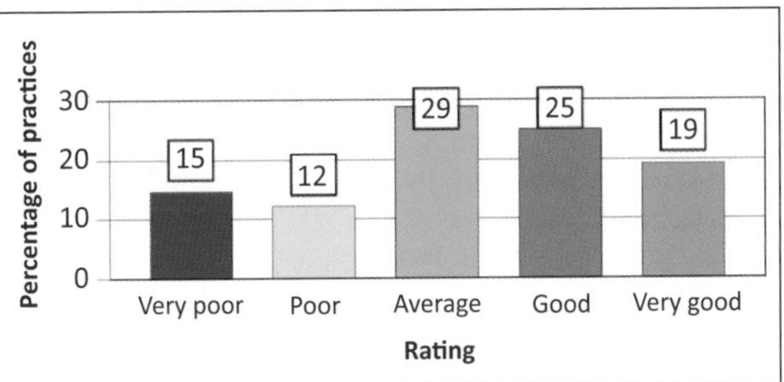

5.24 Client ratings for clarity of price marking, showing percentage of practices rated in each category. (Source: aggregated national Onswitch data to June 2011)

Many different types of display are available, ranging from cardboard 'dump bins' or half-pallet wraps provided by sales representatives for the promotion of offers on specific branded lines, to hanging stands that can spin round, optimizing available space. Countertop displays, peg boards, large modular metal shelved units or glass-fronted lockable cabinets (for more valuable items or POM-V products; Figure 5.25) are also widely used. Any or all of these different displays can be used successfully around the practice, as space allows, as long as they are all of a complementary style and do not give an impression of clutter.

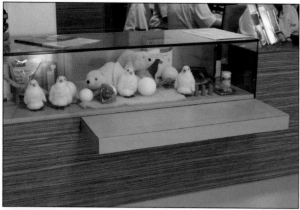

5.25 Glass counter areas can be useful for seasonal or high-value items.

Merchandising does not have to involve expensive display items (Figure 5.26); a colourful hand-drawn poster hanging over a tidy stack of dry dog food by the reception desk can be just as effective as a minimalist acrylic stand with integral spotlights and sound.

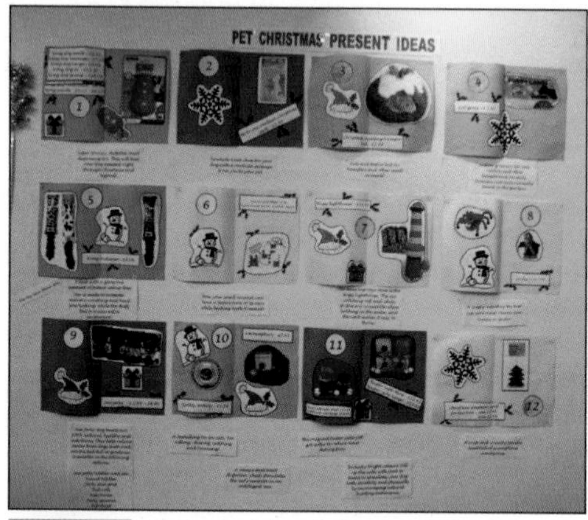

5.26 A seasonal wall display can raise awareness and increase sales.

Careful consideration should be given to the siting of retail products:

- More products will be sold if the merchandising area is clearly visible and the items are displayed and placed in such a way that encourages purchase
- Placing a display in the eyeline of clients in the waiting area will help to maximize sales, but care must be taken that it does not cause an obstruction
- Secondary siting of key lines can be very successful, such as in a small counter-top display which will boost sales, especially if accompanied by a special offer or promotion.

Clients will generally not ask if they cannot find what they need and the practice will lose a potential sale. One way to overcome this is by segmenting products into areas, such as cats/dogs/other pets, or a food section and then a toys and accessories section.

Many clients will not ask the price if it is not immediately obvious, fearing that they will be pressured into buying products they do not really want. Instead they will go somewhere else where they can see the price on the edge of the shelf, or clearly marked on the product, resulting in a lost sale to the practice. Prices can be fixed to the shelf edging, or products can be labelled with a pricing gun. One advantage of price labels is that if they carry the name and phone number of the practice this will encourage repeat purchases. If it is easy for owners to get all the necessary products for their pets in one place (i.e. at the practice, whilst they are there anyway), and at a fair price, then there is a high chance that they will do so.

KEY POINT

Organize stock clearly so that customers can find exactly what they need, and see at a glance how much it will cost.

The practice merchandising area should be re-evaluated regularly:

- Is it tidy?
- Does it look interesting and invite browsing?
- Are all the items 'faced up', i.e. neat with labels facing the right way?
- Are there obvious gaps?
- Can prices be seen easily?
- Is everything easy to find?
- Is the packaging scruffy and bashed about?
- Is there any slow-selling dusty stock?

As with so many areas of veterinary customer care, this requires staff to stop and look at things through the eyes of a client, and see things from their perspective.

Ethical considerations

Some veterinary surgeons raise ethical objections to selling products in a clinical environment. However, pet owners do need to buy food for their animals, and certainly should also be worming and de-fleaing their pets.

Royal Canin studies in 30 French practices in 2002 found that where food was sold, significantly higher volumes of shampoos, wormers and flea treatments were also purchased by clients (Moreau and Nap, 2010).

This has numerous benefits to all concerned:

- Pets receive more, regular and better preventive healthcare
- Owners develop a strong bond with the practice as the source of expertise and care
- Practice profits are boosted.

Selling high-quality products at the practice is beneficial to pet, owner and practice, and is therefore a sound commercial and ethical option for every practice.

Medicines

The current regulations controlling POM-V medicines prohibit their display for self-service. Such products can be displayed in locked cabinets or on shelves behind the reception desk (although they would then be difficult to see), or cardboard mock-ups of the packs can be used instead. No direct advertising for any such products should be displayed to the public, although price lists are permitted. As the Veterinary

Medicines Regulations are reviewed annually, any displays and promotions should always be compliant with the current regulations.

Easy steps to successful merchandising

- **Choose strong products.** Do not be swayed by fancy packaging or exaggerated product claims; with knowledge of which products work and what clients need, lines that will sell quickly can be stocked. Offering clients a choice, such as a top-of-the-range product and a cheaper alternative, will help increase sales; therefore, if space allows, a couple of brands should be chosen and the best-selling lines from each should be stocked (wholesalers and sales reps can help here). If there is a high profit margin on a product that only sells a couple of bags a year, it would be false economy to stock that product line. It is often more financially beneficial to stock a product that is a big seller, even if the profit margin is slightly less. However, if the profit margin is too small, the volume of sales required to make it worthwhile may not be achievable and it would not therefore be worth stocking. Chapter 24 has further guidance on mark-up and profit. Practices need to know the market and offer the right product at the right price; otherwise it will not sell.
- **Optimize space.** Smaller items should be placed on the top shelves and larger items on the bottom shelves. As well as being more aesthetically pleasing, this will assist in complying with any health and safety considerations regarding lifting heavy items (see Chapter 22). Displays should always look full, and this can be achieved by pulling merchandise forward. Big bags of dry foodstuffs will take up most of the available space if allowed. Instead, some big cards with brand names, varieties and, most importantly, prices on them can be printed out. Customers can take these to the reception desk and exchange them for an actual bag, carried to their car for them.
- **Change products to reflect seasonal variations.** Examples would include: Christmas gift boxes; grooming items in summer; puppy and kitten foods in spring.
- **Do not let slow-selling lines languish** on the display for any length of time, as that will give the impression that all stock is old and out of date. Run a promotion to get rid of such stock: 'buy one get one free', give it away with another more valuable line, or just cut the price. Mark it up as a special offer for a limited time only, to help it on its way.
- **Displays should be visibly appealing and grasp the shopper's attention.** For easy accessibility, best-selling and high-profit items should be placed in the 'line of sight' (between eye and waist level). This will be normally be about two thirds of the way up the display unit. Such items should be highlighted using eye-catching signs, such as arrows or starburst cards ('shelf-talkers').
- The retailing industry has spent millions of pounds on research and technology to understand how people shop from a fixture. The salient facts are these:
  - People's eyes are drawn to the upper centre of a display
  - Right-handed people will instinctively pick items just to the right of the central 'hot spot'
  - Colour sells – it is what customers see first (Figure 5.27).
- **Train staff.** The products stocked are quality ones that have been chosen carefully to meet the clients' needs and preferences, and also to generate income and increase footfall for the practice. The final step is to ensure that all staff feel comfortable promoting the products, and that everyone is fully trained regarding the products' features and benefits, so that any questions a client may ask can be answered.
- **Run a virtual shop.** This can either be online via the practice website or via a catalogue in Reception. Clients can pre-order and collect, or smaller items can be posted out or delivered for a small fee.

> **KEY POINT**
>
> Merchandising should be about offering clients a product or a service that they need and will therefore ultimately be of benefit to their pet.

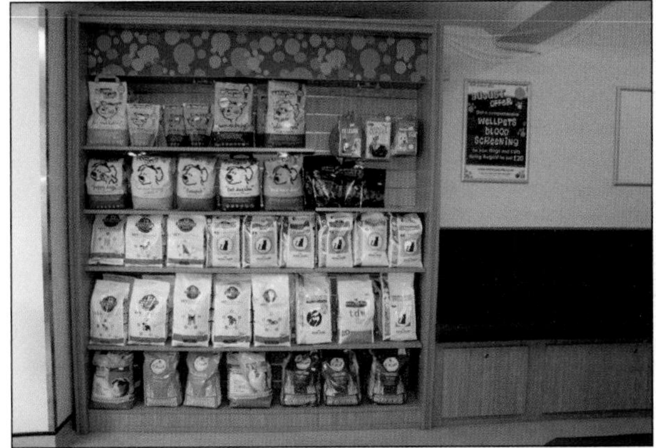

5.27 Colour sells: colour-block brands and packaging if space allows.

Planning and managing changes

Before embarking on changes within the reception and waiting areas, advice should be sought from a good designer or space planner, and clients should be involved. They should be asked for their thoughts on what works at the moment and what could be improved. A simple questionnaire online or a comments box can be helpful. All staff, particularly those who work in reception on a regular basis, should be consulted in order that any problems they face in day-to-day working, both from their point of view and from that of the clients, are revealed and can be addressed. In order to get some ideas, to help benchmark and to see what has worked well in other reception areas, it is advisable to visit and talk to other veterinary practices and also to professionals in other businesses, such as opticians or dentists.

Where areas for improvement in design have been identified, it is imperative not only to implement robust processes to manage these changes, but also to ensure that these are understood by everyone at the practice. Specific considerations might include the following.

- Consider the practice's core values, or mission statement, and ensure that these fit with the plans.
- Take note of practical issues such as whether lights, power sockets or telephone points need installing or moving. Any new equipment staff have requested could be installed at the same time, to minimize disruption, e.g. a photocopier or document scanner. Consider the best place to install these, taking into account ease of access and frequency of use.
- Think about places for forms, leaflets, and handouts. Will they be printed out on demand or do they have to be stored? Where can clients pick up leaflets of general interest?
- Look at what impact the proposed changes will have on the rest of the building. The client flow might be routed elsewhere, which may mean other areas might also need to be spruced up.
- Try to ensure that the reception area will still meet the demands of the practice 5 years from now.
- The help of specialists can be enlisted when designing the reception area, covering the practical needs and feelings of both staff and clients.
- Communicate plans to clients, and show them the perceived end benefits. A newsletter detailing exactly what is happening, and why, along with notification of any changes to parking, phone numbers and emergency cover, etc. whilst the work is underway will ensure that clients understand the end result will be worth any short-term disruption along the way.

KEY POINT

Do not be afraid of change, when it is necessary. It is not a problem if managed correctly (see Chapter 18).

Acknowledgements

The author and editors gratefully acknowledge the following practices, images of which appear in this chapter: All Creatures Healthcare Ltd; Ark House Veterinary Surgery; Bridge Veterinary Practice Ltd; Broadland House Veterinary Surgery; Elands Veterinary Clinic; Goddard Veterinary Group; Mill House Veterinary Surgery and Hospital; Nuvet; Pennards Veterinary Group; Pool House Veterinary Hospital; Sterkliniek, Rotterdam.

References and further reading

Catanzaro T (2007) *Design it Right, 4th edn*. AAHA Press, Lakewood, CO

Moran M (2004) *An Introduction to Veterinary Practice Client Care*. Veterinary Business Development, Peterborough

Moreau P and Nap R (2010) *Essentials of Veterinary Practice: An Introduction to the Science of Practice Management*. Henston Publishers Veterinary Publications, Peterborough

Wilson J and MacConnell C (1995) *The Veterinary Receptionist's Training Manual*. Priority Press; available from AAHA Press, Lakewood, CO

Consulting rooms

6

Pam Mosedale

The consulting area is the main area of contact of veterinary surgeons and veterinary nurses with clients and their pets (Figure 6.1). It is where small animal first-opinion veterinary surgeons usually spend 4 or 5 hours a day and should be an area where vets, nurses *and* clients can feel comfortable and relaxed. It needs to be a hygienic and well maintained environment where effective communication can occur.

A dog will be more relaxed if the room is at a comfortable temperature and the floor covering is not slippery. A cat will be more relaxed (Figure 6.2) if it can be examined with little restraint, if the table has a non-slip surface, and if it is allowed to go back into the safety of its basket without unnecessary delay. The use of pheromone 'plug ins' can also help to make a more relaxing and less fearful atmosphere for pets.

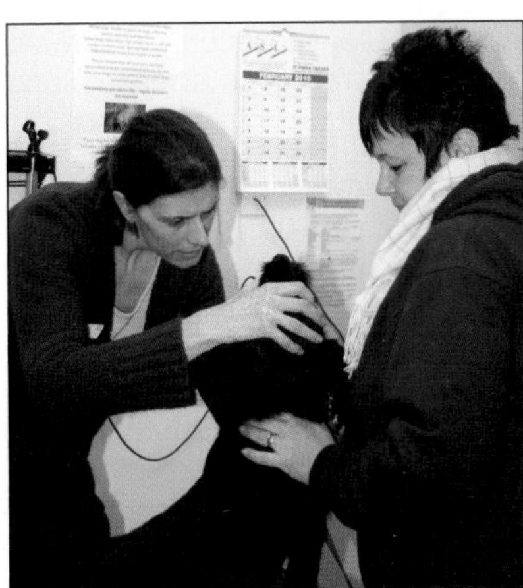

6.1 The consulting room should be a comfortable relaxed environment for clients, vets and pets.

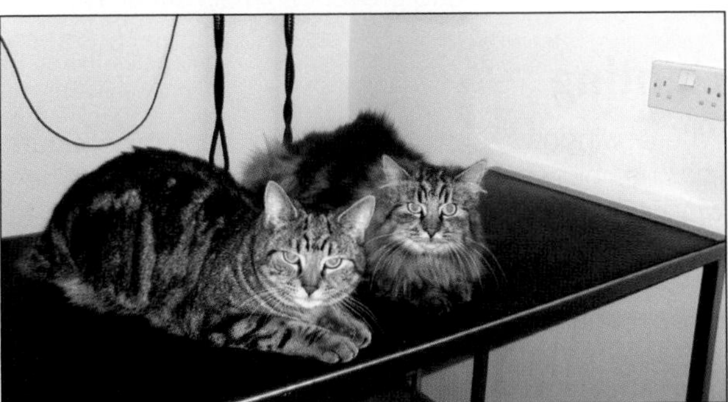

6.2 Cats will be more relaxed on a non-slip table with minimal restraint.

> **KEY POINT**
>
> In many practices clients only see the reception/ waiting area and consulting room, so the impression formed here will affect their view of the whole practice.

Consulting room design

Time spent thinking at the planning stage of any new build or refurbishment (see Chapters 1 and 3) should pay dividends. Staff who will be using the room should be involved at the design and planning stage, to help ensure that the room is ergonomically designed to be suitable for the personnel and procedures involved.

Practical features to consider when planning a new consulting room or refurbishing an existing facility include:

- Proximity to other practice areas
- Storage
- Hand-washing facilities
- Seating
- Positioning of computer terminals.

Privacy is important and soundproofing is vital, both to prevent clients in reception overhearing and to stop staff conversations from disturbing consultations.

The consulting rooms should ideally open directly from the waiting area and be immediately adjacent to the dispensary, to provide easy access to both medicines and reference information (Figure 6.3). Sliding doors are often used between consulting rooms and the dispensary to reduce congestion and save space. It is possible to conceal sliding doors within the wall space (Figure 6.4), to maintain a neat look and maximize the available wall area.

Number and size

It is desirable to have as many consulting areas as possible, as this contributes to efficient use of the veterinary surgeons' and nurses' time. The size of each consulting room, however, should not be compromised to create extra areas (Figure 6.5).

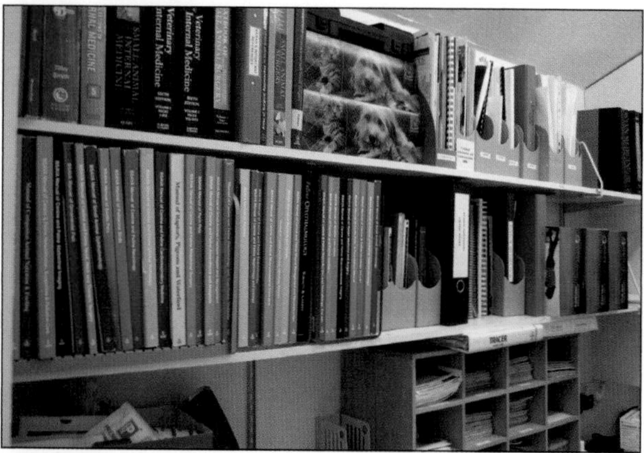

6.3 Reference materials can be kept to hand in an adjoining dispensary.

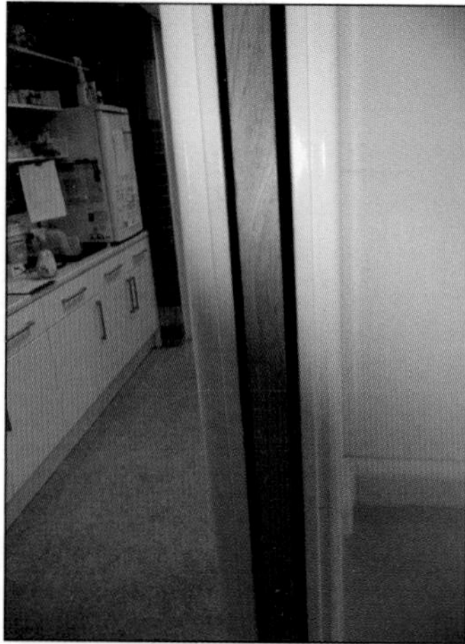

6.4 The door between the consulting room and dispensary has been concealed within the wall for a neater look.

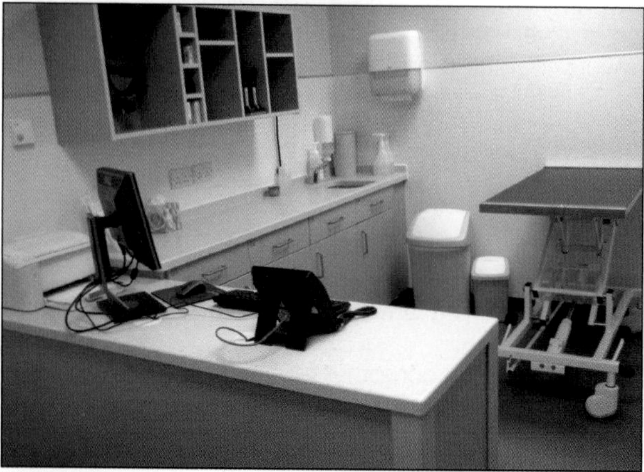

6.5 A large consulting room showing storage, computer wiring through the benchtop, and a hands-free tap.

A spare consulting room allows one room to be taken up by time-consuming procedures such as dressing changes. If space is available, a quieter, less clinical-looking room for euthanasia, where clients can spend time with their pets before and after the procedure, is an added bonus; this room can also be used for confidential discussions without the pet, leaving other rooms still available for consultations. Small security peepholes can be installed into solid consulting room doors to allow staff to check whether rooms are in use when doors are closed. Signs instructing clients not to use mobile phones are helpful (Figure 6.6).

It is preferable to have at least one consulting area that can accommodate a large dog with the family on

6.6 Clear signs on consulting room doors help reduce interruptions from clients' mobile phones during consultations.

a school holiday visit. In a cat-only practice consulting areas can be smaller and less 'clinical' in their feel.

In the USA the trend is to have larger 'exam rooms' because veterinary technicians usually hold or restrain animals rather than owners, to prevent injuries to owners from pet bites and scratches, and to decrease the risk of pets falling off the table. This may be a future trend in the UK, as professional indemnity insurers advise that offering owners the option of having a trained member of staff to restrain their pet will minimize the likelihood of such accidents occurring.

If support staff perform procedures in the consulting room while the veterinary surgeon talks to the client, the room may need to accommodate the owners, two veterinary nurses/technicians and the veterinary surgeon.

Heating and ventilation

There must be adequate heating and ventilation in the consulting area, appropriate to the work undertaken. It is very important to have a comfortable environment for staff, clients and patients. Adequate room air changes are essential both for biosecurity (following examination of patients with infectious diseases) and to remove unpleasant smells.

With the luxury of a new build, ventilation and heating/cooling throughout the building will be incorporated from the start (see Chapter 2). When refurbishing existing premises, air conditioning should be considered (see Figure 6.20), with active air extraction from the consulting room. Consulting rooms often have no external walls, and when fitting extraction fans it is important to consider where the extracted air is going. Air from potentially dirty areas, like the consulting room, must not be directed into clean areas.

If windows are used for ventilation, they should have security guards fitted to prevent animals escaping.

Lighting

Where windows or light wells are available, natural light is beneficial in the consulting area. Where windows are present, blinds should be fitted for privacy and to reduce heating from direct sunlight. It is advisable, for ophthalmological examinations, that at least one examination area is able to be darkened.

Many consulting areas rely on artificial lighting. A good, directable source of light is useful for detailed investigations, as is magnification; additional lighting can be wall- or ceiling-mounted (Figure 6.7). Not all

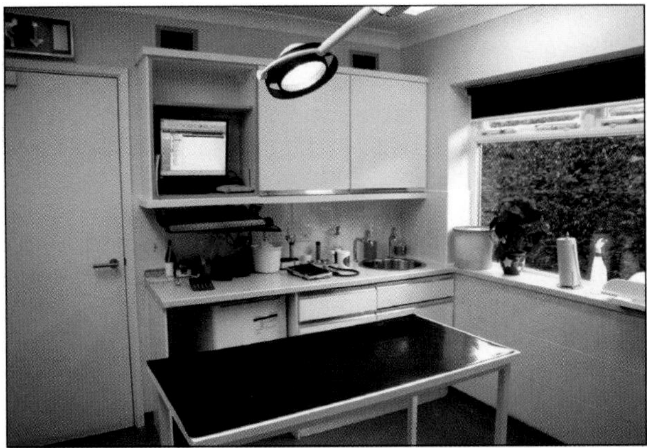

6.7 This examination room has a ceiling-mounted examination light, blackout blind and the computer keyboard mounted under the wall cabinetry to keep the worktop clear. As the veterinary surgeon currently needs to turn their back to the client whilst inputting data, a worktop extension is planned to the left so that the screen and keyboard can be mounted at right angles to its current position.

examinations occur on the consulting table. On many occasions large dogs are examined on the floor of the consulting room, so lighting needs to be good at this level too. It is important to check this when specifying lighting for a new build or renovation (see Chapter 2).

For RCVS-accredited veterinary hospitals, emergency lighting must be provided to allow the hospital to function in the event of a power cut or electrical failure, and this should be a consideration in any practice planning. This is in addition to emergency background lighting, which generally facilitates the safe evacuation of the premises. The fire risk assessment for existing premises will often highlight the need for background emergency lighting, which should be tested regularly.

Finishes

Work surfaces should be impervious, cleanable and kept free of clutter.

Door furniture should be easily cleanable. Lever handles should be avoided, as dogs often try to jump up and open them. Doors and architraves must be well maintained and have an impervious surface to facilitate thorough cleaning and disinfection.

Floor coverings

Floor coverings in consulting rooms must be impervious to fluids (e.g. urine, spillages) and cleanable. Adequate disinfection must be possible following presentation and examination of potentially infectious cases in the rooms. Particular care must be taken to ensure that corners and areas around pipework and cabinetry are kept clean.

The floor covering should be non-slip:

- To ensure the health and safety of clients and staff
- To reduce the risk of a patient slipping or falling
- To help dogs feel more secure.

There is a trade-off between non-slip properties and cleanability. Some floors with extremely non-slip surfaces can be very difficult to clean, and commercial scrubbing machines may be needed. Floor coverings that have heat-welded seams and are continued up the wall, or have set-in coving, make a very good cleanable surface, but ceramic tiles or other impervious surfaces are also suitable (see Chapter 3 for details).

Hand-washing

There should be a sink, either in the consulting room (Figure 6.8) or immediately adjacent to it, so that staff can access it without touching and contaminating door handles. Hands-free taps (Figure 6.9) are desirable to minimize cross-contamination. The intended use, for both hand-washing and cleaning instrumentation and surfaces, should be considered in the design and location of sinks. Hand-washing facilities should be positioned so that they are accessible to both the clinician and clients.

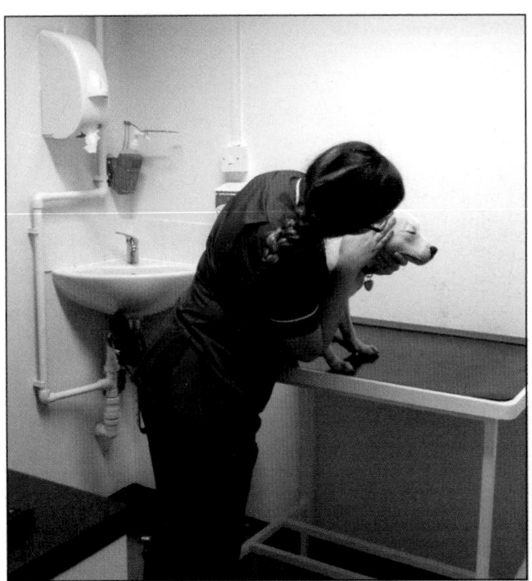

6.8 A dedicated nurse consulting room is a useful addition to the practice.

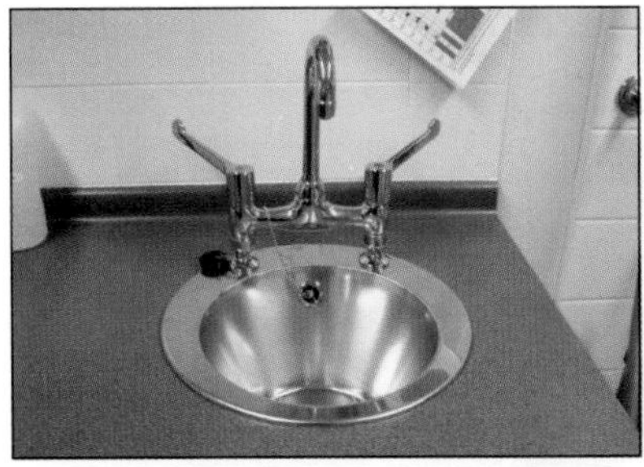

6.9 A small hand basin in the consulting room; note the hands-free taps.

> **KEY POINT**
>
> Effective biosecurity is essential, as the consulting room is an area in which infection could easily spread from one patient to the next.

Furniture and fittings

Consulting tables

Tables can be fixed or of the fold-down variety. In a small consulting room a fold-down table can be a useful space saver (Figure 6.10a,b) as it can be stowed out of the way. Tables with wheels, that can be moved to the side of the room, may be useful in these circumstances and can also be used as a trolley for transporting animals into wards or the preparation room.

Tables that can be adjusted, either hydraulically or electrically, to different heights ('lifting tables'; Figure 6.10c,d) are extremely useful in the consulting room. They avoid the need for manual handling and lifting, and for bending over, allowing the patient to be examined at the ideal height, regardless of patient size or the height of the veterinary surgeon or nurse. It is also possible to buy consulting tables with a built-in weighing facility.

Stainless steel tables maintain their appearance and cleanability longest. Painted metal tables will need regular maintenance; and wooden tables are not advisable for a clinical setting.

The table surface should be non-slip and easily cleanable. Rubber mats are generally used to prevent slipping; these must be replaced if damaged or torn. Mats should be secure on the table: they can be fixed at either end using angled stainless steel clips (Figure 6.11); or a gripper sheet can be placed under the mat. Mats should be removed regularly to allow cleaning underneath – at least at the end of each consulting session. For mats fixed permanently to the table, their edges must be well sealed to prevent dirt accumulating.

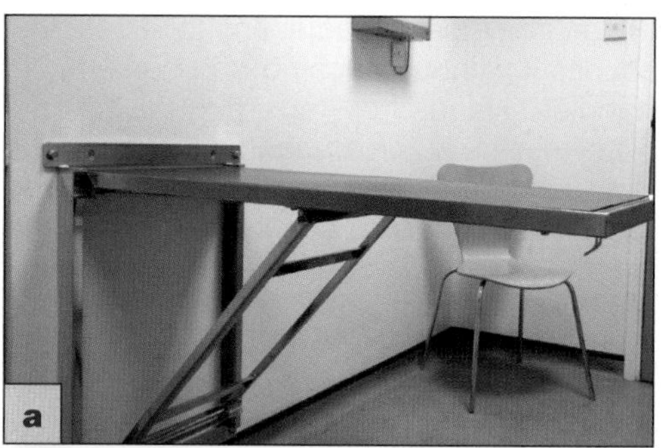

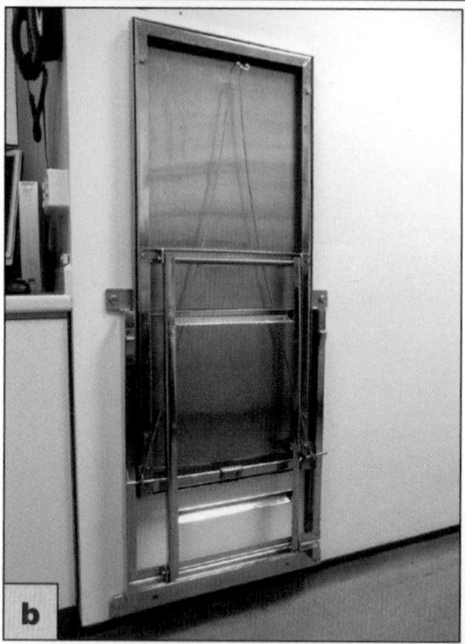

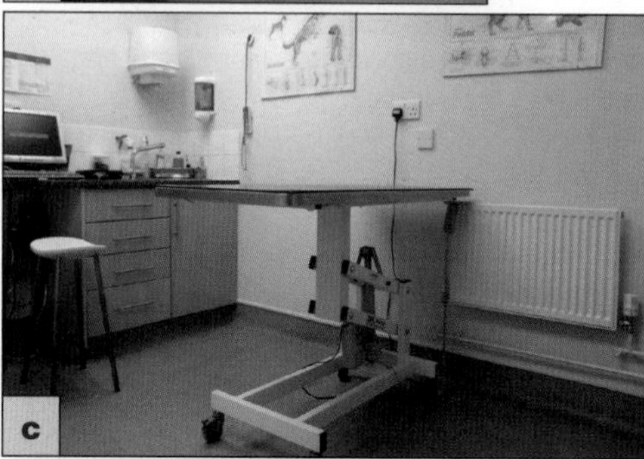

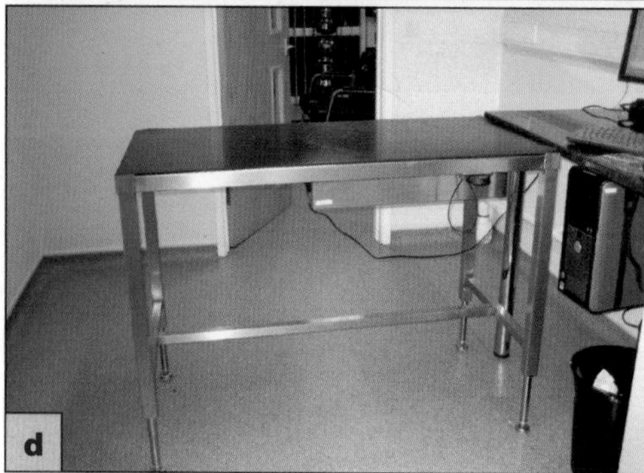

6.10 Examination tables: **(a)** A fold-down consulting table can be useful in a small consulting room and **(b)** can be folded up when out of use. **(c)** A 'lifting table', adjustable to a range of heights. **(d)** This stainless steel table is electrically height-adjustable and easy to clean. The rubber mat is held in place by raised corners.

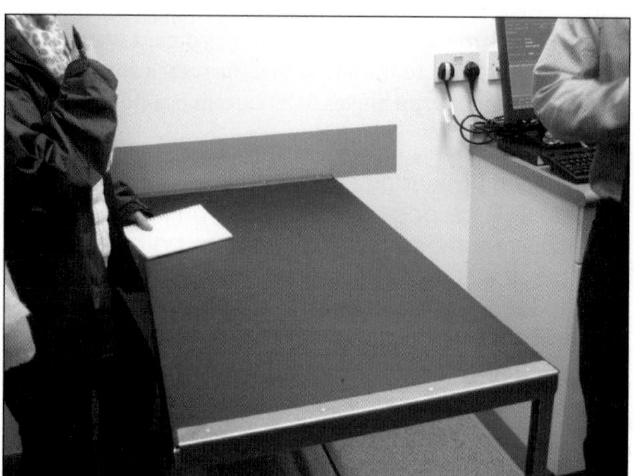

6.11 Angled strips can be attached to each end of a rubber mat to hold it in place on the examination table, allowing easy removal for cleaning. Note the protective strip on the wall to reduce damage to paintwork and facilitate cleaning.

Attention should be paid to the rubber or adjustable feet of both tables and chairs; these can wear, resulting in cutting through of vinyl flooring and in rust staining, which may be impossible to remove. Replacement rubber feet and castors are usually obtainable for metal furniture.

Seating

Consideration should be given to whether to have seating for vets and/or clients in the room (Figure 6.12). This may make the space less flexible but, particularly for longer consultations (e.g. referrals) and in the case of clients less able to stand, it can be desirable. One solution in a compact consulting room can be bench seating along a wall, with storage underneath.

Storage

There should be adequate storage for disposables such as gloves, syringes and needles (unless stored in the dispensary), and for equipment used in consultations. All items should be stored inside cupboards, or preferably in drawers, so that they do not accumulate dust and make the room difficult to keep clean. A list of items kept in each cupboard should be created to assist staff in finding them and to help with stock control.

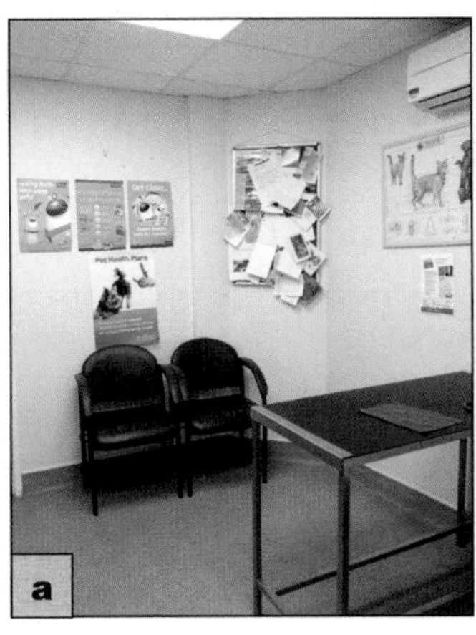
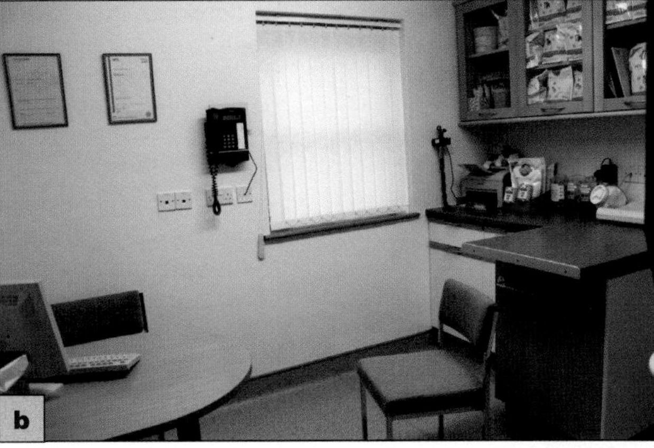

6.12 **(a)** In this consulting room chairs are available for veterinary staff and/or clients. **(b)** A large consulting room with space for seating for clients and staff.

Cupboards can be built in under the work surface. Any top cupboards should be designed so that they reach to the ceiling and do not have any high-level surfaces that need to be kept clean (a source of infection and a potential hazard working at height to clean them).

In a new build or renovation, if all consulting rooms open on to a common dispensary this precludes the need for doubling up of equipment or for storage of any drugs in the consulting room, hence allowing more efficient stock control. It also means that there is no need for refrigeration in the consulting room, as all vaccines can be kept in a fridge in the dispensary. Unfortunately, this cannot be achieved in many practices. If drugs *are* stored in the consulting room they must be kept securely in drawers or cupboards (Figure 6.13a) and not on public display, nor accessible to children. If refrigeration is required, small desktop fridges or refrigerated vaccine dispensers (Figure 6.13b) are available. In all cases, temperatures must be monitored in cupboards and fridges to ensure that veterinary products are kept in accordance with manufacturers' recommendations (see Chapter 15).

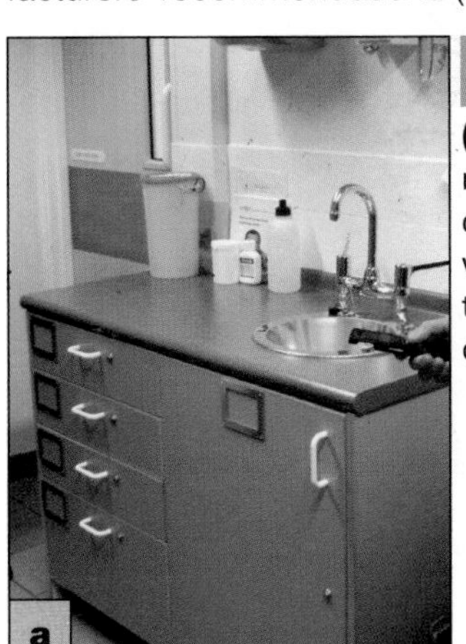

6.13 **(a)** Lockable cupboards. **(b)** A wall-mounted refrigerated vaccine dispenser is useful to keep vaccines at the correct temperature in the consulting room.

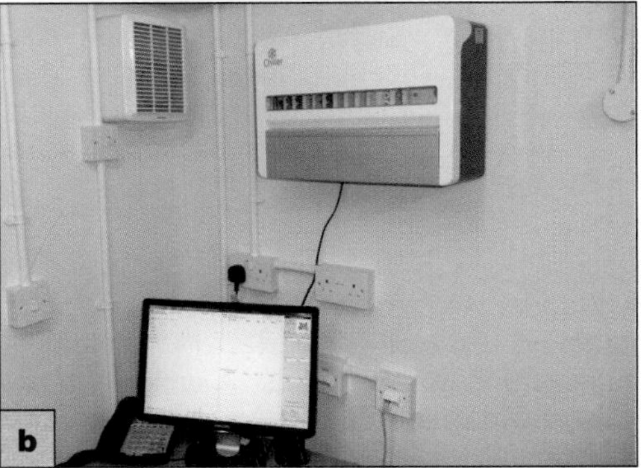

Equipment

General

A selection of scissors and basic forceps is helpful in the consulting room, as is a range of nail clippers varying from heavy duty (Great Dane) to tiny (canary).

It is helpful to have a set of quiet electric clippers in the consulting room. The smaller quieter clippers are particularly useful and upset animals much less than standard clippers. Cordless clippers are more practical and do not present a trip hazard. All clippers should be cleaned thoroughly and disinfected between patients.

Equipment for taking samples (e.g. swabs, blood tubes, sample containers), microscope slides and coverslips should all be to hand.

Examination gloves should include non-latex gloves for any members of staff with a latex allergy.

Weighing scales

Weight tables/charts and scales to allow accurate weighing of the full range of species routinely treated should be available in the practice. Large walk-on electronic scales are usually positioned in the reception area (see Chapter 5), the preparation room or the consulting room. If in the reception area, clients can easily access the scales and staff can weigh each pet before the consultation.

- Large scales should be carefully sited so that they are not in a thoroughfare or causing a trip hazard.
- Smaller scales suitable for cats (Figure 6.14a) are better kept in the consulting room to reduce the risk of escape if removing cats from their baskets in the client waiting area.
- There should also be accurate scales suitable for small and exotic pets (Figure 6.14b); these are also convenient for accurate weighing of food for inpatients.

The scales can be powered from the mains or use rechargeable batteries. They should be checked regularly for accuracy.

KEY POINT

It is good practice to maintain a weight record for patients on every visit, both for accurate drug dosing and to show trends in weight loss or gain of patients.

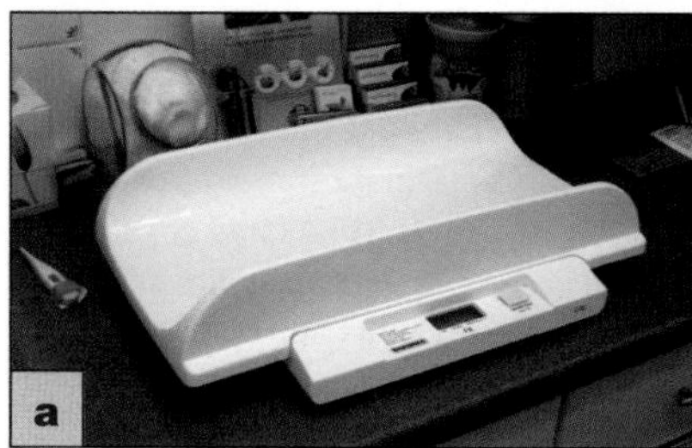

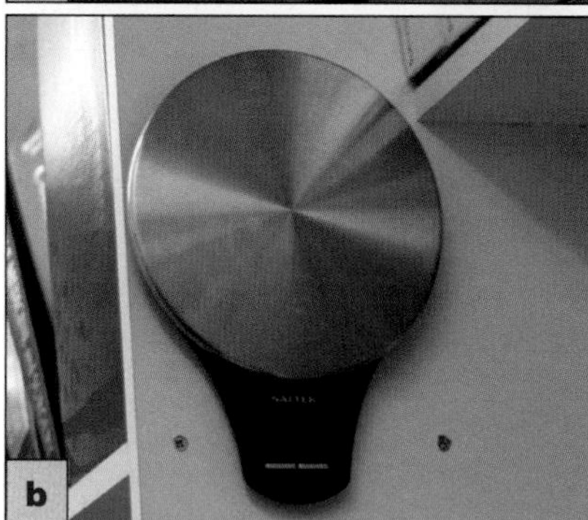

6.14 **(a)** Small scales suitable for weighing cats. **(b)** A set of digital scales for small pets (and medications or food) can be hung on the wall when out of use.

Diagnostic equipment

Basic diagnostic equipment should be available (see below for examples) but can be shared between consulting rooms.

Thermometers

These can be of the traditional **glass and mercury** type, although they will require a risk assessment and plans for mercury disposal in case of breakage. They must be thoroughly cleaned and disinfected between patients. **Digital rectal thermometers** are accurate and easy to read, and are usually supplied with sterile single-use disposable probe covers to avoid cross-infection (Figure 6.15a). **Ear thermometers** can also be used and suitable models are now available for most small animals (Figure 6.15b). These also use disposable covers to prevent cross-infection. It is better to continue to use the same type of thermometer when monitoring the temperature of an ongoing case, as there can be significant differences in readings between rectal and ear thermometers.

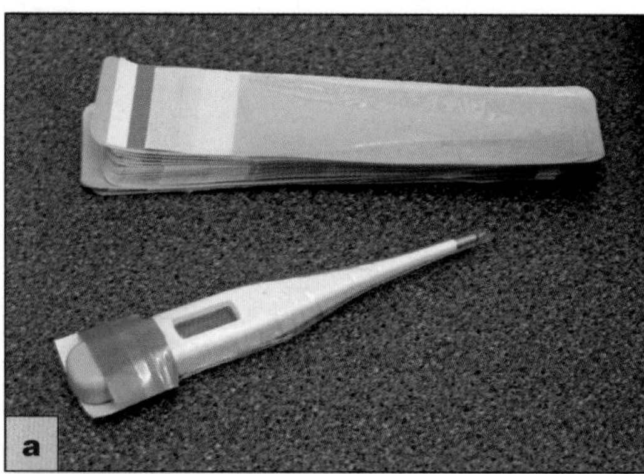

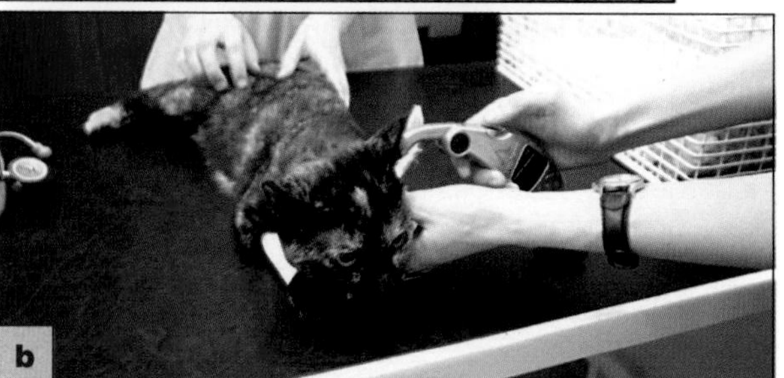

6.15 Thermometers. **(a)** Digital rectal thermometer and sleeve. **(b)** Use of an aural thermometer in a cat. (b, photograph by J. Bosley; © Quantock Veterinary Hospital)

Stethoscopes

Stethoscopes are usually very much a personal choice of the consulting veterinary surgeon, but good-quality stethoscopes are essential, and it is always useful to have a paediatric stethoscope available too. Digital stethoscopes, using earpieces instead of tubing, are also available.

Ophthalmic and aural examinations

For ophthalmic examinations a pen torch or Finhoff transilluminator is useful; a hand lens, fluorescein strips and tear test strips should also be to hand in the consulting area.

Ophthalmoscopes and auriscopes should be cleaned and checked regularly. Ophthalmoscope and auriscope sets can be either mains- or battery-operated. Wall-mounted mains-operated sets in each consulting room (Figure 6.16) are easy to use, look neat and tidy, are always available, and have the added advantage of never having a flat battery, but attention should be paid to the extending wires.

Battery-operated sets are more portable, can be shared between rooms and taken out on visits, but they need regular checks and supplies of spare batteries available (unless rechargeable batteries are used). They are also easy to leave on, leading to flat batteries, although handsets that come on when they are picked up and automatically switch off when they are put down are now available.

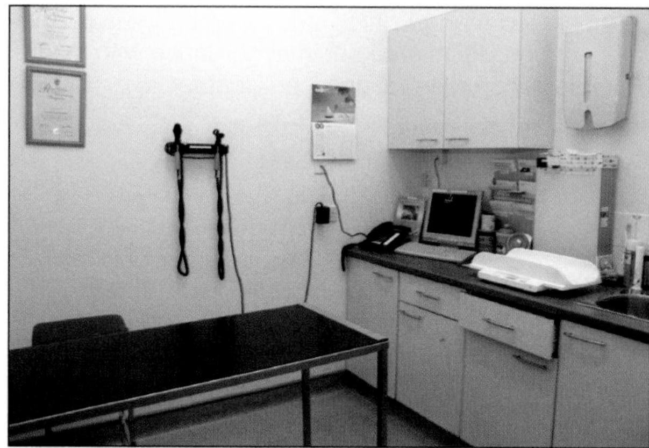

6.16 This consulting room has plenty of storage space, a wall-mounted auriscope/ophthalmoscope, an X-ray viewer and small scales.

RCVS-accredited veterinary hospitals must also have equipment for measurement of intraocular pressure available, which can be either a Schiøtz tonometer or an electronic tonometer such as a Tonopen or Tonovet (Figure 6.17).

Other

Keeping a Woods' lamp in the consulting room that can be darkened is helpful for both dermatological and ophthalmological examinations. A urine refractometer and urine dipsticks are also useful to have for use during consultations.

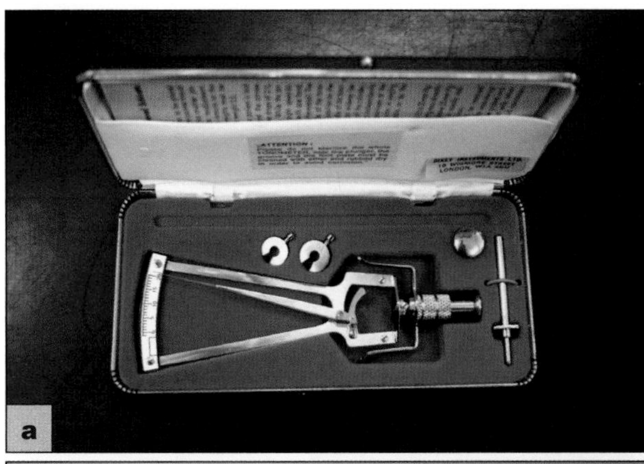

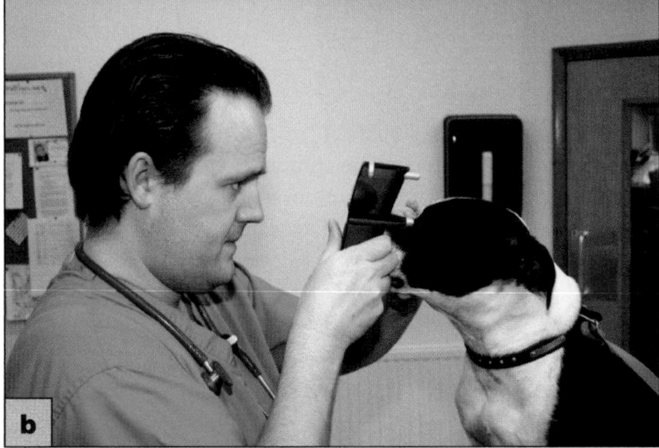

6.17 **(a)** The Schiøtz tonometer may look more awkward to use, but is still useful for measuring intraocular pressure where an electronic tonometer is not available. **(b)** Electronic tonometers such as the Tonovet (seen here) or Tonopen are easy to use and accurate. A tonometer is a Practice Standards requirement for veterinary hospitals.

Emergency equipment

If the consulting room is at a small satellite branch surgery with consulting-only facilities, it is worth considering keeping an 'emergency box' at the branch. This can be similar to the anaesthetic crash kit (see Chapter 8), along with intravenous fluids and catheters, endotracheal tubes, and even a small oxygen cylinder and reducing valve (Figure 6.18), to deal with an emergency that might come in and to stabilize a patient prior to transport to the main surgery.

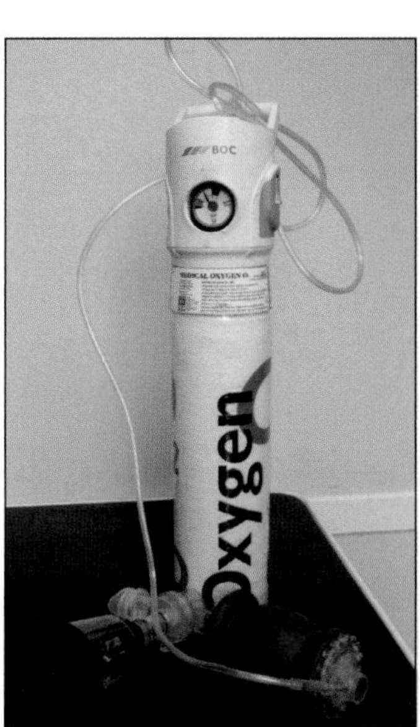

6.18 A small emergency oxygen cylinder with reducing valve can be useful at small branch surgeries.

Communication aids

The principles of communicating with clients are covered in detail in Chapter 17. Staff should be clearly identified or introduced to clients so that they know whom they are dealing with.

The consulting room should be a calm quiet environment for examining the patient and discussing all treatment options with the client. Interruptions should be kept to a minimum, and staff should avoid noise and disturbance in the consulting area. However, telephone extensions are useful in consulting rooms for outgoing calls and intercom use, although outside lines should not be set to ring in this area.

Printed information, leaflets, postoperative instructions, website addresses, etc., should be readily to hand to support the consultation. This can either be as hard copy or printed off the computer. If leaflets are used, they should be neatly stored in racks (Figure 6.19) or drawers. Large whiteboards, or similar, are an excellent tool to help explain complex procedures, as are anatomical models and/or atlases. Alternatively, notepaper can be used for drawing or for clarifying explanations; the client can then take this away.

KEY POINT

Take care not to leave confidential information or messy notes on whiteboards, and thorough cleaning will be needed regularly.

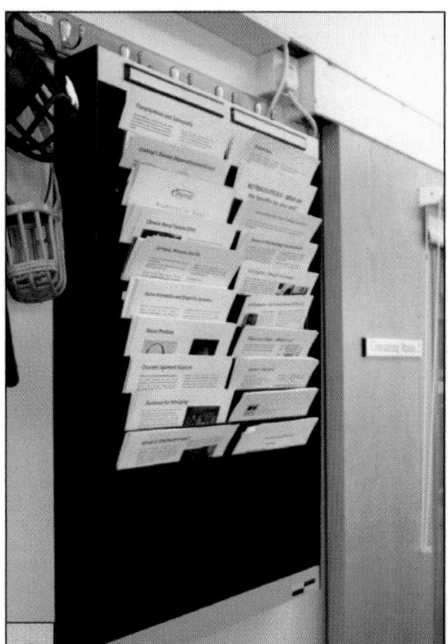

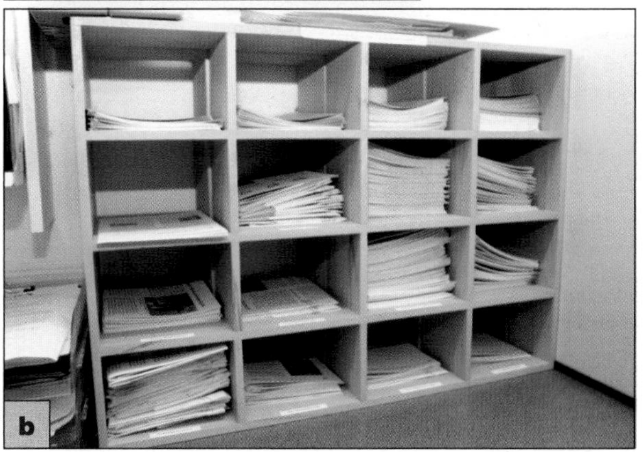

6.19 **(a)** A4 leaflet racks are available. Alternatively, information can be printed on demand, but must be of professional quality. **(b)** Pigeonhole units can be used for smaller or folded leaflets.

If the information is available on the practice computer system, then a large clear computer screen that can easily be positioned for client viewing is necessary (see below). Internet access may be desirable in the consulting room if used routinely for information or for registering microchips, for example.

Posters and displays can be effective in a consulting room, but can become messy and dirty, so care should be taken in maintaining the wall space. Posters should be laminated or framed.

There should be the ability to display radiographs in the outpatient area. Films will require an illuminated viewer (Figure 6.20) but digital images can be shown on the computer screen (see Chapter 13). Those practices that have digital radiography but do not have the means to display the images on their practice software can use laptop computers or digital photo frames to display images in the consulting room.

Some practices use CCTV cameras to record consultations. If this is to be done, the practice must comply with the Data Protection Act 1998 and there must be notices in the waiting room informing clients of recording. Records of consultations may be useful in the event of complaints and differing accounts of a consultation from vet and client.

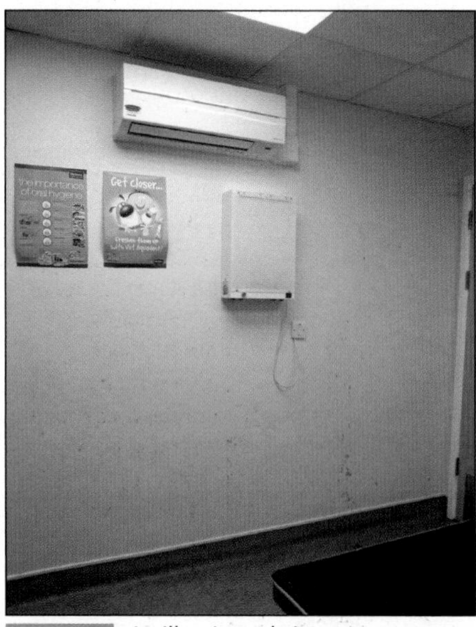

6.20 An illuminated viewer or means to display digital images is useful for radiographs. Air conditioning will make the consulting room more comfortable for people and animals.

Computers

The ideal is to position the screen so that the consulting veterinary surgeon can maintain eye contact with the client. This can be achieved by positioning the screen at an angle to both the vet and client (Figure 6.21), so both can see the screen but the vet does not need to turn his/her back to the client to type in notes. This improves communication and the effectiveness of the consultation.

Keyboard positioning can be problematical, particularly if keyboards are used with the operator sometimes standing, and sometimes sitting down. Where clinicians are seated, knee space is desirable to prevent poor seating posture. This is more important if the consulting room is used for clinicians to catch up with administrative tasks when not consulting. If keyboards are too high or too low, back problems may be more likely. Lighting on the screen is important, and blinds and appropriate lighting can reduce reflections and glare (see Chapter 16).

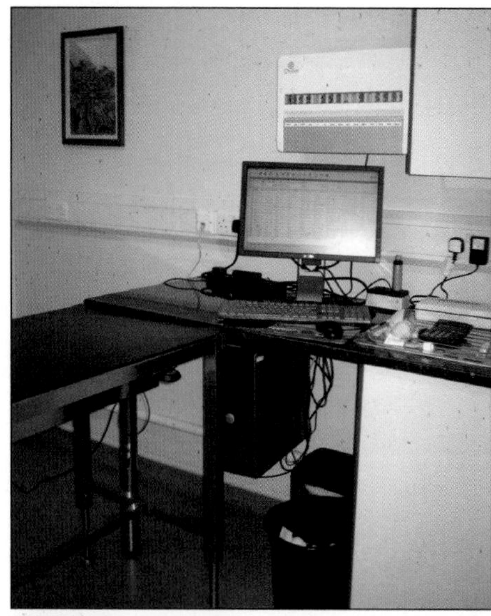

6.21 The position of the computer workstation allows the clinician to input notes and data without turning his/her back to the client. Note the vaccine fridge on the wall.

Wireless technology can be used to make positioning of keyboards and screens more flexible and allows the use of laptops in different areas around the practice. Wireless or compact computer equipment will also minimize the clutter and hazard of electrical wires. If wired equipment is used, positioning should be considered at the design stage so that wires can be hidden away wherever possible and holes made in worktops where necessary.

The number and positioning of electrical power sockets, both for computer equipment and for other electrical items (e.g. scales, diagnostic equipment) should be planned to minimize trailing wires. The use of dado-style electrical trunking can allow additional sockets to be added easily, and keeps surface wiring to a minimum (Figure 6.22).

A display screen equipment risk assessment should be carried out for the use of computers in the

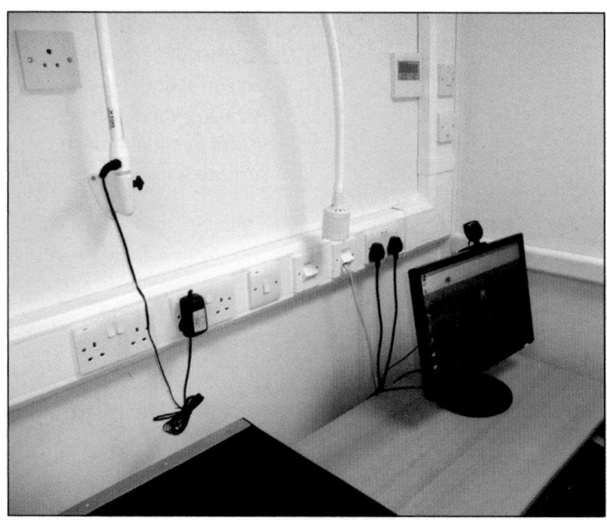

6.22 Electrical trunking keeps surface wiring to a minimum.

consulting room by vets, nurses and other staff. This should include checks to ensure that:

- The screen is readable
- There is no glare from adjacent windows or lights
- The keyboard is in a comfortable position
- Chairs are comfortable and correctly adjusted
- Staff have frequent breaks from the screen.

Good keyboard hygiene is essential, and washable keyboards or keyboard covers are advised, together with frequent cleaning and disinfection.

Animal handling

Animal handling and restraint is one of the main areas of potential risk. This risk needs to be assessed and staff trained in correct animal restraint procedures (see *BSAVA Textbook of Veterinary Nursing*). As discussed above, it is wise to offer owners the option of having a trained member of staff hold or restrain their pet, to minimize the likelihood of accidents occurring.

Any equipment required, such as muzzles (Figure 6.23a), should be readily available and kept clean and disinfected between patients. Other items needed for animal handling, such as crush cages (Figure 6.23b), gloves or even cat and dog catchers (Figure 6.23c), should be stored in a designated area, known to all staff, near to the consulting rooms. Where equipment is used infrequently, e.g. dog catchers, it should be regularly inspected, cleaned and lubricated, and staff refresher training considered.

Biosecurity in the consulting room

Biohazards encountered commonly in the consulting room include kennel cough, parvovirus, feline viral enteritis, ringworm, MRSA (meticillin-resistant *Staphylococcus aureus*) and *Salmonella*. Routes of transmission may include direct contact, contact with body fluids or excretions, inhalation or aerosols, or indirect contact between humans, animals and the environment.

In the evaluation of microbial contamination carried out at The Queen Mother Hospital (Royal Veterinary College) in 2010, standards and techniques used in human hospitals were used to assess environmental hygiene. Slides coated with agar were used to assess staphylococcal load in areas of the hospital. In the consulting room, door handles, floors, examination tables and computer mice were sampled. Human hospital standards were used to assess slides as 'pass' or 'fail'. It was found that consulting tables had the lowest percentage of failed slides, as these were normally cleaned between patients. Half of the samples from door handles and computer mice failed, as these were cleaned less often. Floor samples failed most often, as the floors were cleaned at the beginning and end of the day by cleaners but relied on visual checks by staff for cleaning in between.

Receptionists, nurses and veterinary surgeons must all be aware of biosecurity in the consulting room. Protocols and checklists for consulting room cleaning should be available, be filled in by staff and

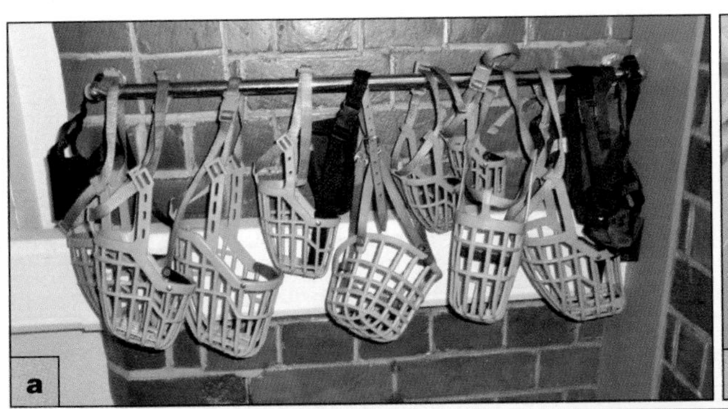

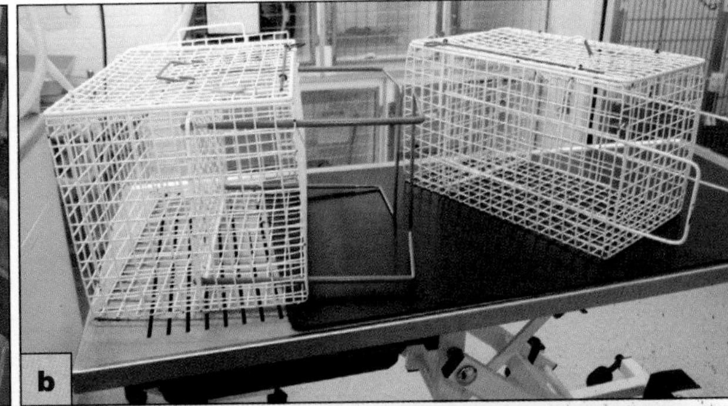

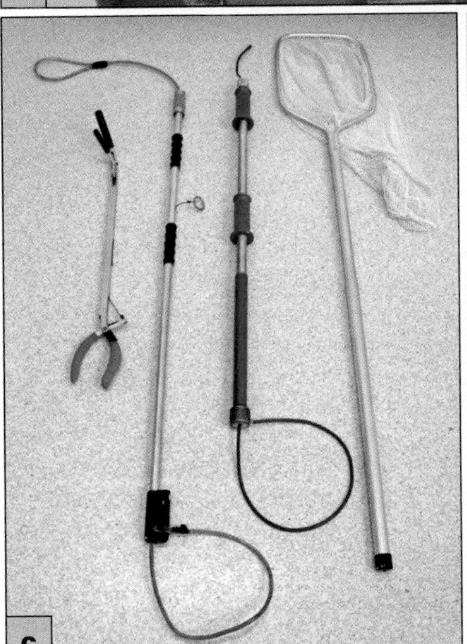

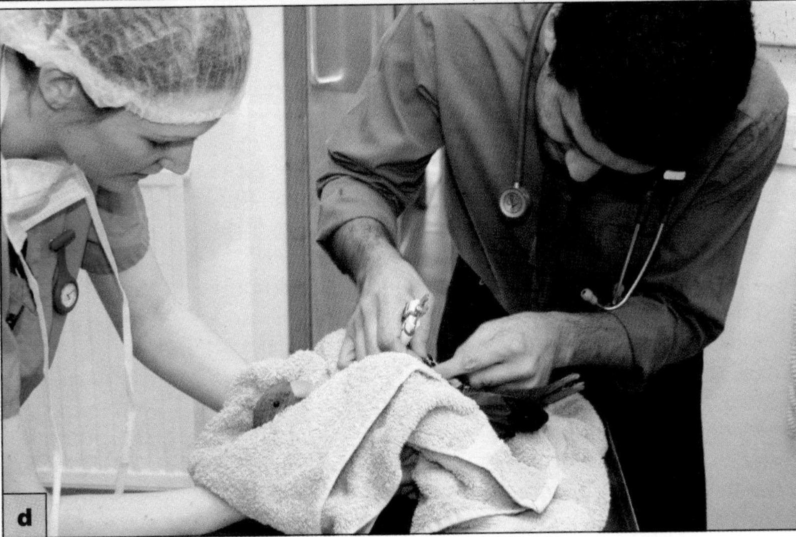

6.23 Animal handling equipment. **(a)** Muzzle rack. **(b)** Crush cages for feral or 'difficult' cats. **(c)** Cat and dog catchers. **(d)** Towels are useful for restraining birds.

be regularly checked and audited. An example of an audit for the outpatient area can be found in Chapter 3. Helpful information is available on the BSAVA website (www.bsava.com).

- Uniforms, scrub tops, overalls or easily changed clothing should be worn in the consulting room by staff, and any soiled items of clothing should be changed as soon as possible. Long sleeves should be avoided and jewellery kept to a minimum.
- Disposable gloves and/or aprons should be worn where a risk of contamination is suspected, and disposed off immediately after use.
- Staff should wash their hands after each consultation, using the hand-washing sinks in or adjacent to the consulting room (Figure 6.24). They should follow the WHO method for hand-washing (see Chapter 7), use disinfecting hand scrub and dry their hands on disposable paper towels. Disinfecting hand gels can be used where there is no access to sinks but these are only effective on clean hands, so thorough hand-washing and drying with disposable paper towels is still important.

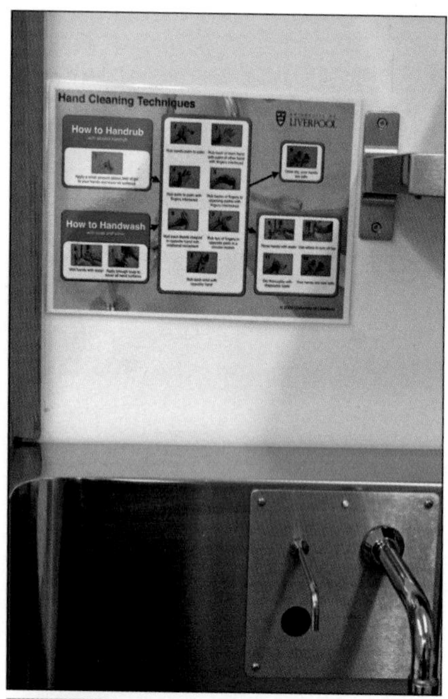

6.24 Thorough hand-washing is an important part of biosecurity in the consulting room.

- Cleaning materials and disinfectants for use in the consulting room should be clearly marked for this area and be close to hand.
- Urine, faeces or any other bodily fluids should be cleaned up immediately, an appropriate disinfectant used and any waste disposed of in either hazardous or non-hazardous streams (see below), as deemed appropriate by the veterinary surgeon.
- The table should be cleaned and then sprayed with viricidal disinfectant (at the correct dilution) between consultations.
- Equipment should be cleaned and disinfected after each use. Ophthalmoscope and auriscope handles, stethoscopes, and other diagnostic equipment should be cleaned at least daily and thoroughly dismantled and cleaned according to manufacturers' recommendations regularly. Auriscope heads can be effectively cleaned in desktop 'scrubbers' (Figure 6.25) and can be autoclaved before use if made of suitable material. The scrubbers must be disinfected regularly.

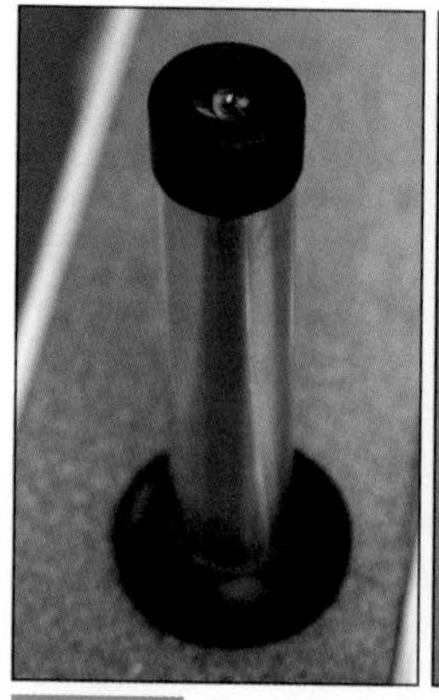

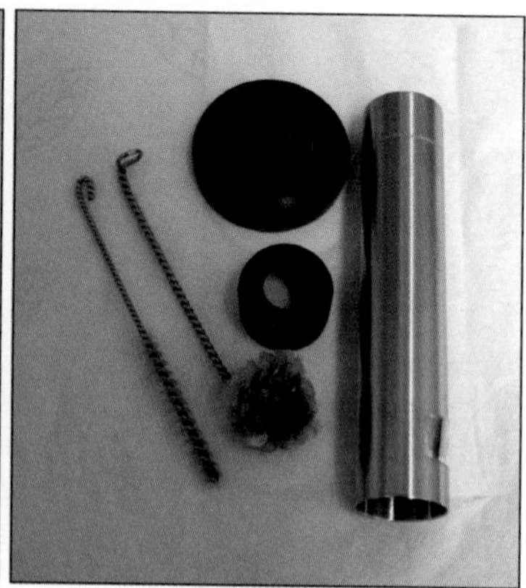

6.25 Purpose-built auriscope head cleaning units, containing detergent and disinfectant, are handy in consulting rooms. Regular dismantling and thorough cleaning of the 'scrubber' unit is necessary to prevent build-up of debris.

- Telephones and computer keyboards, mice and covers must be cleaned and disinfected frequently during the day to prevent spread of infections, including MRSA. A soft bristle brush can be useful for thorough moist cleaning of uncovered keyboards, with frequent replacement when necessary.
- Door handles and edges and worktops should be wiped regularly throughout the day.

Waste disposal

The principle of waste disposal in the consulting area should be that waste is handled as little as possible, is segregated at point of production, and goes to its final destination in the practice as quickly as possible. Categories of waste are defined in Chapter 3.

The practice may have bins for Domestic Waste, Offensive Waste and Pharmaceutical Waste in the consulting room as well as for 'sharps' (see below). Practices should carefully consider the size and design of these bins with regard to ease of use and emptying, aesthetic appearance, and ease of cleaning. Bins must be clearly labelled and secure from investigation by pets and children.

It is also good environmental practice to separate out recyclable materials such as cardboard.

Sharps

Correct tamper-proof sharps containers must be used, positioned either on worktops or inside cupboards, out of reach of clients. Particular attention should be paid to making sure that all needles go into a sharps bin *immediately after use* to avoid needle-stick injuries. They should not be resheathed first. A risk assessment for sharps disposal should be drawn up to avoid the risk of needle-stick injuries. Needle-stick injuries in practice (22% of reported accidents in one veterinary hospital (Mosedale, 2009)) are a real risk, not only to veterinary surgeons and nurses, but also to clients who might get in the way of the needle whilst restraining a fractious pet. An American survey of such injuries in female vets showed effects ranging from mild and localized problems to systemic illness, with one report of spontaneous abortion following accidental self-injection of a prostaglandin (Wilkins and Bowman, 1997).

Ideally, the whole syringe and needle should be placed immediately into the correct sharps container (Figure 6.26); this is the Environment Agency advice. In the UK, waste removal contractors have encouraged practices to separate syringes from needles for disposal, and there can be a cost benefit to this, but if this is done a comprehensive risk assessment of this procedure and staff training should be carried out. Empty vaccine vials and drug bottles are treated as Pharmaceutical Waste and must be disposed of accordingly (see Chapter 3).

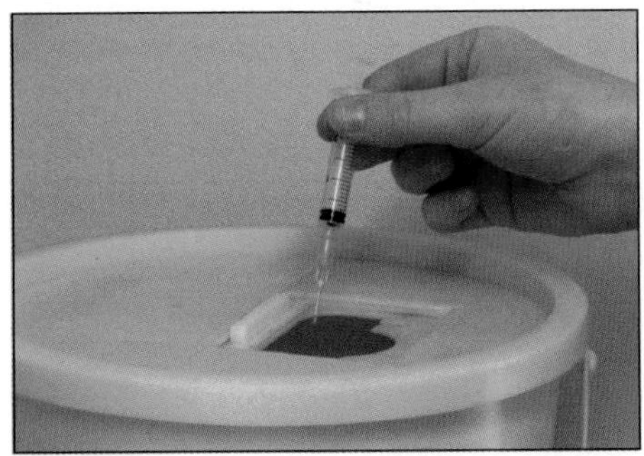

6.26 Ideally the whole syringe and needle should be placed immediately after use into the correct sharps container.

KEY POINT

It is important for biosecurity and health & safety reasons to maintain practice discipline in the consulting area. Consulting room users should clear away all used syringes, needles, pharmaceuticals and other litter and clean surfaces before leaving, so that rooms are safe and ready for use. Convenient bin and cleaning material locations will encourage this.

Acknowledgements

The author and editors gratefully acknowledge the following practices, images of which appear in this chapter: All Creatures Healthcare; Bridge Veterinary Practice Ltd; Elands Veterinary Clinic; Mill House Veterinary Surgery and Hospital; PDSA; Penmellyn Veterinary Group; Willows Veterinary Centre and Referral Service; Woodcroft Veterinary Group.

References and further reading

Aksoy E, Boag A, Brodbelt D and Grierson J (2010) Evaluation of surface contamination with staphylococci in a veterinary hospital using a quantitative biological method. *Journal of Small Animal Practice* **5**, 574–580

Mosedale P (2009) It shouldn't happen to a vet. *Journal of Small Animal Practice* **50**, 264

Wilkins JR III and Bowman ME (1997) Needlestick injuries among female veterinarians: frequency, syringe contents and side-effects. *Occupational Medicine* **47**, 451–457

Wards and inpatient areas

7

Deborah Roberts

The inpatient areas of the practice primarily contain patient accommodation, generally as cages and kennels, as well as space for support activities and cleaning, together with an isolation area where space allows. Larger practices may have separate rooms for the different inpatient activities; these should be close together to reduce movement of patients and staff. Smaller surgeries with space limitations will combine activities into one or two areas. It is important to take time to consider what requirements are essential if space is limited.

Design and layout

More detailed information on design and layout can be found in Chapter 3. The following should be considered when designing or enhancing the inpatient areas:

- Separate wards for cats/dogs/exotic species
- Separate wards for medical/surgical patients
- Minor procedures room
- Critical care/intensive care unit
- Anaesthetic recovery area
- Isolation area, with changing room and independent exit to isolated walking area
- Ward preparation area for support activities
- Wet room/shower area for bathing patients
- Storage space
- Weighing area
- Kitchen/food preparation area
- Laundry room
- Cleaning store (each area in the practice should have individual identifiable cleaning equipment)
- Space and convenient locations for segregated waste bins, including possible hazardous waste from infectious patients, and chemotherapy, sharps, pharmaceutical, offensive and trade waste (see Chapter 3)
- Exercise area.

Ideally, several smaller ward areas are preferable to one large space (Figure 7.1), as the increased wall area will allow installation of more caging, and multiple areas will aid biosecurity, as well as the separation of different species. Although it is tempting to fit in as many kennels and cages as possible, it is important to accommodate sufficient support equipment, as well as hand and equipment washing facilities, in each ward area (Figure 7.2).

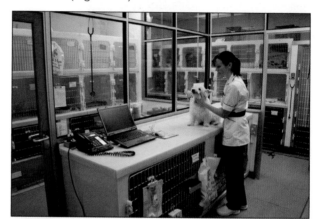

7.1 Several smaller ward areas are preferable to one large space. In this example, glass partitioning keeps the areas light and allows easy observation of all the patients.

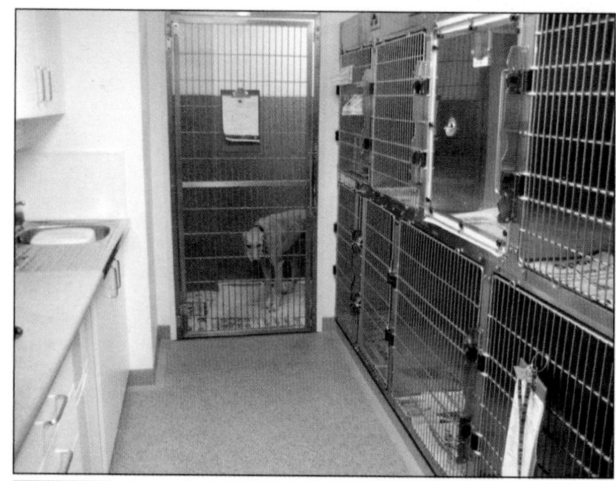

7.2 Dog ward with vinyl flooring, walk-in kennel, plenty of storage and sink with drainer.

Location

The wards should be conveniently located, close to the preparation, theatre, radiography and admittance/discharge areas, in order to make the environment as user-friendly as possible and to allow a smooth passage of work. Where patients are hospitalized close to public areas, effective soundproofing is essential to avoid disturbing reception, consultations and other working areas.

Lighting, ventilation and heating

Daylight improves the working and patient environment, so windows are recommended. Windows in ward areas should be kept shut to prevent escape of patients, ensure privacy and reduce transmission of noise outside the practice. If windows are required to open for ventilation purposes, a grille should be installed to prevent escape. Good controllable negative pressure ventilation is essential in each ward area, and air conditioning is advisable (see Chapter 2).

Additional lighting may be needed and thought should be given to lighting the inside of cages and walk-in kennels for effective patient assessment. Lights should be dimmable (or a separate circuit installed) to permit low-level light at night.

Figure 7.3 shows recommended ambient temperatures for housing dogs and acts. Underfloor heating should be considered if possible, although radiator central heating is often used. Underfloor heating, which can be continued into kennels and improve consistency of temperature, should be considered where possible. Although radiator central heating is often used, radiators are notoriously difficult to keep clean, and ward areas generally have little spare wall space for mounting them.

Species or area	Recommended ambient temperature
Adult dogs	7–26°C Should not drop below 7°C Sleeping area should be at least 10°C
Adult cats	10–26°C
Hospital and isolation kennels	18–23°C
Whelping/kittening and neonate accommodation	Parturition area: 18–21°C Neonates: First week: 26–29°C Second week: 21–26°C Until weaning: 20°C

7.3 Environmental temperatures for housing dogs and cats.

Walls and flooring

Walls should be easy to clean, e.g. tiled, or clad with an impervious coating or hard paint finish. Flooring should be easy to clean and non-slip; although tiles are often used, a vinyl floor (see Figure 7.2) is easier to clean, warmer and quieter. See Chapter 3 for more details.

Doors

Double doors are advisable between the ward area and all other areas:

- The inner door should be a 'pull' door, so that animals are unable to push their way out; alternatively, it could have a manually operated push button security system to release it
- The outer door should remain latched, to prevent patients pushing their way out.

Door knobs rather than levers should be considered, as some dogs can work lever-style handles (a lever fixed upside down can overcome this problem).

The security of personnel is an important consideration and **under no circumstances should any fire door be propped open**. Fire doors on trolleying routes can be held open by an electromagnetic catch which releases when the alarm sounds (see Chapter 2). Vision panels in doors to wards are recommended, and should be full length or include high- and low-level windows so that people each side of the door can see a person and/or patient on the other side.

Electricity

Sufficient electrical sockets are required and circuit breakers should be fitted. Sockets should be located to be accessible for each use, for example above cages or ceiling-mounted (Figure 7.4) for patient equipment and wall-mounted for cleaning equipment. Trailing leads must be avoided.

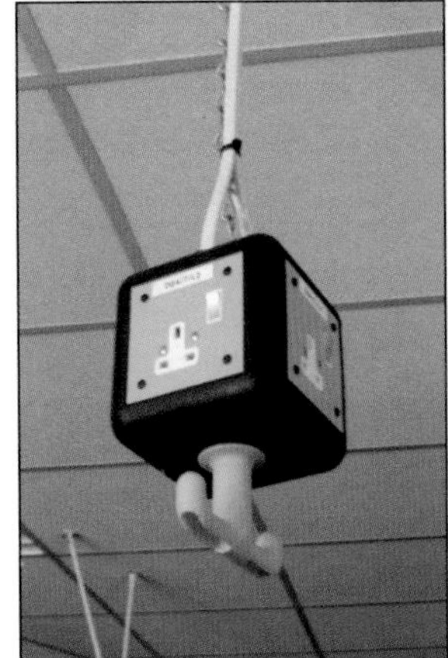

7.4 Ceiling socket unit with hooks for trailing leads.

Oxygen supply

A piped oxygen supply can be wall- or ceiling-mounted, and can make use of space above banks of cages (see Chapter 2). Alternatively, portable oxygen concentrators can be used, but space must be available for these.

Equipment and storage

As well as patient accommodation, the following essential requirements should be considered within wards and ward preparation areas:

- Animal handling and restraint equipment (dog/cat catchers, crush cages, muzzles) (see Chapter 6)
- Tub table/examination table
- Stretcher(s) or trolleys
- Sink(s) for hand-washing and equipment cleaning (Figure 7.5)
- Hand-drying facilities – preferably paper towels, but air dryers can be used
- Towels for drying patients
- Patient incubator
- Appropriate bins for healthcare waste, including 'sharps' (see Chapter 3)

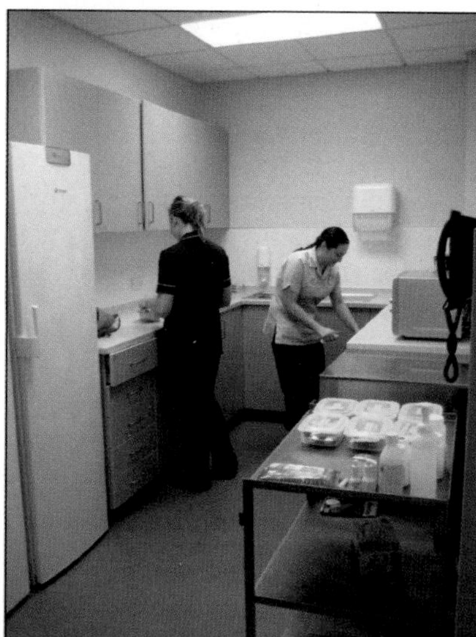

7.5 This ward preparation area contains a fridge, a microwave, a sink, plenty of bench and storage space, and a trolley for individual patient treatments and for carrying food.

- Storage for cleaning equipment
- Storage for PPE (gloves, plastic aprons, etc.)
- Storage for ward supplies: patient bedding, cat baskets, leads, collars, grooming equipment, bandages, protection collars, disposables (e.g. cotton wool, incontinence pads), medications, intravenous fluids, infusion equipment, infusion pumps, patient warming devices (e.g. heat pads or hot air body warmers), cat litter trays, cat litter
- Fridge, microwave, dishwashing facilities and food storage (these may be in a separate ward kitchen)
- Safe steps or kick-steps if cages are too high to reach safely.

It is important, when designing a ward, that caging does not take up all of the available wall space. Items that can make good use of wall space in the ward area include:

- Brackets for intravenous infusion pumps and fluids (see Figure 7.31)
- Clippers (Figure 7.6a)
- Stretcher stations (Figure 7.6b)
- Wall-mounted dog tie
- Weighing scales
- Storage facilities for mattresses and rubber mats used to line slippery kennels
- Apron storage
- Storage units for medication dispensed to inpatients (Figure 7.7)
- Controlled Drugs cupboard
- Nurses' station/work surface for updating records
- Telephone
- Computer terminal
- White board/noticeboard for staff information and messages to aid communication
- Storage facilities for patient case files and practice paperwork (Figure 7.8).

Wall space is also generally needed for:

- Examination/procedure table and/or tub table
- Hoist, electric or manual lift table for large/heavy dogs.

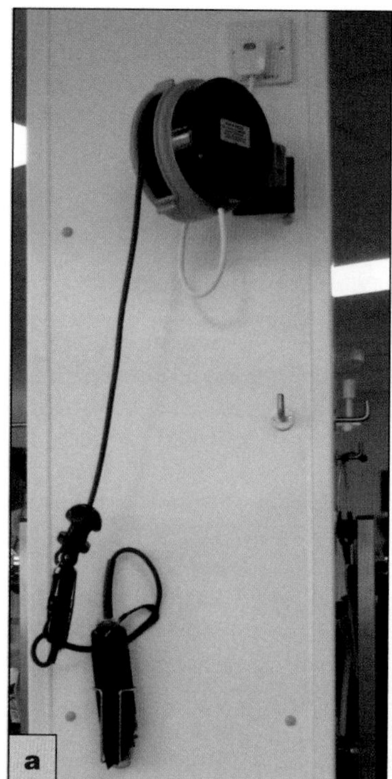

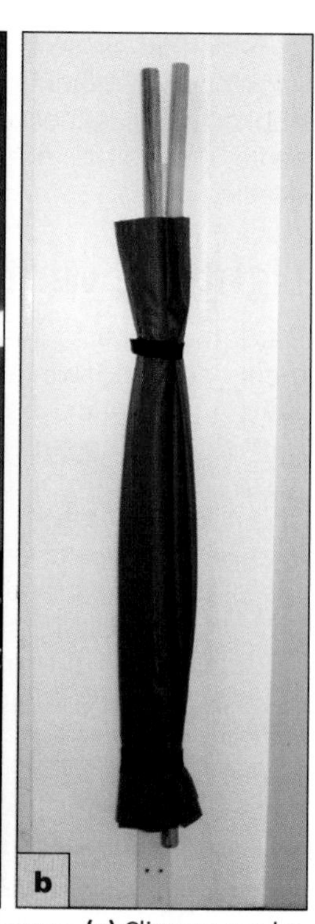

7.6 Making good use of wall space. **(a)** Clippers can be wall-mounted on an extension reel. **(b)** Stretcher stations located in choice places around the practice will encourage use.

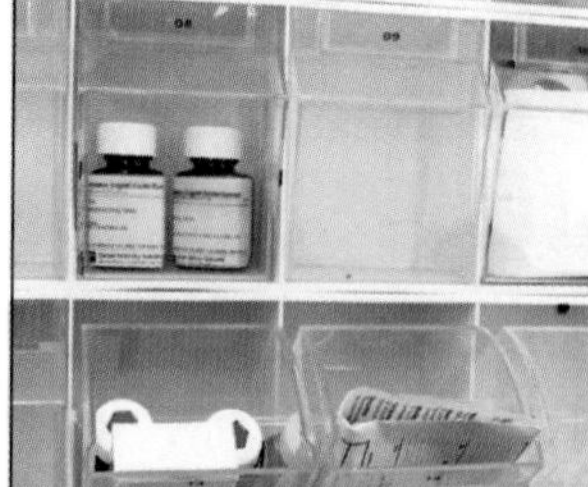

7.7 Inpatient medication should be stored safely and with easy access for nurses. Individual drawers are ideal.

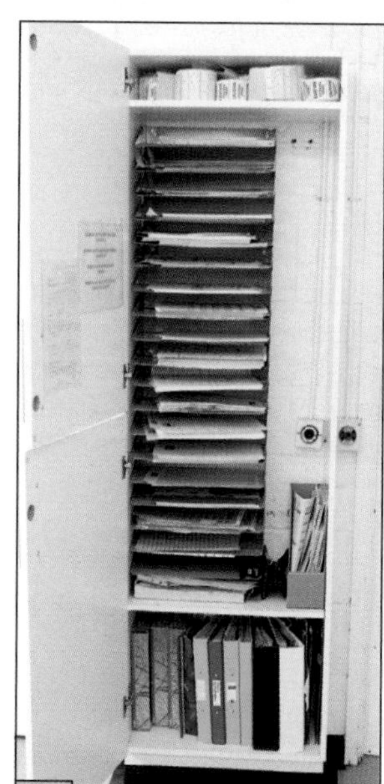

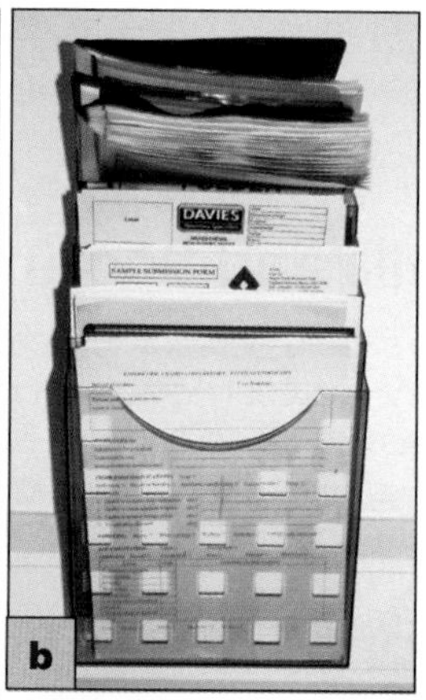

7.8 **(a)** Metal filing trays are useful for storing paper records and bulk blank forms, and keeping them accessible. **(b)** Wall-mounted racks can also be used for storing blank forms.

As space is usually limited, it is best not to admit personal belongings that are not kept with the patient (e.g. pet carriers, leads, spare bedding), thus making storage for these unnecessary. However, a box for uncollected items, clearly labelled, is useful, particularly for inpatients that are euthanased or die in the practice.

Patient accommodation

Accommodation must look smart and provide a safe environment for patients and nursing staff. Insulation of the surrounding walls is important for noise levels and temperature control. Kennel and cage manufacturers may be willing to measure up and design the ward layout in conjunction with the practice. Overall, cage design and arrangement should consider ease of use, visibility, strength, durability and quality.

Kennel design and materials

Cages and kennels should be designed to suit the patients hospitalized. Shorter-stay patients will manage with less room than those staying several days. It is important to ensure that the Five Freedoms (Figure 7.9) are met whenever a pet is hospitalized. The *BSAVA Textbook of Veterinary Nursing* contains more detail on patient accommodation and the clinical aspects of inpatient nursing.

- **Freedom from hunger and thirst** – through ready access to fresh water and a diet to maintain full health and vigour
- **Freedom from discomfort** – through providing an appropriate environment including a comfortable resting area
- **Freedom from pain, injury or disease** – through prevention or rapid diagnosis and treatment
- **Freedom from fear and distress** – through ensuring conditions and treatment that avoid mental suffering
- **Freedom to express normal behaviour** – through providing sufficient space, proper facilities and company of the animal's own kind (where appropriate)

7.9 The Five Freedoms.

All patients need to be comfortable:

- Dogs and cats need to be able to turn around and stand in their space, as well as to lie stretched out during recovery
- Large/giant-breed dogs and longer-stay patients should ideally be hospitalized in a walk-in kennel
- Even where space is limited, preference should be given to accommodating cats separately from dogs
- Rabbits, rodents, birds and other exotic species have particular hospitalization requirements and should be housed away from predator species
- In addition, space within and around the cages must be adequate for nursing observations and safe handling.

The partition walls of dog kennels can be built of brick, blockwork or studwork, or can be made from fibreglass, PVC or stainless steel partitioning (Figure 7.10). Gates are best manufactured from stainless steel, although galvanized and painted metal gates can be successful if well maintained. Glazed stainless steel frames or toughened glass can work well, but ventilation should be considered carefully (Figure 7.11), and may need to be installed separately. Wood

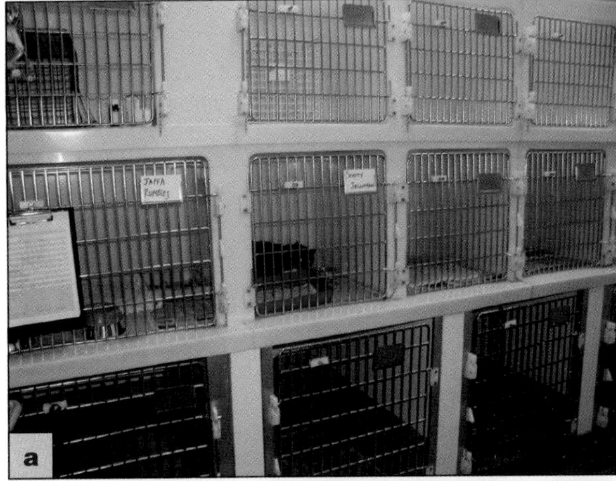

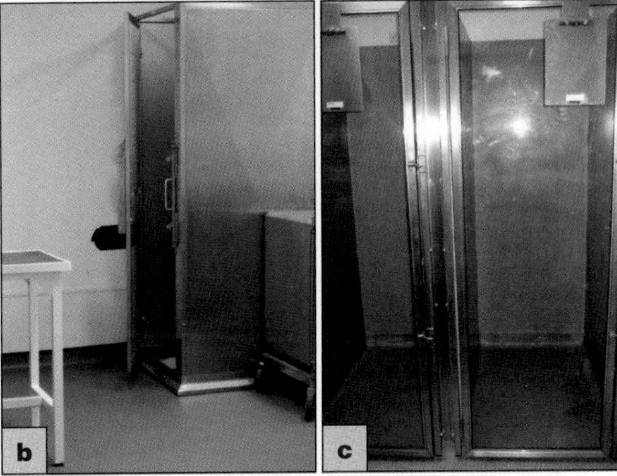

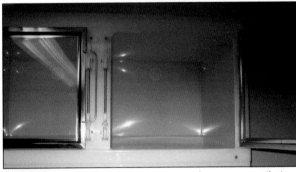

7.10 Dog kennels may be made from a range of materials. **(a)** PVC cages over blockwork kennels. **(b)** Walk-in kennel with stainless steel walls. **(c)** Walk-in kennel with glazed stainless steel doors.

7.11 These glazed-door PVC cages have rear ventilation grilles. With extraction ventilation, anaesthetic gases can be ducted away and humidity reduced.

is not recommended, as it is readily chewed.

The internal lining of any cages should give an easy-to-clean surface, with no dirt-collecting corners. Epoxy finishes with rounded corners can work well, as can coved and sealed vinyl as long as it is well laid and maintained (Figure 7.12). Ceramic tiling is often used but can be difficult to keep clean. There are a number of well known installers of kennel systems in both stainless steel and plastics who will help design a new ward area, and who can often produce bespoke cages for difficult areas. Non-slip rubber mats can be purchased and are useful in kennels housing patients that need to be in a non-slip environment; veterinary bedding with rubber backing can be used but the backing will break down with repeated washing.

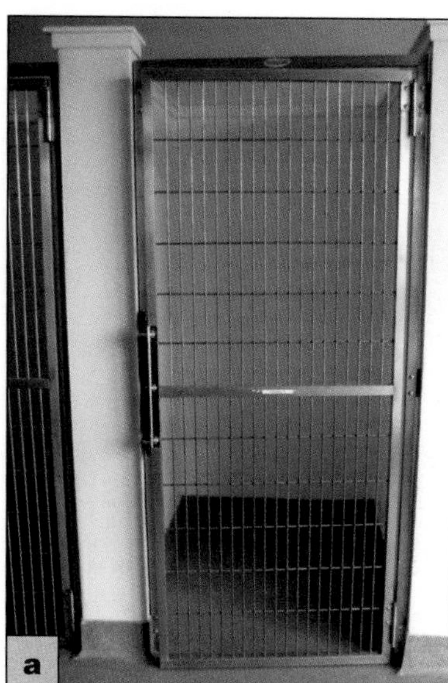

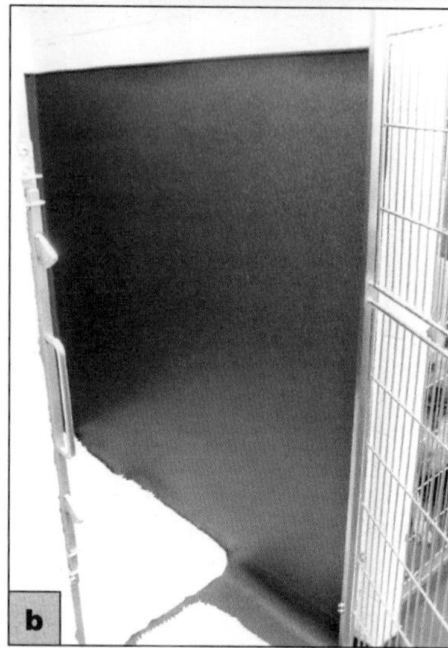

7.12 **(a)** Walk-in kennels built of blockwork with stainless steel gates and epoxy flooring. **(b)** These walk-in kennels have vinyl flooring material both on the floor and vertically, with heat-welded seams.

Cage doors and gates should be chosen to minimize the risk of escape by smaller patients and of entrapment of paws, claws and mandibles. Close supervision of patients in all accommodation is essential. Although cage doors are often used for hanging notes and other items, care should be taken not to obstruct the view of the patient unnecessarily. It may be helpful, however, to have screens available for increasing privacy for disturbed or nervous patients; alternatively, blankets or towels placed over cage doors can be helpful. Network or web cameras can be useful for observation of these patients.

Species considerations

Dogs

Kennels can be banked in two rows, with smaller dogs above. Kennels with floors that slope to the rear can be used, to reduce the likelihood of fluids passing down to the lower tier. It is always recommended to incorporate at least one full-height large kennel (Figure 7.13) for giant breeds and longer-stay patients.

It is advisable to fit a secure collar to each dog in the wards, unless there is a medical reason not to do so. Dogs that 'kennel-guard' can usually be handled safely if a lead is left attached and picked up so that the dog can be led out of the kennel.

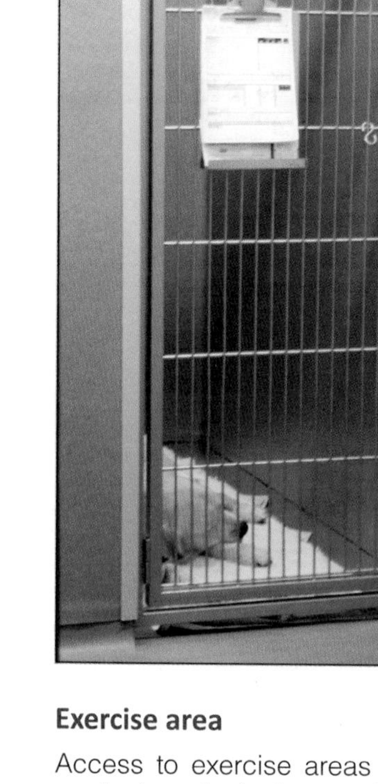

7.13 Walk-in kennels should be available for large or giant breeds.

Exercise area

Access to exercise areas for dogs must be considered when designing wards. Ideally, an exercise area would be an enclosed flat area with a variety of textures and trees to please patients. This is often not possible, however, and communal areas or the garden (Figure 7.14a) or car park may have to suffice. For safety and security, lighting of the outside area is required. Faecal waste bins should be located in areas convenient for staff, and members of the public if the area is not enclosed. These bins should be lined with bags for offensive waste and must be emptied regularly. A supply of bags or a shovel to pick up faecal waste should be within easy reach (Figure 7.14b).

An enclosed secure run allowing patients to be left outside in the better weather can be a pleasant alternative to the patient's kennel, particularly for ambulatory long-stay patients, though patients must remain

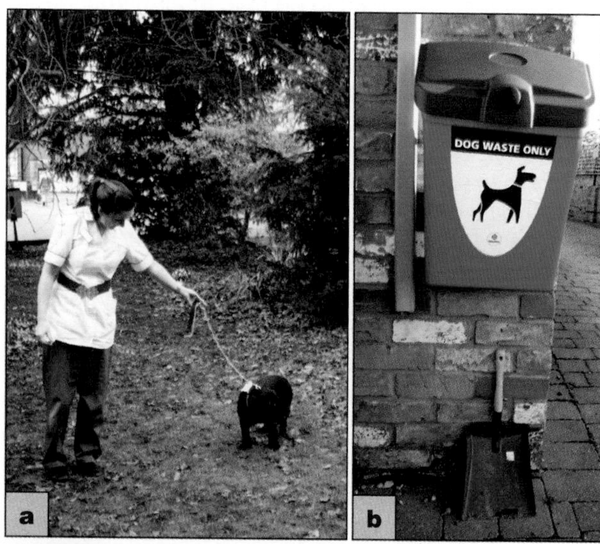

7.14 **(a)** When walking patients in a non-enclosed area, a secure named collar and lead are essential. **(b)** Faecal waste bins should be emptied regularly and a supply of bags or a shovel should be close to hand.

visible to staff at all times. It is essential to ensure that any outside area is fully enclosed and that only permitted staff can enter. Shelter from the elements needs to be provided and surfaces should be easily cleanable.

Cats

A selection of larger and smaller cages is recommended for cats, and provision of higher level perches (Figure 7.15) is appreciated by long-stay feline patients. Where cat cages are to be tiered, it is best to incorporate a row of cupboards on the floor – as cats prefer to be up high; this also minimizes the need for staff to bend down (see Chapter 3). Two rows are recommended: a higher, third, row of cages might increase the risk of scratching and injury to staff handling the top-tier cats.

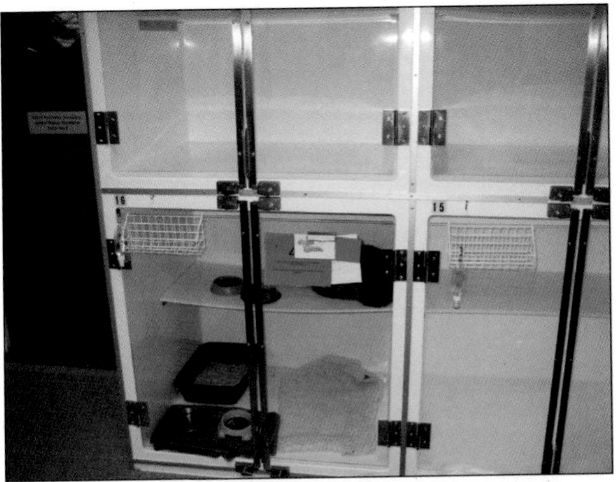

7.15 A raised area for cats to sit on is appreciated, particularly by longer-stay patients.

Considerations for a cat-friendly ward

A separate ward for feline patients is a great asset for any practice and will appeal to cat owners. Feline patients will also benefit from a feline-friendly hospital environment, which will reduce anxiety and aid their recovery. Some measures to consider are listed below; more ideas can be found on the Feline Advisory Bureau (FAB) website www.fabcats.org.uk.

- The layout of cages in a cat ward should be planned so that they all face in the same direction, as cats prefer not to see other cats. If the cats have to face each other, there should be a full cage height impervious 'sneeze barrier' in place to avoid transfer of airborne disease.
- Cats feel safer at a height; locating cat kennels at waist height or above is optimal for a cat-friendly practice, but they should not be positioned at face level or they will become a danger to staff.
- Screens between cages and a screen between the cage bank and examination table can reduce stress.
- Boxes (Figure 7.16) or enclosed 'igloo' types of bed can be used to allow the cat a place to hide.
- A variety of litter trays and types of litter should be available, including an enclosed type of tray.
- Fountain-type water bowls (Figure 7.17) are available for cats that prefer to drink running water.
- A variety of feeding bowls should be available.
- FAB advises that there is evidence to suggest that playing classical music as soft background music provides a relaxing environment for both cats and their carers.
- Small, quiet clippers (Figure 7.18) should be used for cats.
- Synthetic pheromone diffusers and sprays may help reduce stress.
- Long-stay cats may enjoy an elevated shelf or platform on which to relax, but thought should be given to the reason for admission: a cat with a fracture should not have anything to jump on to.

A feline isolation area should also be made available for cats with suspected contagious disease.

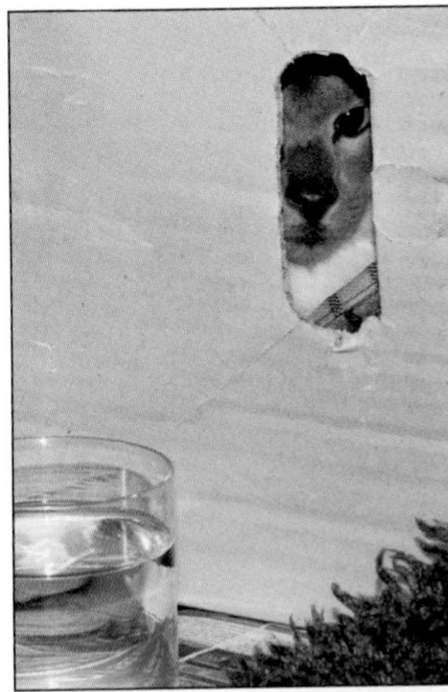

7.16 An old cardboard box makes a good hiding place for a cat and makes them feel more secure.

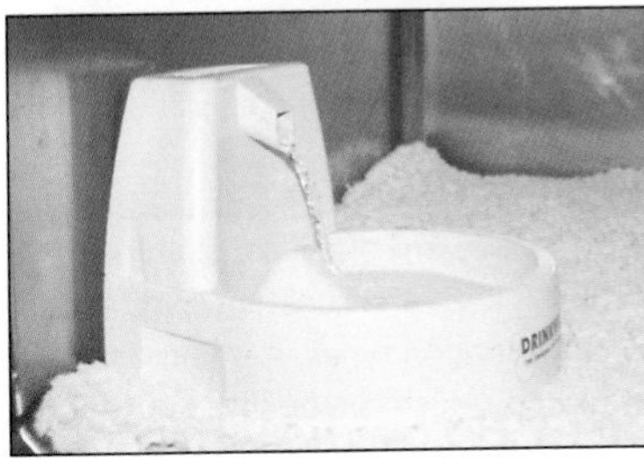

7.17 A water fountain will encourage some cats to drink.

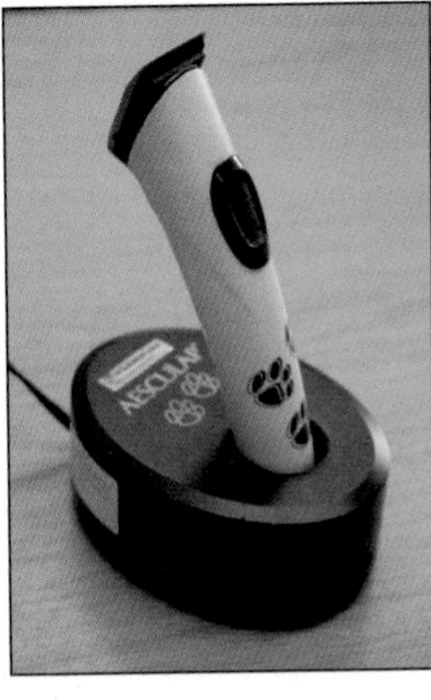

7.18 Small quiet clippers are useful for clipping hair on conscious cats.

Other species

Rabbits should ideally be hospitalized in larger pens on the floor, with room to move about freely (Figure 7.19). Rodents and other small pets should be hospitalized in escape-proof cages, which should be portable. For practices with a high exotics workload, some vivaria with appropriate heating and lighting are advised (Figure 7.20) along with deep shelf space for placing owners' cages should this be necessary.

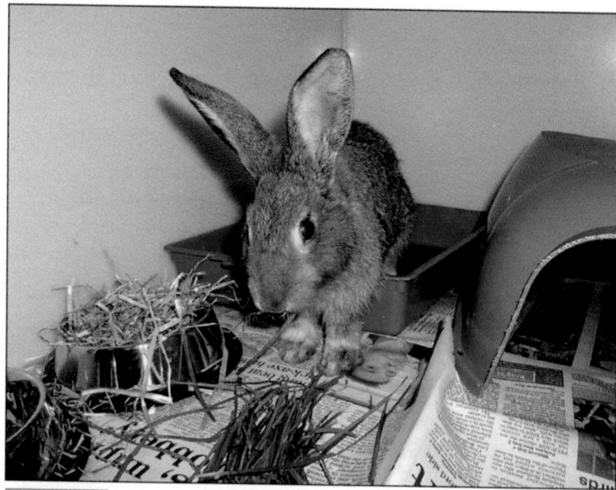

7.19 Hospitalized rabbits need space for several hops, and height to stand on their hindlegs. A private area, toileting area and appropriate fresh food are essential.

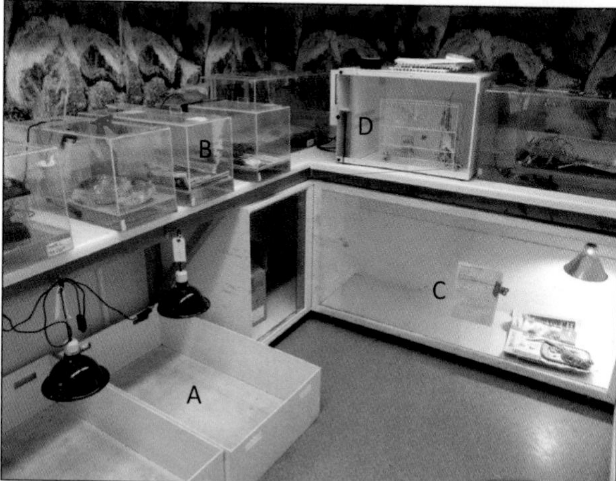

7.20 The avian and reptilian ward of an exotic animal practice. The room is kept at a constant 25°C and has a range of different accommodation types. **A** marks a tortoise tray, made of light plastic, which can be lifted out for cleaning. A full-spectrum light hangs over one end on a cord, so that its height can be varied to adjust the temperature at the basking area. **B** marks a bank of Aquabrooder units, where the animal accommodation is surrounded by thermostatically controlled heated water. **C** is one of three large, traditional-style vivaria in the ward; these are more suited to large reptiles. **D** is an intensive care unit; the temperature and humidity can be set on this unit, which can also be used for critical care of collapsed small mammals. © Avian and Exotic Animal Clinic.

Birds can often be admitted in their own cages; an appropriate selection of toys, perches and accessories should be available.

Bedding

A range of bedding materials should be available, appropriate for species likely to be admitted.

- Veterinary fleece bedding is a comfortable material that draws moisture away from the patient, and is easily washed and disinfected. Alternatives may need to be used for individuals that are inclined to chew fleece bedding.
- Washable quilts and blankets are useful to maintain temperatures of patients recovering from anaesthesia/surgery. Bubble wrap and 'survival' blankets (Figure 7.21) can be used as disposable coverings to maintain warmth.
- A rolled-up towel in a circle can be used to make a small dog feel at ease.
- A blanket on top of veterinary bedding can allow a large dog to arrange its own comfort.
- A supply of cardboard boxes for makeshift shelters and hiding places is useful for cats, and for nervous and smaller patients.
- For small mammals, shredded paper and absorbent paper waste can be useful; sawdust and wood shavings are best avoided.

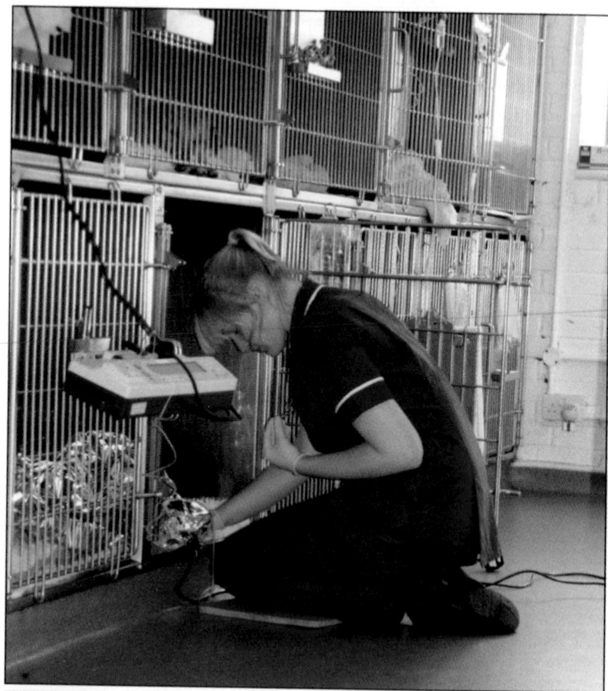

7.21 A disposable recovery (survival) blanket in use. Note also the syringe driver fixed to the cage door and the use of a kneeling pad by the veterinary nurse.

Specific ward areas

Recovery area

Ideally, the recovery area will be situated away from the busy kennel area but in close proximity to the theatre and preparation areas (see Chapter 8). Most practices do not have a separate recovery area for patients recovering from anaesthesia and surgery but use part of the preparation area (Figure 7.22) or the ward area. The principles remain the same:

- A quiet environment
- Thermostatically controlled heating
- Adequate ventilation, to minimize the exposure of staff to the potentially higher levels of exhaled anaesthetic gases from patients during the initial recovery period following gaseous anaesthesia
- Lighting with a dimming facility.

KEY POINT

The area should be staffed at all times and patients should be monitored continuously and closely throughout their recovery period.

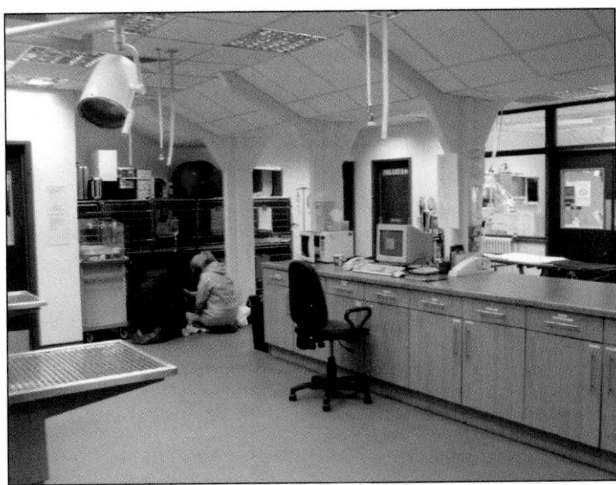

7.22 Recovery cages can be situated in the 'prep' area. Note the blue physiotherapy balls on top of the cages.

In addition to the standard equipment in the ward and preparation area, the following should be available:

- Crash cart (see Chapter 8)
- Suction machine (Figure 7.23)
- Incubator.

Mobile monitoring equipment is beneficial for some patients (see later).

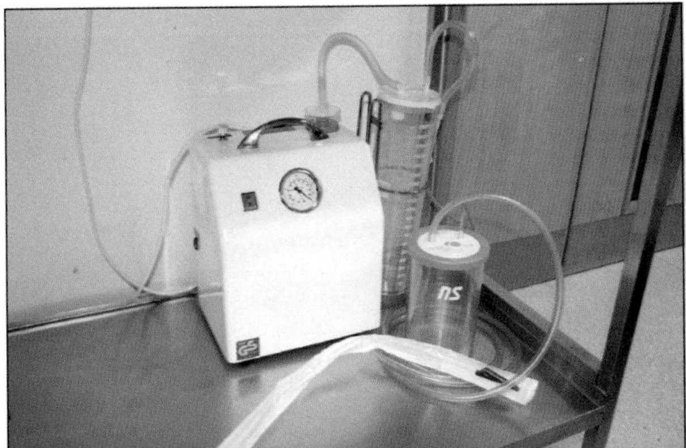

7.23 A portable suction machine should be ready at all times, with sterile tubing and attachments ready for use.

> **KEY POINT**
>
> Anticipation of potential problems is key; the recovery area must be well stocked and maintained.

Intensive care unit

An intensive care unit (ICU) can be incorporated into the recovery area or may be in its own allocated area. It should be designed for the range of patients likely to be hospitalized.

Accommodation

Not all patients will require cages whilst in the ICU, and different patients will have different needs.

- A cat requiring oxygen therapy can be housed in an incubator (Figure 7.24); alternatively, a purpose-made or converted cage can be used as an oxygen cage.
- A dog recovering from surgery can be placed on a waterproof mattress on the floor (Figure 7.25), whilst supervised, and secured by a lead or harness if necessary when fully recovered. Waterproof kneeling mats (Figure 7.26) should be provided for the comfort of attending staff.
- Intensive care beds with drop-down sides are available for veterinary patients, but care must be taken that a patient does not injure itself attempting to jump out.
- Stainless steel kennels can be fitted into an ICU area and will provide safe effective housing, but they may give limited access for intensive care monitoring and frequent nursing interventions. They may also be noisy if patients have excessive voluntary or involuntary movement.

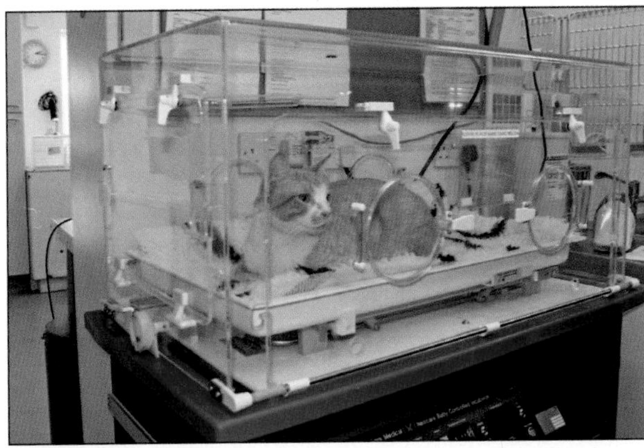

7.24 A cat requiring oxygen therapy can be housed in an incubator.

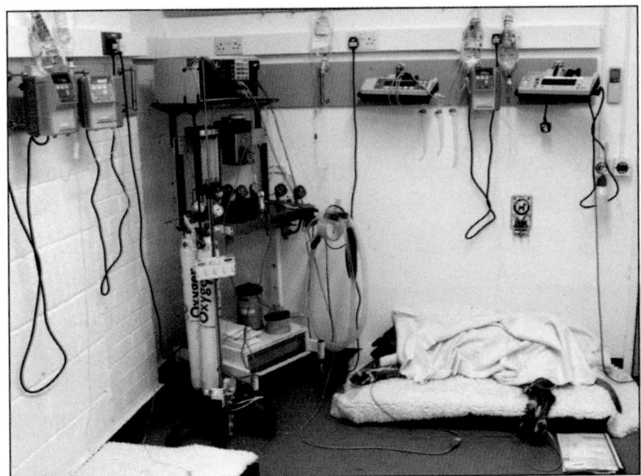

7.25 Intensive care area in use. Note the patient on a floor mattress, the dog parking hook and monitoring equipment.

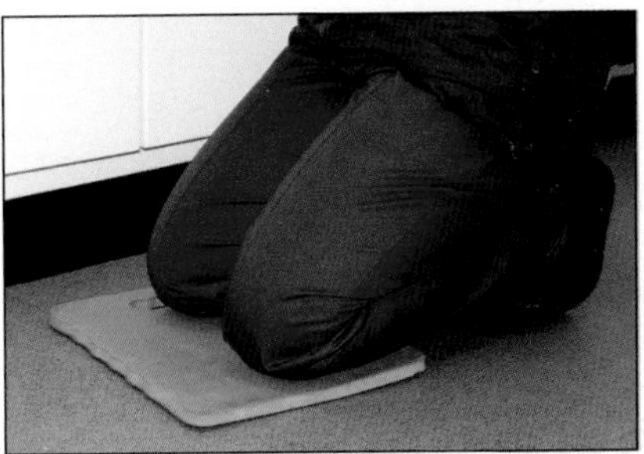

7.26 Kneeling pads situated in convenient places throughout the practice will encourage use and protect nurses' knees.

Equipment

In addition to the standard equipment and requirements for ward areas, the following should be considered for an ICU:

- More points for oxygen supply
- Crash trolley, containing essential drugs (see Chapter 8)
- Anaesthetic machine, with a supply of various breathing systems (see Chapter 8)
- Monitoring equipment: ECG (see Chapter 11); pulse oximetry, capnography, invasive/non-invasive blood pressure monitoring (see Chapter 8)
- Suction machine
- Access to basic in-house laboratory facilities (see Chapter 14)
- Blood gas analyser, glucometers
- Ventilators appropriate to the size of patients
- Incubator or oxygen therapy cage, and delivery systems for large patients
- Computer terminals for access to case records and Internet resources might be useful
- Equipment for urgent intravenous infusions; warming units for intravenous fluids.

Oxygen therapy

Oxygen can be supplied via a pipeline system from a central cylinder source (see Chapter 2), via individual cylinders supported on an anaesthetic machine (see Chapter 8), or from an oxygen generator (Figure 7.27). Oxygen generators are compact, mobile, require little maintenance and eliminate the safety risks of handling cylinders. Their disadvantages are: high initial purchase cost; they can be noisy (check before purchase); and only one can be used per patient. The oxygen concentration in the output of these machines should be checked regularly, using a meter or a patient monitor. The advantage of not having to worry about running out of oxygen usually results in more frequent use of oxygen therapy; with an appropriate fee scale for use, the purchase cost can therefore often be recouped very quickly.

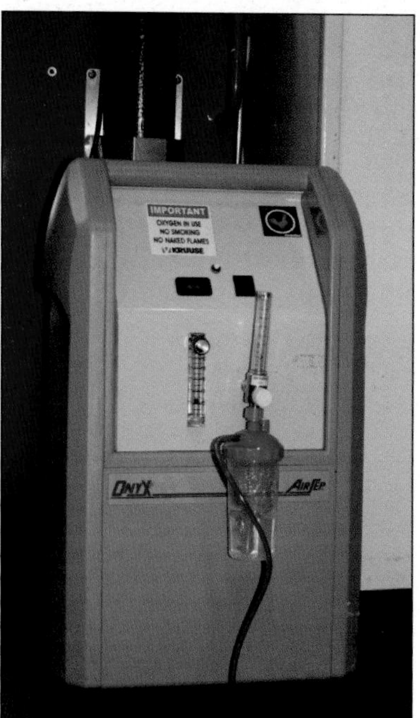

7.27 A mobile oxygen generator.

> **KEY POINT**
>
> Oxygen generators are particularly useful where frequent or long-term oxygen therapy is likely to be required, as there is no worry for staff about running down oxygen stocks, such as over a weekend or a Bank Holiday.

There are a number of ways to supplement the patient's oxygen intake (Figure 7.28):

- Oxygen cage: Kennels can be converted into oxygen cages by the replacement of the kennel door with a closer fitting clear glass or perspex door, allowing for patient observation. This door

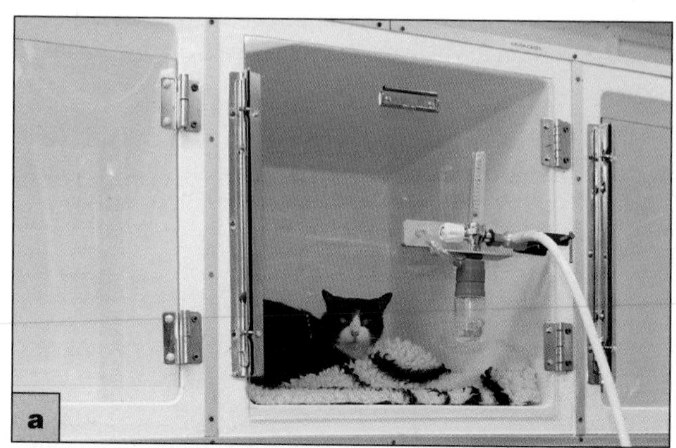

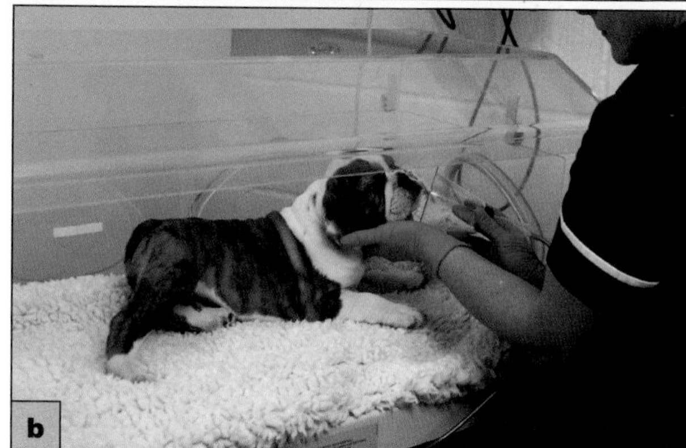

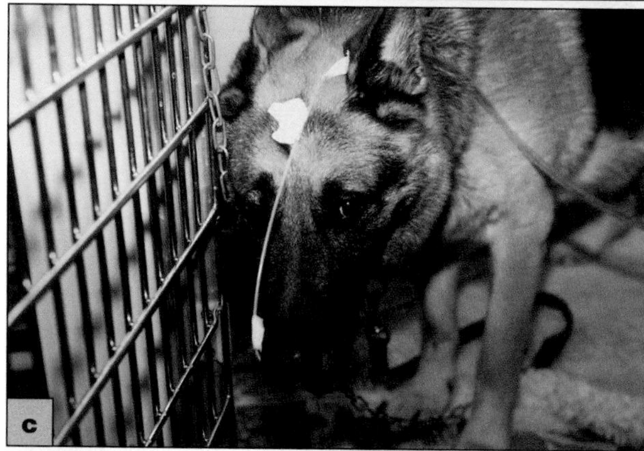

7.28 Oxygen therapy. **(a)** This simple oxygen therapy cage has an overlapping glass door with a delivery unit and flowmeter attached to the front. The oxygen level in the cage can be monitored by a patient multi-parameter anaesthetic monitor with oxygen module. **(b)** Ex-hospital incubators can be very useful for warming and for oxygen delivery. Care is needed in dismantling, cleaning and reassembling. **(c)** Intranasal oxygen is useful for larger patients, though can be poorly tolerated.

can be made through competent DIY; a number of designs are also commercially available, often supplied with flowmeters that enable a regulated flow of oxygen
- Incubator
- Veterinary intensive care cage
- Facemask
- Flow-by oxygen: e.g. nasal prongs
- Intranasal oxygen: useful for larger patients, but can be poorly tolerated
- Tracheotomy tube or endotracheal tube: for intensive care patients.

Oxygen should be humidified if it is to be administered directly for more than a few hours, in order to maintain the airway mucosa. This can be done using: ambient-temperature water vapour; heated water vapour; a nebulizer; a heat and moisture exchanger (HME).

KEY POINT

Oxygen therapy should always be available, ready for any emergency.

Intravenous infusions

Practices admitting inpatients should maintain an adequate stock and range of crystalloid and colloid fluids for routine or emergency intravenous administration. Fluids can be stored for short periods in a thermostatically controlled heated cabinet or incubator so that they are ready for immediate use (Figure 7.29). Blood and blood products may be stocked and will need accurate temperature- controlled storage.

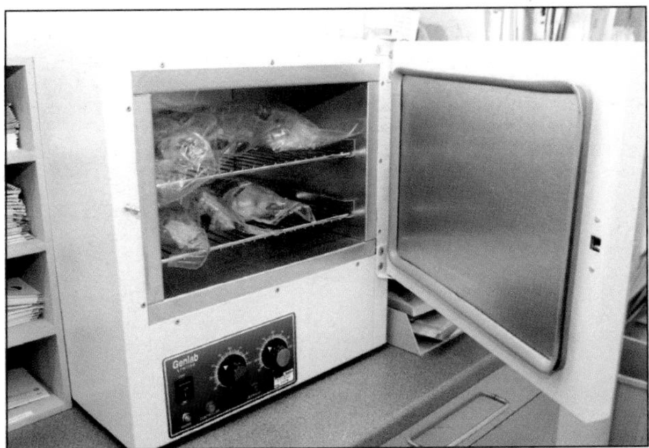

7.29 Small bench-top incubator for warming intravenous fluids before administration.

Manual administration sets ('giving sets') can be purchased in different lengths and designs, depending on use; when selecting a giving set, the position and number of additional ports may be important. Giving sets for transfusing blood have an additional filter. A selection of extension sets, three-way taps and T connectors will also be useful.

Regulating the flow of fluid into the patient can be achieved by moving a roller clamp on the tubing and observing the drip rate in the drip chamber. More accurate flow-control giving sets are available, and burette giving sets are useful for infusing small volumes more accurately. Increasingly, practices are relying on infusion pumps and syringe drivers, as these are more accurate and reliable and will maintain flow even when a patient changes position, which may block the flow with a manual system.

Infusion pumps (Figure 7.30) can administer a rapid accurate bolus of fluid to a patient or simply maintain fluid therapy for the time required. Volumetric pumps force the fluid into the vein under pressure at a rate set by the operator; some models have pressure-sensitive devices to reduce the possibility of tissue damage from inappropriate administration. Most pumps in veterinary use are small portable units with battery back-up and simple controls, although ex-hospital units can be good value for money if servicing and repair is available. Infusion pumps will need to have the correct giving set for the machine or be calibrated to the practice's brand of compatible giving set.

Syringe drivers (Figure 7.30) infuse small volumes of fluid accurately, and are useful for small patients or for when medication needs to be administered over a short period of time (e.g. constant rate infusions for pain management). They can be purchased new but are easily available second-hand. Some units take standard syringes, but others need special syringes designed for the pump. Some pumps can accept syringes of varying sizes. Use of the incorrect syringe or drip line on a pump could affect the accuracy of the infusion, and periodic calibration may be advised. It is helpful, for the avoidance of dosing errors, to have clear instructions for fluid rate and dilutions when using syringe drivers, particularly if more than one type is in use.

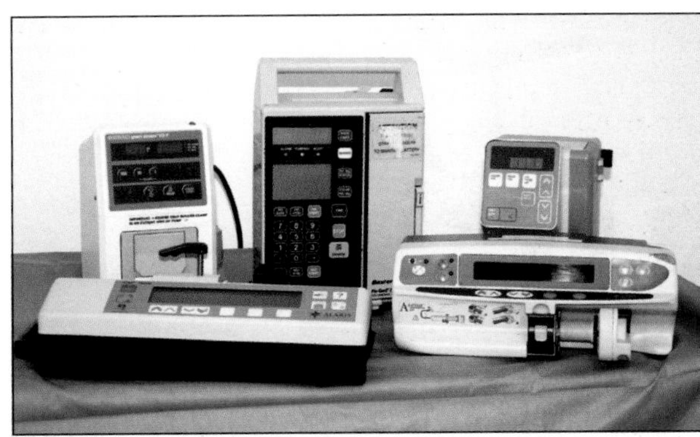

7.30 A selection of infusion pumps (back) and syringe drivers (front).

Both infusion pumps and syringe drivers have an audible and visual alarm in the event of an occlusion or a machine failure. Staff should understand the action needed when an alarm sounds and should monitor closely any infusion.

There should be a pole clamp on the back of these machines to secure the pump to a drip stand, mounting bar (Figure 7.31) or the kennel door; a number of fitments are available for kennel door mounting. If mains-fed, the unit must be positioned so that the patient cannot access the electrical wiring. Care should be taken with siting drip stands, as they can become a trip hazard. Mounting the infusion pump, warming equipment (see Chapter 8) and syringe driver on one stand can reduce clutter in the ICU (Figure 7.32).

Users should ensure that the manufacturer's operating instructions are followed and that servicing is regular, to ensure the accuracy of the equipment.

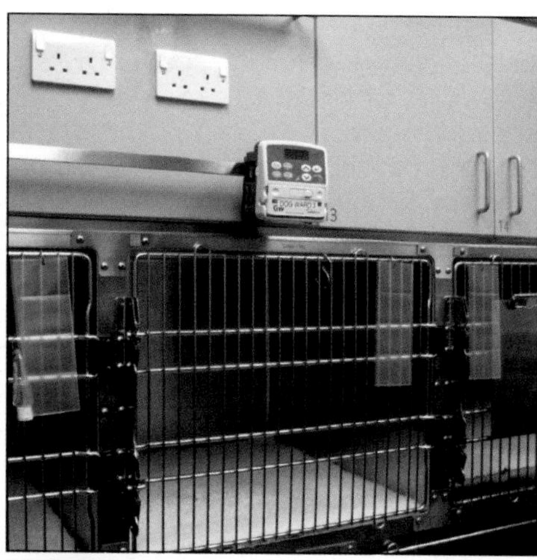

7.31 Infusion pumps can be mounted on wall bars above caging.

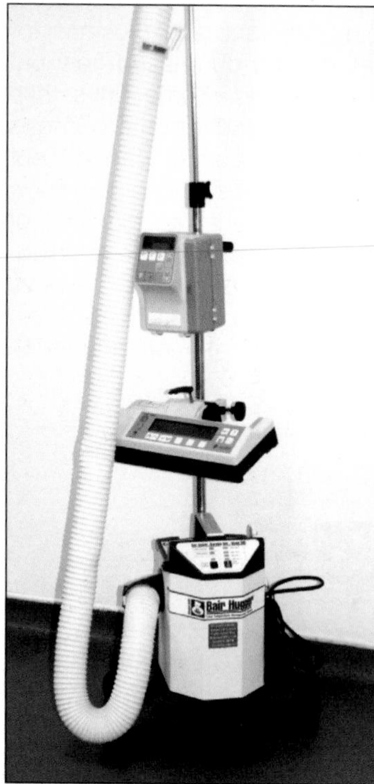

7.32 Infusion pump, warming equipment and syringe driver mounted on one stand.

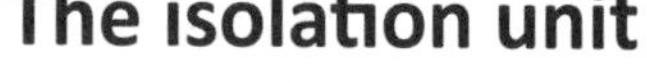

The isolation unit

Although all cases seen in veterinary practice have the potential to transmit infectious disease, those known to be at a higher risk of spreading infection should be nursed in a self-contained isolation unit, ideally with a separate entrance and exit and outside access for exercising isolated dogs. Because practices will generally not encourage the presence of infectious animals on their premises, most patients that are admitted to isolation facilities will require intensive nursing, and this point should be borne in mind when designing and locating the isolation facility.

The unit needs to be easily accessible, for intensive nursing, and a reinforced glass viewing panel is useful to enable staff to watch patients without having to enter the isolation facility. The unit should have separate air space, with negative pressure ventilation allowing the exhausted room air to be vented outside. Any open drainage should be separate to prevent cross-contamination. If there is an outside run, a water supply for a power hose is useful. A sink suitable for washing equipment and hands must be inside the unit, and facilities to wash the patient are very helpful. Clear signage (Figure 7.33), accessible protective clothing and well organized storage are essential for maintaining biosecurity (see later).

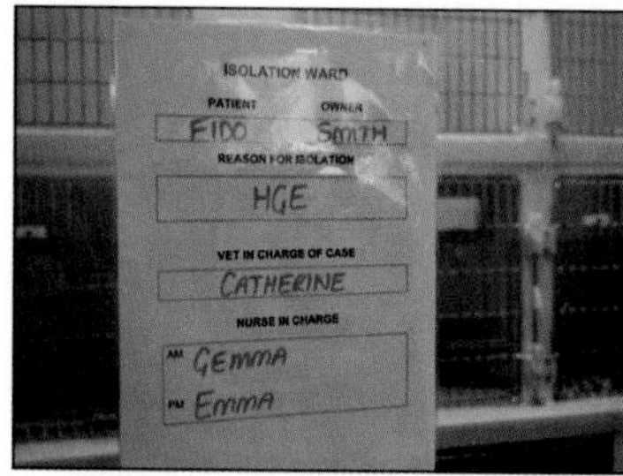

7.33 Clear signage, including clinical and nursing care responsibilities, are essential when hospitalizing patients with suspected infectious disease.

Practices should consider including a variety of kennel sizes, with at least one walk-in kennel. Adequate space must be allowed for intensive care nursing. An isolation unit needs to contain all the equipment that is required in wards. Disposable food bowls and bedding (Figure 7.34) can be used, according to patient need. Non-disposable items can be colour-coded for isolation unit use (Figure 7.35).

> **KEY POINT**
>
> The kennels and equipment in an isolation unit must be easily cleanable and should not be shared with other areas of the practice.

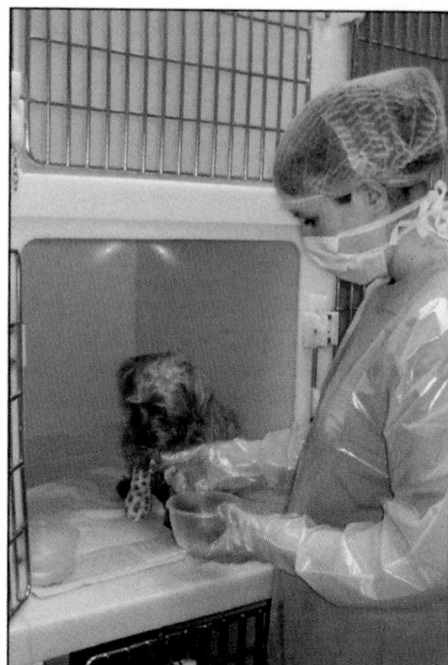

7.34 Disposable bedding and protective clothing can be used in the isolation unit and disposed of securely.

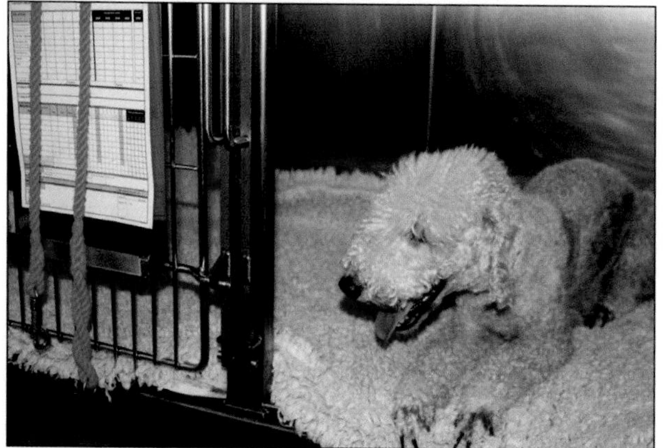

7.35 In this isolation unit, red leads and pink bedding and hospitalization sheets indicate that this patient is being barrier-nursed.

Disposable protective clothing should be worn by nursing staff (see Figure 7.34). There must be space and facilities to disinfect or discard footwear and clothing when leaving the unit.

Other inpatient areas

Minor procedures area

If space allows, a ward preparation area or minor procedures room, where staff can carry out minor procedures such as the cleaning and checking of wounds or placing intravenous catheters, is invaluable. An examination table is essential and a tub table beneficial in this area.

Animal weighing area

Scales should be available for weighing both inpatients and outpatients; in smaller practices these will usually be shared with and sited in the public areas of the practice. Scales should be easy to use, of a size that will accommodate larger patients, and easily accessible if a patient is non-ambulatory. To ensure accuracy, cat scales or, for the smaller patients, digital kitchen scales can be used, and these are best sited in the ward area.

Kitchen/food preparation area

The inpatient food preparation area (see Figure 7.5) should be easily accessible from the ward and, if possible, should contain:

- A sink, with hot and cold water
- Storage for a variety of foods used regularly, including airtight containers for open dry food
- Storage for tinned food that facilitates stock control
- A refrigerator for fresh foods and partly used tins. A freezer is useful for storing a selection of frozen meats
- A blender (for patients requiring liquidized food) or a supply of liquidized food
- A microwave
- A dishwasher: bowls should be washed by hand first and then on a hot wash in the machine
- Food and water bowls, in suitable storage. Stainless steel bowls are preferred as they are easier to clean and disinfect and, if required, can be autoclaved. A selection of different types of bowl may be useful to satisfy individual patient preferences, particularly for cats
- Scales for correct measurement of food (note that volume measures, such as those supplied by food suppliers, are not sufficiently accurate).

Laundry room

Although outside laundry services are available, and can be useful for washing staff uniforms and bedding, most practices use in-house laundry facilities for ward laundry. Ideally there should be a separate laundry room, and consideration needs to be given to the amount of laundry that will be generated and how dirty laundry/bedding is managed. Where a large quantity of patient bedding is generated, and space allows, industrial machines that include a disinfecting agent such as ozone are preferable (Figure 7.36). Although

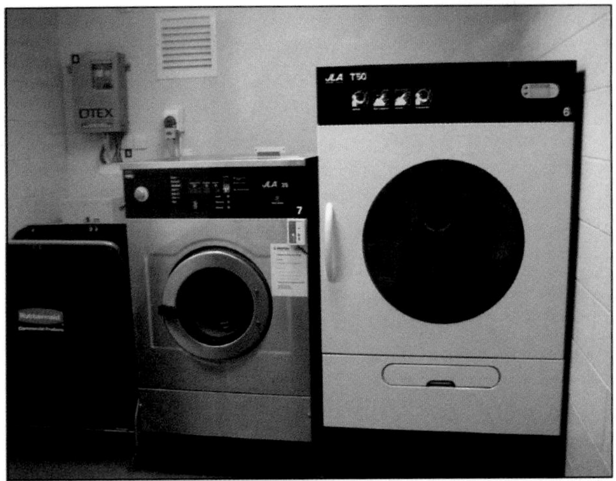

7.36 Large machines that use a disinfecting agent such as ozone are preferable for practices with large quantities of laundry and sufficient space.

initially expensive, ozone disinfection uses cold water, which is cost-effective and environmentally friendly. Alternative methods of processing contaminated bedding would be by way of a commercial or domestic machine using a 90°C wash, or including a measured amount of disinfectant according to manufacturer's instructions. Where veterinary bedding is routinely washed, large-load tumble dryers are advantageous.

The laundry room can also double as a cleaning store/supply room. The room should have non-slip easy to clean flooring and be well ventilated. A sink would be a useful addition to this room, particularly to facilitate washing of hands following handling of contaminated laundry.

Laundry facilities within inpatient areas

Where laundry machines are used within a ward area, machines should be chosen for their quietness and minimal vibration. Many practices manage well with domestic washers and tumble dryers, which can give good service if well maintained. As most do not satisfy water regulations for veterinary practices (see Chapter 2), a separate compliant cold water header tank and pump will usually be necessary. Tumble dryers are best vented to the outside; condenser dryers inevitably raise humidity levels and require more attention. Outside drying facilities or an indoor warm drying area can be beneficial if space allows and will reduce energy consumption.

Cleaning equipment store

Cleaning equipment, such as brushes, brooms, mops and buckets, should be stored in a central or convenient location. Consideration should be given to the provision of separate equipment in each ward area. A low sink can be useful for filling and emptying buckets (see Chapter 3). Safe storage should be available for both in-use bottles and dispensers for cleaning and disinfecting agents, and for any bulk stock.

Grooming and bathing facilities

Grooming is an essential part of the care delivered to inpatients during their stay and appropriate equipment is essential. This should include:

- A suitable table
- A range of brushes and combs, which can be easily cleaned. Different coat types require different equipment (see *BSAVA Textbook of Veterinary Nursing*)
- A bath/shower area (Figure 7.37)
- Drying facilities, such as a wall-mounted dryer (Figure 7.38) or handheld hairdryer.

The bathing area should be easily accessible and non-slip for both patients and staff. It needs to be big enough so that staff using it have room to manoeuvre without reaching or bending in awkward positions that could cause them harm. The area should be easily cleaned afterwards.

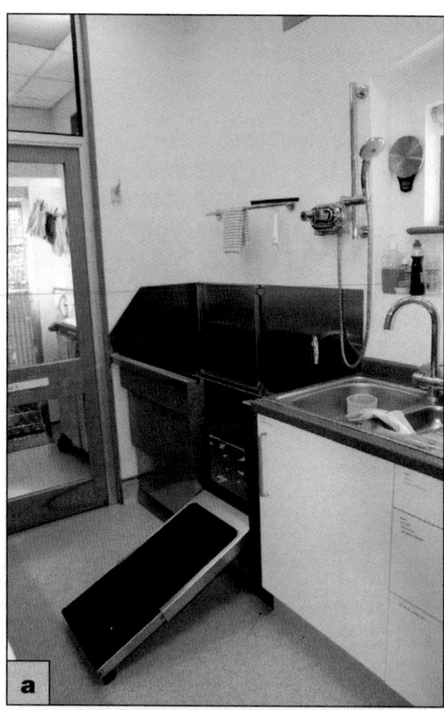

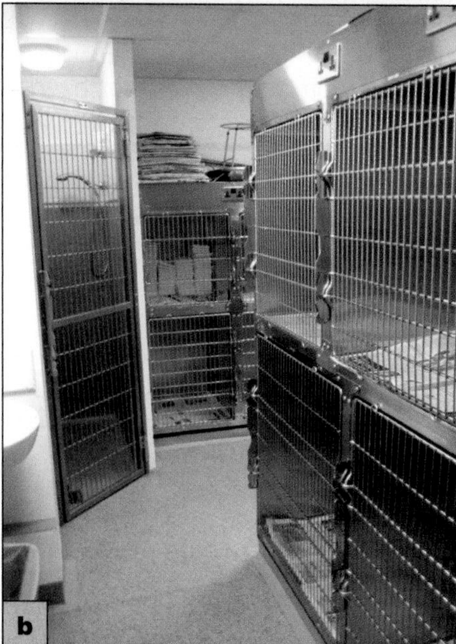

7.37 **(a)** This custom-made dog bath has a non-slip ramp to reduce the need for lifting, and a fold-down platform for showering smaller dogs. **(b)** A shower and drainage can be installed inside a walk-in kennel or wet room if space is at a premium.

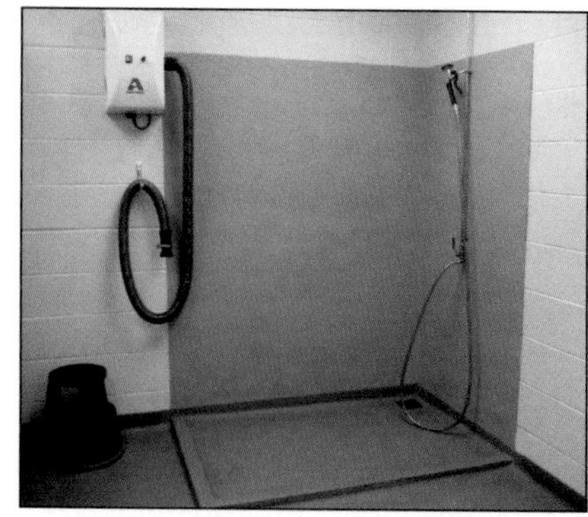

7.38 This purpose-made shower area includes a wall-mounted dryer.

A separate area with raised bath (e.g. a tub table) and/or shower tray unit could be shared with the preparation area or a hydrotherapy unit for larger patients. A large multi-purpose sink can be used for smaller patients.

Physiotherapy and hydrotherapy facilities

Physiotherapy can be beneficial to the treatment of recumbent or recovering patients, and facilities provided will be determined by the type of clinical work carried out in the practice. Depending on the cases seen, an area for physiotherapy might be appropriate, with a selection of floor mats, therapy tables, balls and wobble boards, and specialist equipment such as ultrasound and heating/cooling therapies.

Hydrotherapy can take place in a pool or using an underwater treadmill (Figure 7.39). In both cases, constant supervision by trained staff is essential, and staff costs should be considered as well as the considerable set-up costs of adding or incorporating these facilities in general practice. Underwater treadmills are increasingly seen in veterinary practices with a high orthopaedic caseload. Generally, a dedicated wet room will be needed with space for the filtration and pumping equipment as well as the unit itself. Pools require more space and a changing area for staff.

Further information on physiotherapy and hydrotherapy equipment can be found in the *BSAVA Manual of Canine and Feline Rehabilitation, Supportive and Palliative Care: Case Studies in Patient Management.*

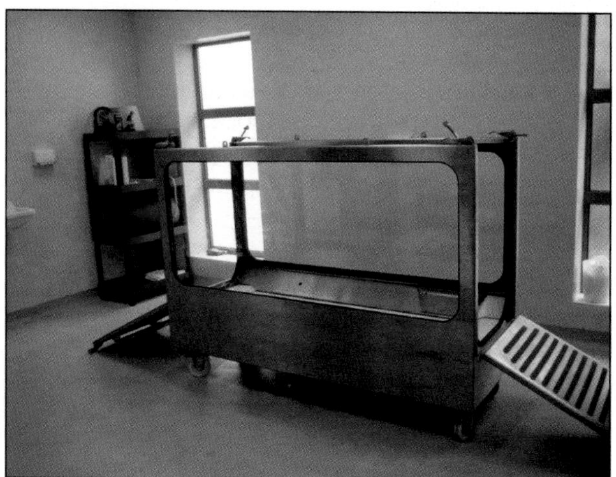

7.39 Underwater treadmills are increasingly seen in practices with a high orthopaedic caseload.

Managing the ward areas

Hygiene and biosecurity

Maintaining biosecurity is essential in all ward and related areas. Particular attention should be paid to:

- Maintenance of the integrity of all surfaces so they remain cleanable
- Keeping work surfaces clear
- Sink and automated equipment available for washing any items that have been in contact with patients
- Designated hand-washing sink with hands-free control in each patient area
- Hand-washing posters (available from www.bsava.com), changed regularly, to act as visual reminders (see Chapter 6)
- Wall-mounted dispensers for gloves and aprons, to encourage use
- Provision of disinfectant hand wipes throughout the practice
- Provision of alcohol gel dispensers
- Each area should have a schedule for cleaning (Figure 7.40)
- Laundering mop heads after each use, or considering disposable ones
- Colour coding of cleaning equipment for different areas of the practice
- Where possible, minimize personal belongings admitted with patients
- Foot-operated bins to prevent hand contamination (Figure 7.41).

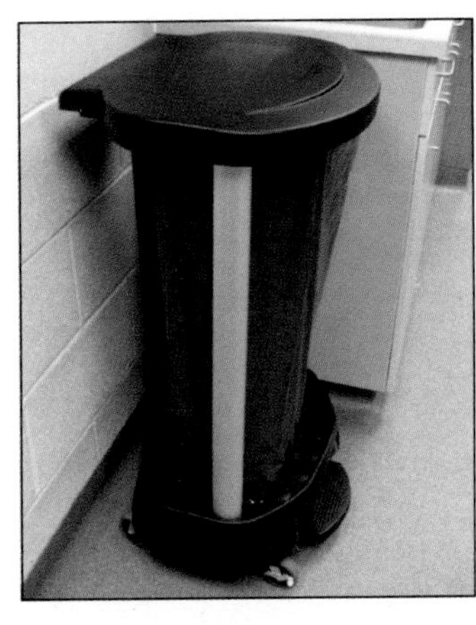

7.41 Bins in ward areas should have hands-free operation such as this mobile, pedal-operated sack bin.

Hand-washing and hand care

The World Health Organization (WHO) has set procedures on hand hygiene in healthcare. Hands should be washed (if necessary) and disinfected:

- Before and after touching a patient
- Before and after touching a patient's surroundings
- Before gloving
- Before any clean or aseptic task
- After any risk of exposure to contaminated fluids or tissues.

It may be necessary for staff to consider washing their hands at intervals *during* a procedure.

Hand-washing facilities should be easily accessible within each ward area, without having to open doors or overcome other barriers. Sinks can be 'automatic',

Date: Week commencing		Monday	Tuesday	Wednesday	Thursday	Friday	Saturday	Sunday
Clean tub table, scales & laundry bin	Daily							
Sweep & mop dishwasher area	Daily							
Clean microwave & fridge	Daily							
Lunchtime sweep & mop	Daily							
Clean phones, keyboards & door handles	Daily							
Empty faecal waste bin	Daily							
Restock fluids	Daily							
Replace pheromone refills	Monthly							
Deep clean ward floors	Weekly							
Fold & tidy isolation scrubs and area	Weekly							
Tidy & clean food & stock areas	Weekly							
Restock paper & inco pads	Weekly							
Clean air-conditioning units	Weekly							
Clean & restock First Aid boxes	Weekly							
Clean walls in ward prep	Weekly							
Clean all doors in wards	Weekly							
Clean medicine pots	Weekly							
Sweep/tidy bin area ROTATE BINS	Weekly							
Recycling rubbish	Weekly							

7.40 Cleaning schedules should be clear and kept in an accessible place so they can be completed immediately. Charts can be pre-printed or laminated and revised as required. More detailed charts can be prepared for new staff and when systems change.

operating via a sensor, or may be activated by foot control, both minimizing cross-contamination between staff. Sinks with elbow taps are an alternative but correct user compliance may be poor. If conventional taps are used they should be disinfected regularly throughout the day. A recommended hand-washing process is available for BSAVA members to access at www.bsava.com, together with a hand-washing poster (Figure 7.42) and video for training and reminding staff of correct procedures.

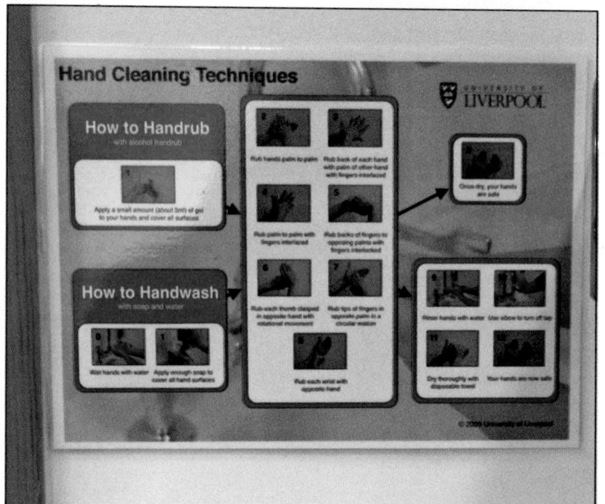

7.42 Hand-washing posters, such as this one produced by the University of Liverpool, are helpful memory aids for staff.

To facilitate training and encourage compliance, products are available that, when applied to hands and viewed under ultraviolet light, act as an invisible marker to demonstrate areas of inappropriate cleaning. To encourage a culture of good practice, staff should be prepared to correct others when poor hand hygiene behaviour is observed.

KEY POINT

Every member of staff has an obligation to their patients and to their colleagues to maintain good hand hygiene.

Hand preparation increases the effectiveness of decontamination:

- Nails should be kept short, clean and polish-free
- Jewellery and wristwatches should be avoided in the clinical area
- Cuts and abrasions should be covered with a waterproof dressing
- Staff should adopt a 'bare below the elbow' rule in all clinical areas of the practice.

Moisturizers and barrier creams may be helpful to maintain healthy skin.

Gloves

'Occupational dermatitis' is recognized as a common condition, which can particularly affect workers in the healthcare sector. It is therefore better to aim to minimize its occurrence rather than treat it once present. The best protection is to avoid direct contact with any chemical or substance that might affect the skin. If this is impossible, gloves can be used to protect the hands. Disposable gloves, in a variety of sizes, located in all clinical areas will also contribute to minimizing the potential spread of infection.

To select and use gloves correctly, it is important to consider the wearer, the workplace conditions and the glove:

- Always select gloves which fit and are suitable for the task
- Use disposable gloves
- Discard gloves immediately if they become damaged or punctured
- Remove contaminated gloves safely so that no contact is made with the contaminant
- Always wash hands before and after wearing gloves
- The use of a barrier cream or moisturiser before and after work is recommended.

If gloves are too large, there is a greater likelihood of contaminants entering them and remaining in contact with the skin; this might even cause greater exposure than if the gloves had not been worn at all. Wearing gloves for extended periods can cause excessive moisture on the skin, which can act as an irritant. An allergic reaction to gloves made of natural rubber (latex) is experienced by some people, as is a reaction to the powder some gloves contain.

KEY POINTS

- If gloves are taken off temporarily, hands could then become contaminated from handling them again and this could transfer infection. It is therefore better practice to dispose of gloves on removal and use a new pair.
- Remember when disposing of gloves that they will be contaminated.

Cleaning and disinfection agents

Cleaning agents and disinfectants must be used at the manufacturer's recommended temperature and dilution rate, and systems must be in place to ensure this. Measuring devices, or plumbed-in automated dispensers can be very useful. Garden-type spray bottles should not be used for dispensing disinfectant solutions, as the nozzles can harbour bacteria and correct dilution is not always achieved. Aerosolization and inhalation of disinfectants can cause discomfort in some staff, and adequate ventilation must be in place whenever disinfectants are used. Solutions should be made up daily.

For day-to-day housekeeping, a detergent made to the correct dilution and the physical act of scrubbing is satisfactory. If disinfectants are used routinely, a detergent should first be used to remove dirt and other organic material, and then the disinfectant applied and allowed to remain in contact with the surface for the required contact time.

Kennel and cage cleaning

A clear protocol must be in place for sweeping, cleaning and disinfecting kennels and cages after occupation, and for cleaning occupied cages. It is not good practice to move patients from one cage to another unless absolutely necessary.

Cleaned and disinfected cages and kennels must be clearly distinguished from those awaiting cleaning or temporarily vacant while a patient is under treatment, in surgery or being exercised. This can be done by clear labelling of the cage door, or using a simple system of, for example, placing the fleece bedding in place upside down in clean cages.

Buckets, brushes, dustpans, vacuum cleaners and mops must all be kept scrupulously clean to prevent the spread of disease. Mopheads can be machine-washed daily.

Laundering bedding

Bedding should first be shaken to remove cat litter, hair and grit; a decontamination area is best for this, but if this is not available bedding can be shaken out inside the individual kennel.

It is vital that washing machines are not overloaded and that they and their filters are regularly descaled if necessary and cleaned. Staff training and a checklist is recommended for maintaining discipline. Regular hot washes in domestic machines, combined with careful use (not over-use) of cleaning and softening agents, will prolong life. Water softeners can be useful. Trolleys or containers for soiled laundry must be kept clean, or disposable bags can be used.

KEY POINT

Theatre clothing and cloth drapes should be washed separately from pet bedding to avoid cross-contamination. Ideally a separate washing machine should be used.

Managing the isolation area

The isolation ward should be prepared and ready for patient admissions at any time of the day.

Details of patients admitted to isolation or barrier-nursed in the wards should be recorded. Where surgical cases are nursed in isolation, keeping a record of bacteriology results may highlight a pattern.

Patients that are unvaccinated, immunosuppressed or receiving cytotoxic medication also require barrier-nursing but may not need to be isolated. These patients could still have colour-coded bedding and leads. In addition, using hospital charts of different colours will act as a visual reminder to highlight to staff the requirement for barrier-nursing. An SOP similar to that discussed below for communal areas would apply.

Admitting potentially infectious cases

If a patient is showing clinical signs of a disease that could be infectious to other patients or is potentially zoonotic (infectious to humans), the animal must be isolated immediately. Practices should have a written policy for dealing with such cases and for commonly seen infectious conditions, such as kennel cough (Figure 7.43), and this should be known to all members of staff.

Dealing with an outbreak of kennel cough

Kennel cough can be caused by Bordetella bronchiseptica or other infectious agents. It is important to recognize an outbreak: this usually starts with an owner reporting a dog coughing on arriving home, or the ward nurse reporting an inpatient coughing.

The following measures should then be taken:

- All dogs housed in the same area as the coughing dog should be treated as if they are infectious
- All these dogs should be barrier-nursed, and all surfaces cleaned and disinfected
- If possible all these dogs should be confined to one area
- New patients should not be associated with these patients
- All staff in contact with infected or suspect dogs must ensure they follow strict hygiene procedures for themselves and their clothing.

To prevent future outbreaks:

- Ask the reception staff to advise all owners coming in with a coughing dog to leave it outside or in the car until the veterinary surgeon is ready to examine it, thus avoiding dog-to-dog contact in the outpatient area. Patients with a suspected infectious cough can then be seen in a designated place or even outside if weather allows
- As far as possible, minimize the number of hospitalized dogs sharing the same airspace, and consider vaccination
- Maintain good biosecurity throughout the inpatient and outpatient areas.

7.43 An example of a practice policy for dealing with an outbreak of kennel cough.

A potentially infectious patient should ideally be admitted directly to isolation and not through the normal outpatient area. If this is not the case, the consulting room that was used for examination of the patient prior to admission, and other common areas of the practice such as the waiting room, should be disinfected as soon as possible after the infected animal has been admitted, in order to minimize the potential for spread of infection.

Nursing potentially infectious cases

The points below can be adapted to create a specific standard operating procedure (SOP) for nursing infectious cases in an individual practice.

- Infectious or potentially infectious cases should be admitted to the isolation ward *[define area]*.
- All patients in this ward must be barrier-nursed at all times, by a limited number of clearly identified staff.
- Details of the type of infectious disease should be communicated to staff with clear instructions for entry.
- The staff should wear distinctive isolation 'scrubs', which can be made available in a different colour from those worn in other parts of the practice.
- Impermeable protective clothing (i.e. disposable long-sleeved gown and gloves) should be worn over the scrubs, and the scrubs should be washed after each visit to the isolation unit. In cooler weather nurses should wear a washable outside coat assigned to each patient, and not their own coats. Ample supplies of protective clothing must be available.
- Protective disposable overshoes should be worn, or shoes should be dipped into a disinfectant footbath at the entrance to the isolation area. The footbath must be regularly maintained or it may become a reservoir for microorganisms.

- Bedding and leads, harnesses, etc., should be designated for isolation patients and colour-coded (see Figure 7.35).
- Disposable bedding and food bowls should be used where possible. Alternatively, all items leaving isolation must be securely bagged before disinfection.
- Use of a hospital chart of a specific colour will enhance visual awareness and act as a reminder that these patients require barrier-nursing.
- The kennel should be cleaned and disinfected with *[enter product and dilution here ...]* as required and at least daily, using a new cleaning cloth which is then disposed of with the kennel waste.
- The floor should be cleaned and disinfected twice a day while the isolation area is in use.
- Protective clothing should be discarded into the kennel waste bag prior to leaving the isolation area.
- All patient, kennel and protective clothing waste should be double-bagged within the isolation area and disposed of according to the veterinary surgeon's risk assessment (see Chapter 3). This may mean segregation as hazardous waste.
- Isolation scrubs must be securely bagged and laundered according to the current disinfection protocol.
- Effective and appropriate disinfectants for the infectious agent suspected should be used for all items. All organic matter must be removed before disinfectants are used.
- Reference should be made to the current COSHH (Control of Substances Hazardous to Health) risk assessment (see Chapter 22) and guidance for infectious and zoonotic microorganisms.

The COSHH risk assessment

Zoonoses are diseases that can be transmitted between animals and humans. The risk assessment should consider the common zoonoses that are likely to be encountered in the ward and isolation area, including infections that can cause gastrointestinal upset (e.g. *Campylobacter*, *Salmonella*, *Escherichia coli*), skin disease (e.g. ringworm) and systemic disease (e.g. toxoplamosis, tuberculosis, rabies (European bat lyssavirus (EBL-2)). All staff should understand the risk and routes of transmission of infectious disease and how to prevent spread of infection. Any additional risk to pregnant workers should be communicated to all staff of childbearing age.

Although patients with a pyothorax are not often isolated, it is recommended that when flushing and draining chest drains, employees wear a mask. Until culture results are available, pathogens and infectious agents will be unknown. Surgical masks are rarely required except in potentially zoonotic cases where infectious aerosols may be inhaled, such as birds with ornithosis, or where tuberculosis is suspected.

Visiting patients in isolation

Visiting of isolated inpatients should be discouraged, although certain consideration needs to be given to those patients who are critically ill. Should an owner need to visit, or want to be present if the patient needs to be euthanased, then they must be made aware of the infection control protocols with regards to barrier-nursing – whilst still being treated sensitively.

Isolating patients in a communal ward area

If purpose-built isolation is not available, infectious patients should only be admitted where absolutely necessary, and must be barrier-nursed in wards using a strict technique. An SOP must be in place, even if a policy of non-admission is maintained, as there will always be situations where a patient has to be admitted on welfare grounds or where a patient starts to show signs of infectious disease some time after admission.

The SOP for barrier-nursing in communal ward areas should cover the following:

- House the patient as far away as possible from other inpatients and in an area that is not crossed by staff or patients *en route* to other areas
- Use signs and floor markings to highlight an isolated case (Figure 7.44)
- Protective clothing must be worn by any member of staff when handling the patient. Protective clothing should be a disposable long-sleeved apron and gloves
- Disinfect the entire area regularly throughout the day
- Ensure the patient has its own equipment, food bowls, thermometer and stethoscope
- Where specific isolation nurses are not available, the patient should be the last patient to be handled, and the examination area must be disinfected immediately afterwards
- Disposable bedding must be used, or laundry should be dealt with immediately and washed and disinfected separately from other bedding
- Disinfect outside exercise areas immediately after use
- Dispose of all waste according to risk assessment in separate secure bags.

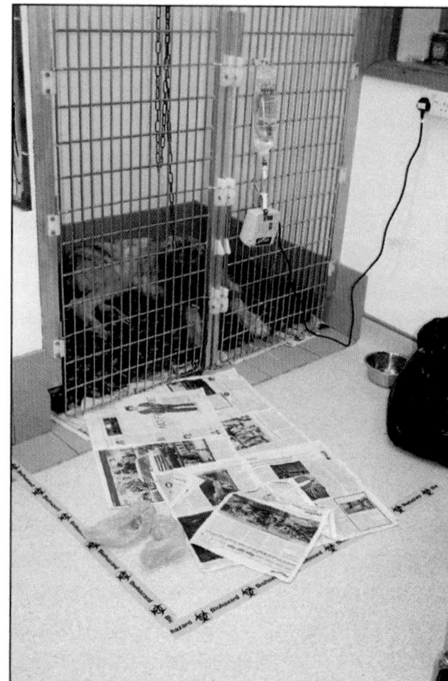

7.44 Barrier-nursing a patient in a communal area is always a challenge and a compromise, but a clear protocol and demarcation of the area helps.

Discharge from isolation

On discharge, the patient should be taken out of the isolation exit and straight to the client's car, avoiding the waiting room. Owners should be informed if the patient could still be shedding microorganisms, so that they can minimize risk to other pets and to people.

The isolation unit and all equipment must be thoroughly cleaned, using a detergent, and allowed to air-dry before being cleaned with a disinfectant at the approved dilution for the agent involved. Reusable equipment must be sterilized if appropriate. The isolation area should then be prepared ready for the next admission.

Animal handling

Instructions should be set for restraint of animals and followed by all staff. Commonly used restraint equipment is illustrated in Chapter 6.

Dogs

Leads, collars and harnesses

Dogs should be restrained appropriately by slip leads or a well fitted collar and lead. There should be an agreed level of restraint for walking dogs in an unsecured area, including the practice policy on leads, harnesses and collars and whether double restraint is necessary. Clear identification must be in place. Two people will be needed to exercise strong, lively or aggressive dogs. Even dogs such as a Labrador can be strong enough to pull someone over, especially if it is wet or icy.

Harnesses: Some patients may need to be exercised on a harness during their stay. Harnesses can slip, however, especially if the patient backs up; it is therefore advisable to use a system of double leads and to have a slip lead on the patient for security (Figure 7.45); there will be no tension on this lead unless the patient escapes from the harness, thereby allowing the handler to remain in control.

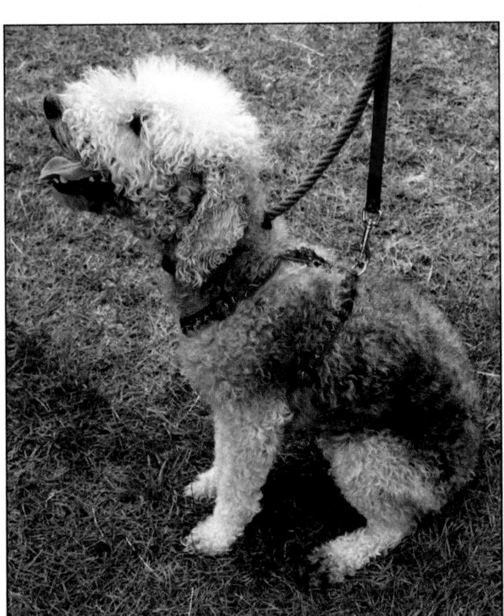

7.45 A dog that requires a harness for exercising should also wear a neck lead to ensure maximum safety.

Leads: The type of lead to be used in the practice should be considered, as this may differ from that normally used by the owner. It is imperative that the handler in the practice has complete control while exercising the dog. Worn correctly, a slip lead will tighten around the patient's neck should it start to struggle; worn incorrectly, the lead may well slip over the patient's head. Extendable leads have their place in practice, such as when exercising a dog that is not used to toileting on the lead; however, they can be very thin and are not always advisable for a boisterous dog.

Collars: Where collars are used, they should be adjusted to fit correctly on admission, so they cannot slip over the dog's head.

Aggressive dogs

Suitable muzzles should be used if temperament is doubtful and dogs should be sedated where appropriate. In extreme circumstances, the use of a 'dog catcher' (see Chapter 6) may be required. An experienced member of staff should handle this patient.

KEY POINT

Under no circumstances should risks be taken when dealing with potentially aggressive animals.

Cats

Disinfected wire baskets should always be used to transport a cat, even if it is unconscious. Cats should be sedated where appropriate. A crush cage can be used in extreme cases and, if absolutely necessary, a 'cat catcher' (see Chapter 6). Difficult or frightened cats should only be handled by experienced personnel. Care should be taken to avoid cats becoming upset by seeing or hearing other cats and dogs. In particular, if species are separated, dogs should not enter a cat ward, and changing clothing after handling dogs should be considered prior to handling cats. Pheromone diffusers can be helpful to reduce stress (see earlier).

Other species

Nursing staff should be confident and familiar with handling all the species normally hospitalized by the practice. Where species are handled infrequently, individuals with more experience could be assigned to nurse those cases. The *BSAVA Manual of Exotic Pets* is a useful resource.

Manual handling

Working in the wards inevitably means a lot of bending down, and lifting and moving large or difficult patients. Appropriate manual handling aids, such as stretchers and trolleys, should be available and used. Manual handling guidance and training should be given to all staff, to cover the following areas:

- Lifting and team lifting
- Pushing and pulling
- Assisted walking for inpatients
- The use of trolleys and stretchers
- Transferring patients from trolley to table
- Transporting the recumbent or unconscious patient
- Patient restraint for various procedures
- Working with high-level kennels, steps (Figure 7.46) and step stools.

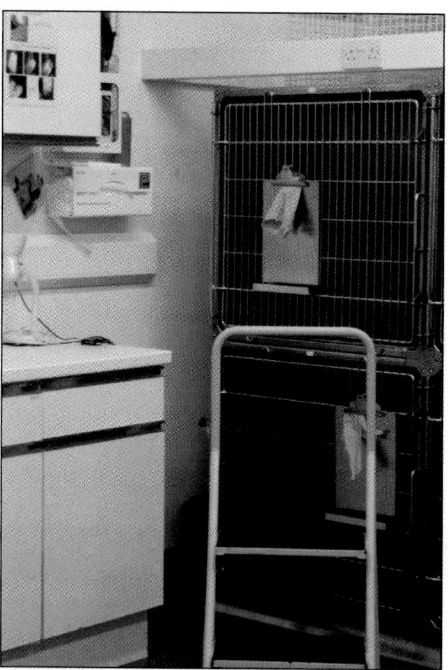

7.46 Where animals or equipment are to be handled at a high level, a risk assessment should be in place. Secure steps with a handrail should be used. These should be non-slip, checked regularly and maintained in good condition.

Nursing team management

The team approach to providing veterinary care for patients will undoubtedly result in smoother and shorter recovery periods. The care of hospitalized patients is the responsibility of the veterinary nurse, under the direction of the veterinary surgeon. Good planning and time management help to ensure that veterinary nurses and their nursing team have time to plan and adapt individual care, monitor vital signs, exercise, feed (Figure 7.47) and medicate the patients, and communicate effectively with the owner.

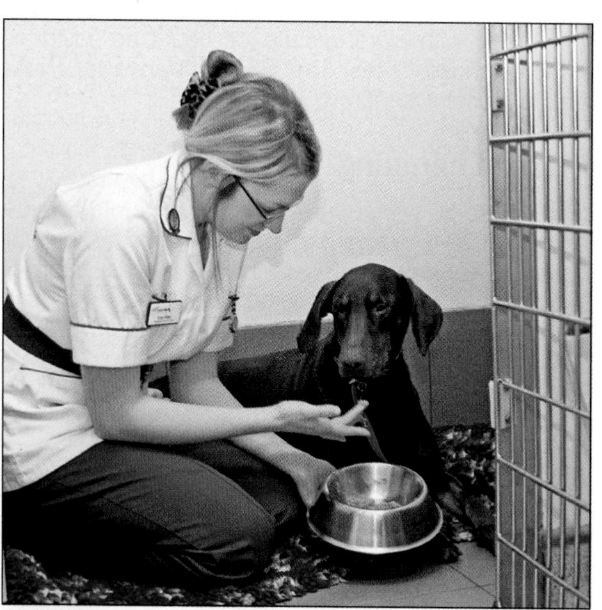

7.47 Nurses must have sufficient time to support patients with feeding, and to plan and adapt individual care.

Continuity of care

Where possible, nursing shifts should be planned to enable the same veterinary nurses to be in charge of the ward environment for a period of time, in order that they may get to know their patients and gain their trust. This also enables the nurse to build a relationship with the client, and is particularly helpful for student nurses completing case assignments.

KEY POINTS

- It is important that the client is made aware of how to contact the nurse who is caring for their pet.
- Written comments should be made regarding all contact with owners, recording how the update was received, and ensuring that comments are initialled by the member of staff who took or made the call.

Ward rounds

Time should be put aside, by means of daily 'rounds', to enable the veterinary surgeons and nurses to share information about the inpatients and to plan appropriate care. This should ideally happen at the beginning of the day, before staff telephone clients with an update regarding their pet, and also at any times when care of patients is handed over to other clinicians or nursing staff.

At the morning rounds with the ward nurses, a care plan (see later) should be agreed for each patient for that day. The veterinary surgeon should give clear concise instructions of what is expected for each patient, and the veterinary nurses should use this opportunity to express concerns, giving their thoughts on how the care plan might be amended with regard to nursing interventions.

Admitting patients

The issue of client consent is discussed in Chapter 21.

Admission questionnaires and client support materials

Before a planned admission, the client should be asked to fill out a questionnaire about their pet (see examples at the end of this chapter). This can help the ward staff in planning appropriate nursing care and making the patients feel less anxious. In terms of customer care this is invaluable, as it also indicates to the client the level of care that the practice is delivering in order to make their pet feel more content in their altered environment.

A variety of support material, such as admission information and postoperative care sheets designed to hand out to clients, should be used as required. This can be provided as preprinted booklets or leaflets, in letter format or as a merged document with specifics added in directly from the computer by the nurse or clinician according to individual needs. Information must be reviewed and updated regularly. Suggested items to consider in written client information on or before surgical admission are given in Figure 7.48. It is important to indicate to the owner the level of care the patient will receive, particularly outside normal working hours.

Procedure and anaesthesia
■ Explanatory information ■ Safety issues ■ Risks ■ Ongoing care needed ■ Reassurance ■ Invitation to ask further questions ■ Expected costs (estimate), what is and is not covered (e.g. consultations, check-ups, complications) ■ Payment arrangements (when and how), insurance claim arrangements
What to do before admission
■ Feeding and water instructions ■ Toileting ■ Any specific preparation ■ Things to bring with the pet ■ Things to have ready at home for recovery ■ Lead/collar/harness, bedding, toys, etc. ■ Instructions for current medication (give or withhold before admission) ■ Pre-anaesthetic blood tests if suggested
Arrangements for admission
■ Where to come and when ■ Preview of consent form ■ Any arrangements for pets kept together (e.g. joint admission and hospitalization)
What happens on the day
■ Timings – procedure, recovery and expected collection ■ What actually will happen ■ Who will be caring for the pet? – named surgeon and nurses if possible ■ Contact phone number, best times to call ■ Possibility of alternative contact methods, e.g. e-mail, SMS text ■ Arrangements for overnight and level of care if applicable ■ Visiting arrangements

7.48 Items to consider when writing client support materials for use before a planned surgical admission.

Patient identification

Security and identification of patients is essential, and patients should be clearly identified on admission to the practice. Practices may seek to rely on keeping the patient's notes with the animal, secured to the cage or in a linked file, but mistakes can be made.

Disposable patient identification collars can be purchased for use around the patient's neck (or hock, depending on the reason for admission). They should be clearly labelled with:

- Name of the animal
- Practice name
- Practice phone number.

> **KEY POINT**
>
> Thought should always be given to the worst-case scenario – were a patient to escape from the practice, would it be identifiable?

Possessions

The practice should have clear guidelines regarding allowing owners to leave personal belongings. During procedures, collars are likely to be removed and could then be misplaced. Beds will get soiled and then could be misplaced during the laundry process. On the other hand, patients may be less stressed when hospitalized with familiar items.

- It is important that if a possession comes into the practice with the patient it is correctly labelled. The client is paying for a professional service and will expect the practice to take care of all belongings.
- If cat carriers are admitted with inpatients, practices should consider space requirements and whether carriers can be stored with adequate biosecurity.

Admissions for surgical procedures

Consideration should be given to provision of drinking water to patients, particularly if surgery is delayed, and veterinary instructions regarding withholding of food and water should be followed, as species needs vary.

The veterinary surgeon may discuss with owners of certain long- or heavy-coated breeds the benefits of arranging for the patient to be professionally bathed and clipped before admission for elective surgeries. This may reduce infection risks and also the time the patient is under anaesthesia.

> **KEY POINT**
>
> Permission for cutting or clipping hair for a procedure should be obtained from the owner.

Pre-anaesthetic health checks should be recorded in the patient notes or anaesthetic record. Following premedication all species of patient should be monitored closely and appropriate bedding provided to prevent hypothermia.

Recording patient weight

Any patient admitted for anaesthesia must have an accurate weight recorded. However, it is beneficial to have a recorded weight for all patients at each visit to the practice. Inpatient weight should be recorded daily and scales should be checked regularly for accuracy.

The practice should have a standardized system for assessing and recording body condition score (BCS); clear guidance on the system used should be available everywhere animals are weighed and assessed. It is good practice to record basic parameters (temperature, pulse and respiration rate) on admission.

Formulating a care plan

It is important that carers understand what preserves life and provides comfort for patients, and that they can systematically assess each patient as an individual and cater for that individual's needs. A good care plan should address these points and prevent further problems from developing.

> **KEY POINT**
>
> A holistic approach to patient care is required, focusing on all of the patient's needs and not just the medical aspects of its care (see *BSAVA Manual of Canine and Feline Rehabilitation, Supportive and Palliative Care: Case Studies in Patient Management*).

Ability areas to consider in formulating a simple care plan	Possible interventions
Ability to eat	Encouragement, feeding tube, syringe feeding
Ability to drink	Encouragement, intravenous fluids, feeding tube
Ability to breathe	Ventilation, oxygen therapy, rest
Ability to hear	Guidance, reassurance, calm environment
Ability to see	Guidance, reassurance, calm environment
Ability to maintain body temperature (stay warm or cool)	Warming, cooling, insulation
Ability to move	Regular turning, physiotherapy
Ability to groom and keep clean	Bathing and drying, brushing and coat care
Ability to urinate and defecate normally	Opportunity to toilet, catheterization, enemas
Ability to behave normally	Interaction, removal of fear triggers, routine
Ability to relax and sleep	Opportunity for sleep (e.g. timing of medication), comfort

7.49 Care planning: areas for nursing support or intervention. These areas need to be considered in the context of the animal's normal lifestyle and in its current condition as a sick patient. For example, does a patient normally only drink water from a running source, and what is its normal intake?

Such a holistic approach to care is taught to student nurses during their training. Whereas the veterinary surgeon will, in general, take a disease- and medicine-focused approach to history taking and planning care, the nurse can gather more information from the client and from patient observation to support this holistic approach and can tailor nursing support to the individual animal and its particular needs. It is also vital that staff continue to communicate with owners throughout the patient's stay, asking relevant 'open questions' regarding their pet. This will assist the staff in updating the care plans.

Nursing models and care planning are huge topics beyond the scope of this book, and are well covered in modern textbooks of both human and veterinary nursing. Practices should develop their own care plans and supporting documentation to ensure that the necessary information is gathered, and that it is acted upon and communicated within the veterinary and nursing teams. To illustrate the issues, examples of areas to consider in care planning are summarized above in Figure 7.49.

Calculating energy requirements

A patient's basic energy requirements (resting energy requirement, RER) should be calculated on admission, using standard formulae. The use of a feeding chart enables staff to demonstrate clearly how much food has been consumed by the patient and provides an objective assessment of how well a patient is eating; an example is given at the end of this chapter.

Admitting patients from surgery – case handover

Each surgical patient will require a care plan for their recovery period, highlighting any potential problems envisaged. Thought should be given to species, breed, size, weight, age, patient compliance and any pre-existing conditions.

The severity of an elective procedure will be known in advance, so in these cases veterinary surgeons and nurses can prepare requirements for recovery. By their nature, emergency surgeries cannot be planned for, but having a designated recovery room/space will enable nursing staff to accommodate cases at short notice.

- It is essential that the surgical nurse gives a clear and detailed verbal handover to the recovery/ward nurse, in addition to ensuring that clear written instructions have been recorded.
- Information should be obtained from the veterinary surgeon regarding details of the procedure, medication used and prescribed, and instructions regarding intravenous fluids, analgesia, drains, wound management and feeding.
- A clear postoperative recovery plan should be written on the patient's hospitalization sheets, and all anaesthetic records should be complete before the surgical nurse leaves the recovery area.

The ward nurse should record the time the patient returned to the recovery area and include information regarding temperature, pulse and respiration, and how responsive the patient is. The patient should be closely observed and clinical parameters should be monitored until the patient is ready to return to the main ward (Figure 7.50). The frequency of monitoring will depend on the patient and procedure. Observation should continue until the patient is able to move around the cage in a controlled manner.

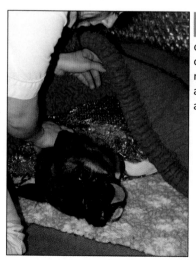

7.50 The patient should be closely observed and clinical parameters monitored until it is able to move around in a controlled manner.

Inpatient care

The level of care and frequency of nursing interventions will be decided by the clinical team, communicated in the care plan, and recorded in detail in the hospitalization records.

> **KEY POINT**
>
> Close observation of all patients is essential to assess whether they are comfortable in their accommodation or whether adjustments (e.g. different bedding) or further enrichment (e.g. toys) are needed.

Hospitalization records

The type of cases the practice routinely admits will determine the style of the hospital record sheets and the level of information recorded. Examples of hospital charts are given at the end of this chapter.

Staff should record appropriate information in a professional manner. **It is vitally important that any persons coming into the ward environment should be able to read the kennel sheet and care plan and continue care of that patient.**

- The patient details should be clear and include name, owner's surname, gender, breed, weight, identification to the practice (case number), contact phone numbers for the owners, and date.
- The responsible veterinary surgeon and nurse for each day should be made clear (Figure 7.51).
- It may be helpful to make the gender of the patient clear on the records to avoid errors (him/her) when talking to clients, particularly where the pet name gives no clues.
- The reason for admission and the basic care plan should be clear.
- Patient observations should be recorded at the time, along with the identification of the observing nurse.
- The timing of all staff interventions and procedures carried out and medications administered should be recorded and these actions initialled. Medication instructions should also carry the initials of the prescribing veterinary surgeon.

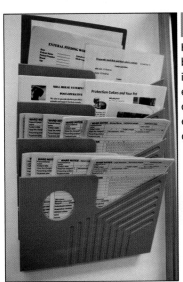

7.51 Hospitalization forms can be designed and printed in house. In this rack, each clinician has forms of a different colour for easy identification of case responsibility.

- All procedures and consumable items used should be recorded, so that the owner can be invoiced accordingly; each practice will develop its own system. A separate charge sheet could be used for each patient on a daily basis, and staff can list chargeable items and procedures, which can then be itemized on the client's invoice. It may also be worthwhile asking a senior member of staff to check the price sheets against the hospitalization sheets on a daily basis to ensure that all consumables have been charged for.

Fluid therapy must be recorded clearly in the hospitalization record. A specific fluid therapy chart and calculation aid may be helpful for recording and planning intravenous fluid therapy.

> **KEY POINT**
>
> It should be noted that hospital charts can be construed as legal documents and that they may be used as evidence of the care provided. An owner may request copies of such documents should there be a complaint regarding the care their pet has received.

Prominent coloured alert or reminder labels (Figure 7.52) are useful for hospitalization records or to label patient accommodation.

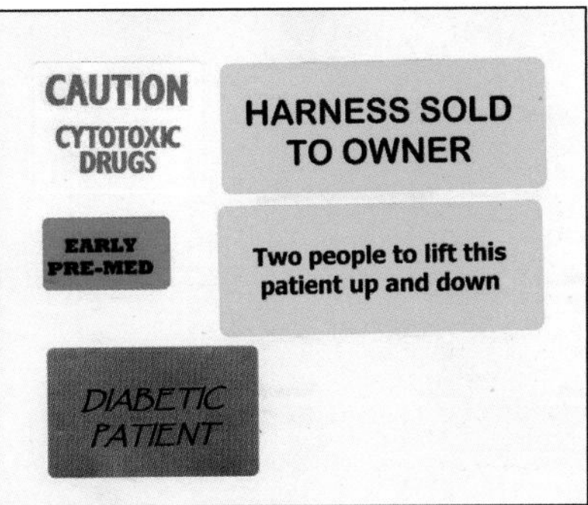

7.52 Coloured alert or reminder labels can be helpful on hospitalization records and accommodation.

Grooming

Grooming keeps the patient clean and enables nursing staff to inspect any bony prominences, skin folds, eyes and ears for early recognition of potential problems. Grooming and spending time with the patient will also build the nurse–patient relationship, aiding recovery. It is beneficial to have connections with a professional groomer, as certain cases may need above-average care. The practice must be aware that permission from the owner will need to be obtained and in some cases the owner may prefer to use the groomer of their choice. Grooming equipment should be kept clean and in good condition.

Bathing is often necessary (Figure 7.53) and convenient showering, bathing and drying facilities for all sizes of patient make the job easier (Figure 7.54). Owners very much appreciate their pet returning home clean and smelling fresh. Care should be taken to avoid slipping on wet floors in and around bathing areas. Non-slip flooring and washable absorbent mats are helpful.

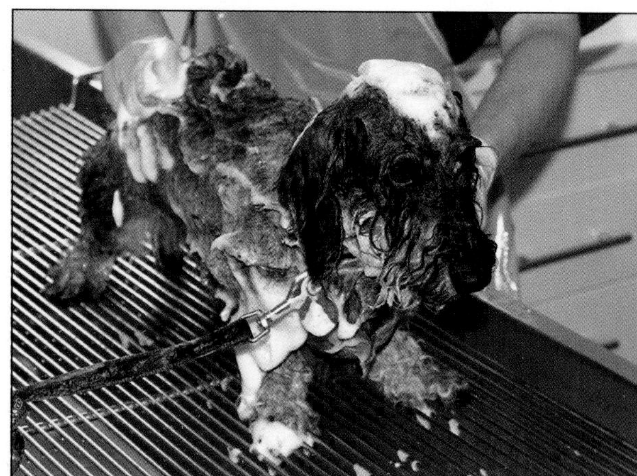

7.53 Bathing a patient when necessary is an integral part of patient care. Gloves should always be worn when bathing patients.

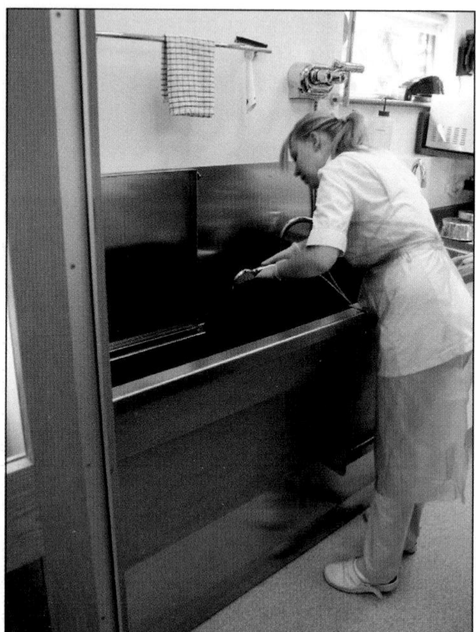

7.54 A raised dog bath minimizes bending and makes bathing easier.

Overnight care

Different practices offer different levels of care for patients overnight. This can range from no in-house hospitalization, or care via a third-party provider, to 24-hour in-house nursing care. The level of care and supervision offered by the practice regarding pets kept in overnight must be clearly communicated to clients, who otherwise may make incorrect assumptions. Information on out-of-hours care can be included in a practice information leaflet or on the practice website.

> **KEY POINT**
>
> It is imperative that the client knows the level of care their pet will be receiving, which will be determined by the veterinary surgeon according to the clinical needs of the patient and where the patient is hospitalized.

It is essential that inpatients receive appropriate care, but they must also have an opportunity to sleep; so lighting and noise levels should be considered. The use of CCTV, web or network cameras enables staff to monitor patients while not having to enter the kennel environment. Simple network cameras can be connected to the wireless or cabled network and fixed to a drip stand to allow observation of particular patients (Figure 7.55). Models that work in low light and can also record sound are beneficial.

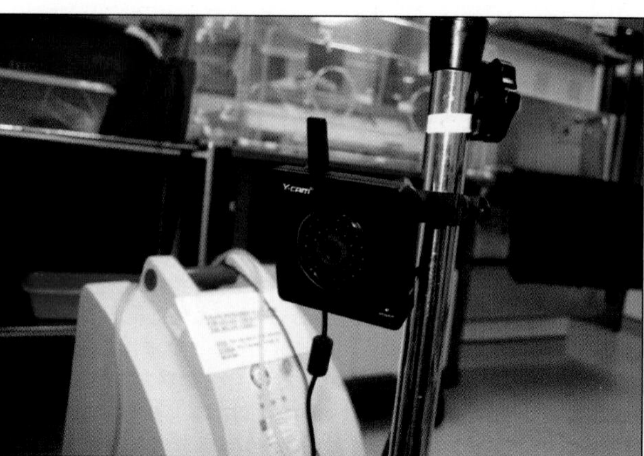

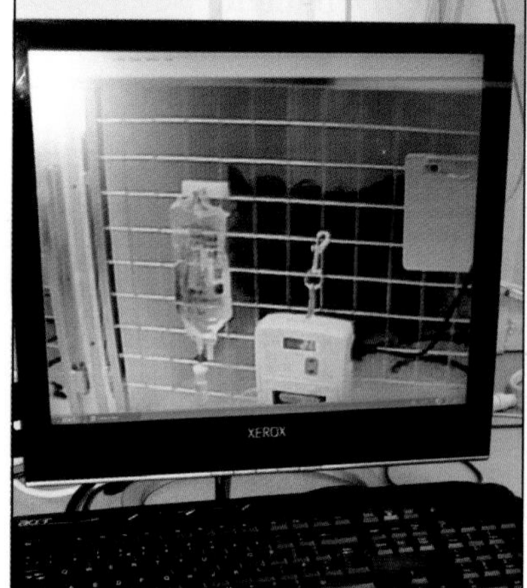

7.55 Remote observation. A camera can be attached to a drip stand and moved to the best position to observe the patient. The patient can then be observed throughout the building on any networked computer.

Any hospitalized patient will require checking on at intervals during the night. It is advisable to have written guidelines regarding what is expected of the clinical team during a night shift. For example:

- Frequency of checks and procedure for calling a veterinary surgeon if appropriate
- Communication with the client
- Regular comments should be recorded and initialled on the patient's hospitalization sheets
- Ambulatory dogs, especially those that are polydipsic, should be taken outside to allow them the opportunity to pass urine or faeces
- Staff must ensure patients receive relevant medication, including analgesia, and that intravenous fluids are running
- Although patients often eat when alone, their food should be removed during the night so that it does not become stale
- Responsibility for general tidiness and cleanliness
- Care and maintenance of equipment – what must be kept ready at all times.

An example of a 24-hour routine is given in Figure 7.56.

7.00 am	Early staff arrive. Night staff hand over to early staff, giving relevant information regarding each inpatient. Early staff continue to exercise the patients, measure TPR, check dressings and wounds, re-dress and flush intravenous catheters.
8.00	Start to feed and medicate the patients.
8.30	Morning rounds: veterinary nurses and veterinary surgeons.
9.00	Clinical team phone owners to update them on their pet's progress.
10.00	Finish feeding and medicating. Start physiotherapy sessions, bathing, grooming and administering premedicant drugs to patients as required. Administer medications at relevant times throughout the day.
11.00	Start walking out the dogs and grooming the cats. Receive any patients back from procedures and monitor their recovery. Discharging inpatients may be required.
11.30	Start nurses' breaks on a rota system. Cover for colleagues on breaks.
12.30 pm	Lunchtime feeds for the patients.
	Late shift nurses start their shift. Begin by doing the inpatient kennel sheets for the next day.
1.30	Early nurses hand over their patients to the evening nurses.
2.00	Afternoon walking out starts and is finished before the early nurses go home.
3.00	Early nurses' shift ends. Late nurses continue to medicate, take patients back from procedures, spend time with the patients and discharge patients going home.
5.00	Start nurses' breaks on a rota system. Cover for colleagues on breaks.
6.00	Start feeding and medicating inpatients.
7.00	Continue general inpatient care.
7.30	Start walking out the dogs. Flush intravenous catheters and check dressings.
8.30	Night staff start their shift. Late nurses start to hand over their inpatients, giving relevant information. While waiting to hand over patients, they need to do general housekeeping tasks, [a] ensuring they leave kennels in a clean and tidy state.
9.00	Late nurses leave. Night staff takes control, administering medication at the times needed.
10.00	General housekeeping duties. [a] Ensure wards are quiet and darkened to enable patients to get some rest.
11.00	Check inpatients and perform appropriate tasks.
Midnight	Night staff take their breaks on a rota system. Cover for colleagues on breaks.
1.00 am	Check inpatients and perform appropriate tasks. Patients on fluids or those with PU/PD will require an opportunity to pass urine.
2.00	General housekeeping duties. [a]
3.00	Check inpatients and perform appropriate tasks.
4.00	Night staff take another break. Cover for colleagues on breaks.
5.00	Checks as above. Once finished, start to walk out the dogs, clean kennels and give clean bedding. Measure TPR and check wounds and dressings. Get the ward ready for the early staff.

7.56 Example of a plan for day and night shift tasks. [a] Housekeeping duties include laundry, stocking up, checking the consulting rooms, and other duties that the practice requires.

Night staff

Night nursing staff should be able to access staff accommodation without going outside, and consideration should be given to ensuring that overnight accommodation is clean, comfortable and that suitable bedding and washing facilities are available. Cooking facilities and food refrigeration facilities may also need to be provided (see Chapter 16).

All staff should have regular training regarding fire safety procedures. Fire alarms must sound in the accommodation should a fire be detected in the clinical areas of the practice. As well as a fire risk assessment, an evacuation plan should have been considered for lone workers so that they do not put their lives at risk attempting to evacuate patients. Adequate zoning and fire doors should minimize risk to staff and patients.

The safety of the staff working the night shift, or lone working at any time, is paramount. Special consideration should be given to the compromise between the ideal patient care and medication plan and the limitations of the duty staff, as determined by skills and risk assessment, particularly if a lone worker is responsible (see Chapters 16 and 22 for more details). Adequate time must be allowed for in-shift changes, for complete handover of each case from the night staff to the day staff, and *vice versa*.

Managing the intensive care unit

The ICU must be kept clean, stocked and ready for use at any point of the day or night.

The patients within an ICU require 24-hour observation and care, and may constitute either medical or surgical emergencies. The room needs to be adaptable should more than one patient be admitted or if different species require intensive care at the same time. Space should be sufficient for the patient and the nursing staff to remain comfortable during long periods of observation and treatment, and equipment, consumable and medication stocks must be adequate to support the care provided without having to leave the unit. Thought should be given as to whether adequate and appropriate intensive care can be provided in house, or whether this service is better delivered by an outside provider. Nurses working in intensive care must be relieved regularly for rest breaks, but effective handover is essential for case continuity. It must be easy for the nurse to call for extra help when required.

Inpatient protocols

It is imperative that all staff know the practice protocols and where to find the SOP manual. This ensures that all members of staff approach every task in the same way and that there is consistency in dealing with situations and scenarios. Some SOPs may seem simple, but a new member of staff may be unfamiliar with procedures and a manual will help. The SOP manual should be regularly checked and updated, and used each time for induction of new staff. Rules should be set, and kept by every member of staff.

Examples of clinical and non-clinical ward procedures for which an SOP could be helpful are:

- Storage and use of Controlled Drugs
- Kennel cleaning (ensure different sort of kennels and isolation have been taken into account, including small mammal/reptile housing)
- Walking patients outside
- Nursing patients on cytotoxic medication
- Administering different types of medication
- Placement and maintenance of a peripheral intravenous catheter
- Care of a central catheter
- Taking a jugular blood sample
- Placement and maintenance of an indwelling urinary catheter
- Management of the patient with a thoracic drain
- Management of the patient with a wound drain
- Management of the patient with a tracheostomy tube
- Management of feeding tubes.

Communicating with owners of inpatients

Having a set time at which owners are asked to telephone for a progress report may work in some practices, especially where large numbers of cases are hospitalized. Other practices may elect to call their owners with an update at an agreed time, thus allowing the veterinary surgeon and nurse time to communicate regarding the daily patient care plan. In terms of client care and best use of staff time, this is preferable to the client having to telephone the practice for an update, particularly as duty staff may be attending to another patient when the call comes in.

KEY POINTS

- Time should be set aside for staff to contact clients and this should be taken into consideration when planning shift patterns.
- Owners of critically ill patients will require more frequent updates.

The practice may consider having a designated telephone line or number for the ward area nurse(s), which could divert to the main practice number or an answering machine to take a message should the ward nurse be unavailable. A mobile phone or handset could also be useful. Some clients may prefer e-mail or text, particularly if they are at work or out and about. The client should be asked what form of contact would be most appropriate when their pet is admitted.

Staff who answer the phones should have a list showing the inpatients' names, the veterinary surgeon in charge of the case, and who will be speaking to the client. This is especially important when staff have planned leave; a clear precise handover and summary of the case needs to be given to the veterinary surgeon taking over the case, and owners need to be made aware of the change in case responsibility.

KEY POINT

It should be standard practice that all inpatient enquiries are passed on to a member of the clinical team, and ideally a member of staff that has been attending to the patient. It is unprofessional to ask the receptionist to relay an update back to the client, even if it is good news, all is well and a discharge appointment just needs to be booked. Inevitably clients are worried, will want more details and will have further questions which a non-clinical member of the team may not be in a position to answer.

Although the veterinary surgeon and/or nurse will have spoken to the client throughout the day, the night nurse might make an unplanned call to the owners of patients that have had surgery that day, in order to give progress reports.

Visiting

A consistent visiting policy should be in place, preferably meeting owners' expectations for access to their pet. The guidelines should be clear regarding visiting times, and should take into account that clients are anxious and worried and therefore will need frequent reassurance regarding their pet's progress. Ideally, visiting times should be at a mutually convenient time. The patient will often benefit from a visit (Figure 7.57), though on occasions visits can be detrimental if the patient becomes more anxious once the owners leave. In this event the issue should be discussed with the owner in a professional manner.

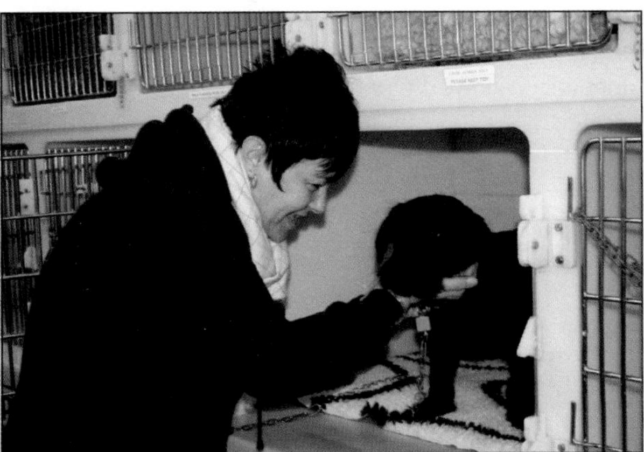

7.57 Where possible, owners should not be discouraged from visiting their pets, and wards should be managed to accommodate this.

KEY POINT

- At all times the client should be aware of who is in charge of the care for their pet, the level of care their patient is receiving day and night, and how to contact the vet or nurse. If possible this should also be provided in written form.
- The client should be kept aware of the ongoing account for the services provided, so that fees are not a surprise.

Discharging patients

For all patients being discharged, an effort should be made to ensure that they go home clean and smelling pleasant. It is unacceptable for a patient to be discharged with dirty eyes or with faecal matter attached to its coat, and this will not go unnoticed by the owner. Removable dressings should be taken off and the patient examined thoroughly before discharge. Owners of patients that have a poor temperament tend to understand if the patient's coat has not been kept up to the owner's standards while hospitalized, but an explanation is usually helpful. Any such conversation should be recorded in the patient's notes.

Patients may be discharged by the veterinary surgeon or nurse, according to practice policy and the individual case. It is often best to discuss treatments, findings and ongoing care without the patient present, to prevent distraction (Figure 7.58).

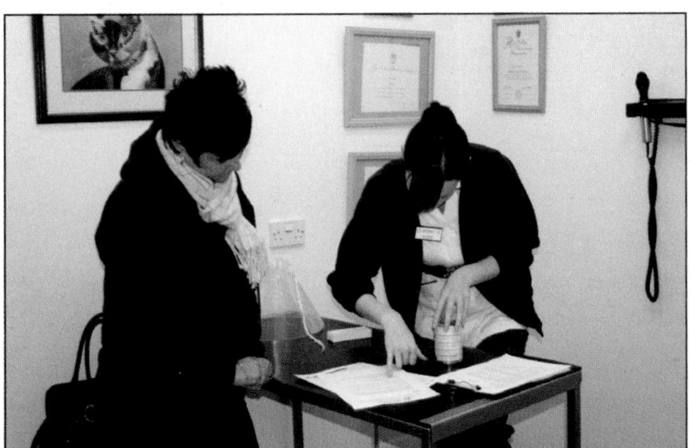

7.58 Discharge explanations and instructions should not be rushed, and should be supported by written materials which should be explained. It is often better if the patient is not present.

Clear explanations should be supported by written materials to take home and clear instructions should be given for medications and specific homecare (Figure 7.59). A follow-up appointment should always be made to check progress and the practice telephone number and a contact name should be given in case the client has any further questions.

- Procedure and anaesthesia:
  - Explanatory information of what has been done
  - Explanation of clipped areas, sutures, etc.
  - Any available results
  - Additional unexpected issues
- Expected progress of recovery
- Common complications or problems to look for
- Medications: what they are; how often and when to give
- Protection collar guidance (if applicable); other aids for preventing wound interference
- How to recognize pain at home and what to do/whom to call
- Emergency and non-emergency team contact numbers
- Any results awaited (e.g. histopathology) and expected timescale and route of contact
- Exercise, feeding and drinking guidance
- Reassurance
- Follow-up appointment schedule

7.59 Items to consider when writing client support materials relating to discharge.

Follow-up

Another added-value service that is appreciated by clients, benefits clinicians and nurses, and improves patient care is the next-day call. Phoning owners the day after discharge to see how things are going is a very positive way to make sure discharge instructions were clear, that the patient is doing well and that no further action is needed before the next re-examination.

A set format should be established for the call to include:

- Enquiring after demeanour, eating, drinking and elimination
- Asking whether medication has been given successfully
- Asking whether the patient is showing any signs of pain or discomfort
- Asking whether the owner has any further questions.

This is an excellent opportunity for the nurse to follow up on the discharge post-hospitalization care plan and to support the owners in their continuing care of their pet.

Retaining records after discharge

Requirements depend on the nature of the practice and the species cared for (short or long lifespan). Guidance from the Royal College of Veterinary Surgeons and Veterinary Defence Society suggests that records should be retained for at least 6 years, and practices are advised to seek professional advice. Records can be kept in hard copy or scanned electronically and filed in date order or attached to individual records for easy reference.

Physiotherapy and hydrotherapy

All nurses should be able to employ a range of massage and physiotherapy techniques according to the care plan agreed with the veterinary surgeon. Physiotherapy includes both therapy carried out in house and appropriate advice to owners for ongoing support of their pet. Where more intensive physiotherapy is required, e.g. for post-orthopaedic surgery and rehabilitation, it is advisable to seek advice and further training from a qualified animal physiotherapist. The Association of Chartered Physiotherapists in Animal Therapy (ACPAT) will advise regarding the location of qualified animal physiotherapists.

Patients that have undergone orthopaedic surgery or have neurological disorders often benefit from hydrotherapy once surgical wounds have healed. It is essential that the veterinary surgeon in charge of the patient has recommended hydrotherapy.

There are now a number of physiotherapy and hydrotherapy courses for veterinary nurses which can be undertaken as continuing professional development.

Acknowledgements

The author would like to thank: Liz Branscombe, for her continued support; Jerry Davies, for suggesting that I should do this; and my dogs DD (Bedlington) and Tommy (Dach) for their patience during photo shoots. The author and editors gratefully acknowledge the following, images from which appear in this chapter: All Creatures Health Centre; Animal Health Trust; Davies Veterinary Specialists; Dovecote Veterinary Hospital; Mill House Veterinary Surgery and Hospital; Nottingham Veterinary School; Pool House Veterinary Hospital; Willows Veterinary Centre; Wilson Veterinary Group.

References and further reading

Aggleton P and Chambers H (2000) *Nursing Models and Nursing Practice, 2nd edn*. Palgrave, Hampshire

Andrews-Jones B and Boag A (2008) Management of the critical care unit. In: *BSAVA Manual of Canine and Feline Advanced Veterinary Nursing, 2nd edn*, ed. A Hotston Moore and S Rudd, pp. 103—113. BSAVA Publications, Gloucester

Dallas S, Jones M and Mullineaux E (2007) Managing clinical environments, equipment and materials. In: *BSAVA Manual of Practical Veterinary Nursing*, ed. E Mullineaux and M Jones, pp.76–85. BSAVA Publications, Gloucester

Jeffrey A and Ford-Fennah S (2011) The nursing process, nursing models and care plans. In: *BSAVA Textbook of Veterinary Nursing, 5th edn*, ed. B Cooper *et al.*, pp. 346–365. BSAVA Publications, Gloucester

Lindley S and Watson P (2010) *BSAVA Manual of Canine and Feline Rehabilitation, Supportive and Palliative Care: Case Studies in Patient Management*. BSAVA Publications, Gloucester

Monsey L and Devaney J (2011) Maintaining animal accommodation. In: *BSAVA Textbook of Veterinary Nursing, 5th edn*, ed. B Cooper *et al.*, pp. 277–304. BSAVA Publications, Gloucester

Hamilton J (2007) Nursing the patient in recovery. In: *Anaesthesia for Veterinary Nurses*, ed. L Welsh, pp.247–270. Blackwell Science, Oxford

Wilson J (2006) *Infection Control in Clinical Practice, 3rd edn*. Elsevier, Oxford

Sample questionnaires, care plan and hospital charts 

Client questionnaire – Canine patients

It would be helpful if you could take a few minutes to tell us a little bit about your dog. Coming into hospital can be stressful a time, and some dogs will develop behaviours or signs that can affect our interpretation of their recovery from disease or surgery. By knowing more about your dog's general routines and personality, we will be able to care more for his/her individual needs during his/her stay with us.

Dog's name: .... **Your surname:** ....

Personality

How does your dog get on with people? ....

How does your dog get on with other dogs? ....

Is your dog shy at home? ....

Does your dog get stressed easily? ....

Other comments: ....

Toilet habits

Where does your dog prefer to urinate at home? .... Anywhere ❑ Grass ❑ Gravel ❑ Bushes ❑

Will your dog go to the toilet when walked on lead? .... Yes ❑ No ❑

Toilet command (if any) ....

Other comments: ....

Diet

What is your dog's normal diet? ....

What is your dog's favourite snack? ....

Would you be surprised if your dog chose not to eat while in hospital? .... Yes ❑ No ❑

How often do you feed your dog? ....

Other comments: ....

Vaccinations

Are your dog's vaccinations current? Yes ❑ No ❑

When did your dog last receive a kennel cough vaccine (given into the nose)? ....

Client questionnaire – Feline patients

Coming into hospital can be a stressful time, and some cats will develop behaviours or signs that can affect our interpretation of their recovery from disease or surgery. By knowing more about your cat's general routines and personality, we will be able to care more for his/her individual needs during their stay with us.

We try and provide our cat patients with an environment which attempts to reduce the stress they may experience while in hospital. They are kept in a ward away from dogs, and noise in the ward is kept to a minimum. Soft classical music is also played, as this has been shown to have a calming effect. Timid cats may have a box in their cage where they can hide away if they wish.

Feline pheromone sprays and 'plug-ins' are used throughout the ward as these have also been shown to reduce anxiety.

It would be helpful if you could take a few minutes to tell us a little bit about your cat.

Cat's name: .... **Your surname:** ....

Personality

How does your cat get on with people? ....

What type of bedding does your cat prefer? ....

Does your cat like being groomed? ....

Other comments: ....

Toilet habits

Will your cat use a litter tray? .... Yes ❑ No ❑

What type of cat litter does your cat prefer? .... Soil ❑ Woodchip ❑ Gravel ❑

Other comments: ....

Diet

What does your cat normally eat? ....

Does your cat prefer to be offered single meals, or does it prefer to 'graze' throughout the day? ....

Would you be surprised if your cat chose not to eat while in hospital? .... Yes ❑ No ❑

What is your cat's favourite treat? ....

Does your cat drink out of a water bowl? .... Yes ❑ No ❑

When did your cat last eat? ....

Other comments: ....

Vaccinations

Are your cat's vaccinations current? Yes ❑ No ❑

Medications

Please list current medications ....

Examples of pre-admission client questionnaires for canine and feline patients.

Nursing care plan	Patient details/date		Presenting problem/diagnosis Clinical status Investigations required			
Nursing considerations	**Assessment of patient problem Current/Potential**	**Nursing goal (measurable)**	**Nursing intervention**	**Review date Initial**	**Reassess/evaluate care given**	**Date Initial**
Nutrition Weight/BCS Feeding Requirement						
Hydration status Fluid balance requirements Normal losses Abnormal losses						
Elimination Urination – catheterization Defecation – enema						
Respiratory O_2 therapy? Handling considerations Temperature						
Cardiac Heart/pulse rate differences? Arrhythmia Blood pressure						
Temperature Warming methods Cooling methods Diphasic						
Behaviour Demeanour Grooming Security/ social interaction						
Mobility Exercise requirement Exercise limitations Sleep/Rest Accommodation Physiotherapy						
Hygiene Zoonoses Infectious / contagious Chemotherapy Wounds						
Pain Pain score assessment CRI Nociceptive Accommodation adaptations/ considerations						

An example of an abbreviated nursing care plan. (Courtesy of Mill House Veterinary Hospital)

WARD NOTES **Vet:**		**Admission weight:**	**Admission Date:**	
Patient/Owner name			Case number	
Today's date	/ /	Today's weight kg	+/- from previous: kg	
Hosp fee charged?		Vet examined - initial		O informed of costs?
Presenting problem				
Treatment plan				

MEDICATION	freq	am 6	7	8	9	10	11	pm 12	1	2	3	4	5	6	7	8	9	10	11	am 12			
		☐	☐	☐	☐	☐	☐	☐	☐	☐	☐	☐	☐	☐	☐	☐	☐	☐	☐	☐	☐	☐	☐
		☐	☐	☐	☐	☐	☐	☐	☐	☐	☐	☐	☐	☐	☐	☐	☐	☐	☐	☐	☐	☐	☐
		☐	☐	☐	☐	☐	☐	☐	☐	☐	☐	☐	☐	☐	☐	☐	☐	☐	☐	☐	☐	☐	☐
		☐	☐	☐	☐	☐	☐	☐	☐	☐	☐	☐	☐	☐	☐	☐	☐	☐	☐	☐	☐	☐	☐
		☐	☐	☐	☐	☐	☐	☐	☐	☐	☐	☐	☐	☐	☐	☐	☐	☐	☐	☐	☐	☐	☐
		☐	☐	☐	☐	☐	☐	☐	☐	☐	☐	☐	☐	☐	☐	☐	☐	☐	☐	☐	☐	☐	☐

Obs every.................... Mins/Hrs (time/initial)										
Temp°C – ....times/day										
Pulse/heart rate/min										
Respiratory rate/min										
CRT/mm colour										
Urine										
Faeces										
Vomit										
Demeanour										
IV Fluids type/rate ml/h										
Cannula maintenance/ date due to change										
Walked?										
Nutrition & amount given										
Appetite										
Water given/mls										
Water consumed										
Comments/consumables										

An example of a hospitalization chart. (Courtesy of Mill House Veterinary Hospital)

DAVIES
Veterinary Specialists

Today's date:	
Hospital Day No:	
Kennel No:	
Admit Weight:	
Today's weight:	
Intrac status: A B C	Vet X-rays: ❑ Vet CD: ❑	Day Case: Yes ❑ No ❑

Standard Hospital Chart

Reason for admission:	Admitted with:
Known Allergies/Drug reactions:	Normal Diet:
Diagnosis/Procedures performed:	Cautions:

Time of Event							Overnight Observations 2300	0100	0300	0500	Pre-rounds 0700
Clinical assessment											
Temperature (°C)											
Pulse rate / character											
Respiratory rate											
Pain Score (see chart)											
Time taken out											
Faeces											
Urine											
IV catheter care	Size			Location				Day No			

Today's Evaluation:

Today's Plan:

Medication (BID/TID treatments shaded) Name of Drug	Freq.	Dose	Route	07 00	08 00	09 00	10 00	11 00	12 00	13 00	14 00	15 00	16 00	17 00	18 00	19 00	20 00	Overnight Medications 21 00	23 00	01 00	03 00	05 00
Fluid Therapy Rate	Fluid Type																					
Flush IV: am ❑ pm ❑	Fluid Additives																					

Anaesthesia	Premed drug1	Dose	Given? ❑ (Time/Sign)	Pre-op drugs
Starve? Yes / No	Premed drug 2	Dose:		
Anaesthesia Warnings:				See anaesthesia chart ❑

Daily Task List	Orders for (pre-rounds)
Check wound:❑ (comment over):	Starve? YES / NO
Speak to owner (circle): Vet / Nurse	

An example of a standard hospital chart. (Courtesy of Davies Veterinary Specialists)

Label

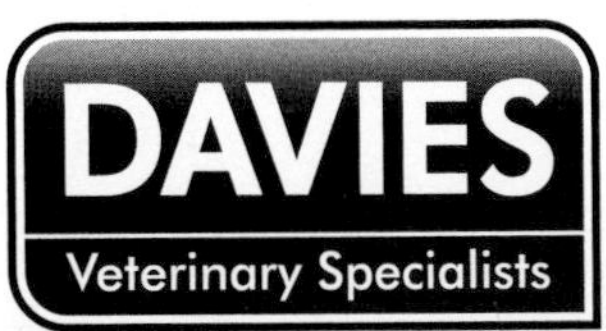

Kennel No:____________

IN PATIENT FEEDING CHART

Admission weight:	Date admitted:	Normal Diet:

Feeding Calculation Area

Diet Selected:______________________ Illness factor:________________ Daily Energy Requirement (RDI):________________

Daily amount to be fed:________________ Number of feeds:______________ Quantity of food req'd (each meal):________________

Daily food intake chart (indicate amount eaten e.g. ◕ = ¾ eaten)

Mealtime		Admit Day						
Comments (e.g. NBM, Sx, Procedures)								
1	% eaten	○	○	○	○	○	○	○
Time ____	Food type							
2	% eaten	○	○	○	○	○	○	○
Time ____	Food type							
3	% eaten	○	○	○	○	○	○	○
Time ____	Food type							
4	% eaten	○	○	○	○	○	○	○
Time ____	Food type							
% RDI eaten								

Comments: ____

An example of an inpatient feeding chart. (Courtesy of Davies Veterinary Specialists)

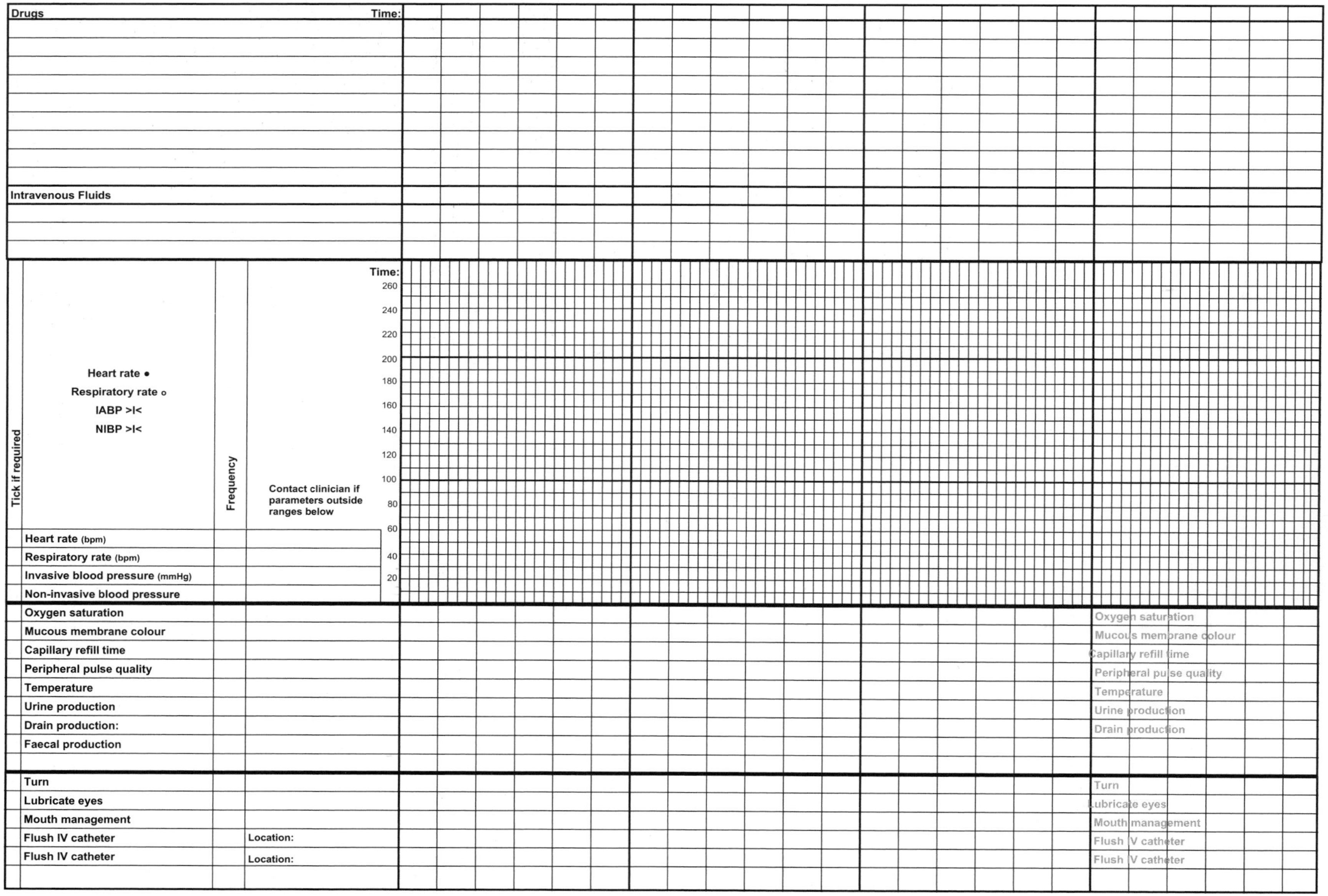

Drugs	Time:
Intravenous Fluids	

Tick if required	Heart rate ● Respiratory rate o IABP >I< NIBP >I<	Frequency	Contact clinician if parameters outside ranges below	Time: 260 240 220 200 180 160 140 120 100 80 60 40 20
	Heart rate (bpm)			
	Respiratory rate (bpm)			
	Invasive blood pressure (mmHg)			
	Non-invasive blood pressure			
	Oxygen saturation			
	Mucous membrane colour			
	Capillary refill time			
	Peripheral pulse quality			
	Temperature			
	Urine production			
	Drain production:			
	Faecal production			
	Turn			
	Lubricate eyes			
	Mouth management			
	Flush IV catheter		Location:	
	Flush IV catheter		Location:	

Oxygen saturation
Mucous membrane colour
Capillary refill time
Peripheral pulse quality
Temperature
Urine production
Drain production
Turn
Lubricate eyes
Mouth management
Flush IV catheter
Flush IV catheter

An example of a hospital chart for an intensive care patient. This should be used with a supplementary narrative chart for patient observations and interactions. (Courtesy of Davies Veterinary Specialists)

The surgical suite

8

Amy Bowcott

Preparation and surgical areas in a veterinary practice can vary greatly – from multi-function rooms in a lock-up branch practice, to multi-theatre suites in purpose-built specialist referral centres. No matter the size or financial constraints of the veterinary practice concerned, excellent aseptic technique and high operational standards must still be achieved. Small changes can improve time management, improve patient outcomes, increase profitability, reduce waste and increase client satisfaction. The management of this crucial area is vital for patient safety and maintenance of the standards and reputation of the practice.

Design considerations

Surgical areas should be well designed, well illuminated and, ideally, situated away from general traffic flow (see Chapter 3).

Preparation room

The preparation ('prep') room is an extremely versatile room that facilitates induction of anaesthesia, initial surgical preparation of patients (including clipping), bladder management prior to surgical procedures, and other associated procedures. It should be separate from the operating theatre but, for easy transfer of patients, it should be close to the theatre(s), radiography facilities and recovery areas.

The layout of tables in the preparation room should be considered carefully. One anaesthetic machine per table is a standard layout, and ideally each table would have a task light overhead to assist with examination or procedures taking place prior to transportation into the operating theatre (Figure 8.1). Each anaesthetic machine should have a gas scavenging system, either passive or active (see Chapter 2).

If surgical instruments are being decontaminated and reprocessed in the preparation room rather than in a separate kit preparation room or sterile service department, the traffic flow of contaminated instruments should be such as to prevent contamination of clean instruments. The packing area for the clean instruments should be kept clean and organized.

Not every practice has space for a large preparation area, and compromises may be needed (Figure 8.2).

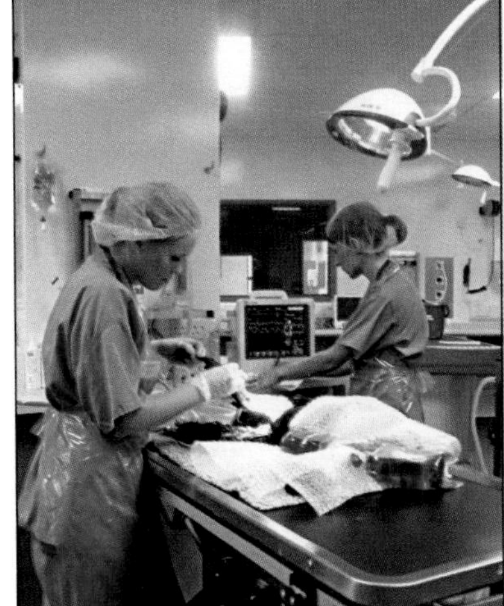

8.1 Lightweight manoeuvrable task lights are ideal for prep areas. Note the multi-parameter monitor in use for this patient.

KEY POINT

Keeping the instrument packing area clean and tidy can be as simple as organizing different trays for 'clean' and 'contaminated' instruments.

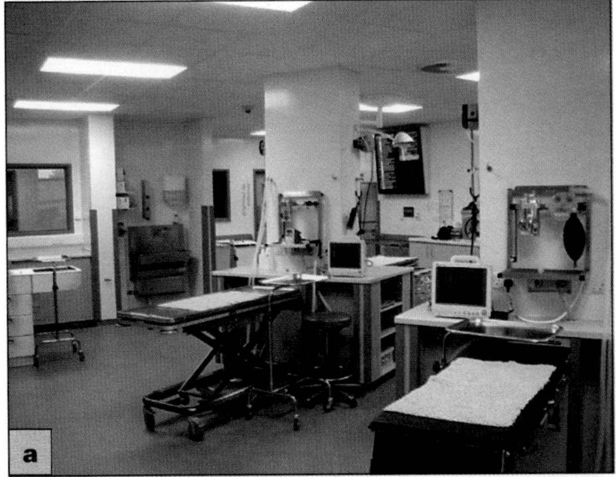

8.2 Preparation room layout will be determined by the space available and the number of stations required. **(a)** This large prep area has tables arranged for easy access to theatre and for staff, with wall-mounted anaesthetic machines and clippers. Note the computer message board on the far wall. (continues) ▶

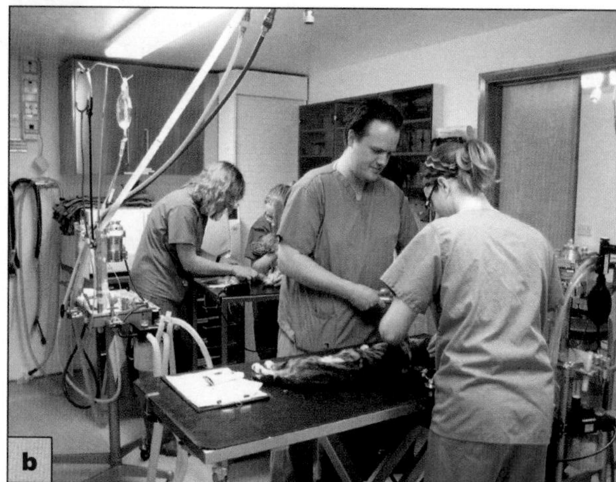

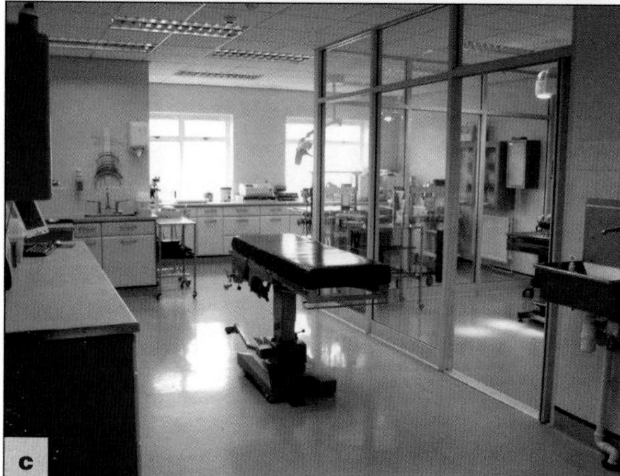

8.2 (continued) Preparation room layout will be determined by the space available and the number of stations required. **(b)** In this small busy prep area, best use is made of limited space with two trolley tables and small manoeuvrable anaesthetic trolleys. **(c)** Here a theatre has been formed using glass partitioning to leave an L-shaped prep room, with good visibility throughout the area.

Central workstations

In larger practices, a centrally located nurse station or computer base with a telephone is beneficial (Figure 8.3). Ideally, the workstation has an open view to all the tables within the room. The coordinator for the day is usually based at the workstation so he/she can oversee the day's activities and the progression of the patients. This enables communication throughout the practice. A whiteboard, or hospitalization/surgery day-book (paper or computer-based), is also a good method of communication in a preparation room; one staff member can be given the responsibility to maintain the whiteboard, date the messages entered, and remove old messages when needed.

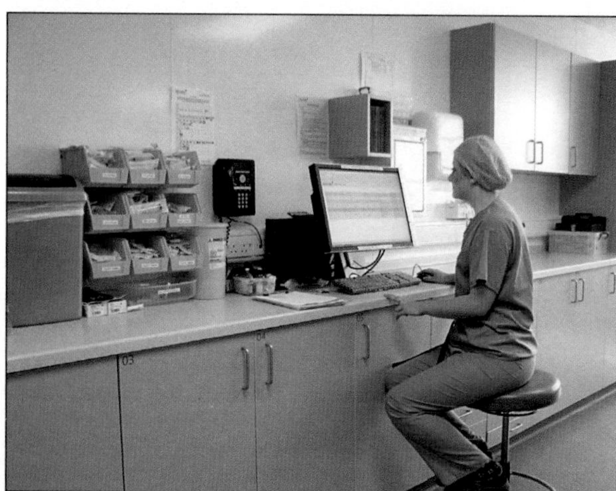

8.3 A central nurse station, with computer and telephone, is essential and should preferably afford a clear view of the preparation area.

Surgical changing rooms

Ideally, a changing room is located close to the surgical environment so that personnel can change into the correct attire before entering the surgical area. In the changing room it is useful to have:

- Closed, numbered or named cabinets for clean storage
- Individual lockers for team members to store their own 'street wear' clothing and personal belongings (Figure 8.4a)
- Containers for soiled linen and scrub suits (Figure 8.4b)
- A separate surgical shoe receptacle for soiled surgical shoes.

When choosing receptacles for storing soiled clothing, it is important to consider how personnel will lift them and how they will be cleaned. Receptacles on wheels are ideal for moving into laundry rooms with ease (see Chapter 7).

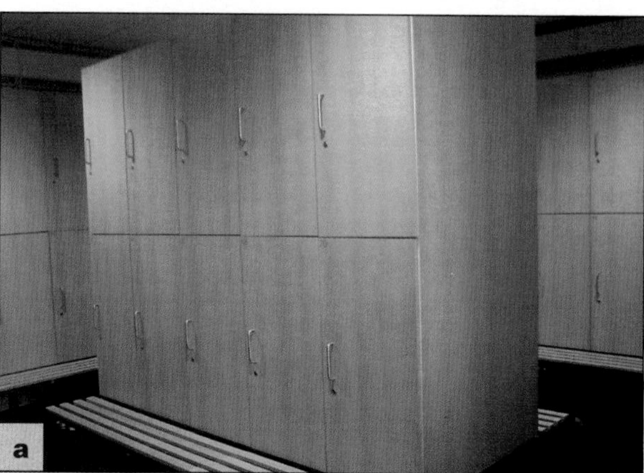

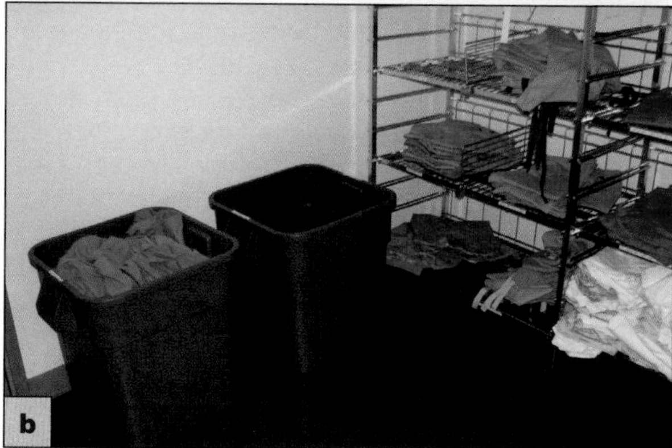

8.4 **(a)** Secure lockers for 'streetwear' and storage for surgical attire should be situated in a changing area close to the surgical suite. **(b)** Separate receptacles for soiled clothing and soiled clogs are useful. Clean, laundered scrub suits can be stored on shelving; these shelves have been designed to allow dust to fall through.

The operating theatre

An operating theatre should be available in every veterinary practice for conducting aseptic surgery. It is also beneficial to have a separate operating theatre dedicated to performing 'dirty' operations or minor procedures. This can be a small room, adjacent to the preparation room, which is used for a variety of procedures including biopsy, wound management procedures, dentistry (see Chapter 9) and endoscopy (see Chapter 10). Larger practices may have the space to provide more than one operating theatre, with each designed for certain types of procedure classified with reference to the National Research Council's wound classification system (Figure 8.5).

Classification	Criteria
Clean wound	No break in asepsis Respiratory, gastrointestinal and genitourinary tracts not entered Non-traumatic, non-inflamed operative wounds
Clean–contaminated wound	Minor break in asepsis Respiratory, gastrointestinal or genitourinary tract entered but spillage or spread of contamination did not occur A clean wound in which a drain is placed
Contaminated wound	Major break in aseptic technique Traumatic wounds without purulent discharge Surgical procedures where gastrointestinal contents or infected urine is spilled Wounds with severe inflammation
Dirty wound	Traumatic wounds with purulent discharge Wounds with devitalized tissues or foreign bodies Procedures where a viscus is perforated Faecal contamination

8.5 NRC surgical wound classifications.

KEY POINT

An operating theatre should not be used for any purpose other than performing surgical procedures.

The operating theatre should be a closed room without through traffic. The door to the operating theatre should be kept closed at all times; laminated signs on the outside of the door can remind staff of this. Doorways should be wide enough to allow passage of patient trolleys, which ideally should be dedicated to the surgical area.

Regardless of the number of theatres, equipment should be kept to a minimum to avoid contamination. The operating theatre should be uncluttered, with no dust traps. The floor should be constructed from an impervious, washable material with no gaps or cracks and should have coved joints where it meets the wall (see Chapter 3). The size of the room should allow for the surgical team members to move around without contaminating the surgical field. Overcrowding can increase the risk of accidental contamination of sterile areas or instruments by unscrubbed members of the surgical team. Even if members of the surgical team do not come into direct contact with sterile surfaces or areas, they will still shed microscopic skin fragments contaminated with bacteria, which could potentially settle in a wound or on one of the operating team or instrument trolleys. Ideally, the anaesthetic equipment should be positioned near to the door of the operating theatre to prevent staff having to walk past the surgical site during handover periods.

There should be no clear view of the interior of the operating room to the general public from outside the premises. Glass windows can be frosted or blinds can be fitted. Windows should be sealed units to prevent opening and contamination. Some surgical procedures (when viewing diagnostic images on a monitor or via an operating microscope) may benefit from having the room darkened, and blackout blinds are ideal for this. The material for the blinds should be water-resistant to allow for cleaning and should tolerate the repeated use of disinfectants.

Recovery areas

Depending on the size of the practice, the recovery room or intensive care unit should also be near to the preparation room and the operating theatre(s). More information on recovery areas can be found in Chapter 7.

Traffic flow

Surgical areas should be well identified and a system of 'clean', 'clean-contaminated' and 'contaminated' areas should be used to alert staff of contamination dangers.

- **Clean rooms** include operating theatres, sterile supply rooms, sterilization rooms and scrub sink areas.
- **Mixed areas** include corridors where patients are transported from preparation rooms to operating theatres, non-sterile supplies store rooms and instrument reprocessing rooms.
- **Contaminated areas** include the preparation room, staff changing areas and offices.

Traffic flow should minimize contamination. For example, cross-contamination could occur if soiled, contaminated instruments were taken to the instrument reprocessing room through the sterilization room. Doors between clean and contaminated areas should be kept closed. A simple mapping system which is colour-coded could be designed to define the area risks and encourage correct traffic flow.

Identification could use simple signage such as 'Surgical area – ensure correct attire prior to entering'. In larger practices more advanced methods of personnel and visitor traffic control can also be used, such as door access control (personnel have pre-programmed fobs to allow only approved individuals to enter certain areas).

KEY POINT

Identify areas clearly and arrange traffic flow to minimize contamination.

Lighting

Good lighting in the surgical suite, along with other clinical areas, is essential. General lighting and lighting specific to tasks (examination, surgery) should be considered. It is advisable to look at the system in use and assess the field coverage and colour rendition, and to consider reliability and serviceability before deciding which lighting system is best for individual requirements.

Lights should be easy to clean and tolerate the repeated use of disinfectants. Safety, efficiency and economy are important considerations. It is important that little heat is produced by the light as heat can dry exposed tissues and make the environment uncomfortable for the surgeon and scrubbed assistants. The main lighting supply in a surgical suite is generally by means of overhead fluorescent lights in the ceiling. Track lighting should be avoided, as this can become a dust trap that could lead to contamination.

The 'colour temperature' of lighting is measured on the Kelvin (K) scale and is a characteristic of visible light. For general lighting, 5000 K would be an ideal bulb choice, as this is close to daylight (5500 K). This is beneficial for accurate assessment of patient colour (e.g. mucous membranes). Dimmable lighting may be useful for interpreting radiographs or other images; fluorescent lights should have dimmable ballasts. Ideally general lighting would be 500 lux at floor level, in case a patient needs assessing on the floor.

In veterinary hospitals and emergency service clinics lighting should continue to function even in the event of loss of power. A generator, or an uninterruptible power supply such as a battery-powered light source, may be needed in order to complete a surgical procedure; lighting level should be maintained without having to switch to different units if power fails during a procedure.

Examination lighting

Examination lights are lightweight manoeuvrable task lights that can be mounted on the ceiling, wall or floor, over patient examination tables (see Figure 8.1) or when additional lighting is required, for example for:

- Dental procedures
- Intravenous catheterization
- Induction of anaesthesia
- Clipping.

Theatre lighting

Overhead ceiling-mounted lights are preferable, and two sets are ideal for shadowless illumination; re-sterilizable handles provide the surgeon with the best control over light position (Figure 8.6). Shadowing can be problematical during surgery if the surgeon's head and the assistant's hands and shoulders cast shadows over the surgical site. Modern lighting may contain microlenses, which reduce shadowing. Some systems also enable adjustment of colour temperature to suit the surgeon's personal preferences depending on the structures being visualized.

Halogen was previously the bulb of choice due to the reduced amount of heat produced and the pale bluish light, which assisted in preventing eye fatigue.

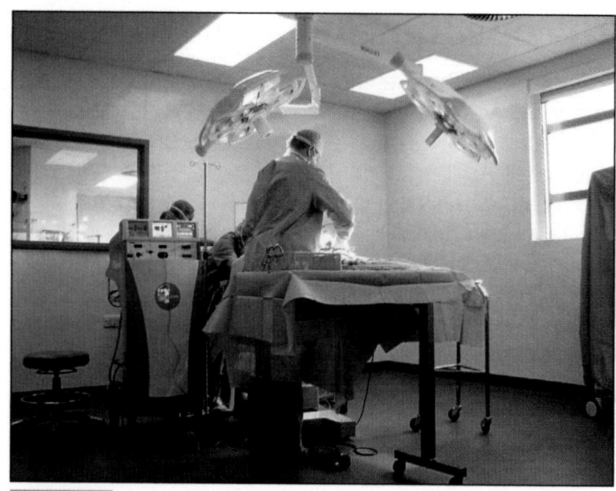

8.6 Operating lighting with built-in camera function and sterilizable handles. Note the draping of the equipment just visible on the right of the picture.

Halogen bulbs tended to require a filter to reduce the amount of the heat produced by the tungsten filament and to direct heat upwards rather than towards the surgical site. LED lights are more expensive than halogen lamps but are more reliable, produce less heat and are more energy-efficient. Halogen bulbs, however, have a track record of serviceability.

Second-hand theatre lights are often available. However, with any light installation, the structure of the ceiling or walls must be capable of bearing the weight, and the ceiling height assessed to ensure that lights designed for a large theatre will fit into the smaller rooms used in most practices. Availability of spares and bulbs should also be checked.

Lights should also be aerodynamic and compatible with the type of ventilation system employed (see below). Some lighting systems can be equipped with high-definition cameras to record the surgical procedure, which can aid teaching, teleconferencing and documentation. Systems can be remotely controlled and may incorporate illumination adjustments and bulb replacement indicators on wall-mounted panels.

Head-mounted light sources (Figure 8.7) can allow surgeons to assess deep cavities without shadowing and are ideal for procedures involving joint cavities and fine, detailed work such as ophthalmic extra-ocular surgery, when they can be combined with a binocular loupe for magnification (Figure 8.8). They can be battery-powered and so continue to function in the event of a power cut.

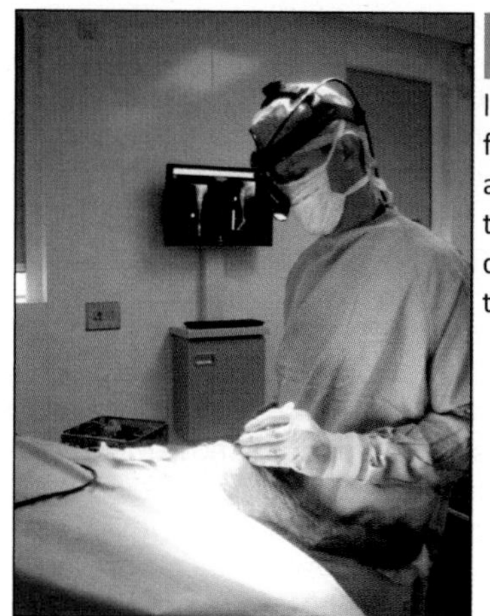

8.7 Head-mounted light sources are useful for lighting cavities and awkward angles. Note the digital screen displaying radiographs in this theatre.

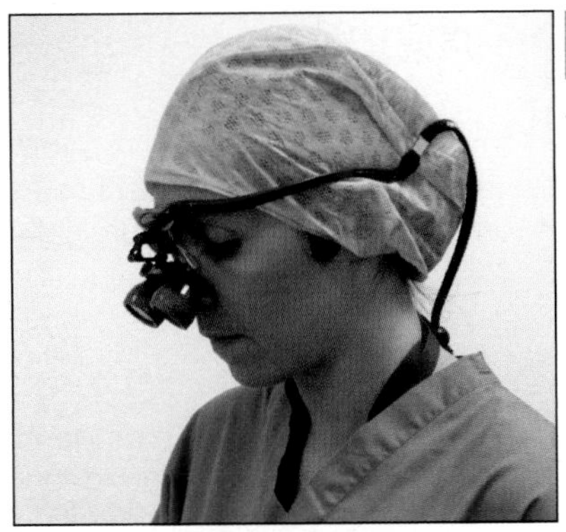

8.8 A binocular loupe is useful for detailed work and may also have a light source.

Ventilation

Ventilation within the surgical suite is important to control room temperature and humidity. The normal room temperature to provide the most comfortable environment for patients and the surgical team in a surgical suite should be approximately 21°C. This can be monitored by wall-mounted thermometers or by digital ventilation-related displays. It is difficult to maintain the patient's normal body temperature if the room temperature is below 21°C (24°C for very small patients).

Ideal relative humidity is 50% (Hobson, 2003). Controlling humidity is hugely expensive and requires a massive externally housed plant.

Ventilation also serves to reduce contamination due to:

- Microorganisms (which can be introduced into the environment by patients and staff)
- Naturally occurring condensation (which can lead to microbial growth)
- Odours
- Surgical smoke (plume) from diathermy or laser surgery
- Aerosols
- Anaesthetic gases.

To achieve optimal air quality and a safe working environment for the surgical team and the patient, air changes should ideally occur at relatively high frequencies but cause minimal turbulence of the air. Ventilation should be designed to provide positive air pressure within the operating theatre and lower air pressure within the corridors, so that when the door is opened the air flows out of the room rather than into it.

KEY POINT

Ventilation systems should ensure that air flows from areas of least contamination ('clean' operating theatres) to corridors and rooms classed as 'contaminated' (e.g. prep room). Positive pressure ventilation in operating theatres should maintain a pressure gradient that forces air from 'clean' areas (with higher air pressure) to 'contaminated' areas (with lower air pressure).

Different ventilation systems have different dimensions, applicability and airflow dynamics. Ventilation performance can be divided into:

- Filtration efficiency: how efficient the filtration system is at removing microorganisms and pollutants
- Ventilation rates: how many air changes per hour
- Pressure control: the pressure and air turbulence a system produces.

Ideally, a minimum of 25 air exchanges per hour is recommended if the air is recirculated, or 15 air changes per hour if the air is exhausted to the outside environment (Hobson, 2003). Each air change reduces airborne contamination to approximately 37% of its former level (Emmerson, 2011). Although ideal, this requires expensive plant and machinery, especially if bacterial filtration is included. Ventilation systems can be hugely expensive to install, run and maintain.

Ventilation systems must be correctly maintained, as filters can easily harbour microbes and a poorly maintained system can spread contamination, leading to surgical site infections (SSIs). However, even the highest quality ventilation system cannot prevent SSIs, and high standards of aseptic technique are of paramount importance. In general practice, most systems can be simple and aim to draw 'clean' (preferably filtered) air in from outside, maintaining positive pressure in the theatres so that air passes from clean to contaminated areas. Care should be taken with extraction ventilation to consider the direction of resultant air flow between several rooms. Further information on ventilation systems is given in Chapter 2.

Two main types of advanced theatre ventilation system (Figure 8.9) are commonly used in human operating theatres, but they are rarely used in veterinary general practice as they are expensive to install and maintain.

Plenum

- Atmospheric air is initially filtered to remove dust and debris, then travels through a bacterial filter positioned in the inlet grille
- Plenum systems maintain approximately 20 air changes per hour
- Some air may be recirculated and an exhaust system removes air to the outside

Laminar airflow

- Provides 'ultra-clean' air for orthopaedic operating and ultra-clean procedures, such as joint replacements
- A continual flow of highly filtered air is recirculated under positive pressure
- The system incorporates several air HEPA filters, which filter the air before it enters the operating theatre
- When the air enters the operating theatre it is circulated in certain directions, depending on the type of laminar airflow system – horizontal or vertical
- Laminar airflow systems may operate at >300 air changes per hour

8.9 Advanced theatre ventilation systems.

Finishes

All sinks and wash basins in clinical areas should ideally have elbow/knee-controlled or sensor-activated mixer taps (Figure 8.10). This prevents recontamination of hands when the taps are turned off, and also reduces water consumption. Scrub sinks for surgeons should be sited close to, but not in, the operating theatre and should be deep, stainless steel sinks set at waist height to minimize splashing.

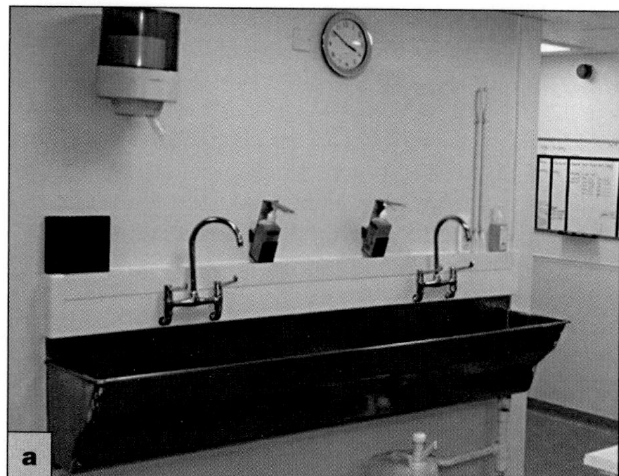

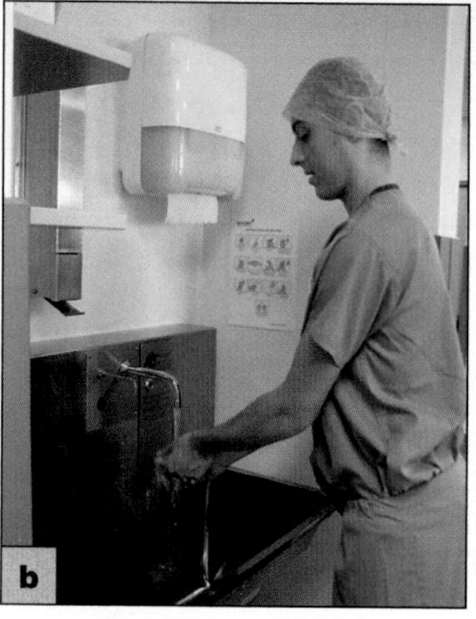

8.10 **(a)** A double scrub sink with elbow-operated taps. Note the wall clock, which is useful in timing pre-surgical hand preparation, and the whiteboard on the wall to the right, which is used to organize the surgical list. **(b)** A hand-washing station with sensor-activated scrub solution and taps.

All surfaces should be easy to clean, with flush fittings where possible, and not damaged by the repeated use of disinfectants. Within the clinical areas, computer keyboards and telephones should be easily cleaned with a disinfectant solution. Waterproof keyboards are commercially available; alternatively, keyboard covers enable disinfection of the keys without penetrating the actual unit.

Storage for important surgical items can be achieved using fitted pass-through supply cabinets with tightly fitting doors. The doors may be made from a transparent material to enable staff to view the contents of the cupboard. Shelving and other permanent fixtures should be kept to a minimum in the operating theatre.

A non-slip floor finish is essential.

Communication systems

Telephones or other communication systems should be available in each room to enable important information to be conveyed without the need for team members to open the door and walk to other areas. Telephone systems with announcement facilities are invaluable for alerting staff when emergencies occur. Standardized call-outs should be used to ensure that all staff are alerted correctly, clearly and efficiently and without confusion. An example of this is in a 'patient crash' situation, when a suitable brief announcement should call available staff to the area immediately; announcements should be repeated for clarity. Handsets should be selected for durability and ease of cleaning. For more information on telephone systems see Chapter 4.

Preparation room equipment

Equipment for sterilizing instruments, etc., is discussed later, in the section on 'Maintenance of a surgically clean environment.'

Tub tables

A tub table can be used to carry out a wide range of procedures, such as bladder evacuation, wound lavage, bathing, endoscopy, and patient preparation before surgery (e.g. enemas, skin preparation). If space is not a problem, the tub table would ideally be kept within a 'dirty' or minor procedures room, to minimize contamination in the preoperative preparation area where patients are prepared for clean procedures. Tub tables are illustrated in Chapters 7 and 9.

Equipment for skin preparation

Clippers

The majority of patients require hair removal prior to surgery. Clipper blades are available in a selection of sizes: the higher the blade number, the shorter the remaining hair will be. Mains-operated or rechargeable electric clippers with size 40 clipper blades are commonly used. Mains-powered clippers can be mounted on recoilable extension cables (Figure 8.11). Small clippers for use with nervous patients are illustrated in Chapter 7.

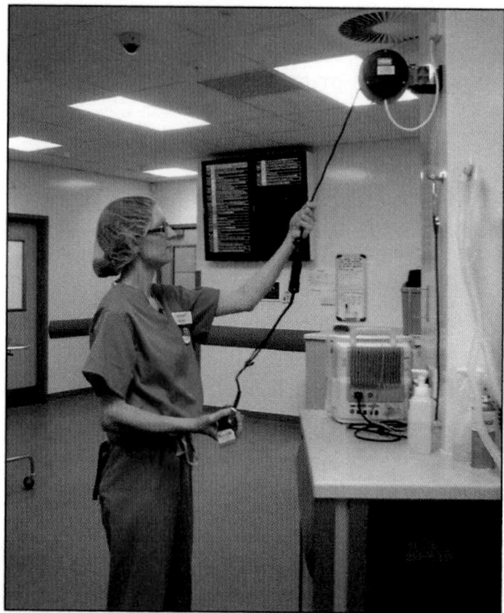

8.11 A wall-mounted cable reel device provides a permanent neat and flexible solution to storing clipper cables safely. The clipper handpiece can be stored separately.

Careful maintenance of clippers and blades is essential to prevent micro-lacerations and skin irritation ('clipper rash') that could promote infection. Correct clipping technique is also essential, and all staff should be trained in the correct use and care of clippers. Lubrication is essential. A 'two-stroke' clipping technique should be used for the majority of patients: first, the bulk of the hair is clipped in the direction of hair growth; the second stroke is when a closer clip is undertaken by shaving the hair in the opposite direction. Patients with long dense hair, if they allow it, may benefit from being pre-clipped immediately prior to the induction of anaesthesia, using a size 10 clipper blade, to reduce clipping time under general anaesthesia. Photographs of routine procedures can be used to indicate the degree of hair removal required. A neat finish is essential for owner satisfaction.

Blades must be cleaned and disinfected after every patient (Figure 8.12). They should be sharpened regularly and blades replaced when necessary. An SOP for clipper care and cleaning is given at the end of this chapter. For more information on clipping techniques and maintenance of clippers and blades see *BSAVA Manual of Canine and Feline Surgical Principles: A Foundation Manual.*

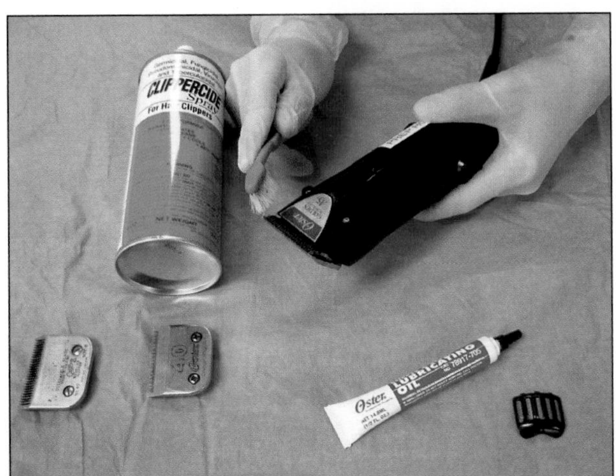

8.12 Clippers must be cleaned between patients. It is important to clean both the blades and the clipper body, particularly the head area. The spray used is bactericidal, fungicidal and viricidal; a COSHH risk assessment is required for its use. Note the spare blades (left); replacements are fitted as required, following the manufacturer's instructions, and pushed down into place with the clippers running. A spare clipper filter is also shown (bottom right); filters should be in place before use to prevent hair build-up within the internal mechanism of the handpiece.

Vacuum cleaners

Vacuum cleaners are useful to remove the clipped hair. These can be hand-held portable units, cylinder cleaners or central units. Hand-held portable units can be difficult to keep clean. Cleaning and disinfection of vacuum units should be included as part of a daily maintenance checklist. Lint rollers can be rolled gently over the clipped site to remove any stubborn hairs and skin squames.

Skin preparation

Antiseptic solutions are required for preoperative skin preparation. Options include iodophors (povidone–iodine agents), busdiguanides (e.g. chlorhexidine), alcohols and alcohol-based solutions. Chlorhexidine followed by an alcohol spray is most commonly used because of the synergistic effect. A small spray bottle for the alcohol is helpful to minimize wetting and thus patient cooling. Pooling of liquid on the table surface must be avoided; alcohol is highly flammable and this could constitute a fire hazard.

A standard procedure should be used for patient preparation (see *BSAVA Manual of Surgical Principles*). Sterile non-gauze swabs should be used to apply the solution. Preparation packs containing sterile dishes, swabs, towel or sponges, and sponge-holding forceps can be made up and sterilized in advance, ready for use. The person performing the surgical preparation should wear gloves in order to prevent cross-contamination; a selection of disposable gloves of different sizes should be readily available in the preparation area. A kick bin close by is handy for disposal of dirty swabs, and a clock is useful to ensure adequate contact time with the agent used.

KEY POINT

Items such as collars and harnesses should be removed following induction of general anaesthesia and prior to transportation to the operating theatre, labelled, and kept safely to avoid loss or mix-ups.

Transporting patients

A suitable means of transporting heavy patients is important. Mobile tables with wheels, castors and mechanical lifting/tilting and lowering functions can be very beneficial and can reduce manual handling risk, allowing easy movement and transportation of anaesthetized patients throughout the practice. Buffers prevent damage to walls and door frames while the tables are being transported, and reduce the risk of finger trapping.

Mobile anaesthetic trolleys are commercially available (Figure 8.13). These have an anaesthetic machine, oxygen cylinder (usually F size) and breath-

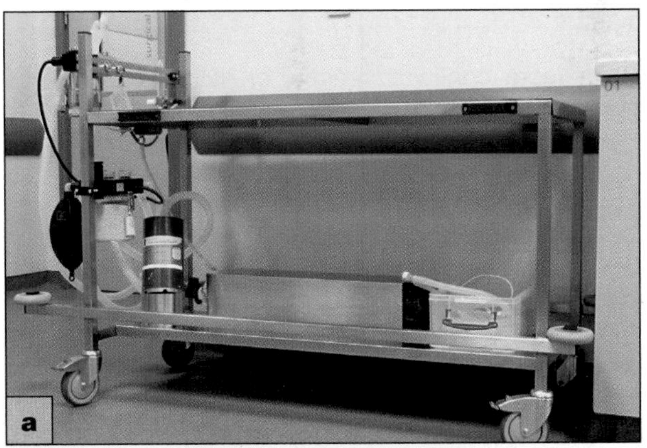

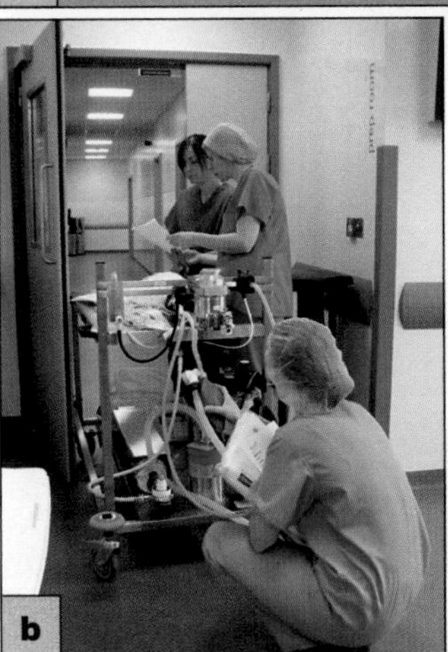

8.13 **(a)** An anaesthetic patient trolley for transporting anaesthetized patients. Note the buffers to prevent finger trapping and damage to walls and door frames during transport. **(b)** A non-surgical team member handing a patient over on an anaesthetic trolley to a coordinator at a cross-point between the preparation room and the non-surgical clinical areas.

ing system(s) built on to them, and are particularly useful for larger premises and emergency use. These trolleys can also carry or store patient monitoring equipment, scavenging systems, ventilators and suction devices. Staff should be aware of the risk of trapping fingers (and patients' extremities) against a wall with some trolleys and should undergo training on how to transport patients correctly. Storage space for trolleys can be an issue, so multipurpose table/trolleys are ideal in most general practices.

Where inpatient or surgical areas are situated on the first floor, a patient lift (Figure 8.14) should ideally be large enough to accommodate the patient trolley, any ancillary equipment and the monitoring personnel.

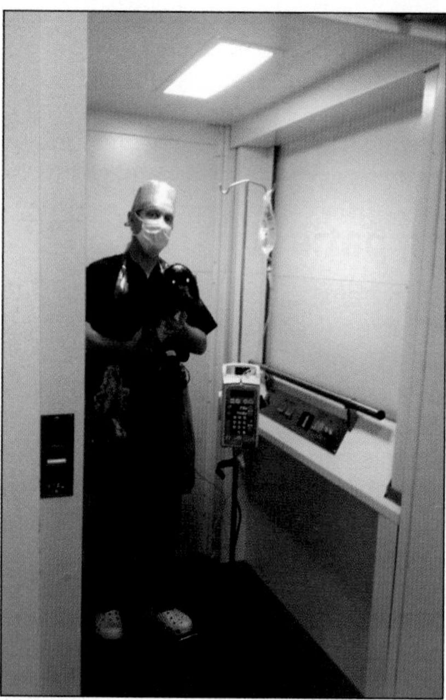

8.14 A patient lift should ideally be large enough to accommodate the patient trolley, personnel, and any ancillary equipment such as drip stands.

In more confined spaces, or if the practice has stairs within clinical areas, stretchers can be used to transport patients. Stretchers (some with wheels) are commercially available and can be manufactured from rigid or flexible materials. Team communication is vital when using stretchers (Figure 8.15) and one team member should take the lead to coordinate the carrying team. Stretchers should be stored or hung safely in an accessible place (see Chapter 7).

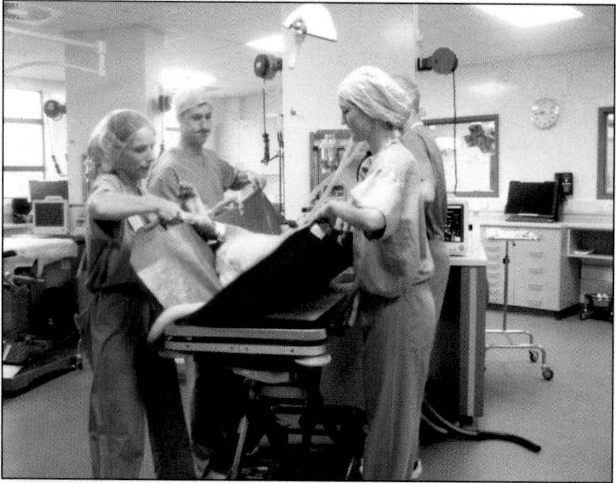

8.15 Transporting a large patient on a stretcher. Effective team coordination is vital.

Surgical attire and PPE

Surgical attire (Figure 8.16) provides a barrier that protects the patient from microorganisms shed into the environment from the skin and hair of surgical personnel and also protects the outside environment from theatre contaminants (see later).

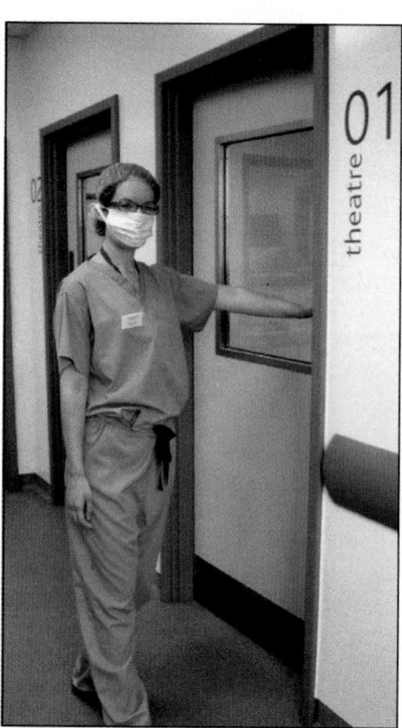

8.16 The correct surgical attire should be worn by all personnel entering an operating room or the surgical suite.

> **KEY POINT**
>
> Surgical attire should be worn by all personnel entering an operating room or the surgical suite, regardless of whether surgery is being performed.

Personal protective equipment (PPE) is also an important health and safety consideration for staff when working within a surgical suite. PPE will include: gloves; eye and ear protection; facemasks; additional clothing, such as aprons; and head protection. Staff should be able to access a variety of PPE of the correct size and type during their working day in order to suit the tasks that are to be carried out.

Surgical scrub suits

A two-piece cotton or cotton-mix suit comprising a top and trouser combination ('scrub suits', 'surgical scrubs') should be worn in the surgical areas. The trousers should have a drawstring or elasticated waist. The top should be tucked into the trousers to prevent shedding of skin squames into the environment, and the sleeves should be short enough to allow hands and arms to be cleaned and scrubbed.

> **KEY POINT**
>
> Hands must be washed before donning scrub suits.

Wearing scrub suits outside the surgical environment increases the microbial contamination of the suit. If a surgical team member is entering a contaminated area from a clean area, a long protective gown, laboratory coat or boilersuit should be worn *over* the clean surgical scrubs. Upon re-entering the clean area, the contaminated clothes should be removed and laundered. If visibly soiled or wet, the suits should be changed immediately. Scrub suits should be laundered between uses, preferably on site (to prevent domestic microbial contamination).

Surgical hats, caps or hoods

Personnel should also wear surgical caps when in clean areas, *regardless of whether surgery is being performed*. The scalp can carry *Staphylococcus aureus*, which can be transported on hair. Complete coverage of the hair (including any beard and/or moustache) is necessary to prevent shedding; beard covers are commercially available. The nape of the neck should also be covered; surgeons' hoods with a longer neck cover can be used.

Facemasks

The use of facemasks is a frequently debated topic: masks can rub off skin squames from the face, resulting in contamination of the surgical environment; masks can quickly become saturated, which will reduce their resistance to the passage of microorganisms significantly; and microorganisms can also pass around the sides of the facemask upon exhalation. However, masks do prevent direct expulsion of larger droplets from personnel during talking, sneezing and coughing. In human operating theatres, masks are worn by anyone who is in close proximity to the operating field.

- Masks are generally constructed from a lint-free material that contains a hydrophilic filter. If wet or contaminated, the mask should be changed immediately, as the filtering efficiency is decreased.
- Masks should be fitted over the mouth and nose (the top of the mask should be shaped around the bridge of the nose) and are used to filter and prevent microorganisms being expelled from the mouth and nasopharynx. Microorganisms are expelled from the nostrils and mouth during coughing, talking and sneezing. For this reason excessive talking should be discouraged in the operating room.
- Masks with a visor incorporated are available (see Chapter 9) and can be useful when power tools are being used and for certain procedures where eye protection is required. These masks are more comfortable than goggles.

Facemasks worn by anaesthetists or theatre staff who are not directly within the operating field are unproven at reducing the risk of infection to the patient, but may contribute to theatre discipline.

Gloves

Surgical gloves should be worn during all aseptic surgical procedures. Surgical, sterile gloves are used as a barrier between the surgical team member and the patient.

A wide range of pre-sterilized surgical gloves is commercially available; some examples are shown in Figure 8.17. It is important to choose a high-quality surgical glove that is hardwearing, in order to reduce

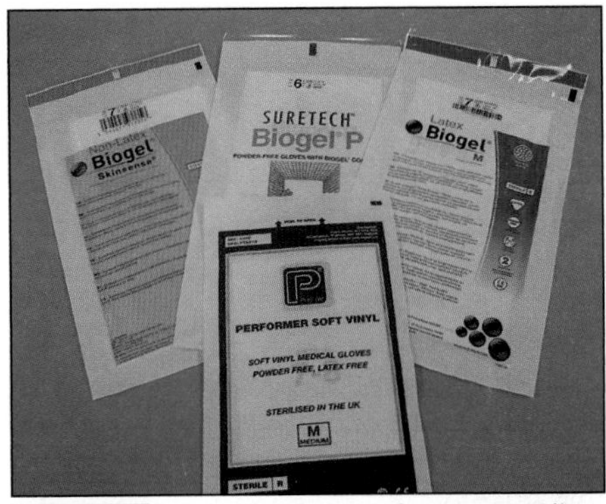

8.17 Some examples of commercially available sterile gloves, including non-latex gloves for staff with latex allergies. The Biogel M gloves are designed for extra grip and touch, which is useful for grasping delicate, fine instruments for ophthalmic or neurological surgery.

the likelihood of accidental punctures or perforations. Even though surgical gloves form an effective barrier, there may still be small holes in up to 1.5% of them (this is the quality control standard). Gloves can also be damaged and punctured in up to 13% of surgical procedures. Therefore, wearing sterile gloves is not a suitable substitute for proper hand-scrubbing methods. If the glove of a correctly scrubbed hand is punctured during a surgical procedure, it is rare for bacteria to be cultured from the punctured glove.

Gloves should fit closely to the hands to reduce baggy pouches around the fingers which could lead to punctures being undetected. Therefore a wide range of sizes to fit different personnel may be required. The correct gloving techniques should be used (see *BSAVA Manual of Surgical Principles*). Double-gloving techniques decrease the risks of accidental punctures but can reduce the surgeon's sensitivity.

Latex gloves have elastic properties, which allow them to conform to the surgeon's hands and stretch with movement. Gloves made from latex only can be difficult to put on, so a lubricating agent such as magnesium silicate (talcum) or cornstarch is added; these agents can, however, be associated with the development of latex allergies. Powdered gloves have now been removed from all UK human hospitals. Powder-free gloves coated with hydrogel should be used for known latex allergy sufferers and should be considered for all staff.

Surgical footwear

Surgical clogs should be non-slip, easily washable (ideally autoclavable) and antistatic. They should only be worn within the surgical areas. If it is impossible to change them to visit other locations within the practice, disposable overshoes should be worn to prevent contamination. Some instrument washers have specially designed footwear cycles and specially designed secure racks so that clogs can be easily washed (Figure 8.18).

> **KEY POINT**
>
> Check the drying temperature if using a washer/disinfector to clean and wash surgical clogs. Some clog brands can only withstand certain temperatures and may shrink with extremes of heat.

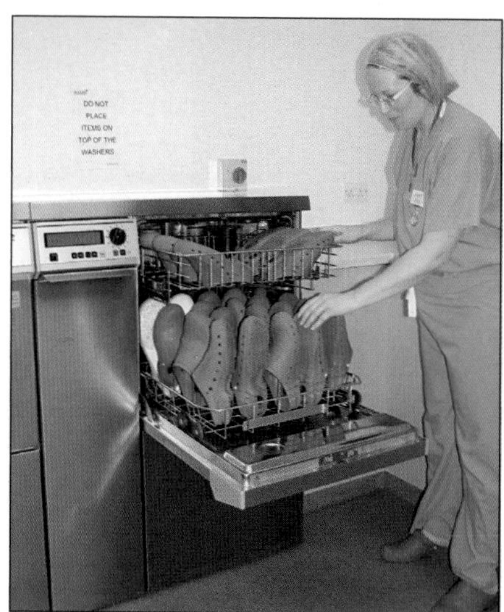

8.18 Surgical clogs can be washed on special cleaning racks within a washer/disinfector.

Other

Other important items for a preparation room include:

- Sinks with hands-free taps
- Monitoring equipment
- Syringes, needles and intravenous catheters (these can be stored in wall-mounted containers for quick access, although containers can harbour dust and therefore require regular cleaning)
- A selection of swabs
- Dressing materials
- 'Sharps' containers and bins for various waste categories.

A refrigerator is useful for storing drugs, solutions and other products.

Equipment for anaesthesia

General anaesthesia induction and recovery often take place in the preparation room, and monitoring equipment is required. More detail on anaesthetic systems and their use can be found in the *BSAVA Manual of Canine and Feline Anaesthesia and Analgesia* and in the *BSAVA Textbook of Veterinary Nursing*.

Emergency equipment

General anaesthesia can be a high-risk procedure, and adequate emergency equipment should be available, including:

- Medications
- Laryngoscopes (with a selection of blade sizes and spare batteries)
- Suction machine and tubing
- Mobile crash trolley
- Defibrillator
- Oxygen supplementation equipment
- A selection of needles and syringes.

The crash trolley (Figure 8.19) or emergency box should be easy to access and well organized, containing an agreed range of emergency drugs and consumables, including endotracheal tubes, tracheostomy tubes, needles, syringes and catheters, and also clear dose rate charts and guidelines for emergency resuscitation. A contents list and audit sheet for checking (including all drug expiry dates) should also be present.

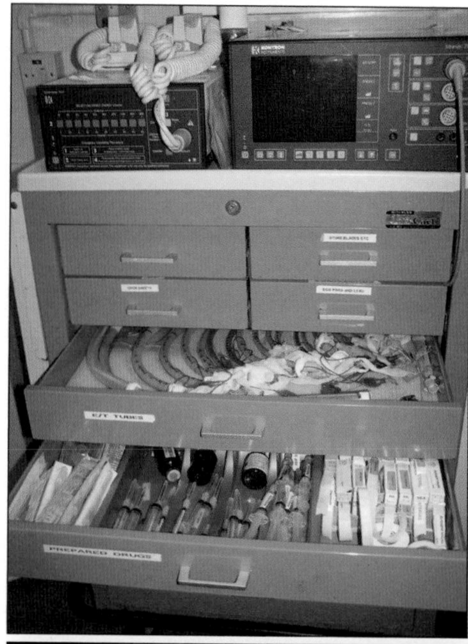

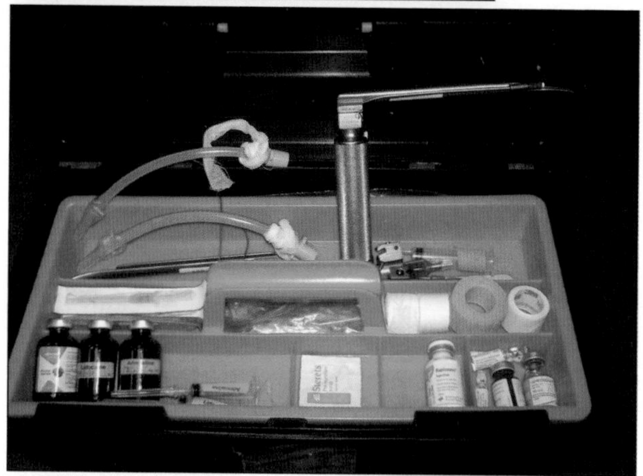

8.19 Example of a crash trolley from a large veterinary hospital and a crash box from a smaller practice. A variety of endotracheal tubes, intravenous catheters, drugs and monitoring equipment is present.

Anaesthetic machines and breathing systems

Every veterinary practice should be able to administer oxygen and maintain anaesthesia safely. Anaesthetic equipment should be maintained professionally, according to the manufacturer's recommendations, and records of regular servicing should be kept for production during inspection for the RCVS Practice Standards Scheme.

The anaesthetic machine takes the supplied carrier gas, regulates the pressure if necessary to a usable level, and passes it to the flowmeter (rotameter) block (see Figure 8.20), which is used to adjust the flow of gases to the appropriate level for the patient. The gas is then delivered to a vaporizer containing the volatile agent (usually isoflurane or sevoflurane); the vaporizer is used to control the level of volatile anaesthetic delivered to the patient. The gaseous mixture is delivered to the animal via the anaesthetic system and an endotracheal tube or facemask. The anaesthetic machine should have an emergency oxygen flush, which can take oxygen directly to the breathing system and patient, bypassing the flowmeters and vaporizer.

KEY POINTS

- Staff should understand the construction and performance of anaesthetic machines.
- Staff must check all anaesthetic machines and breathing systems, of whatever type, prior to each patient use.
- Training and refresher sessions are essential, as anaesthetic machines can be dangerous to patients and staff if they are not used, checked and maintained properly.

Anaesthetic machines

When purchasing a new anaesthetic machine the following features are desirable:

- Low-oxygen warning devices
- Automatic cut-out of nitrous oxide in the case of falling oxygen supply
- Over-pressure relief valve
- Emergency air intake valve.

Free-standing, moveable anaesthetic machines (Figure 8.20) are commonly used.

- Second-hand units, adapted to suit veterinary requirements from human hospital sales, can be cheaper than purpose-built small animal machines and often have more sophisticated safety features. However, they tend to be older and it may therefore be difficult to purchase components.
- Purpose-built anaesthetic machines for small animals often have patient breathing systems built on to them. These machines can be expensive and may lack some of the safety features incorporated within ex-human hospital anaesthetic machines. Some of these systems may not be suitable for birds and small mammals or reptiles.

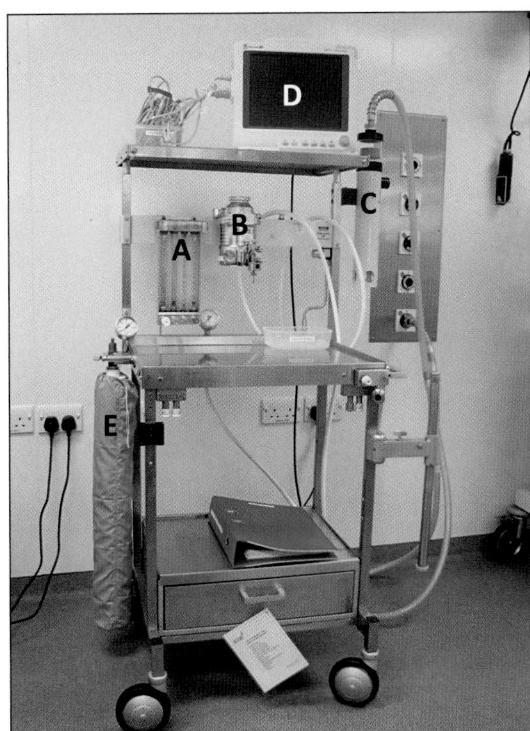

8.20 A freestanding mobile anaesthetic trolley. A = flowmeters; B = vaporizer; C = Barnsley air break receiver attached to scavenging tubing; D = patient monitor; E = spare gas cylinder (size E).

Wall-mounted anaesthetic machines (Figure 8.21) save space, can be economical and are convenient to use. As they are fixed to the wall they are less flexible than mobile machines, although some can be fitted to universal brackets located in different places and moved as necessary to suit workload. They usually do not have a spare oxygen cylinder attached.

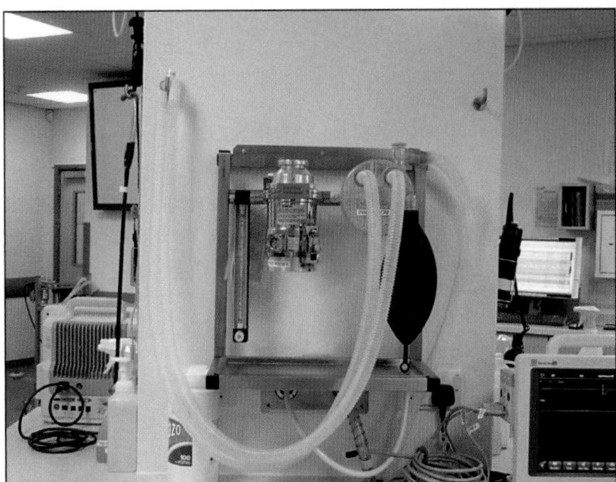

8.21 Wall-mounted anaesthetic machines can be mounted on brackets, allowing them to be moved to different locations according to need. Brackets can be purchased separately. This machine has a circle rebreathing system in place.

Vaporizers

Most inhalational anaesthetic agents are liquid at room temperature and pressure, and undergo vaporization before being delivered to the patient using calibrated vaporizers. There are several types.

Temperature-compensated plenum vaporizers (vaporizers out of circuit; VOCs) are the most common type used in the UK. They are made of copper and so are very heavy, and are fitted to the back bar of the anaesthetic machine (Figures 8.20 and 8.21). They are accurate under varying conditions of temperature, gas flow rate, back pressure and the volume of liquid within the chamber. They must only be used for the agent for which they have been calibrated, and they work under the positive pressure of gas delivered from the flowmeters, which are positioned 'upstream'. Agent-specific key fillers are commercially available and allow staff to fill the vaporizer with reduced risk of errors or inhaling the agent used (Figure 8.22).

Draw-over vaporizers (vaporizers in circuit; VICs) work under negative pressure produced by the patient's own inspiration and are used, for example, with Komesaroff and Stephen's machines. They are not temperature-compensated and their performance can be affected if the system is contaminated with

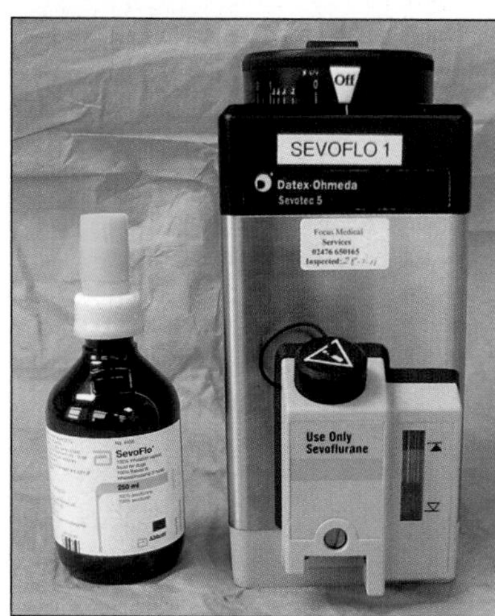

8.22 A TEC 5 sevoflurane vaporizer. Note the 'key-filler' which will only accept the tip of the sevoflurane bottle shown alongside the vaporizer.

water vapour. These machines are similar to circle breathing systems, require experience to use, and can result in anaesthetic overdose if intermittent positive pressure ventilation (IPPV) is carried out.

Inhalational anaesthetic agents

These are volatile liquids that evaporate easily at room temperature. The agent is added to a carrier gas that is breathed in by the patient. Isoflurane and sevoflurane are commonly used in veterinary practice, and halothane may still be occasionally used. Desflurane is also available but is not authorized for use in small animals.

- **Isoflurane** has an unpleasant odour and is slightly irritant to the respiratory mucosa. It is non-explosive but highly flammable and therefore bulk stock should be stored safely away from sources of ignition.
- **Halothane** is becoming less frequently used. It contains thymol as a preservative, which can build up within the vaporizer and affect its function; this is a particular problem with older mark 2 vaporizers, although these are rarely used now. Halothane is a non-irritant, non-explosive agent and non-flammable (in the concentrations usually used). It is a chlorofluorocarbon (CFC) and causes environmental pollution. It must be stored in dark glass bottles as it is decomposed by ultraviolet light.
- **Sevoflurane** is a modern, expensive inhalational agent, commonly used in human anaesthesia and authorized for use in dogs. It produces a rapid induction and recovery. Sevoflurane does not require any preservative but can decompose when used with soda lime to produce compound A (this has been found to be nephrotoxic in rats but this does not appear to be clinically relevant). Sevoflurane has a less pungent smell than isoflurane and so is generally more tolerated for mask inductions.

Anaesthetic breathing systems

Anaesthetic breathing systems connect the patient to the anaesthetic machine and should be chosen carefully, assessing each patient as an individual. A selection of anaesthetic systems should be available, suitable for the range of patients that are routinely treated. When choosing which systems are best for the individual practice, consideration should be given to the very small, to paediatric patients and to the giant breed dogs that may be presented.

The anaesthetic system chosen should allow intermittent positive pressure ventilation (IPPV). The simplest way of achieving IPPV is by intermittent, controlled squeezing of the reservoir bag against a closed or semi-closed adjustable pressure limiting (APL) valve in an appropriate breathing system. This can be labour-intensive, and it can be difficult to measure the correct, consistent inspiratory pressure and volume, which can lead to over- or under-ventilation. A mechanical ventilator is preferred to manual IPPV for the following situations:

- For prolonged ventilation associated with general anaesthesia and neuromuscular blockage
- For long-term management of respiratory disease or thoracic trauma
- For short-duration intensive respiratory care.

Mechanical ventilators are discussed in detail later in this chapter.

Anaesthetic systems are classified in many different ways depending on the following factors:

- Whether they contain an absorbent agent for carbon dioxide (anaesthetic systems which do not contain a carbon dioxide absorbent were classified by Mapleson in 1954 in classes A to F)
- According to their function: open, semi-open, semi-closed or closed.

Two breathing systems are pictured in Figure 8.23; further descriptions of commonly used breathing systems can be found in the *BSAVA Textbook of Veterinary Nursing* and *BSAVA Manual of Canine and Feline Anaesthesia and Analgesia*.

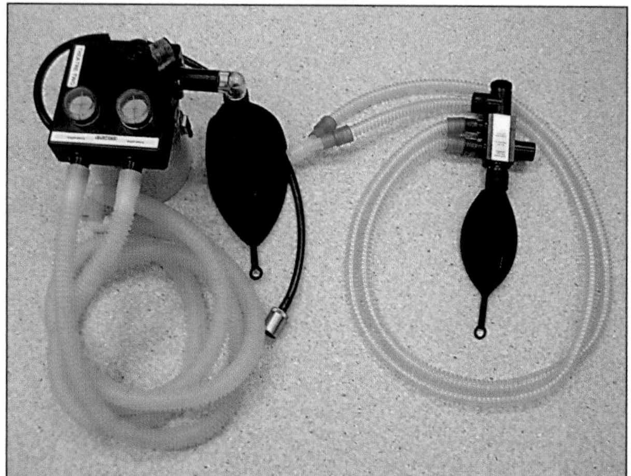

8.23 A rebreathing system (left) for larger patients and a mini-Lack (right) for smaller patients. Either system is suitable for IPPV.

It is useful to classify the most common anaesthetic breathing systems employed in veterinary practices as either 'breathing systems without carbon dioxide absorbent agent' or 'breathing systems with carbon dioxide absorbent agent'. The advantages and disadvantages of these types are discussed in Figure 8.24.

System	Advantages	Disadvantages
Without carbon dioxide absorbent		
Magill	Low resistance. Inexpensive to purchase. Inspired gas content similar to that set at anaesthetic machine. Rapid change in level of anaesthesia. Allows IPPV. Simple. Easy to clean and sterilize. Used for patients >10–60 kg	High volatile agent consumption costs. High running costs. Expired moisture and heat lost. Inconvenient position of Heidbrink valve results in difficulty of use during head and neck surgery and can increase system 'drag'. Gas flow rates for larger patients may exceed flowmeter capability
Coaxial Lack	Lightweight. More efficient than Magill. Long system, which allows the anaesthetic machine to be positioned away from the surgical site. Less drag than Magill (due to absence of valves at patient end). Allows IPPV. Easy to clean and sterilize	Stiff and inconvenient to use in small patients. Cannot see inner tube to detect whether kinked, broken or disconnected
Parallel Lack	Designed to overcome the problems with the coaxial Lack. Lower resistance. Paediatric versions can be used for patients >5 kg	Additional bulk is created with the two hoses. Increased drag
Mini-Lack (see Figure 8.23)	Smaller version of the standard Lack. Suitable for patients <10kg. Allows IPPV	
Bain	Inspired gases from the inner limb are warmed to a degree by expired gases in the outer (expiratory) limb. Used in patients 10–20 kg. Can be used for IPPV	Tube diameters may cause too much resistance in large dogs with spontaneous breathing. Inner tube can become kinked, disconnected or twisted, leading to hypercapnia
Jackson Rees-modified T-piece with closed reservoir bag and APL valve	Allows IPPV. Bag movement acts as respiration monitor. System of choice for patients <10 kg. Very low resistance. Can be used safely with nitrous oxide	
With carbon dioxide absorbent		
Circle	High gas efficiency. Mechanical deadspace remains unchanged during use. Bronchiolitis unlikely. Warms and moistens inspired gases	Difficult to clean. Difficult to sterilize. Some models expensive. Complex, so malfunctions more likely. Bulky. Staff time to replenish CO_2 absorbent. Reaction of inhalants with CO_2 absorbent can cause production of toxic compounds. Inspired gas content may be significantly different to that shown on the vaporizer
To and fro	High gas efficiency. Good heat conservation. Low resistance (compared to circle). Good control of gas concentration. Bidirectional gas flow improves absorbent's ability to absorb CO_2. Denitrogenation rapid. Warms and moistens inspired gases. Simple design and construction. Inexpensive. Easy to clean and sterilize. Portable	Considerable drag. Inconvenient during head and neck surgery. Difficult to perform IPPV due to pressure relief valve position. Bronchiolitis may occur from CO_2 absorbent dust. Mechanical deadspace increases during time of general anaesthetic due to absorbent becoming exhausted. Channelling of gas over CO_2 absorbent can occur if Waters canister is not correctly filled. Hyperthermia can occur in high ambient temperatures. Reaction of inhalants with CO_2 absorbent can cause production of toxic compounds. Inspired gas content may be significantly different to that shown on the vaporizer

8.24 Advantages and disadvantages of commonly used breathing systems without carbon dioxide absorbent.

Breathing systems should be kept clean inside and out, and allowed to dry completely between use; hanging is useful. Re-breathing bags should be hung when not in use and checked regularly for damage and perishing, particularly at the neck. Any rubber or plastic components showing signs of wear or deterioration should be replaced.

Mechanical ventilators

The use of a mechanical or electronic ventilator enables the anaesthetist to be free to monitor a wide variety of parameters rather than concentrating on manual ventilation. The initial cost of ventilators can be high, although basic mechanical 'Manley' ventilators (see Figure 8.31) are available second-hand at low cost for larger patients. Mechanical ventilators may not be suitable for smaller patients but there are several electronic ventilators specifically designed for veterinary patients on the market. Ventilators are controlled by either volume or pressure.

Endotracheal tubes

KEY POINT

The correct placement and fit of the endotracheal tube is a vital part of patient and personnel safety in theatre, and should be routinely checked. Over-inflation of cuffed tubes can damage the tracheal mucosa and may occlude the tube.

A good range of endotracheal (ET) tube types and sizes should be available, depending on the expected workload and considering paediatric patients, rabbits or other exotics, brachycephalic breeds and large-breed dogs. Supraglottic airway devices may also be considered. Tubes often need to be shortened to the correct length to minimize deadspace (some types are not suitable for shortening). Commonly used veterinary ET tubes are made from red rubber, PVC (plastic) or silicone (Figures 8.25 and 8.26).

Feature	Red rubber ETT	Plastic ETT	Silicone ETT
Irritant?	Can irritate trachea	Non-irritant	Non-irritant
Malleability	Rigidity can result in occlusion very easily upon flexion of neck or head, although tubes can soften with use	Soften and 'mould' in place after a period of time	Clear straight tubes that may require a stylet to form curvature to ease intubation. Mould to patient's contours when warmed
Cuffs	Inflate with spherical contour, leading to less contact with, but increased pressure on, tracheal mucosa.Low-volume, high-pressure. More likely to cause mucosal trauma. Pilot balloon not self-sealing	Inflate to rectangular outline, which spreads pressure better over tracheal mucosa. High-volume, low-pressure. Self-sealing pilot balloon – syringe required to deflate	Low-volume, high-pressure. Self-sealing pilot balloon – syringe required to deflate
Relative cost	Small sizes inexpensive; larger sizes can be expensive	Often inexpensive	Expensive
Sterilization	Can withstand autoclave sterilization	Disposable tubes that cannot withstand autoclaving	Can withstand sterilization by autoclaving
Notes	Use with care in cats as high-pressure low-volume cuff carries higher risk of damage to sensitive feline tracheal mucosa. Cannot easily see inside tube to check for obstructions	Disposable tubes designed for human patients can be used	Kits available for minor repairs to cuff, balloon and inflation tube

8.25 Characteristics of different types of endotracheal tube.

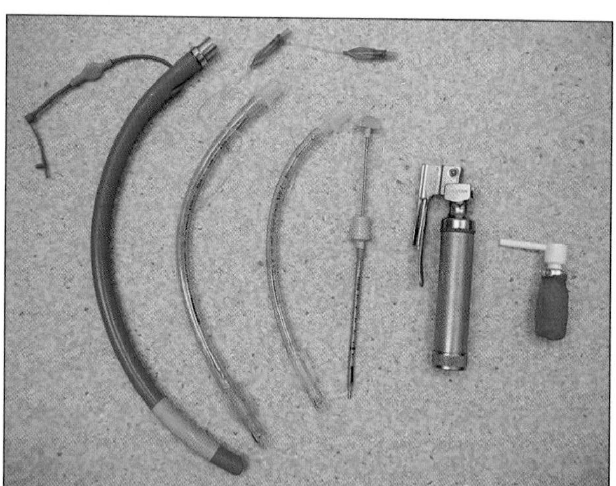

8.26 From left to right: rubber Magill endotracheal tube; two PVC cuffed tubes; uncuffed PVC tube with metal stylet to aid insertion (note the stylet would be drawn back so as not to protrude from the end of the tube during insertion into the patient); laryngoscope; local anaesthetic spray for preparing the airway for insertion of the tube (note that the bottle is wrapped to protect it from light).

- Murphy pattern tubes (Figure 8.27a) have an oval hole just proximal to the distal tip to allow the anaesthetic gas to continue to flow in the event of the distal opening of the tube becoming positioned against the wall of the airway.
- Magill pattern tubes are available for oral and nasal use. The oral versions are cuffed or plain uncuffed and have thicker walls than the nasal versions. The cuffed version has an external inflation pipe.
- Armoured tubes (Figure 8.27b) have a steel wire or nylon coil embedded in the wall of the tube to prevent kinking and occlusion of the tube during positioning. They are useful for patients undergoing head, neck or ophthalmic procedures.
- Cuffed ET tubes reduce contamination of the environment from waste anaesthetic gases and reduce the risk of aspiration of saliva, regurgitated stomach contents or irrigation fluids.

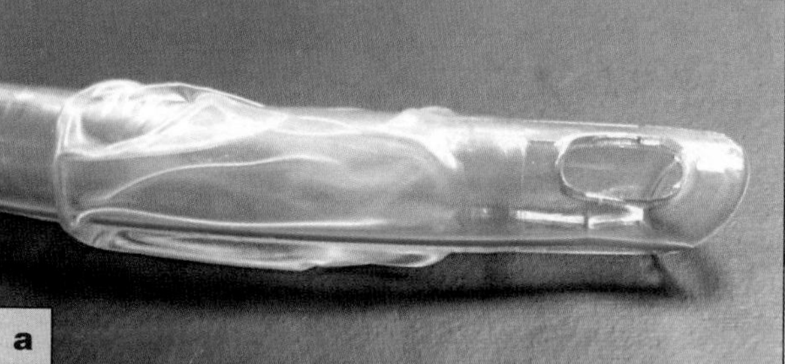

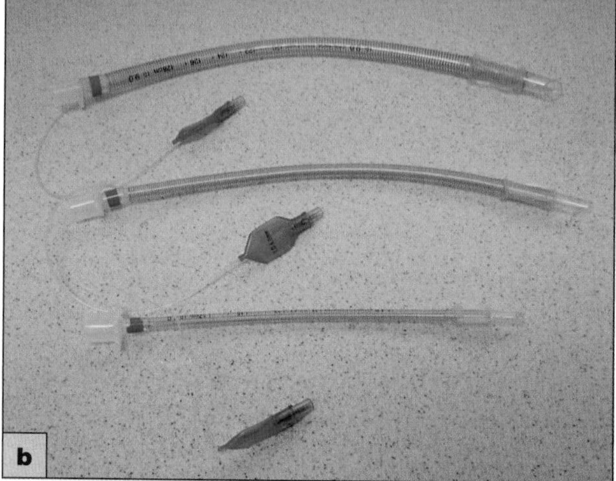

8.27 **(a)** Murphy pattern endotracheal tube with an oval hole just proximal to the distal tip. **(b)** Armoured tubes.

KEY POINTS

- Endotracheal tubes should be washed and dried thoroughly after use.
- They should be stored in closed drawers to prevent dust contamination and damage from light. They should not be stored within an operating theatre and open wall racks are not recommended.
- They should be inspected (inside and out) and checked thoroughly before use.

Patient monitoring equipment

Monitoring machines

Patient monitors are increasingly reliable and are used in addition to observation of the patient's mucous membrane colour, eye position, palpebral reflex, palpation of proximal and distal pulse points, and respiratory pattern and effort. A wide variety of monitors is commercially available, both new and second-hand.

Multi-parameter monitors are becoming more common, with alpha-numeric and graphical display screens (Figure 8.28). Not every piece of monitoring equipment is required for each procedure; monitors should be selected on the basis of a risk assessment, which should take into account the individual patient and nature of procedure to be performed, as well as the technical skill of the staff member involved.

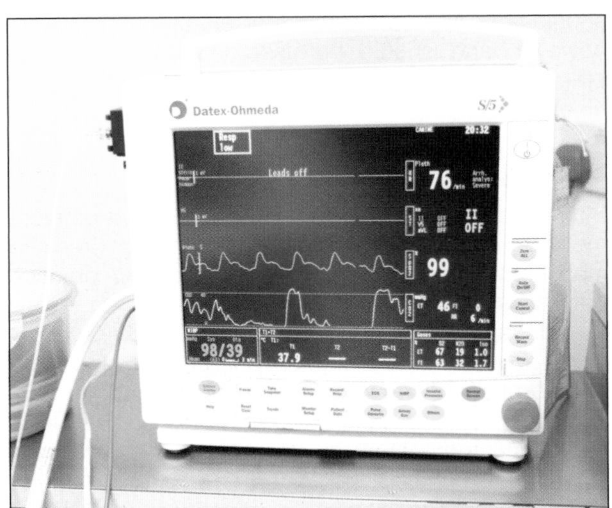

8.28 A multi-parameter monitor showing pulse oximetry and capnography traces. The ECG leads are not being used. Along the lower part of the screen (left to right) are measurements for blood pressure, body temperature and gases (oxygen, nitrous oxide and isoflurane).

It is important with all electrical monitors that the patient leads are isolated from the mains supply. This is usually achieved using optical isolators in the preamplifier of the monitoring unit. Patient leads and the monitors themselves must be kept clean and disinfected between patients. Staff should be thoroughly trained in how to use and interpret the monitoring equipment available; SOPs for equipment usage are beneficial for staff and ensure patient care is not compromised.

Oesophageal stethoscopes

Oesophageal stethoscopes (Figure 8.29) are inexpensive and simple to use for monitoring patients during surgery and the perioperative period. They should always be used in conjunction with other means of assessment, such as palpation of the peripheral pulses, direct patient observation and observation of the reservoir bag. They allow the person monitoring the anaesthetic to listen to the heart and respiration rates and sounds, without the need to disturb the draped patient. They function in the same way as a standard stethoscope and are connected to an earpiece or a dedicated amplifier. A selection of different sizes is essential for any practice.

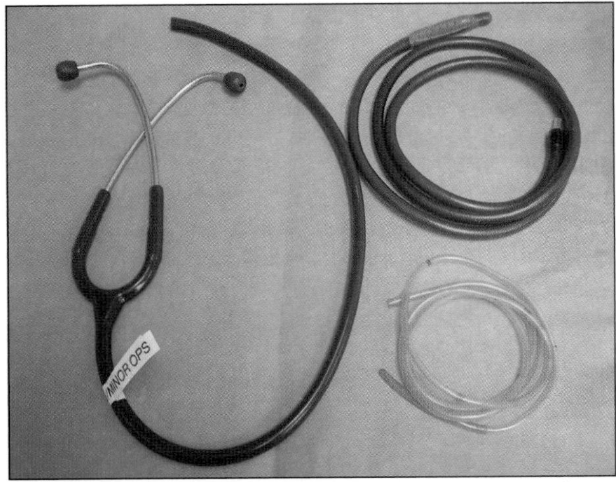

8.29 An oesophageal stethoscope is simple and reliable. The appropriate size should be selected for each patient and the tubing cleaned and disinfected after use.

Pulse oximeters

Pulse oximetry is a non-invasive method of measuring blood oxygen saturation (to provide warning of hypoxaemia) and pulse rate (which gives an indication of the rate of effective stroke volumes of the heart). Pulse oximeters are commonly used in practice and are easy to use. They are available as mains-powered or rechargeable battery-powered units. Most are hand-held, small and light, and can be easily transported. A red and infra-red light signal from a probe is transmitted through tissue, measuring the pulsatile volume changes that occur and calculating the percentage of haemoglobin that is saturated with oxygen. There are many different sensors (patient probes) available (Figure 8.30). Probes incorporate light-emitting diodes

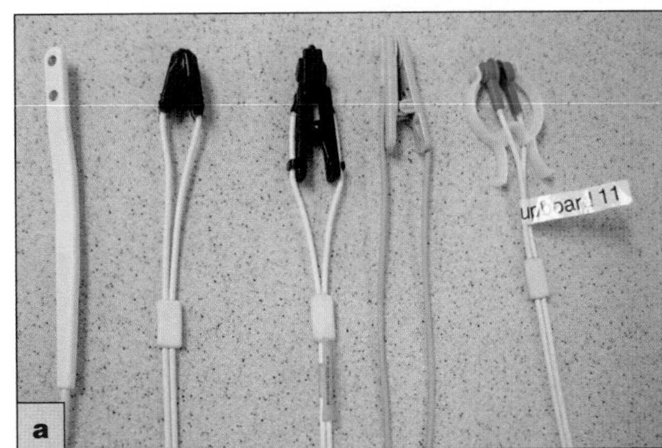

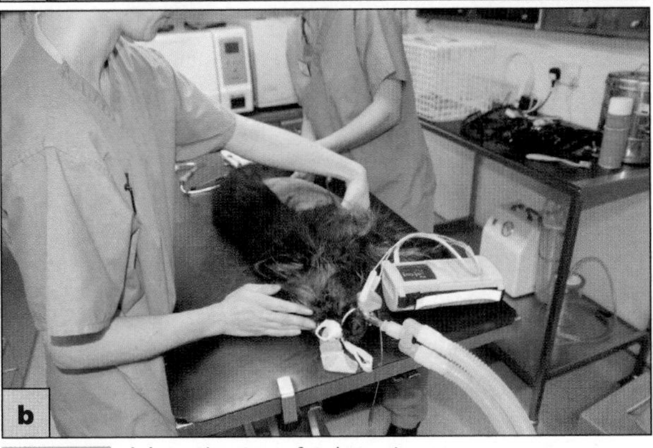

8.30 **(a)** A selection of pulse oximeter sensors. **(b)** A pulse oximeter in use. This model has a rubber jacket to protect it from damage.

(LEDs), which emit light at specific wavelengths, and a photodetector (photocell, transducer). They are fragile and expensive, so should be handled and cleaned with care. Periodic replacement is necessary. Disposable sensors are available and may be preferable where cross-contamination is a concern. An electrical cable attaches the sensor to the console/monitor and cables from different manufacturers should not be used interchangeably.

Pulse oximeters usually have an audible beep to indicate pulse, and this is a helpful alerting feature, although inaccuracies can occur in the event of shivering. Pulse oximeters also display the pulse rate. One of the disadvantages of pulse oximetry is that the operator cannot check the calibration, although there are now devices on the market that can be used to test pulse oximeters.

Capnographs

Capnography (Figure 8.31) is easy to apply, non-invasive and provides valuable information on a patient's ventilation system and cardiac output. A capnograph produces a graphical representation (capnogram) of carbon dioxide levels throughout the patient's respiratory cycle. Information may be displayed on a screen (see Figure 8.28) and/or printed out. The monitors can also display the respiration rate, end-tidal carbon dioxide levels and inspired carbon dioxide levels. Use of capnography can increase deadspace from sampling connectors.

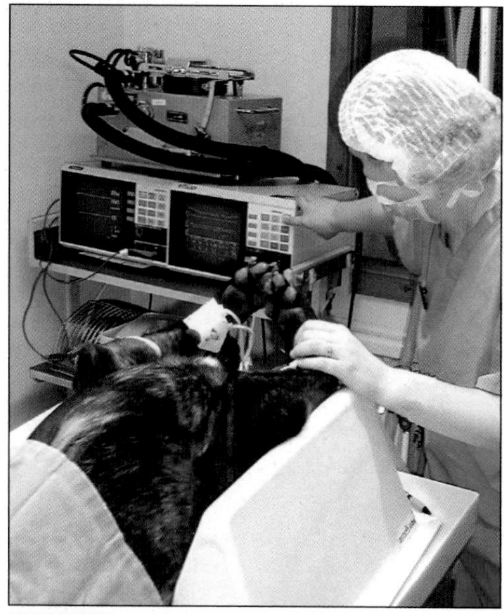

8.31 Older style multi-parameter monitors showing capnography, pulse oximetry, ECG, blood pressure, oxygen and anaesthetic gas monitoring. Note the Manley ventilator on top of the monitors.

Mainstream sampling is the most accurate method and measures gas directly from the airway using a sensor located within the breathing system. Many capnographs, however, utilize sidestream sampling, where the sensor is in the monitor and gas is removed from the breathing system, usually via a small sampling connector located close to the endotracheal tube, increasing the deadspace. In this case, the capnography sampling line must always be connected to a scavenger to avoid polluting the room air.

Staff should be trained in how to use and interpret the capnogram correctly. It is beneficial to have an information sheet of the most frequently seen capnography traces, for staff to refer to. If not used correctly, capnography can increase the risk of leaks within the breathing system and of contamination of the environment with anaesthetic gases. Sampling lines and connectors should be disinfected following use, as cross-contamination could occur between patients.

Capnography is becoming more common in general practice as monitors are more readily available. Monitors can still be expensive, although they are becoming cheaper, both new and second-hand.

Electrocardiography

Many monitors display a three-lead electrocardiogram (ECG), which can be useful to detect physiological abnormalities and changes in heart rhythm. The ECG should not be relied upon to indicate cardiac function, however, and should be used in conjunction with other patient monitoring devices. Further details on electrocardiography can be found in Chapter 11.

Blood pressure

Blood pressure can be measured using two different methods: indirect or direct. Indirect blood pressure measurement is more common in general practice but is less reliable.

Arterial blood pressure can be measured indirectly using a variety of techniques based on the occlusion of blood flow to an extremity (any of the limbs or tail): a blood pressure cuff (also known as an occlusive cuff) is inflated until all flow through the artery ceases and is then deflated until blood flow returns. Indirect blood pressure monitors give intermittent readings of blood pressure. Correct selection of the blood pressure cuff is important, as the width and position of the cuff affect the result. An experienced operator and quiet surroundings facilitate a more accurate measurement and the procedure can often be delegated to veterinary nurses.

- The oscillometric technique (Figure 8.32a) detects the flow of blood by pulsatile changes within the blood pressure cuff, and readings are recorded automatically by the machine. Oscillometric methods can be difficult to use in small patients.
- The Doppler technique (Figure 8.32b) uses an ultrasound probe and audible signal detected (generally through headphones) by a manual operator. Doppler monitors tend to be cheaper and are extremely useful for hypertensive cats. Doppler monitors are mainly used to measure systolic blood pressure; diastolic pressure can be measured but this can be unreliable.

If cost is not an issue it may be beneficial for the practice to invest in both oscillometric and Doppler blood pressure monitors.

Direct blood pressure measurement involves the placement of an arterial cannula into a peripheral artery; although useful, this is less frequently used in general practice. Arterial cannulation can be difficult to achieve and it is extremely important that patients with indwelling arterial cannulae are clearly identified, such as by clear labelling on the dressing.

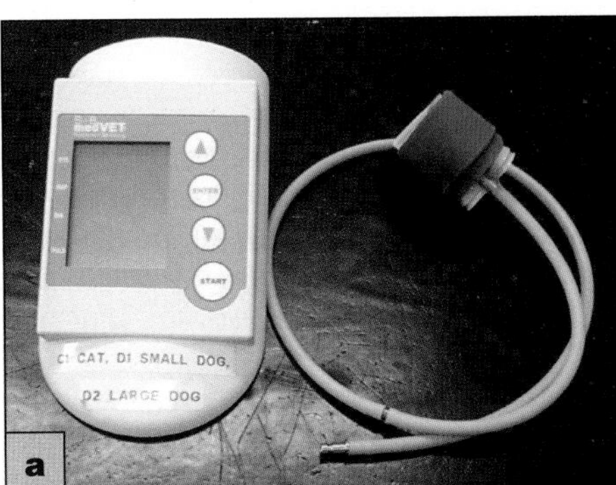

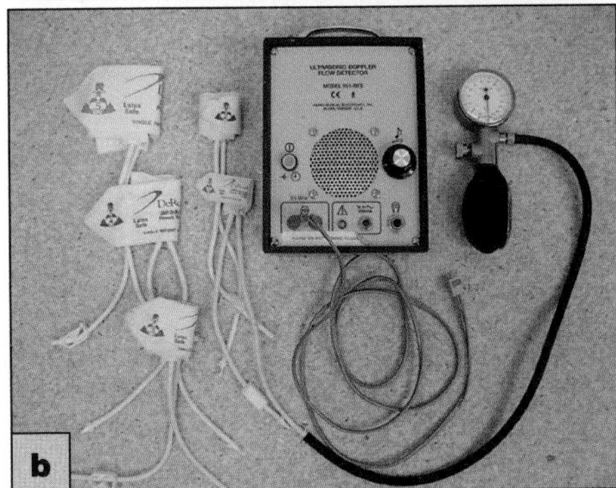

8.32 Indirect blood pressure monitors: **(a)** oscillometric; **(b)** Doppler.

Temperature probes

Rectal or oesophageal probes are available for use with stand-alone or multi-parameter monitors and are invaluable for ensuring body temperature is maintained during procedures.

Patient warming

Maintaining body temperature is an important aspect of anaesthesia, particularly if a surgical procedure is being carried out. Small patients have a large surface area-to-volume ratio and rapidly lose body heat due to surgical preparation, contact with cool surfaces (stainless steel table tops), breathing of dry cold anaesthetic gases, and evaporation and heat loss through any open surgical site/body cavity. Large patients are also at risk of hypothermia. Regardless of patient size, every effort should be made to keep them within their normal physiological temperature range, and preparation times should be minimized. Hypothermia can result in prolonged recovery times, reduction in tissue oxygenation and cardiac arrhythmias, and may also reduce the patient's innate resistance to bacterial infections.

KEY POINTS

- Patient warming equipment should be available in the 'prep' area, operating theatre and recovery area, and applied immediately following the induction of general anesthesia in most patients.
- Devices will be less effective if patients are not kept dry.
- It is important to ensure that any devices used are functioning properly; application of heat over the skin can result in thermal injuries to the patient, and extreme care and continuous observation should be employed when using any heating aids.

External warming aids

External warming aids can vary from cheaper means of preventing heat loss, such as bubble wrap, survival or 'space blankets', insulating blankets and socks, to more expensive controllable electrical warming devices (Figure 8.33). Insulating the patient from the floor or table is as important as covering them to keep them warm. Heated towels, home-made 'hot hands' (gloves or fluid bags with warm water inside them) or hot water bottles are all quick and easy to prepare, and microwaveable heat pads can be useful if care is taken not to overheat them.

KEY POINT

Electric heated pads must be used under close supervision only, and care taken to ensure the patient is dry and that overheating of certain areas does not cause burns.

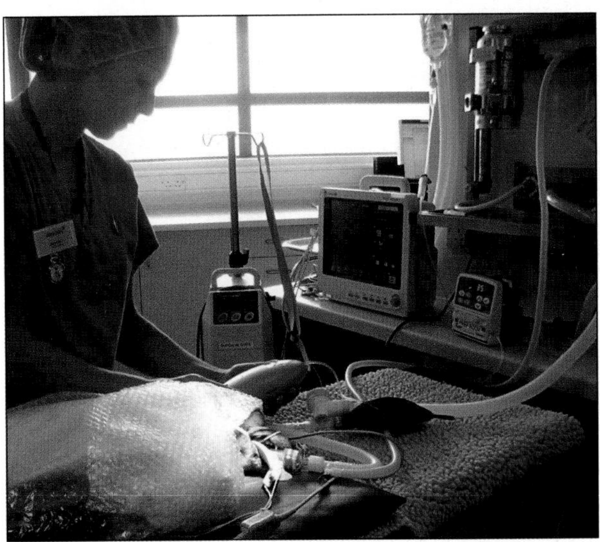

8.33 This patient's body temperature is being maintained using several methods: it is lying on a black thermal mattress (control unit fixed to drip stand); bubble wrap is being used as an insulator; the intravenous drip line is being passed though a line warmer (in the nurse's hands) and a thermovent is in place between the breathing system and the endotracheal tube. The infusion pump can be seen on the worktop to the right. The patient is being monitored with a multi-parameter monitor (on worktop to left); the pulse oximeter probe is visible attached to the tongue.

Operating tables and recovery cages are available with electrically heated surfaces. Padded beds with electronic thermostatically controlled heating (Figure 8.34) are expensive but are easy to maintain, very durable and do not carry the risk of thermal burns associated with many electric heated pads. A variety of sizes is available.

Circulating warm-air blankets can be used: a hot-air blower unit with a flexible hose is attached to disposable paper blankets that hold the warm air next to the patient (Figure 8.35). The blankets are available in a variety of sizes. It is important to ensure the warm air is flowing into the blanket rather than into the environment. Because they are expensive, the blankets are often re-used, but this is not ideal for infection control purposes. With both warm air and warm water

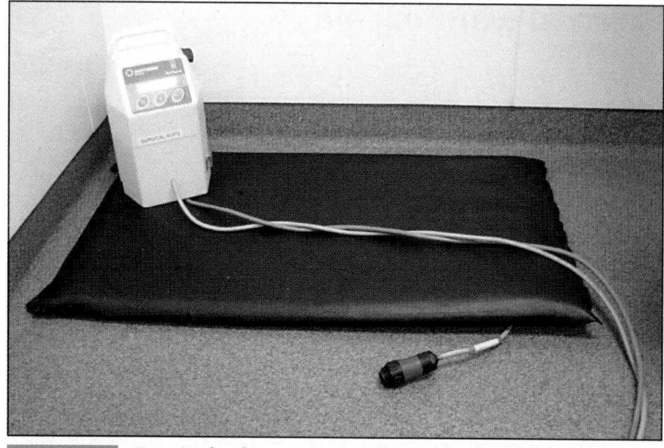

8.34 Precisely thermostatically controlled heated padded beds are expensive but are easy to maintain, very durable and do not carry the risk of thermal burns associated with many electric heated pads. A variety of sizes is available.

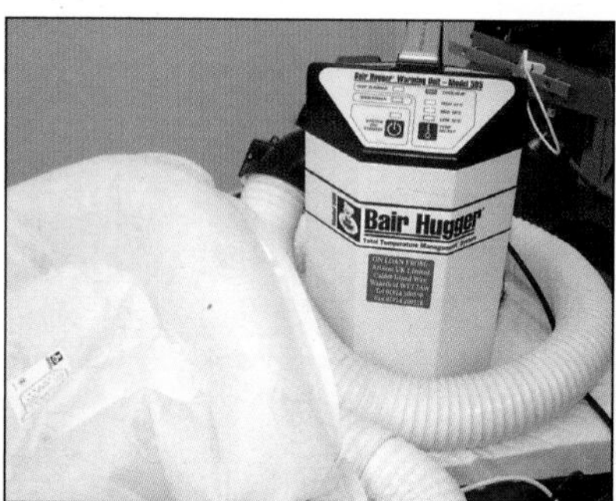

8.35 A circulating warmed air system is an efficient way to provide supplementary warmth, but has some disadvantages in the surgical environment.

units (see below) it is important that they are maintained correctly using the manufacturer's recommendations. These units require close observation of the patient and can be noisy during use. They can also contribute to excessive air movement within the surgical field, though modern versions have antibacterial air inlet filters.

Circulating hot-water blankets, generally used under the patient, are also available in a variety of sizes. A thermostatically controlled water circulating unit is attached to a reusable plastic mattress with multiple water channels. The mattresses are expensive and are vulnerable to puncture, but are usually made from reusable materials that are easy to clean. Water in recirculating units should be monitored and treated with a fungicide and algicide to maintain function.

Other measures

Other methods of maintaining body temperature during and after surgery include:

- Warming intravenous and other fluids (e.g. for lavage) before use with electrically operated warmers or by passing fluid lines through beakers of warm water
- Using disposable heat moisture exchangers (HMEs, 'thermovents') between the endotracheal tube and the breathing system, to conserve heat from exhaled breath and use it to warm inhaled gases
- Using circle breathing systems at moderate or low fresh gas flow, rather than non-rebreathing systems
- Pre-warming the patient before surgery.

Theatre equipment

Further information on theatre equipment and instrumentation can be found in the *BSAVA Manual of Canine and Feline Surgical Principles: A Foundation Manual* and the *BSAVA Textbook of Veterinary Nursing*.

Operating tables

The operating table should be chosen carefully.

- The height of the table should be adjustable; this can be mechanical, foot-pumped or electronic.
- The table should ideally be able to tilt in many directions, as certain procedures (e.g. laparoscopy) benefit from the use of tilting during the procedure in order to alter the position of the patient. Other means of tilting the patient are available, such as the use of positioning boards; however, this can be time-consuming and it is sometimes difficult to achieve the desired results.
- Tilting devices are available; these are secured on to the operating table and facilitate secure patient tilting, such as during laparoscopic procedures (see Chapter 10).
- Table attachments are available to create a 'tent' with the drapes, allowing the anaesthetist to monitor the patient without contaminating the surgical field. Alternatively, hand-made wire-framed structures can be used (bent cooling trays are handy for smaller patients). In the author's experience this is valuable for both nurses and anaesthetists to aid close monitoring of the patient.
- Attachments can also be purchased that allow instrument stands, drip stands and limb supports to be attached to the operating table.
- If fluoroscopy is to be used, the table should be radiolucent.
- As noted above, tables are available with heated surfaces to facilitate patient warming (Figure 8.36).

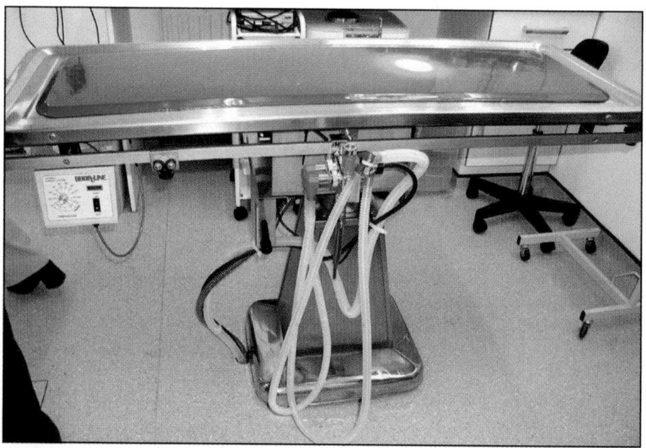

8.36 Thermostatically controlled heated operating tables can be useful for maintaining patient body temperature. This picture also shows gas scavenging routed under the floor.

Positioning aids

Positioning aids for surgery can include:

- Sandbags
- Rope ties
- Vacuum-activated bean bags

- Cradles
- Tapes
- Orthopaedic limb positioning devices
- Table attachments, overhead bars and hooks.

Positioning aids should be maintained, cleaned and used correctly. They carry a high risk of contamination and so should be reserved for use within the theatre.

Stools

Adjustable mobile seat or saddle stools, particularly if they are of ergonomic design, can be useful for the anaesthetist and surgeon. Stools used in the surgical area should be easy to clean and in good repair.

Radiograph viewers

There should be a means of displaying radiographs in the operating theatre. This could be a mobile lightbox viewer or computer display screen for digital images (see Figure 8.7 and Chapter 13). If fluoroscopy or a mobile radiography machine is to be used in the operating theatre, consideration should be given as to where in the theatre this equipment is to be stored. This can be problematical, with reduced floor space increasing the chance of non-sterile personnel contaminating the sterile field, and increased dust traps becoming a source of microbial contamination. If equipment such as this has to be stored in an operating theatre, washable protective covers can be made to measure (see Figure 8.6). The risks associated with ionizing radiation must also be considered (see Chapter 13).

Surgical instruments

Practices should have a range of surgical instruments, appropriate to the species and patient sizes treated and for the procedures normally carried out. It is useful to have standard kits or sets of instruments, with additional instruments added for particular procedures. Using a standard kit reduces problems at surgery and the risk of leaving an instrument undetected inside a patient (instrument count sheets can be used if this is a significant concern, e.g for deep abdominal procedures).

KEY POINT

A standard surgical kit instrument list should be agreed with the team and written down. Photographs of complete kits with instruments identified are useful for training purposes.

Instruments in the veterinary market tend to be manufactured from chromium-plated carbon steel, as they are cheaper than stainless steel. However, they are less hardwearing and will rust, pit and blister quickly when they come into contact with blood, irrigation fluids and chemicals. Instruments made from stainless steel are more resistant to corrosion and have greater strength. Some instruments made from stainless steel have tungsten carbide tips, e.g. scissors and needle holders. These are more expensive than standard tips but are harder and more resistant to wear. These instruments are easy to identify as they have gold-coloured handles (Figure 8.37).

Care of instruments and their sterilization are covered later in the chapter.

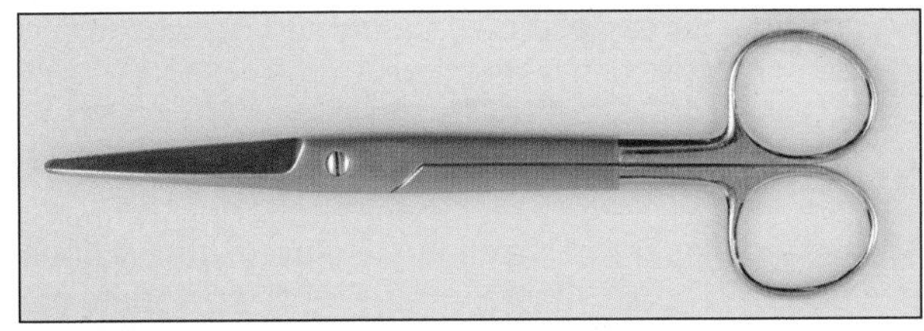

8.37 Instruments with tungsten carbide tips have gold-coloured handles.

Electrosurgery

Electrosurgery, also referred to as diathermy, vessel-sealing or electrocautery, is commonly used in veterinary practice for tissue dissection and coagulation during surgical procedures. It is extremely useful for controlling haemorrhage during surgery and thus reducing surgical time. Electrosurgery utilizes the passage of a high-frequency alternating electrical current (AC) through the tissues, and can be 'monopolar' or 'bipolar' (Figure 8.38):

- Monopolar diathermy is the most frequently used method and offers a greater range of tissue effects. The patient forms a large proportion of the electrical circuit. An active cable from the electrosurgery unit carries current to the monopolar electrode (handpiece plus forceps/tip). The current then spreads through the tissue to the patient plate or return electrode (earthing plate), which is placed in direct contact with the patient. It is extremely important that the patient plate electrode is correctly positioned. The electrosurgical unit can be either handpiece- or foot-activated
- Bipolar electrosurgery forceps incorporate two electrodes, either of which returns the current. The current just passes between the electrodes (generally the two tips of a pair of forceps), and no patient plate electrode is needed.

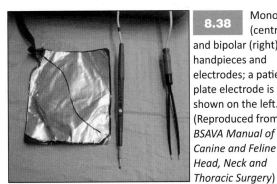

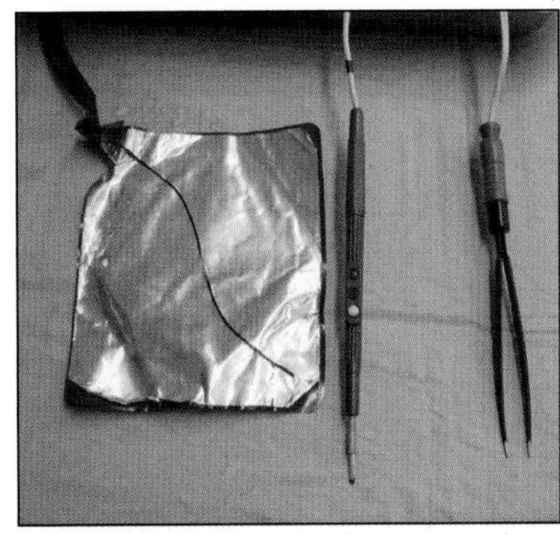

8.38 Monopolar (centre) and bipolar (right) handpieces and electrodes; a patient plate electrode is shown on the left. (Reproduced from *BSAVA Manual of Canine and Feline Head, Neck and Thoracic Surgery*)

A number of units are available for the veterinary market, or new or reconditioned human machines are readily purchased. Intended use, size and species of patient, space available and costs are all significant considerations in the choice of unit.

An SOP should be created for the safe use of the electrosurgery unit within the practice. Routine daily checks of the electrosurgery unit should be limited to external checks of the unit but should include all accessories and cables. Before the machine is used it should undergo a visual check to ensure no cables are damaged and that switches are working correctly. Routine maintenance should be carried out according to the manufacturer's instructions.

Surgical lasers

The use of lasers in veterinary surgery can reduce postoperative pain, haemorrhage and postoperative swelling.

Lasers are expensive and some older models can be cumbersome, though modern models are now commercially available which are portable and compact (Figure 8.39). The disadvantages of laser surgery are mainly the purchase cost of a laser unit and the health and safety considerations.

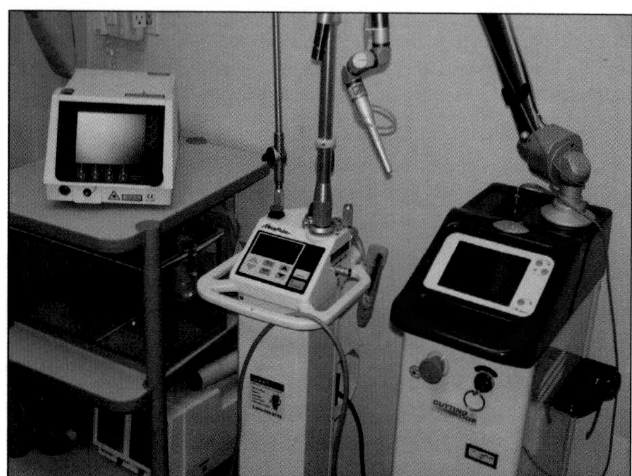

8.39 Three common commercially available surgical lasers: (left to right) Accuvet 25D-980 Diode Surgical Laser; Novapulse 20 watt CO_2 laser; Cutting Edge ML030 30 watt CO_2 laser.

Lasers can be of various types:

- Gas lasers (carbon dioxide laser; wavelength 10,600 nm)
- Liquid lasers (generally rhodamine dye; tunable from 100 nm to 1000 nm)
- Solid crystal lasers (neodymium:yttididium–aluminum–garnet laser (ND:YAG); wavelength 1064 nm)
- Diode lasers: (wavelengths ranging from 590 nm to 980 nm or higher). This type does not produce light in a lasing chamber but emits light when an electric current is passed through a solid-state chip. Semiconductor diode lasers can be used for trans-scleral cyclophotocoagulation in the treatment of glaucoma, treatment of iris cysts and tumours, and retinopexy.

When looking to purchase a laser unit, a long warranty (ideally 3 years) is beneficial and should cover the entire unit, including energy transfer apparatus and focusing device; technical support and cover should be clarified. Second-hand units are commercially available, but caution should be exercised when purchasing these, and a re-certification from either the manufacturers or a certified repair company should be obtained, which should be to the same standards as a new unit; an extended warranty is also useful. The Veterinary Surgical Laser Society (VSLS) can provide more information on surgical lasers and staff training programmes.

Suction

Suction is used for removing fluids from surgical fields and for emergency airway clearance. A suction machine should be available for use within the operating theatre and support areas, and can be portable or piped in (Figure 8.40). Piped-in systems tend to have the main unit situated in a separate plant room, as it is bulky and noisy. These units have outlets in the theatre into which compatible machines can be plugged using a specially designed hose. Disposable or re-usable fluid collection bottles can be used; when choosing between these options, thought should be directed to ease of cleaning, reliability and cost-effectiveness. Noise may also be a factor. Suction machines often have filters which are disposable items. When purchasing new suction machines, the costs of the filters as well as of the overall unit should be considered.

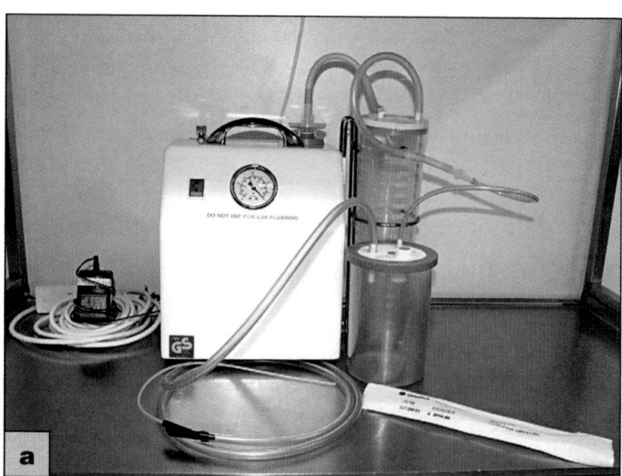

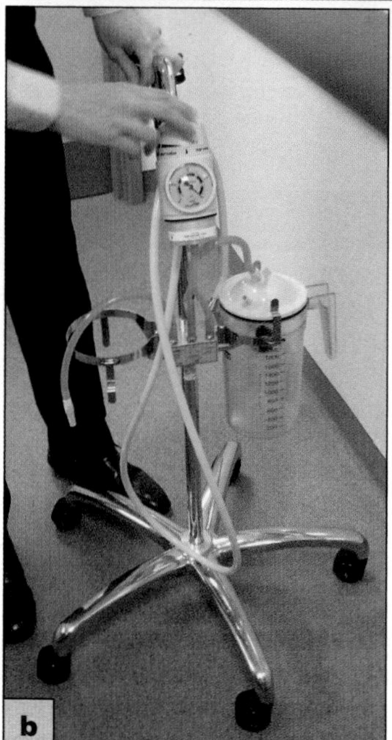

8.40 **(a)** A portable suction machine should be ready to use at all times in case of emergency. The disposable filter is fitted where the suction tubing enters the machine on the top. **(b)** A mobile suction unit for attachment to a central suction source.

Gowns and drapes

Factors to consider when purchasing drapes and gowns are detailed in Figure 8.41.

Gowns

The 'ply' category of an operating gown (the number of layers a material contains) can be used to determine whether it is suitable for a certain procedure. General suggestions to assist in choosing a surgical gown are as follows (Humes and Lobo, 2009):

- One-ply gown: suitable for surgeries of <2 hours and where <100 ml blood loss is expected and lavage fluids will not be used
- Two-ply reinforced gowns: used for longer procedures (2–4 hours), where 100–500 ml blood loss is anticipated, or the chest or abdominal cavity is being entered
- Impervious gowns: suitable for procedures lasting >4 hours.

Drapes

Pre-sterilized disposable drapes are available with a variety of characteristics. Customized drape packs are available that may be useful for routine surgical procedures, reducing the number of individual disposable products that need to be opened and presented to the surgeon. These save time and may be a worthwhile consideration, depending on usage and price.

Re-usable gowns and drapes should be inspected visually to ensure they are not damaged prior to packing. They will withstand around 50 reprocessing cycles before becoming damaged and it is important that wash cycles are traced to prevent over-use. Small fabric charts are available to attach to the fabric; these are ticked or dotted after each use in order to trace the number of times the drapes or gown has been reprocessed and used.

Ancillary equipment

Other important equipment for use within an operating theatre includes:

- Anaesthetic machines and supplies (see above)
- Patient monitoring equipment (see above)
- Intravenous fluid stands
- Intravenous fluid pumps and syringe drivers (both are important, particularly for very small patients or those receiving constant rate infusions) (see Chapter 7)
- Mayo instrument stands
- Instrument tables (large enough to accommodate all the necessary instrumentation)
- Kick buckets on wheels (to allow ease of movement)
- Height-adjustable instrument trays/tables (fit over the top of the operating table and patient during surgery)
- Absorbent pads
- Selection of needles and syringes
- Laboratory sample collection equipment (e.g. swabs, pots, microscope slides, tissue transport containers and baskets)
- Mouth gags and pharyngeal packs
- Personal Protective Equipment (PPE).

The operating room should also have a clock which is visible from the room itself, with a sweeping second hand. A stopwatch is also useful for critical procedures such as when occluding vasculature.

Requirements	Reasons	Comments
Resistant to penetration by blood or other body fluids	To minimize strikethrough and potential personnel contamination	Microorganisms can be transferred through barrier materials by wicking of fluids. Pressure exerted by leaning on flooded areas can lead to wet and dry penetration by microorganisms if the pressure exceeds the level of resistance ('barrier quality') provided by the material
Maintain integrity; durable	To prevent the passage of microorganisms and fluids between sterile and non-sterile areas	Gowns and drapes should be resistant to tears, punctures and abrasions. Items in use must be free from holes and other defects
Low linting	Bacteria can attach to lint particles, which could result in SSIs. Lint particles can dissipate into the environment	Lint can be used as a transport vehicle (fomite) for microorganisms
Suitable for sterilization	To ensure the drape or gown is completely sterile prior to use	Disposable products are mostly provided in a sterile package. Reusable materials should have the ability to be sterilized and should not be damaged by repeated washing, drying and sterilization
Resist combustion	To provide a safe environment for staff and patients	The operating theatre contains many fire hazards.There are many combustible materials and potential ignition sources
Comfort; maintenance of the wearer's body temperature	To provide a comfortable isothermic environment for surgeons and patients	Drapes that result in discomfort to the surgeon or the patient are suboptimal
Limited 'memory'; conform to patient contours	Ease of working for the operating team. Prevents contamination	Drapes with 'memory' can spring back easily into their original shape. The handling quality of materials should be taken into account

8.41 Factors to consider when purchasing drapes or gowns.

Pressurized gases and liquid nitrogen

Anaesthetic gases such as oxygen and nitrous oxide, as well as compressed medical air and carbon dioxide (for laparoscopy), are used frequently within the surgical suite.

Compressed gas storage

Most veterinary practices store gases in compressed form in small portable (size E) cylinders, in larger cylinder banks (size J and G) connected to a pipeline system (Figure 8.42), or a combination of the two.

Small-volume 'E' size cylinders attach directly to the hanger yokes on the anaesthetic machine (see Figure 8.20). It is important to carry out constant pressure checks, and changing the cylinder can be tedious, so this system is problematical when gas consumption is high. For cost-effectiveness and convenience, a piped gas system is preferable and the machine-mounted cylinders should act as a reserve supply.

Small-volume 'C' size cylinders of medical air or carbon dioxide, with a regulator attached, are often used to power tools or supply insufflation for laparoscopic equipment, respectively.

KEY POINT

Understanding the correct handling and use of these gases, as well as the risks associated with them, is essential for patient safety and the health of the surgical team (see later).

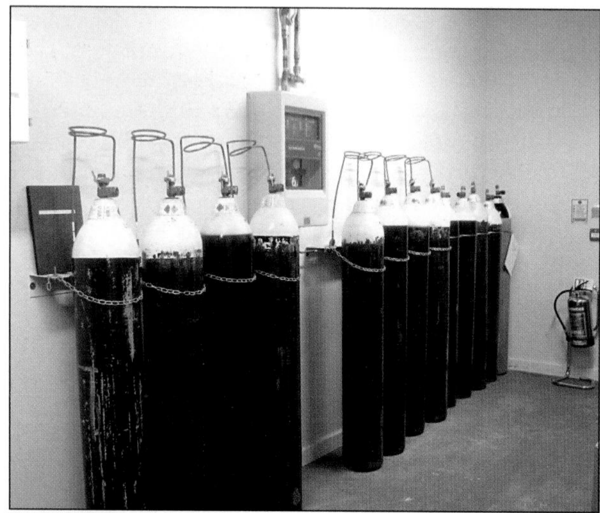

8.42 An oxygen cylinder bank in a large practice.

Oxygen

Oxygen can be stored in liquid form or as a compressed gas. Liquid oxygen is stored in vacuum-insulated evaporators (VIEs) and this is the most economical way to store and supply oxygen, as cylinders are no longer required; however, it is only practical for very large hospitals. Most veterinary establishments store oxygen in compressed form in cylinders, although oxygen generators can prove more economical in some practices (see Chapter 2).

Nitrous oxide

Nitrous oxide (N_2O) gas is commonly used during anaesthesia as a carrier gas, in part for its analgesic (pain-relieving) qualities, and it allows the anaesthetist to reduce the amount of volatile agent administered to the patient. The use of nitrous oxide is potentially hazardous in low-flow or closed systems (see later), as the uptake of oxygen and nitrous oxide will occur at different rates, reducing the relative oxygen content.

Nitrous oxide is a greenhouse gas and depletes the ozone layer more than other anaesthetic gases. It can be potentially dangerous to staff and should only be used with an active scavenging system or with passive scavenging vented directly to the outside atmosphere (see Chapter 2). Nitrous oxide is non-irritant and odourless, which increases the risk of accidental exposure. Regular (at least annual) exposure monitoring is essential (see later).

Compressed air

Compressed air may be required to operate surgical power instruments/equipment, and also occasionally patient ventilators. See Chapter 2 for further details.

Liquid nitrogen

Freezing tissue with liquid nitrogen (cryosurgery) is often performed within a surgical suite; living tissue is destroyed by the controlled application of cold temperatures. Pyrometer probes are available to monitor the temperature of the surrounding tissues during the procedure, and it is now possible to purchase cryoprobes with these pyrometers built into them. COSHH regulations should be followed and an SOP produced for the safe storage of liquid nitrogen. All storage containers must be labelled with the appropriate hazard signs and warnings and liquid nitrogen should be stored in a dry, well ventilated area, usually away from the clinical area. The operator and team members assisting with the procedure should wear PPE in the form of heavy-duty gloves, protective eye goggles and aprons.

Maintenance of a surgically clean environment

The importance of infection control in the surgical suite cannot be overestimated. Reinforcing surgical discipline, and reminding and educating staff of the vulnerability of the patients within their care are important aspects to managing a highly productive, safe surgical suite.

Hand and personal hygiene

Although most contaminants during surgery come from the patient (endogenous), surgical personnel are a major cause of microbial contamination during surgical procedures. The principles of good hand hygiene are covered in Chapter 7.

KEY POINT

Regular observational assessments of the team's practice of hand hygiene is the best way of checking compliance.

The preparation of the surgical team and environment is vitally important. Nails should be kept short, and nail varnish and false nails should not be worn. Hand and wrist jewellery interfere with hand hygiene and therefore surgical team members should have a 'bare below the elbow' protocol to ensure high standards are maintained. The maintenance of the surgical environment should be part of the overall biosecurity policy of the practice. More details and a framework for compiling this policy can be found in Chapter 7 and on the BSAVA website.

Surgical site infections

Surgical site infections (SSIs) are infections related to surgical procedures that affect the surgical wound or deeper tissues which have been handled during the surgical procedure. The majority of these infections involve endogenous microbial flora such as *Staphylococcus* and *Streptococcus* species. Antibiotic resistance increases the difficulty of treating SSIs and prevention is therefore paramount. Correct thorough patient preparation and high standards of aseptic technique can all play a part in reducing the likelihood of patient morbidity and mortality.

> A study in human healthcare reported that 65% of nurses who had performed patient care activities on patients that had MRSA (meticillin-resistant *Staphylococcus aureus*) in a wound or in their urine had contaminated nursing uniforms or gowns (Boyce *et al.*, 1997). This highlights the importance of wearing correct personal protective equipment (PPE). Wearing the correct, clean attire when entering a surgical environment will reduce, though not eliminate, microbial contamination. MRSA can survive for up to 90 days on various types of worn scrub suits (Neely and Maley, 2000).

Surgical patients generally undergo initial preparation for surgery within the 'prep' room. The skin and coat of each patient is a source of potential wound contamination and, although it is impossible to *sterilize* the skin prior to the surgical procedure, the aim of patient preparation is to reduce the bacterial population significantly and to remove dirt and debris. It is useful to bathe excessively hairy or dirty patients with an antibacterial shampoo prior to certain procedures to remove loose hair and dirt; patients should be dried thoroughly to prevent hypothermia.

> **KEY POINT**
>
> Patients should not be clipped in an operating room as the clipped hair and shed skin squames can transport microorganisms that can become airborne, travel around the theatre environment, and lead to surgical site infections.

The presence of microorganisms in a wound does not necessarily mean that there will be an infection; all wounds will become contaminated to some degree. Wound infection depends on the virulence (disease-causing ability) of the bacteria entering a wound, the level of contamination, the wound environment and immune response of the patient. Each surgical patient will have a different ability to overcome the contamination, but the following points can have an impact on the likelihood of an SSI developing:

- The status of the patient
- The length of the procedure
- Body temperature
- Aseptic technique
- The surgical technique and the skills of the surgeon
- Experience of the surgical team.

Cleaning the surgical suite

Cleaning is an extremely important aspect of infection control. Cleaning equipment should be colour-coded or labelled so that it is only used within the surgical suite, to reduce contamination. Clear protocols should be in place for cleaning and disinfection before, during and after working in the surgical suite (see example of protocol for maintaining a surgically clean environment at the end of this chapter).

Disinfection

Disinfectants should be used at the correct dilution and water temperature. Incorrect dilutions can prevent disinfectants from working adequately, may result in concentrated disinfectants damaging surfaces, and can be wasteful. Automatic dispensers and measuring devices are commercially available. Charts that display the recommended dilution rates for frequently used disinfectants are beneficial.

Sterilization

The sterilization process is designed to destroy all microorganisms that may be present on any item that is to be used during surgery. There are several different methods of sterilizing surgical instruments and other equipment:

- Steam (steam under pressure autoclave; most common)
- Dry heat (hot air oven)
- Chemicals (gas or liquid)
- Plasma
- Ionizing radiation.

The method(s) chosen for each practice will depend on the type of equipment that requires sterilization and on financial constraints, space available and cycle times to process the item in question.

Autoclaves

Autoclaves are usually situated in a sterilizing room or in the preparation area. In smaller practices, it may prove necessary to keep an autoclave within the operating theatre. In this case, there should be a written SOP for maintaining asepsis within the operating theatre.

European standard EN13060 specifies the performance requirements and test methods for small steam sterilizers used for hygiene and infection control in medical and veterinary establishments. Autoclaves are classified as follows:

- Type N units (often called gravity displacement autoclaves):
  - Do not use a vacuum pump to remove air from the sterilization chamber; air removal from the chamber is achieved by a fractionated gravity displacement
  - Suitable for solid and unwrapped items only (not hollow instruments)
  - Should not be used to sterilize peelable pouches as there is no vacuum to remove air pockets
  - Not suitable for porous loads
  - Items cannot be stored following sterilization, they should be handed to the surgeon as soon as the cycle is completed.
- Type B units:
  - Use a vacuum pump to remove air from the sterilization chamber in a pulsed negative/positive style or 'fragmented' vacuum, prior to the heating up process for sterilization
  - Use a vacuum drying cycle
  - Are always fitted with a steam generator
  - Provide medical-grade sterilization for solid, porous, hollow, unwrapped, bagged, single- or double-wrapped items
  - Can be used to sterilize items that can be stored for future use
  - Can be benchtop or larger units (Figure 8.43).
- Type S units:
  - Use a pre-vacuum and post-vacuum but not a pulsed vacuum
  - Suitable for sterilizing items as specified by the manufacturer (i.e. will not sterilize the full range of items that a B class autoclave can handle)
  - May be suitable for single- or double-wrapped items, depending on manufacturer's instructions.

When selecting an autoclave, hollow instruments for sterilization are classed as: hollow load type A (hollow instruments with cavity length-to-diameter ratio more than 5); or hollow load type B (instruments with cavity length-to-diameter ratio between 1 and 5).

KEY POINT

Following steam sterilization, items should be allowed to cool on drying racks and should not be placed on top of each other during this period as condensation could occur, resulting in strike-through contamination.

Dry heat sterilization

Hot-air ovens tend to be small units, which are economical to run. They are not generally used, due to their high operating temperature (150–180°C) and the limited range of items that can be sterilized. The door to the unit must be fitted with a safety device to prevent it being opened before the chamber contents are cool. Long cooling times are required before items can be used.

Chemical sterilization

Chemical sterilization, with gaseous or liquid chemicals (see below), is useful for heat-sensitive items such as endoscopes (see Chapter 10), plastics and power cables.

Liquid chemicals (cold chemical sterilization)

This method refers to soaking equipment/instruments in a disinfectant solution. It is not an effective sterilization method but more a means of disinfection, although some manufacturers guarantee sterility following long immersion times. It is used for sterilizing/disinfecting endoscopes, bronchoscopes and cystoscopes, and several different agents are commercially available. Instruments with multiple parts should be disassembled prior to immersion and it is important that immersion times suggested by the manufacturer are adhered to. Ideally, a closed cold chemical sterilization chamber should be used to prevent contaminants entering the solution. Following immersion, items should be rinsed thoroughly with sterile water to avoid contact with patient's body tissues. PPE should be worn by staff when preparing cold sterilization solutions.

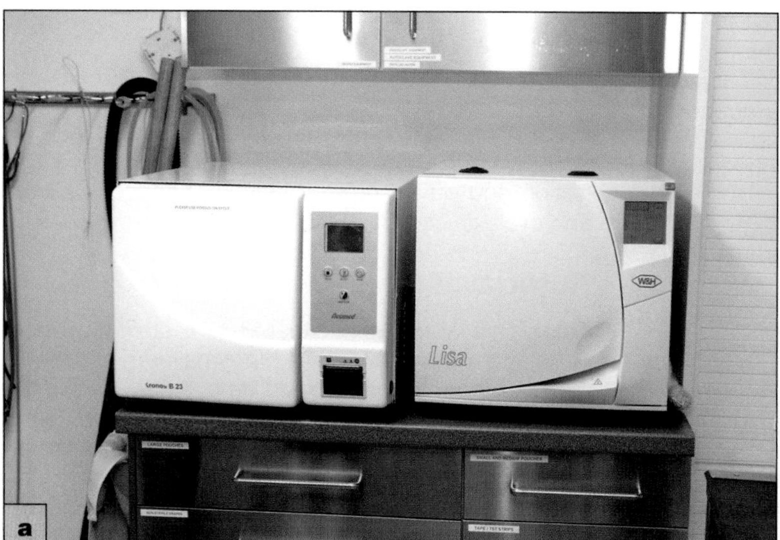

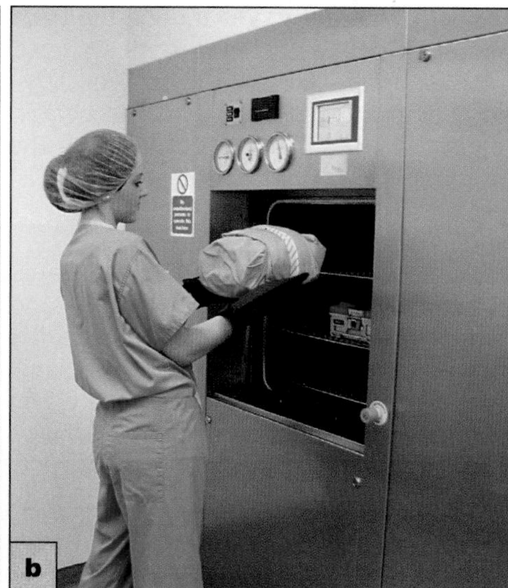

8.43 **(a)** Two benchtop type B autoclaves suitable for general practice. Although some benchtop vacuum autoclaves will fit well on to standard depth worktops, increasing the depth to 700 mm or more is advisable. **(b)** A large type B built-in autoclave.

Ethylene oxide (gas sterilization)

Ethylene oxide (EtO) kills microorganisms by alkylation. Its effectiveness depends on:

- Gas concentration
- Temperature (optimum temperature range 20–60°C)
- Exposure time
- Humidity (optimum humidity range 30–95%).

Ethylene oxide sterilizers are commercially available and often used in veterinary practices (Figure 8.44). Cycle times vary, depending on the chamber temperature and the items being sterilized. Items are packed and the ethylene oxide vial(s) broken open within the bag before it is secured within the sterilizer unit. The items are aerated after sterilization and before they can be removed from the cabinet.

KEY POINT

Items made from PVC can absorb ethylene oxide, and so should undergo additional aeration periods. This is particularly important if PVC items are coming into close contact with sensitive tissues such as the eye, gastrointestinal tract, wounds or operation sites.

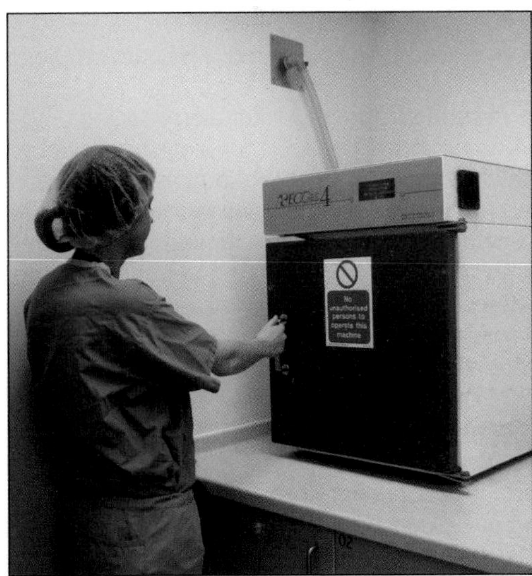

8.44 An ethylene oxide sterilization cabinet. A sign on the door warns that only trained operators should use this equipment.

Hydrogen peroxide–gas plasma sterilization

This method of sterilization is becoming more popular within human hospitals and is the sterilization method of choice for heat-sensitive items. It is expected to become available for veterinary practices in the future. The method incorporates the synergism between hydrogen peroxide and low-temperature gas plasma, which is activated using radiofrequency energy. A sterilization chamber is used and a vacuum created. During the cycle there are two phases: the diffusion phase and the gas phase. This method does not require aeration and benefits from reduced cycle times (approximately one hour).

Hydrogen peroxide liquid is an irritant to skin and can cause eye injuries following direct contact. The sterilization system has several safety features that prevent the operator coming into contact with hydrogen peroxide: the process occurs at low pressures, which reduces the chance of leakage into the environment: the hydrogen peroxide is sealed within a cassette, which is wrapped in plastic and has a leak indicator on the outside; following the process, all the vapour is removed by a filter that decomposes hydrogen peroxide into water and oxygen; and the radiofrequency can only be turned on when the chamber door is closed and is under vacuum.

Ionizing radiation

Pre-packaged sterile items such as syringes, gowns and drapes, which are available directly from manufacturers, tend to have undergone this method of sterilization using cobalt 60. The process is extremely expensive and for this reason is limited to commercial use.

Monitoring sterilization

Sterilization indicators assist in monitoring the effectiveness of the sterilization process. Failure to achieve sterility may be caused by any of the following factors:

- Improper cleaning method
- Mechanical failure of the method used
- Improper use of equipment
- Incorrect wrapping technique
- Incorrect loading technique
- Human/team errors.

The correct indicator should be chosen for the method of sterilization in use, or incorrect results could occur.

Chemical indicators

Chemical indicators are available for most methods of sterilization and are generally paper strips with a material that changes colour (Figure 8.45). The colour change occurs when a certain temperature, pressure or humidity is reached, depending on the type of chemical indicator used.

Examples of chemical indicators are:

- **Bowie Dick tape (BDT/autoclave tape):** Beige tape with a chemical strip that turns dark brown in temperatures over 121°C. It is useful for sealing wrapped packs but should not be relied upon heavily as it does not ensure the temperature has been maintained for a set time. When used on metal or plastic containers it can leave a hard to remove residue
- **Browne's tubes:** Small glass tubes that change colour (usually from red to green) on autoclaving. They should be stored in a cool, dry place. Different tubes work at different temperatures and are identified by a spot on the end of the tube.
- **Time, steam, temperature (TST) strips:** Paper strips that are used at specific temperatures and/or pressures (usually indicated on the strip itself). When the indicator has been exposed to the correct temperature and pressure, the two dots on the strip should match.

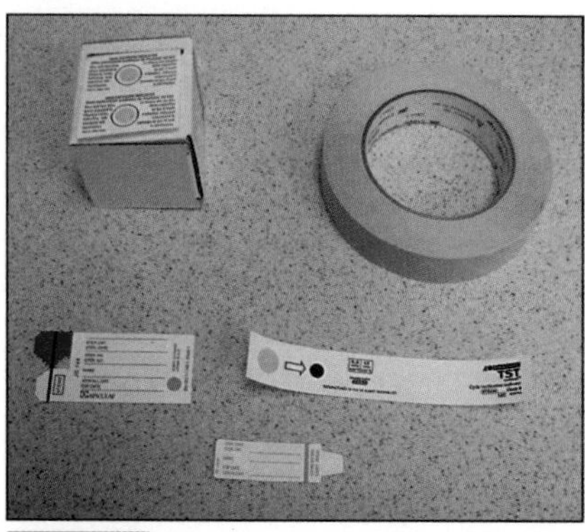

8.45 Sterilization indicators. Clockwise from top left: ethylene oxide chemical indicators; Bowie Dick tape; TST strip; small and larger versions of chemical indicator stickers for surgical containers.

KEY POINT

Indicators should be placed in the centre of packaged items or kits *and* on the outside of the item. This will indicate that the pack has been penetrated successfully by the method employed. It is important that surgeons remember to check the indicators inside each surgical kit.

Chemical indicators are available as stickers, tapes, and strips. It is useful to keep these items on record by attaching them to the patient records or theatre checklists; these can be useful in tracking any problems that can arise. The colour change does not reflect the duration of exposure, and therefore chemical indicators do not indicate sterility *per se*, but only show that certain conditions have been achieved.

Biological methods

These are accurate but time-consuming. They incorporate a strain of highly resistant non-pathogenic bacterium within a glass vial, or dried spores on a strip of paper. *Bacillus stearothermophilus* is used for steam sterilization and *Bacillus subtilis* for dry heat, gas plasma and ethylene oxide. Following the cycle, the indicator is cultured (in the medium provided) using incubation at room temperature for 72 hours. Any growth of microorganisms indicates inadequate sterilization. Ideally, this method should be employed on a weekly basis to ensure the method of sterilization is effective.

Mechanical methods

Modern autoclaves provide paper printouts that include information on the temperature and time scales of each load, which is gained from thermocouples inside the sterilization chamber. These can be kept for future reference. Some machines also have an alarm within the machine to indicate failed cycles, for example when the pressure chamber is 1°C under the ideal temperature.

Wrapping for sterilization

Prior to sterilization most instruments (and other equipment) will require packing and/or wrapping to enable storage after sterilization. The procedure for wrapping items is based on facilitating sterilization and preserving sterility of the item. Correct packing is essential for effective steam or gas sterilization; for example, complex instruments should be disassembled prior to sterilization when possible, and containers and bowls should have the open end facing downwards or horizontal. Instruments should be placed so that they can be removed with the handles first when the kit is opened. Instruments with sharp tips should have sharp ends covered to prevent blunting and stop them piercing packaging.

The ideal wrapping material is permeable to steam and gas, but not to microorganisms, and returns to a flat position easily. It should be flexible and resistant to damage when handled.

- **Autoclave film bags** can be either heat-sealed bags or sealed with autoclave tape. They are made of nylon or nylon and paper. Some materials can be re-used but small cracks and micro-holes can occur. Sharp items may puncture these bags.
- **Peelable (peel-and-seal) pouches** are quick and easy to use. They are made from nylon and paper and have a self-seal tab at one end that enables the operator to remove a strip of paper and seal the end down. It is important that the ends are sealed along the identified strip, as holes can occur if they are not sealed correctly and this renders the pouch unsterile. One side remains transparent, whilst the paper side has a built-in chemical indicator. These pouches are easily punctured by sharp items. They are single-use items.
- **Cotton muslin wraps** are available at 140- or 270-thread counts. They are durable, re-usable and easy to handle. Prior to use they should be checked for micro-holes by holding them up to a window or a light; any wraps with holes should be discarded. A disadvantage of cotton muslin is that it provides a shorter storage time than other wraps. Muslin wraps should be used double-layered, and two wraps should be used for each pack. They should be placed so that they are easy to unwrap without breaking asepsis.
- **Non-woven surgical paper** is used for wrapping items such as containers prior to sterilization. It cannot be re-used but is inexpensive. It is not moisture-resistant, and can be awkward to handle as it retains its folds. Surgical paper can be used in single or double layers, but a single layer gives a shorter storage time.
- **Corrugated plastic boxes** are re-usable, re-sterilizable boxes that are useful for larger items such as gowns and hand towels. They are sturdy and not easily damaged.
- **Surgical containers** are modern, easy-to-use containers that incorporate a bacterial filter within the lid. They have an outer container and an inner basket(s) which the surgeon can lift out. They are expensive but over time can reduce costs of wrapping materials and also staff time. They have a section located on the outer container for a chemical indicator strip. They also require the use of safety (tamper-proof) tags, which indicate the kit has not been tampered with following the sterilization cycle. Tamper-proof tags are available with or without a chemical sterilization dot.

Different methods of wrapping and packing allow different storage times, but the wrapping must be suitable for the sterilization method. For example, instruments to be sterilized in a type N autoclave cannot be wrapped, as this type of autoclave should only be used for unwrapped instruments. Items that are intended to be sterilized using ethylene oxide should be wrapped in heat-sealable nylon bags, peelable pouches or muslin wrap. Items that are intended to be sterilized using plasma sterilization should be wrapped in heat-sealable Tyvek–Mylar pouches or polypropylene wraps.

KEY POINT

A type N autoclave should only be used for sterilizing unwrapped instruments.

Labelling

All packs for sterilization should be labelled with the following details:

- Date the item/kit was packed (Figure 8.46)
- Name of the item/surgical kit (e.g. 'cat spay kit 1')
- Name of the person who packed it
- Whether the pack contains a sterilization indicator
- Expiry date of the item/surgical kit (i.e. when it will no longer be regarded as sterile).

Items should be labelled on the outside of the pack, e.g. on the autoclave tape for wrapped items, or on the chemical sterilization strip (which has a space for this) on surgical containers.

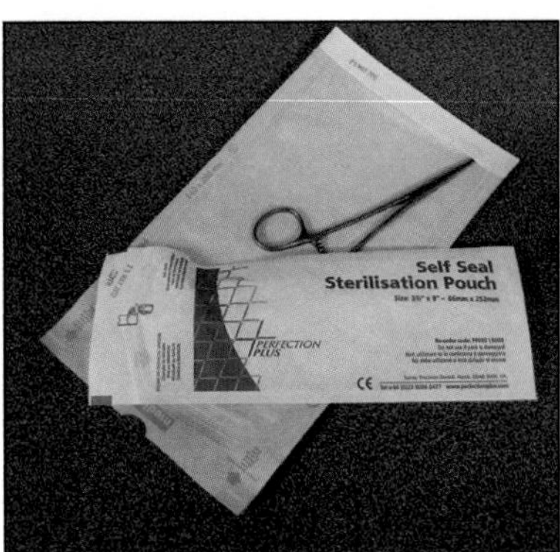

8.46 Sterile packs should be dated and initialled (see top left corner of the pouch).

Storing items following sterilization

All items, regardless of the method of sterilization, should ideally be stored in closed cabinets rather than on open shelves, and away from heat-producing lights, ventilation ducts and sprinkler systems. Excessive handling should be avoided.

Double-wrapped items that are not intended to be used within 24 hours should be wrapped in a 'post-sterilization' or 'dust' wrap, which is a waterproof, heat-sealable plastic dust cover that prevents exposure to dust-borne bacteria and moisture. Plastic dust covers should be removed prior to transportation into the operating theatre.

The sterile shelf-life of sterilized items can be controversial. Events, rather than time, can lead to contamination of items, e.g. excessive handling or dropping items on the floor. The following factors are taken into account to judge the shelf-life:

- The type and configuration of packing materials
- Number of times an item is handled
- Number of personnel who have handled the item
- Storage facilities, e.g. open or closed shelves
- Condition of the storage area (how clean; environmental factors)
- Method of sealing the pack
- Whether dust covers were used.

KEY POINTS

- A storage rotation system should be in place to ensure that items sterilized first are used first.
- The surgical team should routinely check for pack entirety prior to moving it into the operating theatre.
- If there is any possibility that a pack is damaged it should not be used.

Care of surgical instruments

Surgical instruments are expensive but if cared for correctly and handled carefully can last for many years:

- Do not drop them into sinks or trolleys
- Regularly sharpen instruments with cutting edges
- Clean all instruments immediately after use to prevent blood and irrigation fluids drying on them and causing corrosion.

Before packing or sterilizing, instruments should be inspected using a magnification lamp (Figure 8.47) or magnifying glass to ensure that the instrument is completely clean (paying attention to joints and teeth), any teeth function smoothly, and the instrument is not damaged or corroded.

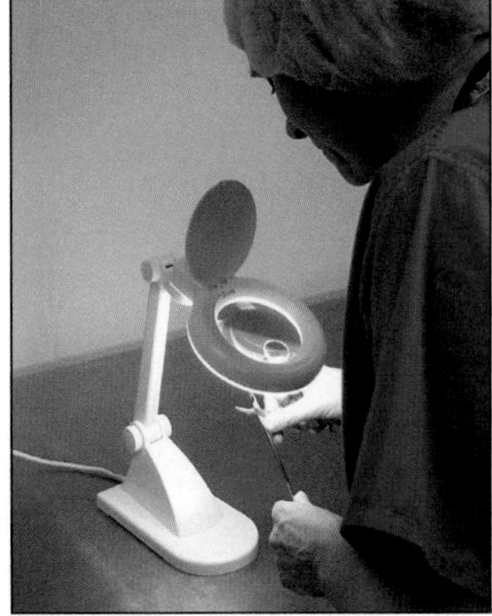

8.47 An illuminated magnification lamp is useful for close inspection of instruments prior to packing and sterilization.

Cleaning

Surgical instruments should be rinsed in cold water as soon as possible after surgery, in order to prevent coagulation of plasma proteins and aid removal of blood stains. If blood has already been allowed to dry on the instruments, they should be soaked in warm water with a detergent. Delicate instruments should not be left in sinks where heavier items could be put on top of them.

Manual cleaning

Abrasive agents should not be used, as these can damage the instrument surface. Standard soap can cause an insoluble alkali film on the instrument surface, which can trap bacteria and lead to ineffective sterilization. Following manual cleaning, instruments should be rinsed in cold water and then dried carefully. Inadequate drying, and water becoming trapped within joints, can lead to corrosion and discoloration.

Instrument washers

Instrument washers and disinfectors are commercially available; these are expensive but save staff time and clean and disinfect instruments more effectively than manual cleaning. They look very similar to domestic dishwashers and can have several racks (Figure 8.48), which enable, for example, hollow items to be flushed and surgical clogs to be cleaned. Smaller racks are for delicate instruments such as ophthalmic items. Instruments should be loaded carefully into the appropriate tray, ensuring that joints are opened. Often these machines have a drying cycle, which saves more staff time as instruments are retrieved from cleaning in a dry state, ready to be inspected and packed.

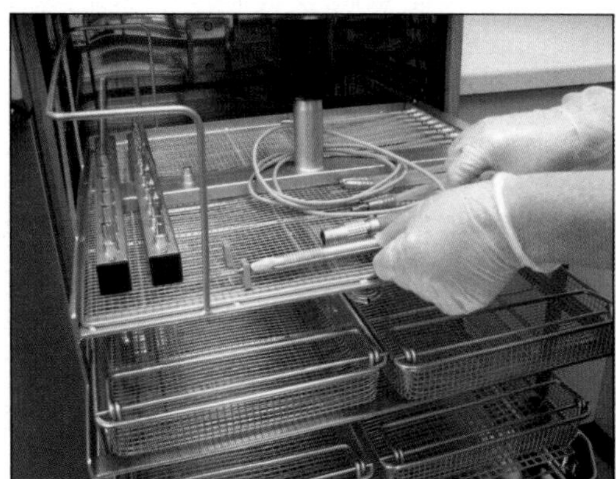

8.48 An instrument washer/disinfector, with racking and location points for delicate instruments.

Ultrasonic cleaners

Ultrasonic cleaners are extremely efficient at removing debris from areas inaccessible to manual cleaning. They are convenient, tending to be small benchtop units.

> **KEY POINTS**
>
> - Ultrasonic cleaners should be used in conjunction with instrument washing and do not replace the washing process.
> - Instruments should be soaked in cold water prior to ultrasonic cleaning.

Ultrasonic cleaners work through the production of sinusoidal energy waves with a frequency of over 20,000 vibrations per second. The cleaning process involves 'cavitation'. Ultrasonic energy produces tiny bubbles; these form on the surface of instruments and expand until they become unstable. Bubbles implode almost as soon as they are formed, which creates small vacuum areas. This process dislodges any debris on the instrument surface, which is then dissolved by the ultrasonic cleaning solution. Ultrasonic cleaners use a specially designed detergent. The instruments are placed into a wire basket or tray and submerged into the cleaner. Instruments with joints should be opened when the tray is loaded. Gloves should be worn when loading the cleaners as the detergent used may be irritating to the skin. Eye protection may be necessary in case splashes occur. During the ultrasonic cycle, the lid of the cleaner should be closed; modern units have sealed lids and cannot start the cycle until the lid is closed. The manufacturer's instructions should be adhered to, and all dilutions should be measured carefully.

The majority of ultrasonic cleaners have timers; the standard cycle time is 15 minutes. More advanced cleaners are now available, which combine a cycle selection time with a heating element that heats the chamber during the cleaning process.

> **KEY POINT**
>
> Electrolysis may occur if different types of metals are mixed during cleaning. This can be seen by damage to instrument surfaces. Following the ultrasonic cycle, instruments should be rinsed thoroughly in cold water to remove any residual detergent.

Equipment maintenance

The surgical areas contain many different, expensive and potentially hazardous materials and pieces of equipment. All staff that use any piece of equipment must be authorized and trained to do so, and safety alert signs are available to remind staff of this (see Figure 8.44). Risk assessments should be carried out on any equipment that poses a potential risk to the operator or patient, and portable appliance testing (PAT) should be carried out as required (see Chapter 22).

Standard operating procedures and operator manuals

It is important with any piece of equipment that the manufacturer's recommendations are followed, and that the staff members responsible know how to look after it properly and are aware of potential hazards. Some manufacturers will be willing to visit a practice and provide training for the employees; user manuals should be readily available for training and for reference. SOPs should be available; additional information sheets, which include troubleshooting tips, can also be created.

Service contracts

Service contracts are available for most equipment and are beneficial as they can provide:

- Financial benefits
- Reduced down-time of equipment
- Loan equipment to ensure patient procedures are not compromised
- Fixed maintenance costs
- Properly maintained products
- Rapid call out in event of breakdown.

KEY POINT

Records of services and faults should be kept for future reference and to prove that the service has taken place. It is beneficial to have a computerized document as a reminder when services should be booked.

Managing the surgical team

Surgical team roles and responsibilities

The 'surgical team' refers to every member of staff who is present at the time of a surgical procedure. Depending on the nature of the practice, and the type of surgery being performed, the surgical team can include:

- Veterinary surgeon
- Second (assistant) surgeon
- Veterinary anaesthetist
- Circulating nurse
- Scrub nurse.

KEY POINTS

- All personnel should be trained in good aseptic technique and in how to behave in an operating theatre.
- This includes preventing excessive air movement and minimizing personnel entering and leaving during a surgical procedure.
- Non-sterile surgical personnel should be aware of the surgical field, taking care to create distance when walking past sterile trolleys, and ensuring they do not walk between two sterile surfaces.

Every member of the surgical team should understand their role and responsibilities (Figure 8.49) in order for the day to run efficiently. It is essential that the theatre is set up properly to reduce anaesthetic time, as longer anaesthetic time leads to increased patient risk, e.g. from hypothermia or infection. Planning which team members assist with certain procedures is an important consideration. Nurse planners can be as simple as a diary or more advanced, such as a dedicated computer system which is available for all staff to look at. Managers or nurse coordinators (see below) should decide which nurse would be most suitable for assisting with certain procedures; for example, a more experienced nurse would be required to assist with a thoracotomy than with a cat castration. Managers should also ensure that nurses are getting regular exposure to a wide variety of procedures, so that they do not become de-skilled in a particular area. Training, continuing professional development (CPD), clinical discussions, and reading about new protocols and techniques should be arranged and recorded for all surgical team members.

Lead surgeon
■ Direct the operation ■ Perform the majority of the operation ■ Liaise with the anaesthetist on the up-and-coming surgical events ■ Overall responsibility for safety in theatre
Assistant surgeon
■ Assist the surgeon ■ Swab the surgical field ■ Apply lavage and suction ■ Retract tissues ■ Cut suture material
Anaesthetist (Vet)
■ Check anaesthetic equipment prior to use ■ Induce and maintain anaesthesia, and supervise recovery
Nurse monitoring anaesthetic
■ Check anaesthetic equipment prior to use ■ Maintain anaesthesia under the veterinary surgeon's direction ■ Supervise recovery
Scrub nurse
■ Prepare and receive sterile instruments from circulating nurse ■ Manage and set up the instrument trolley ■ Hand instruments to surgeon and assistant surgeon ■ Keep instruments clean during surgery by wiping or rinsing in sterile saline ■ Perform swab count (verbally confirming for safety checklists); keep account of needles and suture packs
Circulating nurse
■ Prepare the theatre for surgery ■ Ensure all instrumentation and consumable items are prepared ■ Complete theatre checklist ■ Prepare the patient ■ Open instrument packs and present to members of the operating team so that they can lift out the sterile contents ■ Attend to non-sterile items (e.g. suction, electrosurgery, power supply units, plug in medical air for power tools) ■ Complete laboratory forms and safe keeping of samples obtained ■ Fetch supplies if necessary ■ Liaise with coordinators in recovery areas

8.49 Roles and responsibilities of the surgical team.

Nurse coordinators

Nurse coordinators play an important role in larger practices; with adequate training, the responsibility of the coordinator role can be shared among the nursing team. The coordinator for the day should oversee each procedure and organize the day's cases, ensuring that patients receive premedication at correct times, are anaesthetized on time, and undergo surgical preparation to fit the necessary theatre slots. A good coordinator can ensure the operating theatre is used to its full potential throughout the day and can facilitate communication with the rest of the practice. Coordinators should be easy to identify to other staff and visitors; simple means of identification, such as wearing a different colour of surgical scrub suit or cap (Figure 8.50), is useful. Team members should have an idea of how long surgical preparation should last to help minimize anaesthetic times; for example, preparing a patient for routine orthopaedic surgery should not take longer than 20 minutes. Coordinators should monitor preparation times and provide assistance when required.

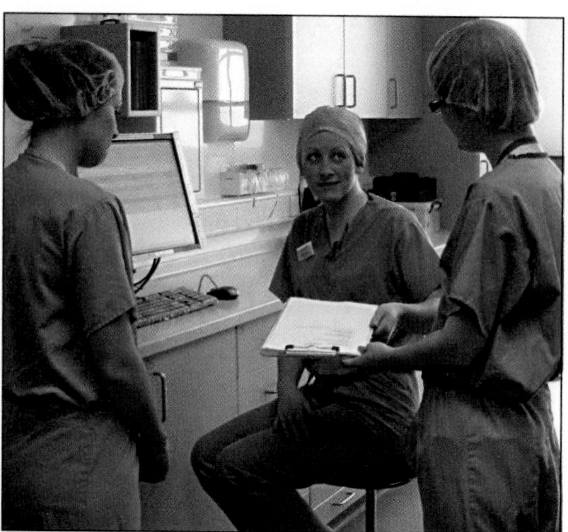

8.50 The nurse coordinator is identified by a pink surgical cap.

Delegated tasks

Delegating jobs can be beneficial to any practice. The tasks can range from weekly deep cleans of an operating theatre to checking the function of, and maintaining, the endotracheal tubes. It is useful to produce a task list for individuals that may be working certain shifts, giving them clearly defined times to complete certain tasks, which can be indicated on a tick list so that the coordinators or senior staff can ensure that certain tasks have been completed. Documents ranging from simple wall charts to computerized lists can be created for traceability. Delegation boosts team morale and is vital to smooth everyday running and efficiency within the practice.

Organizing the surgical list

A well run surgical list can make a difference between an organized busy fulfilling day (for staff involved) or a hectic disorganized stressful day (which can reduce staff morale). This can have an effect on the care that patients receive.

In smaller practices, surgical lists may be simple handwritten day lists (Figure 8.51). However, in larger hospitals a computerized list can help all staff, from receptionists to nurses and veterinary surgeons, keep up to date with the ongoing caseload and details of an individual patient's progress through the hospital. This allows staff to provide clients with updates if necessary, or to transfer callers to nurses or veterinary surgeons with ease, without entering the surgical areas.

Booking the surgical list

It is worth having guidelines as to how many surgical procedures should be booked in routinely per day, and how this may vary if a procedure is booked in that may take up more of the surgeon's time. Consideration should also be given to potential emergency procedures that may be admitted. A simple chart with timescales for a variety of surgical procedures may help support staff understand associated timescales; e.g. a bitch spay is estimated at 40 minutes of theatre time whilst a TPLO (tibial plateau levelling osteotomy) may take an hour or more. Turnaround time for the theatre and the availability of

Patient name	Patient surname	Age	Breed	Weight (kg)	Premedication	Procedure	Vet	Medications	Comments	Imaging?	Stay or home?
Sidney	Bowcott	8 years	X-breed	20.3	0.01mg/kg ACP 0.1mg/kg methadone	GA castration and microchip		Propofol Isoflurane Carprofen		No	Home at 4.00pm
Narla	Tildesley	2 years	DSH	4.3	0.01mg/kg ACP 0.3mg/kg buprenorphine	GA cat spay and nail trim		Alfaxan Isoflurane Meloxicam		No	Home at 5.00pm
Frankie	Griffin	9 years	X-breed	14.4	0.01mg/kg ACP 0.3mg/kg methadone	GA amputate right hind limb		Propofol Isoflurane Carprofen Fentanyl patch 50mcg Compound sodium lactate	IVFT at 5 ml/kg/h	Yes CT	Stay
Bella	Dalvensa	10 years	Italian Spinone	30.6	0.01mg/kg ACP 0.3mg/kg buprenorphine	GA dental scale and polish ,poss extractions		Alfaxan Isoflurane Meloxicam Compound sodium lactate	Heart murmur IVFT at 4 ml/kg/h	YES X-ray	Home at 6.00pm

8.51 An example of a basic handwritten day list for surgical procedures.

surgical instrumentation should also be considered when establishing how many surgical procedures can be performed during one day. The number of more specialized procedures booked in may depend upon surgeon availability, particularly in referral practices where more non-routine cases may be presented.

Managing the surgical list

Where possible the surgical list should be organized using the National Research Council (NRC) wound classification system. This system classifies surgical wounds into four different classes (see Figure 8.5) according to the degree of contamination and the likelihood of infection developing. Ideally any 'clean' procedures should be performed first in the day, followed by 'clean-contaminated', then 'contaminated' and, finally, 'dirty' procedures. There are exceptions to this system: any critical patients who will require emergency surgery or are anticipated to require intense monitoring following the procedure may need to be dealt with first on the day's operating list. Examples include patients undergoing airway or thoracic surgery, and paediatric patients where pre-operative fasting may result in hypoglycaemia. In multi-vet practices, having more than one operating theatre is extremely valuable under such circumstances. Where several operating tables are in one theatre, in order to reduce the potential for SSIs, orthopaedic operations should not be carried out at the same time as other procedures.

Using checklists and SOPs

Checklists are important for maintaining supplies, opening (Figure 8.52) and closing rooms at the start and end of the day, ensuring equipment works correctly and making sure that staff are performing the checks consistently. Checklists and SOPs can be designed for any room within the practice, and could include:

- Checking and setting up anaesthetic machines and scavenging (see example SOP at end of chapter)
- Cleaning, checking and setting up clippers, ensuring new blades are attached (see example SOP at end of chapter)
- Checking and setting up anaesthetic trolleys
- Laying out monitoring equipment
- Checking and replenishing the patient crash cart/box
- Turning on all computers.

KEY POINT

Standard operating procedures and protocols should be available for all staff to read, including a written protocol for how to maintain a surgically clean environment (see example at the end of this chapter). Regular review is essential.

Record-keeping and clinical governance

Theatre/instrumentation checklists

Theatre checklists aid staff when setting up an operating theatre for certain procedures. They range from small laminated cards detailing the surgical instrumentation required for the procedure, to more detailed computerized printouts detailing requirements for all aspects of theatre set-up. Computerized theatre

Task	Tick when completed
Damp-dust all surfaces with a disinfectant solution	
Disinfect all high-risk cross-contamination areas: door handles, computer keyboards, telephones, etc.	
Carry out a spot check on all walls, ceiling and equipment to ensure there is no visible soiling. If soiling is detected, this should be cleaned immediately with a disinfectant solution	
Turn on all computers and load the necessary programs	
Gas scavenging: ■ Turn on active system and check it is working properly ■ For passive systems, check tubing and connections, and carry out daily weighing check on charcoal adsorbers	
Check all patient monitoring equipment is in good working order	
Carry out daily safety checks on anaesthetic machines and anaesthetic systems	
Check all sharps containers; when three-quarters full, discard and replace with a new container	
Ensure all bins are clean and have the correct waste bags inside them	
Ensure all clippers have clean blades and are in good working order	
Ensure all tables have bedding materials on ready for patients	
Set up patient tables with intravenous cannula equipment, monitoring equipment, skin preparation materials, anaesthetic equipment and patient warming aids	
Ensure cupboards are stocked fully; replenish if necessary	
Check crash cart has not been broached (re-stock if necessary)	
Mop the floor with a disinfectant solution (remember wet floor signs)	

8.52 Example of a checklist for opening up a preparation room at the start of the day. An example of an SOP for checking anaesthetic equipment prior to use is given at the end of the chapter.

checklists can be printed out and double up as an audit record for the individual surgical procedure.

It is important to keep an **audit** of each surgical procedure, detailing:

- Surgical instrumentation used (and whether any problems were encountered)
- The sterility of the instruments
- Any problems encountered during the surgery (such as a break in asepsis).

These records provide traceability and can assist in completing clinical audits for SSIs, instrument problems or other morbidity and mortality issues. Consumable items (e.g. disposable gowns and drapes) usually have traceability stickers, which can be attached to the theatre audit record for traceability and pricing purposes.

Patient safety checklists

Maintaining and managing an efficient surgical suite is challenging. Surgical safety checklists, designed to ensure several checks occur between colleagues, are invaluable in ensuring communication and preventing avoidable risks. Specific checks are undertaken for each surgical patient at different stages of the patient's progress through the surgical suite. In 2007 the World Health Organization undertook a global challenge to address surgical safety and provide safer surgical procedures to human patients across the world. One of the initiatives was the WHO Safe Surgery Checklist (see their website for details). Safety checklists (see example at end of chapter) can be adapted to suit the individual practice. Staff training and compliance are vital.

General anaesthesia

Prior to each use, the anaesthetic machine and breathing system should undergo a thorough check, according to a set protocol (see example at end of this chapter). **The operator's manual should be referred to for a complete check procedure, as no universal checklist is appropriate for all anaesthetic machines.** Further checks should be carried out for function and to ensure there is no gas leakage when the patient is connected to the machine. It is also important not to allow gas or anaesthetic agents to pass into the atmosphere during connection and disconnection of the patient and whilst setting up, filling and cleaning the equipment. Particular attention should be paid to all connections on the machine and components, checking that the flowmeter block is vertical and that all rubber parts are in good order with no signs of perishing.

KEY POINT

All general anaesthesia must be induced and maintained by a veterinary surgeon if the induction dose is either incremental or to effect.

A member of staff adequately trained in monitoring patients under general anaesthesia must be present throughout the procedure. A listed or registered veterinary nurse is the ideal person to monitor anaesthesia, but if an unqualified person assists, suitable training should be recorded. The person monitoring the patient should not be distracted by other tasks during the procedure.

Record-keeping

Patient monitoring during anaesthesia (see earlier) is paramount to ensure patient safety.

KEY POINT

A comprehensive anaesthetic record should be made for every patient and for every procedure, however brief. This will facilitate effective monitoring and assist communication about the case from admission through to recovery. It forms part of the clinical record and should be retained.

The anaesthetic record should include:

- Date
- Personnel involved (surgeon, anaesthetist)
- Procedure undertaken (e.g. surgical, investigation)
- Premedication details and any significant findings of the pre-anaesthetic check, e.g. risk assessment
- Anaesthesia and procedure start and finish times
- Induction agent
- Maintenance agent
- Regular observations of vital signs and any changes in anaesthesia protocol
- Any anaesthetic complications or significant events.

Standard charts are available in many textbooks (Figure 8.53) and may be obtained from some anaesthetic suppliers. An alternative example is given at the end of this chapter.

Reviewing performance

In larger practices there may be several disciplines working together. Weekly 'rounds' or group meetings within each discipline can be invaluable, as they give all team members an opportunity to discuss interesting or problematical cases and to gain advice from more experienced colleagues (see Chapter 28). These reviews are beneficial to progressing and improving future cases, writing additional protocols and ensuring high standards of care. They give an opportunity for the team to discuss problems that may have been encountered, and suggestions can be made on how to avoid problems arising in the future. It is also important to discuss any SSIs that may have arisen. With any SSI, morbidity or mortality, the individual case should be reviewed and any actions, amendments or policy changes implemented. Following non-routine procedures it is a good idea to review the case once the procedure has finished and the patient has recovered. A basic template can be created, which gives areas to discuss such as:

- Time management
- Surgical instrumentation
- Surgical procedure
- Anaesthetic considerations
- Nursing considerations.

An example of a procedure review form is given at the end of the chapter.

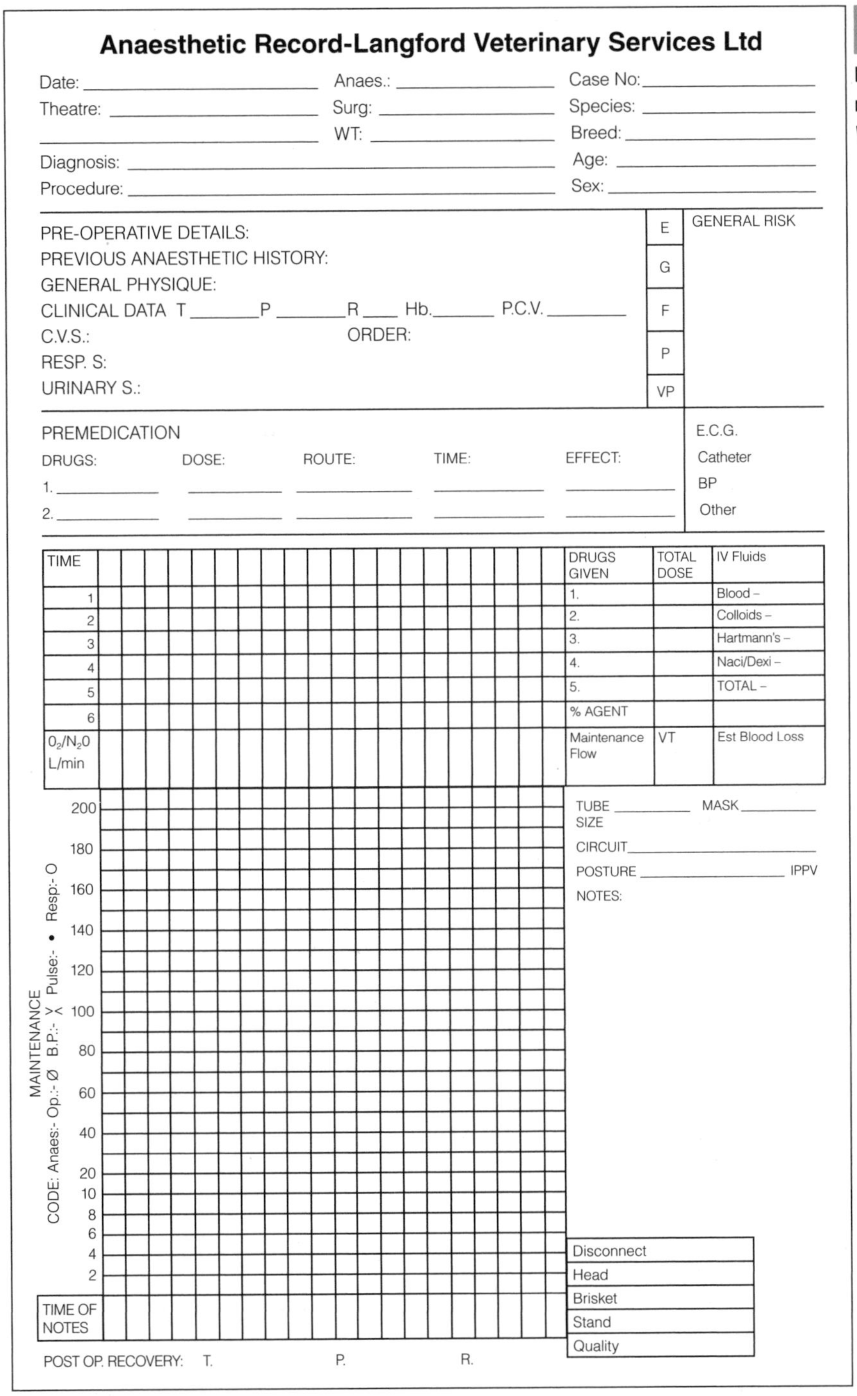

Anaesthetic Record-Langford Veterinary Services Ltd

Date: ______ Anaes.: ______ Case No: ______
Theatre: ______ Surg: ______ Species: ______
______ WT: ______ Breed: ______
Diagnosis: ______ Age: ______
Procedure: ______ Sex: ______

PRE-OPERATIVE DETAILS:
PREVIOUS ANAESTHETIC HISTORY:
GENERAL PHYSIQUE:
CLINICAL DATA T ______ P ______ R ____ Hb. ______ P.C.V. ______
C.V.S.: ORDER:
RESP. S:
URINARY S.:

	GENERAL RISK
E	
G	
F	
P	
VP	

PREMEDICATION

DRUGS:	DOSE:	ROUTE:	TIME:	EFFECT:
1.				
2.				

E.C.G.
Catheter
BP
Other

TIME	DRUGS GIVEN	TOTAL DOSE	IV Fluids
1	1.		Blood –
2	2.		Colloids –
3	3.		Hartmann's –
4	4.		Naci/Dexi –
5	5.		TOTAL –
6	% AGENT		
O_2/N_2O L/min	Maintenance Flow	VT	Est Blood Loss

CODE: Anaes:- Op.:- Ø B.P.:- V Pulse:- • Resp:- O

MAINTENANCE

200, 180, 160, 140, 120, 100, 80, 60, 40, 20, 10, 8, 6, 4, 2

TIME OF NOTES

TUBE SIZE ______ MASK ______
CIRCUIT ______
POSTURE ______ IPPV
NOTES:

Disconnect
Head
Brisket
Stand
Quality

POST OP. RECOVERY: T. P. R.

8.53 An example of an anaesthetic monitoring chart. (Courtesy of Langford Veterinary Services Ltd and reproduced from the *BSAVA Textbook of Veterinary Nursing, 5th edn.*)

Safety issues in the surgical suite

Principles of health and safety management are covered in Chapter 22; a number of hazards specific to the surgical suite are mentioned here.

KEY POINT

It is important to remind team members that they have an obligation under the Health and Safety at Work etc. Act 1974 to ensure they adhere to the protocols and SOPs that have been created to provide a safe working environment for other team members and patients.

Hazardous substances

Employers have a duty under the Control of Substances Hazardous to Health (COSHH) Regulations 2002 to carry out risk assessments and control workplace exposures to all hazardous substances.

Anaesthetic gases

All inhalational agents and nitrous oxide gas are subject to maximum exposure limits (MELs; see www.hse.gov.uk) and risk assessments should be completed under COSHH regulations. The MEL refers to a time-weighted average level of exposure to environmental contamination. Monitoring of anaesthetic gas pollutants in operating and recovery areas should be carried out on an annual basis unless anaesthetic equipment or breathing systems are changed. Monitoring is generally done on a time-weighted average basis, using a returnable monitor; personal dosimeters can be worn for a recorded time and analysed off site. Real-time monitors are available but are expensive. Anaesthetic agent exposure should be checked against the MEL and results kept on file; any higher than usual results should be acted upon and rechecked. More information on anaesthetic pollutant monitoring and the current workplace exposure limits for agents used can be found on the RCVS, HSE and BSAVA websites.

Ethylene oxide

There are many environmental and safety hazards associated with ethylene oxide. It is a highly flammable explosive liquid and should be stored in a fireproof cabinet (see Figure 8.59). It is also irritating to the skin and mucous membranes, and there is some concern that it may be carcinogenic and cause birth defects. Exposure to ethylene oxide and its byproducts should be avoided. Ethylene oxide sterilizers should be located in well ventilated rooms and have an exhaust to the outside environment. It is extremely important that manufacturer's recommendations are followed; some manufacturers provide staff training, tests and certificates to ensure that staff are trained to operate the sterilizer. COSHH regulations should be referred to. Personnel monitoring badges and hand-held detection units are commercially available which detect exposure levels. For more information on approved workplace exposure limits see the HSE website.

Bone cement

Polymethylmethacrylate (PMME; otherwise known as bone cement) is mainly used for orthopaedic procedures and certain neurological procedures and is classed as an implant. It is important that a COSHH assessment is carried out on this product. The surgeon should undergo specific training on how to mix the liquid and powder to achieve the best results and how to avoid mixing errors that can occur and lead to implant failure. Adequate ventilation is important, and mixing chambers with a ventilation system incorporated are commercially available. It is recommended that handlers wear double gloves. The product is also highly flammable, and therefore members of the surgical team should be aware of the nearest fire extinguisher during its application.

Electrosurgery

Surgical smoke (plume) is produced during the use of electrosurgery. This can contain potentially harmful substances which can cause health problems to surgical staff if inhaled. It is important to provide effective ventilation within the operating theatre to remove the smoke, unless a dedicated smoke evacuator (commercially available) is used. Some surgical smoke particles measure less than 5 μm; these are unlikely to be filtered effectively through surgical masks and are capable of travelling through the respiratory tree to the alveolar level. High-filtration facemasks are commercially available to minimize inhalation. More information can be found at www.hse.gov.uk.

Physical hazards

Autoclaves

The main hazards of autoclaves are: impact from a blast or explosion; release of compressed liquid; contact with released steam; and contact with hot shelves and contents. Autoclaves are covered by the Pressure Equipment Regulations 1999 and the Pressure Safety Regulations 2000. All autoclaves should be serviced regularly by a qualified engineer to ensure they remain safe and in good working order. There should be a suitable maintenance programme for each autoclave; under the Pressure Safety Regulations 2000 a written scheme of examination is required for most pressure systems, which should be provided by the manufacturer. More information can be found on the HSE website.

Surgical instruments

Following a surgical procedure, the surgical instruments should be removed from the operating theatre in a safe manner.

- All sharp items such as scalpel blades, needles, saw attachments and drill bits should be disposed of inside a designated 'sharps' bin or secured suitably prior to transport. Sharps bins should be available within both the operating theatre and the preparation room.
- Sterile adhesive pads are commercially available for procedures where several sharp items may be used; the sharps are then attached to the sticky pads by the surgeon and the pads disposed of directly into the 'sharps' container.
- Scalpel blade removers are commercially available; these attach to scalpel blades to aid safe removal.
- Mobile trolleys with several closed drawers can be used to transport dirty instruments into the correct area for cleaning (Figure 8.54).
- Gloves should always be worn when handling dirty instruments.
- Staff should be trained in the necessary actions to take following a 'needle stick' injury.

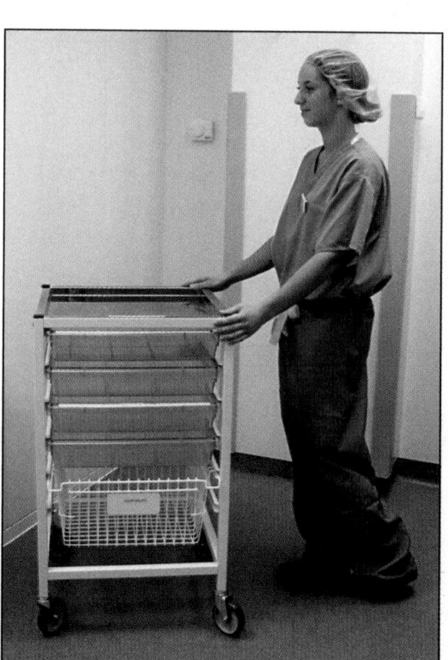

8.54 Mobile trolleys are useful for transporting dirty instruments safely to the cleaning area.

Gas cylinders

It is important that team members are trained in cylinder safety; manual handling regulations should also be considered. Cylinder trolleys are commercially available (Figure 8.55).

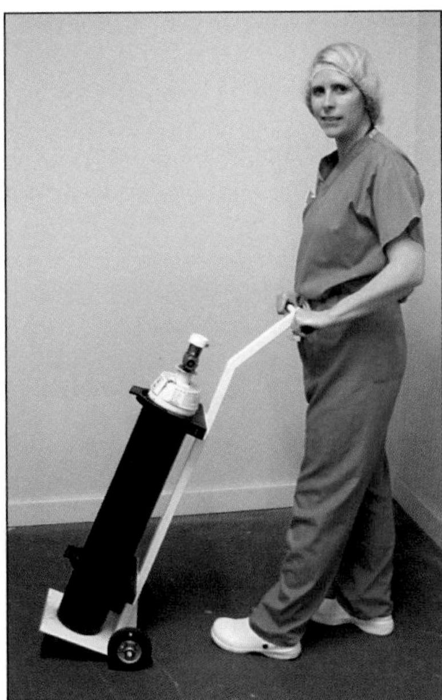

8.55 Gas cylinders should always be moved safely using a dedicated cylinder trolley.

For piped-gas installations there should be a daily check of the storage area to ensure that the system is working correctly; the alarm system in place to show low oxygen levels should also be checked. Staff should be trained in how to store certain cylinders and in stock rotation methods:

- E size and smaller cylinders should be stored horizontally
- F size and larger cylinders should be stored vertically in concrete-floored pens (Figure 8.56)
- Cylinders should be stored in a dry, clean, well ventilated area, away from the working environment, under cover, and not subjected to extremes of heat or cold
- The storage area should display warning notices, prohibiting smoking and naked lights
- Industrial and non-medical cylinders should be stored separately and full and empty cylinders should also be stored separately
- Cylinders should be properly secured to prevent falling, exploding and injuring personnel
- It is important to inform the emergency services of the location of the cylinder store and the nature of the gases kept inside it
- Full cylinders should be used in order of the date, i.e. earliest date used first to prevent cylinder contents reaching expiry date.

Safety checks on cylinders are carried out by the manufacturers. These tests include impact, pressure and tensile testing. Colour-coded plastic discs around the neck of the cylinder indicate when the next tests are due to be carried out. Cylinders should all have identification labels usually located on the neck of the cylinder. Further information such as tare weight, chemical formula of the contents, test pressure and testing dates may be found on the valve block.

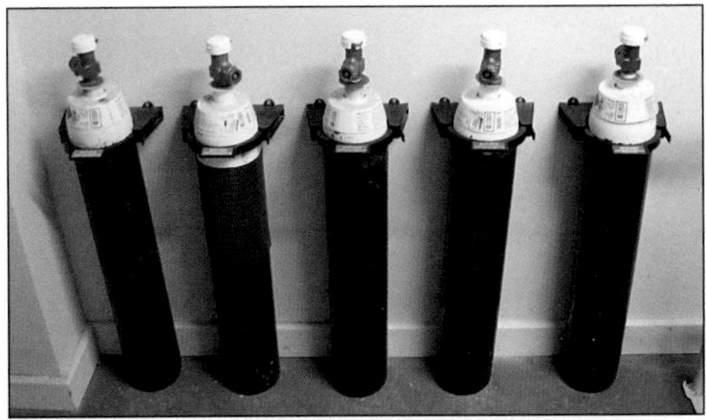

8.56 Size F and larger cylinders should be stored vertically and restrained securely, such as with cylinder locks as shown here.

Surgical lasers

Lasers are potentially dangerous. Prior to use, the surgeon and the surgical team should learn the basic laser principles and have a good, clear understanding of laser safety and safety precautions, to ensure that the patient and the surgical team are protected from injury. Risk assessments should be carried out and an SOP created dictating safe use. Potential hazards will depend on the type of laser, the operating environment and the personnel involved. Lasers are classified by the International Electrotechnical Commission into four classes, representing the degree of hazard the laser presents to human patients.

- A warning sign should be displayed on the operating theatre door.
- The risk of fire is high, and all members of the surgical team present should be aware of the nearest fire extinguisher and fire procedures.
- Every member of the surgical team should wear the wavelength-appropriate laser safety goggles (Figure 8.57a), as reflections can cause corneal burns and retinal damage.
- Surgical instruments used in laser surgery should have a dull or ebonized finish to minimize reflections.
- Patients' eyes can be protected by several moistened gauze swabs or commercially available eye shields.
- Laser surgery produces smoke (similar to electrosurgery but in larger quantities), so ventilation should be sufficient to remove plumes; commercially available smoke evacuators are recommended. Laser-safe masks with a very fine

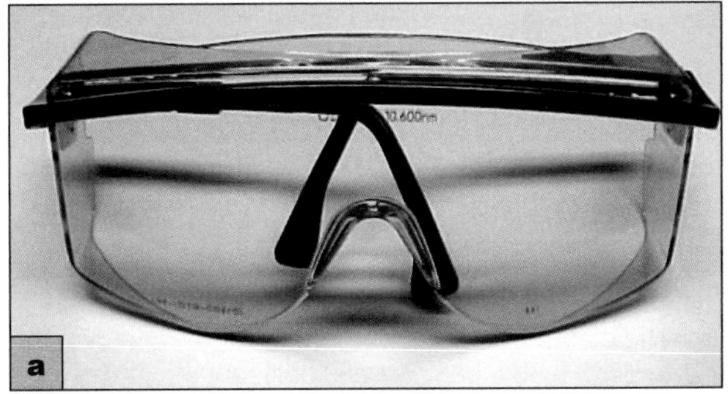

8.57 PPE for laser surgery. **(a)** Protective goggles for CO_2 laser surgery use. The pair shown are rated OD6 because they reduce the intensity of 10.6 μm laser light by a factor of 10^6. (continues) ▶

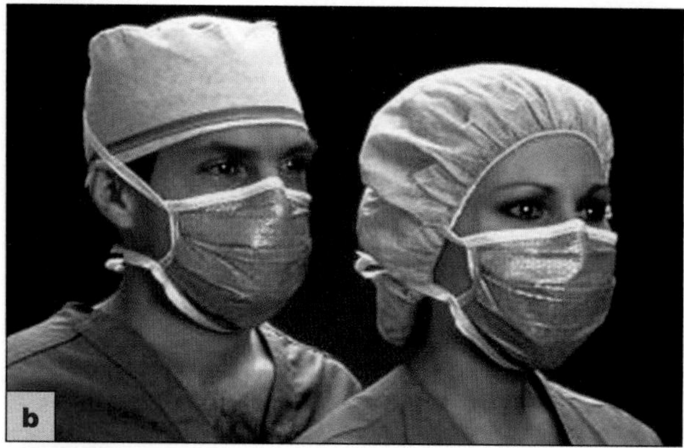

8.57 (continued) PPE for laser surgery. **(b)** High-filtration particulate surgical masks have a pore size of <1 µm. This small diameter protects the surgeon and assistant from inhaling heavy plume material.

filtration system (Figure 8.57b) are available to minimize inhalation of plume material that has not been removed by the smoke evacuator.
- Laser equipment should be serviced regularly according to the manufacturer's recommendations.

Slips and trips

Floors may be wet following mopping, which can lead to slipping and potential injury to team members. Ideally, floors should be mopped when there is little traffic to reduce the chance of someone slipping, but this is not always possible. 'Wet floor' signs should be used (Figure 8.58) and team members should be trained in how to display these correctly. Signs should be removed as soon as the area dries, to prevent them becoming a trip hazard – or being ignored. More information on how to mop floors correctly and how to prevent slips and falls can be found on the HSE website, which also provides training videos, e.g. on correct mopping techniques.

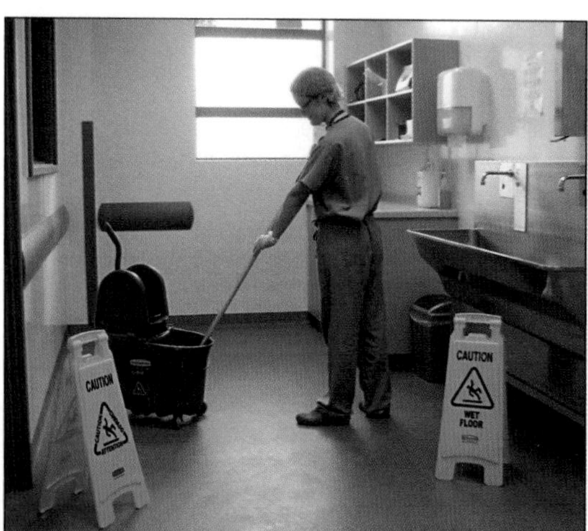

8.58 Where floors have to be mopped whilst an area is in use, clear warning signs should be used.

Good housekeeping should reduce trip hazards from equipment and supplies being left in circulation areas.

Trailing leads can be a significant hazard in the surgical suite, and care should be taken to prevent electrical wires, patient drip lines and monitoring leads from crossing walking routes and circulation areas, particularly at low levels where they are not easily seen.

Fire safety

The surgical suite contains many fire hazards and potential sources of ignition. For example:

- There are highly flammable anaesthetic volatile agents and gases which support combustion. These should be stored in appropriate containers (Figure 8.59)
- The majority of veterinary patients are covered in hair, which burns readily
- Electrosurgery (diathermy) machines are capable of producing sparks that could cause fuel to ignite.

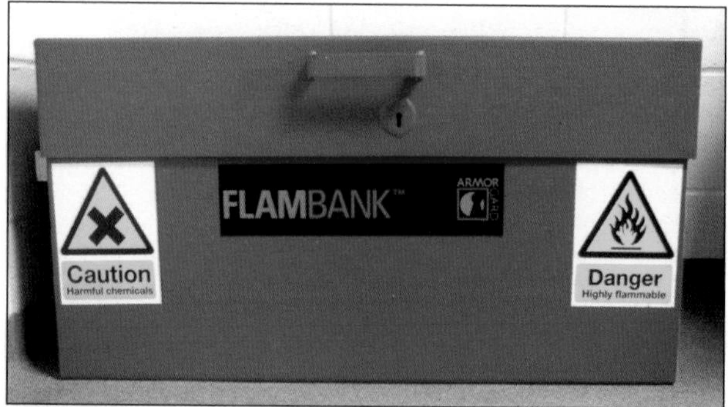

8.59 Fireproof box for storing flammable liquids such as ethylene oxide vials.

A selection of fire extinguishers (see Chapter 2) should be positioned near to the operating theatre, and staff should undergo training on how to use these. All staff should be trained in fire safety and how to reduce the chance of a fire occurring. During the training session hazard signs should be discussed. Several DVDs which cover the basic principles of fire safety are commercially available.

A protocol should be created on how to evacuate the building should a fire occur. Protocols are based on individual practice guidelines, but the following points should be considered:

- Staff (human) safety
- Patient safety
- What would happen to anaesthetized patients or patients that are undergoing surgery at that time?
- Fire escape routes
- Security of patients if taken to the outside environment
- Who would call the fire brigade?
- Important details to give the fire brigade, e.g. pressurized oxygen cylinders located within the building and the use of gases that support combustion; whether the practice has an MRI scanner on site
- Roll call (who would take charge in this situation?)
- Fire call points
- Safety handouts for the fire brigade (local fire services often carry out familiarization visits to local businesses where there may be a greater risk of fire occurring).

It is important to have discussed and agreed fire action protocols for the surgical suite because of the difficulties in evacuating patients from this area. It is vital that staff do not put themselves at risk if patients cannot be evacuated. Regular refresher training should be carried out.

Acknowledgements

The author would like to thank Jenny Tubb, Stephen Baines, Malcolm McKee, Peter Renwick, Karen Walsh and Alessandra Mathis for their help and advice with this chapter. The author and editors gratefully acknowledge the following practices, images of which appear in this chapter: Copeland Veterinary Surgeons; Elands Veterinary Clinic; Holly House Veterinary Hospital; Mill House Veterinary Surgery and Hospital; Wheelhouse Veterinary Centre; Willows Veterinary Centre and Referral Service.

References and further reading

Baines S, Lipscomb V and Hutchinson T (2012) *BSAVA Manual of Canine and Feline Surgical Principles: A Foundation Manual.* BSAVA Publications, Gloucester

Berger N and Eeg PH (2006) *Veterinary Laser Surgery – A Practical Guide*. Blackwell Publishing, Oxford

Boyce JM, Potter-Bynoe G and Chenevert C (1997) Environmental contamination due to methicillin resistant *Staphylococcus aureus*; possible infection control implications. *Infection Control and Hospital Epidemiology* **18**, 622–627

Emmerson T (2011) Surgical facilities – design, management, equipment and personnel. In: *BSAVA Manual of Canine and Feline Surgical Principles: A Foundation Manual*, ed. S Baines *et al.*, pp. 1–7. BSAVA Publications, Gloucester

Fossum T (2000) Preparation of the operative site. In: *Small Animal Surgery*, ed. T Fossum, pp. 23—26. Elsevier, USA

Hobson HP (2003) Surgical facilities and equipment In: *Textbook of Small Animal Surgery, 3rd edn*, ed. D. Slatter, pp. 179–85. WB Saunders, Philadelphia

Humes D and Lobo D (2009) Antisepsis, asepsis and skin preparation. *Surgery* **27,** 441–445

Maker VK, Elseth KM and Radoservich JA (1995) Reduced in-vivo local recurrence with contact neodymium:yttrium-aluminum garnet (Nd:YAG) laser scalpels. *Laser Surgery and Medicine* **111,** 290–298

McCormick PW (2008) Bovie smoke: a perilous plume. *Neurosurgeon* **17**(1), 10–12

McHugh D, Young A and Johnson J (2011) Theatre practice. In: *BSAVA Textbook of Veterinary Nursing, 5th edn*, ed. B Cooper *et al.*, pp. 738—773. BSAVA Publications, Gloucester

Murrell J and Ford-Fennah V (2011) Anaesthesia and analgesia. In: *BSAVA Textbook of Veterinary Nursing, 5th edn*, ed. B Cooper *et al.*, pp. 663–737. BSAVA Publications, Gloucester

Neely AN and Maley MP (2000) Survival of enterococci and staphylococci on hospital fabrics and plastic. *Journal of Clinical Microbiology* **38**, 724–726

O'Riley M (2010) Electrosurgery in preoperative practice. *Journal of Perioperative Practice* **20**, 329–333

Seymour C and Duke-Novakovski T (2007) *BSAVA Manual of Canine and Feline Anaesthesia and Analgesia, 2nd edn.* BSAVA Publications, Gloucester

Slade L (2012) Supraglottic airway devices in cats undergoing routine ovariohysterectomy. *The Veterinary Nurse* **3**(1), 30–35

White JM, S I Chaudhry, J J Kudler *et al.* (1998) Nd:YAG and CO_2 laser therapy of oral mucosa lesions. *Journal of Clinical Laser Medicine and Surgery* **16,** 299–304

Examples of SOPs and charts ▶

SOP No ....

Clippers: care and cleaning

Cleaning clippers

Disinfectant cleaner spray (e.g. Clippercide) must be used on clippers AFTER EVERY PATIENT. There should be a can and toothbrush with every set of clippers.

Stage 1: Routine clean – after *every* use

1. Remove the blades. With the clippers turned OFF, blades are removed by depressing the blade hinge lock at the base of the blade and pushing up from the toothed end to swing the blade away from the head. The blades are then lifted off the blade hinge, which should stay open at an angle.
2. Use the toothbrush to remove loose hair from the casing and from the blades themselves.
3. Replace the blade set on to the blade hinge and then switch clippers ON. Snap the blade gently back down into place with the clippers running.
4. Hold the clippers sidewards over a piece of paper towel and aim a jet of cleaning spray through the gap where the two half blades attach; then gently wipe the sides on the paper towel. Any loose hair/debris will be removed on to the paper towel.
5. Hold the clippers up to the light and look through the gap between the blades to ensure that the clippers are free from hair and debris. If not, repeat stage 4 or deep clean.

Stage 2: Cleaning more soiled blades

1. Follow Stage 1 instructions for routine cleaning.
2. Partly fill a small plastic dish with the special clipper blade wash, ensuring there is just enough liquid to submerge the blades while still attached.
3. With the clippers running, immerse the blades into the blade wash. CAUTION: DO NOT GET ANY OTHER PART OF THE CLIPPERS WET!
4. Remove the clippers from the wash solution and wipe off any excess with a paper towel.
5. Using the special clipper oil, trickle a small amount along the blades. Turn the clippers ON to run oil into the blades and then turn OFF again. ALWAYS OIL BLADES AFTER WASHING.

Stage 3: Cleaning heavily soiled blades

1. Follow Stage 1 and Stage 2 (steps 1 to 4) above, as appropriate.
2. Remove the blades again and place them in an ultrasonic cleaner or, if covered in pus, blood, etc., wash them in disinfectant such as Hibiscrub. Rinse in water and then dry immediately.
3. Replace the blades with the clippers running.
4. Using the special clipper oil, trickle a small amount along the blades. Turn the clippers ON to run oil into the blades and then turn OFF again. ALWAYS OIL BLADES AFTER WASHING. Do not leave for any time without oil as they will rust.

Troubleshooting

1. Ensure clipper blades are free from all hair and debris.
2. Check both parts of the clipper blades are moving when the clippers are running; if they are not, the blades could be seized together due to rust, dirt, pus, not enough oil, etc. OSTER BLADES ONLY can have the upper blade slid to one side, without loosening the tension spring or removing the blade completely; the surfaces can then be carefully wiped, the upper blade slid to the other side, and the process repeated. Check the clipper blade drive for wear.
3. Ensure the smaller top blade is aligned parallel to the larger bottom blade and check that the smaller blade runs approx 2 mm back from the larger blade. This can be adjusted if required by taking the blades apart (as above), realigning them and screwing back together again.
4. Check for broken blade teeth. These cannot be repaired in house.
5. If the blades are still not cutting, they may be blunt and will then need to be sent away for sharpening.
6. If the clippers are not working at all, check to see if the clipper blade motor is running whilst the blades are removed. If so, try replacing the blades and check that they are definitely clean. If not, then check for an electrical fault, e.g. loose or damaged cable. Report any such fault immediately and remove the clippers from use.

General maintenance (to be performed by the area nurse)

- Once a week: Lubricate blades in use with clipper oil and generally check them over; clean and check filters.
- Once a month: Refresh the rechargeable battery, if applicable.
- Every 6 months:
  (OSTER CLIPPERS ONLY) Inspect the carbon brushes and replace as necessary to maintain performance and motor life expectancy.
- Check stored blades (see below).

Note: Spare clipper equipment/toothbrushes, etc., are kept in prep room, above the sink.

Storage and maintenance of spare blades

- Spare clipper blades must be clean initially and free from rust. They are well lubricated with clipper oil, wrapped in wax or greaseproof paper, and stored in an airtight container. The last date they were checked, and their size, should be clearly written on the outside of each wrapped blade.
- Any blades not in use should always be checked for correct alignment (see Troubleshooting step 3) before using, and re-oiled.
- Please ensure the area nurse is informed when blades are received back from the repairers, and complete the repair tracking form.

An example of an SOP for cleaning and maintenance of clippers with removable blades.

SOP No ....

Checking anaesthetic equipment

This SOP should be followed at the start of each working day. In addition, steps 2, 11, 16 and 20–33 should be completed prior to each new patient being connected to the system.

1. Take note of any information or labelling on the anaesthetic machine referring to the current status of the machine. Read service labels and pay attention to the last service date.
2. Check all monitoring devices are functioning and ready for use: pulse oximeter, blood pressure, capnograph (check sampling lines are properly attached and free from obstructions).
3. Ensure flowmeters are turned off.
4. Press oxygen flush valve until no gas flows through the common gas outlet.
5. Check all flowmeters and pressure gauges are at zero.
6. Ensure the reserve oxygen cylinder is securely connected to the hanger yoke.
7. Open the reserve oxygen cylinder valve slowly, anticlockwise. Take note of the registered pressure.
8. Replace the cylinder if the gas content is low.
9. Label the cylinder as 'in use' or 'full' depending on its contents.
10. Turn off the emergency cylinder and ensure the pressure gauge returns to zero.
11. Connect the Schrader probe of the piped oxygen supply to the corresponding gas supply terminal outlet, giving a gentle tug to ensure they are connected correctly. A safety alarm may sound when piped oxygen is connected and disconnected (this is a safety feature to indicate low oxygen pressure).
12. Check that the pipeline pressure gauges (if applicable) on the anaesthetic machine indicate 400 kPa (kilopascals) (4 bar).
13. Open and then close the oxygen flowmeter to ensure it is working smoothly and that the bobbin (or ball) is spinning and is not sticking to the side of the flowmeter. Check the vaporizer to ensure that it contains enough liquid anaesthetic agent; replenish if necessary, ensuring that it is not overfilled.
14. Check that the vaporizer is correctly seated and locked on the back bar.
15. Adjust the control spindle on the vaporizer, ensuring it turns smoothly.
16. Turn the vaporizer to the 'off' position.
17. Check that the filling port on the vaporizer is closed correctly.
18. Select the breathing system required for use, based on the patient's bodyweight, the procedure to be performed and whether IPPV is intended.
19. Visually inspect the system for correct configuration and soiling. Replace or clean if necessary.
20. Visually inspect the patient-end tubing, ensuring no blockages are present.
21. Connect the breathing system to the common gas outlet of the anaesthetic machine.
22. Close the adjustable pressure limiting (APL) valve on the system, ensuring it closes smoothly and correctly without cross-threading.
23. Perform a pressure leak test on the breathing system by occluding the patient-end tubing (using a thumb or occlusion cap) and pressing the emergency oxygen flush valve to fill the reservoir bag. (Be careful not to overfill the reservoir bag, as this could cause damage and create micro-holes.) Systems with modern APL valves may release pressure at this point; this is a safety feature of the modern systems, although the reservoir bag should still remain distended and not collapse.
24. If the system has a pressure manometer incorporated within it, fill the reservoir bag until the manometer reaches 20 cmH_2O.
25. Observe the bag closely and ensure it remains distended for 30 seconds, or the manometer remains at 20 cmH_2O.
26. Gently compress the reservoir bag (for coaxial Bain system checks see Step 27).
27. To check a co-axial Bain system:
    i. Follow steps 22 to 26.
    ii. Inspect the inner inspiratory tubing for any blockages or damage.
    iii. Set the oxygen flow at 2 litres/minute.
    iv. Briefly occlude the inner inspiratory tube using an occlusion cap (or a 2 ml syringe plunger).
    v. Back pressure from the occluded inspiratory tubing should cause the flowmeter (bobbin) to drop.
    vi. Compress the bag gently. Any leaks should be detected at this point.
28. Open the APL valve to release the pressure within the reservoir bag. *Systems with CO_2 absorbent should not have the occlusion cap removed to reduce pressure in the reservoir bag as this could force dust from the absorbent into the breathing tubing, which could be inhaled by the next patient.*
29. Check the correct operation of all valves, including unidirectional valves within a circle system, and ensure they are not sticking.
30. Check all exhaust valves for correct operation.
31. Check that the anaesthetic gas scavenging system is switched on and functioning correctly.
32. Check the scavenging tubing is attached to the appropriate exhaust port of the breathing system and the scavenging system (either active or passive).
33. Check the APL valves to ensure they are not cross-threading or sticking, and are left in an open position.

Example of an SOP for checking anaesthetic equipment prior to use. This SOP is designed for practices with a central piped gas system and anaesthetic machines with one reserve oxygen cylinder fitted to the hanger yoke and a single plenum vaporizer. It can be adapted to suit individual practice requirements.

SOP No ....

Protocol for maintaining a surgically clean environment

At the start of each day:

1. Ensure you are wearing the correct surgical attire and any PPE required for the task in hand.
2. Damp-dust all surfaces with a disinfectant solution. Paying particular attention to high-risk cross-contamination areas, such as door handles, computer keyboards, computer mouse, the operating table and telephones.
3. Wipe over the anaesthetic machine and patient monitors with a disinfectant solution (following the manufacturers' guidelines)
4. Mop the floor with a disinfectant solution (remember wet floor signs).

During a surgical procedure:

1. Limit the number of personnel entering the operating theatre to those necessary for the surgical procedure. The microbial level in the operating theatre is directly proportional to the number of people moving about in the theatre.
2. Avoid excess talking and moving around.
3. Keep the operating theatre door closed except as needed for passage of equipment, personnel and the patient.
4. Establish and maintain a sterile field.
5. Do not walk between two sterile surfaces.
6. Non-sterile personnel should not walk too closely to the surgical field.
7. Non-sterile personnel should not reach across the surgical field.
8. Sterile personnel should not reach across unsterile areas or touch unsterile items.
9. Be conscious of where your body is at all times (this applies to both sterile and non-sterile personnel).
10. Sterile items should not be placed near open doors.
11. When in doubt about the sterility of an item or an area, consider it contaminated.

Following a surgical procedure (between patients):

1. All 'sharps' should be removed and disposed of in the correct containers. Sharps containers should be removed when they are three-quarters full and replaced.
2. Soiled items should be removed from the operating theatre in a covered container and taken to the decontamination room for cleaning.
3. All waste bags should be removed from the operating room and put into the necessary storage areas.
4. All linen should be placed into laundry baskets and removed for cleaning (and re-processing if necessary).
5. All windows should remain closed.
6. All surfaces should be damp-dusted using a disinfectant solution (paying particular attention to high-risk cross-contamination areas such as door handles, computer keyboards, computer mouse, the operating table and telephones).
7. Monitoring equipment should be wiped with a suitable disinfectant solution.
8. The floor should be mopped with a disinfectant solution (remember wet floor signs).
9. A spot check should be carried out on all walls, ceiling and equipment to ensure there is no visible soiling; if soiling is detected this should be cleaned immediately with a disinfectant solution.
10. The anaesthetic machine and system should be cleaned, and safety checks carried out; volatile anaesthetic agents should be replenished if necessary.
11. Change your surgical scrub suit if it is soiled (or if you have been assisting with a known infectious or zoonotic case).
12. Prepare the operating theatre for the next patient by gathering, checking sterility and recording any instrumentation or equipment required (see Theatre checklist).

At the end of the day:

1. Wet wash all surfaces with a disinfectant solution (paying particular attention to high-risk cross-contamination areas such as door handles, computer keyboards, computer mouse, the operating table and telephones).
2. Wipe the nozzles of spray bottles with a disinfectant solution and check hazard and product labels; re-label if necessary.
3. Clean all windows with a disinfectant solution; finish with a specialist window cleaning agent.
4. Check sharps containers; remove and replace if three-quarters full.
5. Clean the anaesthetic machine and system, according to manufacturer's instructions. Carry out safety checks and replenish volatile anaesthetic agents if necessary.
6. Clean monitoring equipment according to manufacturer's instructions, and put it away neatly.
7. Replenish stock of suture materials, syringes, needles, sterile swabs, incontinence pads, dressing materials, etc., as required.
8. Turn off the computer.
9. Turn off the active gas scavenging system (or if passive system carry out daily weighing checks of adsorbent canisters).
10. Mop the floor with a disinfectant solution (remember wet floor signs).

PTO

Protocol for maintaining a surgically clean environment. (continues) ▶

Once weekly (or following a dirty procedure):

1. Carry out a thorough 'deep clean' of the operating theatre: *(continued)*
   - Remove all equipment
   - Wet wash all walls and surfaces with a disinfectant solution, starting from the farthest point and working towards the door
   - Disinfect all equipment (including wheels by rolling in a tray of disinfectant solution)
   - Clean all windows with a disinfectant solution, and finish with a specialist window cleaner
   - Empty all storage shelves/cupboards; wipe with a disinfectant solution and re-stock
2. Check stock of consumables for integrity and expiration dates, and replenish as necessary.
3. Clean monitoring equipment thoroughly with a suitable disinfectant solution, according to manufacturer's instructions.
4. Clean the anaesthetic machine and system thoroughly, according to manufacturer's instructions, and repeat safety checks.
5. Clean and maintain the ventilation system in accordance with the manufacturer's instructions (e.g. recommended checks on filters/air flow, etc.).
6. Empty any bottles of disinfectants, alcohol sprays, etc., and check product and hazard labels. Clean and sterilize bottles, and replenish.
7. Clean active gas scavenging ABR receivers thoroughly, per manufacturer's instructions; re-assemble and check they are functioning correctly. If scavenging is passive, carry out a weighing check on charcoal adsorbents.

(continued) Protocol for maintaining a surgically clean environment.

WILLOWS

Anaesthetic Record

Page no: _____

Date:		Patient name:		Owners Name:	
Clinician:	Species:	Breed:	ASA: 12345 E	ID No:	
Anaesthetist/nurse monitoring:			Sex:	Age:	Weight: Kg

Pre-operative Assessment			**Time:**
Temp: °C	Pulse: bpm	RR: bpm	Catheters: 1. 2. 3.
PE and presenting problem:			
Procedure:			Special considerations:

Premedication			**Effect:**			
Agent	Dose (mg/kg)	mls	Checked by	Route	Time	Initials

Anaesthetic Induction and Pre-Op drugs						
Agent	Dose (mg/kg)	mls	Route	Quality	Time	Initials

ET tube:	Cuffed/ Uncuffed	Breathing system:		Fluids:
Empty Bladder		Time:	Circulating volume (dogs 80ml/kg; cats 60ml/kg)	
Adrenaline 0.01mg/kg	mls	Atropine 0.04mg/kg	mls	Lidocaine 1-2mg/kg mls

Recovery		
Anaesthesia finish:	Extubation time:	Sternal Recumbency:

Recovery considerations:	**Anaesthetic complications:**
Frequency of observations: 5/10/15/20/30 mins (Please circle)	Obs required: Temp/ pulse/ respiration/ mm colour/ CRT/ SpO2/ NIBP/ Pain score (please circle)

Parameter										
Time										

Fluid Plan:

Analgesia plan:

Empty Bladder	Size 0/1/2/3	Surgery Time:
Bandage cannula		Anaesthesia Time:

An alternative example of an anaesthetic monitoring chart (see also Figure 8.53). (© Willows Veterinary Centre and Referral Service) (continues)

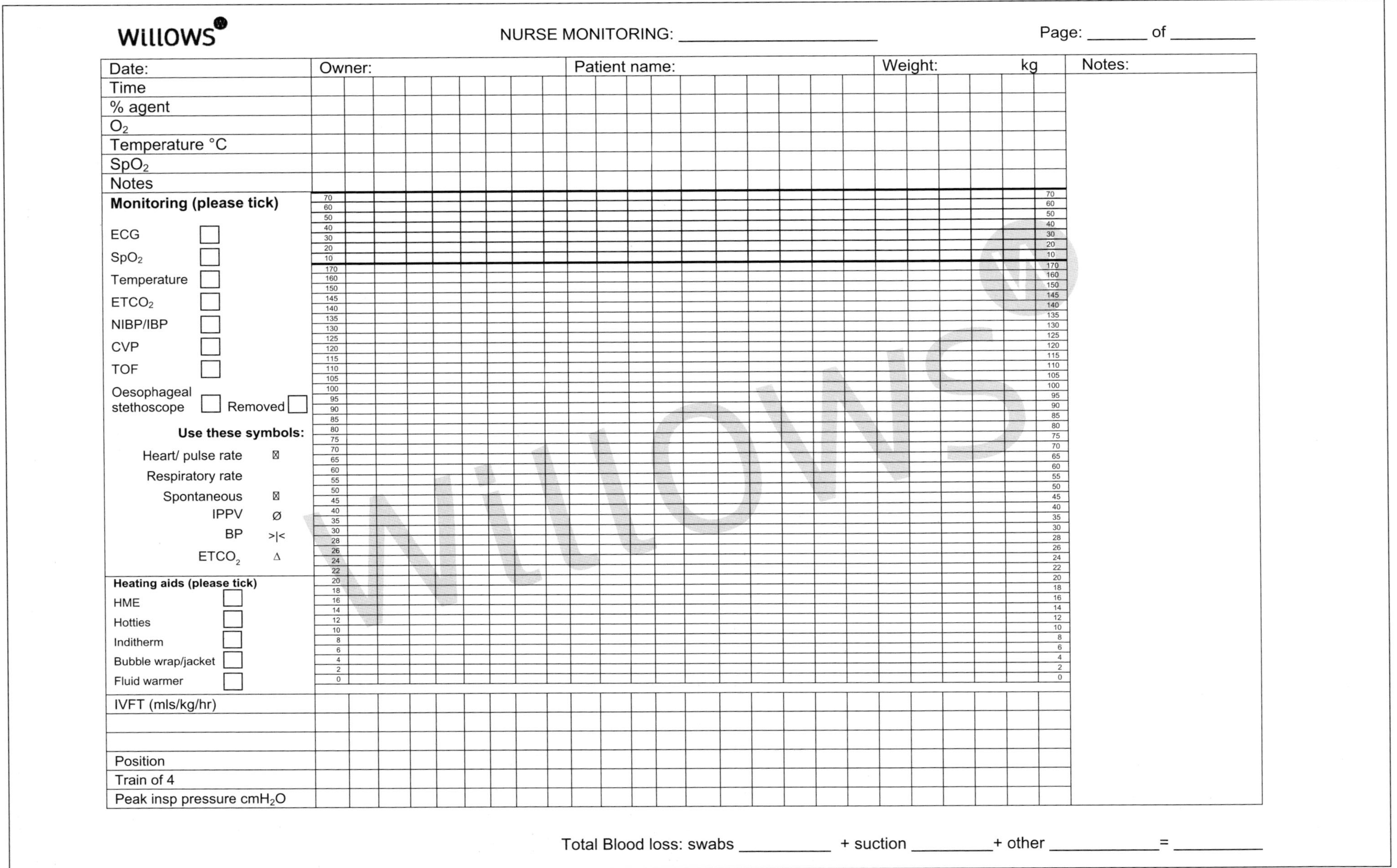

WILLOWS

NURSE MONITORING: ____________________ Page: ______ of ________

Date:	Owner:	Patient name:	Weight: kg	Notes:
Time				
% agent				
O_2				
Temperature °C				
SpO_2				
Notes				

Monitoring (please tick)

ECG ☐

SpO_2 ☐

Temperature ☐

$ETCO_2$ ☐

NIBP/IBP ☐

CVP ☐

TOF ☐

Oesophageal stethoscope ☐ Removed ☐

Use these symbols:

Heart/ pulse rate ⊠

Respiratory rate

Spontaneous ⊠

IPPV Ø

BP >|<

$ETCO_2$ Δ

Scale: 70, 60, 50, 40, 30, 20, 10 / 170, 160, 150, 145, 140, 135, 130, 125, 120, 115, 110, 105, 100, 95, 90, 85, 80, 75, 70, 65, 60, 55, 50, 45, 40, 35, 30, 28, 26, 24, 22, 20, 18, 16, 14, 12, 10, 8, 6, 4, 2, 0

Heating aids (please tick)

HME ☐

Hotties ☐

Inditherm ☐

Bubble wrap/jacket ☐

Fluid warmer ☐

IVFT (mls/kg/hr)

Position

Train of 4

Peak insp pressure cmH_2O

Total Blood loss: swabs ________ + suction ________ + other ________ = ________

(continued) An alternative example of an anaesthetic monitoring chart (see also Figure 8.53). (© Willows Veterinary Centre and Referral Service)

WiLLOWS
veterinary centre & referral service

Safety checklist flowchart

Committed to excellence

Patient name	
Breed	
Age	
Procedure	
Date	

Theatre set up (if necessary)	Tick	Initial
Suction		
Anaesthesia check		
Audit check		
Hanging limbs for orthopaedic		

Induction/prep room (to be read out loud and confirmed)	Tick	Initial
Patients' name/ID band		
Procedure		
Procedure site		
Anaesthetic machine/circuit checked		
Laryngoscope/endotracheal tubes prepared		
Drugs prepared		
NSAIDS		
Is your time plan correct?		
Check IVFT, rate, type, labelled		
MRI checklist confirmed and passed to radiographer		

Before start of intervention (to be read out loud and confirmed)	Tick	Initial
Patient name/id band		
Procedure		
Procedure site		
First prep confirmed		
Antibiotic prophylaxis confirmed		
Final prep confirmed		
Sterility of instrumentation confirmed		
Swab count (pre surgery)		
Temperature control devices (if needed)		
Correct imaging displayed (where necessary)		
Bladder management		
Diathermy earthing plate in correct place under patient & plugged in		

Sign out before any member of team leaves theatre (to be read out loud and confirmed)	Tick	Initial
Swab count (where appropriate)		
Remove mouth gag/pharyngeal pack		
Sharp count		
Samples labelled		
Postoperative medications confirmed		
Any equipment problems to be addressed		
What are the key concerns for recovery?		
Bladder management instructions (if necessary)		

Any problems encountered? Need for clinical audit? Enter details below and inform line manager

An example of a patient safety checklist flowchart. Each section is completed as the patient's care/procedure progresses. Each section should be read out loud and confirmed. The chart can be adapted for particular procedures. (© Willows Veterinary Centre and Referral Service)

Name of procedure:

Date performed:

Surgeon:

Scrubbed assistant required?

Nurse (s) present:

Anaesthetic considerations

- ASA score for patient:
- Premedication drugs used and route of administration:
- Vascular access required (detail the location of access):
- Anaesthetic induction, agents used and any problems encountered:
- Intubation details, size and type of endotracheal tube used, problems encountered?
- Breathing system used/IPPV required?
- Anaesthetic drugs required (or on stand-by), dose and route of administration:
- Perioperative anaesthetic problems/is there a point in the procedure that is particularly high risk or painful?
- Recovery period, were any problems encountered?
- Patient temperature management (were additional heating aids required)?
- Pain management, was the patient's pain managed sufficiently?

Preoperative preparation

- Surgical clip details:
- Preoperative skin preparation (type of agent(s) used):
- Prophylactic antibiotics required, if yes, give details of route of administration and dose:

Surgical procedure

- Surgical approach, give details:
- Haemorrhage encountered, how was this controlled?
- Any problems encountered, give details:

Time management

- Time taken to prepare patient for surgery (minutes):
- Total surgical time (minutes):
- Recovery time (minutes):
- Duration of hospital stay:

Surgical instrumentation

- Surgical instrumentation noted initially as required:
- Surgical instrumentation requested as additional items during procedure:

Equipment used:

- Equipment used and any problems encountered?
- Need to calibrate equipment, purchase new bulbs, batteries etc?
- Need to re-order equipment, power tool blades, implants, staples, etc?

Nursing considerations

- Postoperative nursing care required, give details (e.g. feeding tube management, physiotherapy, TPR, nutritional support):
- Bladder management instructions (if applicable):
- Postoperative drugs, dosage and route of administration:
- Key concerns for recovery/any problems encountered?

Further actions needed

For example: SOPS, further staff training, purchase of new equipment or instrumentation, need to review pricing for procedure, ideas for future improvements

Procedure review form. An example of a template that can be completed when reviewing a new surgical procedure. ASA = American Society of Anesthesiologists

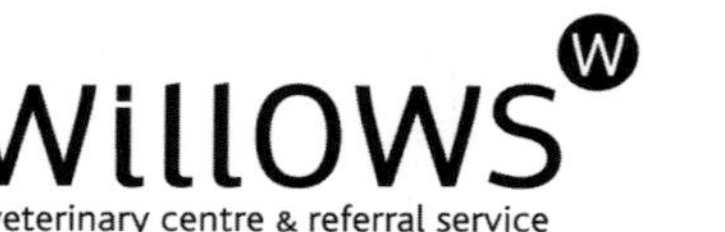

Primary procedure theatre checklist

Pyometra and bitch spay

PATIENT NAME:		DATE:		PATIENT AGE:	
NURSE:		ASSISTANT?:		SURGEON:	
PROCEDURE SITE:		PROCEDURE:	Pyometra and bitch spay	CLIPPING/LASH TRIM DETAILS:	
CONDITION OF SURGICAL SITE (POST CLIP):		SITE PREPARATION AGENTS TO BE USED:			
SITE PREPARED BY (NURSE'S NAME):				THEATRE:	4

ANAESTHETIC CONSIDERATIONS:	Ventilator set-up (in case required)			
PRE-EXISTING ILLNESS?:	Pyometra			
PATIENT POSITIONING:	Sandbag selection required in kick bin at end of table	Blue tie selection required	Dorsal recumbency	

EQUIPMENT REQUIRED:	TICK WHEN READY:	EQUIPMENT REQUIRED:	TICK WHEN READY:	EQUIPMENT REQUIRED:	TICK WHEN READY:	EQUIPMENT REQUIRED	TICK WHEN READY:
Heated bed		Suction set-up and checked		Diathermy unit set up		Sandbags	

Committed to excellence

An example of a theatre set-up sheet, detailing equipment needed for a particular procedure. This form can also act as an audit sheet, to which sterilization indicators can be attached for traceability. (© Willows Veterinary Centre and Referral Service) (continues)

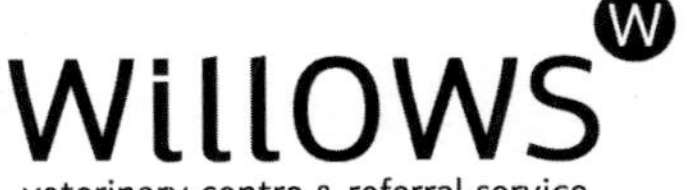

CONSUMABLE ITEMS REQUIRED	TICK WHEN READY:	CONSUMABLE ITEMS REQUIRED	TICK WHEN READY:	CONSUMABLE ITEMS REQUIRED:	TICK WHEN READY:
20ml syringe					
Scalpel blades size 10 & 15					
Biogel P gloves size 7.0					
3/0 Ethilon x 2 packets					
Sodium chloride (warmed) 1 litre x 2					
Inco pads x 5					
Additional gauze swabs pack of10 x 5					
Buster drape x 1					
Primapore dressing					
Incise spray					

RE-USEABLE ITEMS REQUIRED	PACKED BY:	DATE PACKED:	METHOD OF STERILIZATION:	COMMENTS:
Gown and Drape Pack				
General Kit				
Bitch Spay Kit				
Bipolar Diathermy				
Sterile Prep Bowl				
Sterile Kidney Dish				
Balfour Retractor (check size of patient)				

Committed to excellence

(continued) An example of a theatre set-up sheet, detailing equipment needed for a particular procedure. This form can also act as an audit sheet, to which sterilization indicators can be attached for traceability. (© Willows Veterinary Centre and Referral Service)

Dentistry

9

Amy Bowcott

Veterinary dentistry ranges from basic scaling, polishing and tooth extraction procedures to include more advanced methods of conserving teeth. The dental equipment required varies with the individual requirements of the practice, client needs and expectations, and financial constraints.

The dental room or area

A dedicated room with negative pressure ventilation is ideal (Figure 9.1). Practices often have to compromise, however, by using an area of the preparation room (Figure 9.2) or another multi-function room, perhaps shared with imaging or endoscopy (Figure 9.3). In shared areas, dental procedures should be carried out last on the surgical list.

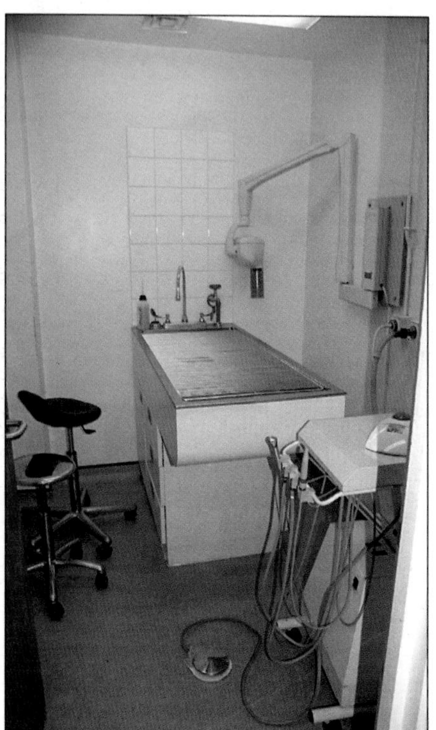

9.1 A dedicated dental room with a fixed-height tub table with grille and drawer storage for dental instruments, wall-mounted dental X-ray machine, air-driven dental unit and an adjustable stool.

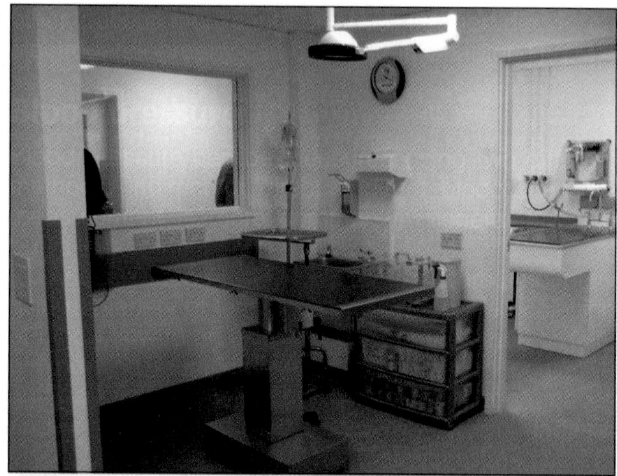

9.2 This dental room (on the right) leads off the 'dirty ops' area of the preparation room.

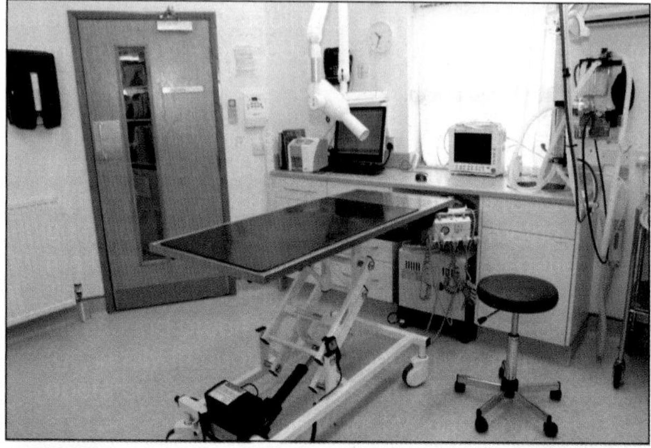

9.3 This dental area is situated in a room also used for endoscopy. Note the electrically adjustable table, with inbuilt grid area for fluid drainage. The adjustable stool aids operator comfort. This room has a wall-mounted dental X-ray unit with a digital CR processor. Dedicated dental cabinetry has been used, with purpose-built drawers for instruments and a hands-free enclosed waste bin under the sink.

KEY POINT

To maintain a surgically clean environment, dentistry should never be performed within an operating theatre.

- Dentistry is best performed in a seated position with the table and patient's mouth at elbow height and close to the table edge. A stool of adjustable height (see Figure 9.1) allows the operator to keep their back straight.
- Fixed-height tub tables are often used; however, tables with gridded tops or adjustable-height tables with gridded trays on top allow height adjustment as well as allowing fluid to drain away during the procedure.
- Suitable lighting (preferably an overhead task light) should be provided (see Figure 9.10).
- Sterile instrument sets should be available for each dental procedure. For information on hand-held dental instruments please see the *BSAVA Manual of Canine and Feline Dentistry*. The range of instruments should include sets and gags suitable for dogs, cats, rabbits and rodents.
- A dental radiography machine *within the dental area* (see Figure 9.3) is convenient, will reduce the need to move the anaesthetized patient and will improve service standards by facilitating the taking of dental radiographs to aid decision-making.

Equipment

Dental radiography

Dental X-ray machines are fairly economical, can be trolley- or wall-mounted, and have arm extensions, allowing precise positioning for specific views (see Figures 9.1 and 9.3). Exposures are obtained at a short focal film distance.

Many automatic film processors will not allow processing of the tiny film sizes required for some of the specialized dental views (Figure 9.4a), so a purpose-built benchtop dental wet processor (Figure 9.4b), or some other form of wet processing for dental films, e.g. polaroid film pouch or similar, will be needed.

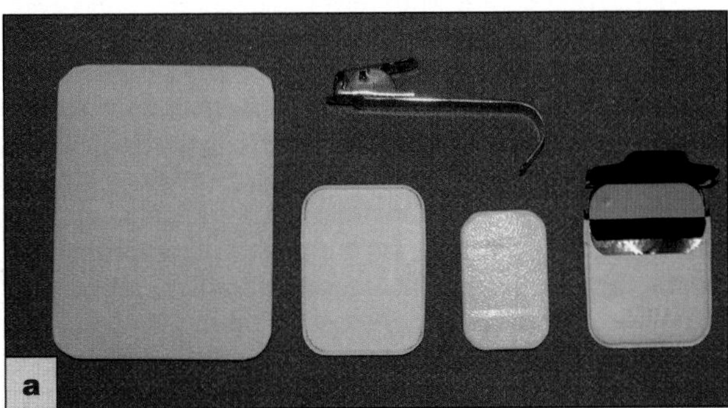

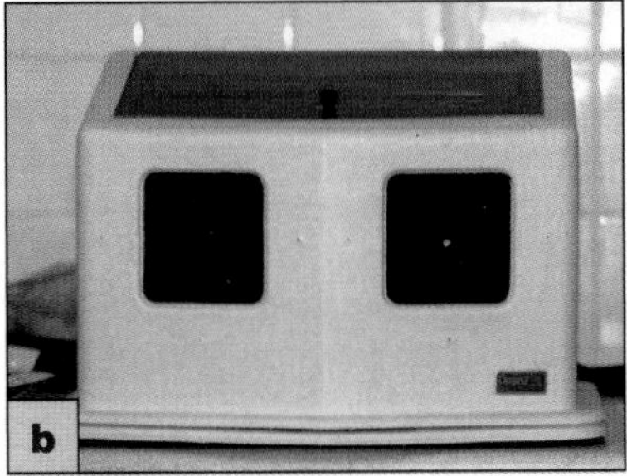

9.4 **(a)** The dental X-ray films commonly used in practice are, from left: occlusal, adult periapical, paediatric periapical. An opened film envelope reveals the film (green), lead backing sheet, and black protective paper. Also shown is an X-ray film clip. **(b)** A chairside 'darkroom' is convenient for processing dental X-ray films.

Direct digital radiography (DDR) sensors are available for oral work (Figure 9.5a) and can be wired directly to a laptop or desktop computer (with the appropriate software) in the dental area. The sensors are relatively bulky and are expensive to replace, but are the major cost of the system as any computer with a reasonable specification can usually be used. Computed radiography (CR) film (Figure 9.5b) is cheaper but the film reader (Figure 9.5c) will be more costly. CR film is more manoeuvrable than oral DDR sensors and is cheaper to replace.

If the practice is using its main radiographic facility for dental work and considering switching to a digital unit for its main radiographic needs (see Chapter 13), this will have implications for dental imaging. A different method for intraoral views will be needed if an integrated table/DDR main unit is purchased.

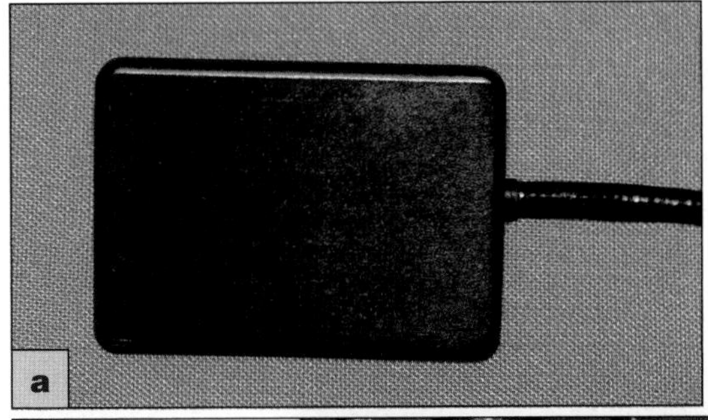

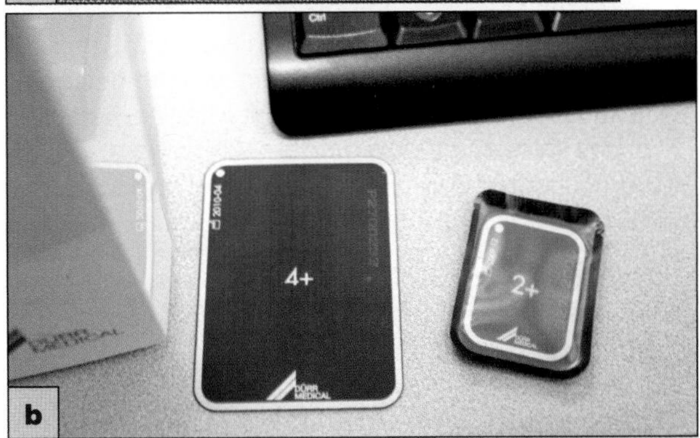

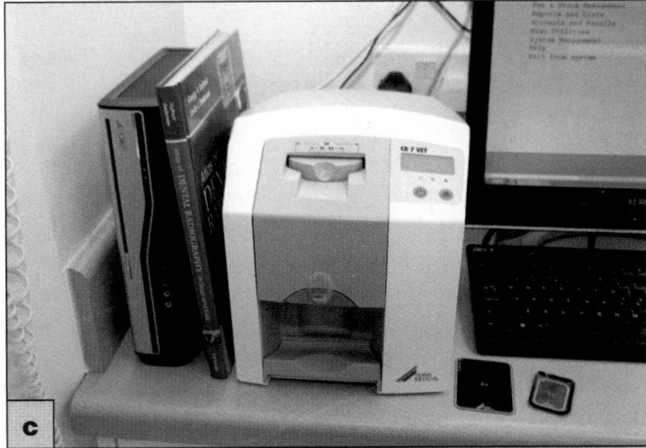

9.5 Digital dental radiography. **(a)** This transducer is used to take digital dental radiographs using the direct technique. The image is displayed almost immediately on a computer screen. **(b)** The digital CR film is small and easy to manoeuvre; sizes 2 and 4 are shown here. The film is protected in a clear disposable pouch, which is discarded when the film is inserted into the processing machine. **(c)** A digital CR dental radiography processor, which reads specific dental film to display on a PC.

Dental machines

Dentistry machines can be powered either electrically or by pressurized air. All power equipment will generate heat, so water irrigation is mandatory to prevent damage to the teeth, soft tissue and bone.

Electrically driven units

Electrically driven units use a micromotor attached directly to the dental handpiece to drive the burs. Most electrical units are classed as 'low speed', as the motor speed is less than 35,000 rpm. A micromotor unit is often referred to inaccurately as a 'polishing unit'. Electrical units take a variety of slow handpieces. 'Speed-increasing handpieces' can be purchased; these increase the bur speed, by up to five times, through a gearing system in the handpiece.

If it is intended to use a micromotor for sectioning teeth or cutting bone, irrigation is needed. Where handpieces do not have integral tubing, an external source such as a syringe or giving set is required for water irrigation of the bur.

- Units and handpieces intended for sectioning teeth have irrigation capability, allowing irrigant to the tip of a bur via internal or external tubing. A speed of 30,000–40,000 rpm (with a 1:1 handpiece; higher where a speed-increasing handpiece is used) allows cutting of teeth with the appropriate bur.
- Units designed for cutting bone have a 1:1 handpiece and no dental scaler, and are designed to be used with sterile irrigant, e.g. saline via a pump and integral tubing. They are used at 30,000–40,000 rpm to remove bone and section teeth (e.g. surgical extractions).

Micromotor units will be damaged if there is water or oil ingress or they are slowed by heavy use, and replacement motors are expensive. Handpieces for both electrically and air-driven units need to be oiled after cleaning and then stood upright to allow excess oil to drain off before they are reattached to the motor unit.

Air-powered units

Air-powered dental machines use pressurized air or nitrogen, from a medical air cylinder or air compressor. The gas is directed into an air turbine, which is either in the head of a high-speed handpiece or within a low-speed motor to which a variety of handpieces can be attached. High-speed handpieces are also known as air turbines. When the tooth surface is contacted, rotational speed is easily reduced and these units therefore require a very light touch. Air-driven units are usually equipped with water irrigation, which comes from the tip of the high-speed handpiece. Compressors can be fixed to the machine trolley or can be located away from the dental area, with reduced noise and machine footprint (Figure 9.6). A combination air and water syringe is available on all air-driven machines, and is used for rinsing and drying areas to examine. Suction is also available on some machines, which aids fluid and debris removal (see Figure 9.10).

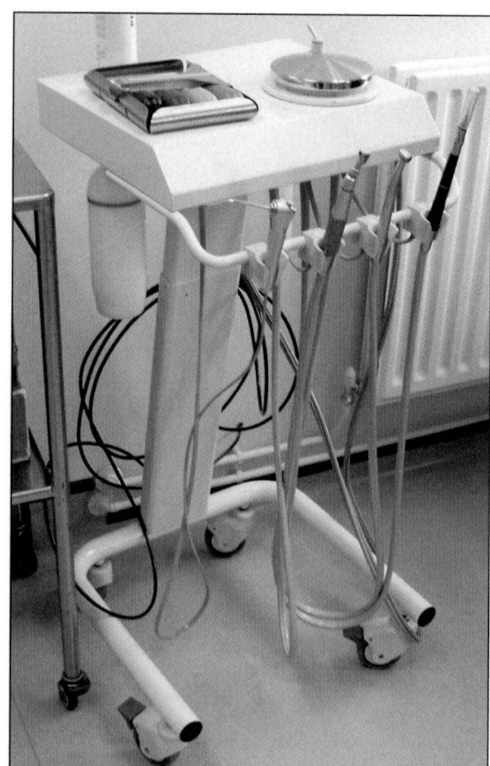

9.6 An air-driven dental machine can have an integral compressor (see Figures 9.1 and 9.10) or the compressor can be located elsewhere, as in this example, which makes the unit easier to move and reduces noise and clutter in the dental area.

Choosing a machine

When looking at dental machines, 'torque' should be considered: this is the ability of the handpiece to keep rotating when the working tip is pressed against the tooth surface. Modern electrical units can produce more torque than can air-driven machines.

Air-powered machines are relatively expensive but are preferred for their flexibility and range of functions. Whilst a single electrically driven slow handpiece for polishing can be sufficient for much small animal dentistry, the investment in an air-driven unit with high- and low-speed handpieces and additional attachments broadens the range of functions, particularly cutting. For practices that perform more than the occasional dental work, despite the initial capital expense, this machine ultimately provides better value.

Where finances are limited or the low number of dental procedures may not justify the expense of an air-powered machine, such as at a branch surgery, an ultrasonic dental scaler with a micromotor drill unit (ideally with integral water coolant) is a suitable alternative (Figure 9.7). Although cutting teeth is slower, such a unit is more than satisfactory for routine dentistry (including on small mammals) in a first-opinion small animal practice. It is also compact and therefore ideal if space is limited. It is important that the unit of choice has an integral water supply going through the drill and scaler. One main disadvantage of these units is the lack of a three-way (air and water) syringe for rinsing and drying teeth. It is not always necessary to have the scaler and micromotor in one unit; they can be separate machines. A combination unit may be cheaper to buy, but repair and replacement costs may be lower for separate scaler and drill units.

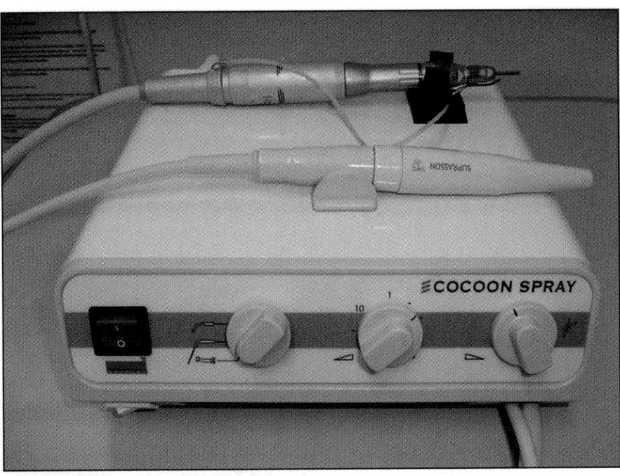

9.7 An example of a dental combination unit.

Dental handpieces

- **High-speed handpieces:**
  - Usually air-powered and water-cooled and operating at 300,000 to 400,000 rpm.
  - Used to section teeth
  - A wide selection of bur sizes is available. Burs are held in the handpiece by a friction-grip (FG) mechanism within the turbine head. These burs are called FG burs (Figure 9.8a,b).
- **Low-speed handpieces:**
  - Powered by a directly attached external motor – electrically (micromotor) or air-powered (air motor). The motor speed is dependent on the air pressure supplying it (in the latter type)
  - The handpieces may have no gearing, or may have speed-increasing or speed-reducing gearing
  - For cutting bone, a low-speed handpiece should be used with integral tubing for an external irrigant source, to which a giving set can be attached. A lower specification alternative is to have an assistant, with saline bag, giving set and three-way tap attachment, provide constant irrigation of the bur
  - Straight, contra-angle, prophylaxis angle and oscillating head handpieces are available for low-speed motors:
    - The straight handpiece is usually used with burs to remove bone and for adjusting rabbit cheek teeth, but also can accept a mandrel to hold diamond and sanding discs and finishing stones. The shafts of the burs are designated handpiece type (HP; Figure 9.8e,f)
    - The contra-angle handpieces can have a variety of heads, which accept either latch (right-angled (RA); Figure 9.8c,d) or FG type burs but not both
    - The prophylaxis angle is used to carry out polishing. The cups used for polishing can be latch grip, screw-in or push-on cups. To-and-fro prophylaxis heads are available which produce less heat and reduce the chance of hair entrapment; these tend to be more expensive than rotating prophylaxis angle handpieces. (The oscillating polishing heads tend to be disposable; other types are usually non-disposable.)

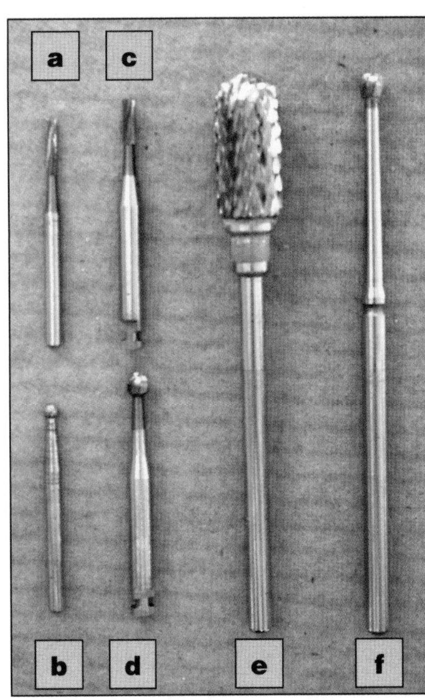

9.8 Different types of bur. **(a)** FG fissure bur (TC). **(b)** FG round bur (diamond). **(c)** RA fissure bur (TC). **(d)** RA round bur (TC). **(e)** HP acrylic trimmer bur (TC). **(f)** HP round bur (TC). FG = friction-grip; HP are for straight handpieces; TC = tungsten carbide. (Reproduced *from BSAVA Manual of Canine and Feline Dentistry, 3rd edn.*)

Some handpieces have a fibreoptic light fitted to them, to illuminate the cutting area (Figure 9.9).

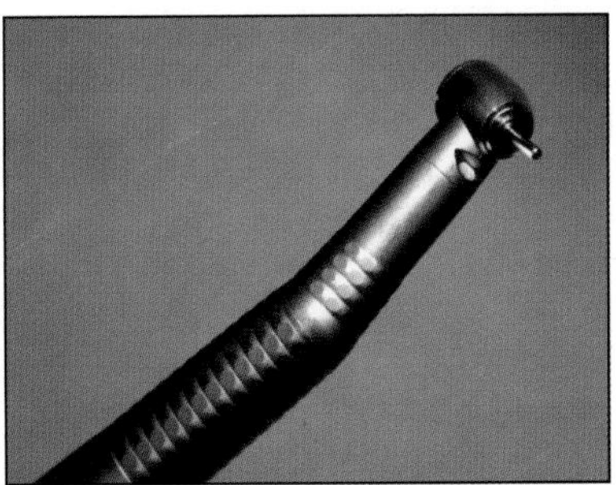

9.9 This handpiece is fitted with a fibreoptic light for illuminating the tooth.

Scaling and polishing

Powered scalers are not essential, as dental scaling can be performed using hand instruments; however, powered units make the scaling procedure quick and easy and are therefore recommended. Caution should be taken, as they can cause damage to the teeth and surrounding tissues due to the heat produced. Roto pro burs should never be used for scaling teeth.

There are two types of powered scaler used in veterinary dentistry:

- **Sonic scalers:** These are attachments (handpieces) for air-driven dental uints. They oscillate at a sonic frequency that is lower than ultrasonic; they are considerably slower at removing tartar and relatively expensive
- **Ultrasonic scalers:** There are two types of ultrasonic scaler mechanism – magnetostrictive and piezoelectric. They act to disrupt calculus (tartar), and are generally designed for scaling the tooth surface above the gumline, although they can be used with care just below it. Subgingival tips may damage teeth and surrounding tissues.

Following scaling, teeth should be polished to remove plaque and ensure that the tooth surface is smooth. Using a coarse or gritty paste will increase roughness by scouring. Polishing can be carried out using the low-speed contra-angle handpiece with 'prophy' paste. A new disposable polishing cup (see Figure 9.11) should always be used for each patient. Caution should be taken with 'prophy' paste in bulk containers, as cross-contamination could occur when refilling the cup.

Management considerations

Radiation safety

The practice's Radiological Protection Advisor (RPA) should be consulted regarding the arrangements for radiography. Because of the lower radiation doses involved with dental radiography equipment, radiation protection measures advised by the RPA may be less stringent than for the main radiography room. A controlled area must be clearly signed and Local Rules must be in place. A detailed record of exposures should be kept and the X-ray machine checked and serviced annually. See Chapter 13 for more details on radiation safety.

Biosecurity

The oral cavity contains a wide array of bacteria, which become airborne when ultrasonic scaling is undertaken. It is important for staff members to wear personal protective equipment (PPE; Figure 9.10) when carrying out or assisting with dental procedures, to prevent aspiration of bacteria and also to protect the eyes from fluid, aerosols or debris. A facemask (available with pre-attached visor for ocular protection), eye safety goggles, aprons and disposable examination gloves should be worn.

The patient's mouth should be rinsed with an antibacterial (chlorhexidine) mouthwash prior to treatment to reduce the bacterial load in any aerosol produced. Ventilation or air cleaning within the room is essential but is difficult to achieve to an adequate standard in many premises.

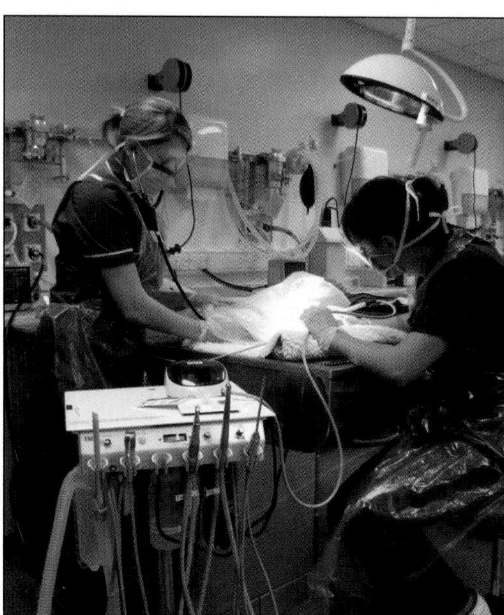

9.10 PPE must be comfortable and easy to wear and work in. Facemasks are available with clear plastic splash guards. Note also the overhead lighting and the blue suction handpiece on the dental machine.

> **KEY POINT**
>
> A zone of at least 2 metres around the dental table should be considered as a contaminated zone.

Patient safety

Pharyngeal packs (Figure 9.11) should be available to prevent aspiration of fluid or debris by the patient, but extreme caution should be used to ensure that they do not block the airway. It is vitally important that all team members communicate clearly when the pack has been placed and ensure that it is removed before the recovery period. This can be included in safety checklists. Long ties (ideally made from a bright material) should be placed securely around the pack; forceps can then be attached to the ends of the ties, to ensure that staff are visually alerted to the pack being in place and to ensure its prompt and safe removal.

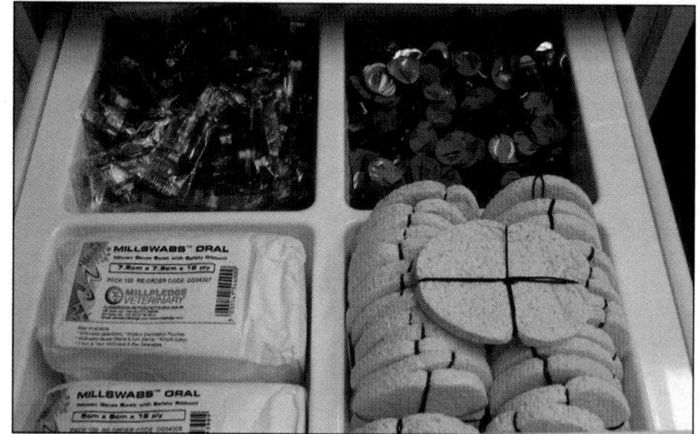

9.11 Dental unit drawer containing (clockwise from bottom right): pharyngeal packs with black ties; oral swabs with ribbons; prophy cups for polishing teeth; and individual cups of prophy paste.

Patients undergoing dental procedures should be monitored closely, including body temperature, as for any animal under general anaesthesia. Because of the nature of dental procedures and their length, patients may be at higher risk of hypothermia, so insulation (Figure 9.12) and patient warming (see Chapter 8) are essential.

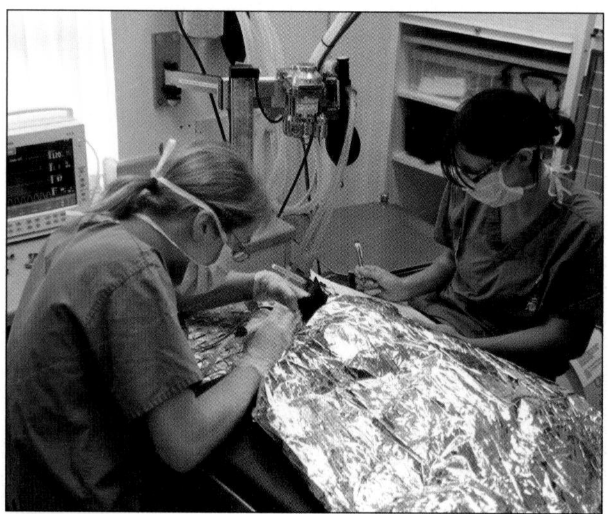

9.12 A survival blanket has been employed to keep this cat warm during the dental procedure.

Dental charts

Charts assist in planning treatment and ensure documentation of the examination that can be used to track a patient's progress. There are many different charts available, which can be adapted to suit the individual practice's requirements; some examples are given at the end of this chapter. The dental chart should be easy to use and staff must be trained to complete the chart correctly (see *BSAVA Textbook of Veterinary Nursing*). Where the charts do not incorporate explanations of abbreviations, etc., it is helpful to have these printed out and laminated so they can be referred to if needed.

Completed charts (Figure 9.13) can be scanned into patients' computerized records or filed away physically. Clients may appreciate a copy of the chart as a reminder of the treatment performed. Dental charts are also useful support for nurses to use during patient discharge; added notes can indicate any advised homecare treatment the patient should receive to maintain the condition of the teeth. Detailed homecare guidance notes are useful for clients, and encourage concordance and compliance with the ongoing dental treatment and care plan.

Equipment and instrument maintenance

Dental machines should be maintained according to the manufacturer's instructions. If a dental machine has an air compressor of more than 250 bar litres, it will require a written scheme of examination and a certificate of inspection under the Pressure Systems Safety Regulations 2000. Compressors must be kept clean and air inlets free of hair and debris.

Staff should be trained in how to care correctly for the dental instruments.

- Any instrument with sharp edges should be sharpened with a sharpening stone and oil (Figure 9.14). Dental scalers and curettes need to be sharpened frequently, i.e. after a couple of uses. Extraction instruments only need to be sharpened if they have become damaged. Staff should only sharpen instruments after being trained in the correct techniques.

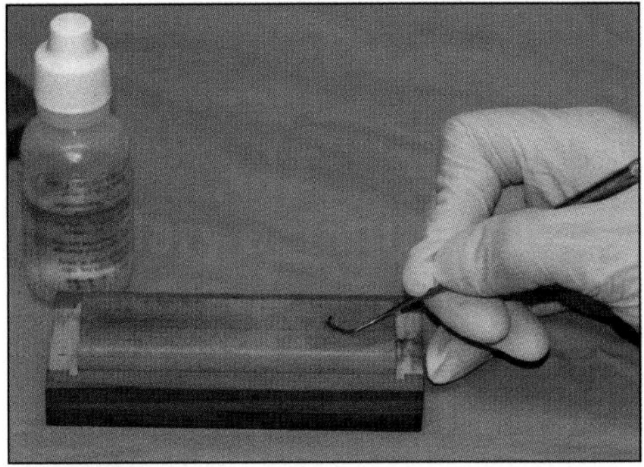

9.14 Sharpening a subgingival curette on an Arkansas stone.

- Following dental procedures the instruments, handpieces and attachments used should be cleaned, disinfected and, where possible, sterilized using the appropriate method. The dental machine should be cleaned with a suitable equipment wipe or disinfectant, such as an alcohol-based hard surface disinfectant.
- Handpieces should be lubricated after cleaning, and stored correctly according to manufacturers' instructions.

Training

Specific practical dental technique training is important for all clinicians carrying out small animal dentistry, and particularly where advanced restorative dentistry is needed. Where veterinary nurses are carrying out dentistry procedures under Schedule 3 of the Veterinary Surgeons Act 1966, appropriate training in both theoretical and practical aspects, and a competence assessment, should be clearly documented and communicated to all directing veterinary surgeons. Veterinary nurses are not permitted to carry out extractions except in the case of simple digital extractions of loose teeth. There are a number of practical and theoretical training courses, and some distance learning material, available.

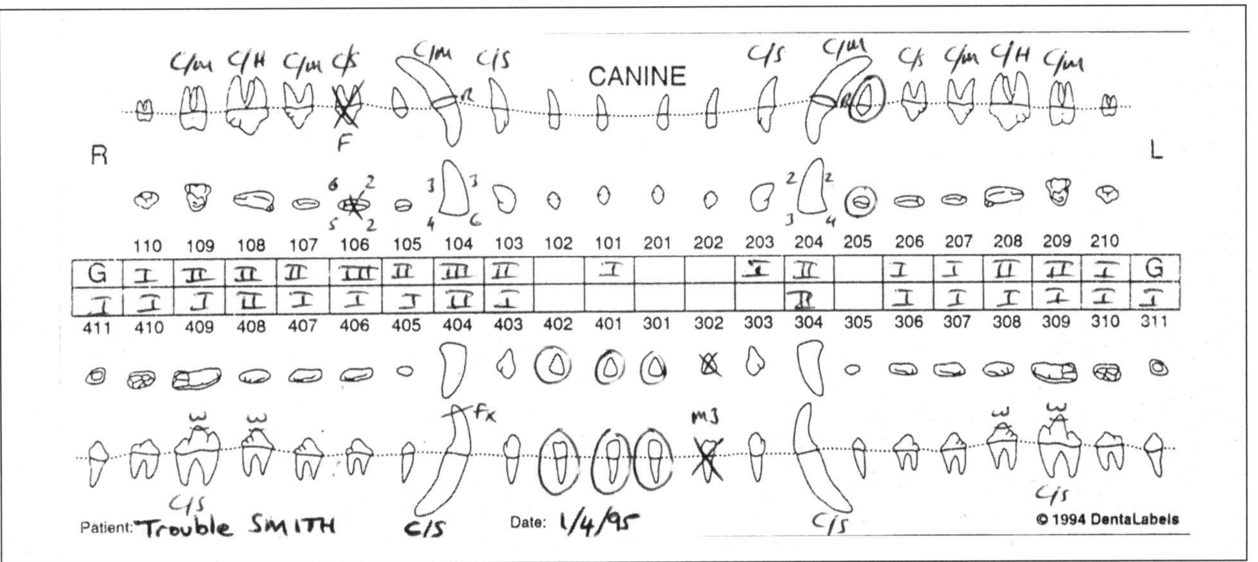

9.13 A small canine dental chart completed for a patient. © DentaLabels, John Robinson.

Follow-up

Veterinary nurses are well placed to advise and support clients with dental homecare, and the enthusiasm and ability of owners to carry out homecare should be an important factor in planning dental treatment. These issues can usefully be discussed before the dental procedure, after discharge and at regular follow-up appointments.

Acknowledgements

The author and editors are grateful to the specialist veterinary dentists who have advised on this chapter. The author and editors gratefully acknowledge the following practices, images of which appear in this chapter: Astonlee Veterinary Hospital; Mill House Veterinary Surgery and Hospital; Pool House Veterinary Hospital; Willows Veterinary Centre and Referral Service.

Further reading

Gorrel C, Hennet P and Verhaert L (2001) *Clinical Handbook of Veterinary Dentistry*. Virbac

Milella L and Helm M (2008) Dentistry. In: *BSAVA Manual of Canine and Feline Advanced Veterinary Nursing, 2nd edn*, ed. A Hotston Moore and S Rudd, pp. 175–194. BSAVA Publications, Gloucester

Robinson J (2007) Dental instrumentation and equipment. In: *BSAVA Manual of Canine and Feline Dentistry, 3rd edn*, ed. C Tutt *et al.*, pp. 67–76. BSAVA Publications, Gloucester

Tutt C, Deeprose J and Crossley D (2007) *BSAVA Manual of Canine and Feline Dentistry, 3rd edn*. BSAVA Publications, Gloucester

Tutt C and Vranch S (2011) Dentistry. In: *BSAVA Textbook of Veterinary Nursing, 5th edn*, ed. B Cooper *et al.*, pp. 881–900. BSAVA Publications, Gloucester

Examples of dental charts 

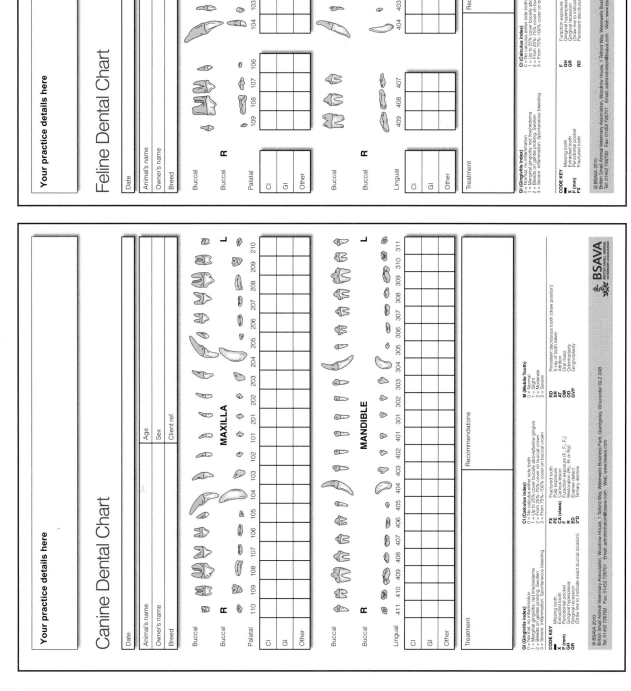

Your practice details here

Canine Dental Chart

Date	
Animal's name	Age
Owner's name	Sex
Breed	Client ref.

Buccal

Buccal **R** **MAXILLA** **L**

Palatal	110	109	108	107	106	105	104	103	102	101	201	202	203	204	205	206	207	208	209	210
CI																				
GI																				
Other																				

Buccal

Buccal **R** **MANDIBLE** **L**

Lingual	411	410	409	408	407	406	405	404	403	402	401	301	302	303	304	305	306	307	308	309	310	311
CI																						
GI																						
Other																						

Treatment	Recommendations

GI (Gingivitis index)
0 = Normal; no inflammation
1 = Marginal gingivitis; red line/oedema
2 = Bleeds on gentle probing. Swollen
3 = Severe inflammation. Spontaneous bleeding

CI (Calculus index)
0 = No calculus either side tooth
1 = Up to 25% cover bucally above/below gingiva
2 = From 25%–75% cover on buccal crown
3 = From 75%–100% cover on buccal crown

M (Mobile Tooth)
0 = Normal
1 = Slight
2 = Moderate
3 = Severe

CODE KEY

▬	Missing tooth
X	Extracted tooth
P (mm)	Periodontal pocket
GH	Gingival hyperplasia
GR	Gingival recession (Draw line to indicate exact buccal location)
FX	Fractured tooth
PE	Pulp exposure
CA (class)	Carious lesion
F	Furaction exposure (F_1, F_2, F_3)
R	Restoration (Rc, Ri or Ra)
ED	Enamel defect
3*D	Tertiary dentine
RD	Persistent deciduous tooth (draw position)
XR	X-ray of tooth taken
AT	Attrition
OM	Oral mass
OD	Odontoplasty
GVP	Gingivoplasty

British Small Animal Veterinary Association, Woodrow House, 1 Telford Way, Waterwells Business Park, Quedgeley, Gloucester GL2 2AB
Tel: 01452 726700 Fax: 01452 726701 Email: administration@bsava.com Web: www.bsava.com

BSAVA BRITISH SMALL ANIMAL VETERINARY ASSOCIATION

Your practice details here

Feline Dental Chart

Date	
Animal's name	Age
Owner's name	Sex
Breed	Client ref.

Buccal

Buccal **R** **MAXILLA** **L**

Palatal	109	108	107	106	104	103	102	101	201	202	203	204	206	207	208	209
CI																
GI																
Other																

Buccal

Buccal **R** **MANDIBLE** **L**

Lingual	409	408	407	404	403	402	401	301	302	303	304	307	308	309
CI														
GI														
Other														

Treatment	Recommendations

GI (Gingivitis index)
0 = Normal; no inflammation
1 = Marginal gingivitis; red line/oedema
2 = Bleeds on gentle probing. Swollen
3 = Severe inflammation. Spontaneous bleeding

CI (Calculus index)
0 = No calculus either side tooth
1 = Up to 25% cover bucally above/below gingiva
2 = From 25%–75% cover on buccal crown
3 = From 75%–100% cover on buccal crown

FORL'S (FORL – state type and class eg FORL 2/4) Requires X-ray
Type 1: Focal resorption in crown/roots. Most of root/PL intact
Type 2: Total resorption of roots & replacement by bone
Class 1 = 0.5 mm lesion in enamel
Class 2 = penetration into dentine
Class 3 = penetration into pulp
Class 4 = major destruction of tooth
Class 5 = crown lost/roots retained

CODE KEY

▬	Missing tooth
X	Extracted tooth
P (mm)	Periodontal pocket
FX	Fractured tooth
F	Furaction exposure (F_1, F_2, F_3)
GH	Gingival hyperplasia
GR	Gingival recession (Draw line to indicate exact buccal location)
RD	Persistent deciduous tooth (draw position)
XR	X-ray of tooth taken
AT	Attrition
OM	Oral mass
OD	Odontoplasty
GVP	Gingivoplasty

British Small Animal Veterinary Association, Woodrow House, 1 Telford Way, Waterwells Business Park, Quedgeley, Gloucester GL2 2AB
Tel: 01452 726700 Fax: 01452 726701 Email: administration@bsava.com Web: www.bsava.com

BSAVA BRITISH SMALL ANIMAL VETERINARY ASSOCIATION

Full-size downloadable charts are available for BSAVA members at www.bsava.com

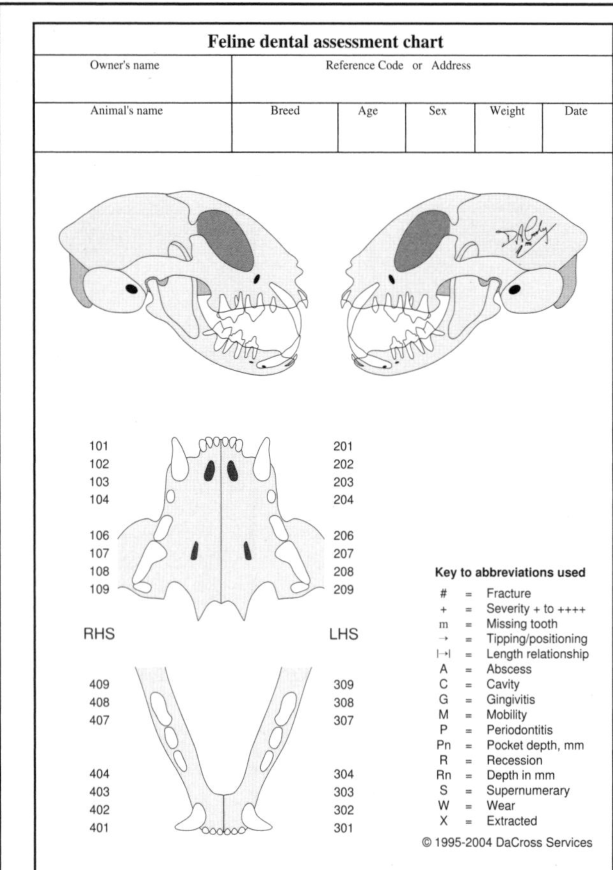

Dental procedures

Performed		Required
{ }	Pre-anaesthetic checks	{ }
{ }	General anaesthesia	{ }
{ }	Radiography	{ }
{ }	Occlusal assessment	{ }
{ }	Supra-gingival scaling	{ }
{ }	Subgingival scaling	{ }
{ }	Root planing	{ }
{ }	Polishing	{ }
{ }	Gingival lavage	{ }
{ }	Gingival surgery	{ }
{ }	Extraction	{ }
{ }	Periodontal splinting	{ }
{ }	Crown height reduction	{ }
{ }	Occlusal adjustment	{ }
{ }	Endodontic therapy	{ }
{ }	Restoration	{ }
{ }	Orthodontic treatment	{ }
{ }	Oro-facial surgery	{ }
	Homecare program	{ ✓ }

Assessment by quadrant
(graded +, ++, +++, ++++)

	1 (RU)	2 (LU)	3 (LL)	4 (RL)
Plaque	:	:	:	:
Calculus	:	:	:	:
Gingivitis	:	:	:	:
Periodontitis	:	:	:	:
Occlusion	:	:	:	:
Tooth wear	:	:	:	:

Other comments

Routine Home Dental Care

The efficient daily use of a soft bristled toothbrush, with an appropriate animal toothpaste, is still the only proven method for long term control of plaque and gum disease.

Chewing exercise is beneficial as it stimulates natural tooth cleaning and protection mechanisms. In general hard chewing objects are not a good idea as many animals damage their teeth and gums on them, and swallowed pieces can cause serious problems. Avoid feeding soft sticky foods and never give items containing sugar or oil/fat as treats.

Specific Instructions

(Courtesy of David Crossley)

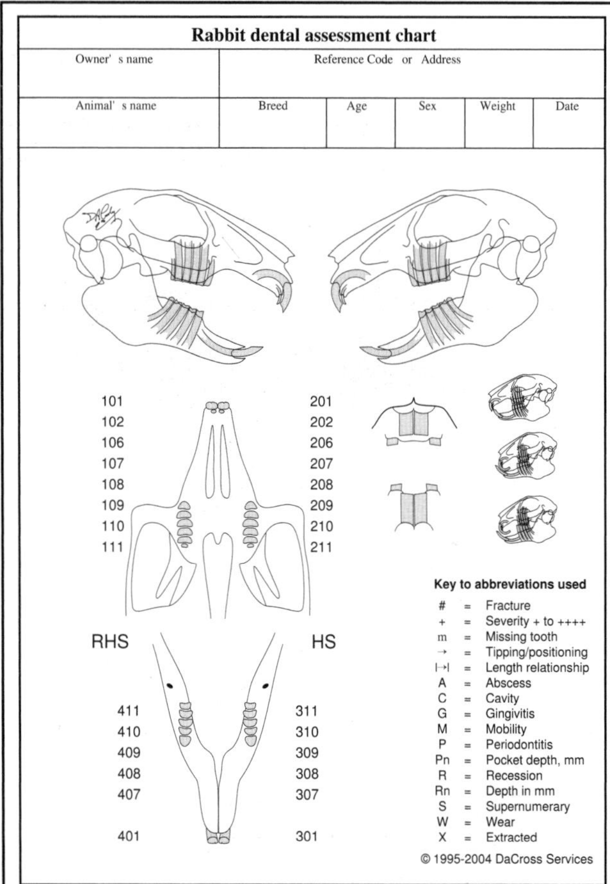

Dental procedures

Performed		Required
{ }	Pre-anaesthetic checks	{ }
{ }	General anaesthesia	{ }
{ }	Radiography	{ }
{ }	Occlusal assessment	{ }
{ }	Supra-gingival scaling	{ }
{ }	Subgingival scaling	{ }
{ }	Root planing	{ }
{ }	Polishing	{ }
{ }	Gingival lavage	{ }
{ }	Gingival surgery	{ }
{ }	Extraction	{ }
{ }	Periodontal splinting	{ }
{ }	Crown height reduction	{ }
{ }	Occlusal adjustment	{ }
{ }	Endodontic therapy	{ }
{ }	Restoration	{ }
{ }	Orthodontic treatment	{ }
{ }	Oro-facial surgery	{ }
	Homecare program	{ ✓ }

Assessment by quadrant
(graded +, ++, +++, ++++)

	1 (RU)	2 (LU)	3 (LL)	4 (RL)
Plaque	:	:	:	:
Calculus	:	:	:	:
Gingivitis	:	:	:	:
Periodontitis	:	:	:	:
Occlusion	:	:	:	:
Tooth wear	:	:	:	:

Other comments

Routine Home Dental Care

Herbivores naturally wear their teeth by prolonged chewing. To compensate for this the teeth continue erupting. If they do not have enough natural food the teeth get longer and develop sharp spikes which injure the cheeks and tongue. Chewing exercise is also beneficial as it stimulates natural tooth cleaning and protection mechanisms. In general hard and artificial chewing objects are not a good idea as many animals damage their teeth and gums on them, and swallowed pieces can cause serious problems.

Provide the bulk of the diet as growing grass or hay. Avoid feeding soft sticky foods and never give items containing sugar or oil/fat.

Specific Instructions

(Courtesy of David Crossley)

Endoscopy

10

Philip Lhermette

Flexible endoscopy has been used for many years for investigation of the respiratory and gastrointestinal tracts, and in recent years rigid endoscopy has become much more widely used for routine procedures in general practice, including laparoscopic ovariectomy and cryptorchidectomy.

The decision to invest in endoscopy equipment should not be taken lightly. The cost of equipment over the whole of its operational life includes purchase/leasing, maintenance, repair and disposal costs, as well as the cost of consumables. Training in effective use of the equipment is essential, and nursing staff will also need training in its care, cleaning and storage. Maintenance costs and, ultimately, replacement costs should also be factored in. Once the operational costs are known, it is possible to forecast the financial impact on the practice for the projected caseload. The purchase decision should be made with a realistic view of operational profits that may be generated. This should take into account the practice location and client demographics, the types of patient and cases seen, demand for the procedures on offer, and the willingness and ability of practice staff to learn new procedures. Intangible benefits should also be appreciated, such as an improved working environment, improved clinical satisfaction and better services for clients, as well as the increased ability to attract and retain staff through broader facilities. The reputation of the practice will also be enhanced and fewer cases may need to be referred.

Consideration should be given to the number of staff who will be able to use new equipment. This will have a bearing not only on training costs but also on the income received. The loss of trained staff from the practice may leave too few clinicians able to use the equipment to maintain a reasonable profit. If only one person is trained, their departure may mean that the equipment is left unused. It is, unfortunately, common to find that a new ultrasound machine or flexible endoscope has been purchased for an enthusiastic assistant who then moves on and the expensive equipment sits in a cupboard gathering dust. In-house training can sometimes be arranged, to include most or all of the clinical team. This enables more usage of the equipment, and can also increase staff retention by broadening clinical experience and adding new skills.

Equipment

If purchasing new equipment, most manufacturers or re-sellers will recommend a basic range to suit individual needs. Advice should be sought from several manufacturers, and also from more experienced colleagues, to ensure that the best range is selected, not only for immediate needs but also so that equipment can be added as experience progresses.

Planning a purchase so that equipment is compatible can save a considerable amount of money. A complete new set-up for rigid rhinoscopy, otoscopy, urethrocystoscopy, laparoscopy, thoracoscopy and arthroscopy can cost around £12,000 to £15,000. If the light source, suction and camera systems are compatible, adding flexible endoscopes will only require the cost of the endoscopes themselves rather than a whole new system.

KEY POINT

Much of the equipment required can be used for both rigid and flexible procedures, e.g. light source, suction, camera system and video capture systems (Figure 10.1).

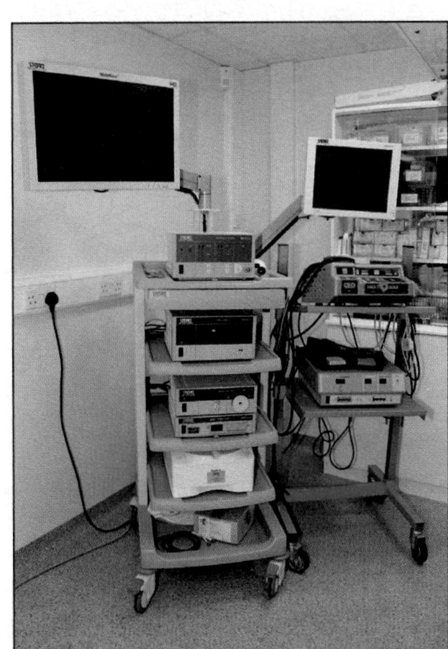

10.1 The grey trolley houses endoscopy equipment with two monitors, electronic insufflator, image capture system, xenon light source, camera system and printer. The blue trolley contains equipment for electrosurgery.

Endoscopes

The choice of rigid or flexible endoscopes – or both – will be governed by the caseload and interests of the individual practice. Often a basic system will be purchased with a view to adding to it as experience grows.

Flexible endoscopes

Flexible endoscopes are complex instruments, consisting of a long flexible insertion tube, operated via levers or rotating wheels on the handpiece, and connected to a light source by an umbilical cord that also carries air and water channels (Figure 10.2).

The type of endoscope purchased will depend on the anticipated workload.

- For **gastrointestinal** work a duodenoscope with four-way tip deflection is required. This should have a tip deflection in one plane of at least 180 degrees (Figure 10.3). No single flexible endoscope is suitable for all patients, but the most widely used endoscope will have an outside diameter of around 7.8–8 mm and an insertion tube length of 140–150 cm. This will enable the endoscopist to intubate the pylorus of most cats and also to reach the duodenum of giant-breed dogs. This endoscope can also double as a bronchoscope in medium to large breeds of dog. Specific veterinary endoscopes are now being manufactured to meet these needs, as most flexible human duodenoscopes only have an insertion tube length of 100 cm.
- For **tracheobronchoscopy**, an endoscope with a two-way tip deflection, an outside diameter of around 3.7 mm and an insertion tube length of 54 cm is adequate for most cats and small to medium dogs This should also have a tip deflection in one plane of at least 180 degrees, and is usually operated by a lever on the handpiece (Figure 10.4).
- **Instrument channels:** The largest size possible should be selected. Channels normally range from 2 mm to 2.8 mm in gastroduodenoscopes. A large channel enables the passage of larger instruments and therefore permits larger, more diagnostic, biopsy samples to be taken.
- **Fibreoptic** *versus* **video**. Video-endoscopes smaller than about 6 mm in diameter are not available due to constraints imposed by the size of the video chip (CCD). A fibreoptic endoscope is considerably cheaper to purchase and can be used with the same camera system as rigid endoscopes. However, the image quality is considerably poorer than with video-endoscopes as the fibreoptics create a pixellated image (Figure 10.5). Wherever possible, a video-endoscope should be considered; if chosen from the same manufacturer, it may connect to the same camera console as the separate camera for the rigid endoscopy system (see Figure 10.10).

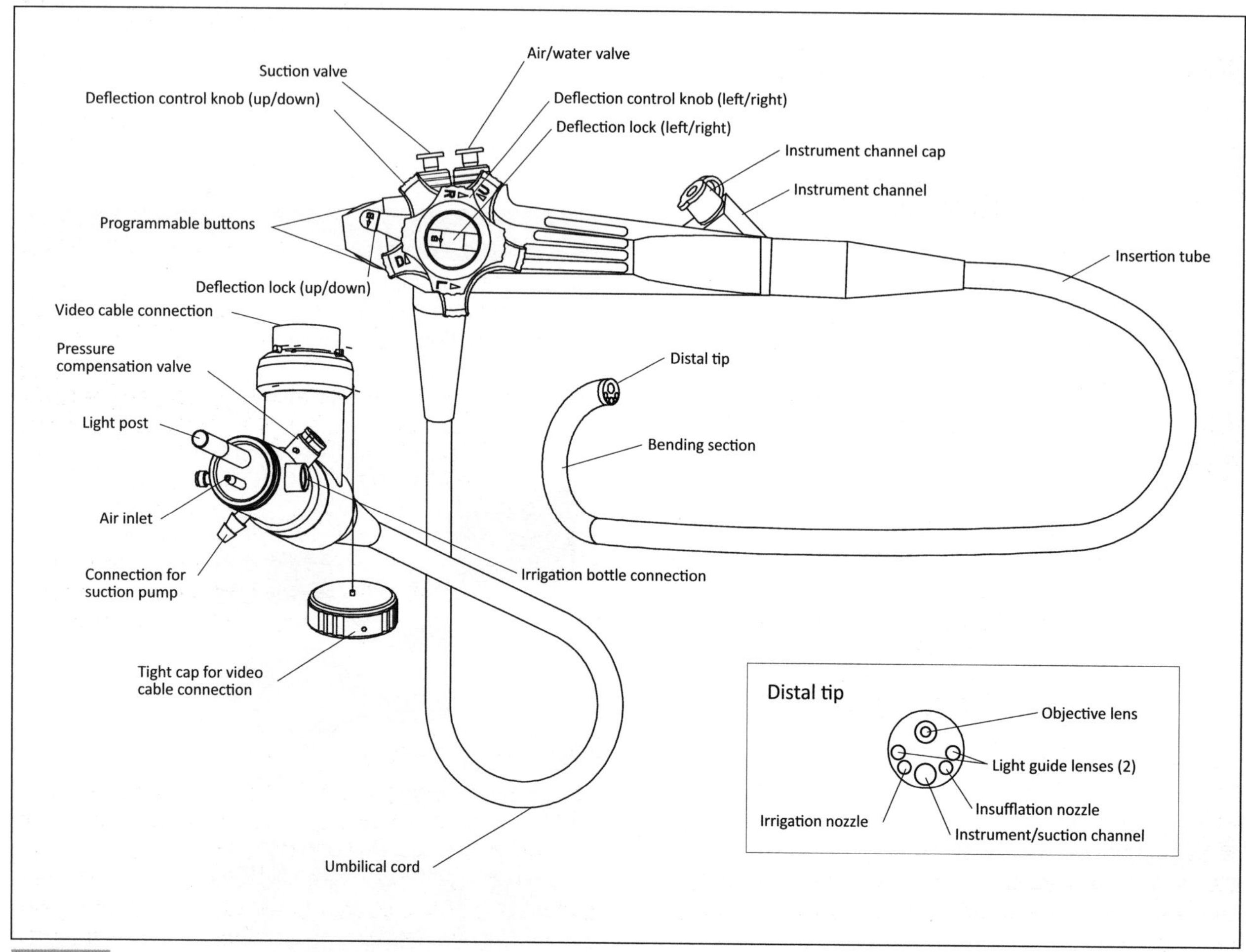

10.2 Diagram of flexible endoscope. (Reproduced from the *BSAVA Manual of Canine and Feline Endoscopy and Endosurgery*)

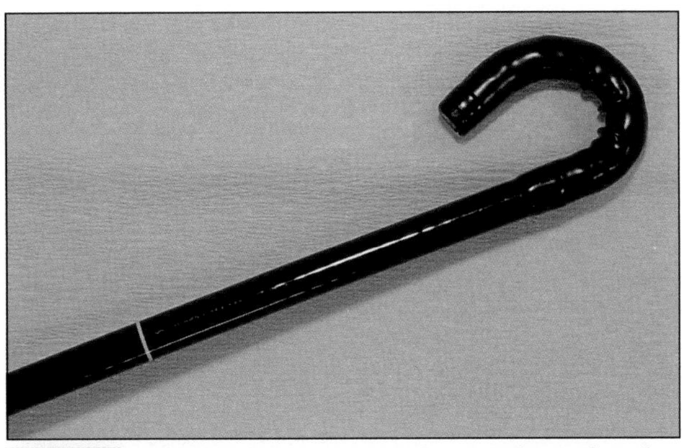

10.3 A flexible duodenoscope, showing the tip flexed at 180 degrees.

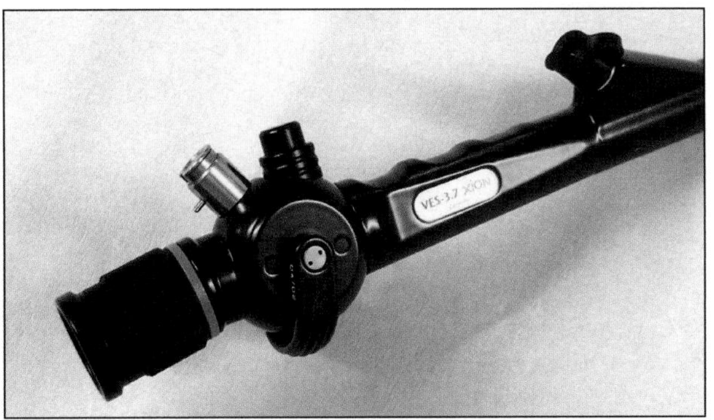

10.4 Bronchoscope handpiece with a lever to operate the two-way flexible tip.

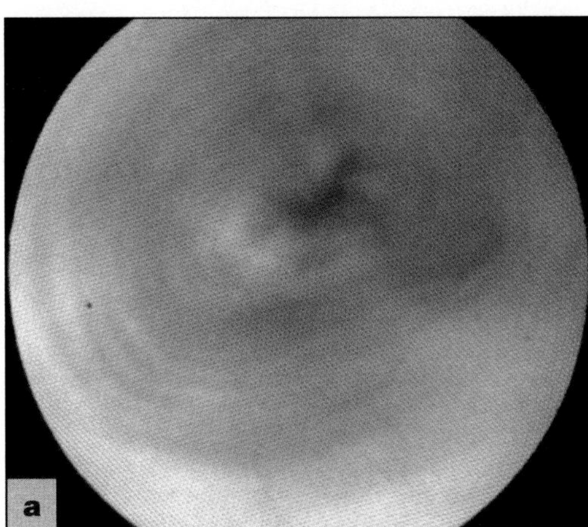

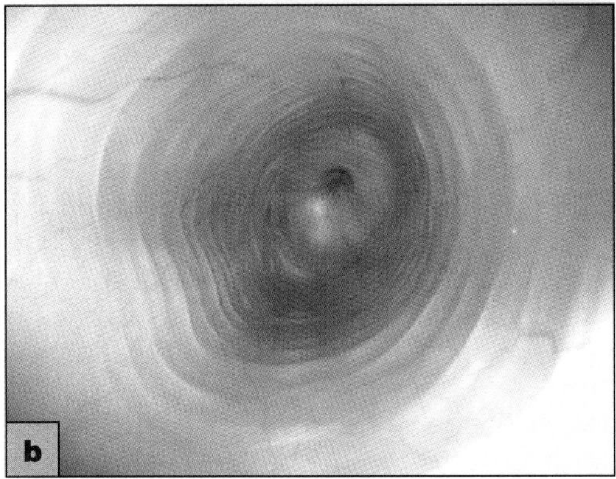

10.5 Images of a cat's oesophagus. **(a)** With a fibreoptic flexible endoscope, pixellation can be reduced by using a filter system in the camera, but the image is still less sharp. **(b)** Image quality is considerably better with a video-endoscope.

A range of ancillary instruments will also be required (Figure 10.6) and these are tailored to the diameter of the instrument channel and the length of the insertion tube.

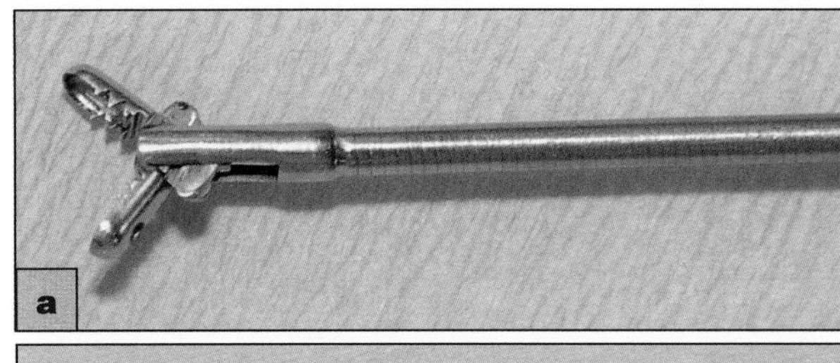

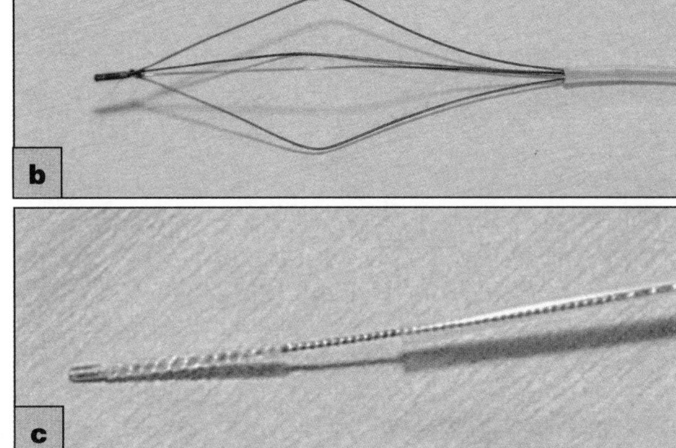

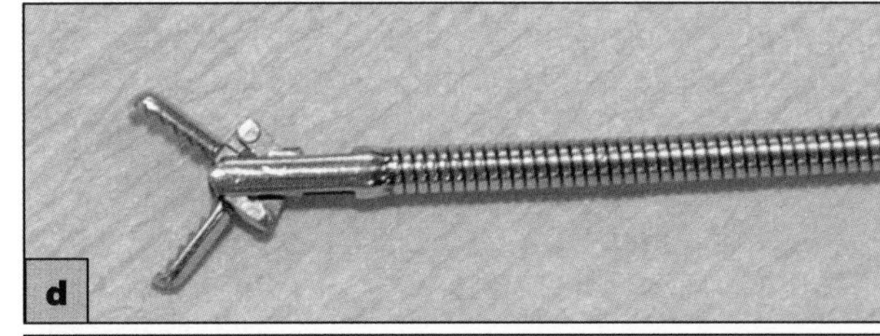

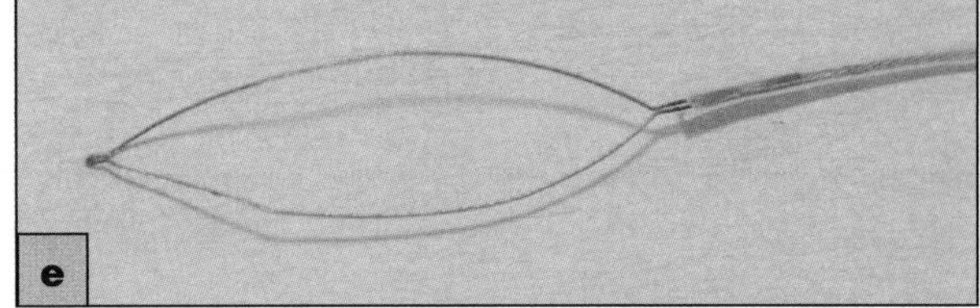

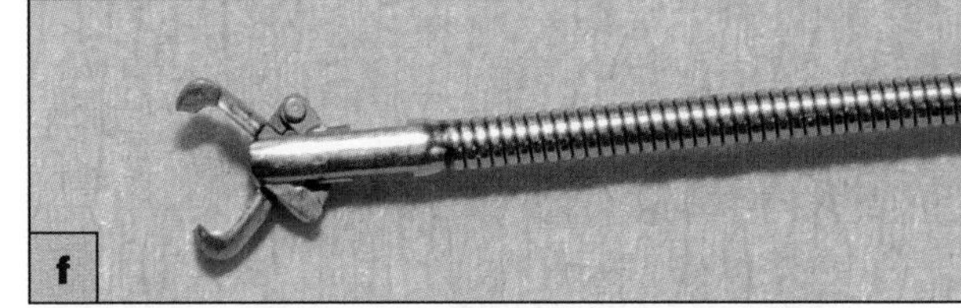

10.6 Examples of ancillary equipment for flexible endoscopes. **(a)** Biopsy forceps – oval perforated cup with serrated edge; **(b)** basket forceps; **(c)** cytology brush; **(d)** grasping forceps; **(e)** loop snare; **(f)** rat-toothed forceps.

Rigid endoscopes

Rigid endoscopes (Figure 10.7) are relatively simple, short steel tubes containing lenses, with an eyepiece at one end that is usually connected to a clip-on camera, and a light guidepost that is connected to the light source via a fibreoptic light guide cable. They are used for laparoscopy, thoracoscopy, rhinoscopy, urethrocystoscopy and arthroscopy, and various other procedures that do not require entry into a tortuous channel.

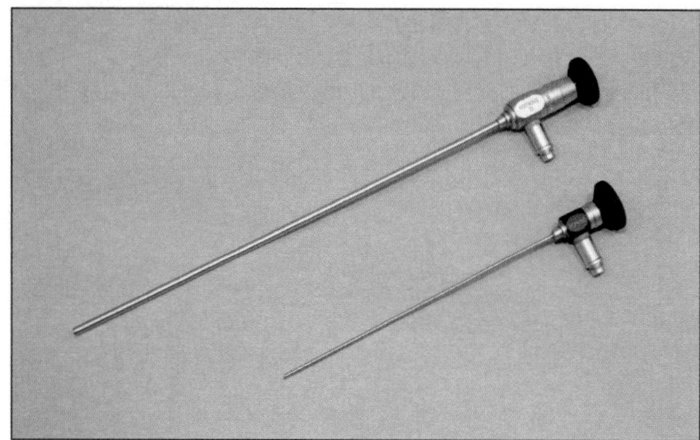

10.7 Rigid endoscopes with diameters 5 mm and 2.8 mm.

The most versatile rigid endoscope for use in general practice is the 2.7 mm 30 degrees 18 cm telescope. This is 18 cm long and has an insertion tube of 2.7 mm and an angle of view that is at 30 degrees from the long axis of the insertion tube, directed away from the light guidepost (Figure 10.8). This permits the veterinary surgeon to look over the top of organs or to widen the range of view in a tight space by rotating the telescope around its long axis. The length of the insertion tube, and the lower light transmission relative to the 5 mm or 10 mm rigid endoscopes, limits the telescope's use in laparoscopy to small patients or small spaces. This is a fragile instrument that is always used in a protective sheath. This endoscope can be used for:

- Small exotic pets
- Rhinoscopy, urethrocystoscopy and otoscopy in all dogs and cats
- Arthroscopy in large dogs
- Laparoscopy and thoracoscopy in cats and small dogs
- Exploration of fistulae and penetrating injuries.

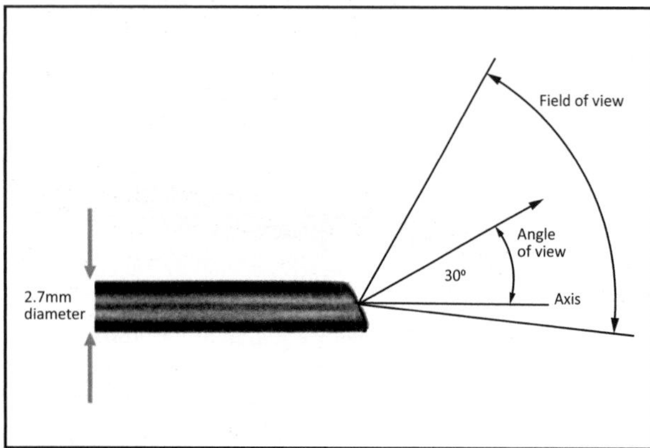

10.8 Field of view of a 2.7 mm 30 degrees arthroscope. The field of view delineates the margins of the image that can be seen. The angle of view is the centre of direction of view in relation to the long axis of the endoscope. In this case the centre of the field of view is at 30 degrees to the long axis.

A 5 mm 0 degrees 30 cm telescope is a more robust instrument and is used for laparoscopy and thoracoscopy in medium to large dogs. A suitable range of equipment for most rigid endoscopy procedures is listed in Figure 10.9.

Basic equipment: suitable for urethrocystoscopy, rhinoscopy, otoscopy, laparoscopy and thoracoscopy in cats and small dogs, and for use in exotic pets

- Camera system (single chip)
- Monitor
- Light source (preferably xenon)
- Light guide cable
- 2.7 mm 18 cm Hopkins 30 degrees endoscope
- 14.5 Fr cystoscopy sheath with 5 Fr instrument channel
- 7 Fr 40 cm biopsy forceps
- 7 Fr 40 cm grasping forceps
- 3 mm rigid biopsy forceps
- 3 mm protection sheath
- 3.9 mm laparoscopic cannula (ternamian-tipped or with sharp trochar)

Additional equipment for laparoscopy or thoracoscopy

- CO_2 electronic insufflator
- Electrosurgery generator
- Surgical suction pump
- Veress needle
- Sterile insufflation tubing
- 5.0 mm 29 cm Hopkins 0 degrees endoscope
- (5.0 mm 29 cm Hopkins 30 degrees endoscope)
- 6 mm laparoscopic cannula (ternamian-tipped or with sharp trochar) (x3)
- 11 mm laparoscopic cannula with sharp trochar
- 6 mm disposable thoracic cannulae with blunt obturator
- 11/6 mm reducing valve
- 5 mm endoscopic biopsy forceps (cup and/or punch type)
- 5 mm endoscopic grasping/dissecting forceps
- 5 mm endoscopic Babcock's forceps
- 5 mm curved endoscopic scissors (monopolar)
- 5 mm palpation probe with centimetre markings
- 5 mm suction probe with monopolar hook dissector
- Bipolar coagulation forceps

Additional equipment for arthroscopy

- 1.9 mm, 2.4 mm and 2.7 mm 30 degrees endoscopes
- Arthroscope sheaths to fit above endoscopes
- Pressure bag or arthroscopic irrigation system
- Selection of operating cannulae and switching sticks
- Hand burr
- Right-angled palpation probe 1–3 mm
- Curette 2.5 or 3 mm
- Sickle knife, hook knife or forward cutting knife
- Grasping forceps
- Arthroscopic shaver system

10.9 Equipment required for rigid endoscopy procedures.

Camera

A basic camera system is essential for most endoscopy (Figure 10.10). A simple one-chip camera is perfectly adequate for general surgical use, although three-chip, HD and digital cameras are available at a considerable price premium. 3D cameras are also in development. A single-chip camera can be attached to both rigid endoscopes and fibreoptic flexible endoscopes, although an adapter may be required for the latter (Figure 10.11). The use of a camera and monitor will greatly enhance the diagnostic capability of the endoscopist by providing a large magnified image on screen. In the author's opinion, peering through the oculus of a fibreoptic or rigid endoscope should never be encouraged.

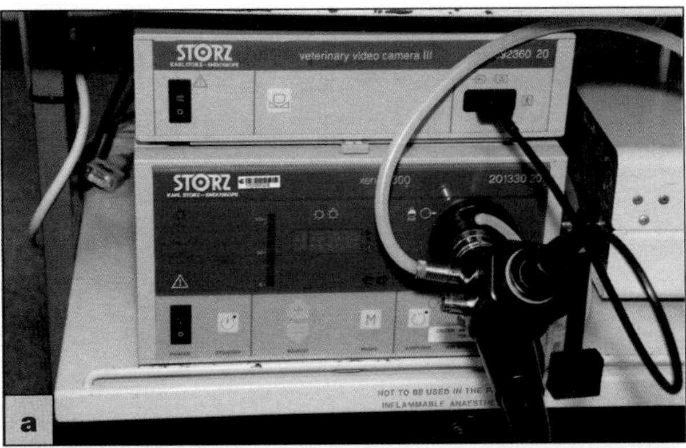

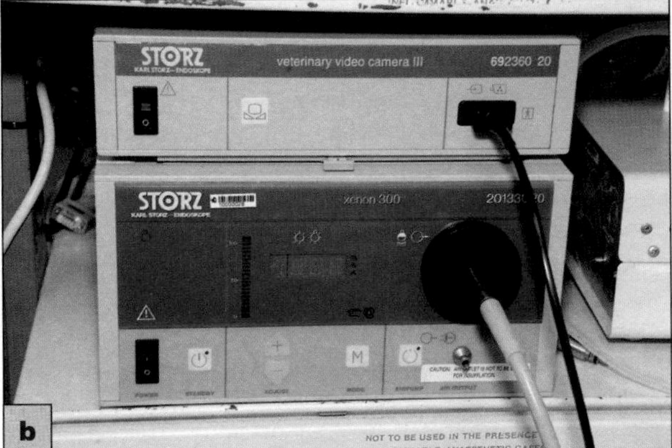

10.10 **(a)** Video camera connected to console. **(b)** Rigid endoscopy camera connected to console.

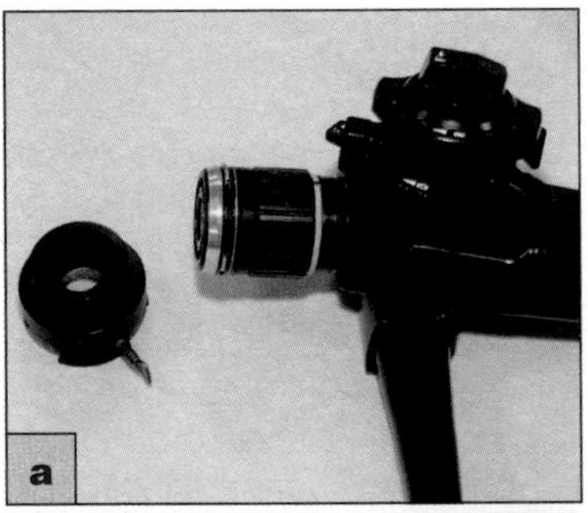

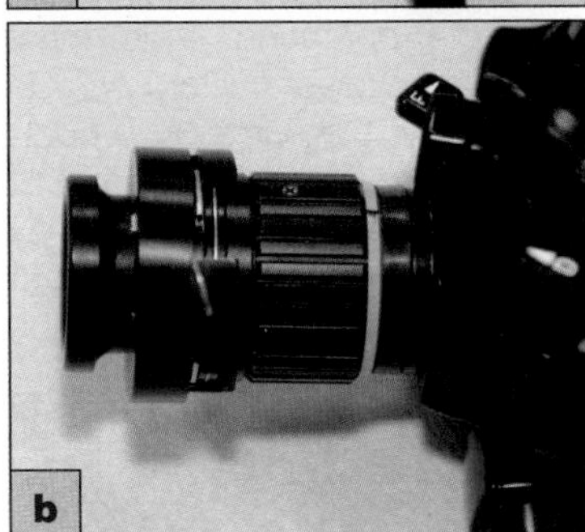

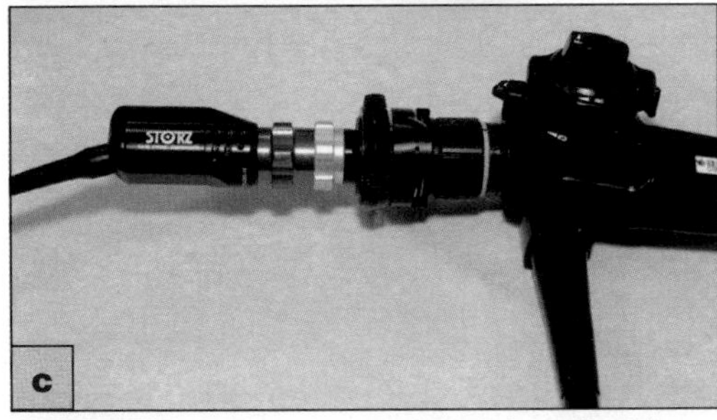

10.11 Using a camera adapter for a flexible endoscope. **(a)** Camera adapter and endoscope handpiece. **(b)** Adapter in place on oculus of handpiece. **(c)** Camera attached to handpiece with adapter.

> **KEY POINT**
>
> An additional benefit of using a camera and screen is that other members of the team can also see the image, which increases involvement and the enjoyment of the procedure.

Other equipment

A tub table or large tray with a gridded top (Figure 10.12a) is required for rhinoscopy and urethrocystoscopy, where copious fluid irrigation is used. An operating table that tilts in four directions is useful for laparoscopy and thoracoscopy but is not essential. Alternatively, the patient can be rotated on the table, or a tabletop tilting cradle (Fig 10.12b) can be purchased.

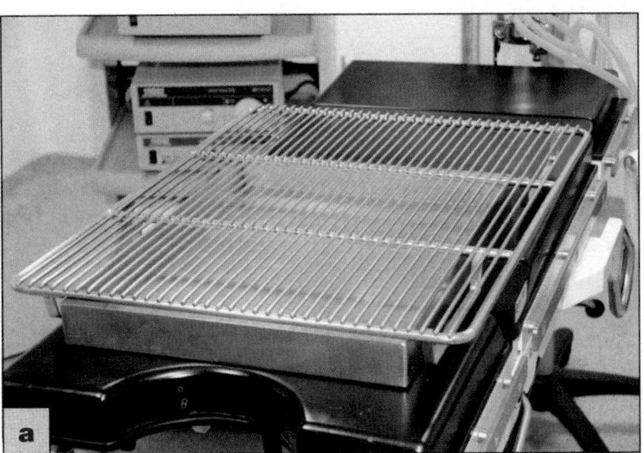

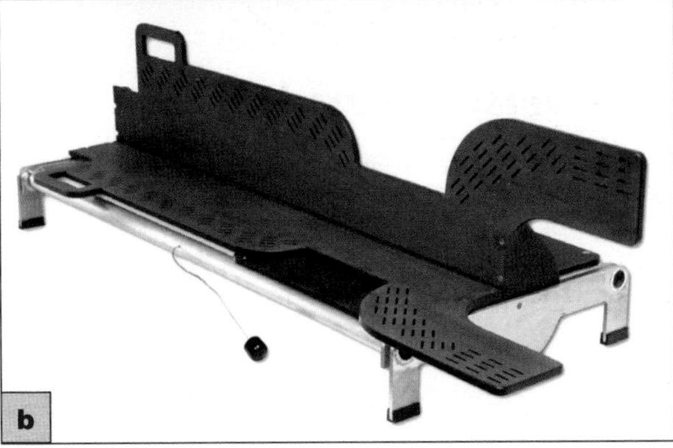

10.12 **(a)** A gridded table is useful for collecting saline and fluids during rhinoscopy, otoscopy or cystoscopy. **(b)** A rotating cradle is useful for moving the patient during laparoscopy, to allow gravitational movement of abdominal contents away from the operative field.

Other equipment that will be required includes a long plastic bath for cold sterilization of instruments (Figure 10.13) and an endoscopy trolley or stack system, on which to place the equipment (see Figure 10.1). This will include a light source (metal halide or preferably xenon), carbon dioxide automatic insufflator, suction machine, camera system and monitor. A medical flat screen monitor is preferred as commercial flat screen monitors have lower resolution and tend to lose details in the highlights. The insufflator will usually incorporate a cradle at the back for housing a small carbon dioxide cylinder although this may be attached to the stack system trolley instead. The cylinder is connected to the insufflator via a standard pin index system and pressure hose.

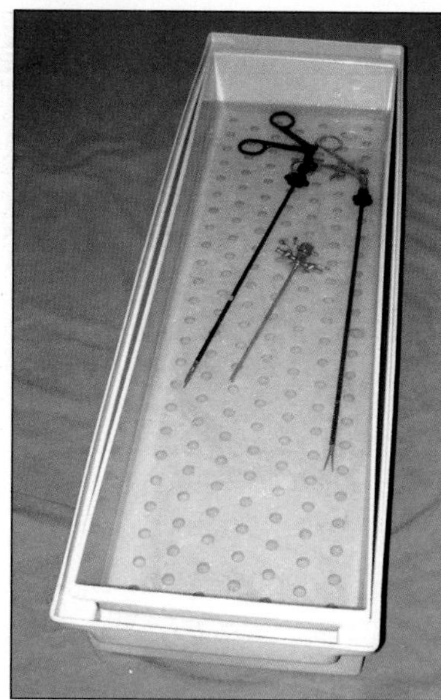

10.13 Cold sterilization bath with removable tray, suitable for rigid instruments.

Small integrated units can also be purchased and are suitable for consulting rooms or moving between premises. These will usually incorporate a screen, light source, air pump and camera system and may even include an image capture capability. An image-capturing system for recording video and still images is also extremely useful. Consumer products from the high street (e.g. DVD or hard disk recorders) are often suitable and considerably more cost-effective than bespoke medical units.

Purchasing options

New *versus* second-hand

In some cases it may be preferable to purchase second-hand equipment. Hospital auction houses, medical equipment re-sellers and even online purchase sites may be used to source both endoscopic and ultrasound equipment, and there are bargains to be had. However, the following should be borne in mind:

- Equipment has been retired from hospitals for a reason
- Often it is found to be faulty or near the end of its useful life
- Spares may no longer be available
- Repairs may be expensive or impossible
- Equipment from abroad may be incompatible with UK standards (120V *versus* 240V electrical supply or NTSC *versus* PAL video standards) and may also be incompatible with other equipment in the practice.

The more complex the equipment, the riskier it is to buy second-hand. Flexible endoscopes, for instance, can look fine on cursory examination but may harbour faults that make them completely uneconomical to repair. It is always better to buy new if at all possible, as this guarantees a reasonable life during which spares will be available. New equipment will also usually have a warranty. Furthermore, most equipment companies will provide some free training for staff in care and maintenance of the equipment, and this can be invaluable.

Warranties

When buying any equipment a warranty should always be given; if it is not offered, it should be requested. Second-hand equipment will often have only a 3-month warranty at best, and sometimes has no warranty at all. Faults may only become obvious once the equipment is in use and the purchaser should always insist on at least a minimum period during which the equipment can be returned if faulty.

Trials

There is no better way of seeing whether a particular piece of equipment or system suits the practice needs than to use it on real cases in the practice. When buying new equipment, it is useful to arrange for similar models from different manufacturers to be loaned to the practice on a trial basis for a period of time sufficient to allow assessment. If several trials can be arranged consecutively, so much the better, as comparisons are more easily made if the previous trial is fresh in the mind. The equipment must suit not only the practice's clinical needs but also the realistic aims for the future and the individual's personal preferences.

Managing the endoscopy service

Space considerations

Both flexible and rigid endoscopy will require space within the practice. Space must be allocated for an endoscopy tower system that contains the light source, insufflator, suction and video system as well as ancillary equipment. This will normally be placed in an operating theatre for rigid endoscopy, although a separate area is preferable for non-sterile procedures such as flexible GI endoscopy and rhinoscopy. Adequate space around the operating table must be provided such that the whole tower system can be moved around the table to allow the surgeon to operate from either side with the monitor positioned directly opposite (Figure 10.14). Alternatively two monitors may be used. There must also be provision for power supplies to the endoscopy tower and ancillary equipment,

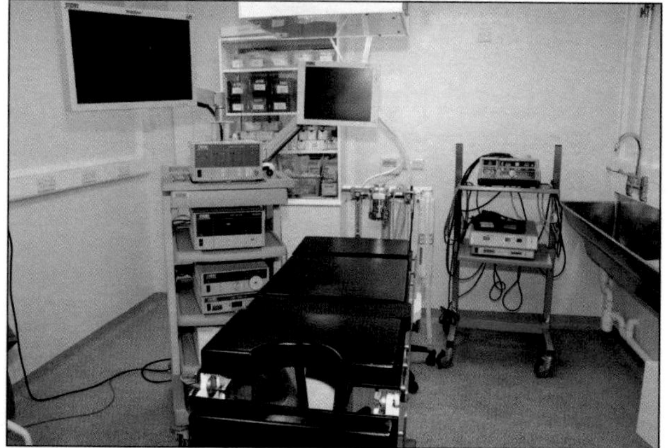

10.14 Typical theatre set-up to show positioning of endoscopy trolley and and electrosurgery units, and space required for equipment.

although many endoscopy trolleys carry a transformer and several extension sockets that supply all the equipment on the trolley.

Where endoscopy is being used in a sterile environment, it is important to maintain the equipment in a very clean condition and, preferably, to cover as much as possible with dustproof washable covers to minimize contamination of the area. Only equipment that is necessary for the conduct of sterile procedures should be present in the operating theatre.

KEY POINT

Carbon dioxide gas cylinders are pressurized and therefore may constitute a hazard, especially in the event of a fire. Spare cylinders should be stored away from main areas of the practice and preferably in a locked container on the outside of the building (see Chapter 2).

Maintenance

It is important that equipment, particularly any electrical equipment, complies with current relevant health and safety legislation, and that its use does not present a risk to staff. All electrical equipment will require regular testing and equipment should be regularly inspected for signs of wear or deterioration. SOPs should be drawn up for the use and cleaning of any endoscopic equipment, and should include who is qualified to use the equipment. Endoscopes are fragile instruments and are easily damaged. All equipment should be covered by the practice insurance for breakage and replacement costs, and if necessary, hire of a replacement instrument during repair. This may increase the overall cost of the practice insurance policy. A maintenance contract with the manufacturer or supplier should be in place to ensure a thorough inspection is carried out annually. When cared for properly, endoscopic equipment should last many years. An example SOP can be found at the end of this chapter.

KEY POINTS

- It is essential that only trained staff are permitted to clean and handle endoscopes, as mishandling can very easily lead to expensive repairs.
- Training in care and sterilization will often be provided by the manufacturer free of charge and should be taken advantage of.

Flexible endoscopes

Leakage and pressure testing

Flexible endoscopes can develop leaks through damage to the seals around the lenses (Figure 10.15) or wear on the instrument channel. Annual servicing will help prevent this and a maintenance contract should be taken out with the manufacturer or supplier.

KEY POINT

Flexible endoscopes should be pressure-tested before each procedure and *before cleaning*.

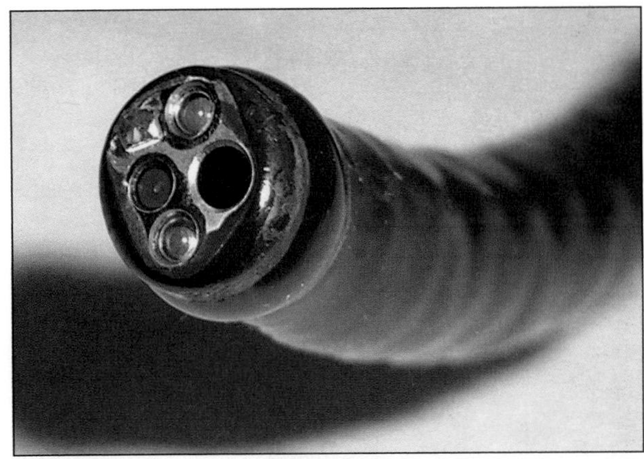

10.15 Close-up of a flexible endoscope lens, showing wear and tear.

The sealing cap should be screwed in place to cover and seal the electronic terminals of a video-endoscope, and then the leakage tester should be attached to the pressure compensation valve at the light source end of the umbilical cord. A leakage tester is a small rubber bulb and pressure gauge, which enables the operator to pump up the pressure inside the endoscope to a pre-set pressure recommended by the endoscope manufacturer. This prevents fluid entering the internal structures of the endoscope and causing irreparable damage and detects any damage to the integrity of the endoscope, in particular the bending section and instrument channel.

Cleaning and storage

Flexible endoscopes should be cleaned, sterilized and dried (see the SOP at the end of the chapter). All channels should be flushed through with enzymatic cleaner, water and cold sterilizer. A cleaning bath with channel attachments and pump (Figure 10.16) facilitates this. A bespoke automatic endoscope washer is ideal but takes up more space and typically must be plumbed in to the water and waste supplies. A large plastic tub can also be used for manual cleaning. After cleaning, the endoscopes should be hung up, with the insertion tube and umbilical cord vertical and the junction of the handpiece and the umbilical cord at approximately 90 degrees (Figure 10.17). The buttons should be left out so that all the channels are open to the air and can dry thoroughly.

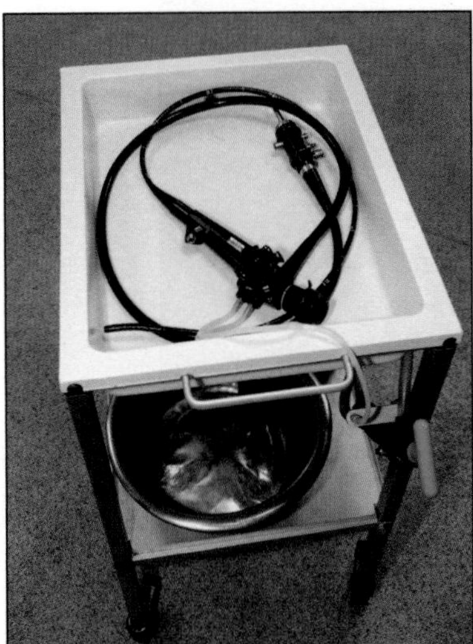

10.16 A cleaning bath for flexible endoscopes.

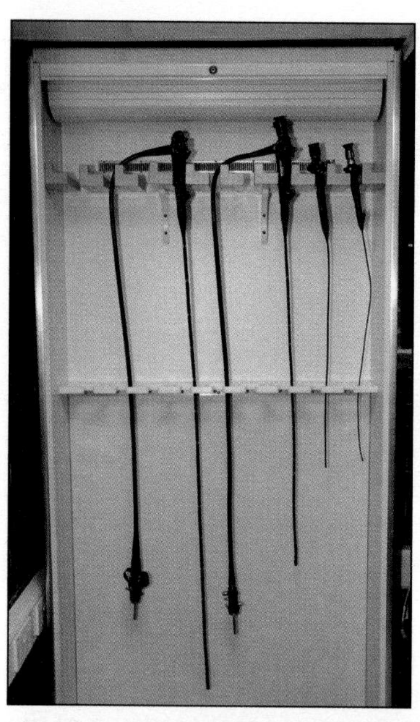

10.17 Storage of flexible endoscopes.

> **KEY POINTS**
>
> - Flexible endoscopes should never be stored in the case in which they were purchased. This is for transport only.
> - Storage in a case allows bacteria to multiply within the endoscope channels and optical fibres are more prone to breakage as they retain a memory effect when coiled.

Rigid endoscopes

Although less complex, these are also prone to damage, especially during arthroscopy where delicate telescopes are levered between bones. An allowance for replacement or repair costs should be made.

A plastic bath is less likely to damage delicate instruments during cleaning (Figure 10.18). Rigid endoscopes should be cleaned, sterilized and dried (see the SOP at the end of the chapter) before storage in padded drawers; preferably with dividers. A toolbox designed for car maintenance tools can provide an ideal storage box (Figure 10.19), as the drawers are long enough to accommodate laparoscopic instruments.

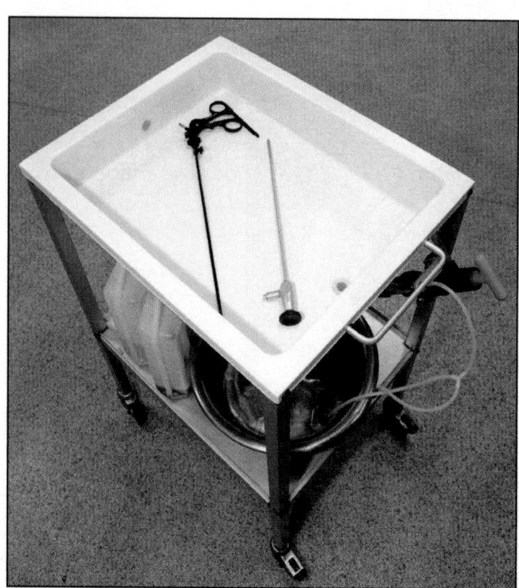

10.18 A plastic bath is suitable for rigid endoscopes.

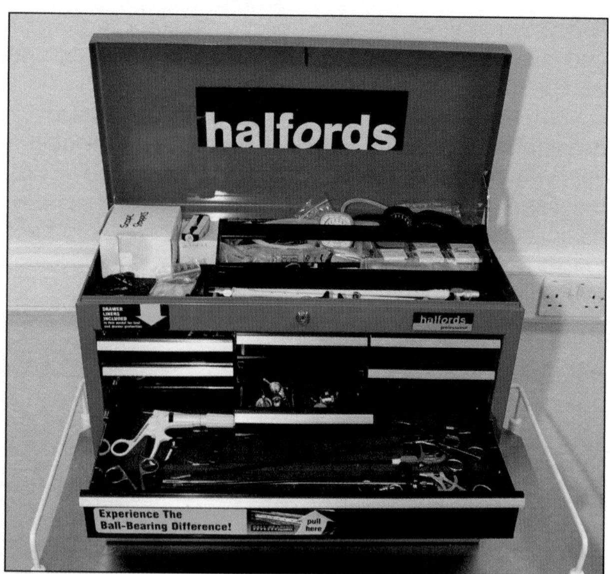

10.19 A storage box suitable for rigid endoscopes.

Pricing the service

Cleaning and disinfection of endoscopes is a lengthy process, often taking an hour or more and the nurse's time should be costed out carefully. Endoscopes also require specialized cleaning solutions and possibly gas sterilization facilities, and adequate space must be available to accommodate everything. An endoscope usage fee should be calculated (Figure 10.20) to offset the operational costs and provide a reasonable profit margin. This will obviously vary according to the individual set-up and practice costs and can be charged out as an endoscopy theatre set-up fee.

Item	Annual cost
Equipment: £15,000 over 5 years	£3000
Servicing	£1000
Replacement	£1000
Gas sterilizer: £2000 over 5 years	£400
Sterilization costs:	
■ Consumables	£500
■ Nurse time	£1500
Insurance	£100
Consumables	£500
Total (A)	**£8000**
Number of procedures per annum (B)	156
Cost per procedure (A ÷ B)	**£51.28**
Add 50% profit margin	**£75 endoscope usage fee**

10.20 Calculation of an endoscope usage fee, assuming three procedures per week.

Training

Endoscopy requires considerable training and practice for the operator to become proficient. Attendance at 'wet labs' and other practical courses is essential, not only to acquire the basic handling skills and techniques but also to become acquainted with the range of instrumentation available and to decide what is most appropriate for the practice. Advice on handling, cleaning and care of the instrumentation is also usually given on courses and by manufacturers.

RCVS Practice Standards Scheme Inspectors may require evidence of suitable training in the use of endoscopy equipment.

Inevitably, further training will be required to maintain skills and to practise advanced techniques. Training aids such as plastic gastrointestinal tracts for flexible endoscopy and laparoscopic trainers containing abdominal organs are available, at a price. A simple laparoscopic training box can be made from a plastic storage box with holes drilled in the top, overlaid by paper drape. This enables the endoscopist to carry out a variety of training exercises and manipulations using beads, sugar lumps and dried pulses, or even viscera or chicken thighs. Training videos for both flexible and rigid endoscopy are also available commercially and are constantly being updated. There are also web-based training videos; several sites such as www.websurg.com and www.or-live.com offer large archives of recorded procedures from human hospitals, many of which show techniques or procedures relevant to veterinary surgery.

Further reading

Chamness CJ (2008) Instrumentation. In: *BSAVA Manual of Canine and Feline Endoscopy and Endosurgery*, ed. P Lhermette and D Sobel, pp. 11–30. BSAVA Publications, Gloucester

Lhermette P and Sobel D (2008) An introduction to endoscopy and endosurgery. In: *BSAVA Manual of Canine and Feline Endoscopy and Endosurgery*, ed. P Lhermette and D Sobel, pp. 1–10. BSAVA Publications, Gloucester

McCarthy TC (2005) *Veterinary Endoscopy for the Small Animal Practitioner*. Elsevier Saunders, St. Louis

Tams TR and Rawlings CA (2011) *Small Animal Endoscopy, 3rd edn*. Elsevier, St. Louis

Examples of SOPs

SOP No..........

Preparation and use of endoscopy equipment

NOTE: All endoscopy equipment should only be handled by trained staff.

The following staff are trained to use flexible endoscopy equipment:

The following staff are trained to use rigid endoscopy equipment:

The following staff are trained to care for and clean endoscopy equipment:

The endoscope tower

- The endoscope tower must be plugged in and tested prior to a procedure:
- Turn on the light source and check that the bulb illuminates. Note: The light source should not be turned off between procedures as this shortens bulb life. The brightness setting may be turned down instead.
- Check the camera and monitor to ensure that all connections are correct and a picture is displayed.
- Turn on and check the video and still image software/equipment.

Other equipment

- For laparoscopy, open the carbon dioxide cylinder and turn on the insufflator. Ensure there is sufficient gas left in the cylinder by checking the gauge on the insufflator. Ensure a spare carbon dioxide cylinder is available.
- Check the suction machine is functioning and providing a vacuum, and that the reception vessel is clean and empty.
- Turn on the radiosurgery unit and/or bipolar vessel sealing/cutting device. Ensure the return electrode is in place for monopolar electrosurgery.
- Check all rubber grommets and seals for damage that could allow gas leakage from ports.

Endoscopes

Sterilization:

- Place all instruments, light guide cables, endoscopes and camera to be cold sterilized in the cold sterilizer bath at least 15–30 minutes before the procedure (see manufacturer's recommendations). Do not soak the electrical connector for the camera.
- Make sure sharp objects are not placed near light guide connectors or camera cables in the bath as these are easily damaged. Make sure no objects are placed on top of the endoscope in the bath.
- Total soaking time should never exceed 1 hour for endoscopes, light guide cables and cameras, as prolonged soaking may damage the seals and result in damage to the instrument.
- Many instruments are autoclavable – check with the manufacturer.
- 'Autoclavable endoscopes' are designed to be autoclaved in a human hospital autoclave, which typically has a slow heat and cool cycle. Veterinary autoclaves are 'flash' autoclaves, which heat and cool rapidly and will shorten the life of the endoscope. Cold sterilizing or gas sterilizing is therefore the method of choice in most veterinary practices.
- 'Single-use' instruments and plastic ports can often be cleaned and then gas-sterilized for re-use

Preparation:

- All flexible endoscopes must be pressure-checked before each procedure. (See SOP no....)
- For flexible endoscopy, all biopsy forceps, graspers, biopsy pots and other ancillary equipment should be placed on a trolley within reach of the endoscopist.
- Position the monitor appropriately for the procedure, directly in front of the surgeon where possible.
- Ensure all ancillary instruments are available for the designated procedure.
- Ensure a general surgery kit is available in case of conversion to an open technique.

Use:

- Prepare warm sterile deionized water for rinsing the endoscope and instruments prior to use. Note: Bronchoscopes should be sterilized immediately before each procedure.
- 2.7 mm diameter and smaller endoscopes must always be used in a protective sheath to avoid damage. There are no exceptions to this.
- For upper GI endoscopy, a mouth gag must always be used.
- Light guide connectors and flexible endoscopes must not be kinked or coiled tightly.
- All endoscopy equipment must be cleaned immediately after the procedure (see SOP No. .....).

An example of an SOP for preparation and use of endoscopy equipment.

SOP No...........

Cleaning flexible endoscopes

NOTE: All endoscopy equipment should only be handled by trained staff.

The following staff are trained to care for and clean endoscopy equipment:

All flexible endoscopes should be cleaned immediately after use to prevent drying on of proteinaceous residues and blockage of channels.

- Handle endoscopes with care.
- Avoid knocking the tip on hard surfaces and avoid excessive coiling or bending, which may damage the fibres.
- Never force an instrument through the channels and only pass instruments and brushes through the instrument channel with the tip in the straight, forward-pointing position to avoid damage to the channel lining.

Note: Video-endoscopes have a watertight cap to cover the camera's electronic contacts and cable attachment on the light guide connector. This must be firmly screwed in place before attempting to clean the endoscope.

1. Attach the leakage tester to the pressure compensation valve on the light guide connector and pressurize the endoscope to the recommended pressure.
2. Remove the leakage tester, keeping the endoscope pressurized.
3. Observe for 2 minutes for a drop in pressure. If there is a pressure drop DO NOT IMMERSE THE ENDOSCOPE IN FLUID OR FLUSH THE CHANNELS. Simply wipe with a damp cloth and send the endoscope for repair. If there is no drop in pressure, go to Step 4.
4. Flush enzymatic detergent (as recommended by the manufacturer) though the suction channel of the endoscope by attaching a syringe to the instrument channel. Alternatively, with the endoscope attached to the suction machine, suck detergent through the endoscope until it runs clear.
5. Remove the cap from the instrument channel and both buttons from the suction and irrigation channels, and soak them in enzymatic detergent.
6. Wipe the insertion tube with a damp cloth soaked in detergent to remove major contamination.
7. Place the endoscope carefully in the endoscope bath or a plastic tub filled with enzymatic detergent.
8. Carefully insert the cleaning brush into the instrument channel and pass it right through until it exits at the tip. Clean the brush between your fingers and then withdraw it back up through the endoscope. Never use a back-and-forth motion inside the channel as this can damage the lining.
9. Place the brush into the suction channel and direct the tip down towards the instrument channel.
10. Place the brush into the suction channel and direct it straight down the umbilical cord until it exits from the suction port. Clean the brush as before and pull it back though the endoscope.
11. Attach the cleaning adapters supplied with the endoscope or cleaning bath to the suction, irrigation and instrument ports, and flush enzymatic detergent into all the channels until they are completely filled. Leave for 10 minutes.
12. Drain all the enzymatic detergent and rinse the endoscope thoroughly in deionized water, flushing all the channels as before to remove any detergent.
13. Fill the endoscope cleaning bath with an appropriate cold sterilizer (as recommended by the manufacturer). Flush all channels as before and leave the endoscope immersed for 30 minutes.
14. Drain all the cold sterilizer and rinse the endoscope thoroughly in deionized water, flushing all the channels as before to remove any cold sterilizer.
15. Blow air through the channels using a large syringe to remove any residual water and then remove the cleaning adapters.
16. Dry the outside of the endoscope with a soft, dry lint-free cloth.
17. Clean the optical lenses with 70% alcohol. Channels may also be flushed with 70% alcohol to assist drying.
18. Attach the leakage tester and release the pressure from the endoscope.
19. Remove the leakage tester and hang the endoscope in a safe dry place (preferably an endoscope cupboard) with the insertion tube and umbilical cord hanging straight down and all buttons and caps removed.
20. Rinse and dry the instrument channel cap and channel buttons and store safely in a dry place.

Note that:

- Total soaking time should never exceed 1 hour, as prolonged soaking may damage the seals and result in damage to the instrument.
- Flexible endoscopes may also be gas-sterilized. In this case the pressure compensation cap should be in place to allow exposure of the inside of the endoscope to the gas. THIS CAP MUST NEVER BE LEFT IN PLACE WHEN THE ENDOSCOPE IS IMMERSED IN FLUID AS THIS WILL DESTROY THE ENDOSCOPE.
- Flexible endoscopes should never be stored coiled in a transport case. This can damage the light guide and optical fibres as they retain a memory of their shape over time and can break on straightening. A travel case also provides an ideal environment for bacterial growth within the endoscope if it is not completely dry on storage.

An example of an SOP for cleaning flexible endoscopes.

SOP No...........

Cleaning rigid endoscopes

NOTE: All endoscopy equipment should only be handled by trained staff.

The following staff are trained to care for and clean endoscopy equipment:

All rigid endoscopes should be cleaned immediately after use to prevent drying on of proteinaceous residues.

1. Rinse all instruments and ports under running water to remove gross contamination.
2. Clean endoscopes separately to prevent damage. Never place instruments on top of the endoscope.
3. Disassemble all instruments and ports and remove all rubber grommets prior to placing in a plastic endoscope-cleaning bath. Remove adapters from the light guide post of the endoscope and open all taps on the ports.
4. Fill the bath with enzymatic detergent (as recommended by the manufacturer) and carefully brush through all channels and ports with a pipe-cleaning brush. Soak for 10 minutes.
5. Endoscopes, light guide cables and cameras should be soaked for 10 minutes and then cleaned with a soft cloth or swab.
6. Most metal instruments and ports can be cleaned in an ultrasonic bath. NEVER PUT ENDOSCOPES, LIGHT GUIDE CABLES OR CAMERAS IN AN ULTRASONIC BATH.
7. Drain all the enzymatic detergent and rinse the endoscope and instruments thoroughly in deionized water, flushing all the channels to remove any detergent.
8. Fill the endoscope cleaning bath with an appropriate cold sterilizer (as recommended by the manufacturer). Flush all channels as before and leave the endoscope and instruments immersed for 15 minutes.
9. Drain all the cold sterilizer and rinse the endoscope and instruments thoroughly in deionized water, flushing all the channels as before to remove any cold sterilizer.
10. Dry the outside of the endoscope with a soft, dry lint-free cloth. Clean the optical lenses and light guide post with 70% alcohol.
11. Dry the instruments carefully with a soft lint-free cloth or paper towel and leave to dry on an absorbent paper towel before storage in a padded drawer.
12. Particular care should be taken with storage of endoscopes, especially those of 2.7 mm diameter and smaller. These should always be stored in a protective sheath to avoid damage

Note that:

- Total soaking time should never exceed 1 hour for endoscopes, light guide cables and cameras, as prolonged soaking may damage the seals and result in damage to the instrument.
- Many instruments are autoclavable – check with the manufacturer first. ‘Autoclavable endoscopes’ are designed to be autoclaved in a human hospital autoclave which typically has a slow heat and cool cycle. Veterinary autoclaves are ‘flash’ autoclaves which heat and cool rapidly and will shorten the life of the endoscope. Cold sterilizing or gas sterilizing is therefore the method of choice in most veterinary practices.
- ‘Single use’ instruments and plastic ports can often be cleaned and then gas sterilized for re-use.

An example of an SOP for cleaning rigid endoscopes.

Electrocardiography

11

Stephen Collins

An electrocardiogram (ECG) is a recording of the electrical activity of the heart, providing definitive information about heart rate and rhythm. ECG recording is indicated when investigating cardiac arrhythmia, heart disease or collapse. ECG monitoring is indicated during higher-risk anaesthesia and for critically ill animals.

Cardiac rhythm disturbances *cannot* be investigated without an ECG; therefore an electrocardiography machine should be considered an essential piece of equipment for the majority of veterinary practices. The ability to record an ECG is a mandatory RCVS Practice Standards Scheme requirement only for Veterinary Hospitals.

Recording an ECG is a simple skill, easily performed by vets or nurses, and requires minimal training. ECG *interpretation* can be challenging, however, and this sometimes limits the use of ECG in practice. Interpretation services are offered by many veterinary cardiologists and are useful for clinicians reluctant to interpret their own ECG recordings. Many practices charge the client a fee for recording an ECG and a second fee for specialist interpretation.

Electrocardiography machines

There are a variety of machines available for ECG recording and monitoring. Although some machines are marketed specifically for veterinary use, many are principally designed for use in humans and therefore some features, such as interpretation modules, are not useful.

General features

Lead systems and channels

- All electrocardiography machines use standard lead systems (typically leads I, II, III plus aVr, aVl and aVf) when recording ECGs (Figure 11.1). The lead II recording (Figure 11.2) is most commonly used for interpretation.
- Single-channel machines record from one lead at a time, whereas multi-channel machines (usually three- or six-channel) record from leads simultaneously, making interpretation easier.
- Many ECG machines come supplied with four limb leads and six chest leads. Although chest leads are not routinely used in veterinary patients, this does not preclude use of these machines on animals.

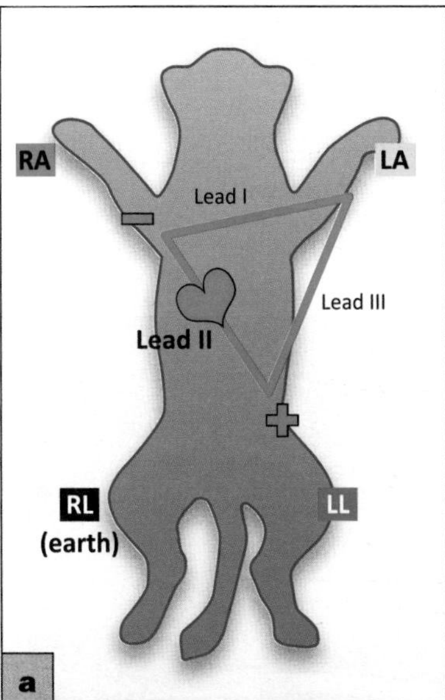

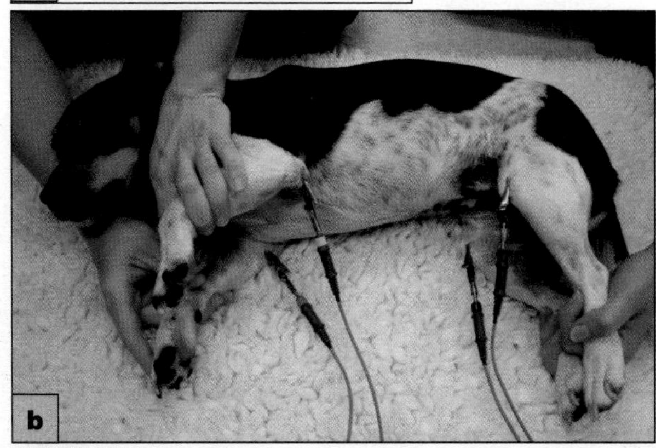

11.1 **(a)** Standard leads for electrocardiography. RA (right 'arm') – attach to right elbow; LA (left 'arm') – attach to left elbow; LL (left leg) – attach to left stifle; RL (right leg, earth lead) – attach to right stifle. **(b)** Patient positioning and restraint for a resting ECG. (b, Courtesy of Simon Dennis. Reproduced from *BSAVA Manual of Canine and Feline Cardiorespiratory Medicine, 2nd edn*).

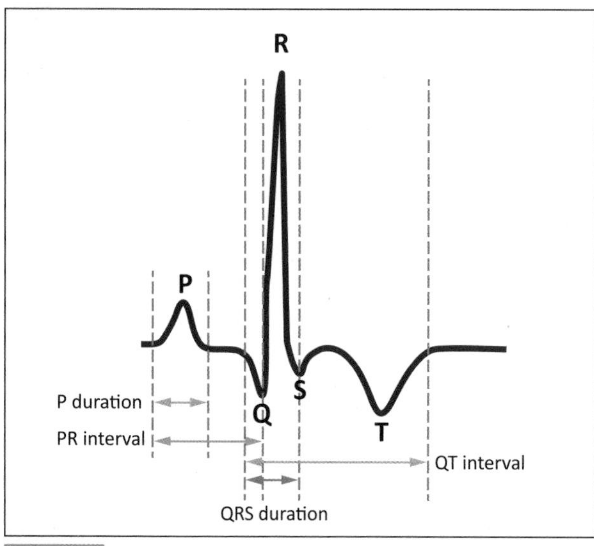

11.2 Lead II trace for interpretation.

ECG controls: paper speed, sensitivity, filters

- Paper speeds are typically 25 or 50 mm/s; however, 10 mm/s and 100 mm/s are useful features if available.
- Voltage sensitivity may be adjusted automatically but should also be manually adjustable for optimal recording quality.
- Most machines have electrical and muscle tremor filters. It is important that these can be *switched off* for veterinary patients, particularly for cats, to avoid filtering out important information, such as P waves.
- QWERTY keyboards are useful for entering patient data.

Electrodes

There are a variety of electrodes available for connecting the patient to the machine. Metal crocodile clips are standard but are often poorly tolerated by the patient, creating movement or tremor artefact; they should be filed flat for comfort (Figure 11.3a). Ideally, atraumatic ECG clips (Figure 11.3b) or adhesive electrodes (Figure 11.3cde) should be used.

Automated interpretation

Some ECG machines offer an interpretation capability, but they are usually calibrated for humans. Although waveforms may be measured accurately using this interpretation, rhythm diagnoses are extremely unreliable.

Recording methods

RCVS Practice Standards require that veterinary hospitals must file and store ECG recordings.

Paper recorders

The most common method for recording ECGs uses a paper recorder. The ECG is recorded and transcribed in real time on to special paper, forming a permanent record at the time of examination (Figure 11.4).

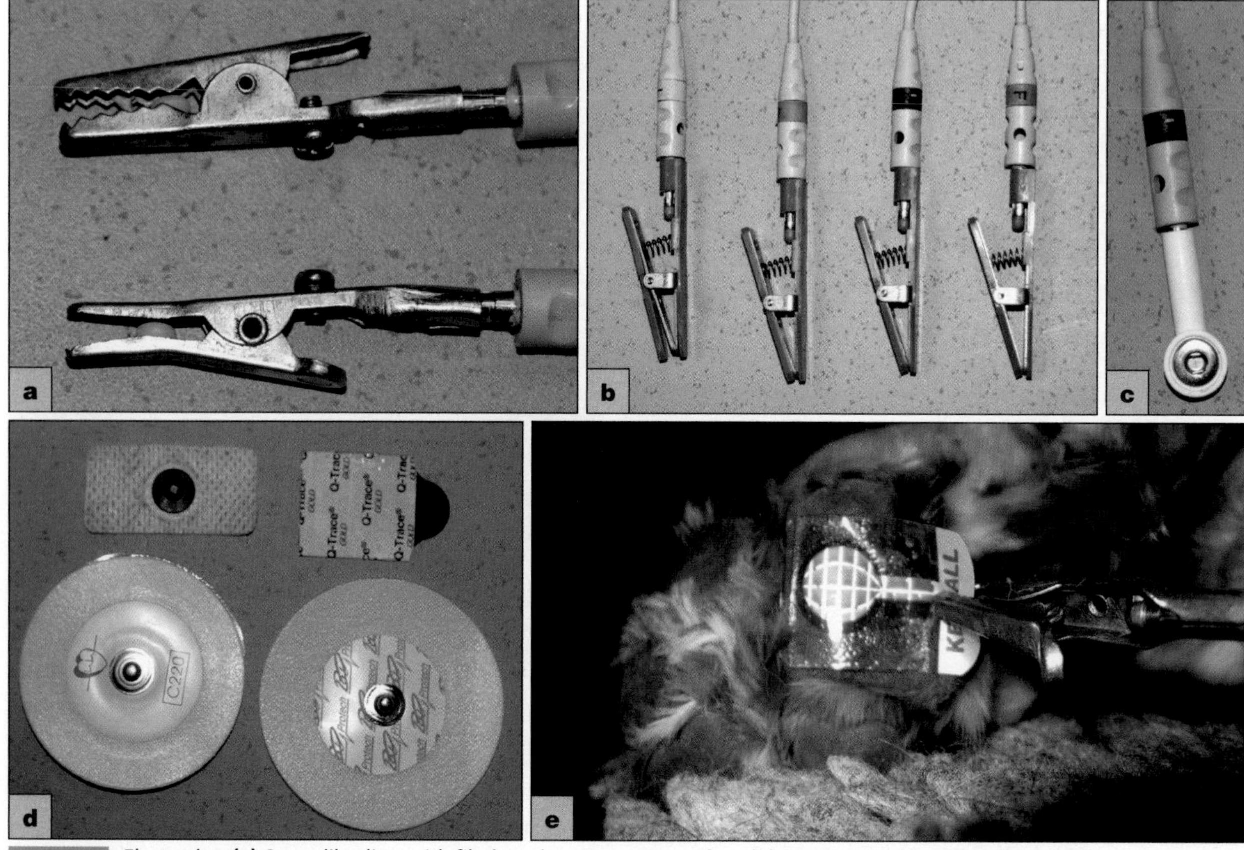

11.3 Electrodes. **(a)** Crocodile clips, with filed teeth to improve comfort. **(b)** Atraumatic clips. **(c)** Button clip for use with adhesive electrodes. **(d)** Adhesive electrodes. **(e)** Clip attached by an adhesive pad to prevent skin trauma. (e, Courtesy of Ruth Willis. Reproduced from *BSAVA Manual of Canine and Feline Cardiorespiratory Medicine, 2nd edn*).

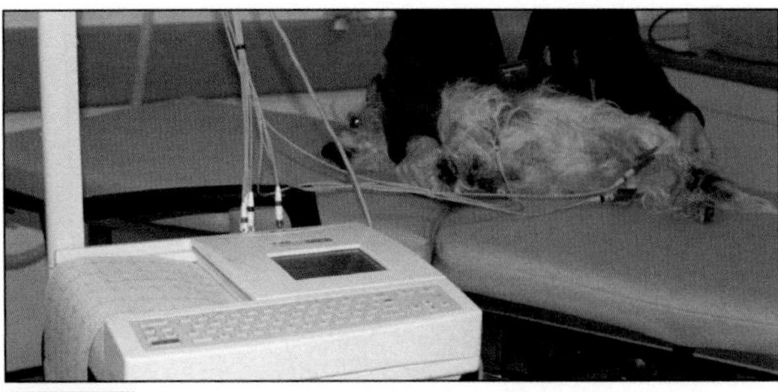

11.4 The ECG is recorded and transcribed on to the paper in real time.

ECG paper is heat-sensitive and is preprinted with high-quality fine gridlines. The ECG is transcribed by heated electrodes, producing a high-quality waveform which is easily viewed (and measured). ECG paper is inexpensive. The small premium for prefolded (Z-fold) paper is worthwhile, as it is easier to manage during recording and is more easily stored than rolls of paper. A4 ECG pages are significantly more expensive than standard three-channel paper, but are easier to store and copy.

There are a variety of excellent paper recording machines available. An LCD screen is a useful additional feature and allows the operator to view the ECG without transcribing it to paper, making it a handy ECG monitor, useful for monitoring arrhythmias in practices where dedicated ECG monitors are not available. Some machines have electronic module options, allowing electronic storage of data to computer as well as paper recording.

Advantages:

- Paper recordings can be attained rapidly, especially if the ECG machine is set up on a dedicated trolley ready for use (Figure 11.5)
- ECG recordings can be analysed quickly, which is important in an emergency situation.

Disadvantages:

- ECG recordings usually span several pages of non-standard size paper, making it awkward to file and time-consuming to copy electronically
- Faxed or scanned copies sent for specialist interpretation are often of poor quality, making interpretation difficult
- ECG tracings on paper fade with time.

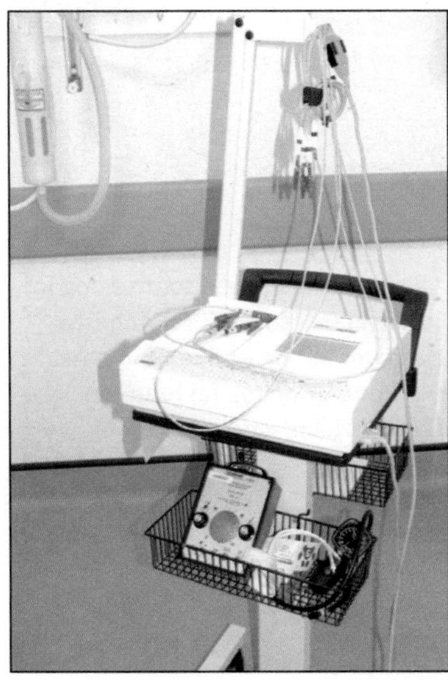

11.5 ECG trolley ready for use.

Electronic recorders

Electronic ECG recorders display ECGs on a PC (or laptop) screen. ECG recordings can be stored electronically and/or printed on standard A4 paper if required.

Advantages:

- Smaller ECG machines are more portable and more easily stowed
- ECG recordings can be stored electronically, particularly useful for practices with 'paperless' record systems
- Files can be easily e-mailed for further interpretation if required
- No paper cost.

Disadvantages:

- Require a computer:
  - Potential compatibility issues and IT glitches
  - Can be a frustration in an emergency situation
- Digitally recorded waveforms can be more time-consuming to analyse when using digital calipers. ECG recordings printed to standard paper are sometimes poor quality.

Telephonic systems

The ECG is recorded and transmitted telephonically to a distant ECG receiver/printer.

Advantage:

- ECG is printed (and interpreted) by an experienced cardiologist, making this system a good starting point for practices that prefer not to interpret ECG recordings.

Disadvantages:

- ECGs cannot be analysed on site
- All ECGs will incur an interpretation fee.

Anaesthetic monitors

Most multiparameter anaesthetic monitors provide digital ECG recording, and some will print ECGs on a single channel or capture images using a data logger. These machines are used to monitor cardiac and respiratory function during anaesthesia, by measuring arterial blood pressure, pulse oximetry and end-tidal carbon dioxide concentrations.

Advantage:

- They are valuable monitors for practices with a high anaesthetic caseload.

Disadvantages:

- Expensive
- Limited utility as ECG recorders.

Radiotelemetry systems

Radiotelemetry systems are ideally suited to veterinary hospitals. A small transmitter worn by the patient transmits the recording to a receiver, and the ECG is displayed on a PC (or portable laptop) screen (Figure 11.6).

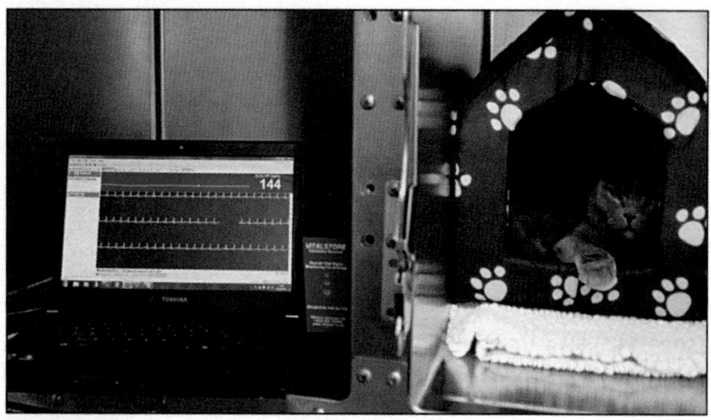

11.6 ECG recording and display via a telemetric system.

Advantages:

- Monitoring of up to six hospitalized patients at the same time
- The transmitter is worn by the patient, thereby avoiding potential damage to expensive cables and inconvenience of a bulky monitor in kennels.

Disadvantages:

- Cost
- All the disadvantages of electronic recorders (see above).

Holter monitors

These are invaluable for the investigation and management of collapse and arrhythmia. A small recording unit worn by the patient (Figure 11.7) records continuously on three channels for up to 48 hours, or on two channels for up to 7 days. Data are stored digitally and must then be processed using specialist software. Both hardware and software are expensive, and purchasing a Holter system is rarely cost-effective in first-opinion practice. Holter monitors can, however, be rented from Holter Monitoring Service (www.holtermonitoring.co.uk), who also provide a Holter interpretation service by a veterinary cardiologist in the UK.

Choosing an electrocardiography machine

Perhaps the most important consideration when choosing an electrocardiography machine is how frequently it will be used.

- In small practices, ECGs may be recorded infrequently and staff members may be unfamiliar with using the machine; therefore, the ideal machine should be easy to use, reliable and inexpensive.
- In larger practices and veterinary hospitals, ECG recording and monitoring is likely to be more routine; it is therefore important to consider carefully the particular requirements of the practice to avoid purchasing unsuitable equipment.

The reader may wish to refer to Figure 11.8 as a starting point; other models may also be available. Recommendations are based on likely use and financial viability.

Basic machines are inexpensive and incur minimal running costs; therefore investment should be easily returned, even with minimal use. Additional features incur more expense, but are often justified with improved utility, especially in larger practices. High-quality second-hand machines can often be purchased for minimal cost at medical auctions, or through used medical equipment merchants. ECG consumables are inexpensive and do not constitute a significant cost, even when heavily used. Electrocardiography machines are generally very reliable and service contracts are usually not cost-effective. Second-hand machines are a relatively safe investment, although repair costs can be high. New machines will carry a standard manufacturer's warranty.

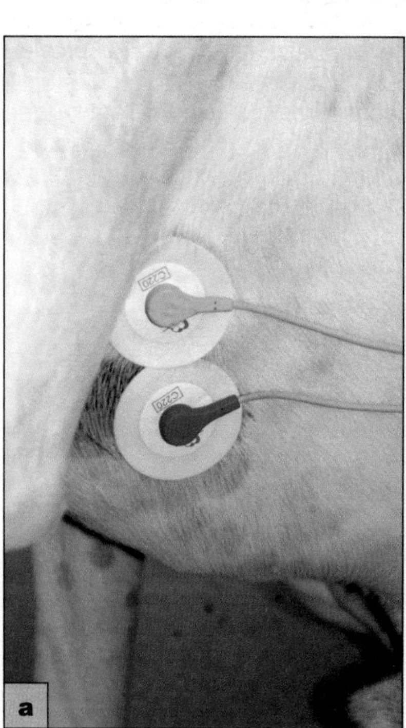

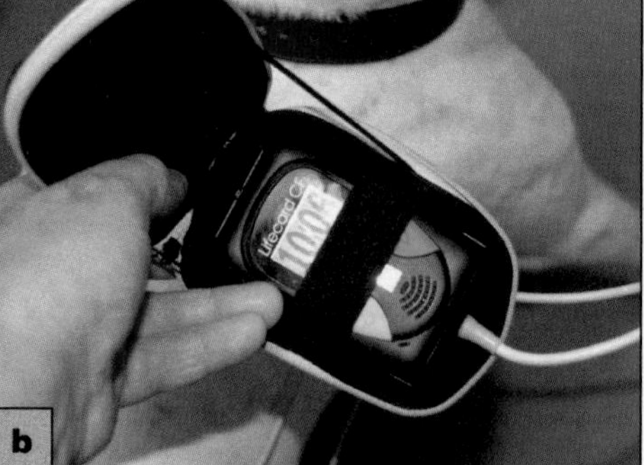

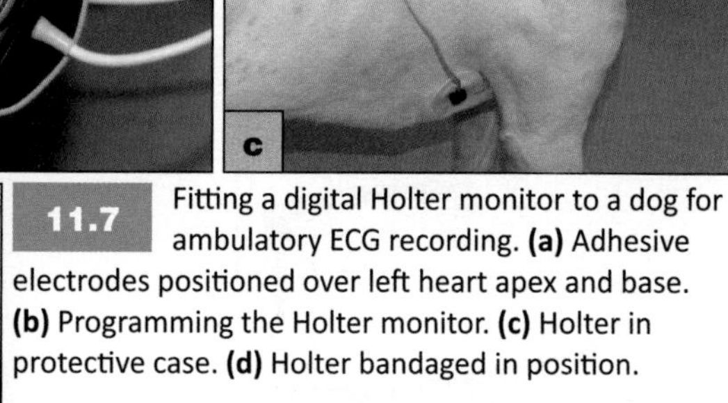

11.7 Fitting a digital Holter monitor to a dog for ambulatory ECG recording. **(a)** Adhesive electrodes positioned over left heart apex and base. **(b)** Programming the Holter monitor. **(c)** Holter in protective case. **(d)** Holter bandaged in position.

Machine type and examples of models	Estimated purchase cost (£)	Small animal general practice				Small animal specialist practice	
		1–2 vets	3–5 vets	6+ vets	Hospital	Emergency clinic	Referral practice/hospital
Single channel, paper (e.g. Edan VE-100)	400	◆◆	◆	X	X	X	X
Telephonic	325 40 per ECG	◆◆	◆	X	X	X	X
Three channel, paper (e.g. Imotek CT3000i, Edan VE-300 (electronic recording module option), Cardipia 200)	600–1100	◆◆◆	◆◆	◆◆	◆◆	◆◆	◆
Three channel, paper plus LCD (e.g. Fukada FX-7102, Imotek/ Seca CT8000i, Nihon Kohden ECG-9620)	1200–1650	◆	◆◆	◆◆◆	◆◆◆	◆◆◆	◆◆◆
Six channel, paper (e.g. Imotek/Seca CT6B)	1800	X	◆	◆	◆	◆	◆
Six channel, paper plus LCD (e.g. Cardipia Vet 400, Imotek/Seca CT6i/Pi (electronic recording module option), Fukada FX-7402, Nihon Kohden ECG-1250)	800–2400	X	◆◆	◆◆◆	◆◆◆	◆◆◆	◆◆◆
Electronic (e.g. Seca CT110 Cardioconcept, Edan VE-1010, Vetronic Cardiostore)	900–1400	◆	◆	◆	◆	◆	◆
Holter (e.g. Lifecard CF Digital Holter, Novacor Systems)	1800 (excl. software)	X	X	X	◆	◆	◆◆◆
Holter monitoring service (external)	Price on application	◆◆◆	◆◆◆	◆◆◆	◆◆◆	◆◆◆	◆◆
Radiotelemetric (e.g. Vetronic Sapphire, Kruuse Televet 100)	1800	X	X	X	◆	◆◆	◆◆◆
Multiparameter monitor (e.g. Surgivet Advisor, Vetronic Vitalstore Multimonitor)	800–6000	◆	◆	◆	◆◆	◆◆	◆◆◆

11.8 A buying guide for ECG recorders and monitors. Please note that the examples given do not constitute an exhaustive list of machines available on the veterinary market, nor do they imply any endorsement. ◆ = Consider; ◆◆ = Recommended; ◆◆◆ = Strongly recommended; **X** = Not recommended.

Further reading

Martin M (2007) *Small Animal ECGs: An Introductory Guide, 2nd edn.* Blackwell Publishing, Oxford

Phibbs B (2006) *Advanced ECG: Boards and Beyond, 2nd edn*. Saunders Elsevier, St Louis

Ware W (2007) *Cardiovascular Disease in Small Animal Medicine*. Manson Publishing, London

Willis R (2010) Electrocardiography and ambulatory monitoring. In: *BSAVA Manual of Canine and Feline Cardiorespiratory Medicine, 2nd edn,* ed. V Luis Fuentes *et al.*, pp.67–73. BSAVA Publications, Gloucester

Ultrasonography

12

Philip Lhermette

Proficiency in basic ultrasonography within the practice will enhance diagnostic capabilities and reduce the need for referral. Ultrasonography can also be extremely useful in acute situations such as whelpings or cardiac tamponade, where referral is not an option. Machines are inexpensive enough to be afforded by most practices but training requires considerable time and effort, as well as cost. Ultrasonography will undoubtedly benefit the practice by improving the range of clinical services provided and the financial return, but only if staff are sufficiently trained to operate the equipment effectively. It can take several years for an operator to become proficient. The impact of the new equipment on the use (and therefore profitability) of existing facilities should also be considered, for example increasing expertise and use of ultrasonography may mean that fewer radiographs are taken. If staff are well trained, an ultrasound scanner will be used on an almost daily basis for many types of cases and will provide a good return on investment.

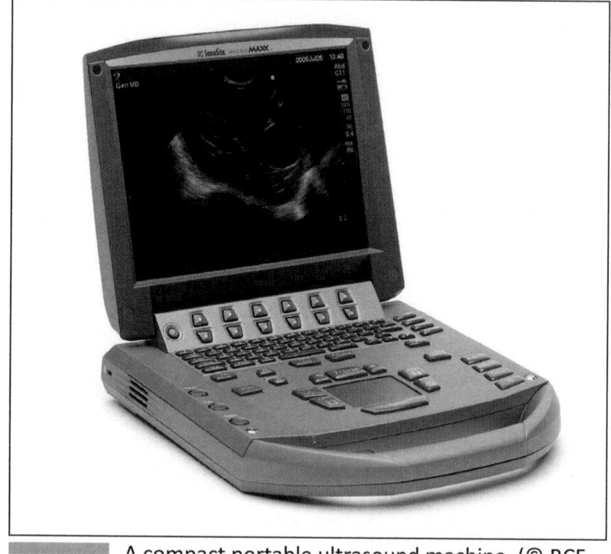

12.1 A compact portable ultrasound machine. (© BCF Technology)

Equipment

There are many types of ultrasound machine available and the facilities on each will vary. No one machine is ideal for both small and large animals; indeed, different transducers (probes) are required for different purposes and different sizes of dogs and cats. It is therefore important to plan for the expected caseload and purchase a machine that meets the needs of the practice.

The ultrasound machine

If space is at a premium a compact portable machine (Figure 12.1) may be the best option. Larger machines on a trolley (Figure 12.2) can be more immediately available but take up more space; if stored in a tight space, cables and transducers projecting from the side of the machine (Figure 12.3) can be easily damaged.

Advice should be taken from several different manufacturers and from experienced colleagues in order to understand which features best suit the individual practice. The following should be considered:

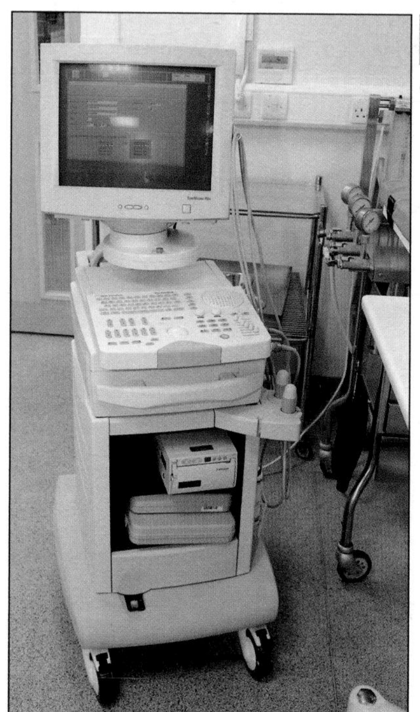

12.2 A larger machine on a trolley.

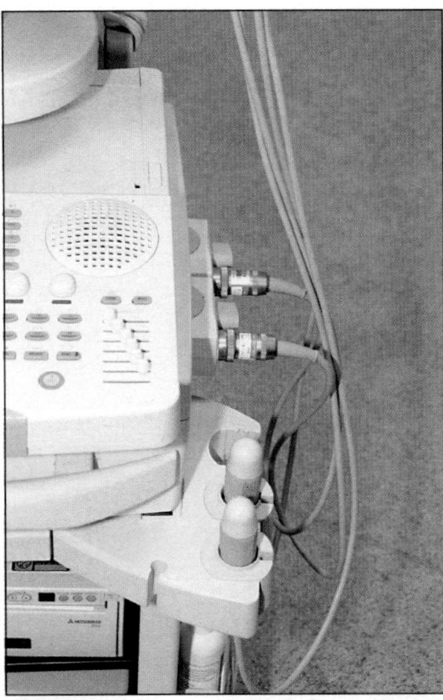

12.3 Cables and transducers projecting from the side of the machine can easily be damaged.

- What budget has been set?
- What will the machine be used for?
  - Predominantly abdominal scans in dogs and cats?
  - Cardiology? Will continuous-flow Doppler or colour-flow Doppler be required? These can add considerably to the cost of the machine, but in many cases can be added at a later date if required.
- Does the practice have digital radiography facilities with a DICOM server or PACS? If so, digital ultrasonography with DICOM may be preferred so that images can be stored on the network.

It is important to estimate the cost over the whole of the machine's operational life, including purchase, running and end-of-life disposal costs. Consumables such as gel and printing paper are relatively inexpensive. Replacement costs must also be considered. Ultrasound technology improves over time and today's top-of-the-range machine will become obsolete in a few years. Realistically, a 5- to 10-year lifespan is the norm, although more specialist ultrasonographers may need to upgrade more frequently.

Ultrasound machines need regular servicing, testing and adjustment to maintain optimum quality. A service contract is often available from the manufacturer or supplier, and the cost of this should be borne in mind when contemplating purchase. Transducers (see below) are expensive, delicate and easily damaged and a reasonable amount for the cost of replacements or repairs should also be factored in. Consideration should also be given to the additional cost of insurance, as items with high capital costs may need to be insured separately.

Second-hand *versus* new

Second-hand ultrasound machines are often available from human hospitals or re-sellers (see Figure 12.6b). These are frequently optimized for one particular function, such as obstetrics or echocardiography, and may not be suitable for general veterinary use. In addition, the software will be set up for human patients and will be unsuitable for dogs and cats. Also, many ex-hospital machines are too large for the average veterinary practice. Some companies are able to refurbish ex-hospital machines and install veterinary-specific software. These machines can be an economical choice but, as always with second-hand equipment, the availability of spares and servicing needs to be checked before purchase as this may have been a factor in retiring the equipment. A bespoke veterinary ultrasound unit with veterinary-specific software is often a better choice, particularly for the inexperienced user. It is useful to set up a list of priorities, considering factors such as those in Figure 12.4.

- Manufacturer choice
- Price
- Size
- Veterinary-specific software
- Transducers (probes)
  - Linear, microcurved, phased or mechanical sector annular array
  - Single-frequency, multiple-frequency or broadband
- Cine loops
- DICOM compatibility
- Tissue harmonics
- Colour Doppler
- DICOM
- 2D, 3D or 4D
- Versatility (good at one or two applications, or a multitude of applications?)
- Warranty
- Training
- Upgradability

12.4 Factors to consider when buying an ultrasound machine.

Transducers

Whatever machine is chosen, a selection of transducers will be required to cater for the widest variety of cases. Ultimately the image quality obtained will depend on the transducers used and it is important to get the best advice possible on the types available that suit the practice's particular requirements.

- Lower-frequency transducers are required to investigate deeper lesions or large dogs, whereas high-frequency transducers give more detail in superficial tissues.
- Some transducers are single frequency and some have dual frequency (e.g. can be switched between 5.5 and 7.5 MHz).
- Broadband/Ultraband transducers operate over a range of imaging frequencies such as 2–4 MHz.
- Linear transducers (Figure 12.5a) are less easy to use between ribs but provide excellent abdominal images, whereas microcurved transducers (Figure 12.5b) provide better access between ribs.
- Phased-array transducers (Figure 12.5c) have no moving parts, are technically more advanced, give better images and are more robust than the old mechanical sector annular array transducers (Figure 12.5d), but are more expensive.

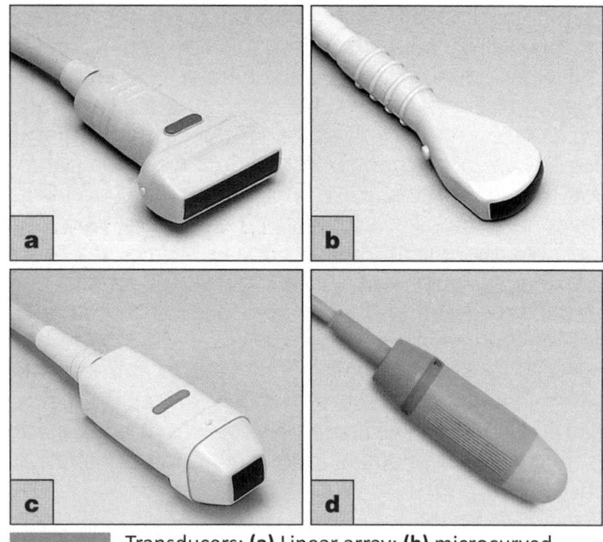

12.5 Transducers: **(a)** Linear array; **(b)** microcurved array; **(c)** phased array; **(d)** mechanical sector annular array. (Reproduced from the *BSAVA Manual of Canine and Feline Ultrasonography*)

KEY POINT

Not all types of transducer will be available for all machines, and individual transducers may be specific to the individual manufacturer or model. It is important to check the range of transducers available for any machine, taking into consideration future requirements.

Adaptors can be purchased for individual probes to facilitate guidance of a biopsy needle into tissue in line with the ultrasound beam. These devices may be helpful if ultrasound-guided biopsy is done infrequently, but they do restrict the operator to a specific trajectory. With practice, freehand needle insertion gives the operator more flexibility in placing the needle.

Tables

A good scanning table is extremely useful and should have a cut-out section (Figure 12.6) so that the transducer can be introduced from underneath the patient; often multiple cut-outs of different sizes are provided. The height of the table should be adjustable; for larger dogs, support staff will need to lean over the table some distance to maintain adequate comfortable restraint and this can be difficult if the table is too high. An adjustable-height mobile chair or saddle stool (Figure 12.6b) is required for the operator, particularly if long examinations are carried out. Reverse-friction castors, which move easily but fix in place when weight is applied, can be helpful.

There is also a wide range of tabletop scanning benches available. In smaller practices, it is useful to have a table that can also be used for other purposes; these may have an infill for the cut-out section. Alternatively, a specially made top can be placed on an adjustable-height table (Figure 12.6). Where an ultrasound scanning bench is removable, it should be light enough to manoeuvre into place easily, and space should be allocated in the scanning area for safe storage.

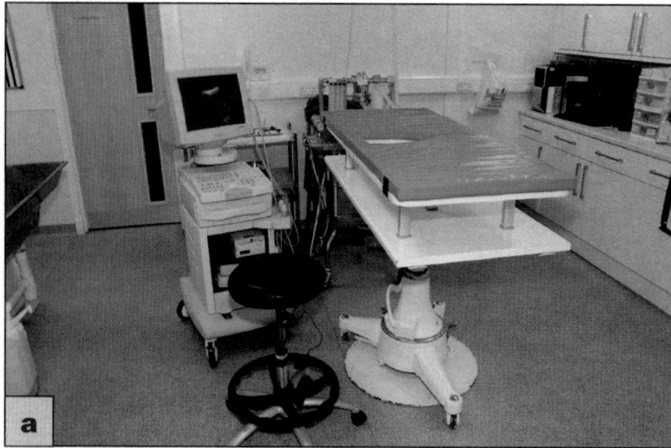

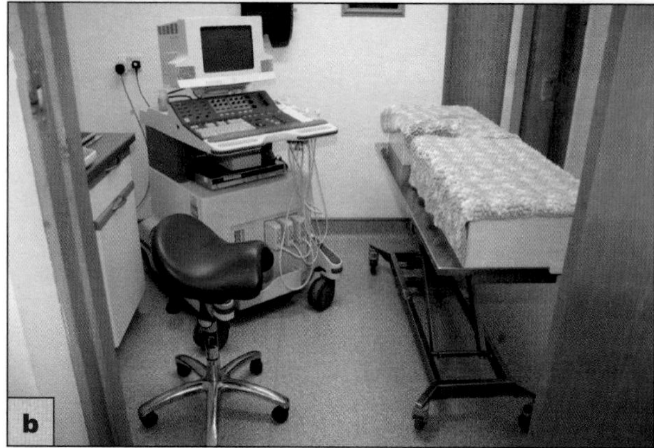

12.6 Adjustable-height tables fitted with removable tops with cut-out sections facilitate scanning (especially echocardiography) and offer flexibility for other uses. Mobile stools improve ergonomics and operator comfort. **(a)** The padded table improves patient comfort. **(b)** A narrower trolley table is useful for moving patients. The ergonomic saddle stool aids posture to reduce operator back problems and has reverse-friction castors to give stability whilst scanning.

Stand-offs

A stand-off is a non-echogenic block of material that is used to separate the transducer from superficial structures being imaged. This brings the point of interest into the focal zone of the transducer and moves it away from the near field, where there are intense echoes due to transducer reverberation which may obscure structural detail. Commercial stand-offs can be purchased (Figure 12.7) but a simple stand-off can be made by filling a surgical glove with water or ultrasound gel.

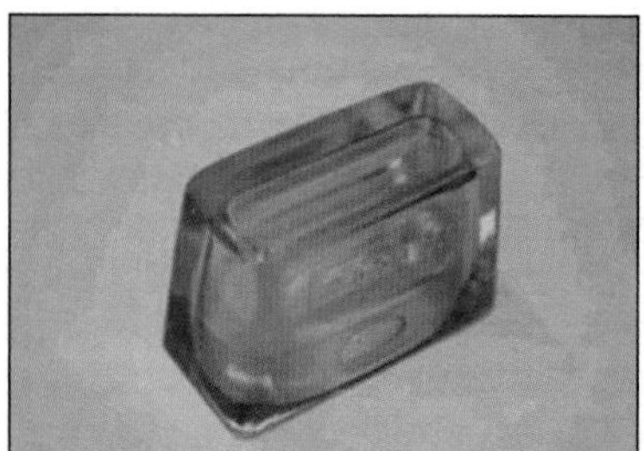

12.7 A stand-off pad for use with linear array transducers. (Reproduced from the *BSAVA Manual of Canine and Feline Ultrasonography*)

KEY POINT

It is helpful to warm ultrasound gel before application. This can be done by placing the gel bottle in a warm water bath or electric baby bottle warmer.

Image viewing and storage

Most ultrasound machines come with an adequate monitoring screen, but larger screens can be added to many machines if preferred. It is important that ambient lighting, reflections and glare do not make the image difficult to interpret.

The practice may wish to purchase an image recording device for still or video image storage. It may be helpful to send a video of the examination to a third party for a second opinion; however, even video images can be difficult to interpret by a third party who does not have the benefit of personal interaction with the patient and knowledge of the exact placement of the probe.

Video, DVD or hard-drive recorders can be used, and images can be stored on DVD or optical discs, or on hard drives if sufficient space is available. Some machines are able to export to a USB memory stick for transfer to a standalone PC or server. Network compatibility makes transfer into the practice management system easier still and if the machine is DICOM-compatible, images can be transferred and stored on a DICOM or PACS server alongside digital radiographs. In this case patient details and dates are also stored for easy retrieval.

Printers are available for still images and are not usually prohibitively expensive. Still images are less frequently used, however, now that moving images are routinely recorded, but can be useful for showing salient points to clients and for recording measurements for future comparison.

Managing the ultrasonography service

Although ultrasound scans can often be performed as outpatient procedures, and pregnancy scans and simple assessments can be performed relatively quickly, it is usually essential to book time for more thorough and diagnostic abdominal, chest and specific scans, which may take 45 minutes or longer, and so tie up staff and the ultrasound room.

The scanning room

The area provided should be quiet and away from distractions and electrical interference. A bespoke imaging room is ideal, and ultrasonography can be combined with the radiography suite if there is adequate space for a second table. If the radiography room is not large enough, the preparation room or even a consulting room may be used, but scanning should be scheduled for a time when these areas are not in use for other purposes. If owners are permitted to stay with their pet during the procedure, there should be sufficient space to allow for this. The ability to darken the room should be considered, as this greatly enhances the ability to read the image (Figure 12.8). Air conditioning is helpful as it reduces panting during thoracic scans. Facilities for sedation and monitoring are useful for detailed abdominal scans, as these may be lengthy procedures.

It is often necessary to scan unconscious or anaesthetized patients undergoing other procedures or admitted in an emergency. Smaller mobile scanners or portable units can be moved to the patient. For large ultrasound machines it may be more convenient to move the patient to the scanning room, and an adjustable-height mobile ultrasonography table can be very useful (see Figure 12.6b). Where sterile procedures are planned, e.g. ultrasound-guided biopsy, the room must be appropriately situated and arranged to satisfy the criteria for working with a sterile field (see Chapter 8).

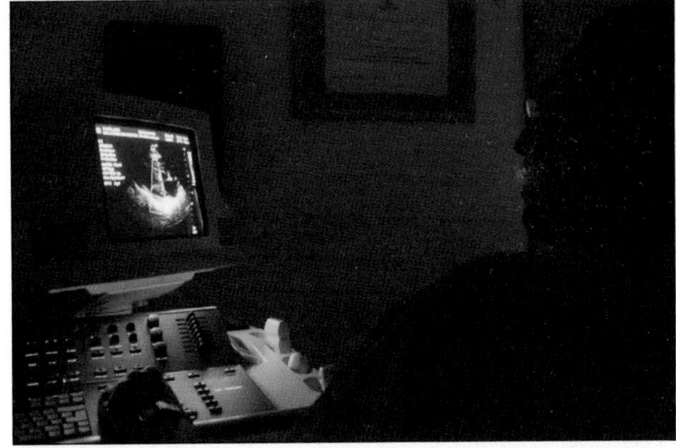

12.8 Darkening the room is very helpful for interpreting images, particularly for colour-flow Doppler.

Patient and staff preparation

Most patients are scanned without the use of sedative or anaesthesia, and it is important to reduce stress to a minimum to ensure that the patient remains calm and still. Restraint (Figure 12.9) will require one or two support staff, and their time must be factored into the overall cost of the procedure. The table should be adjusted to a suitable height to enable staff to hold the patient comfortably for the duration of the examination without causing undue strain (Figure 12.10).

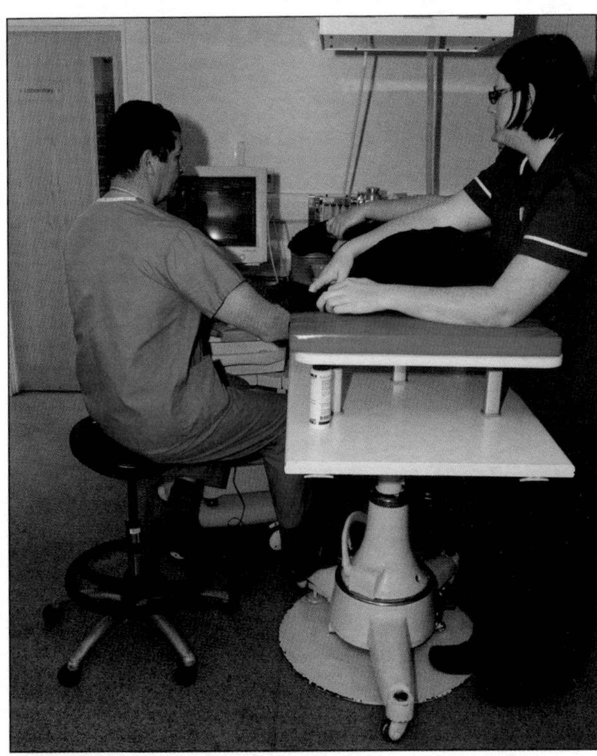

12.9 Calm effective restraint is key to a successful examination.

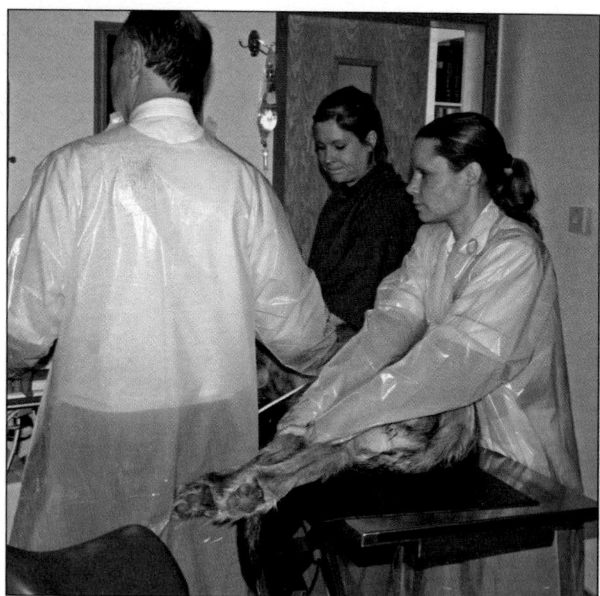

12.10 Practices seeing a significant number of giant-breed dogs may need an extra long, narrow table with lower height adjustment to accommodate the dog effectively in lateral recumbency. Two nurses are often needed to restrain larger dogs for scanning.

It is usually preferable to clip hair from the area to be examined, and clients should be warned of this prior to the procedure. In show animals, or where clients will not allow clipping, it may still be possible to carry out an examination if the hair is not too thick and is saturated with gel.

Biopsy

Ultrasound-guided biopsy procedures should be carried out in a sterile manner and surgical preparation of the area to be sampled will be required. The probe is placed in a sterile sleeve made for the purpose, but if this is not available a sterile surgical glove makes a suitable alternative. The surgeon should also scrub up and wear surgical gloves.

Equipment care and maintenance

It is important that equipment, particularly any electrical equipment, complies with current relevant health and safety legislation, and that its use does not present a risk to staff. An SOP should be drawn up for the use and cleaning of any ultrasound equipment, and should include who is competent at using the equipment. An example of an SOP can be found at the end of this chapter.

The ultrasound machine

Ultrasound scanners have many apertures in which dust and hair can build up and cause problems. A dust cover should be placed over the machine to provide protection when the machine is not in use. Regular vacuuming is recommended, with special attention paid to the air intake filters, which can usually be removed for thorough cleaning.

Transducers

Transducers are extremely delicate and may be irreparably damaged if dropped. Wrist bands can be purchased to help prevent expensive accidents, or the lead may be draped around the operator's neck during use. The transducers should be cleaned after use with a paper towel and clean water. Surgical spirit should generally not be used as it can damage the delicate transducer head.

KEY POINT

It is important to check with the manufacturer before using any cleaning or sterilizing agent on transducers.

Transducers are generally stored on a hook or in a rack on the system trolley (Figure 12.11). Care should be taken that the machine is stored away from busy areas where the transducers could get knocked.

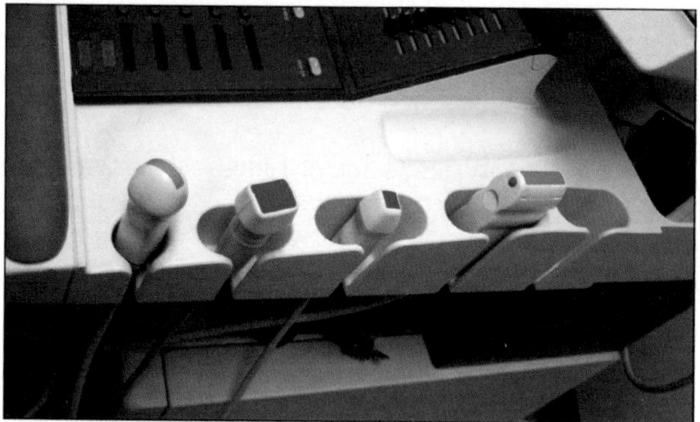

12.11 Transducer probes stored in a rack on the ultrasound machine.

Training

The main limitations of ultrasonography are the ability of staff to use the equipment and to interpret results correctly, together with the long examination times needed, particularly when gaining experience and confidence with the technique. Adequate training, at considerable cost, and hours of practice over several years are essential to become really proficient. The learning curve is steep and effective diagnosis requires considerable experience. It is therefore vital to ensure that adequate provision for training is made and that trained staff are retained or replaced by others with similar skills where possible. RCVS Practice Standards Scheme Inspectors require evidence of suitable training in the use of ultrasound equipment. This can be by external courses or in-house training and self-development with appropriate resources, including practising with healthy pets.

Further reading

Barr F and Gaschen L (2011) *BSAVA Manual of Canine and Feline Ultrasonography.* BSAVA Publications, Gloucester

SOP example follows ▶

SOP No ....

Preparation, use and cleaning of ultrasound equipment

NOTE: All ultrasound equipment should only be handled by trained staff.

The following staff are trained to use ultrasound equipment:

The following staff are trained to care for and clean ultrasound equipment:

Preparing the machine for use

1. Remove the dust cover.
2. Plug in the machine and switch on.
3. Enter client and patient details, complete all fields.
4. Select probe.
5. Select settings appropriate to study.
6. Ensure machine is within easy reach of operator but not so close to patient that it may get knocked.
7. Attach foot pedal and place on floor near operator chair.
8. Ensure printer has sufficient paper and is turned on.
9. Insert USB stick or turn on video recorder.

Patient preparation

- Warm gel before use in water bath.
- Clip the area to be scanned with clippers (unless the client has not agreed to this).
- Clean skin with surgical spirit on cotton wool unless there are open wounds, abrasions or clipper rash.
- Never place a probe or clippers on the table where a patient may dislodge them.
- Apply warm gel to skin.

Procedure

- A wrist band must always be used when handling probes.
- Ensure adequate restraint of the patient; this will often require two assistants.
- Always use a padded table: a comfortable patient is less likely to struggle.
- Maintain a calm atmosphere and subdued lighting.
- If the patient is still anxious, consider sedation.
- Adjust the table and operator's chair to suitable heights to prevent fatigue.
- Have adequate paper towels to hand at all times.
- Prepare biopsy needles and pots beforehand and arrange on a side table within reach.
- **Do not operate the controls with gel on your hands, especially the roller ball, as this will damage the machine**.

At the end of the procedure

1. Ensure all video has been recorded or moved to the USB stick as required.
2. Turn off the power switch.
3. Remove the footswitch and place in the drawer provided. Unplug the machine from the mains and coil the power lead around the hooks provided.
4. Wipe all probes with clean damp paper towels. **Use only clean water not soap or surgical spirit as this can damage the probe.**
5. Replace the probes in the probe carrier, with the leads over the hooks provided.
6. Replace the dust cover.
7. Move the machine to the corner of the ultrasound room, with the probe carrier facing towards the wall where it cannot get knocked.

Cleaning the ultrasound machine

- Never clean the machine when it is powered on or plugged in.

1. Remove the dust cover.
2. Using a cleaning nozzle on the vacuum cleaner, clean all around the keyboard.
3. Remove the cover of the air intake vent by unscrewing the lock nuts on the corners.
4. Remove the filter and vacuum to remove hair and dust.
5. Wipe the screen and keyboard with appropriate screen cleaning tissues, paying special attention to the roller ball.
6. Wipe all probes and leads with paper towel dampened with clean water.

Example of an SOP for the use and cleaning of equipment for ultrasonography.

Radiography

13

Victoria S. Johnson

The radiography department of a small animal practice is an important area, both in terms of facilitating accurate clinical diagnosis and with respect to essential legal requirements. Practices must be able safely to produce radiographs of diagnostic quality for all species being treated as well as to ensure that clinicians can accurately interpret the images. Diagnostic quality embraces correct patient positioning, and exposure, development and viewing of the image. A carefully designed and well run radiography department is a worthwhile investment and will realize benefits for years to come. The advent of digital systems has brought potential advantages, and this chapter will look at the decision-making process on whether to change over from film-based systems. More details on the physics of radiography and radiographic equipment may be found in the *BSAVA Textbook of Veterinary Nursing.*

Dental radiographic equipment may be in a separate location to the main radiographic equipment; if this is the case, then separate Local Rules (see below) must be agreed with the Radiation Protection Advisor (RPA). Dental radiography is discussed in Chapter 9.

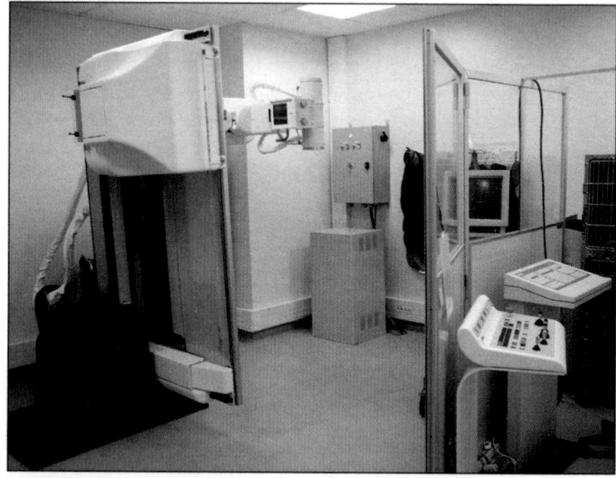

13.1 The controlled area. Normally the whole of the room in which the X-ray tube (shown here in an upright position) is situated is designated a controlled area. The controlled area must be described in the Local Rules, physically demarcated and have sufficient signs. Ideally there should only be one entrance. In this room the X-ray machine controls are situated behind a protective screen.

Controlled areas

Areas where X-rays are used must be designated 'controlled areas' (Figure 13.1). A controlled area has a very precise definition in legal terms but in most small animal practices constitutes the room where the radiographs are taken. Advice should be sought from the RPA as to the exact nature and size of the required controlled area in the practice. If an X-ray area is being designed for a new or existing practice, then a good understanding of the requirements of a controlled area is advisable before proceeding with plans and development.

The controlled area exists at all times when the X-ray machine is connected to the electrical mains supply. Once a controlled area has been defined, it must be described in the Local Rules (see later), physically demarcated and provided with sufficient signs to indicate that is it a controlled area due to the presence of X-ray radiation.

KEY POINTS

Warning signs and lights required to be provided at each entrance to the X-ray room:

- A warning sign incorporating the trefoil radiation sign and wording such as 'X-RAY CONTROLLED AREA. DO NOT ENTER WHEN LIGHT IS ON' (Figure 13.2)
- A red warning light which is illuminated automatically when X-rays are being generated (Figure 13.3)

Design of controlled areas

Often the controlled area is already designated within a practice, but on occasion there may be a need for a new controlled area to be built or converted. In this case, there are some important considerations to take into account.

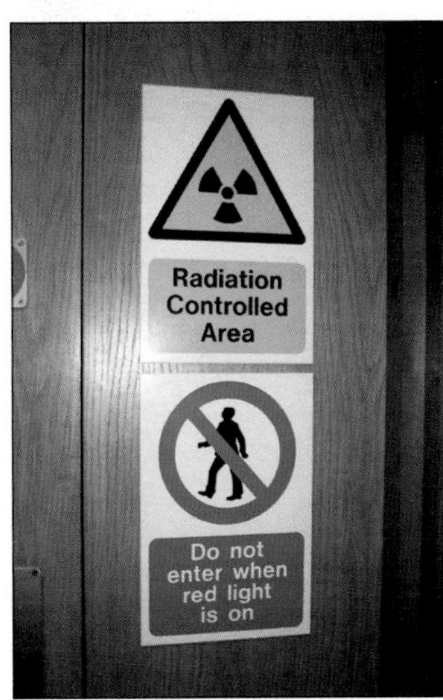
Radiation
Controlled
Area
Do not
enter when
red light
is on

13.2 A warning sign incorporating the trefoil radiation sign and wording such as 'X-RAY CONTROLLED AREA. DO NOT ENTER WHEN LIGHT IS ON' must be provided at each entrance to the radiography room.

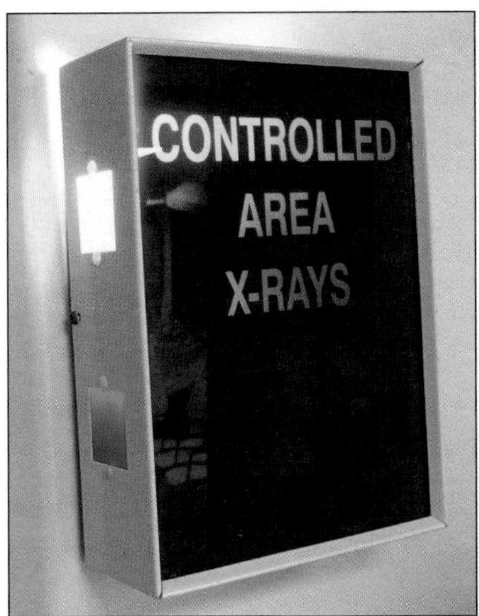

13.3 Warning lights must be provided at each entrance to the X-ray room. In this example, the controlled area light illuminates when the equipment is connected to the power supply, and an additional red light becomes visible below the yellow wording when radiographs are being taken and states 'DO NOT ENTER'.

- **Location:**
  - A specified room *must* be provided for radiography
  - Ideally, this room should only be used for radiography
  - Normally the whole of the X-ray room is defined as the controlled area
  - It is very important to consider the current use of areas above and below the X-ray room. The X-ray beam is usually angled vertically downwards; hence, the degree of protection afforded by the floor must be considered if there is access to an area below.
- **Entrances and thoroughfare:**
  - When the controlled area exists (usually defined as when the X-ray machine is connected to the electrical supply), the room must only be used for radiography and must *not* be used as a thoroughfare
  - It is best if there is only one entrance, to aid control of access
  - Each entrance must have suitable warning signs and lights as described above.
- **Size:**
  - The room should be of adequate size to ensure that everyone present during radiography can remain behind a protective screen or other suitable barrier, or be at least 2 metres from the beam during exposures.
- **Shielding:**
  - The RPA should be consulted on all issues of shielding
  - In most cases the shielding of the physical boundaries (walls) will be adequate if the barriers subjected to scattered radiation have a lead equivalence of 0.5 mm (single brick or high-density block) and those subjected to the primary beam have a lead equivalence of 2 mm (double brick or double high-density block)
  - Unshielded doors, walls and windows may be acceptable if the radiographic workload is minimal (<10 exposures per week) and the primary beam is only used vertically downwards (must consult the RPA)
  - Additional shielding can be employed where required, e.g. a door incorporating a lead sheet sandwich 0.5 mm lead equivalent.

Radiography equipment

X-ray machines

X-ray machines vary in their features and benefits (Figures 13.4 and 13.5).

There are many considerations when purchasing an X-ray machine for small animal practice. The most important of these concern safety features:

- Accurate electronic timer
- Adequate primary beam filtration
- Suitable warning features and an exposure button that allows safe operation from outside a suitable barrier

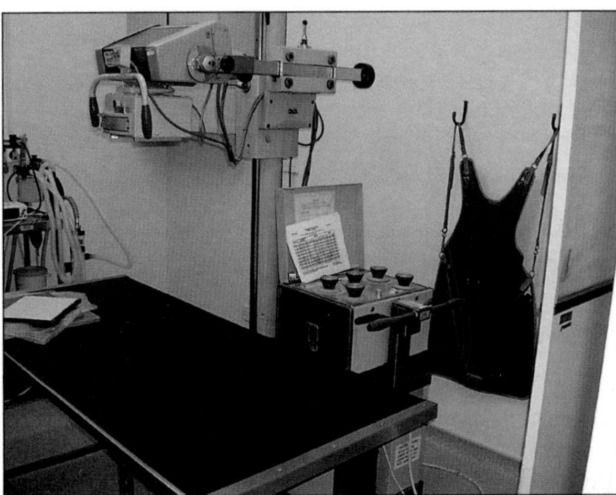

13.4 A simple X-ray machine of the mobile variety. The tube head has been mounted on a vertical stand, which enables variation of FFD (film focal distance) but the tube cannot be moved over different areas of the table. A moveable table can be helpful with this type of set-up.

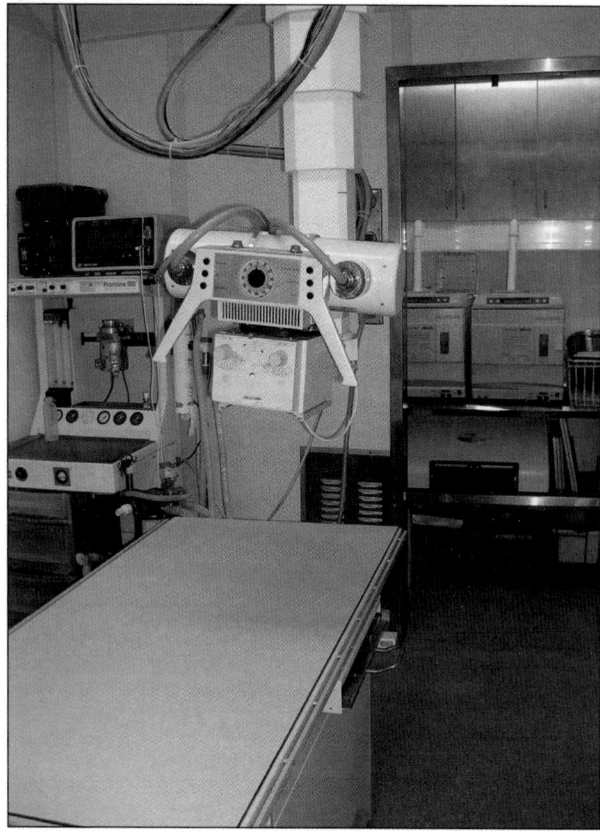

13.5 A ceiling-mounted X-ray tube head. This type of mounting provides much greater flexibility in manoeuvring the tube. The tube shown here is tilted for an angled exposure; this can be helpful for obtaining intraoral views, decubitus views and oblique skeletal radiographs.

- Light beam diaphragm (LBD): the LBD light shows where the primary beam will fall, and accuracy should be checked regularly to enable thorough collimation (restriction of the primary beam to the minimum area required for the area of interest).

Although these features are fairly standard in modern machines, they are particularly important if considering purchasing a second-hand machine:

- X-ray machines should be checked in accordance with the advice of the manufacturer, supplier and/or RPA, particularly with respect to radiation leakage from the tube housing
- Regular service records or safety certification should be inspected.

Installation is subject to regulations and it must be verified that safety features and warning devices operate correctly.

Other practical features to consider are:

- Increments of exposure factors (kV, mA, time) available
- Automatic presets for different anatomical areas; can be useful if designed for veterinary use
- Dual focus: A smaller focal spot (the source of the radiation from the tube head) can be selected to improve image resolution; a larger focal spot size is used for thicker body parts where a greater intensity of X-rays is required
- Ability to angle the beam; can be employed to obtain oblique views and horizontal beam views, all of which can be helpful in diagnosis of specific conditions. *Note: when the beam is angled away from a vertical downwards direction, it is important to consider the radiation implications and the beam should only be angled at a suitably shielded barrier*
- Ability to vary the film focal distance (distance from the tube head focal spot to the film cassette)
- Type of mounting: wall-, table- or ceiling-mounted for dedicated small animal radiography; stand-mounted if X-ray machine is mobile or shared by ambulatory equine practice. The quality of the mounting is important, both for accurate positioning and for minimizing movement of the tube head during exposure
- Power requirements: X-ray machines vary in their power requirements; practices will need to consider whether the existing practice electrical supply will need to be upgraded before purchasing
- Warranties, servicing and service contracts: service intervals should be regular and should not exceed one year. Service contracts may be available and the exact terms of what is included and covered should be noted. Warranties should be examined carefully, as replacement parts can be very costly.

Tables

It is strongly recommended to use a purpose-built radiography table rather than a normal examination table. Radiographic tables can be 'floating' or fixed. A floating table is one that, once unlocked, can be freely moved in any direction in the horizontal plane; this is very helpful as it allows smooth, controlled movement of the patient during selection of the area to be exposed. These tables are used with cassette trays beneath the table, which are usually self-centring. Some techniques may require tilting of the table or patient (e.g. myelography), so this may be a consideration.

It is also useful to have methods of patient restraint incorporated into the table. Cleats around the edge of the table can be helpful, but a system of grooved metal plates with locking cleats is now available (Figure 13.6).

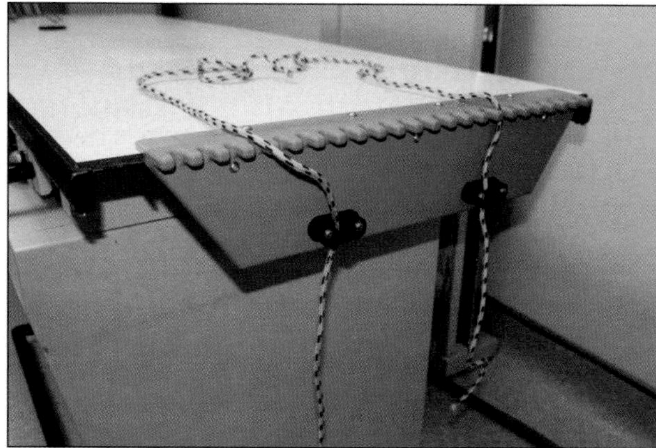

13.6 Special devices can be attached to the end of the radiography table to facilitate patient positioning and restraint. One such device uses a system of grooved metal plates and locking cleats which are used to secure thin ropes.

This is fixed at each end of the radiography table and can be extremely helpful for patient positioning.

If a non-purpose-built radiography table is used, a sheet of lead or lead rubber (of 1 mm lead equivalence and larger than the maximum beam width employed) should be placed on the table under the cassette. This is important to limit radiation scatter.

Patient positioning aids

It is a legal requirement that no animal should be held for radiography unless there are clinical reasons why it cannot be restrained by other means.

KEY POINT

It is vital to have a good protocol for sedation and anaesthesia for radiography, and appropriate systems for safe and comfortable restraint.

A range of positioning aids should be available, including:

- Sand bags: generally long, thin bags are the best, as they can be easily wrapped around a patient's legs (Figure 13.7a)
- Foam wedges (Figure 13.7a): can be covered with wipe-clean fabrics to preserve their longevity and prevent absorption of body fluids and contrast media
- Thin washable rope ties (see Figure 13.6)
- Radiolucent cradles: at least three sizes should be provided (small holes can be drilled into the base for wall hanging; Figure 13.7b)

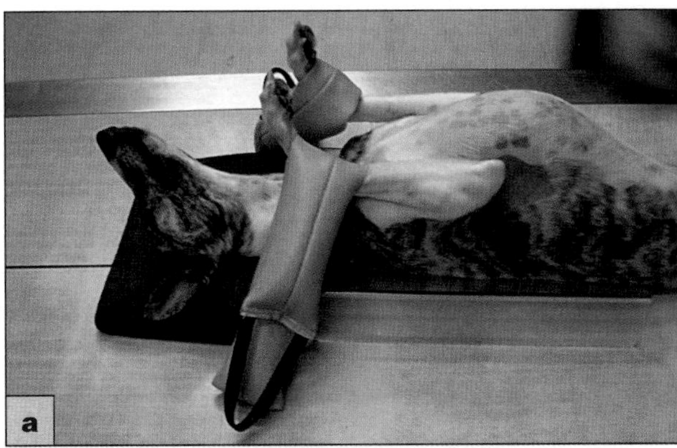

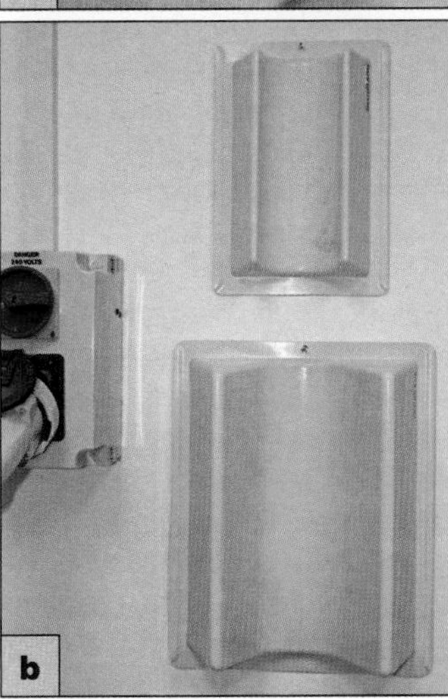

13.7 **(a)** A dog positioned in a trough. Sandbags have been used to pull the forelimbs cranially, and there is a foam wedge under the dog's head for comfort. **(b)** Positioning troughs can be stored by means of a simple hook on walls within the radiography area. (a, reproduced from *BSAVA Manual of Canine and Feline Thoracic Radiography*)

- Cardboard box (Figure 13.8) or perspex box with access for oxygen: to obtain conscious dorsoventral views of stressed or dyspnoeic animals
- Atraumatic clothes pegs: can be used on the scruff region to restrain puppies and kittens.

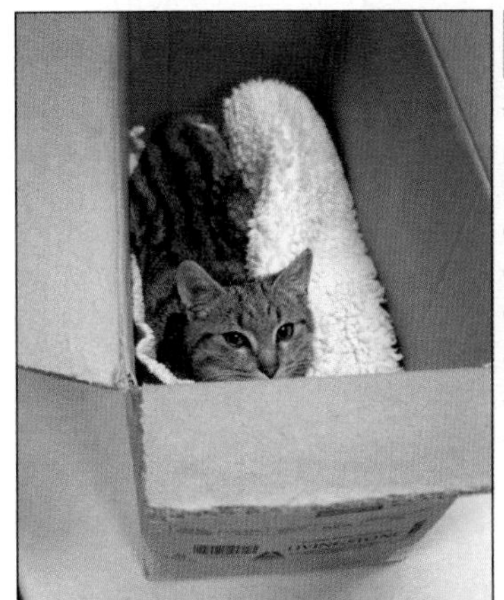

13.8 If essential for a dyspnoeic or stressed patient, a screening radiograph can be obtained through a cardboard box. The lid can be closed (provide airholes or oxygen supply) for further calming effect. (Reproduced from *BSAVA Manual of Canine and Feline Thoracic Radiography*)

Patient identification and positional markers

Where film is used, patient details must be recorded on the film at the time of exposure. This is known as 'primary labelling' and is particularly important for films taken for the BVA/Kennel Club Hip Dysplasia Scheme. Choices are:

- X-ray marking tape (comes on a reel for handwriting with a ballpoint pen and is adhesive)
- Individual lettering (time-consuming and easy to lose letters)
- A light marker (used in the darkroom to transfer written details on to to a non-exposed area of the film before processing).

In digital systems the patient information is entered at the time of registration, before commencing the radiographic examination. It is very important that each animal is registered carefully, according to a standard protocol, otherwise it will be difficult to retrieve images in the future.

A range of positional markers is required to indicate left, right and other positioning details, or sequential numbering/timing for contrast studies if needed. These are available from most radiographic suppliers, and should be placed on the table or cassette for incorporation into the image on exposure. Digital radiographs can be annotated later at the quality control viewing station but this is not ideal and primary positional labelling is preferable.

Measuring devices

Measuring callipers (Figure 13.9) (or at least a ruler) should be supplied to determine the thickness of the body part being radiographed and used in tandem with a technique chart to optimize exposures.

A long rule or tape measure should be available for accurate assessment of the film focal distance (see earlier) if this is variable and measurement is not incorporated into the X-ray machine.

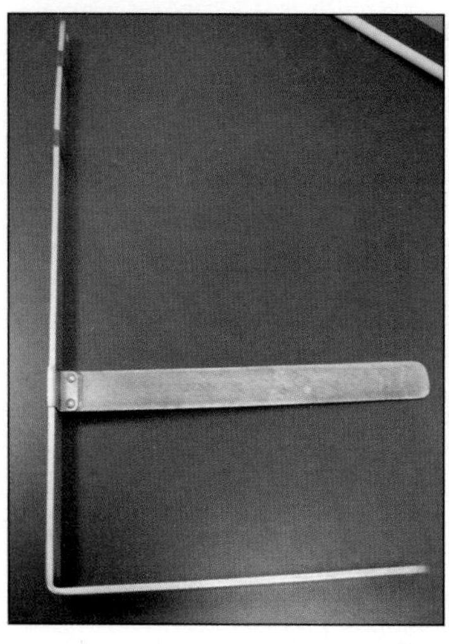

13.9 Callipers are extremely helpful to measure the thickness of the body part being radiographed and should be used in combination with a technique chart.

Contrast media

Various contrast media should be available. The type required will depend on the caseload, but as a minimum, a non-ionic iodinated contrast medium and a barium-based contrast medium should be provided. It should be noted that both iodinated contrast and barium products have 'use by' dates and careful stock control is vital.

Personal protective equipment

If the presence of a person within the controlled area is essential, they must be provided with suitable protective clothing (Figure 13.10):

- Protective lead aprons, or jacket and skirt (lighter and more comfortable to wear); lead equivalence of not less than 0.25 mm
- Gloves and sleeves; lead equivalence of not less than 0.50 mm
- Advice from the RPA should be sought regarding the need for additional protection, such as thyroid or eye protection.

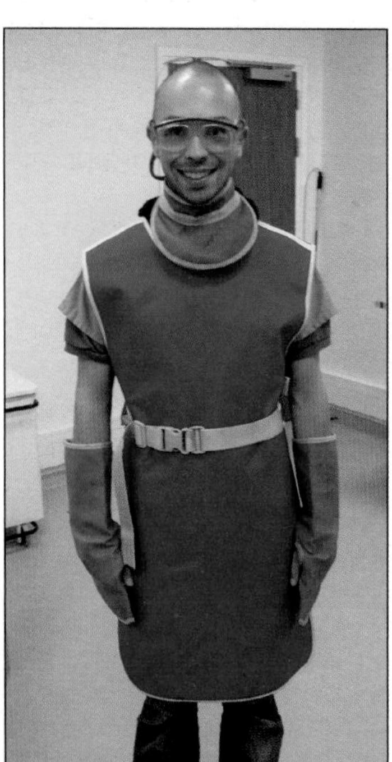

13.10 Personal protective equipment must be available for occasions when the presence of a person within the controlled area is essential. Equipment should be carefully maintained and stored and checked regularly.

KEY POINT

It should be noted that this equipment is not designed to protect the wearer from the primary beam, and therefore *no body part* should enter the exposed area even when protective clothing is worn.

Protective clothing can become damaged when stored incorrectly. A large-diameter hanging rail or a series of appropriate hangers should be available for storage when not in use (Figure 13.11). Clothing should be examined regularly (at least annually) for defects and cracks.

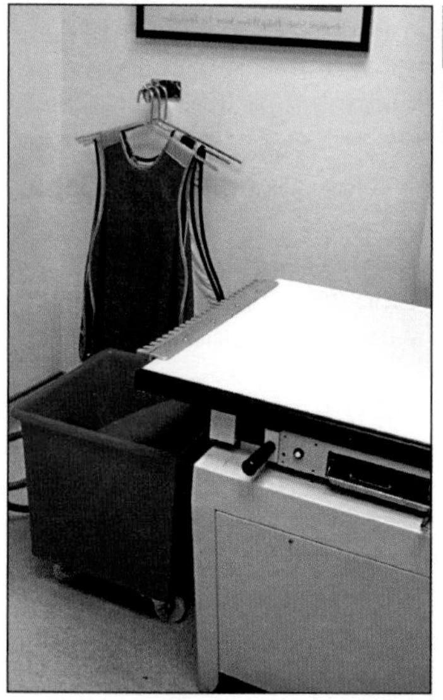

13.11 Lead gowns should be hung on appropriate hangers when not in use.

Film–screen radiography

Films, screens and cassettes

The cassette houses the X-ray film and the intensifying screens. Typically, double-sided film is used and is sandwiched between two screens, although single-sided emulsion film can also be employed with a single screen for more detailed radiographic examinations. The screens incorporate phosphor crystals, which emit light when they interact with X-ray radiation. It is this light which exposes the X-ray film. Cassettes with intensifying screens must be used in film-screen radiography to decrease exposure dose and exposure times. For reasons of radiation protection, the fastest appropriate combination of film and intensifying screens compatible with good radiographic results should be used. Screens must be handled carefully and kept very clean (see later). Many older screens are irretrievably damaged and should be replaced to gain better images. It is vital to match the correct type of X-ray film to the correct type of image-intensifying screen. This is because the screens emit different wavelengths of light depending on the phosphor they contain, and the X-ray film used must be sensitive to the spectrum of light emitted.

It is important to have an adequate range of cassette and film sizes available within the practice (Figure 13.12). For example, radiography of the thorax or abdomen of a large dog requires the use of a

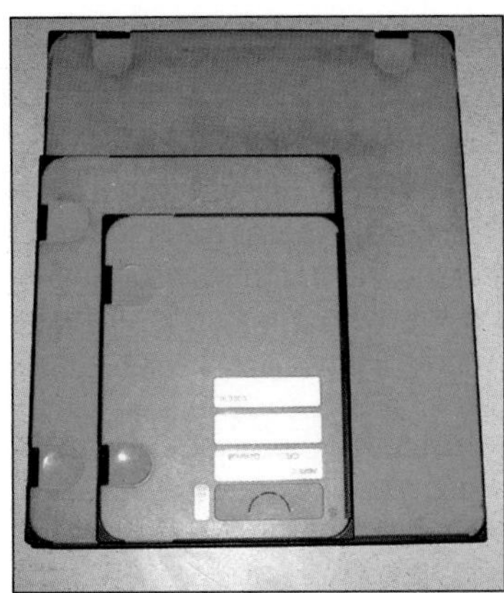

13.12 It is very important to have a wide range of cassette sizes available for small animal radiography. In particular, the large size 35 x 43 cm is required for exposures of the thorax or abdomen in a large dog. Imaging plates for digital radiography also come in a variety of sizes (some are shown here).

30 cm x 40 cm cassette size (preferably 35 cm x 43 cm if available) and it is not acceptable to patch together a collection of smaller images.

Cassettes must be stored carefully, in an upright position, away from extremes of temperature and from sources of radiation. Cassettes can be easily damaged and bent, and should be used with care and inspected regularly.

Grids

A grid is a device used to reduce scattered radiation reaching and exposing a film or imaging plate. A grid should be used when making an exposure of large body parts (usually >10 cm thick; e.g. hips, chest and abdomen of medium to large breed dogs), which generate more scattered radiation. Grids are not recommended when radiographing smaller body areas because the use of a grid necessitates increased exposure factors.

There are many types of grid available. One of the simplest to use is the moving or Potter Bucky grid. These are usually integral to a complete X-ray machine and table system. The grid oscillates during the exposure to remove the appearance of any grid lines on the final image. The cassette is placed *under* the X-ray table to use the grid, and directly *on top of* the table when the grid is not required. These grids do, however, require slightly higher exposures than other grid systems. Some older moving grids can result in table vibration and should be avoided.

A static grid can also be used and is cheaper. Externally it looks like a flat piece of lightweight metal. It is important to have a large size available (at least 30 cm x 40 cm) to correspond with the large cassettes. These grids are simply placed over the X-ray cassette for the exposure and the patient positioned on top. This makes the process of aligning body part, grid and cassette more cumbersome, and patients tend to be less compliant with this set-up. Grids can be set into grid holders that fit snugly over the cassette, and hold the grid in place.

There are different types of static grid, but for most small animal applications a focused grid should be chosen and used with a fixed film focal distance. The exposure chart must note when the grid should be used and how the exposure factors should be varied. The grid must be kept clean, stored carefully and used appropriately (correct orientation to the primary X-ray beam). Grids can be seriously damaged if dropped.

Automatic processors

There is a wide range of affordable automatic processors available, and manual film processing is no longer recommended. Most modern automatic processing units are ideally suited to small animal practices, being compact, requiring minimal or no plumbing, and using a normal 13 amp power supply. Some can be used in daylight, while others require a darkroom. Desirable features include automatic replenishment of chemicals and an internal structure that is easily cleanable to make maintenance easy. Processors should accept all film sizes used in the practice and have a reasonable throughput time.

All automatic processors should be regularly cleaned and inspected, and a maintenance schedule should be used to ensure this is performed. Eye protection, gloves and aprons should be worn for processor maintenance. Images should also be examined on a regular schedule for quality control purposes.

KEY POINT

No matter where the processor is situated, adequate ventilation is required.

Darkroom

Where a darkroom is necessary, the following are important:

- A safelight with filter appropriate to the type and speed of film used, to prevent fogging
- Adequate normal lighting to allow easy maintenance of the processor and general cleaning
- Easy to access safelight and main light switches with no possibility of confusion
- Sufficient safe storage space to store film upright in original boxes and allow clear access to each size of film; a light-tight cupboard or box is recommended
- Space to move about with ease
- Sufficient dry bench area to open cassettes, label film if necessary, and avoid contamination with wet chemicals
- A clear system to avoid inadvertent opening of the door when films are being handled
- Work surfaces, walls and floor of impermeable and easy to clean materials
- Active ventilation with light baffle where necessary to prevent build-up of chemical fumes from developer and fixer.

Lightbox viewer

A lightbox should be used to view radiographs. Using double- or triple-panel viewers means that multiple images can be viewed simultaneously (Figure 13.13) and that lateral views taken with a 35 cm x 43 cm cassette can be examined. The lightbox should be in a quiet area of the practice with low ambient lighting, ideally controlled by a dimmer switch. A hotlight (high-intensity light) should be available for examination of darker areas of the films. These are often incorporated in modern lightboxes but can also be acquired separately.

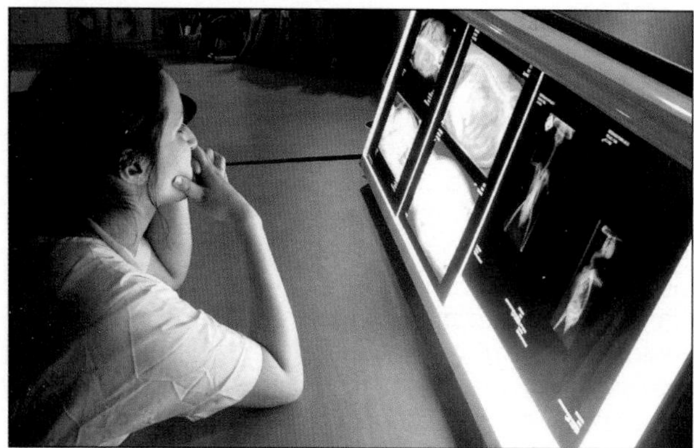

13.13 Lightboxes of adequate size should be available for viewing films. Films should be viewed in a quiet darkened room.

Digital radiography

Many small animal practices are considering changing to digital radiographic technology. There are two types of digital radiographic technology: computed radiography (CR) and direct digital radiography (DDR). Both systems produce a digital image, but there are some differences between them.

Computed radiography

Computed radiography (CR) replaces the normal cassette and its contents with an imaging plate (IP). The IP is used in the same way as a cassette and looks very similar. It can be used under the radiography table with a Bucky grid or on top of the table. Once it has been exposed to X-rays, it is taken to an imaging reader (Figure 13.14) for processing. This is a freestanding or benchtop piece of equipment that reads the IP and produces a digital radiographic image. Only one IP can be read at a time and it takes about 60–90 seconds to produce the image.

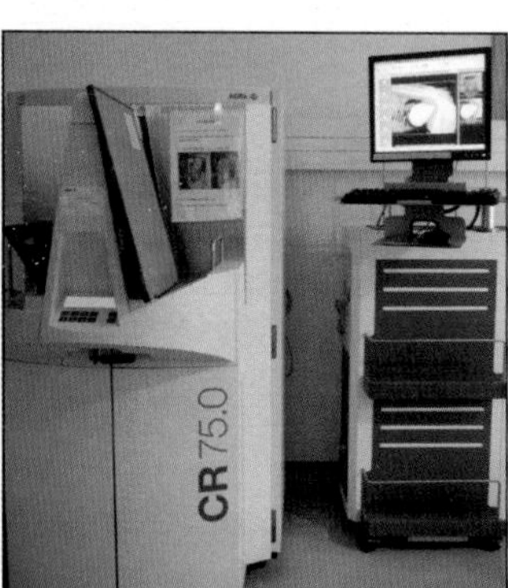

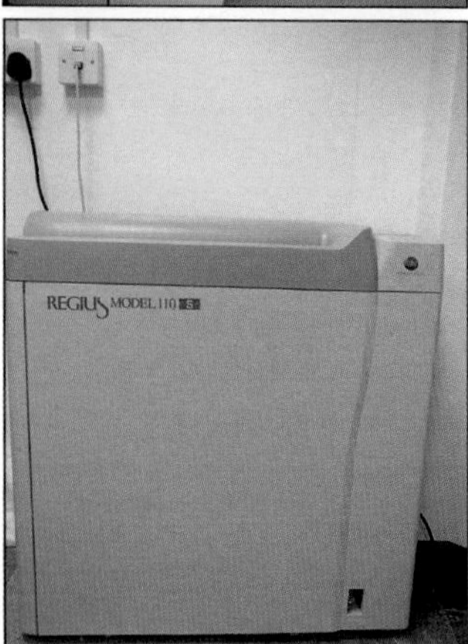

13.14 In CR, an image reader is used to process the imaging plate. These come in various formats, and in large hospitals automatic loading systems can be utilized.

Direct digital radiography

In direct digital radiography (DDR; also known as DR) the traditional cassette is replaced by a digital imaging sensor. This sensor detects X-rays during the exposure and a digital radiographic image is immediately generated. There is no need for a processing step in DDR, and hence the whole process is faster and simpler. Generally, DDR systems are more expensive than CR systems.

In small animal DDR systems the imaging sensor is usually an integral fixed part of the radiographic table. This means that horizontal beam views and intra-oral views can no longer be performed with the DDR equipment.

There are two types of DDR sensor:

- **Flat panel detectors.** In these machines the imaging sensor is a rigid plate, usually affixed to the table. Flat panel detectors can usually be fitted to existing X-ray equipment
- **Charge-coupled device (CCD) detectors.** These are more complex and involve: a type of camera set-up with a phosphor detector, which receives the X-rays; and charge coupled devices that read out the data. The camera is built into the X-ray table design. Most CCD cameras are sold with new X-ray machine equipment.

Flat panel detectors are generally of a high standard. There can be more variability in the performance of CCD cameras and care should be taken in selecting one of these systems. In general, digital systems should be carefully assessed and compared before taking the decision to purchase.

X-ray machines

Most digital radiography systems can be used with the existing X-ray tube and there may be no need to upgrade equipment. There may, however, be an increase in X-ray exposure when using some digital systems, and it is advisable to arrange a specific servicing appointment and to ask the engineer whether the machine will be able to cope with the additional workload.

Grids

Some recent research suggests that grids may be less important in digital radiography, where multiscale or multifrequency processing algorithms are used. Use of grids with digital image processing only led to a slight improvement in image quality when compared to images without a grid. It should also be noted that there is less requirement to increase exposure factors when using a grid with digital processing, as the display greyscale of a digital system is not linked to exposure dose.

Monitors

There are many factors that affect standards of practice in digital radiography and the quality of the monitor used to view the final image is one of these (Figure 13.15). There are two main types of monitor available: cathode-ray tube (CRT); and liquid crystal display

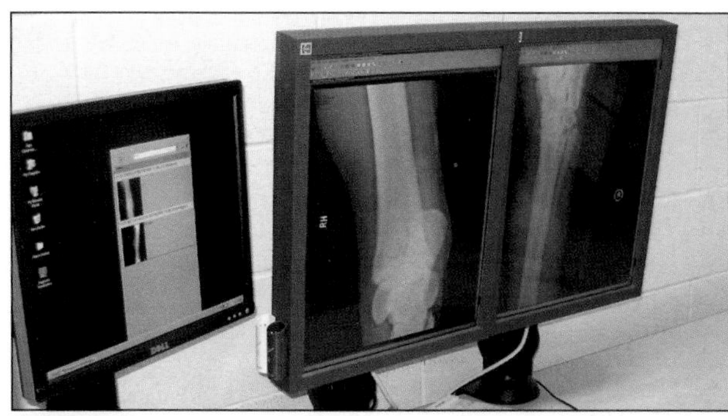

13.15 There are many different types of digital monitor available. This figure shows a standard PC monitor (left) next to two medical-grade monitors. It is important to choose the correct monitor to make a radiographic diagnosis.

(LCD). Though both can be suitable for the interpretation of medical images, LCD monitors are recommended as they: take up less space; do not have image flicker; reflect less ambient light; and show truer shades of black than a CRT monitor.

Monitors can also be divided into consumer-grade and medical-grade. Medical-grade monitors have much higher luminance (brightness) and resolution compared to a consumer-grade monitor, but are more expensive. Medical-grade monitors are usually supplied with a high-quality graphics card and it is possible to perform DICOM calibration, an important feature in viewing medical images.

Finally, monitors can be colour or greyscale. In a greyscale monitor each pixel can only produce shades of grey; in general this leads to better quality display for radiographic images.

KEY POINT

The optimal monitor for making a radiographic diagnosis is:

- Medical-grade
- Greyscale
- High-resolution (3 MP (megapixels) preferably, or minimum 2 MP)
- LCD
- Calibrated for the DICOM greyscale standard display function.

Medical-grade monitors are costly and therefore a compromise is usually reached. A diagnostic workstation (either within the practice, or at a teleradiology location), with at least one high-resolution, greyscale medical-grade LCD viewer should be used to make a radiographic diagnosis. Other monitors (in consulting rooms, theatre, reception, etc.) can be consumer-grade LCD monitors (Figure 13.16).

Ambient lighting at the monitor location should be controlled by a dimmer switch. It has been shown that the ability of the eye to discriminate between grey levels is best when the ambient light level of the room is close to the amount of light coming from the monitor(s). The monitor(s) should be positioned so that no light entering the room (e.g. from a doorway) shines and reflects on the screen. Images should be viewed at eye level.

Quality assurance workstation
■ Often supplied with the digital radiography system. ■ Consists of a computer, consumer-grade monitor (often with a touch screen), keyboard and mouse. ■ Used to enter or retrieve records for a patient, to choose processing algorithms, and to review and manipulate the images once produced. ■ Not designed for diagnosis and should not be used in this way.
Diagnostic workstation
■ Consists of a computer, high-specification (medical-grade) monitor, keyboard and mouse. ■ Designed to facilitate optimal clinical diagnosis. ■ Should be situated in a quiet area of the practice with controlled ambient lighting.
Additional viewing workstations
■ Located around the practice, such as in the consulting rooms or operating theatre. ■ May use lower-specification monitors, provided they are not used for primary diagnosis.

13.16 Workstations in the digital radiography practice.

Monitors should be recalibrated regularly. All monitors deteriorate with time and will need eventually to be replaced.

Changing over to digital radiography

The decision to purchase a digital system should be approached seriously, as the costs are high and there are ongoing fees for maintenance and support. It is important to choose the correct system. Some equipment suppliers will allow in-house trials and this provides an excellent means of assessing whether the system will suit the needs of the practice. Image quality is of prime importance. Trial exposures of different body parts should be performed in various patients and the resultant images compared to the existing film–screen system (the digital images should be better, or at least of comparable quality). Comparisons should also be made with other digital systems.

- Images must be generated in DICOM format (see Figure 13.17); other image formats, such as .jpg, are **not** acceptable.
- The machine should be straightforward to use and the company selling the product should offer a comprehensive support package. It is important to understand the breakdown of the costs of the system and the support package and exactly what is included.
- Beyond the actual radiographic equipment, the monitors used to view the images have an enormous impact on standards. Many systems are sold with a quality assurance workstation, where the monitor is of a standard sufficient to review positioning and exposure, but not to make a clinical diagnosis. An additional diagnostic workstation is recommended.
- Digital radiography will reduce the number of repeat radiographs required due to poor exposure technique. It will *not* alter repeats due to patient movement or positioning errors, and these must be addressed separately.
- The ease of sharing and discussing radiographic images is vastly improved with digital radiography.

The DICOM standard: The digital imaging and communication in medicine (DICOM) standard is a standard protocol for communication between devices that generate, transmit and open medical images. It has been reviewed since its original inception and the current version (December 2011) is DICOM 3.0.
DICOM file/image: A DICOM file is a universal type of file format used in all modern digital imaging equipment. A DICOM file is an image file, but also has a large amount of additional embedded information (e.g. patient name, identification number, date of imaging).
DICOM viewer: A DICOM viewer is a piece of software that can open and manipulate DICOM files.
DICOM workstation: A DICOM workstation is a computer where DICOM files are viewed on a DICOM viewer. Workstations can be for quality control or for diagnosis.
PACS: A picture archiving and communication system (PACS) provides storage, rapid retrieval and access to digital images. It consists of the imaging modalities, a data network, viewing workstations, and storage archives.

13.17 Some terms used in digital radiography.

Financial considerations

The costs of a digital radiography system are not simply limited to the radiographic equipment. Figure 13.18 shows some of the other cost implications that need to be considered when taking the decision to purchase a digital system. Figure 13.19 shows the ongoing costs that should also be factored into the equation.

These costs must, however, be weighed against the potential savings of retiring the current film–screen system. Potential cost benefits of switching to a digital radiography system are shown in Figure 13.20. Note that in order to optimize these benefits a completely filmless system must be used, i.e. no digital films should be printed.

- CR: Purchase of adequate number of imaging plates (IPs); imaging reader; adaptation of existing radiographic facilities to incorporate and use new equipment
- DDR: Purchase of DDR equipment ± new X-ray machine and table set-up (especially with CCD) or adaptation of existing radiographic facilities
- Quality control workstation with monitor in radiography room
- Diagnostic workstation(s) with appropriate monitor(s) around the practice
- Adequate number of software licences if using proprietary software
- IT costs, including installation labour fees, network upgrades, static IP addresses, switches, etc.
- Costs of establishing connections between digital radiography system, PACS and other imaging equipment (may be included in installation fee)
- Server for image storage on site
- Data back-up facility (preferably off site)
- Fees to remove existing equipment (may or may not be charged)

13.18 Potential costs in setting up a digital radiography system.

- Costs of regular software upgrades if using proprietary software
- Broadband Internet fees if sending images beyond the practice
- Servicing contract or regular service costs
- Replacement parts and upgrades to digital radiography system
- Computer upgrades, particularly with respect to storage capacity
- Ongoing IT support

13.19 Ongoing costs of operating a digital radiography system.

- Film costs (including wastage of out-of-date or damaged films)
- Cost of chemicals and hazardous waste disposal/silver trap (significant)
- Cost of automatic processor maintenance, ± costs of darkroom and additional ventilation
- No further need for film envelopes or stickers
- Saved space for storage of films in envelopes
- Saved time spent filing envelopes and searching for old films
- No lost films
- With some digital systems there is increased efficiency in taking images
- Decreased repeat exposures (radiation and time benefits)

13.20 Potential savings when moving to a digital radiography system.

Some suppliers include various services and items in a single package and fee. In this situation it is well worth asking for a specification of the individual items to be aware of exactly what is being purchased. It may be possible to source identical items of hardware (servers, monitors, etc.) elsewhere at reduced costs. There are also some options for free-of-charge open-source DICOM viewing software and PACS systems available on the Internet. This removes the need for licence fees and software update costs, but some IT knowledge is required to set up and network equipment to these systems.

Managing imaging services

Legal and safety considerations

X-rays are a type of ionizing radiation. Exposure to ionizing radiation can cause damage to living tissue, hence rigorous legal requirements exist to limit the damaging effects of X-rays whilst optimizing their diagnostic potential. This section presents an *overview* of legal considerations in the use of ionizing radiations in veterinary practice. The reader is referred to the Further reading section and to their Radiation Protection Advisor (RPA) for definitive legal advice.

Radiation protection with respect to X-rays relies on three principles:

- There should be clear justification for carrying out the X-ray procedure
- Any exposure of personnel should be kept as low as reasonably practicable
- No dose limit should be exceeded.

An organizational infrastructure must be in place to make sure that these principles are upheld in veterinary practice (see below). More details can be found in the *Guidance Notes for the Safe Use of Ionising Radiations in Veterinary Practice (Ionising Radiations Regulations (IRR)* 1999) (Figure 13.21), which should be available to all members of the practice.

Risk assessment

It is a legal requirement that a prior risk assessment is made when a practice contemplates using ionizing radiation. The risk assessment must be sufficient to demonstrate that:

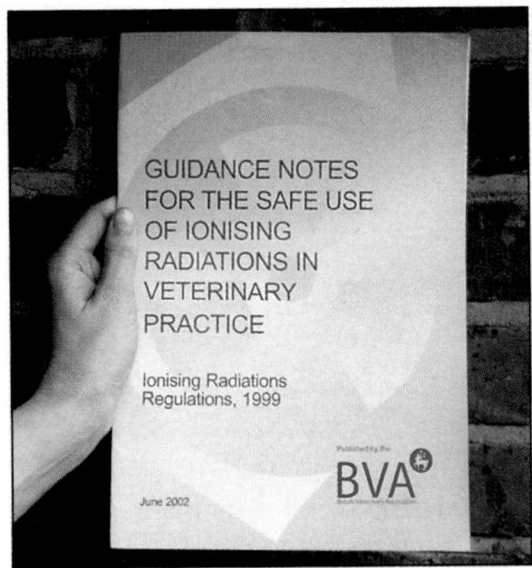

13.21 Guidance notes for the safe use of ionizing radiations in veterinary practice are published by and available from BVA. These notes outline the legal requirements for establishing the use of X-rays within a practice and should be readily available to all members of staff.

- All hazards with the potential to cause a radiation accident have been identified
- The nature and magnitude of the risks have been evaluated.

In practical terms, the hazards in a veterinary practice generally include the X-ray machine itself, and any design features, arrangement, working practice or piece of equipment that could lead to an increased risk of exposure to X-rays from the machine.

Where the risk assessment shows the existence of a risk of a reasonably foreseeable radiation accident, the radiation employer shall take all reasonable steps to:

- Prevent any such accident
- Limit the consequences of any such accident
- Provide employees with such instruction and training as is necessary to restrict their exposure.

If there is any doubt as to what constitutes a potential risk within the practice, the Radiation Protection Advisor (RPA) should be contacted (see below for further information). A sample risk assessment can be found at the end of this chapter.

Notification of work with ionizing radiations

It is a further legal requirement that the Health and Safety Executive (HSE) must be notified in writing at least 28 days prior to commencement of work using ionizing radiations for the first time. The letter should be sent by post or fax to the local HSE office and should include the following information:

- Name and address of radiation employer, with telephone, fax and e-mail details
- Address of premises where the work is to be carried out
- Nature of the business of the employer
- Category of the source of the ionizing radiation (in this case: 'electrical equipment, X-ray machine')
- Whether or not any source is to be used at any premises other than the address of the work premises
- Dates of notification and commencement of the work activity.

A sample letter is shown at the end of the chapter. If any subsequent changes are made (such as a change of premises) to the work with ionizing radiations, these must be notified to the HSE immediately.

As required by Regulation 5 of the IRR 1999, the use of X-ray sets for veterinary diagnostic or investigational purposes is covered by a generic authorization. The conditions incorporated in the generic authorization are designed to ensure that any risk of exposure to ionizing radiation arising from the specified practice is limited. Radiation employers who rely on the generic authorization must comply with the conditions set out in the authorization, and must also comply with all relevant duties under the IRR 1999. The generic authorization can be downloaded from www.hse.gov.uk. An HSE information sheet regarding prior authorization under the IRR 1999 can be downloaded from www.hse.gov.uk.

If a practice has been in business for a number of years and has been using ionizing radiation for some time, then the practice should telephone the HSE to obtain confirmation of registration. The practice should note the name of the individual with whom they spoke and also the date of the call. Additional written confirmation of registration can also be requested. Additional information is available on the HSE website (www.hse.gov.uk).

The Radiation Protection Advisor

A Radiation Protection Advisor (RPA) is a person who has received specific training in Radiation Protection Practice and holds either a relevant valid certificate of competence or a specific National or Scottish Vocational Qualification. A list of RPAs is available from www.srp-uk.org. Note that the RPA selected must be suitable for the working conditions for which he/she is being appointed, and hence must have appropriate knowledge and experience of veterinary work. The practice should make the necessary enquiries.

It is a legal requirement that the RPA is appointed by the practice *in writing* (see end of chapter). The letter must include the scope of the activities on which advice is required (Figure 13.22). The practice does not need to notify HSE of this appointment. The RPA will normally make visits to the practice and will issue reports. The frequency of these visits will be discussed and agreed between the practice and the RPA. If the practice makes a change to equipment, workload or working practice, then the RPA should be informed and will decide whether a visit is necessary or not. Inspectors under the RCVS Practice Standards Scheme will ask to see the last RPA report and evidence that any recommendations have been acted upon. Routine RPA visits are strongly advised by the RCVS Practice Standards Scheme.

The Radiation Protection Supervisor

The Radiation Protection Supervisor (RPS) is generally someone that works within the practice and is present on the premises. They must command sufficient authority to permit them to supervise the work so that it is performed in accordance with the local rules. They must have an adequate understanding of the requirement of the IRR 1999 and know what to do in an emergency. The radiation employer must appoint one or more RPSs *in writing*. The duties of an RPS are outlined in Figure 13.23.

Matters in respect of which an RPA must be consulted by a radiation employer:

- The implementation of requirements as to controlled and supervised areas.
- The prior examination of plans for installations and acceptance into service of new or modified sources of ionizing radiations in relation to any engineering controls, design features, safety features and warning devices provided to restrict exposures to ionizing radiations.
- The regular calibration of equipment provided for monitoring levels of ionizing radiations and the regular checking that such equipment is serviceable and correctly used.
- The periodic examination and testing of engineering controls, design features, safety features and warning devices and regular checking of systems of work provided to restrict exposure to ionizing radiations.
- (Ionising Radiations Regulations, 1999, SI 1999/3232)

In addition the radiation employer is required to seek the advice of an RPA on such matters as:

- Risk Assessment required by Regulation 7.
- Designation of controlled and supervised areas as required by Regulation 16, except where there is good reason to consider that such areas are not required, for example based on advice from the supplier of the radiation source or written guidance from an authoritative body.
- The conduct of various investigations required by the Regulations e.g. should any member of staff exceed, or appear likely to exceed the formal investigation dose level.
- The drawing up of contingency plans required by Regulation 12.
- The dose assessment and recording required by Regulation 21.
- (Work with Ionising Radiations, Ionising Radiations Regulations 1999, Approved Code of Practice and Guidance L121, paragraph 217)

The scope will also include appropriate advice on:

- Provision of training as required by Regulation 14.
- Appointment of Radiation Protection Supervisors as required by Regulation 17.
- Local Rules and written systems of work as required by Regulation 8 and Regulation 17.
- Selection and use of personal protective equipment as required by Regulation 8.
- Arrangements for outside workers as required by Regulation 18 and Regulation 21.

13.22 Duties of the Radiation Protection Advisor.

The Ionising Radiations Regulations 1999, Regulation 17 (4) states that a radiation employer shall:

a. Appoint one or more suitable Radiation Protection Supervisors for the purposes of securing compliance with the Regulations in respect of work carried out in any area made subject to local rules
b. Set down in the local rules the names of such individuals so appointed.

The RPS is the person with 'on site' responsibility for radiation protection matters, ensuring adherence to the arrangements made by the radiation employer and in particular, supervising the arrangements set out in local rules. However the legal responsibility remains with the radiation employer and cannot be delegated to the RPS.
RPSs should receive appropriate training (as required under the Ionising Radiations Regulations 1999, Regulation 14) to fulfil the task adequately, reflecting the complexity of the work undertaken. Training by the RPA may be sufficient in some cases.
They should be directly involved with the work with ionizing radiations, preferably in a line management position that will allow them to exercise close supervision to ensure that the work is done in accordance with the local rules, though they need not be present all the time.
They should:

a. Know and understand the requirements of the Ionising Radiations Regulations 1999 and local rules
b. Command sufficient respect from the people doing the work as will allow them to exercise the necessary supervision of radiation protection
c. Understand the necessary precautions to be taken in the work which is being done and the extent to which these precautions will restrict exposures
d. Know what to do in an emergency.

They will liaise with the Radiation Protection Adviser and the radiation employer on matters of radiation protection.
It is good practice to confirm appointments to the individuals in writing providing them with sufficient information about the role.
Appointment as RPS may prove time-consuming and this should be recognized by allowing suitable time and resources to enable the duties of the role to be met.

The following list of duties includes most of those likely to be required of the RPS:

1. Formulation and revision of local rules and systems of work.
2. Liaising with Radiation Protection Adviser on matters of radiation protection.
3. Coordinating the implementation of advice from the Radiation Protection Adviser.
4. Ensuring that new and existing staff receive adequate radiation protection information, instruction and training and that this is recorded.
5. Implementing the appropriate personnel monitoring scheme within the practice, involving the distribution and collection of dosimeters, maintaining staff awareness of exposure levels and that abnormal dosimeter readings are reported to the Radiation Protection Adviser and investigated.
6. Ensuring that environmental monitors are checked and calibrated regularly.
7. Involved in the preparation of contingency plans and ensure that staff are able to implement these effectively.
8. Ensuring that accidents and near misses involving radiation are immediately reported to the Radiation Protection Adviser and investigated.

13.23 The duties of a Radiation Protection Supervisor. (continued) ▶

The following list of duties includes most of those likely to be required of the RPS (continued):

9. Monitor that:
   a. Adequate precautions are taken regarding any special, existing or new radiation hazard.
   b. Plant equipment and processes are being maintained and records are kept, e.g. servicing records, equipment faults, and radiographic exposures.
   c. A high standard of housekeeping is maintained.
   d. Staff are suitably informed and trained.
   e. Adequate radiation protection records are being maintained as required by statutory provisions or employer policy.
   f. Safe working practices, risk assessments and systems of work are being compiled and complied with.
   g. Personal protective equipment appropriate to the task is available and used.
   h. Appropriate methods of monitoring are implemented (in discussion with the Radiation Protection Adviser) and personal dosimetry is provided, maintained in good repair and used correctly.
   i. Periodically reviewing radiation protection procedures.

The safety organisation should be such that in the absence of the RPS for an extended period, arrangements for providing cover should be implemented so that there is always a nominated person to take on RPS duties.

13.23 (continues) The duties of a Radiation Protection Supervisor.

Local Rules

Once a controlled area has been designated, the radiation employer must write a set of Local Rules, which are appropriate to the radiation risk of X-rays and relevant to the nature of veterinary radiography. The RPA will consult with the employer to assist with this legally required task.

KEY POINTS

- The Local Rules *must* be clearly displayed to all staff, and staff involved with radiography should sign to indicate that they have read and understood the Local Rules.
- The Local Rules must be reviewed once per year or more often if advised by the RPA.
- Note that separate Local Rules are required for any separate dental X-ray equipment.

The Local Rules must contain the following information:

- **General introduction:** This indicates that radiography must be carried out in accordance with the requirements of the Ionising Radiations Regulations 1999 and the Approved Code of Practice 'Work with ionizing radiation – Approved code of practice and guidance' and should follow the advice given in 'Guidance notes for the safe use of ionising radiations in veterinary practice'
- **Radiation Protection Advisor (RPA):** The name, address and telephone number of the person appointed
- **Radiation Protection Supervisor (RPS):** The name of the person appointed and the nature of their duties (to ensure that work is carried out in accordance with the Local Rules)
- **Controlled area:** Identification of the controlled area and how it is demarcated; when the controlled area exists and how access is restricted. Arrangement for environmental monitoring
- **X-ray equipment:** Maintenance arrangements. Procedure for reporting faults
- **Personal protective equipment (PPE):** Arrangements for use, storage and checking
- **Dosimetry:** Arrangements for personal and fixed dose monitoring, including where and when dosimeters should be worn and how they should be stored when not in use. Action to be taken in the event of loss or damage of dosimeters. Annual dose (in mSv) which is not expected to be exceeded by any member of staff
- **Formal dose investigation level:** The dose level at which action will be taken if exceeded must be stated. Action to be taken must be listed
- **Contingency plan:** Action to be taken in the event of any fault or suspected fault with the X-ray machine (this is normally to isolate the machine from the electrical supply) or other incident (e.g. fire). Requirement to report the incident, and action taken, to the RPS for further investigation
- **Workload:** Type of work undertaken. Maximum workload per week (in mAs). Action to be taken if this is exceeded
- **Records:** Details to be recorded for each exposure made
- **Written arrangements:** These should include the following statements:
  - The purpose of the written arrangements is to ensure that persons involved in radiography receive doses of ionizing radiations which are as low as is reasonably practicable
  - Radiography to be undertaken only when clinically indicated
  - Policy for patient restraint to keep manual holding to an absolute minimum
  - Availability and use of positioning aids
  - Restriction of access to the controlled area to the minimum number of persons necessary to carry out the procedure. Those present should stand behind a suitable barrier or at least 2 metres from the path of the primary X-ray beam
  - The need to isolate the X-ray machine from the electrical supply after each radiographic session
  - Unrestricted access is permitted when the X-ray machine is isolated from the electrical supply and the warning sign is not illuminated
  - The radiographer has authority over all persons involved in the procedure and must ensure that the procedure is carried out in accordance with the local rules and written arrangements
  - The sequence of actions to be followed for each procedure.

A sample set of Local Rules is provided at the end of this chapter.

Personal dose monitoring

It is a legal requirement that there is a system of personal dose monitoring for all persons entering the controlled area, as agreed with the appointed RPA. Dosimeters should be worn by any person with access to the controlled areas and this includes temporary staff and visitors to the practice.

> **KEY POINT**
>
> The dosimeter should be worn whilst working in and around the controlled area, but should not be taken outside the practice. Dosimeters must not be exposed to external sources of radiation or heat.

- Dosimeters (Figure 13.24) may be either film badges or thermoluminescent dosimeters (TLDs). A film badge contains a small piece of film sandwiched between various filters (thick plastic, aluminium, and tin with a thin lead foil) to enable the detection of different types of radiation. A TLD generally consists of a small chip of lithium fluoride in a plastic holder. X-rays are absorbed by the lithium fluoride and the dose information can be measured in a dosimetry laboratory.
- Some newer dosimeters contain a USB stick, to enable rapid extraction of dose information in a digital format.
- Dosimeters must be supplied by an approved dosimetry service, and are usually issued for 1–3 months at a time, after which the dose levels are evaluated and a replacement dosimeter supplied.
- Records of the doses must be maintained for at least 2 years, although in practice it is usually advisable to keep them indefinitely. If requested, records must be made available to the person to whom they relate.
- Personal dosimeters should normally be worn on the trunk and should not be repositioned when protective clothing is put on.
- Additional dosimeters may occasionally be recommended (such as extremity dosimeters in the form of a ring to measure the dose to the hands).
- It is vital to prevent any dosimeter being inadvertently exposed to ionizing radiations when not worn by the person:
  - Store carefully when not being worn
  - Never leave inside a controlled area
  - Avoid exposure to excessive heat or sunlight.

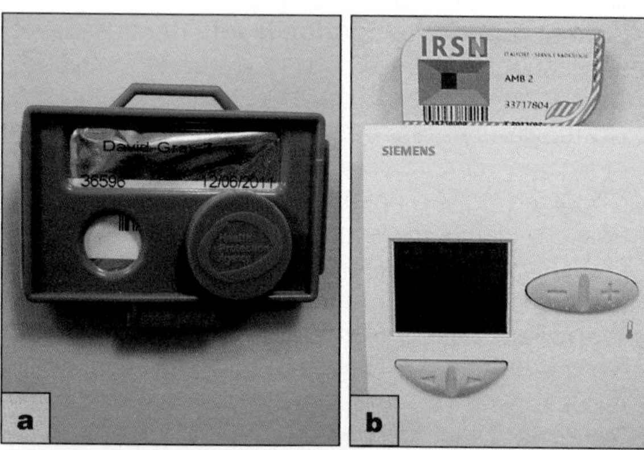

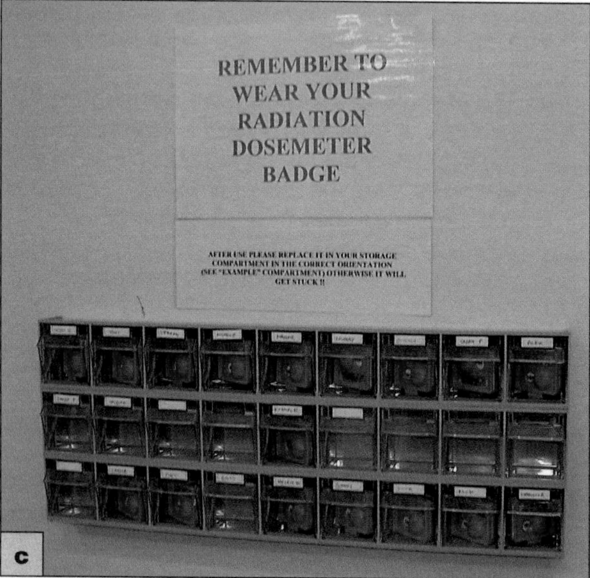

13.24 Personal dose monitoring is a legal requirement. **(a)** A thermoluminescent dosimeter (TLD) is shown here. TLDs are marked with the wearer's name and must only be used by that person. **(b)** In addition a TLD or a film badge (as shown here) can be used to monitor environmental radiation levels within various areas of the room. **(c)** It can be very useful to have a system of pigeonholes or a clipboard area to keep the dosimeters together and facilitate return and replacement after wear. The storage system should be located in an area of the practice sufficiently remote from the controlled area.

> **KEY POINT**
>
> Dosimeters must only be worn by the person to whom they were issued and never shared between staff.

Pregnant and breast-feeding employees

There are several legal requirements regarding pregnant and breast-feeding employees to limit their risks from ionizing radiation exposure. These concern dose limits and potential risks and should be discussed with the RPA. Staff coming into contact with ionizing radiation should be advised to tell the relevant supervisor as soon as they become aware that they are pregnant, in order to limit these risks at an early stage. Advice should be sought from the HSE publication *Working Safely with Ionising Radiations: Guidelines for Expectant or Breast Feeding Mothers*.

Daily and other regular quality control procedures

There are many procedures that must be performed on a regular basis to maintain image quality.

- Automatic processor:
  - Each morning the automatic processor should be given time to warm up and a test film passed through the system. Chemical levels and the temperature of the developer should be checked
  - Any film faults should be investigated as and when identified
  - The automatic processor must be cleaned regularly and according to the manufacturer's instructions; training is often required for this.

- X-ray machine:
  - If recommended by the manufacturer, warm-up exposures should be performed
  - It is a legal requirement that the X-ray machine is serviced annually and written evidence of a satisfactory report must be obtained and archived.
- Screens (non-digital):
  - These require regular cleaning according to level of use and whenever marks appear on the films. Screens should be cleaned gently with a soft lint-free cloth and a solution containing an antistatic agent and a detergent. Individuals within the practice should be identified and trained to perform this correctly
  - The cassette should then be left open to dry in a vertical position
- Imaging plates (digital):
  - These should be erased daily, usually at the start of the day
  - Cleaning may be necessary from time to time, following the manufacturer's recommendations.

The radiography procedure

Many factors at the time of taking the radiographic exposure affect the standards of a practice's radiography department. Good-quality images first time around will improve personnel safety, practice efficiency, and clinical diagnosis. An exposure chart indicating recommended exposures for different examinations and patient sizes should be available and regularly updated.

Key considerations include:

- Appropriate patient restraint and control of respiratory motion for thoracic and abdominal exposures
- Patient positioning to obtain correct radiographic views
- Appropriate choice of cassette
- Careful collimation to include a region of non-exposed film around the edge of each exposed area
- Use of a technique chart and measuring calipers (see Figure 13.9)
- Primary labelling of the image with patient identification and positional markers (see earlier); sticky labels or marker pens are not acceptable as standard forms of labelling
- Assessment of the end result for suitable exposure factors and film faults.

Storing and sharing images

Standard radiographic films

Archiving and storage

Radiographic films are generally stored in X-ray envelopes and then in a shelving system. It is important to institute a reliable method of labelling envelopes to aid retrieval. It is also advisable to give a member of staff responsibility for filing the cases and maintaining a well-run archive. Fire poses a severe risk to a radiographic archive and adequate precautions should be taken.

Digital images

Radiographic images require archiving, just as standard radiographic films need to be filed on a shelf. One of the main advantages of a digital system is the ease of archiving and retrieving radiographs. DICOM images can be large files, however, and it is essential to consider long-term storage requirements from the outset. A secure back-up of all images is required for the RCVS Practice Standards Scheme.

Image data archiving and PACS systems

Digital image archives vary in their complexity, but generally need to include:

- A network to send images from the radiography system to the archive and to retrieve them at various locations within the practice and beyond
- Adequate primary data storage (usually an on-site server)
- A back-up storage system (ideally off site, or at least in a different physical location to the primary system; may be web-based)
- Archiving and viewing software on workstations.

Radiographic images are sent from the digital radiography system to the local server and are also regularly and automatically routed to the back-up system. The local server will use software that allows archiving and retrieval of cases. Images are then retrieved from the local server to be viewed on workstations around the practice. These workstations utilize DICOM viewing software (the DICOM viewer). The combination of all the computer hardware, software and networking to achieve these tasks is collectively known as a picture archiving and communication system (PACS).

Choosing a digital archiving method

It is important to be aware that digital images take up significant space on a server. Each radiographic image is typically 12–20 Mb. The long-term data storage requirements will need to be calculated before investing in an archiving system.

If the practice anticipates a large radiographic caseload, then it is worth investing in a dedicated RAID server, which stores data using an internal back-up. This should stand alone from the practice management system (PMS) server, and IT advice should be sought as to which type of RAID server is appropriate.

KEY POINT

Low radiographic caseloads could be stored in house on external hard drives (with a back-up). CDs and DVDs are not recommended, as they become easily damaged or lost.

In the situation where an off-site data storage company is used to back-up any images, it should be verified that images are being stored in DICOM format and whether any sort of compression is being used. Excessive compression (especially 'lossy compression') can seriously affect image quality.

Another option is not to store any images within the practice at all. All images can be sent to a remote 'cloud-based' PACS and can then be accessed from any location using an Internet browser. This is a relatively new possibility and means that software and hardware costs are dramatically reduced, and that image sharing is easy. It is vital to have a fast broadband system before considering this option, and care should be taken in selecting a provider of a cloud-based system.

Regardless of the archiving system chosen, the legal necessity to keep medical images of all patients for specific periods of time must be taken into account.

Network considerations within the practice

Most practices have an established IT infrastructure for their practice management system (PMS). When considering installing a digital radiography system and establishing a PACS it is important to ask an IT expert to review the network capabilities. It may be necessary to upgrade some areas of performance to avoid compromising the smooth running of the PMS.

Some manufacturers provide image viewing solutions that can be linked to the PMS, allowing access to images at the same time as the medical record. This can be helpful, but is not a necessary requirement. There are many excellent and cost-effective solutions available, whereby access to high-quality radiographic images can be provided on the same computer workstation, using DICOM viewing software rather than via the PMS. Only DICOM images can be used for radiographic diagnosis: image quality remains the most important factor and the type of image file has an important effect on this.

KEY POINT

Including DICOM data in the PMS has the potential to result in a considerable extra burden on the PMS in terms of processor requirements and data storage. Including .jpg image files in the PMS does not allow them to be used for diagnosis but can be useful for demonstrating images to clients in the consulting room.

Sharing images within the practice environment

One of the great advantages of digital radiography is the ability to view the images at multiple locations within the practice and beyond. When establishing a digital system the question of where the images are going to be viewed (consulting rooms, theatre, branch practices, veterinary surgeons' homes, etc.) should be carefully considered. There are many solutions available, including web access to a practice's in-house PACS, a remote 'cloud-based' PACS, direct DICOM send, DICOM query/retrieve functions and file sharing. It is important to consider working practices before making a choice.

KEY POINT

Care must be taken in entering patient data into the different fields when registering a patient for a digital imaging examination. The patient ID number, patient name, client name, etc., must be correctly entered for each examination as this has enormous implications for image retrieval from the PACS at a later time.

Sharing images with clients

Clients are more frequently requesting copies of medical images of their pets. This can be easily achieved by burning a CD or DVD and most PACS have a simple function to do this. Alternatively, some PACS with web access allow password access to a particular case, and the client can be emailed a link to view their pet's radiographs. For client personal use, the DICOM file images can also usually be exported as a compressed format .jpg file, which should be compatible with most home computer software.

Teleradiology and telemedicine

Teleradiology is the practice of transferring digital radiological images and associated data via the Internet between locations for the purpose of interpretation or clinical review. This may include transferring images to a reporting service or to a referral centre prior to sending a patient for a consultation.

Telemedicine broadens the service to include remote interpretation of data such as laboratory results and ECG traces, and also provides other specialist advice on clinical cases (e.g. a surgical opinion, a neurological opinion).

The rapid move to digital imaging in veterinary medicine, coupled with improvements in telecommunications, is leading to increased utilization of remote specialist services. This has the potential to improve patient care and augment collaboration between veterinary colleagues. There are, however, some important considerations for practice standards. Of particular note is that images must be transferred in DICOM format and compression techniques (to reduce file size) must only be used with caution. There are many teleradiology/telemedicine providers available and it is important that the practice knows who it is dealing with, what type of service is offered, and where the provider is located. Location of the provider (UK *versus* overseas) may have legal and licensing implications, and many of these are currently unresolved.

Record-keeping

Careful record-keeping is part of good radiographic practice. A hardback logbook or digital record should be maintained in an accessible position, close to the X-ray control panel. Staff should complete a record for each exposure of each patient:

- Patient identification
- Breed
- Area exposed/view
- Exposure factors
- Type of film/grid/screen
- Date
- Quality of the resultant radiograph
- Names of any personnel present
- A special note should be made if the animal was held or restrained manually.

KEY POINT

Not only is record-keeping important for safety reasons, but over time it will also provide a valuable reference manual when radiographing other patients of similar proportions.

Handling and disposing of chemicals

It is a legal requirement that all film processing chemicals must be stored safely and disposed of in an appropriate manner. Used chemicals should be disposed of as hazardous waste. Unless waste material is disposed of by a registered contractor, the advice of the local water authorities should be obtained and recorded. Silver traps may be used in accordance with guidance/approval from the relevant local water authority.

Staff training

A well run radiography department very much depends on the staff. It is worth investing in regular staff training (in-house or CPD courses) to enable good radiographic practice. Areas of responsibility should be allocated to key staff. Ongoing clinical radiology training is vital for veterinary surgeons and, where applicable, nursing staff in order to achieve accuracy in radiological diagnosis. A selection of good up-to-date reference materials is useful. Teleradiology can also be very helpful in this respect.

Acknowledgements

Victoria Johnson would like to thank the following for their help with the section on Radiography: Anna Williams (Radiographer, Queens Veterinary School Hospital, Cambridge); Tony Butterworth (Radiation Protection Adviser/Laser Safety Adviser/Health & Safety Adviser, University of Bristol); and Kate Bradley (Radiology Department, Langford Veterinary Services, University of Bristol). The author and editors gratefully acknowledge the following, images from which appear in this chapter: Alfreton Park Veterinary Hospital; Buckley House Veterinary Surgery; Clerkenwell Animal Hospital; Ecole Nationale Vétérinaire d'Alfort; Mill House Veterinary Surgery and Hospital.

Further reading

Barr F and Kirberger R (2006) *BSAVA Manual of Canine and Feline Musculoskeletal Imaging*. BSAVA Publications, Gloucester

British Veterinary Association (2002) *Guidance Notes for the Safe Use of Ionising Radiations in Veterinary Practice: Ionising Radiation Regulations 1999*. Available from www.bva.co.uk

Dennis R, Northwood S, Lhermette P, Girling S and Butler J (2011) Diagnostic imaging. In: *BSAVA Textbook of Veterinary Nursing, 5th edn*, ed. B Cooper *et. al.*, pp. 442–507

HSE (2000) *Work with Ionising Radiation: Approved Code of Practice and Guidance*. HSE publication L121. HSE Books, Sudbury, Suffolk

HSE (2001) *Working Safely with Ionising Radiations: Guidelines for Expectant or Breast Feeding Mothers*. Available from www.hse.gov.uk

Johnson VS (2013) Teleradiology: practicalities and implications. *In Practice* **33**, 180–185

Lo WY, Hornof WJ, Zwingenberger AZ and Robertson ID (2009) Multiscale image processing and antiscatter grids in digital radiography. *Veterinary Radiology and Ultrasound* **50**, 569–576

McConnell F and Holloway A (in preparation) *BSAVA Manual of Canine and Feline Radiography and Radiology: A Foundation Manual*. BSAVA Publications, Gloucester

O'Brien R and Barr F (2009) *BSAVA Manual of Canine and Feline Abdominal Imaging*. BSAVA Publications, Gloucester

Royal College of Radiologists (2010) *Standards for the Provision of Teleradiology within the United Kingdom*. Available from www.rcr.ac.uk

Royal College of Veterinary Surgeons. *RCVS Practice Standards Scheme Manual*. Available from www.rcvs.org.uk

Schwarz T and Johnson V (2008) *BSAVA Manual of Canine and Feline Thoracic Imaging*. BSAVA Publications, Gloucester

Sample risk assessment, letters and Local Rules ▶

<table>
<tr><td colspan="2">In accordance with Regulation 7(1) of the Ionising Radiations Regulations 1999, a prior risk assessment must be completed before a radiation employer commences a new activity involving work with ionising radiation for the purposes of identifying the measures required to restrict exposure of employees or other persons to ionising radiation.</td></tr>
<tr><td>Activity/area/task</td><td></td></tr>
<tr><td>Name of assessor(s)</td><td></td></tr>
<tr><td>Date of assessment</td><td></td></tr>
<tr><td>Location of work</td><td></td></tr>
<tr><td>Date work commenced</td><td></td></tr>
<tr><td>Nature of hazard</td><td></td></tr>
<tr><td>Relevant legislation and guidance</td><td></td></tr>
<tr><td>All persons exposed to hazard</td><td></td></tr>
<tr><td>Matters to be considered in risk assessment</td><td></td></tr>
<tr><td>The nature of the sources of ionizing radiation to be used</td><td></td></tr>
<tr><td>Estimated radiation dose rates to which anyone can be exposed (including consideration of pregnant/breast-feeding mothers)</td><td></td></tr>
<tr><td>The results of any previous personal dosimetry or area monitoring relevant to the proposed work</td><td></td></tr>
<tr><td>Advice from the manufacturer or supplier of equipment about its safe use and maintenance</td><td></td></tr>
<tr><td>Engineering control measures and design features already in place or planned</td><td></td></tr>
<tr><td>Any planned systems of work</td><td></td></tr>
<tr><td>The effectiveness and suitability of personal protective equipment to be provided</td><td></td></tr>
<tr><td>The extent of unrestricted access to working areas where dose rates or contamination levels are likely to be significant</td><td></td></tr>
<tr><td>Possible accident situations, their likelihood and potential severity (including dose investigation level)</td><td></td></tr>
<tr><td>The consequences of possible failure of control measures such as electrical interlocks and warning devices – or systems of work (including maintenance and testing schedules)</td><td></td></tr>
<tr><td>Steps to prevent identified accident situations or limit their consequences</td><td></td></tr>
<tr><td>Action/additional control measures required</td><td></td></tr>
<tr><td>Comments</td><td></td></tr>
<tr><td>Date of review and reason (regular interval/significant change/no longer valid)</td><td></td></tr>
<tr><td colspan="2">Duties of Manufacturers etc. of Articles for use In Work with Ionising Radiation
In accordance with Regulation 31(2) of The Ionising Radiation Regulation 1999 where a person erects or installs an article for work, being work with ionizing radiation, he shall:
a. Undertake a critical examination of the way in which it was erected or installed for the purpose of ensuring, in particular, that:
i. the safety features and warning devices operate correctly; and
ii. there is sufficient protection for persons from exposure to ionizing radiation
b. Consult with the RPA appointed by the employer with regard to the nature and extent of any critical examination and the results of that examination
c. Provide the radiation employer with adequate information about proper use, testing and maintenance of the article.
The duty to ensure that the critical examination is carried out rests with the employer who erects or installs the article, not the user.</td></tr>
</table>

An example of a risk assessment for working with ionizing radiation.

Name of radiation employer
Practice address
Practice telephone/fax number
Practice e-mail address

RPA address and contact details
Date

Dear *(insert name of RPA)*

Re: Appointment of Radiation Protection Adviser for *(name of practice)*
Under the Ionising Radiations Regulations 1999, we wish to formally appoint you as the Radiation Protection Advisor for this veterinary practice as of *(insert date)*.

As the appointed Radiation Protection Adviser you will provide advice on matters in respect of which a Radiation Protection Adviser must be consulted by the radiation employer, as detailed in the document attached.

The radiation employer is *(insert name of the practice)* and the address(es) of the premises where your advice will be required is (are) *(include all locations where the advice of RPA will be required)*.

The scope of the activities for which we require advice is: use of X-ray-generating equipment for small animal veterinary radiography.

Yours sincerely
(Insert name and signature of radiation employer)

An example of an appointment letter for a Radiation Protection Advisor.

Name, address and contact details
of radiation employer

Date
Re: Proposed use of Ionizing Radiations at the above premises commencing on
(insert date – at least 28 days hence from the date of this letter)

Dear Sir or Madam,

In accordance with Regulation 6(2) and Schedule 2 of the Ionising Radiations Regulations 1999, I am writing to notify the HSE that it is proposed to commence work with ionizing radiations at the premises *(address, telephone and fax numbers and e-mail address where work will be carried out).*

The business of the radiation employer is veterinary practice for small animal patients. The category of the source of ionizing radiations is electrical equipment (one X-ray generator). The source of ionising radiations will only be used at this address. The date of notification is *(insert date of letter)* and commencement of work will be from *(insert date – at least 28 days hence from the date of this letter).*

Please contact us for further details if required.

Yours sincerely,
(Insert name and signature of radiation employer)

A sample letter to the HSE, notifying them of work using ionizing radiations. This must be sent at least 28 days prior to the start of work with ionizing radiations. Local office details are at www.hse.gov.uk

Local Rules for the Use of Ionizing Radiation

Address of premises: ....

Date: ....

In accordance with the Ionising Radiations Regulations 1999 (IRR99), the purpose of these Local Rules is to set out the key arrangements for restricting exposure, enabling radiography to be carried out safely in the veterinary practice.

Appointments

The appointed Radiation Protection Advisor (RPA) for the Veterinary Practice is *(insert name and contact details).*
The appointed Radiation Protection Supervisor (RPS) for the Veterinary Practice is *(insert name and contact details).*
The radiation employer is *(insert name and contact details).*

Work undertaken

The type of work to be undertaken includes radiography of a wide variety of animal species, excluding humans. The maximum workload per week will be 500 radiographic exposures, with the milliampere second (mAs) in each case varying from a minimum of 4 mAs up to a maximum of 150 mAs.

Identification of designated areas

In accordance with Regulation 16(1)(a) IRR99, the area *(describe)* is designated a Controlled Area when an X-ray generator is located within the room and connected to the electricity supply.
In accordance with Regulation 18(1)(a) IRR99, radiation warning signs shall be placed at each point of access to the controlled area, indicating the nature of the radiation sources (X-rays), and the risks arising from such sources *(for example, an illuminated sign which reads 'Controlled Area – X-rays' and, 'Do Not Enter' during radiographic exposures).*
All work within the Controlled Area(s) should follow the written safe system of work.
The room supervisor in each case is the radiographer in charge, who will ensure compliance with the local rules and safe system of work.

Entry to the Controlled Area

- Entry to the Controlled Area is restricted to personnel who have undergone the radiography induction training at the veterinary practice, (which includes the information on good practice given in the Veterinary Guidance Notes for the Ionising Radiations Regulations 2002), read and understood these local rules and written a safe system of work and signed the declaration indicating they have done so.
- Entry the Controlled Area is restricted to persons aged 18 years old or older.
- Pregnant members of staff must not enter the Controlled Area without prior consultation with the RPS and RPA.
- All persons entering the Controlled Area must wear their personal dosimeter badge in accordance with their instruction and training.
- Every person in the veterinary practice has a duty to observe the Local Rules relating to the Controlled Area and failure to comply may result in disciplinary procedures.

Sources of ionizing radiations – X-ray equipment

- The X-ray equipment may only be operated by suitably trained authorized personnel.
- The X-ray equipment must be isolated from the electrical supply when not in use.
- The X-ray tube head must not be touched or held whilst an exposure is being made.
- Any fault, suspected fault, defect or damage must be immediately reported to the RPS or to one of the radiographers, who will then inform the RPS.
- The X-ray equipment should be regularly maintained in accordance with the manufacturer's recommendations and will be regularly serviced, at least annually.
- If the X-ray equipment is changed, modified, or if the circumstances of its operation alter (e.g. a significant increase in workload) the Radiation Protection Advisor (RPA) must be informed so that radiation protection requirements are reviewed.
- The following details shall be recorded for each exposure made: patient identification, the body part under examination, kV/mAs/FFD, whether or not a grid was used, and the number of exposures taken.

Personal protective equipment

Appropriate lead rubber aprons, lead rubber gloves and mitts, and lead rubber thyroid protectors are available in the radiography room, and must be stored appropriately when not in use. These should be used in accordance with the written System of Work (Appendix 1).
All personal protective equipment will be visually checked for cracks or tears on regular basis by the radiographers and these checks recorded; in addition all lead-based personal protective equipment will be regularly screened for any defects and results recorded.

Radiation dose monitoring

Authorized personnel who are required to work in the Controlled Area must be issued with the appropriate personal dosimeter badge *(list those issued).*

- Badges must be worn in accordance with instruction and training whenever radiography is being performed.
- Badges must be treated with care and returned to the RPS in accordance with protocol *(e.g. on the 1st of each month/each quarter).*
- If a dosimeter badge is damaged, laundered or exposed the RPS must be notified immediately.
- In compliance with Regulation 8(7) IRR99, the dose investigation level is *(state this e.g. 0.2 mSv/3 month period for a whole body badge).* If this is exceeded a formal investigation will be carried out, in consultation with the RPS and RPA.

An example of Local Rules. Proposed dates for, and records of, reviews should be appended to the document. (continues) ▶

Contingency arrangements

In the event of a fault or suspected overexposure to staff or patients:

- The X-ray equipment must be switched off and disconnected from the electrical supply immediately and the RPS informed
- A prominent notice must be fixed to the X-ray machine declaring that it must not be used until further notice
- An account of the incident must be documented including all details of the exposure so that an estimated dose may be calculated if necessary
- The RPA must be informed.

Arrangements for pregnant staff

Female staff should notify their employer in writing as soon as possible if they are, or suspect that they are, pregnant.
In compliance with IRR99 and The Management of Health and Safety at Work Regulations 1999, special consideration must be given to the type of work pregnant members of staff are expected to carry out.
Specific risk assessments must be written for all procedures involving sources of radiation, to ensure the dose limit to the fetus is unlikely to exceed 1 mSv during the reminder of the pregnancy. This is equivalent to a dose of 2mSv to the surface of the abdomen of the pregnant member of staff.
Pregnant members of staff must not enter the Controlled Area without prior consultation with the RPS and RPA.

DECLARATION

I have received, read and understood the Local Radiation Safety Rules for *(insert the name of the Veterinary Practice).*

Print name:..

Sign:.. Date:..............................

CONFIRMATION SIGNATURES OF APPOINTED PERSONS:

RPS.. Date..............................

Approved by the RPA.. Date..............................

Appendix 1

WRITTEN SYSTEM OF WORK FOR THE CONTROLLED AREA

- The purpose of the written system of work is to ensure that persons involved in radiography receive doses of ionizing radiations which are as low as reasonably practicable.
- Radiography is to be undertaken only when clinically indicated.
- The X-ray equipment must not be used for human radiography.
- Only essential authorized personnel may remain within the Controlled Area during an examination.
- The door to the radiography room must be closed during radiographic exposures and the appropriate warning signs displayed/illuminated.
- Every precaution must be taken to ensure that no person present during radiography is exposed to undue risks.
- The radiographer has authority over all persons involved in the procedure and must ensure that the procedure is carried out in accordance with the local rules and written system of work.
- Personnel required to remain in the Controlled Area must make full and proper use of all appropriate personal protective equipment provided (as dictated by risk assessment) in accordance with instruction and training, and all those who are able must stand behind the lead screen for the duration of the exposure.
- Wherever possible animals must be artificially restrained with the use of positioning aids (sandbags, troughs, ties, foam pads and wedges) and appropriate chemical restraint.
- Manual restraint may only be performed if a radiograph is essential for diagnosis before treatment can begin, and if non-manual restraint is not possible. Anyone carrying out manual restraint must be wearing a lead apron, thyroid protector, lead gloves or sleeves and a personal dosimeter. No part of the person, even if protected, must enter the primary beam. Assistants who are or believe that they may be pregnant must not participate in restraint of the patient.
- Good technique consistent with high quality radiographs using minimum radiation exposure must always be used. The exposure chart should be referred to in order to set the correct exposures and suitable grids, screens and films should be used.
- To minimize scattered radiation the area of the primary beam must be collimated as tight as possible using the light beam diaphragm and should never exceed the limits of the cassette.
- If a horizontal beam is used, it must be directed towards the moveable lead screen.
- All exposures (including details of any manual restraint) must be recorded in the exposure record book.
- If a case of overexposure is suspected, the radiographer/RPS will immediately inform the RPA.
- The Controlled Area may be de-designated and unrestricted access allowed when:
  - The X-ray equipment has been isolated from the electrical supply, and
  - All warning signs have been removed.

SIGNATURES OF APPOINTED PERSONS:

RPS.. Date..............................

Appointed RPA.. Date..............................

(continued) An example of Local Rules. Proposed dates for, and records of, reviews should be appended to the document.

Laboratory diagnostic services

14

Roger Powell

Laboratory services in small animal general practice are often provided by external laboratories. There are, however, core tests that are usually offered in house by practices, and many practices have extensive in-house provision. Figure 14.1 lists some typical practice laboratory equipment and its purpose; further details of equipment and its use are given in the chapter.

Equipment	Function
Centrifuge	Separates blood sample into constituents – cells and liquid serum or plasma
Refractometer	Measures a liquid's refractive index to assess urine specific gravity and plasma/serum proteins
Biochemistry analyser	Measures various markers of organ disease such as liver and kidney
Electrodes	Measure electrolytes (e.g. sodium, potassium, chloride, calcium) and pH
Haematology analyser	Measures the number and types of blood cells
Glucometer	Measures glucose levels in whole blood
Microscope	Allows examination of cells, urine and parasites
Coagulation analyser	Measures the clotting times for bleeding disorders
Stains	Assist the microscopic examination of cells and tissues

14.1 Typical practice laboratory equipment and its purpose.

The choice of what to offer may be influenced purely by financial constraints or by clinical needs, but is typically a compromise of both. If a practice provides a test that is prohibitively expensive, due to inherent costs and minimal demand, there could be a pressure to increase the demand, i.e. test more patients. However, if animals are tested without clinical need, ethical considerations come into play. Evaluating all these factors is vital when designing a practice laboratory; decisions should involve as many key personnel as possible. The reader is directed to the *BSAVA Manual of Canine and Feline Clinical Pathology* for a detailed discussion of many laboratory tests and principles.

Assessing the need for in-house testing

The starting point is an honest assessment of what a practice can do and how it could do it, both practically and professionally. Future plans for practice development and expansion should be considered, and both internal (practice) and external (referral) laboratory testing incorporated. Factors to consider include those shown in Figure 14.2. These often overlap to impact on each other.

Internal testing	External testing
Fresh samples	Potential sample deterioration
Faster turnaround (e.g. for critical care or out-of-hours cases)	Variable delay or turnaround
Client appreciation	
Risk of inappropriate analysis	Expertise
Expense	Usually cheaper
Limited test range	Greater test range
Operator should understand test	Interpretive support
Reduced quality control	Independent quality assurance

14.2 Factors to consider when choosing between internal and external provision of laboratory diagnostic services.

Reliability

A good external laboratory will perform more quality control and assessment (see below) and a wider range of tests than a practice laboratory, and the results it produces should therefore always be accurate, precise and reliable. However, practices can achieve similar results, even if not operating in the same strict way.

The control system and monitoring merely indicate that a system is operating as it should be and as expected, so results can be trusted. However, as practice quality control systems are typically performed less frequently, any errors may not be identified as quickly as in an external laboratory. Results produced in this period will therefore be wrong and could lead to misdiagnoses.

Many practice laboratories do not perform daily internal quality control checks. The frequency of control monitoring required relates to the performance of the analyser and the number of tests being carried out. Daily control checks are pointless for a test that is only run once a month. The more frequently control monitoring is performed, the more expensive the test. However, this control 'cost' is spread over the volume of tests, so frequently run tests are typically cheaper. The practice must assess which tests it will run commonly, as these are the most cost-effective. They are also likely to be the most reliable, as operators are familiar with the testing and become more experienced in spotting problems or errors. External quality control schemes for in-house tests can operate on a fortnightly basis; checks should be at least quarterly according to current RCVS Practice Standards guidelines.

Cost

Due to economies of scale, the actual cost of performing any test at a commercial external laboratory will inevitably be much lower than the same test performed in house. For infrequent tests requiring expensive equipment and specialist techniques, and where extensive tests are required for certain diseases, an external laboratory will always be the better option financially. There is also the added benefit of an interpretive back-up being provided with the results. For routine tests that are carried out frequently, because of volume-related cost efficiencies the in-house option can be cost-effective as well as convenient, although more staff and facility resources are needed.

In budgeting costs for in-house testing, the following should be included:

- Staff time, training and development for performing tests, interpretation and recording
- Analyser capital depreciation, maintenance and troubleshooting
- Reagents and controls
- Disposal of waste
- Space, climate control and ventilation costs
- Ongoing quality control costs.

Pricing

External

When using an external laboratory, it is generally more appropriate to charge the client a fixed fee, such as a handling and interpretation fee, rather than a blanket percentage mark-up on the charge made from the laboratory to the practice. This is particularly pertinent for tests that are more expensive. Blanket mark-ups on external tests may be easier to operate but are more difficult to justify. They may also start to impact on client acceptance, as innovative test procedures are inherently expensive and the mark-up could make the test unaffordable. The cost of the veterinary surgeon's interpretation time is significant; ideally, this should be itemized separately for transparency.

In house

Prices charged to the client for tests performed in house should be comparable to the price the client would pay if the test were done externally, although a premium can be justified for instant results and out-of-hours tests. At the same time, the practice must ensure not only that such costs as staff time, training and quality control are covered, plus any direct costs of reagents, but that there is also a return on investment built into the equation.

Profitability

To determine whether or not it is financially feasible to run a test in house, the practice will need to calculate the true cost of each test. This can be difficult, as there are many factors to take into consideration when doing the calculation. Figure 14.3 shows examples of calculating margins for in-house and external testing. Only by inputting individual practice figures will it become apparent whether a practice will find internal testing more profitable than sending tests to an external laboratory. The margin for different analysers will vary enormously, and the extent to which margins will vary according to number of tests performed depends on the individual contract with the external laboratory or machine supplier. Some analyser providers will offer fixed running costs within a range of test numbers; others will have a fixed cost per test.

- **Staff time and facility costs are significant and so must be considered to give the true picture.**
- As a minimum, every practice should record all internal lab diagnostic costs in one group on the purchase ledger, separate from external lab costs.
- All in-house test sales figures should also be in one group on the practice management system (PMS).
- **All calculations shown in Figure 14.3 must include failed and repeated tests and controls.** Tracking the totals as percentages and actual figures is useful for benchmarking, as is breaking down the figures to give separate margins, e.g. for haematology, biochemistry, coagulation analysers.

KEY POINT

A retrospective assessment of practice lab profitability is always advisable, as margin will increase with level of usage, which has to be estimated for new equipment.

Turnaround time

A strong argument for in-house testing is the rapid availability of test results, which can be vital in a medical or surgical emergency, and can offer peace of mind for both the clinician and the owner. This rapidity can increase client loyalty and appreciation, which is difficult to quantify but is often very significant.

Which tests are considered critical is controversial but these could include electrolytes (sodium, potassium), glucose and packed cell volume (PCV). Rapid testing naturally prevents sample deterioration and potential sample variation.

Many tests are not considered critical or immediate. For these, the cost of performing the test in house may not be deemed acceptable. Also, with many

Internal laboratory		External laboratory	
Client charge per test	A	A	Client charge per test
Practice/vet interpretation fee per test if applicable. This may or may not be charged separately or may be part of the consultation fee	B	B	Interpretation fee charged to client if itemized separately; or fee charged by practice if additional
Sample submission/posting fee charged to client (fixed sum or percentage)	–	C	C may be charged per test or be a combined fee for several tests on same patient (NB prepaid postal labels/packages are often available)
Number of tests performed	D	D	Number of tests performed
Total income = (A + B) x D; or from PMS figures *Total income can be:* ■ *For individual tests: income received per test multiplied by the actual (or projected) number of test, or* ■ *The total lab income (all tests) analysed on the PMS (gives a true figure for income as any mischarging and pricing anomalies will be automatically included)*	TI	TI	Total income = (A + B + C) x D; or from PMS figures *Total income can be:* ■ *Income received per individual test multiplied by the actual (or projected) number of tests, or* ■ *The total income analysed on the PMS (gives a true figure for income as any mischarging and pricing anomalies will be automatically included)*
Lab machinery costs (e.g. leasing/depreciation): fixed costs (e.g. just centrifuge)	F	F	Lab machinery costs (e.g. leasing/depreciation): fixed costs (e.g. just centrifuge)
Lab machinery fixed running costs (service contract, consumables for controls, quality controls, calibrators, cleaning where these are not dependent on number of tests carried out, e.g. if a fixed contract is in place for wet biochemistry)	FR	–	–
Quality Assurance Scheme costs	QA	–	–
Total variable costs (for reagent/dry slides, additional controls, etc. – depends on machinery used and number of tests) x D (number of tests)	VR	LF	Lab fee for performing test multiplied by number of tests
Sample tubes and supporting consumables (e.g. deionizer filters)	SP	SP	Sample tubes and supporting consumables, e.g. packaging
Staff costs (variable according to machinery used and routine care and QA needed). Include pay, taxes, PPE, CPD	S	S	Staff costs (mainly preparing and packing samples and admin time, handling results and invoices)
Facility costs – space costs for lab. Calculated as a proportion of overhead and cost of square meterage of space, to include specifics such as climate control	FA	FA	Facility costs – space costs for packing, separating, etc.
Total costs (per test or total): F + FR + QA + (VR x D) + SP + S + FA *Costs can be calculated for each individual test, or the total internal lab costs can be used from the management accounts*	TC	TC	Total costs (per test or total) *Costs can be calculated for each individual test or external lab, or the total external lab fees (costs) can be used from the management accounts. (Staff costs will be limited to interpretation, packaging and sending; requirements for interpretation may be reduced if done by external laboratory)*
Profit = income minus costs	T I – TC	T I – TC	Profit = income minus costs
% Margin overall = profit / income x 100 *Depending on the fixed costs of the equipment versus the variable costs of the tests, the margin will change according to the number of tests carried out*	%	%	% Margin overall = profit / income x 100 *The margin will not vary with the number of tests, unless the lab offers a quantity discount*

14.3 Calculating a margin for laboratory testing. Recording and grouping income (blue) and costs (pink) in the PMS and management accounts allows simple analysis; prices can then be adjusted in order to maintain or improve margins (profitability). This model can also be used for predicting margins when considering purchasing new equipment.

external laboratories now offering next-day delivery of test results via a courier service and/or electronic or telephoned reports, clinical decision-making and therapy are not unduly delayed. Some tests, such as the less common hormone assays, are however only available on a batched basis.

KEY POINT

Keeping the owner well informed of the expected turnaround time is vital.

Trust and expertise

There is no point in being able to offer a test on site if it is not performed correctly. Whilst rapid test results are desired and will generate trust and appreciation, it is very easy to lose these positive benefits if mistakes are made.

In-house test results that appear wrong or unexplained can be rechecked the next day using an external laboratory. However, this approach relies on understanding how testing is done in each individual situation, or how an individual analyser performs. As an example, no automated haematology analyser can provide a complete assessment of an animal's haematological status: assessing a blood smear is essential for the complete picture. All practices should be able to make and examine a blood smear, but this is often not performed well, or not done at all, due to lack of experience and perceived need. Experience can only be built up over time if it is done regularly. As an alternative, an automatic analyser can be used and where problems are highlighted those samples can be further assessed by an external laboratory. This approach can, however, add significantly to the client's expense. As haematology is a specialized area and automated analysis is potentially unreliable and/or misleading, some practices choose to send all haematology assessments away, confining in-house activities to measuring PCV and making good blood smears for external examination.

If sending samples to an external laboratory, the practice should trust that laboratory's expertise and results. Some external laboratories specialize in certain fields, such as infectious disease testing. Others offer an extensive range of tests for many species, acting as a single source for a practice's external laboratory testing. Their service should be backed up by comprehensive interpretive support, so that testing is appropriate and the meaning of the results fully communicated; those principles also apply to in-house testing. Both external and internal testing should be flexible and adaptable, to cater where possible to the variable demands of client circumstances and disease presentations.

Breadth and range

With the huge number of potential tests that can be carried out, another consideration is the time it takes to perform them. Demand and technology have created faster and often more reliable test methods, but speed is not enough without proper technique and understanding. Indeed, the speed of results and the reliability of analysers without significant user input may generate complacency that 'all is well' when erroneous results are in fact being produced and then used. This is especially true if the entire method is not known and understood; for example, incorrect storage of refrigerated reagents or slides may result in sample degradation and incorrect results.

In most practices, laboratory testing is performed by many people – as and when the need arises. This naturally creates analytical variance that will affect results unless managed very well. Having dedicated staff to do the testing may be more expensive but will generally produce more reliable results over time, and can allow expansion of the test repertoire to offset the additional cost. For general practices, current RCVS Practice Standards Scheme guidelines stipulate that the practice should be able to run a minimum of blood glucose, urine specific gravity and PCV. Veterinary hospitals should also offer biochemical analysis (electrolytes, total calcium, total protein and creatinine) on site. Anything more is down to what the practice feels is required and appropriate, given the staff's training and experience.

Discussion about the in-practice laboratory then comes full circle. If honestly appraised, it should allow a streamlined, efficient and seamless combination of internal and external testing. This will ensure the patient's needs are met to diagnose a disease, whilst fulfilling the client's realistic practical and financial expectations.

Designing and installing a practice laboratory

The laboratory area requires a designated impervious bench, with many electrical sockets available. If equipment is small or mobile, the room within which the benchtop is located can be shared with other practice functions, such as patient preparation for surgical or dental procedures (see Chapter 8). However, having a designated laboratory room, even if minimal and box-like, has several advantages:

- A focused approach without distractions is helpful for analysis and lab techniques
- Some analysers and equipment, such as centrifuges, are quite noisy when in operation, potentially impacting on other functions or tasks occurring in a shared room
- Health and safety and COSHH compliance issues (see Chapter 22) can be 'significant' with laboratory material and are much easier to control in a self-contained space
- Analyser operation and laboratory testing is often temperature-dependent and should only be done within a certain temperature range, typically 15–25°C. Analysers and refrigeration can produce a lot of heat, requiring good ventilation and, ideally, air conditioning for temperature control to prevent overheating and incorrect analysis or analyser error.

Figure 14.4 shows some different layouts and use of space for small and larger practice laboratories.

Benches

If only the minimum tests are being performed, a bench that is about 1 metre long may suffice. If biochemical and haematology analysers are required, these will typically be benchtop systems and would need at least another metre to accommodate them both. Whilst not essential, the space provided would ideally be slightly greater, to allow easy access for troubleshooting and reagent changing (1.25–1.5 times the width is a guideline for this).

If haematology and general microscope work are to be performed, having a separate and non-contiguous benchtop for these is ideal. This minimizes inherent vibrations transmitted by analysers and, especially, centrifuges, along the bench and through the floor (if not solid). Working at a microscope also necessitates a seating space below the benchtop and a specific adjustable high chair (laboratory benches are higher than standard desks).

KEY POINT

A separate and non-continguous benchtop for microscope work is ideal where machines nearby produce vibration.

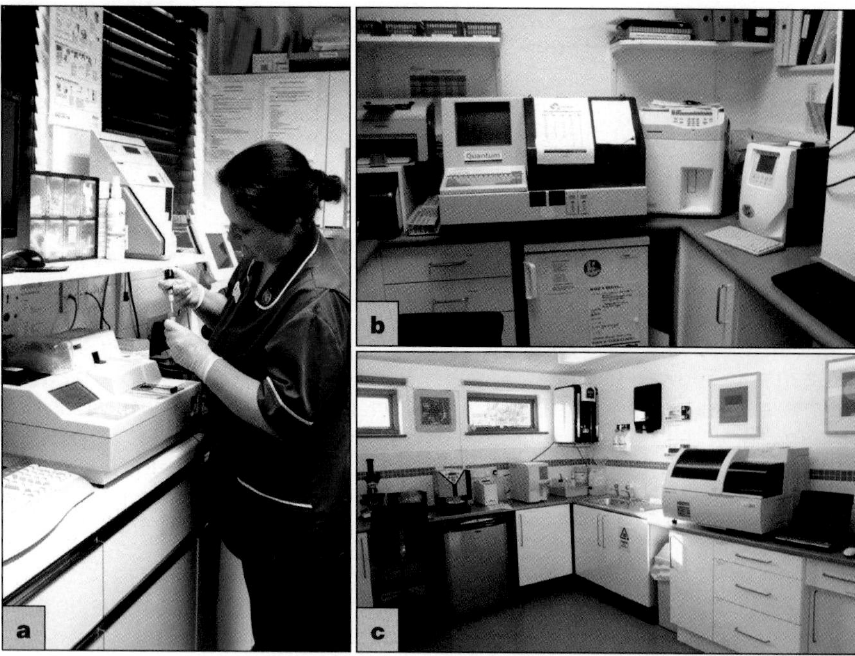

14.4 Laboratory layouts. **(a)** A compact practice laboratory, with efficient use of space for analysers. **(b)** This small practice laboratory is arranged in a U format. **(c)** Larger analysers can only be used where there is sufficient space, preferably in a dedicated laboratory, and often require a deeper workbench than the standard 600 mm.

Sufficient floor or under-bench space will be needed for waste bins, both general and potentially hazardous, including rigid 'sharps' containers (see Chapter 3).

Sinks

As space and provision must be made for hand-washing, the laboratory space will incorporate, or be adjacent to, a sink, possibly with a drainage board. Sink units can be enamel, epoxy or stainless steel, the last being recommended as it is easier to keep clean and maintain. Hands-free taps are recommended.

KEY POINT

Provision must be made for hand-washing in the lab area.

Storage

With a designated room or area, there will typically be sufficient space under the required benching for storing consumables, especially if combined with judicious overhead shelving for books or reference material and cupboards for other consumables. If the space is shared, specific cupboard and shelf space should be dedicated for laboratory material.

Low-level storage requires comfortable space for opening doors and drawers whilst bending. Overhead storage will often necessitate provision of mobile steps for all staff to access these areas. Storage space can be integrated cupboards and drawers, the drawers potentially being removable trays or larger bins on sliding tracks (Figure 14.5). Having a separate mobile unit can be an advantage for certain consumables, such as blood sample tubes, so a combination of fixed and mobile units is recommended.

All laboratories require certain items to be refrigerated; this is usually best achieved with a dedicated under-the-bench small fridge. These often have a small integral freezer unit, which is recommended for samples that require specific handling and rapid freezing. The amount of fridge space required will depend primarily on the type and number of tests being performed internally, especially with regard to the biochemical analyser. The types of perishable reagents and material that can be stored at room temperature are increasing, but many liquid reagents or dry chemistry cartridges and rotors still need, and will

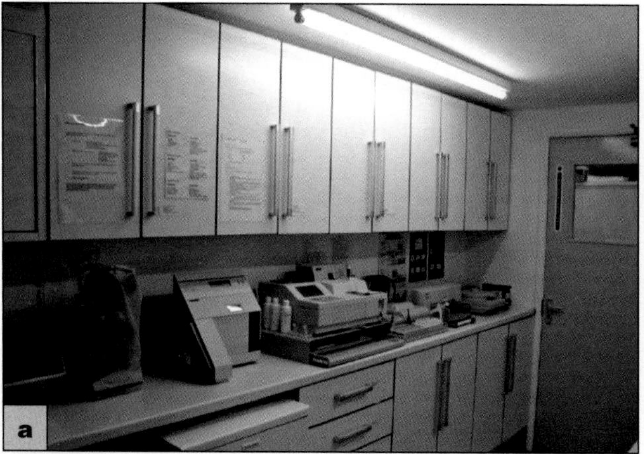

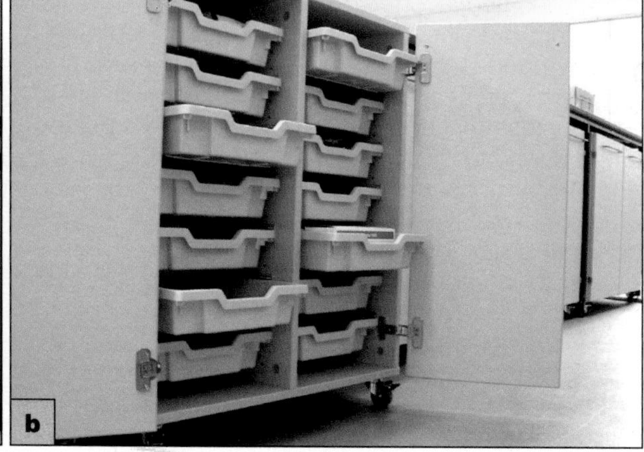

14.5 Laboratory storage often includes a mix of drawers and cupboards. **(a)** Note the lists of contents on these top cupboards. **(b)** Integrated mobile removable drawer units under an impervious benchtop.

continue to need, refrigerated storage for maximum shelf life. Longer storage for reconstituted lyophilized material can often be achieved by freezing aliquots once made up, for intermittent defrosting and quality control analysis.

Some reagents are hazardous and must be stored appropriately with regard to COSHH regulations (see Chapter 22), typically in a lockable, controlled steel cabinet with appropriate labelling (Figure 14.6).

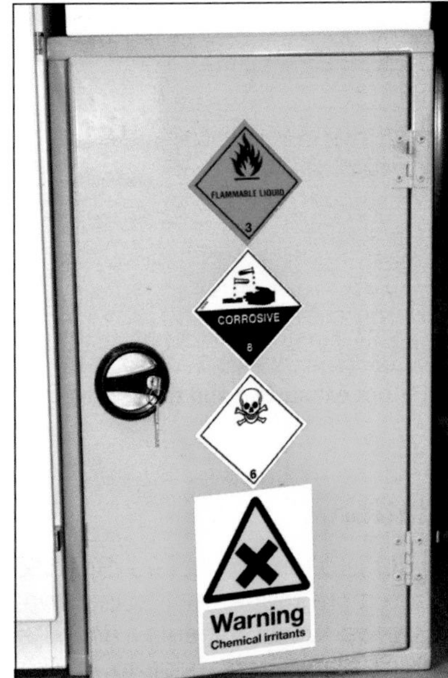

14.6 An appropriately labelled and lockable steel cabinet for storing hazardous chemicals.

Consumables

A list of commonly needed laboratory equipment and consumables is given in Figure 14.7.

- Soap; alcohol cleaning gel
- Disposable hand towels
- Disposable gloves: powder-free, latex
- Disposable lab aprons
- Tissues
- Cotton wool
- Syringes
- Needles
- Blood tubes: EDTA, serum (gel, plain), heparin, fluoride, citrate
- Capillary tubes and sealant
- Centrifuge tubes
- Pasteur pipettes
- Slides – frosted
- Coverslips (18 x 18 mm)
- Permanent marker and pencils
- Liquid paraffin/mounting medium
- Immersion oil
- Swabs – plain, charcoal, viral
- Coplin jars and stains
- Biohazard bags
- Sterile and boric acid universal containers
- Thermometer
- Timer
- Lab coats

14.7 'Consumables' and general equipment required for the practice laboratory. This list is not exhaustive but serves as a guide; requirements will inevitably change over time as tests change or new manufacturers are sourced.

Blood sampling tubes

Given the range of species encountered in practice, a range of sizes from 0.5 to 1.3 ml is advisable, as these tubes are typically designed for a certain quantity of blood, and significant under- or overfilling can dramatically affect subsequent analysis and results. Small animal collection systems are typically open, with blood being taken in a syringe and then transferred from the syringe to the opened blood sample tube after removing the needle. Closed systems such as vacuum suction methods or integral anticoagulated disposable syringes are also available, especially for larger farm animal species.

For many disposable items, such as blood sampling tubes, there are numerous manufacturers, all with varying costs and quality. Whilst these differences may not be clinically significant, discussion with the manufacturers is recommended prior to purchasing. Sample packs can often be provided to try out before committing to a given product.

A number of factors will need to be considered:

- The commonest requirements for in-house laboratories are tubes containing EDTA, heparin or no anticoagulant (serum)
- Fluoride and citrate tubes may also be required, but typically in lesser numbers
- Dry powder or liquid anticoagulant preparations are available, the former requiring more thorough mixing to ensure adequate anticoagulation
- Specific heparin-coated syringes are available for obtaining blood samples to undergo blood gas analysis on electrochemical analysers; these syringes will give the most accurate results by minimizing problems such as heparin excess in the sample
- Specialized anticoagulants or deproteinizing tubes are also available but are only required rarely and will often be provided by the external laboratories to which the sample is to be submitted
- Consideration when selecting blood tubes should also include the practice analyser:
  - Results with heparinized blood and with serum can be slightly different
  - EDTA-based haematology analysers may be based upon a sample with K_2EDTA rather than K_3EDTA
- Certain blood tubes can crack and then leak when centrifuged for plasma and serum separation.

Similarly, if changing the source of a product, such as a pipette or centrifugation tube, communication with the manufacturer about its intended purpose is recommended, as certain tubes or pipettes may not be appropriate for the intended test or may introduce a significant variation and therefore alter the results produced.

Analysers

Communication with manufacturers is vital when contemplating the purchase of, and investment in, an automated analyser. Factors to consider when purchasing an analyser are summarized in Figure 14.8.

Factors	Considerations
Physical	Footprint; plumbing; electricity; noise level
Performance	Accuracy; precision; range; detection limit; interference
Validation	Species – healthy *versus* diseased
Samples	Volumes; types
User-friendliness	Software; touch screen; accessibility
Manufacturer	Technical support; maintenance contract; engineers; loan analyser; warranty
User maintenance and troubleshooting	Moving parts; tubing; electrodes; lamps; robustness
Reagents	Volumes; stability; hazardous?
Flexibility	Open (new tests or profiles can be added as and when) or closed (preset with no additions allowed); ability to run single tests or profiles; can profiles be tailored to needs?
Quality assurance	Control material; frequency; external scheme
Turnaround time	Single or multiple tests; single or multiple samples
Integration with PMS	Result documentation; archiving; record transfer
Expected lifespan	Sample numbers; superseded by new technology?

14.8 Factors to consider when purchasing and assessing an automatic analyser. This list is not exhaustive and the relative merits of the various factors will be both operator- and practice-dependent.

Possibly the four most important factors are: cost, reliability, validation, and dedicated staff time. As mentioned above, exact cost is difficult to evaluate accurately and, therefore, to compare directly between different analysers. Examples of generic capital cost, maintenance and operating costs for different types of analyser (see later) are given in Figure 14.9.

Provision should be made for when the analyser malfunctions. This provision may include technical support from the manufacturer, which may be an on-site engineer or may involve the temporary loan of an analyser whilst the faulty one is sent for repair. Regular maintenance visits can be helpful for ongoing training support and troubleshooting minor or non-urgent faults. Where support is not offered by the manufacturer in a timely or practical way, alternatives must be sought, either via an external laboratory or through agreement with another local practice.

Reliability

The reliability of the analyser is important: the less reliable it is, the more often quality control material will need to be assessed and samples re-run to ensure accurate analysis. This all adds to the expense. An assessment of reliability can come, in part, from the manufacturer but is best garnered via conversation with current users elsewhere and also by an actual trial. Whilst this is time-consuming, the information gathered is very useful and provides a basis for assessing the manufacturer's general support and back-up.

Veterinary validation

Validation of the analyser is often overlooked. Specific veterinary analysers are more readily available nowadays, but quality can be quite variable, and the assessment done by manufacturers prior to launch and selling can often be very limited, or biased. Detailed examination of their figures and the populations used is strongly recommended. For example, interference from haemolysis or lipaemia is often a significant factor affecting analysis and the manufacturer should have assessed these specifically using samples from veterinary species. Manufacturers may quote studies based on human blood samples. This can be a starting point but each species can produce very specific interference that human blood samples do not. Conversely, human samples produce interference, such as high potassium with sample haemolysis, that many small animal species do not.

Similarly, haematology analysers are often assessed on a very limited and therefore biased population, especially if experimental colonies of a single or limited number of breeds have been used. Validation testing on both healthy and diseased populations is crucial, as the analyser may perform well in the former instance but very poorly in the latter.

Purchasers should watch out for reference intervals (ranges of 'normal' results) that are unrealistically 'restricted' in relation to the breadth inherent to the numerous breeds and interspecies variation that veterinary practices have to deal with.

Analyser type	Capital cost (£)	Maintenance (£ per annum)	Cost per example screen/profile (£)	Cost per test (£)
Electrochemical	2,500–5,000	475	11.00 [a]	1.00
Dry spectrophotometry	5,000–10,000	1,200	12.00	0.80
Wet spectrophotometry	13,000–25,000	3,500	2.00	0.10

14.9 Approximate cost estimation for comparison of biochemical analysers, based on illustrative figures. It is important to compare relative costs of purchase, maintenance and operation. [a] NB The electrochemical method cannot assess a full anaesthetic screen with regard to liver enzymes.

Biochemistry and endocrinology

Three general systems are available:

- Electrochemical
- Dry spectrophotometric
- Wet spectrophotometric.

Electrochemical analysers

These are typically handheld point-of-care analysers (Figure 14.10) and are often the cheapest type in terms of capital outlay. They usually provide results most quickly but they are relatively more expensive to run per test, and also more limited with regard to the breadth of tests available (see Figure 14.9). As they inherently calibrate and control with minimal moving parts, they are also usually very reliable. However, fundamentally their analysis is electrical and can involve calculated assumptions that may lead to significant errors and misleading results.

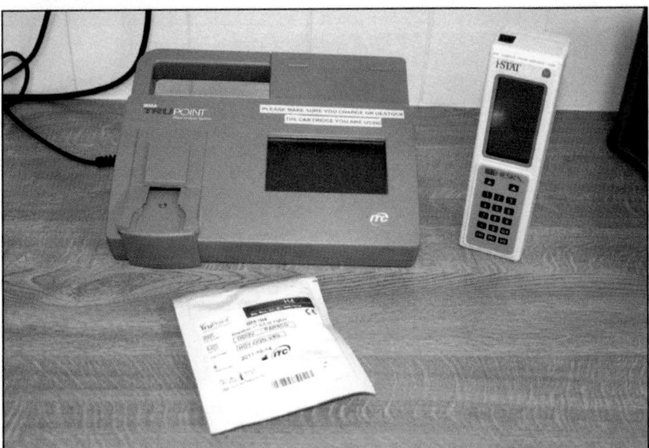

14.10 Digital display electrochemical analysers. Clockwise from top left: Mobile example with built-in thermal printer; handheld example which can be linked to an external printer; single-use sample cartridge package. Cartridges often require refrigerated storage but some can be stored at room temperature; shelf-life is limited.

Spectrophotometric analysis

This involves reagents which, when mixed with the sample, produce a colour change that is measured; the rate or amount of colour change at a certain wavelength relates to the amount of substance in the sample.

Dry methods typically come as prepackaged profiles or various individual analytes. Whilst less flexible, each package is factory-calibrated and controlled, and therefore maintenance is minimal. Presuming that all tests within a package are required, the cost per test is cheaper than with electrochemical analysers, but turnaround is slightly slower. These analysers can measure interference from factors such as haemolysis, potentially suppressing inaccurate results and thereby preventing misinterpretation. Inherent filtering can also be incorporated into the packages to minimize such interference, though this may affect the resulting values.

Wet spectrophotometric analysers are typically much larger and more expensive than dry or electrochemical analysers. They often also create more liquid waste, which requires either collection and intermittent disposal or connection to the practice's drainage pipework. Provision of (certain grade) distilled water is also often a requirement. This can take the form of a bottled supply if of low volume, but larger analysers with greater throughput will typically require a specific distilled water deionizer (Figure 14.11) and exchange system connected between the analyser and the practice's cold water pipe. Such a source can be used for other purposes and equipment, such as autoclaves.

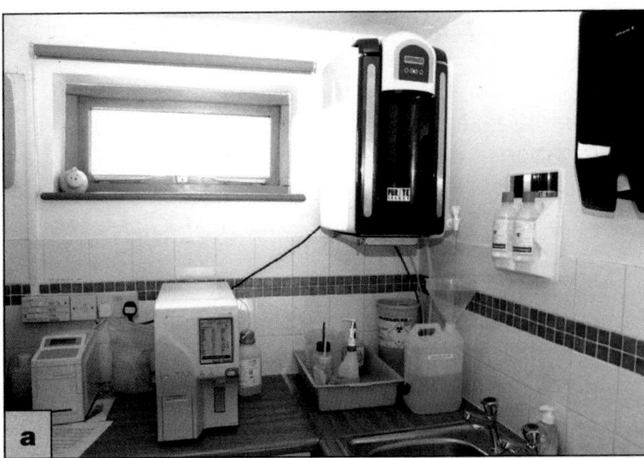

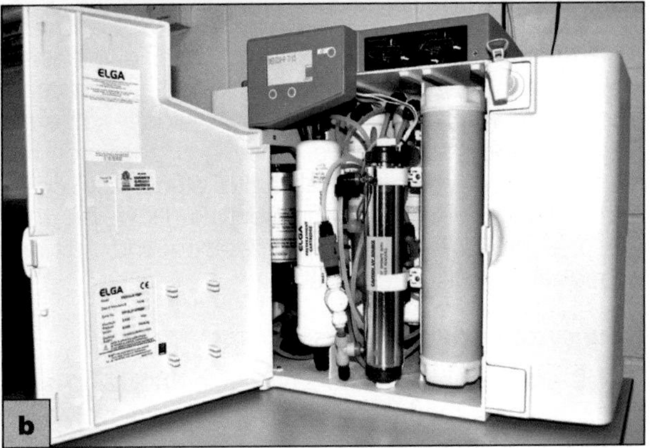

14.11 **(a)** A practice laboratory with a wall-mounted deionizer for producing large volumes of distilled water. **(b)** An alternative deionizer, showing the internal workings.

Whilst the capital cost of wet systems is greater, their running cost can be significantly lower, especially if greater numbers of samples are being tested. Wet analysers are standard for external laboratories but less common in practice laboratories. They require a greater degree of maintenance and quality control but inherently are much more flexible and potentially more accurate and reliable. With this consideration, greater training is likely to be required for their proper operation and dedicated staff are recommended.

Some dry and wet spectrophotometric analysers can also measure hormones, such as thyroxine (T4). Addition of such tests to a practice's repertoire may be desirable, and also more cost-effective. Crucially, the validation of the analyser should be assessed, especially if being used to diagnose hyperthyroidism in cats and hypothyroidism in dogs. The detection limit and linearity (the range within which the results are valid) should be critiqued, as the performance of the analyser and internal analysis may be acceptable for hyperthyroidism but not hypothyroidism, especially as low total thyroxine production in dogs does not necessarily diagnose clinical hypothyroidism (see

BSAVA Manual of Canine and Feline Endocrinology). This form of hormonal analysis is also more prone to artefactual interference, such as from haemolysis.

Endocrinology otherwise typically involves a form of antibody-mediated hormonal detection that requires a specific analyser and therefore high capital investment and maintenance costs.

Haematology

There are three main types of automated haematology analyser:

- Centrifugal or quantitative buffy coat (QBC)
- Impedance or Coulter
- Laser flow cytometry.

QBC

This is likely to involve the lowest capital investment, but is relatively expensive to run and is slower. It provides useful parameters such as PCV and total white blood cell count, but differential counts are unreliable.

Coulter or impedance-based systems

These are probably the most widely used and available, often with a quick turnaround. Specific veterinary models and software are now available. Analysers from different manufacturers have slightly different reliability and performance. They are good for red blood cell parameters, total white blood cell count and, potentially, white cell differentials. However, they are also prone to specific interference and artefact, especially in relation to cell size.

Flow cytometric analysers

These are now more widely available, including specific veterinary models and software. They involve the highest investment, and are the most expensive type to run and maintain. However, they provide the most accurate analysis and automated values, and are the standard for external laboratories. Whilst they are typically large machines, smaller benchtop equivalents are available but their relative expense and the maintenance experience required may preclude their usefulness in practice.

KEY POINT

No matter how expensive, all automated haematology analysers have inherent pitfalls, and assessment of a good blood smear is an absolute requirement for veterinary haematology.

Given sufficient experience and training, a lot of information can be garnered from only a spun PCV (in a capillary tube) and a good blood smear. Complete and accurate haematological analysis requires extensive experience and if done properly is expensive, and time-consuming. For these reasons, some practices choose not to spend time and money in this area.

Other equipment

Whilst automated analysers are often the centrepiece and focus of the practice laboratory, a good practice cannot function without other essential equipment. Practices will need a variable centrifuge, binocular microscope and urine/plasma protein refractometer as core equipment (Figure 14.12). Other point-of-care assessments, such as for lactate and haemoglobin, may form part of a mobile specific rapid laboratory 'suite' or be used as analyser back-up, but are expensive and typically not justified in practice.

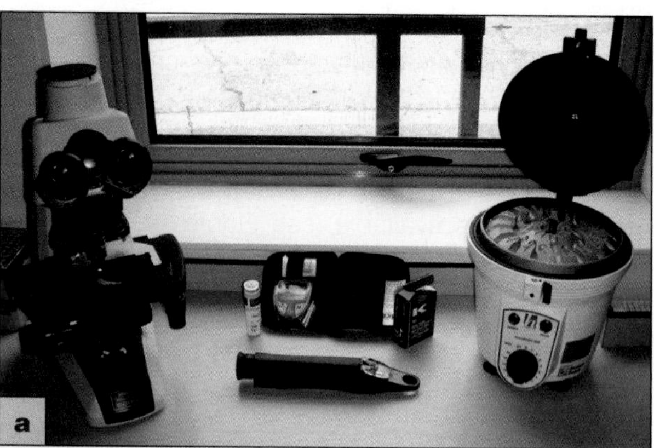

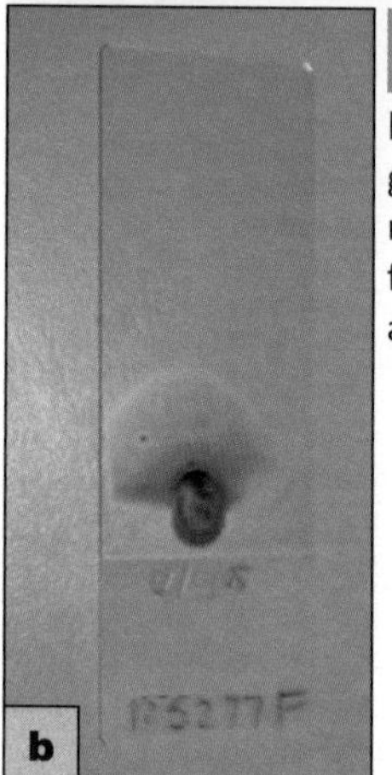

14.12 Core equipment. **(a)** Clockwise from left: binocular microscope; capillary tubes; glucometer; slides; centrifuge; refractometer. **(b)** Glass slides with frosted ends can be labelled quickly and easily with a pencil.

Centrifuges

Specific considerations when purchasing a centrifuge include: variable speed programs with adaptable buckets; or flexible fixed rotor systems. It is very difficult to buy one universal centrifuge that can accommodate both slow speeds for cell and sediment spinning as well as very high speeds for microhaematocrit measurement and plasma or serum separation. Therefore, two centrifuges may be required. Consideration should then include inherent back-up if one should fail.

Microscopes

Binocular microscopes come in all shapes and sizes, with very varying quality. If only wet preparation microscopy and scanning blood smear evaluation is to be performed, a relatively cheap microscope should be acceptable. However, for more prolonged usage and detailed examination of blood smears and cytological preparations, investment in a higher quality microscope is recommended, for both accuracy and stress-free user performance. Understanding the application and appropriate use of the microscope (see below) is more important than being able to describe its physical characteristics such as the Vernier scale. Maintenance contracts for cleaning and troubleshooting can be incorporated into the purchase but are also independently available, alongside sources for purchasing replacement bulbs. A trial assessment is vital before purchasing.

Tissue staining kits

Automated staining is usually not justified in practice, due to the substantial cost and inherent maintenance, although it is standard practice for external laboratories. Staining in practice is typically based upon a form of rapid Romanowsky stain. Staining kits vary slightly in their quality and consistency between batches, so familiarity with the staining pattern of the kit being used is most crucial (see below). If practice cytology is to be pursued in earnest, investment in different stains such as modified Wright's or May–Grünwald–Giemsa, which require longer staining times, may be recommended to maximize the detail obtained.

Refractometers

Refractometers are most commonly generic instruments although specific veterinary models are available. The latter may be recommended as otherwise certain species differences, such as feline reference intervals, will need to be accommodated when interpreting values. They are temperature-dependent, which should be taken into account given the location of their use. Refractometers should be handled with care to avoid scratching and should be regularly cleaned.

Glucometers

Glucometers are widely available, and specific veterinary models are now in circulation (Figure 14.13). Whilst very specific in their use, their relatively low capital and maintenance costs are justified with regard to facilitating the monitoring and assessment of diabetic patients. As with any analyser, care should be given to monitoring and confirming performance, as analytical error can occur due to poor calibration and incorrect procedure.

Glucometers require only a very small quantity of blood to be taken. This, alongside cheaper analysis relative to more fixed electrochemical or dry biochemistry systems on a single analyte makes them very useful, and rapid turnaround is an added bonus.

The relatively low cost of hand-held glucometers makes them very suitable for purchase by, or loan to, owners of diabetic pets; with appropriate training, owners can be supported to monitor their pets at home and even to record regular glucose curves for discussion with the supervising clinician. This is particularly helpful for nervous patients and cats whose stress levels in the practice can significantly affect results when hospitalized.

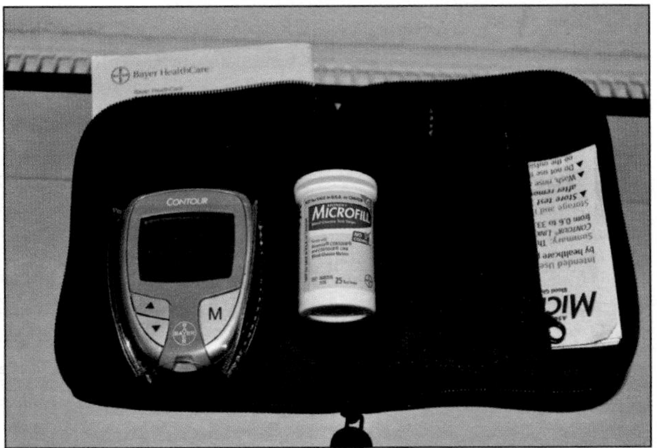

14.13 An example of a glucometer for veterinary use.

> **KEY POINTS**
>
> - As glucometers measure glucose within a different medium to biochemical analysers, they will not produce the same result.
> - Results will also vary from glucometer to glucometer, so it is vital that if clients are using this test at home, the practice and the client use the same method.
> - The glucose value will often be inaccurate if the patient is anaemic or has increased numbers of red blood cells.

Coagulation analysers

Analysers measuring secondary blood coagulation pathways are desirable due to the perceived turnaround advantage and accompanying clinical benefits. Automated analysers can be photo-optical or mechanically based, with lipaemic and haemolysed samples especially often giving falsely high results in the former. Sample handling with regard to the degree of citrate anticoagulant is crucial and often overlooked. Reference intervals are often relatively long in comparison to manual methods, so they may not be as sensitive. When faced with a bleeding dog, having this test available immediately can be useful, but the actual treatment of the dog rarely requires these tests. Such situations are also not common, and having such an analyser sitting and waiting for once-monthly use is expensive, especially as better external reference testing is usually achievable within 24 hours. However, if procedures, such as liver biopsy, that require preoperative coagulation screening are commonly performed in the practice, having an analyser in the practice may be justified. Use of newer, more holistic coagulation testing methods such as thromboelastography (TEG) is not recommended in practice, as it requires much more detailed knowledge of the analytical method, sample handling is more crucial, and specific use in clinical and practical veterinary situations is limited and unclear.

Infectious disease test kits

Infectious disease testing is often done in practice, and many kits for specific infections are now available. These are often a type of modified immunosorbent antigen or antibody test. Each has inherent limitations and applications that should be understood before using. The sensitivity and specificity of infectious disease tests inherently dictate the positive and negative predictive values of a result, and the patient's clinical signs and situation are significant in interpreting the test. Many tests for infectious diseases require expertise and specific dedicated equipment, such as fluorescent microscopy for serology tests and a thermal cycler for PCR (polymerase chain reaction) analysis, and are thus not appropriate for in-house use.

FIV and FeLV kits

Possibly the commonest kits used are for feline immunodeficiency virus (FIV) and feline leukaemia virus (FeLV; Figure 14.14), the former testing for a cat's antibody response and the latter for a virus antigen. These are fundamentally different and so the meaning of a negative or positive result can also be very different for each test; this crucial point must be understood before communicating a result to the owner. The decision as to whether a practice opts to run these tests in house rather than referring to an external laboratory relies upon this understanding. The financial factor often relates to the number likely to be tested compared to the shelf life of the kit. One should not attempt to 'improve' the economics of in-house testing by increasing the number of healthy animals tested, as a positive result can be very misleading.

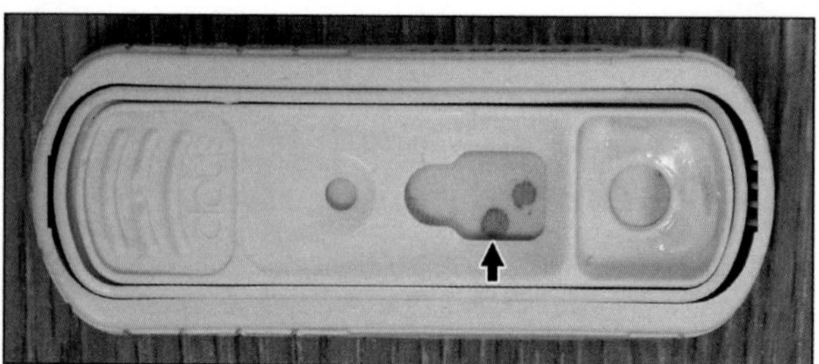

14.14 A positive FeLV test result (black arrow) on an in-house test kit. (Reproduced from *BSAVA Manual of Canine and Feline Haematology and Transfusion Medicine, 2nd edn*).

Microbiology

On a very small scale, a small animal practice may invest in certain kits such as fungal slopes or plates for dermatophyte culture. These are fundamentally similar and, whilst easy to use, require certain experience to ensure that significant isolates are identified rather than non-pathogenic contaminants. The temperature for incubation and the timing of plate reading is crucial and should be monitored, recorded and assessed to ensure accurate results.

Bacteriology kits have recently become available that claim to allow identification of common pathogens from certain sites such as skin and urine. They can include antibacterial sensitivity testing too. Their use has not been thoroughly evaluated, especially in a clinical setting. They do not identify each organism to species level, which can be misleading with regard to the significance of any bacterium cultured. Mixed infections are not accommodated and the sensitivity testing relies on the culturing of only one isolate per sensitivity test, which these kits do not guarantee. This sensitivity testing is also not as accurate as standard disc diffusion or minimum inhibitory concentrations. Use of such kits in practice is not recommended. Bacteriology requires experienced and trained personnel, and specific veterinary experience is very useful. Bacteriology should be performed by trained personnel with a Higher National Certificate in applied biology or equivalent and higher, with a specific person in charge, and typically in small animal practice is not performed in house as such personnel are not available.

If culture and sensitivity testing is to be performed in practice, the space required can be large. A minimum of two incubators, at different temperatures, would be required, with appropriate refrigerated space to store inoculation plates and sensitivity discs. Continued subculturing and use of control bacterial colonies are required to confirm proper technique and ensure accurate results. Specific biochemical or a range of biochemical testing is required to identify the bacterial species. Significantly, the production of infectious agents requires separate waste handling and practice procedures within a designated and controlled environment. Rigorous cleaning and appropriate protective clothing, including gloves, are required and periodic sterilization may be advisable. Specific advice may be obtained in the report from the Advisory Committee on Dangerous Pathogens 1995 and 2000 (see www.dh.gov.uk).

Post-mortem examinations

Facilities for post-mortem examinations should be available, although this can be and often is provided via an external laboratory. When utilizing an external laboratory, specific provision must be made for shipping, with the associated health and safety requirements. Consideration should also be given to the policies of the destination laboratory on subsequent disposal of the cadaver, particularly if an owner wishes to have the body returned.

If in practice a post-mortem examination must be carried out in a clinical area, it may need to be done after the day's work in a contained non-surgical area, such as on a dental table in an area closed to the public. It would be unusual for a practice laboratory room to have sufficient space, and therefore post-mortem examinations are typically carried out in another designated area. Incorporation of this into other practice procedures and protocols is also therefore required. Particular attention must be paid to the zoonotic potential, and personal protective equipment such as gloves, masks, goggles and aprons as well as appropriate gowns or other protective clothing, should be worn. In part dependent on the species involved, air filtration and extraction is also recommended and is a stipulation for certain species such as birds or primates.

Laboratory management

Staffing

A list of people trained in laboratory testing is currently a requirement for the RCVS Practice Standards Scheme. Having designated staff familiar with testing is ideal but may not be practical and can be expensive, especially if employing specific laboratory personnel.

KEY POINT

A designated person should be in charge of the laboratory, both for staff management purposes and also for practical testing and ordering of supplies.

The majority of practices allow many people, especially veterinary nurses, to perform testing as and when needed. This approach can be efficient with regards to time management, but may result in delayed or missed analysis if it is not managed effectively. A specified rota is a possible consideration.

Even if using designated staff, a fundamental and recommended requirement is a system of standard operating procedures (SOPs) for each task (see below). These are particularly useful for members of staff not designated to the laboratory who only perform tests intermittently.

Progression

While the laboratory is operating, provision should be made for maintaining staff training and experience. Specific regular time within the laboratory and training courses are recommended, allowing new skills to be learnt and slowly incorporated into the practice laboratory. Access to literature and textbooks both within the lab area itself and via the Internet is also useful. Staff should be comfortable working in a laboratory that ensures accurate results are produced and morale maintained.

Health and safety considerations

- Hands should be washed after performing tests, followed by alcohol gel rubs if dealing with samples such as urine and faeces.
- Protective clothing should be worn when handling samples and reagents, a minimum being disposable aprons and gloves. Goggles are required if there is a splash risk.
- Risk assessment (see Chapter 22) and health and safety reviews should be performed at least annually. The offering of laboratory procedures, and the necessity to stock hazardous reagents and chemicals, should be decided after careful consideration of clinical need balanced against the risk of harm to personnel using the laboratory.
- Regular staff consultation and familiarity with the Health and Safety at Work etc. Act 1974 and the Management of Health and Safety at Work Regulations 1999 is recommended.

Waste management

All laboratory analysis creates some form of waste. This will often be healthcare waste that can therefore be incorporated into standard practice procedure for this material (see Chapter 3). Hazardous material may need to be catered for separately. Designated and rigid bins are recommended for each specific waste stream. Haematology analysers often have packaged waste material that can be incinerated or appropriately treated before entering the practice's drainage system. Biochemistry analysers are often similar, although wet chemistry analysers typically require a large collection vessel or connection to the actual waste pipe system.

Standard operating procedures

Whilst it may be assumed that everyone's analysis produces the same result, numerous studies have shown that this is not the case and that one of the biggest analytical variables is due to the individual operator. Whenever a sample is analysed, any variation that sample handling and the analysis itself introduces must be minimized, so that results reflect the changes and variations due to the animal and disease. SOPs are designed to achieve this and can be created for any task in the practice.

SOPs can be brief, covering just the fundamentals for a test, especially if users are familiar with the test procedure. In principle, however, the SOP should be sufficiently detailed so that anyone can follow it. In that way, someone performing the test for the first time should be able to produce a result that is just as valid as that from a person who has done the test numerous times. Indeed, this can be a good way to assess whether an SOP works. Once an SOP has been written, all operators should read it and perform the test. If they understand and are deemed competent, they should be 'signed off' as able to do that test. The SOP is kept accessible in the laboratory and is used for training new staff and for quality control processes within the team. It should be updated and modified if the testing equipment or protocol changes.

SOPs can also be applied to automated analysis and handling of the analysers, potentially incorporating the operating manual specific to that analyser.

KEY POINT

SOPs should be written for all laboratory procedures and tests. In theory, the SOP should apply and operate from the time of blood sampling through to logging and reporting the result to the owner.

Some examples

Setting up a microscope

An example of a protocol for setting up an adjustable binocular microscope for an individual user is shown in an SOP at the end of this chapter.

Proper use of a microscope is described in detail in the *BSAVA Textbook of Veterinary Nursing*. Some important things to include in an SOP are:

- As a rule of thumb, the condenser is lowered and its iris closed down for examination of wet preparations such as skin scrapes or urine; conversely, for dried stained preparations requiring greater detail, the condenser is raised to just short of its highest point, with its iris now opened fully
- When using the X40 lens, the slide must have a cover slip to prevent slight blurring of the image
- Do not leave the lamp switched on while the microscope is unattended
- Microscopes must be kept clean and covered when not in use. Gently wiping off any oil from the X100 lens after each user is recommended, with weekly to monthly cleaning of the lenses using isopropyl alcohol and soft lens tissue.

Manual PCV

An example of a protocol for performing a manual PCV measurement is shown in an SOP at the end of this chapter.

Tissue staining

A standardized practice approach should be used to maximize the information gained. Consistent smear production and subsequent staining is required, followed by rinsing in distilled or buffered water. Some important things to consider are:

- Longer staining times, causing greater depletion, will be seen with more usage and thicker preparations, especially if using for cytology
- If submitting blood smears and cytological preparations to an external laboratory, the slides do not need to be stained to be able to assess diagnostic cellularity
- It should also be noted that if automated staining is used by the external laboratory with no variation in this procedure, any material present at the ends of the slide will not be assessed
- Similarly, if the slides are mislabelled and the material is actually present on the other side, this may be missed as common automated systems only stain one side.

Packing and posting samples

For external analysis, samples will need to be posted or collected by a courier. A guideline protocol for preparing, packing and posting samples is shown in an SOP at the end of this chapter, and packaging is illustrated in Figure 14.15. For a comprehensive review of requirements for shipping biological agents, please refer to the website www.dft.gov.uk/vca/dangerousgoods.

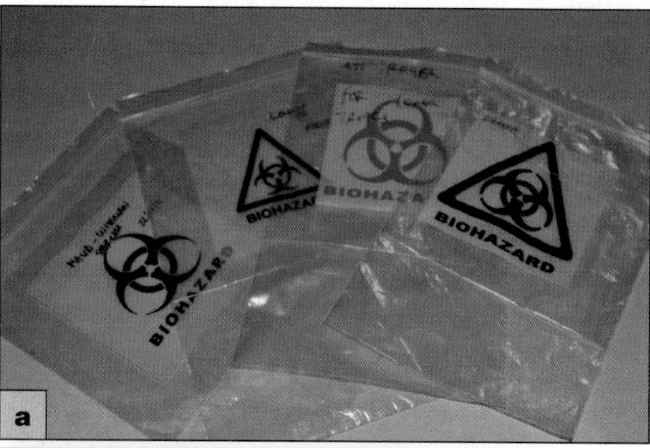

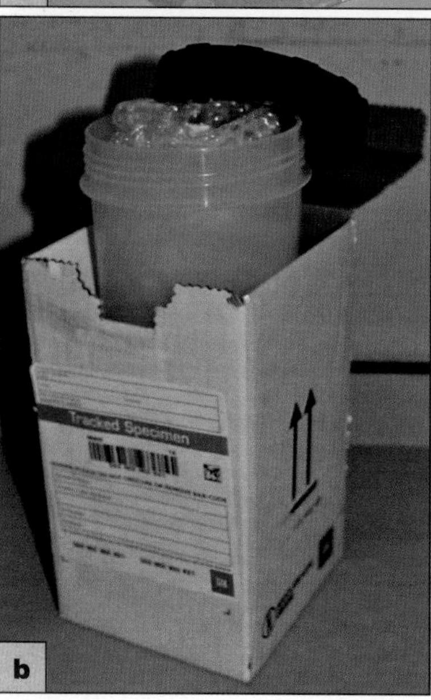

14.15
(a) Biohazard bags. **(b)** Containers of formalin-fixed samples must be placed inside a second rigid container with absorbable material.

Maintenance and monitoring

The laboratory area should be kept clean and tidy.

- The work surfaces and outer cases of all equipment should be cleaned regularly during use and at least daily, with intermittent more thorough cleaning and disinfection according to level of use and the risk from samples handled in the area.
- It is important to pay attention to the insides of cupboards, drawers and bins and to the areas under pieces of equipment where spills and dust can remain unnoticed.
- As with computer equipment, air intakes to fan-cooled devices should be kept clean and free from dust and hair for trouble-free operation.

Equipment maintenance

Analysers typically come with a maintenance schedule and this should be followed. All maintenance and monitoring activity should be documented, both for inspection accreditation purposes and also to identify potential sources of any problems for troubleshooting. Monitoring should include:

- Analyser control and calibration, and reagent changes (see below)
- Daily monitoring of temperature-controlled storage, such as fridge and freezer temperatures
- Refractometer calibration checks (confirming calibration by assessment of distilled water (specific gravity (SG) = 1.000) is advisable at least once a month)
- Changing of stains (with time stains are naturally depleted, become contaminated and potentially crystallize or grow bacteria; they should be filtered and/or replaced regularly, with infrequent cleaning of the staining vessels or Coplin jars. The frequency in part depends upon the usage; a guideline for minimal usage may be every two weeks for replacement, with quarterly cleaning).

With clear maintenance records, everyone can see and be assured that the proper protocols are being followed, ensuring that the laboratory operates efficiently and effectively.

Analyser maintenance and quality control

Obtaining meaningful results from an analyser relies upon it working properly. Testing samples of known composition (controls) and documenting the results proves this, so that results with patient samples can then be trusted. If the results of control testing are not acceptable, patient samples should not be run until the cause is identified and fixed and a repeated control test gives acceptable results.

Features of quality control and quality assessment are noted in Figure 14.16.

Analyser manufacturers should provide reference material (internal control) for regular – typically daily – checks. For dry biochemistry analysers and electrochemical point of care systems, internal control material and testing can be incorporated inherently into each batch of cartridges and rotors.

Periodic checks can use external material sent from an independent assurance scheme, usually on

Quality control (QC)
■ The regular analysis of material or solutions of known composition. This is performed daily when analysers are used regularly (internal) and also more intermittently, such as monthly (external). It involves both calibration and control material. ■ **Calibration:** Material of known value is analysed to 'set' the assay or test reaction. ■ **Controls:** Materials of low and high values are run to check that the assay works for samples with potentially healthy and abnormal levels. ■ **Levey–Jennings charts:** A way of plotting values from control solutions (*y* axis) against time (*x* axis) to assess analytical variation or changes such as those caused by new reagent batches and lots.
Quality assessment (QA)
■ Monitoring and real-time assessment of quality control procedures and results, to ensure that analysis is both accurate and precise, results can be trusted and any errors are detected and corrected quickly. More detail can be found in the *BSAVA Manual of Canine and Feline Clinical Pathology*, with a comprehensive review on various websites (e.g. www.westgard.com). ■ Accuracy: How close the test result is to the actual value. *'Is my value the correct value?'* It measures the test's systematic bias. ■ Precision: The ability of a test to give the same result repeatedly when a sample is analysed several times. *'Can I always get the correct value?'* This is the test's reproducibility and measures random error.

14.16 Features of quality control and quality assessment.

an annual contract. Whilst a veterinary scheme exists that provides some species-specific material, it is limited as to the number of tests and species covered. The majority of schemes used are based on human medicine and use a variety of control and calibrator material derived from both animal and human sources. Whilst species-specific material would be ideal for various reasons, it is realistically and practically impossible to produce such material for each and every species that may be tested using a veterinary practice analyser. Using the available non-species-specific reference material provided by external schemes is valid, recommended and useful, as it proves the method and testing does work against a standardized and validated external scheme, as well as comparing a practice's testing to other similar practices or laboratories. These schemes can identify both human and analyser errors.

A less ideal, but the cheapest, form of external assessment is that of analysing 'paired samples'. Sufficient blood is taken to allow it to be split into two identical samples for analysis both in house and at an external laboratory. To minimise pre-analytical variation, the in-house sample is stored at room temperature to mimic shipping to the external laboratory. Both samples are analysed on the same day and the results compared. This can identify significant analytical bias or poor technique, especially when assessed over time, but can miss subtle clinically significant variation. Because the methods used in the two laboratories are often different, the system does not actually compare 'like with like', and the actual values produced are often therefore naturally slightly different. A biased difference may be acceptable if the reference intervals are also appropriately biased in relation, as the clinical interpretation of the result should not then differ. If values are different, the referral laboratory or analyser manufacturer should be able to offer advice on possible reasons and corrective procedure.

Record-keeping

All laboratory testing should be recorded as part of the clinical record and also so that the relevant charges can be applied. For in-house analysis, a simple request form covering potential tests is an ideal solution, effectively mimicking submission to an external laboratory. An example is given at the end of this chapter. The form, or the results paperwork, should include an area to identify that results have been entered on the patient's clinical record or into the Practice Management System (PMS) and that the client has been notified.

Submission of samples to external laboratories should also be recorded. Information here should include:

- Unique identifiers (such as a client/animal reference number or animal/owner name)
- Date sent
- Tests requested
- Where sent
- The person submitting
- Expected turnaround
- Date of return
- Results recorded
- Results reported to clinician and owner.

KEY POINT

The system should facilitate identification of any lost or delayed samples.

Data storage and retrieval

The format for recording the results, if manually transcribed, should be agreed and universally applied throughout the practice. Different methods may need to be used for internal and for different external laboratory reports.

Results can be entered individually into the animal's consultation record, or the whole report file attached separately as a scanned pdf or text file. Results emailed in from external laboratories may be handled automatically by the PMS, but a clinician alert or automatic printout is essential for timely notification.

If all results, even if unremarkable, are (manually) recorded, this is often time-consuming. However, if only abnormal results are recorded, knowledge of what has been tested should also be noted. Thus, anyone reviewing the patient's record will know what has been tested for and any significant results or changes. It is helpful if results are presented in the same order, and standardized units of measurement are essential. Where different analysers or laboratories are used, the relevant reference ranges should be recorded next to the results for future reference.

Ideally, automated analysis is linked directly to the PMS. This facilitates data transfer and prevents human error during transcription, which can be significant. However, laboratory results must be validated and checked before allowing uploading or transfer to the patient's records.

If a single provider has been used to source the analysers, data transfer can be seamless and integrated but is also much more expensive. Independently sourced and separate analyses can be integrated into most PMSs but would require specific software and physical connections. Such provision is also available but again relatively expensive compared to manual transfer. Internal testing and the associated paperwork needs to be traceable and available for review, if necessary, for an extended period (usually 6–7 years.)

KEY POINT

Old results can be filed in alphabetical or client numerical order, but storing them in date order (most recent on top) is the least time-consuming and most convenient for archiving, and is just as efficient for retrieval.

Communication of results

It is important to ensure that:

- The clinician has seen the results and acted on them
- The client has been charged for the tests, and informed of the results.

It is helpful to discuss with the client before the test is done how they would like to be informed of results if they are not coming back in for a check-up. For example, would they prefer a phone call (NB remember to check contact numbers as they may be at work), a letter, email or text (SMS) message, or would they like to be told face to face?

KEY POINTS

- It is important that clients are given realistic timescales as to when results may be expected.
- It is not fair for the practice to leave an owner anxious and fretting longer than is absolutely necessary. As soon as results are available to the clinician, they should be reported back to the owner without delay.
- A system should be in place for an informed person to communicate results where the clinician is absent.

Acknowledgements

The author and editors gratefully acknowledge the following practices, images of which appear in this chapter: Blythwood Veterinary Group; Mill House Veterinary Surgery and Hospital; Pool House Veterinary Hospital; Wheelhouse Veterinary Centre.

Further reading

Blackwood L and Villiers E (2005) *BSAVA Manual of Canine and Feline Clinical Pathology, 2nd edn.* BSAVA Publications, Gloucester

Burtis CA and Ashwood ER (2001) *Tietz Fundamentals of Clinical Chemistry, 5th edn.* WB Saunders, Philadelphia

Irwin-Porter G (2011) Laboratory diagnostic aids. In: *BSAVA Textbook of Veterinary Nursing, 5th edn*, ed. B Cooper *et al.*, pp. 508–536. BSAVA Publications, Gloucester

Westgard JO (2001) *Six Sigma Quality Design and Control.* Westgard QC, Madison, WI

Willard M and Tvedten H (2007) *Small Animal Clinical Diagnosis by Laboratory Methods, 4th edn.* Saunders Elsevier, St. Louis

Examples of SOPs and forms 

SOP No ....

Protocol for setting up an adjustable binocular microscope without an adjustable field iris diaphragm

NOTE: All microscope equipment should only be handled by trained staff.

The following staff are trained to care for and clean microscope equipment:

1. Turn the lamp on and adjust the brightness for comfort.
2. Adjust the distance between the eyepieces so that only one image is seen.
3. Place a coverslipped slide on to the microscope stage.
4. Ensure the eyepiece focus settings are equal to each other.
5. Using the X10 objective lens, focus on the slide material – using the fine and coarse controls and using your right eye only. Then, using your left eye only, adjust the left eyepiece only so that the image is also focused for this eye.
6. Repeat step 5 with the X40 objective lens to fine tune the microscope to your eyes.
7. Set the condenser to just lower than its highest setting using its focus control knob.
8. Use the desired lens for examination. If the microscope has an adjustable aperture diaphragm on the condenser, this should be set to the same figure as the magnification of the lens (i.e. 4, 10, 40 or 100). Ideally, this aperture should be changed each time the objective lens is changed. If not, a compromise setting for most objective lenses is 40.

SOP No ....

Packing and posting lab samples

1. Ensure that all sample tubes or other containers are labelled appropriately (date, animal and client ID).
2. Where required, centrifuge and separate off plasma or serum into a fresh, plain, sealable, screwtop tube.
3. Seal sample containers tightly and wrap them in absorbent material such as cotton wool or tissue paper before placing and sealing in a biohazard bag. NB Containers of formalin-fixed samples must be placed inside a second rigid container, with sufficient absorbable material to soak up all liquid should it leak during transit.
4. Complete the relevant laboratory request form and place it in the relevant back section of the biohazard bag.
5. Place the filled biohazard bag in a durable padded or rigid outer postage container or bag.
6. Address the outer postage container or bag and label with 'Pathological Specimen – UN 3373'.
7. If not postage-paid, calculate the correct postage and apply frank/stamps to the package.
8. Record the sample details and ID, together with date of posting and destination, in a book or on a computer record.
9. Follow up to ensure that the sample is posted by the last post on that day. If there is a delay in posting, store the package in the laboratory fridge until it can be posted.

Examples of SOPs for use in the laboratory. (continues)

▶

SOP No ....

Packed cell volume – manual measurement

Date effective ....

Background

Blood is a mixture of cells and plasma. The packed cell volume (PCV) is a percentage (%) measurement of the proportion of blood that is made up of red blood cells (RBCs). A manual PCV may be needed to check against an automatic analyser's HCT (haematocrit) measurement, or in order to monitor intravenous fluids and anaemia when assessing therapy.

Materials

- 1 microhaematocrit/capillary tube (in cupboard drawer)
- Soft clay sealant (in cupboard drawer)
- Standard ruler (in cupboard drawer)
- Disposable tissues (on bench top)
- Microhaematocrit centrifuge with additional capillary tube to balance (on lab bench top)
- Labelled patient sample of whole blood in EDTA tube
- Disposable gloves

Method

1. Gently mix the blood sample by inverting and rolling it between your hands for at least 1 minute or placing it on a mechanical mixer for at least 1 minute.
2. Place the end of the microhaematocrit tube into the blood sample tube, at a slight angle, and allow capillary action to draw the blood up until the microhaematocrit tube is two-thirds to three-quarters full.
3. Place one finger over the top of the microhaematocrit tube and remove it from the sample tube. Keep your finger in place, so that the blood stays in the microhaematocrit tube.
4. Wipe off excess blood from the outside of the tube with a tissue.
5. Place the bottom end of the microhaematocrit tube into the tray of clay sealant. Rock the tube and then angle it to seal the tube with a plug of the clay. You can now take your finger off the other end.
6. Place the tube into the microhaematocrit rack in the microhaematocrit centrifuge, with the sealant plug outermost, opposite the balance capillary tube, and close the lid.
7. Spin the tube for 5 minutes.
8. After spinning, place the microhaematocrit tube next to the ruler, with the bottom of the red blood cell column (band B) at zero.
9. Read off the length of band B.
10. Read off the length for the entire column of liquid and cells (B + C + D).
11. Calculate PCV (%):

    PCV (%) = $B / (B + C + D) \times 100$

12. Write the PCV value on the relevant patient's chart and records.
13. Dispose of the tube in the blood-contaminated sharps bin.

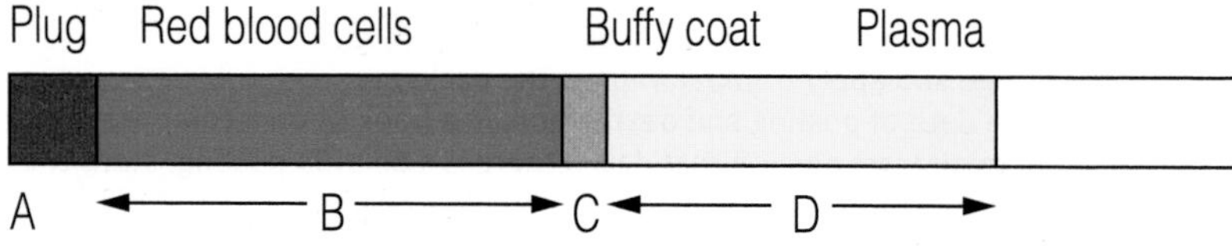

(continued) Examples of SOPs for use in the laboratory.

INTERNAL LAB REQUEST AND REPORT FORM

Date

EDTA	ml	HEPARIN	ml
PLAIN	ml	OTHER	ml

VN to take samples?	YES:	NO:

Animal name
Owner
Species **Age**
Sex **VET**
Ref No:

BLOOD PANELS

☐**BP Biochem Profile Prestige**
albumin, Alk Phos, ALT, creatinine, total protein, urea, globulin, AST, calcium, cholesterol, CK, GGT, glucose, phosphorus including Na, K, Cl (Jokoh)

☐**HPN Haematology**
WCC, Hb, RBC, HCT, MCV, MCHC, MCH, PLT, MPV on Nihon Kohden machine; PCV

☐ **BHP Biochem & Haem Combined Profile**
Haematology profile plus BP

INDIVIDUAL TESTS

Prestige

☐Total bilirubin ☐ Urea
☐Triglyceride ☐ Creatinine
☐ Bile acids ☐ GGT
☐ Mg ☐
☐ ☐
☐ ☐

☐ **EPJ Electrolyte Panel Jokoh only**
Na, K, Cl
Plasma/serum

☐ **IRMA CC Panel**
pH, pCO2, pO2, Na, K, iCa, HCT, HCO3, TCO2, BEecf, BEb, O2sat, tHB
Blood gas syringe

☐ **Lactate (not available)**
Blood gas syringe

☐ PCV
☐ Plasma Protein (refractometer)
☐ **BLSM** Examine Blood Smear +/- WCC

☐ ACT Coag test *ACTT*

WELL PETS ONLY

☐ **PAS Pre-anaesthetic Screen**
Haematology profile plus albumin, Alk Phos, ALT, creatinine, total protein, urea, globulin, calcium, glucose

☐**GS1 Geriatric Simple Screen**
Haematology profile plus albumin, Alk Phos, ALT, creatinine, total protein, urea, globulin, calcium, glucose

☐ **TS Therapy Screen**
Haematology profile plus albumin, Alk Phos, ALT, creatinine, total protein, urea, globulin, calcium, glucose

SNAP BLOOD TESTS etc

☐FeLV /FIV test Combo *FELVF*

☐Premate *PTR / PTR*

☐Parvo test (Speed)*PARVO*

URINE TESTS

☐ **UFE Full Exam**
Includes SG, dipstick, sediment

☐ **UDS Dipstick & SG**
- Glucose Blood
- Protein Bilirubin
- PH Ketones
- SG (Refractometer)

☐ **BUS** Booster Urine Sample or Diabetes Month Urine Sample (= UDS)

USED Sediment microscopy

☐ Wet prep with drop of #3 Rapidiff

☐ Deposit on slide, dry and 3 stage stain with Rapidiff

☐ Plain Smear

☐Cytology *CYTO*

SKIN EXAMINATIONS

☐Scraping for direct examination

☐Scraping for KOH *SKINS*

OTHER TESTS

Sample quality:

	Initials
TESTS PERFORMED BY	
RESULTS ON COMPUTER	
CHARGED	
SSF?	
Prepaid?	
Owner Informed?	
Results Checked By Vet	

An example of an internal laboratory request and report form.

The practice dispensary

15

Pam Mosedale

All veterinary practices that dispense veterinary drugs and medicinal products need an area where drugs are stored and prescriptions dispensed. This dispensary area (Figure 15.1) is a vital hub of the practice, generating income from drug sales. It must:

- Comply with drug-dispensing legislation and best practice
- Store drugs correctly, according to manufacturers' instructions
- Provide a clean tidy environment to facilitate correct handling of medicines and minimize the risk of dispensing errors.

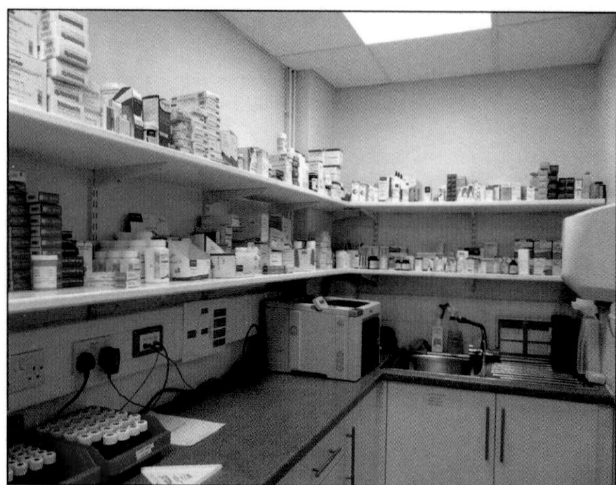

15.1 A clean and tidy dispensary will reduce the risk of dispensing errors.

Legislation and regulation

Premises

All premises where veterinary medicinal products (VMPs) are stored or supplied to clients must be listed on a register as a Veterinary Practice Premises (VPP). This register is currently maintained by the RCVS on behalf of the Veterinary Medicines Directorate (VMD).

VMPs can be supplied by a wholesaler to a veterinary surgeon at non-registered premises, but the veterinary surgeon can only supply VMPs to clients from a registered VPP. The VMD is entitled to inspect these premises. Those practices that are members of the RCVS Practice Standards Scheme (PSS) will not currently be inspected by the VMD inspection and investigation team, as their dispensaries and drug storage arrangements will be inspected as part of the PSS inspection. Inspections by the VMD, or under the RCVS PSS, will include a check on the RCVS registration of veterinary surgeons and premises, as well as the registration and qualifications of any Suitably Qualified Persons (SQPs; Figure 15.2) employed in the practice.

The Veterinary Medicines Regulations (VMR) require practices to keep a record, at their main premises, of all places that they store medicines; this includes practice cars and veterinary surgeons' homes if medicines are kept there for 'on-call' use. This record can be held within the practice management system or

Suitably Qualified Persons (SQPs) are a category of professionally qualified persons who are allowed to prescribe or supply certain veterinary medicines under the Veterinary Medicines Regulations.

SQPs have to pass a base examination on the Veterinary Medicines legislation, plus a species-specific examination. They can register with AMTRA (Animal Medicines Training and Regulation Authority) and are then permitted to prescribe and supply POM-VPS and NFA-VPS medicines from registered premises.

There are different categories of SQP; the relevant categories for companion animals are:

- C-SQP: can prescibe companion animal VPS medicines only
- E-SQP: can prescribe equine and companion animal VPS medicines
- K-SQP: can prescribe farm and companion animal VPS medicines
- R-SQP: can prescribe all VPS medicines.

All SQPs are obliged to undertake CPD accredited by AMTRA.

Veterinary Nurses are not automatically SQPs but they are given credit for their nursing qualification and can do a 'top-up' exam to qualify as an SQP.

15.2 Suitably Qualified Persons (SQPs).

it can be a stock book showing transfers of stock between branches, into cars, or within the practice areas. All medicines should be stored in accordance with manufacturers' recommendations, whether in the practice or in a vehicle (see above).

Veterinary surgeons can prescribe and dispense medicines or they can write a prescription for the client to get their drugs from a pharmacy or another practice (see *BSAVA Small Animal Formulary* for prescription requirements). The RCVS Code of Professional Conduct for veterinary surgeons supporting guidance requires a prominently displayed sign in the waiting room, informing clients that they can obtain a prescription (Figure 15.3) and clients should also be informed of this on an ongoing basis, e.g. through practice leaflets or information on the practice website.

PRESCRIPTION NOTICE

Prescriptions are available from this practice.

You may obtain Prescription-Only Medicines, Category V (POM-Vs) from us OR ask for a prescription and obtain these medicines from another veterinary surgeon or a pharmacy.

A prescription may not be appropriate if your animal is an inpatient or if immediate treatment is necessary.

You will be informed on request of the price of any medicine that may be prescribed for your animal.

The general policy of this practice is to re-assess an animal requiring repeat prescriptions every ...... months, but this may vary with individual circumstances.

The standard charge for re-examination is £......

The standard charge for a prescription is £......

The current prices for the top 10 POM-Vs most commonly prescribed or supplied during *(specify dates of 3-month period)* are:

1 ....
2 ....
3 ....
4 ....
5 ....
6 ....
7 ....
8 ....
9 ....
10 ....

15.3 Example of the content required for a prescription notice.

Veterinary medicines classification

VMPs are classified under the VMR into four groups (Figure 15.4). Medicines for use in certain pet species (aquarium fish, cage birds, ferrets, homing pigeons, rabbits, small rodents and terrarium animals), the active ingredient of which has been declared by the

AVM-GSL *Authorized veterinary medicine – general sales list*

Medicines in the AVM-GSL category may be legally supplied by any retailer, to anyone, without restriction.

NFA-VPS *Non-food animal medicine – veterinarian, pharmacist, suitably qualified person (SQP)*

Medicines in the NFA-VPS category are for companion animals (excluding horses). They must be supplied by a veterinary surgeon, pharmacist or SQP from registered premises. A clinical assessment of the animal is not required for supply of this category of veterinary medicine but the animal owner should be given practical advice to ensure safe and effective use of the product.

POM-VPS *Prescription-only medicine – veterinarian, pharmacist, SQP*

Medicines in the POM-VPS category must be both prescribed and supplied by a veterinary surgeon, pharmacist or SQP. Any authorized supplier may supply in accordance with a written prescription from any authorized prescriber. The medicine must be supplied from registered premises. A clinical assessment of the animal is not required when prescribing this category of veterinary medicine; however, sufficient information about the animal and the way it is kept must be known to the person prescribing so that they can prescribe and supply appropriately.

POM-V *Prescription-only medicine – veterinarian*

Medicines in the POM-V category must only be prescribed by a veterinary surgeon following a clinical assessment of the animal or group of animals, which must be under their care. The veterinary surgeon must also be satisfied that the person who will use the product will do so safely, and intends to use it for the purpose(s) for which it is authorized. The medicine may then be supplied by that veterinary surgeon or in accordance with a written prescription by another veterinary surgeon or a pharmacist. The medicine must be supplied from registered premises.

15.4 The four groups of veterinary medicines.

Secretary of State as not requiring veterinary control, may be marketed under the Small Animal Exemption Scheme. These may be sold by any retailer.

Labelling requirements

In theory, if a medicine is dispensed in the container supplied by the manufacturer with all the information supplied and all information on the packaging is legible, and if it is intended for a condition and species listed on the data sheet, there is no legal requirement for further labelling. However, the RCVS Code of Professional Conduct for Veterinary Surgeons Supporting Guidance advises that all veterinary medical products are labelled appropriately.

The RCVS Practice Standards Scheme requires that labels for POM-V medicines should include:

- The name and address of the registered veterinary practice premises supplying the VMP
- The name and address of the animal's owner
- The date of supply
- The name or description of the medicinal product and its strength
- The dosage and administration instructions
- The words 'Keep out of reach of children' and 'For animal treatment only'
- The words 'For external use only' for topical preparations.

In addition, for medicines supplied for use under the prescribing cascade (see below):

- The name of the veterinary surgeon who has prescribed the medicine (initials may suffice)
- The identification (including the species) of the animal or group of animals
- Plus, unless already specified on the manufacturer's packaging:
  - The expiry date of the medicine
  - Any special precautions
  - Any necessary warnings with reference to the user, target species, administration or disposal of the product.

Record-keeping in the dispensary

The VMR require any veterinary surgeon who supplies a prescription medicine to keep records for at least 5 years for all incoming drugs (from wholesalers) and all outgoing drugs (prescribed and supplied to clients). The following information is required:

- Date and nature of the transaction
- Name of the veterinary medicinal product
- The batch number (in the case of a medicine for a non-food-producing animal, this need only be recorded either on the date the batch was received or the date the batch was first used)
- Quantity received or supplied
- Name and address of the supplier or recipient
- If there is a written prescription, the name and address of the person who wrote the prescription and a copy of the prescription.

The requirement for keeping records of drugs purchased may be met by retaining the invoices or delivery notes from wholesalers.

Batch numbers

Veterinary practices should have an efficient stock control system (see below) to monitor the use of veterinary medicines and to allow for the recall of an individual medicine or particular batch. Veterinary wholesalers record the batch numbers of all medicinal products supplied to the practices on their invoices, and these records can also often be accessed online by the practice. As it is not necessary, with the exception of vaccinations, for small animal practices to record individual batch numbers on an animal's record, if batch numbers are not recorded the first time a drug is used then it must be assumed for the purposes of any product recall that the batch was used from the first day it arrived at the practice. This would mean that in any product recall more clients would be contacted, but within this large group would be the smaller group whose animals actually received the batch in question. This is acceptable to the VMD.

Drugs audit

Practices should be able to carry out a detailed drug audit (Figure 15.5). The VMD states that 'a system linking incoming and outgoing transactions with stock held may provide an ongoing running total which, with the addition of a periodic physical stock count to verify stock held, may meet the audit requirement'.

KEY POINT

Ideally, and at least once a year, a detailed audit should be carried out, where incoming and outgoing medicines are reconciled with the medicines held in stock, and any discrepancies recorded.

The practice should:

- Perform a full stock take of all prescription drugs
- Keep records of all drugs received (e.g. by retaining invoices or delivery notes from wholesalers)
- Keep records of all drugs supplied to clients (e.g. from the practice computer system or by a sales log)
- Record any out-of-date or damaged drugs discarded.

15.5 Elements required in a drug audit.

In practice it is important to know when medicines have been stolen, undelivered or dispensed incorrectly. It is up to the practice to account for discrepancies and decide what level is acceptable. Discrepancies are to be expected in the case of drugs used during procedures and not priced individually (e.g. premedicants, anaesthetics and euthanasia drugs) and with multi-dose injectables where needle hub and uninjected volumes can throw out totals significantly. In order to account for discrepancies, all out-of-date or damaged drugs disposed of need to be accounted for. This is done in many practices by allocating all drugs that have been disposed of to a 'client account' with a name such as 'Out of date' or 'Reception discrepancies'. If computerized stock control is used, this system will allow tracking of shrinkage and assessment of several factors, such as poor recording of consumables use by clinical staff or pilfering of reception stock.

'Off-licence' use of medicines

Medicines must be used in accordance with the legislation commonly referred to as 'the cascade' (Figure 15.6). This is detailed in the VMR and is explained fully in Veterinary Medicines Guidance Note 15 (VMG15) which can be found on the VMD website (www.vmd.gov.uk). Where medicines are imported for specific patients, Special Treatment Certificates or Special Import Certificates are required (Figure 15.7).

If there is no authorized VMP in the UK to treat a condition in a particular species, then a veterinary surgeon may exercise his/her clinical judgement in order to avoid suffering. In the case of any medicine prescribed under the prescribing cascade, the RCVS recommends in its Code of Professional Conduct that informed consent should be obtained from the owners for use in their animal. This includes explaining any special precautions or warnings for the use, administration or disposal of the product.

If there is no authorized veterinary medicinal product in the UK to treat a condition in a particular species, the cascade allows veterinary surgeons to select a product in this order:

1. A veterinary medicine for another animal species or for another condition in the same species
2. If these are not available, the veterinary surgeon may select a medicinal product authorized in the UK for human use or a veterinary medicinal product not authorized in the UK but authorized in another Member State of the EU (European Union) for use with any animal species (if the product is for use in a food-producing animal, then it must be authorized for a food-producing species).
3. Only if there is still no suitable product, a veterinary medicinal product prepared extemporaneously by a pharmacist, veterinary surgeon or person holding a Marketing Authorization can be used.
4. If there is still no suitable product, a veterinary surgeon can apply for a Special Treatment Certificate (STC; see Figure 15.7) to import a suitable authorized product from outside the UK.

15.6 The prescribing cascade for veterinary medicines.

It is illegal to import unauthorized medicines into the UK. Veterinary surgeons may apply to the VMD for products to treat animals under their care, if medicines are available abroad but not in the UK. There are two licences for importing drugs.

- **Special Treatment Certificates (STCs):**
  - For non-European or human medicinal products
  - Initial application in writing
  - Initial application charged for (see VMD website for cost)
  - Subsequent applications can be made online [a]
  - No charge for subsequent applications
- **Special Import Certificates (SICs):**
  - For European medicinal products
  - Initial application online [a] or in writing
  - Initial application charged for (see VMD website for cost)
  - Subsequent applications can be made online [a]
  - No charge for subsequent applications.

[a] For all online applications the VMD must have been notified in writing or by telephone, so that the practice applying can be registered and allocated a specific VMD number.

All applications for either Certificate must contain:
- RCVS number of veterinary surgeon
- Address of veterinary premises
- Owner's name and address
- Patient's name
- Details of the drug and the importer
- Amount of drug, dose and route of administration
- Justification for use.

15.7 Importing medicines into the United Kingdom: STCs and SICs.

- General 'lifelong' consent forms can be used for the treatment of some small mammals, birds, reptiles, amphibians, fish and invertebrates, for which there are few authorized medicines.
- For cats and dogs, a form 'to consent to the administration of a medicine not authorized for the particular use proposed in the treatment of an animal' should be used. If a second drug is used 'off-licence' on a different occasion, a further consent form must be filled in.
- Templates of written consent forms for 'off-licence' drug use can be accessed by Veterinary Defence Society members at their website (www.veterinarydefencesociety.co.uk).

Where possible, written information about the product should be supplied to the owner:

- Summary of product characteristics data sheets (SPCs) for all human prescription-only medicines can be found in the electronic medicines compendium (www.emc.medicines.org.uk)
- Veterinary-specific information can be found by BSAVA members on the BSAVA website, where client information leaflets for commonly prescribed unauthorized medicines can be sourced.

There are also differences in the labelling requirements for 'off-licence' drugs (see Labelling requirements, above).

Adverse reactions

All adverse reactions must be reported under the suspected adverse reaction surveillance scheme (SARSS), whether they are in animals or in humans handling the medicines. They should be reported direct to the VMD online (www.vmd.defra.gov.uk) or to the manufacturer of the medicine. Yellow SARSS forms should be available where Internet reporting is not straightforward. Copies of all reports should be kept and a note made of adverse reactions reported to manufacturers, if they submit the form to VMD. Lack of efficacy of a product should be reported in the same way.

KEY POINT

Practices should have a protocol, known to all staff, on when and how to report adverse reactions. This should include information on how to access forms online (Figure 15.8).

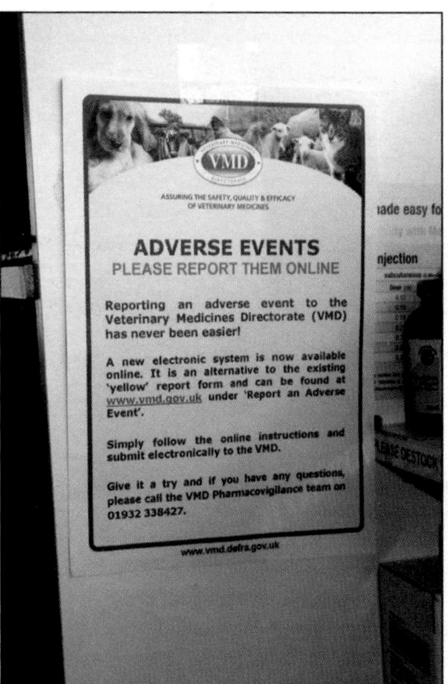
VMD
ASSURING THE SAFETY, QUALITY & EFFICACY OF VETERINARY MEDICINES
ADVERSE EVENTS
PLEASE REPORT THEM ONLINE
Reporting an adverse event to the Veterinary Medicines Directorate (VMD) has never been easier!
A new electronic system is now available online. It is an alternative to the existing 'yellow' report form and can be found at www.vmd.gov.uk under 'Report an Adverse Event'.
Simply follow the online instructions and submit electronically to the VMD.
Give it a try and if you have any questions, please call the VMD Pharmacovigilance team on 01932 338427.
www.vmd.defra.gov.uk

15.8 Staff should be made aware of the online reporting system for adverse reactions to veterinary medicines.

Controlled Drugs

There are five schedules of Controlled Drugs (CDs; Figure 15.9). Where CDs are kept, they must be stored and recorded according to current legislation (Figure 15.10).

Schedule 1
Veterinary surgeons do not have the authority to supply these, as they have no therapeutic value. They include LSD, ecstasy and other hallucinogenic drugs.
Schedule 2
Those used in veterinary practice include etorphine, fentanyl, morphine, papaveretum, pethidine, alfentanil, secobarbital and amphetamines. These drugs are subject to safe custody requirements: they must be kept in a suitable locked cabinet at all times, secured to the fabric of the building. All purchases and each individual supply of these drugs must be recorded in the Controlled Drugs Register.
Schedule 3
These include buprenorphine, butorphanol, the barbiturates, pentazocine and midazolam. These drugs are also subject to safe custody requirements but do not have to be recorded in the Controlled Drugs Register.
Schedule 4
Part 1 – the benzodiazepines; Part 2 – androgenic and anabolic steroids. These are not subject to safe custody requirements. Note, however, that ketamine (Schedule 4, Part 1) is a substance of potential abuse and the RCVS therefore considers that it should be treated as a Schedule 2 CD and recommends in the Code of Professional Conduct that it should be stored in the CD cabinet, with its use recorded in an informal register.
Schedule 5
These include some preparations of morphine and codeine preparations present in medicinal products of low strength. These are exempt from all CD requirements, except that invoices must be retained for 5 years.

15.9 The five Schedules of Controlled Drugs.

Element	CD classification: Schedule					
	2	*2: secobarbital only*	3	4	*4: ketamine only*	5
Safe custody. Store in CD cabinet	Yes	No	Yes	No	Yes	No
Record in Controlled Drug Register	Yes	Yes	No	No	Record in informal register	No
Written requisition to wholesalers	Yes	Yes	Yes	No	No	No

15.10 Requirements for Controlled Drugs.

KEY POINT

Veterinary practices should ensure that they have robust systems in place for the security and recording of all Controlled Drugs used in the practice.

Controlled Drugs cabinet

Schedule 2 and 3 CDs (apart from secobarbital) must be kept in a locked cabinet which is attached to the fabric of the building (Figure 15.11). The Misuse of Drugs Regulations 2001 give specifications for drug safes and Controlled Drug cabinets. Cabinets should conform to British Standards (BS2881: 1989 is the specification for cupboards for storage of medicines in healthcare premises).

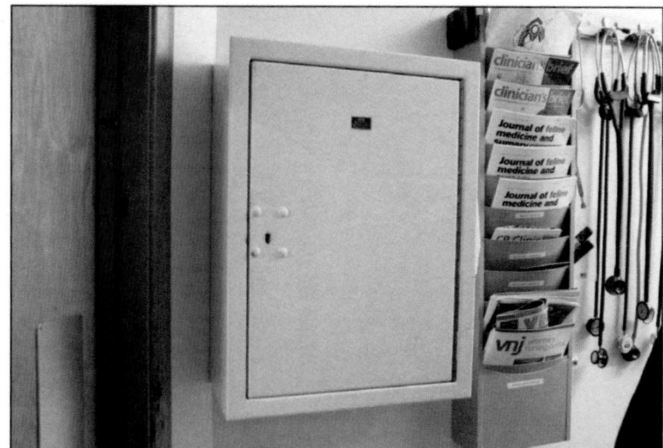

15.11 The Controlled Drugs cupboard should be securely fixed to the wall and large enough to store the entire CD stock.

Access to the CD cupboard should be restricted. The keys to the cupboard should be held only by the veterinary surgeon, or those under his/her strict authorization. If there are multiple keys to the cupboard then each veterinary surgeon can have their own key. If there is only one key, this can be passed from one veterinary surgeon or RVN authorized by the veterinary surgeon to another (this can be recorded in a key register). If this is not practicable, a single key can be kept in a code-operated key safe, with the code known only to the veterinary surgeon or those authorized by him/her. This has the advantage of being able to change the code if there are changes of personnel or if the code becomes known to other staff members.

Whichever method is used, the CD cupboard should only be used for Controlled or hazardous drugs storage and should never be used as a general medicines cupboard, a safe for money, or for any reason which would involve more than the authorized staff having access. The cupboard should never be left unlocked, even during the working day.

KEY POINT

A common non-compliance with both VMD and PSS inspections is that although most practices have locked receptacles for Controlled Drug storage, many are accessible to all staff rather than just to authorized personnel.

Controlled Drugs Register

- Controlled Drugs must be audited continuously.
- All supply and use must be recorded, keeping a running balance in the Controlled Drugs Register (CDR; Figure 15.12), and having a system of regularly reconciling this with stock actually in the CD cupboard (generally weekly).
- Both VMD and PSS inspectors will ask to see a full audit and reconciliation of all Schedule 2 Controlled Drugs (i.e. the Register and the balance of drugs in stock).

Entries made when a Controlled Drug is received					
Date received	Name and address of supplier	Amount received	Form in which received		Running total
Entries made when a Controlled Drug is supplied					
Date supplied	Name and address of person supplied	Name and signature of veterinary surgeon	Amount supplied	Form in which supplied	Running total

15.12 Entries required in a Controlled Drugs Register.

The CDR can be a bound book or a computerized record. A loose-leaf or spiral-bound book is **not** acceptable, as pages can be removed. Entries in the book must be in chronological order, with no alterations. Each drug, and each strength of the drug, must have a separate section in the book.

The Register must be filled in within 24 hours of use of the CD. It is acceptable during a busy day to record use of the drug temporarily on notes or consent forms and to fill the Register in at the end of the day. The veterinary surgeon must sign for each entry in the CDR.

A written requisition to the wholesaler, signed by a veterinary surgeon, is required before Schedule 2 and 3 CDs are supplied to a practice. All incoming Schedule 2 CDs from the wholesaler, and all use or prescribing of Schedule 2 drugs in the practice, must be recorded. Each individual use must be recorded as a separate entry in the CDR and there must be a running balance. The stock in the cupboard should be checked regularly (at least weekly) against the running balance to create a continuous audit of Controlled Drugs.

The ketamine informal register only differs in that it does not have to be signed by the veterinary surgeon, otherwise all details should be as in the CDR. Again, a running balance should be kept and checked against stock at least weekly.

If a computerized CDR is used, safeguards must be built into the software to ensure that the author of each entry is identifiable and that entries cannot be altered. The system must be password-protected and only the veterinary surgeon (and those specifically authorized by him/her) should have access to it.

Disposal of Controlled Drugs

Controlled Drugs must be rendered irretrievable by denaturing before disposal. Denaturing kits are easily available from veterinary wholesalers. This disposal must also be witnessed; this can be by a police officer or by an RCVS PSS Inspector, VMD Animal Medicines Inspector or a veterinary surgeon who is independent of the practice.

Dispensary design

The VMR state that medicines should be stored in a clean and tidy location, in accordance with manufacturers' recommendations. Premises will be inspected to check that they are housed in a permanent and secure building, which does not allow the entrance of birds or vermin, and that the medicines storage areas are designed to allow drugs to be stored at the correct temperature. RCVS Practice Standards inspectors will also check that there are hand-washing facilities, and that toilets and amenities for staff are available but separate from the drug storage areas.

Medicines should not be stored in areas that are accessible to the public. Only AVM-GSL medicines are allowed to be displayed on a self-service basis, so dispensary design should consider accessibility for staff but not for the public, and take security issues into account.

Location

Where the dispensary area is sited will depend on practice size and positioning of other areas. A common dispensary area behind the consulting area, with access from all consulting rooms, is the ideal as there is then no necessity to store drugs in consulting rooms (Figure 15.13). Direct secure access from the reception, inpatient and surgical areas is desirable. This facilitates efficient stock control, as only one bottle of any multidose injectable drug needs to be open at one time, and refrigeration facilities can be in the dispensary and used by all consulting areas.

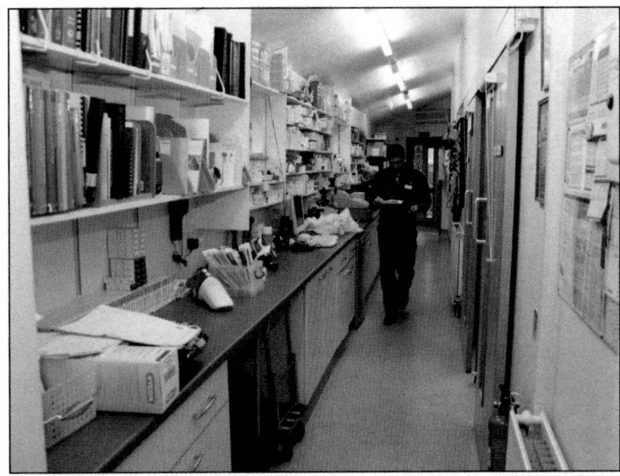

15.13 A dispensary running behind consulting rooms is very convenient, though it can be an extremely busy area. Note the stock trolleys stowed under the bench on the left and bulk orders stored visibly on top shelves. Safe steps are required to access these.

Heating,ventilation and lighting

Medicines should be stored in areas away from excessive light and/or moisture. The dispensary area should have good ventilation and heating or cooling, not only to make it a pleasant area for staff but also to maintain ideal drug storage conditions (see below). Lighting should be adequate for controlling stock, dispensing and reading small print on drug packaging and inserts.

Fitments

Worktop

It is important to have a clear uncluttered and impervious worktop area, which is not shared with other practice functions, to allow organized and hygienic dispensing. There should be space for label printers (Figure 15.14) and computer equipment.

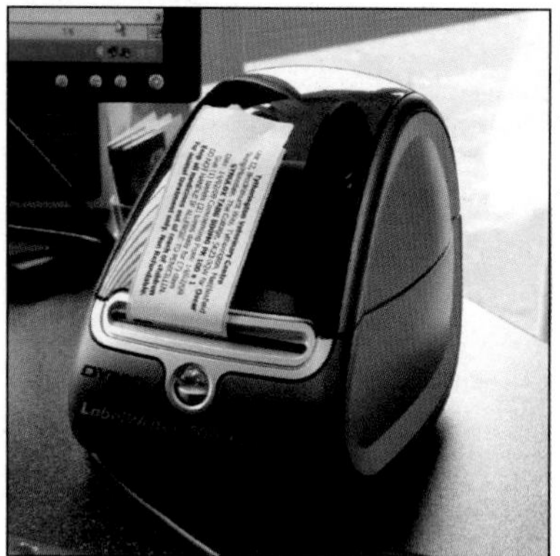

15.14 A label printer should be available within the dispensary.

Shelving and storage units

Shelving should be easily cleanable. Pharmaceutical suppliers can provide pharmacy shelving, which has angled shelves (Figure 15.15) and moveable product dividers to make stock rotation and organization easier. Shelf height is always a compromise but sufficient height should be allowed so that larger pack sizes do not have be stored out of their expected location.

- Medicines should be stored in their original packaging with a copy of their product leaflet or SPC.
- Stock should be organized logically on shelves for efficiency in locating the necessary drug quickly and to minimize the risk of dispensing errors. This will depend on practice preference but there should be a clear and consistent system. For example, drugs can be arranged by:
  - Therapeutic group (e.g. antibiotics, steroids)
  - System affected (e.g. cardiac drugs)
  - Alphabetical order.
- Those products with the shortest expiry date should be positioned at the front of the shelves so that they are used first.
- VMPs with the same batch number should be kept together. It is good practice to record the date of first using a batch of a medicinal product for recall purposes (see above).

Keeping a list, either computerized or manual, of the location of stocks of each drug, and (in larger dispensaries) numbering shelves and cupboards, is helpful both for stock control, and to help new staff or locums locate products. See also Controlled Drugs cabinet, above.

KEY POINT

In the case of a group practice it makes sense to use the same drug locating system at each branch.

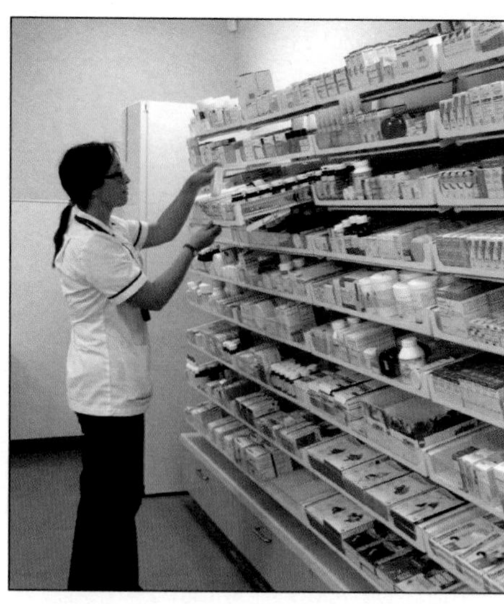

15.15 Angled shelves that pull out make stock rotation easier.

Veterinary dispensaries are often quite small areas, so designing storage to make full use of the space available is important. Accommodation for stacking and handling incoming orders is vital: underbench space can be used (see Figure 15.21), or a secure lobby area.

Storage and temperature control for medicines

The manufacturers' storage recommendations should be checked for all products stocked. This involves looking at the SPC.

- For veterinary authorized products SPCs can be found on the Veterinary Medicines Directorate (VMD) website (www.vmd.gov.uk). At section 6 of the SPC for each drug there is information on any special precautions for storage.
- For unauthorized drugs, such as human POMs, the SPCs can be found on the electronic medicines compendium website (www.emc.medicines.org.uk) in exactly the same format.

Recommendations may state 'Keep out of light' or 'Store in a dry place' or 'Store in original packaging' and will give an indication of the temperature at which the product should be stored. Monitoring should be undertaken *wherever medicines are stored*; this may include reception (for repeat medications awaiting collection), surgical and preparation areas, and vehicles. Any flammable medicines should be stored in a labelled metal cupboard.

The SPC should also be consulted when carrying out risk assessments under COSHH and developing SOPs for handling spillages, accidental self-injection, etc. Stock control, dating broached vials and temperature monitoring SOPs should all be included in staff training for working in the dispensary (see below).

Temperature

- Most product SPCs state 'Do not store above 25°C'.
- For products that require refrigeration, the SPC may state 'Store at +2°C to +8°C; should be transported under recommended conditions'.
- For temperature-sensitive products temperatures need to be monitored regularly.

Although many practices use domestic refrigerators for storage, specific medical or pharmacy units are available (Figure 15.16). Maximum/minimum thermometers should be used to monitor room and fridge temperatures (Figure 15.17). Rather than knowing the ambient temperature in the refrigerator at a particular time, it is important to know that temperatures have stayed within the range of 2–8°C, so that vaccines and other medicines have been kept within their recommended temperature range. Constant monitoring can be provided by data loggers, which can be easily downloaded on to a PC periodically. Data loggers and other thermometers should ideally have some form of alarm or alerting system to indicate when the temperature has gone out of range; otherwise they should be checked at least daily and records, either paper-based or electronic, kept of temperatures (Figure 15.18).

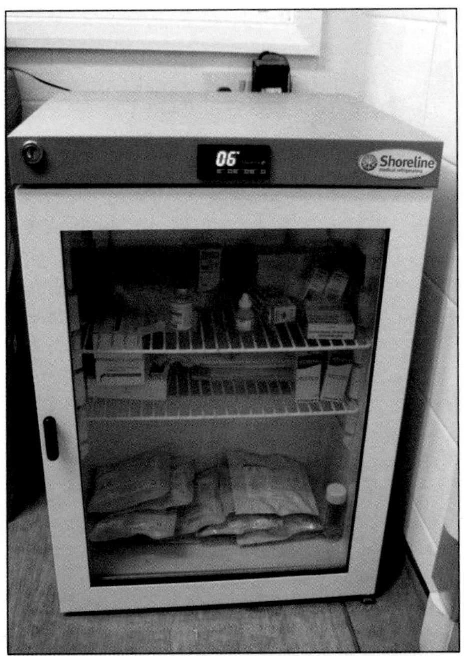

15.16 A pharmacy fridge with the temperature clearly shown on the outside is helpful for monitoring drug storage. These fridges also have a built-in alarm should the temperature go outside the pre-set range.

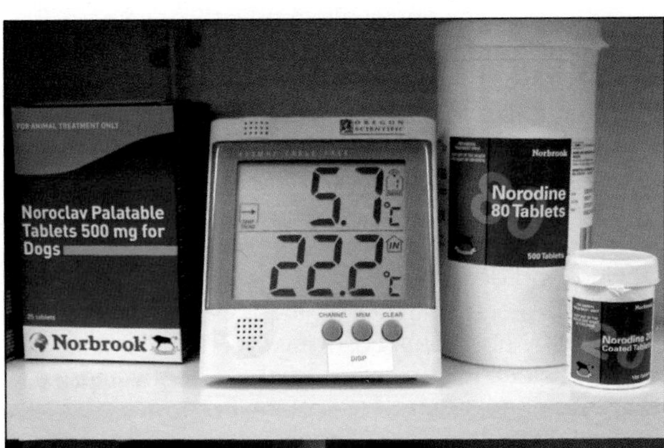

15.17 This electronic thermometer is showing the ambient temperature in the dispensary and in the refrigerator (via a wireless remote probe). The unit will hold maximum and minimum temperature recordings for up to four areas, and the clear display is easy to read.

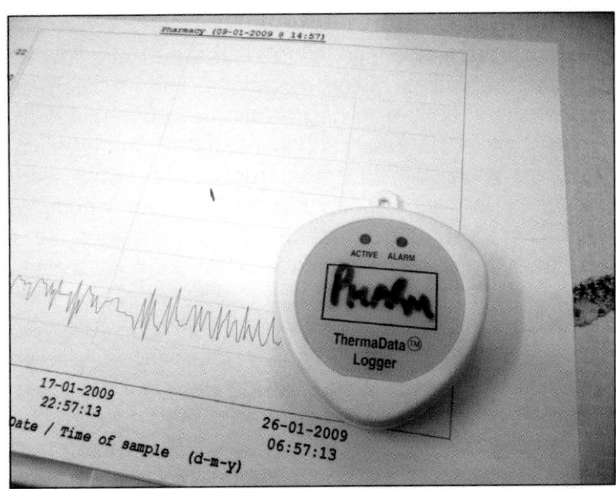

15.18 Data loggers can be convenient to use but should be downloaded regularly and have an audible or visible alarm to indicate temperatures out of the desired range.

There must also be a protocol informing staff of what temperature range they should be looking for, and who they should inform if temperatures deviate from the normal range. Where temperatures have been recorded out of the appropriate ranges, there must be an action plan to remedy such deviations and to deal with affected medicines. It is safest to consult the manufacturers of the drug in question, giving them the relevant information on temperature deviation and duration, and to take their advice on the appropriate course of action, which may be accepting the drug back into stock or disposing of it. If any VMPs are – or appear to have been – frozen, they must be disposed of.

Medicines requiring refrigeration should be moved from any incoming delivery into the refrigerator as soon as they arrive at the practice to ensure cool chain continuity (i.e. the temperature and storage conditions have not deviated from the acceptable range for that product throughout the delivery process).

If the dispensary area has windows, these should have blinds to protect light-sensitive medicines and also to keep dispensary temperatures below 25°C in summer months. Drugs should never be stored on window sills. If temperatures in the drug storage area exceed 25°C, a source of cooling such as fans or air conditioning must be used.

KEY POINT

Consideration must be given to temperatures at nights and weekends when the building may not be occupied, and when fridges remain closed for a longer period.

Shelf life

It is also important to note and abide by shelf life as stated in the SPC and to comply with expiry dates on medicinal products.

KEY POINT

It is illegal to prescribe, dispense or administer out-of-date veterinary medicines.

Most multi-dose bottles or vials of injectable drugs have an 'in-use' shelf life, which is the period following the first broaching of the container. This is because they are susceptible to degradation or contamination, as most do not contain an antimicrobial preservative. Many are marked with the instruction 'Following withdrawal of the first dose, use the product within 28 days. Discard unused material'. The in-use shelf life is not always 28 days; it may be shorter or longer, depending on the drug. Products with an in-use shelf life must be labelled on opening (Figure 15.19a) and discarded after the shelf life has elapsed, to ensure safety and efficacy. Where drugs are drawn up into syringes and not administered immediately, the syringes should be clearly labelled. Pre-printed adhesive labels are convenient (Figure 15.19b). Unidentified drugs should be discarded.

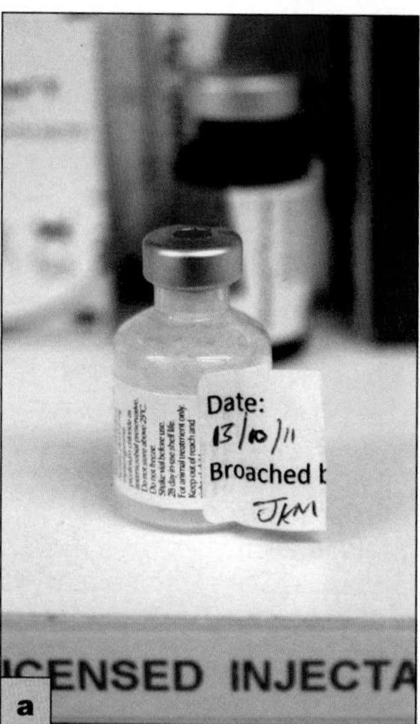

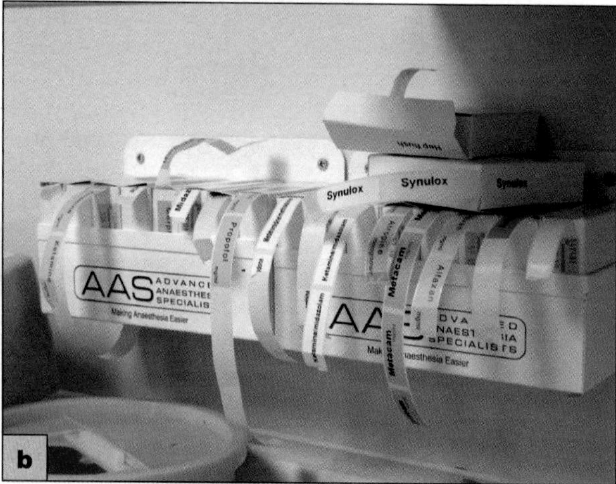

15.19 **(a)** Multi-use injectables should be marked with the date of broaching and must be discarded according to data sheet recommendations. Small labels attached to bottles on arrival can help remind staff to comply. **(b)** Adhesive labels can be useful for labelling syringes into which medicines have been dispensed for use within the practice.

Stock control

Efficient stock control is extremely important: it minimizes the investment in medicines on the shelf, while ensuring that there is always a reliable supply of medicines in the practice. It is good practice to have a designated member of staff who has responsibility for stock control in the dispensary. Stock levels are usually controlled by setting and then monitoring a minimum and maximum stock level of each item.

Setting stock levels

The minimum stock level is the number of items on the shelf at which a replacement order is required.

- For rarely used single items, the minimum stock level can be zero: sell one, then re-order one.
- Where an out-of stock situation is not desirable, such as with drugs needed in an emergency, the minimum would normally be set to one, so there would always be one or two items in stock.
- Where sales are higher, the minimum stock level needs to be set at the usage for the period of time between one order and the next. Thus, if ordering is weekly, in theory one week's stock should be sufficient. In reality, usage (or sales) may not be predictable, so a practice must balance the importance of having stock available with the cost of having too much stock on the shelf and the cost of destroying out-dated stock that has not sold.

Most practice management system software can order automatically from a set minimum, and can also calculate the desired minimum level from the average usage or sales.

Minimum levels should be reviewed regularly and when sales patterns change. Over-stocking costs money, but under-stocking may cause frustration for the clinicians and could drive customers to seek supplies elsewhere, including other practices, other suppliers and the Internet. The cost of holding stock on the shelf is the lost interest from the capital tied up, or the interest paid on the money borrowed to finance the stock. This is easy to calculate and should be compared with the cost of a lost client or missed ongoing sale. To maintain excellent customer service, a certain level of over-stocking may be required to satisfy fluctuating demand, particularly when people bulk buy at a weekend and before holiday periods.

- Where only bulk packs are available (e.g. 'outers' of 20), stock will have to be over-ordered; the minimum level can still be set as above but re-ordering will be less frequent.
- Seasonal variation should be considered; for affected items (e.g. kennel cough vaccine if demanded by local boarding kennels) minimum quantities can be adjusted seasonally. Increased demand from special offers advertised internally or externally (e.g. on TV) should be anticipated with higher stock levels.
- When trying to minimize stock, consideration should be given to reducing duplication of similar medication ranges, to streamlining pack sizes, where possible, and to maintaining an adequate minimum stock to cover normal and weekend demand.
- The cost of maintaining extra stock on the shelf is offset by additional costs involved in having to order stock in specially and client inconvenience in having to return to collect their order.

Monitoring stock levels

Stock levels should be checked regularly, either manually or using barcode readers (Figure 15.20). Wholesaler drug ordering systems are now available, which set up drug lists for different locations in the practice. These systems can also: give live 'out of stock' information; select alternatives; suggest order volumes based on previous ordering; and update prices. Many veterinary wholesalers deliver to practices daily, making it easier to maintain lower stock levels. Ordering can be manual or online (using hand-held barcode readers (Figure 15.20) or palm-top devices).

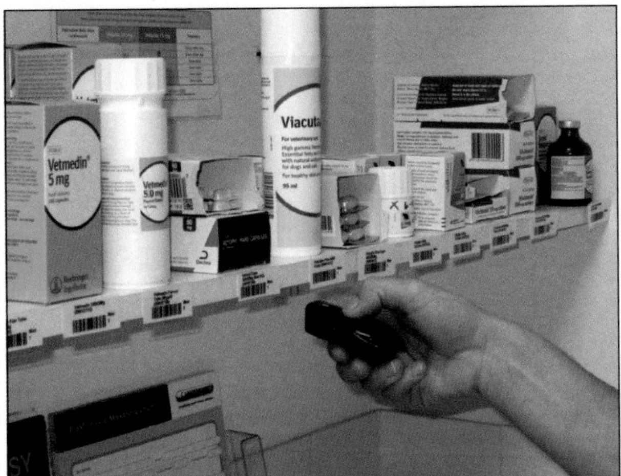

15.20 In this simple stock ordering system, the small scanner reads the pre-prepared barcodes and the operator clicks the number of items needed to get the stock level up to the maximum level indicated. The order is then downloaded on to the PMS.

> **KEY POINT**
>
> When checking stock levels, expiry dates should also be checked. Any-out-of date or damaged stock should be removed, recorded (see above) and disposed of, according to current waste regulations.

Re-ordering stock

An integrated computerized stock control system linked to client records is the most efficient and accurate system but requires discipline and accurate destocking and writing up to be effective. Regular reports can be run to adjust minimum levels of stock. Re-order levels must be set appropriately, so that there is never a need to 'over-ride' the system. The automatically generated order should not be adjusted manually except by adjusting the settings in the individual product record. A lack of discipline in this area is often the main reason for problems experienced in running automated ordering systems.

- Bulk buying can often be advantageous if a supplier is offering discounts or special offers. Again, the financial implications must be calculated carefully and care should be taken to check end dates on stock and ongoing staff prescribing and recommendation behaviours, as over-stocking always carries the risk of stock having to be discarded when out of date. Good deals are often offered when a competitor is about to launch a similar product. Good ongoing records of usage or sales levels will be invaluable in deciding whether bulk offers are worthwhile.
- Shelf space is a significant consideration, as having to store bulk stock elsewhere can add to workload and result in stock being forgotten about.
- Although 'just in time' ordering may seem attractive, the time costs of checking and handling daily small orders should be balanced against the efficiency of less frequent larger deliveries if stock levels seem high but stock is not going out of date.

Choosing a wholesaler

When choosing a wholesaler, it is useful to consider the following.

- **Delivery frequency.** Daily deliveries potentially allow lower stockholding. However, frequency of deliveries can sometimes mask inefficient systems and less frequent deliveries may be less time-consuming to process.
- **Who delivers?** Some companies use couriers, whilst others use dedicated vans with refrigerated storage, or a combination of the two. A regular driver with a cheerful disposition who is familiar with the practice can make a big difference to the level of service the practice experiences.
- **Handling of large items and delivery packaging.** A delivery driver who is willing to carry the delivery through to the unpacking area rather than depositing items in the waiting room can influence the choice of wholesaler. Some wholesalers will also take away delivery packaging, such as cardboard boxes, at the next delivery.
- **Delivery times.** A predictable, regular and convenient drug delivery slot is essential and will allow the practice not only to plan with regards to staffing arrangements, but also to inform clients reliably as to when they may be able to collect any specific items ordered.
- **Ordering arrangements.** With many practices ordering electronically via the PMS, it is important to establish that the wholesaler's IT software will integrate with the practice's system. As well as saving time, ordering electronically reduces the number of order errors and so is encouraged by wholesalers, often by attracting additional discount.
- **Returns policy.** A clear and easy-to-use flexible returns policy for damaged or over-ordered stock, or items ordered in error, can help in reducing any potential staff frustration.
- **Availability of items and handling of back orders.** Practices should be informed of any items which are on 'to follow 'and should be given the opportunity to order an alternative.
- **Minimum order quantities.** It is more cost-effective for practices if multi-packs are broken down for infrequently used products.
- **Expiry dates.** Short-dated items should be flagged and/or be returnable, refundable or replaced.
- **Batch number recording.** For small animal practices, for most drugs batch numbers need only be recorded either on the date of receipt of the batch or on the date a VMP from the batch is first dispensed. However, batch numbers for vaccines, for example, need to be recorded on

individual patient records and therefore some small animal practices choose to track all batch numbers. Data can be supplied by the wholesalers; practices requiring this information electronically will need to ensure that a download is possible via their PMS or that a suitable alternative (hard copy, scanner) is available.

- **Assistance with stock control and minimum stock level setting.** Supplied software and/or hand-held barcode readers may be of interest.
- **Branch surgeries.** The setting up, and subsequent management, of any branch surgery with regards to order processing, acting as a delivery point and as a separate cost centre if required, should be discussed in detail, particularly if discounts (including any from the manufacturers) need to be allocated.
- **Invoicing and delivery note administration.** The ease and manner of checking the order off against the paperwork provided should be taken into consideration. For example, can this be done electronically or by barcode scanner?
- **Special orders and non-discounted items.** A list of the wholesaler's non-discounted and long lead time products (special orders) should be examined, to predict any impact on costs if these are commonly used items.
- **Competitive pricing.** This is particularly relevant for items such as consumables (e.g. syringes, cotton wool, swabs, gloves and cleaning materials). Some wholesalers have a recommended 'value' range; as long as quality is not compromised, this may be of benefit financially to the practice.
- **Overall wholesaler discount and any additional discount for electronic ordering.** Discounts and volume purchased are usually linked. This may be less significant if a practice already belongs to a buying group and benefits from higher discount irrespective of volume purchased.
- **Payment terms.** For a large outstanding amount, the 'payment due' date can have a significant effect on cash flow. Direct debits can reduce the risk of lost discount due to late payment.
- **Management reports to help with purchasing decisions.** Configurable reports available to track spending in different categories, and from different manufacturers, are useful. Practices with branches and/or members of a buying group need to ensure that for discount purposes, their wholesaler can provide an adequate breakdown of purchasing figures. Another point of consideration is whether or not comparative data from other practices or areas are available.
- **Helpline.** An efficient telephone- or web-based helpline is essential.
- **Other benefits.** Training, conversion of current stock data from previous wholesalers, special promotions, etc. are often provided.

Receiving stock

Orders are often received in re-useable plastic boxes, which take up a substantial amount of space and can mark the flooring if dragged. A flatbed trolley that the order can be delivered on to is ideal and helps with moving the stock to its destination (Figure 15.21a). Incoming stock must not be allowed to obstruct fire exits or circulation areas in the dispensary or nearby, and must not present a trip hazard, particularly where animals are also being moved. Checking off (Figure 15.21b) and putting the stock away as soon as it arrives can minimize disruption.

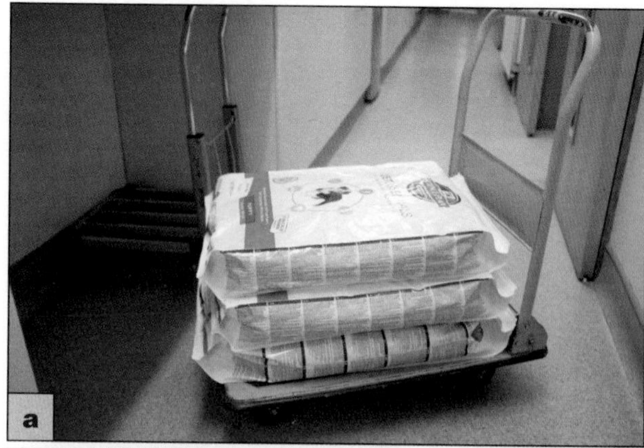

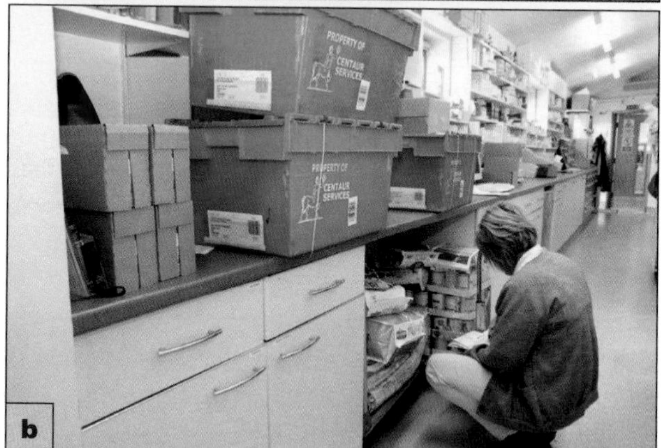

15.21 **(a)** A flatbed trolley that orders can be delivered on to is ideal and helps with moving stock to its destination. **(b)** Checking off each item in the drug delivery against the delivery note or invoice is an important part of accurate stock control. Where space is limited, care should be taken that incoming orders do not block passageways and circulation areas. Smaller drug items are usually delivered in re-usable plastic crates.

> **KEY POINT**
>
> Medicines that have been dispensed to clients should NOT be accepted back into the dispensary for resale, as the conditions of storage are unknown.

Dispensing medicines

Only the minimum amount of drug required for the treatment should be dispensed, as advised by the prescribing veterinary surgeon.

Veterinary authorization

If the veterinary surgeon is not present when the medicine is supplied, for instance when a client rings in to request more medication for their animal, then the vet must authorize each transaction. This can happen in a variety of ways:

- The vet may make a note on the animal's history after the last consultation that repeat prescriptions of a certain drug can be given for 1 month or 3 months, for example
- A member of staff may take a message and put it on a 'repeat prescriptions' list to be checked and authorized by the vet later in the day
- The medicine may be put aside by a staff member for the vet to authorize later
- If there is no vet present and a client calls in for a repeat medication unexpectedly, then the vet can authorize the transaction over the phone; in this case, clear notes should be recorded.

The procedure for ordering medication and the expected timescale for authorization and preparation should be made clear to clients. Practices may consider allowing ordering by phone, email, fax or SMS text, and can use pre-printed order forms or web forms to facilitate the process. The practice should also have a written protocol for repeat prescribing and dispensing (Figure 15.22).

When a client phones up or calls in to request a further supply of a medication their pet is currently receiving:

The receptionist must:

1. Take full details of:
   - The owner's name, address and telephone number
   - The animal's name
   - The name of the medication
   - The dose the animal is currently taking.
2. Check that the client is registered at this practice and has been seen in the last 3 months.
3. Ask the owner how the animal is doing. If the owner has any concerns, note these down for the vet to read.
4. If the animal has not been seen in the last 3 months, politely request that the owner makes an appointment to bring their animal in to see the vet before any more medication is prescribed.
5. If the animal has been seen in the last 3 months, record the full details of the request in the repeat prescriptions book on reception or on the repeat prescriptions list on the computer, and politely inform the owner that the drug has to be authorized by the vet and will be ready for collection in 24 hours. Should the vet not authorize the repeat prescription, a veterinary nurse will ring the owner back to explain the situation.
6. Inform the vet of the request by placing a message on the computer screen or in the book.

The veterinary surgeon must initial the repeat prescribing book or make a note on the repeat prescribing list on the computer if he/she is happy to authorize the medication.

The veterinary nurse on the consulting room/dispensary shift should:

- Check the book/list regularly
- When any drug has been authorized, print off a label and dispense the medication
- Initial the label and ensure that the patient's records are complete.

Double checking:

A veterinary surgeon or another veterinary nurse should double check that the medication is correct and also initial the label.

Collection

- Drugs awaiting collection should be placed in reception (Figure 15.23a).
- The nurse or receptionist giving the drug to the client should check that they have the correct medication and go through the dosage and any special instructions with the client (Figure 15.23b).

15.22 Example of a protocol for repeat prescribing and dispensing.

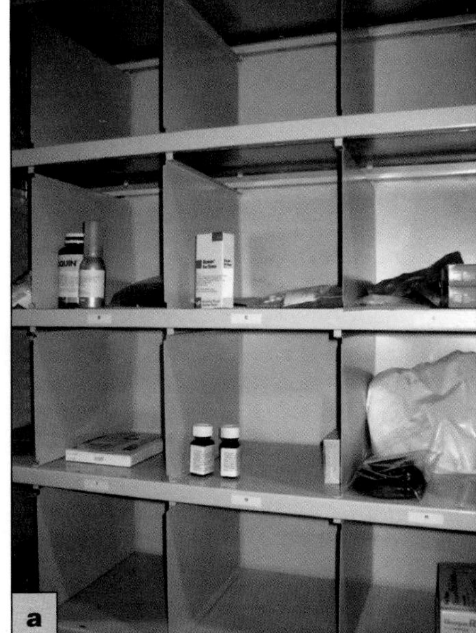

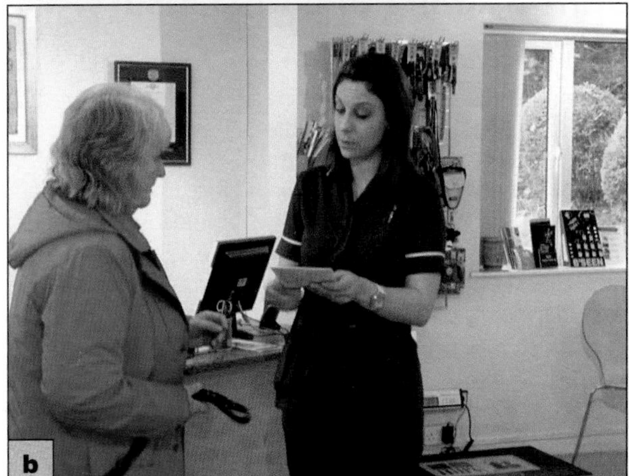

15.23 **(a)** Repeat medicines awaiting collection. **(b)** Staff must ensure that clients understand how to use the dispensed medicines.

Containers and packaging

There are some basic rules:

- Tablets and capsules should be dispensed in moisture-proof and crush-proof containers.
- From a safety point of view, child-resistant containers should be used unless a client requests an alternative.
- Blister-packed medicines and sachets can be dispensed in paper envelopes or cardboard cartons.
- It is not acceptable to dispense loose tablets in paper envelopes.

Drug containers must be labelled appropriately (see above). The information on the label can be handwritten but must be legible and indelible. Label printers linked to the practice management software and programmed to produce labels with precautions for use of each drug are efficient. The label printer should normally be sited in the dispensary so that drugs can be labelled immediately, reducing the risk of dispensing errors. Labels must be securely attached so as not to obliterate any information from the manufacturer on the packaging; this can be challenging.

When veterinary surgeons prescribe and supply POM-V drugs, in a consultation for instance, they must advise owners on the safe administration of the drug and, if necessary, of any warnings or contraindications. The product leaflet or SPC should always be included with the medication. In practice, this means that if packs are split there must be a supply of product leaflets, or they must be photocopied or downloaded by the practice.

KEY POINT

It is good practice for both the medication and the label to be double-checked by a second staff member before being given to the client. For example, a veterinary surgeon may be required to sign the label before the medication is issued.

Staff training and dispensary SOPs

Under the Veterinary Medicines Regulations, veterinary surgeons must be satisfied that the member of staff handing over the medication is competent to do so. This means that all staff involved in handing out prescriptions to clients (including repeat prescriptions) must be adequately trained and able to give the correct directions and advice on storing, administering and disposing of the medication.

Reference material such as the BSAVA's online *Guide to the Use of Veterinary Medicines*, *BSAVA Small Animal Formulary*, the *BVA Good Practice Guide on Veterinary Medicines* and Veterinary Medicines Guidance notes from the VMD should all be available in the dispensary and used when formulating policy and training.

Continuing professional development (CPD) courses are available. For example, BSAVA runs a Dispensing Course twice a year to help practices manage their dispensaries and keep up to date with the Veterinary Medicines Regulations. Details can be found at www.bsava.com, and courses are available for all members of the practice team.

Good SOPs ensure that there is consistency and reliability in dispensary procedures, and reduce the likelihood of dispensing errors. Dispensary SOPs (Figure 15.24) should be drawn up according to practice policy and regularly reviewed to reflect any change in that policy or in relevant regulations. Staff who perform the tasks should be involved in writing the SOPs to make them as simple, up to date, practical and user-friendly as possible. The SOPs should be used in training and should be available to all staff in the dispensary area (Figure 15.25). The *BSAVA Guide to the Use of Veterinary Medicines*, available to all at www.bsava.com, has example SOPs for practices to adapt for their own use. This guide is updated annually to reflect any changes in the Regulations.

Staff should not handle medicines unless they have been made aware of the relevant safety data, have access to the COSHH risk assessment (see Chapter 22) and are familiar with the spillage procedure and First Aid arrangements.

- Dealing with spillages
- Dispensing medicines in consultations
- Dispensing repeat medicines in the absence of a veterinary surgeon
- Disposal of Controlled Drugs
- Disposal of cytotoxic drugs
- Disposing of out-of-date drugs
- Handling and use of cytotoxic drugs
- Handling Veterinary Medicines
- Labelling medicines
- Medicines returned by clients
- 'Off-licence' drug prescribing and dispensing
- Placing a drug order
- Receiving and storing Controlled Drugs
- Stock control and expiry date checking
- Temperature monitoring protocols
- Unpacking the drug order
- Using ampoules

15.24 Useful SOPs to have in place for the dispensary.

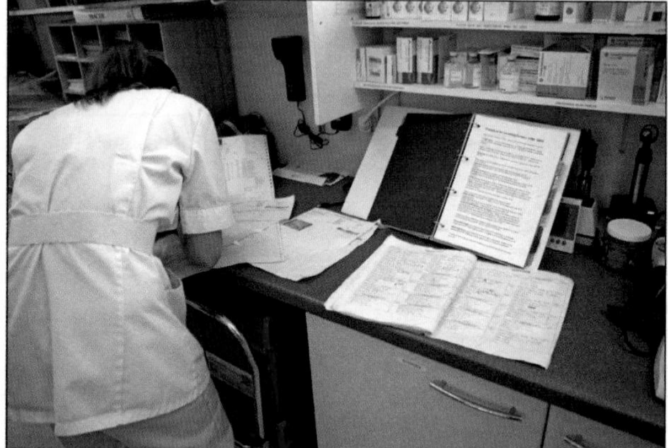

15.25 SOPs can be kept in a folder in the dispensary, ready for use.

'Off-licence' medicines

It is part of good pharmacy management to establish a system of reminding staff about 'off-licence' dispensing (see above). This involves training and maintaining SOPs (an example can be found at the end of this chapter) but can be made easier by clearly distinguishing human POMs. This can be done by:

- Storing them together in one section of the dispensary
- Labelling the shelves where these products are stored with a coloured dot
- Having a list of products in the dispensary or on the practice computer software, highlighting 'off-licence' drugs when they are dispensed, and reminding the clinician of the procedure.

In busy practices it may be difficult to remember to formalize informed consent and to get a form signed during a busy consulting period. Many PMS systems can now be set up to remind the veterinary surgeon when an unauthorized product is being prescribed, and can generate a form at the time.

Responsible use of antimicrobials

Practices should have a policy for the use of antimicrobial drugs in order to decrease the risk of antimicrobial resistance. This should include avoiding inappropriate use, choosing the right drug for the infection being treated, monitoring sensitivity, minimizing prophylactic and perioperative use, keeping accurate records and reporting treatment failures to VMD. This is very well summarized in handy posters available from BVA and BSAVA, and clinicians should ensure they are aware of current guidance in this area.

Health and safety considerations

Hazardous substances

Many potentially hazardous substances are encountered in veterinary practice and some of these are found in the dispensary. Practices are required to make a thorough assessment of the risks to health and safety arising from exposure to veterinary medicines and other hazardous substances used throughout the practice. Risk assessment principles and guidance are outlined in Chapter 22.

The Control of Substances Hazardous to Health Regulations (COSHH) 2002 require that an assessment is carried out regarding exposure to hazardous substances. The purpose of the assessment is to identify the hazards and risks, and to determine whether control measures are adequate. Drugs and all substances should be classified according to risk – low, medium or high.

Low- and medium-risk substances can be grouped by therapeutic group, type, route of administration, etc., and standard measures to control exposure can be used for the whole group. Examples of therapeutic groups include antibiotics, vaccines, injectable anaesthetic agents, inhalation anaesthetic agents, and steroids. Any specific risks within the groups that may cause longer-term health problems must be identified; for example, allergy to penicillin.

High-risk substances must have individual detailed assessment. Examples of high-risk substances found in the dispensary include:

- Oil-based vaccines
- Cytotoxic drugs
- Hormones
- Micotil (Tilmicosin)
- Large Animal Immobilon (Etorphine).

Measures to control exposure to these high-risk substances must be identified to staff, and SOPs drawn up for their use.

Safety data must be available for all drugs stocked. Drug companies no longer have to supply safety data sheets but many companies still do and some can be found in the National Office of Animal Health (NOAH) data sheet compendium available from NOAH or their website (www.noahcompendium.co.uk).

All veterinary authorized products have SPCs, and staff members should know how to access these in an emergency (see above). All veterinary medicinal products currently authorized in the UK, plus homeopathic products and specified feed additives (including a list of suspended or recently expired products) are on the VMD product information database (www.vmd.gov.uk). SPCs of human POMs used under the prescribing cascade may be found at www.emc.medicines.org.uk.

> **KEY POINT**
>
> All staff should have the COSHH assessment drawn to their attention before starting work in the dispensary and know which medicines are particularly hazardous.

Cytotoxic drugs

Cytotoxic drugs can damage healthy as well as cancerous or diseased cells and are a potential health risk to anyone involved in preparing or administering them, or caring for animals undergoing treatment. If cytotoxic drugs are used in the practice there should be a comprehensive risk assessment. They are hazardous substances and should be classified as high risk in the COSHH assessment (see Chapter 22).

Full safety information from the SPC should be available for any cytotoxic drug used, and in a form immediately available to staff in case of spillage or exposure to one of these drugs. Staff should be fully trained in the risks of working with cytotoxic drugs and the precautions they should take when handling them. Suitable protective clothing, gowns, aprons, gloves and eye protection must be available (Figure 15.26).

For inpatients or outpatients receiving cytotoxic drug therapies, consideration should be given to handling the patient and any excreta, vomit, etc. Cages of inpatients on chemotherapy should be clearly labelled, and staff *and owners* informed of the correct procedures for handling the patients and any waste. If oral cytotoxic drugs are dispensed for clients to administer to their animals at home, the owners

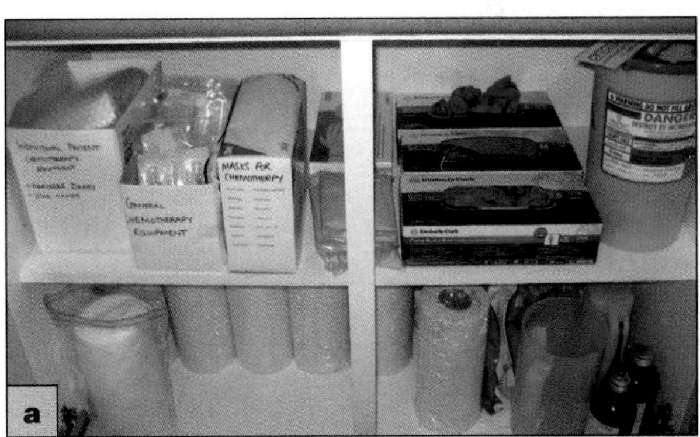

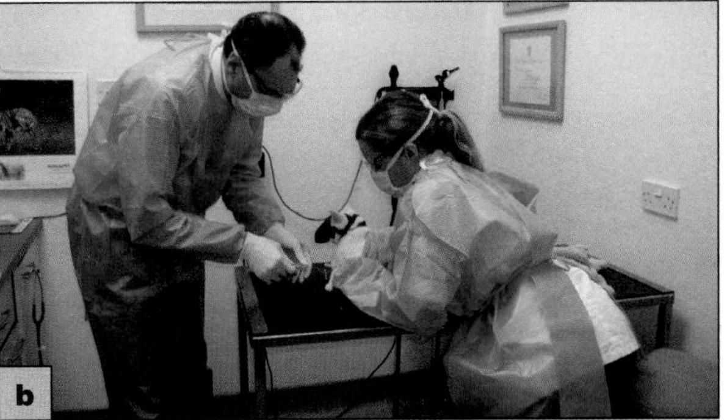

15.26 Handling cytotoxic drugs. **(a,b)** Special equipment and suitable protective clothing, gowns, aprons, gloves and eye protection must be available. (continues) ▶

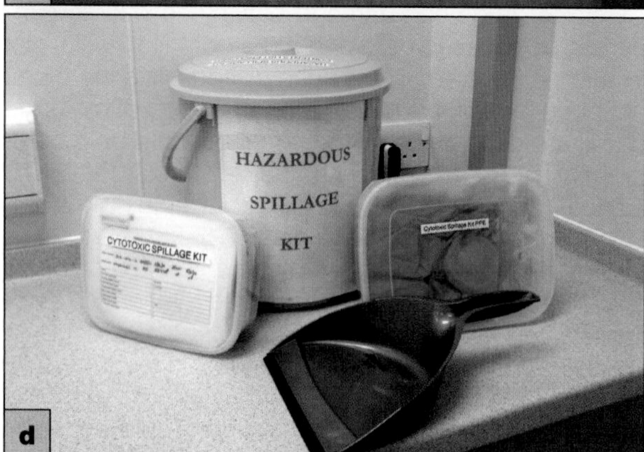

15.26 (continued) Handling cytotoxic drugs. **(c)** A clear sign on the procedure room door, warning other staff of chemotherapy in progress, is helpful to reduce risk from interruptions. **(d)** Spillage kits must be available.

must be fully informed of all risks and of precautions for handling the drugs. Waste is considered hazardous and must be treated accordingly (see below).

Other high-risk drugs

The risks to pregnant women of handling prostaglandins, griseofulvin and other teratogenic drugs should be fully explained. A list of these can be found in the *BSAVA Small Animal Formulary*.

Waste disposal

Pharmaceutical waste is classified (see Chapter 3) as Non-hazardous waste, unless it contains cytotoxic or cytostatic pharmaceuticals, when it should then be classified as Hazardous waste.

Non-hazardous waste

Pharmaceutical waste includes:

- Prescription-only medicines
- Out-of-date or damaged drugs
- Glass bottles that have contained medicines
- Ampoules
- Vaccine vials
- Contaminated syringe bodies.

It also includes Controlled Drugs if they have been denatured (Figure 15.27).

Pharmaceutical waste should be collected in a leak-proof rigid container. Medicines should be kept

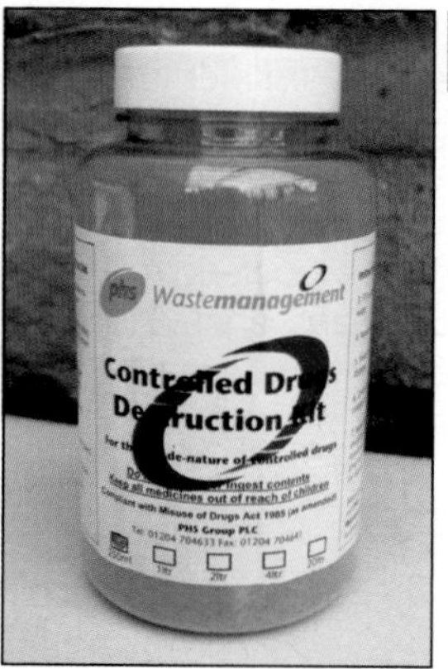

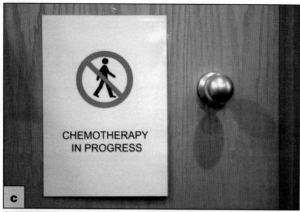

15.27 A denaturing kit used for Controlled Drugs.

in their packaging and solids and liquids not mixed, as this can cause chemical reactions and be a potential fire hazard. A record should be kept of the contents of the bin. This is easily done by creating a client file on the practice management system. It is important for this record to be available to the waste disposal contractor; it is also necessary to account for any whole medicines disposed of in a drug audit.

Hazardous waste

Cytotoxic or cytostatic pharmaceutical waste is in a special category of healthcare waste and is classified as Hazardous waste. Medicines in this category include:

- Chemotherapy agents used in treating cancers
- Antiviral medicines
- Ciclosporins
- Some hormones, including prostaglandins and androgens.

All waste items from using these medications must be placed in the appropriate purple-lidded bin (see Figure 15.26a).

Acknowledgements

The author and editors gratefully acknowledge the following practices, images of which appear in this chapter: Bollington Veterinary Centre; Broadland House Veterinary Surgery; Mill House Veterinary Surgery and Hospital; Orchard Veterinary Group; Pool House Veterinary Hospital; Penmellyn Veterinary Group; Taverham Vets Ltd; Willows Veterinary Centre and Referral Service.

Further reading

BSAVA: *BSAVA Guide to Use of Veterinary Medicines* (website and app, updated annually; available at www.bsava.com)

British Veterinary Association: *BVA Good Practice Guide on Veterinary Medicines*. (available at www.bva.com)

Ramsey I (2011) *BSAVA Small Animal Formulary, 7th edn*. BSAVA Publications, Gloucester (also available to members online and as a smart phone application

Royal College of Veterinary Surgeons: Advice notes regarding Veterinary Medicines Regulations and the RCVS Code of Professional Conduct ; available at www.rcvs.org.uk

Veterinary Medicines Directorate: Guidance notes available at www.vmd.defra.gov.uk

Example of an SOP ▶

SOP No ....

Prescribing and dispensing veterinary medicines 'off-licence'

- If there is no authorized Veterinary Medicinal Product to treat a condition, a veterinary surgeon may select a veterinary medicine for another animal species or another condition. If these are not available, the veterinary surgeon may select a medicinal product authorized in the UK for human use.
- The human medicines available in this practice are:
  - ....
  - ....
  - ....
  - ....
- These medicines are:
  - Marked with a red dot on the dispensary shelf
  - Highlighted on the computer system when prescribed.
- These medicines must be clearly identified to owners by the vet, who must obtain the owner's informed consent for their use.
  - Consent forms are in the drawer in the consulting room.
  - 'Lifetime' consent forms may be used for owners of exotic animals.
  - For cats and dogs, a consent form must be filled in each time a new 'off-licence' medication is started.
  - When a form has been signed, a note should be put in the appropriate box on the clinical records.
- The veterinary surgeon must explain any special precautions or warnings to the owner and, where possible, issue the relevant product information.
- The labels for 'off-licence' medications must include:
  - The name or initials of the vet prescribing
  - The expiry date, if this is not on the packaging (e.g. split packs, loose tablets, liquids).
- The veterinary surgeon, or the member of staff handing over the medication for repeat prescriptions, must check that all these steps have been followed.

An example of an SOP for unauthorized drugs.

16

Offices, administration and staff accommodation

Rita Dingwall

Office space in veterinary practices is often undervalued as a resource. Space, particularly when limited, tends to be prioritized for clinical or fee-generating areas. However, well designed and functional office space, together with an effective administrative and management team (or person in a small practice), will make a huge difference to the health and profitability of a practice. The range of activities carried out in non-clinical and non-public areas reflects the varied nature of the roles undertaken by the practice manager and office staff as well as by clinical staff members:

- **Business strategy:**
  - Support for strategic decision-making – preparation of reports, 'what if?' scenarios, market research
  - Meetings – partners, directors, managers
  - Preparation of business and marketing plans
- **General administration:**
  - Building maintenance and repairs
  - Equipment maintenance and servicing
  - Drafting and implementation of policies, protocols and procedures
  - Updating the staff handbook and the staff manual
  - IT
  - General purchasing
  - Managing utilities, insurance and supplier contracts
  - Managing the vehicle fleet
  - Overseeing all aspects related to practice accommodation
  - Staff rotas, including out-of-hours arrangements
  - Overseeing all aspects of security relating to staff and to the building
  - Insurance claim administration
  - Other general administration that could be done in reception but is often best relocated to the office area to avoid distraction and unsightly clutter
- **Communications:**
  - Handling incoming and outgoing post, faxes and e-mails
  - Referral letters and other professional correspondence
  - Telephone calls – many practices try to keep phones away from the reception area to enable receptionists to focus on their client-facing responsibilities
  - Organising, planning and recording meetings of clinical and non-clinical staff
  - Meeting with sales representatives
  - Customer surveys and feedback
  - Dealing with and responding to complaints
- **Marketing**:
  - Regular client mailings
  - Vaccination and other client reminders
  - Newsletters
  - Open days
  - Launching new products or services
  - Promotional campaigns, merchandising materials
  - Local and directory advertising
  - Articles for the local paper
  - Maintaining practice website and social media activity
- **Clinical administration:**
  - Veterinary surgeons and nurses returning telephone calls and writing letters
  - Ordering stock
  - Research and reading
  - Writing clinical articles and practice information
- **Storage:**
  - Archiving
  - Organizing stocks of stationery and preprinted material
  - Organizing and maintaining office equipment – printers, copiers, franking machines, laminators, folding machines, computers
- **Financial:**
  - Financial performance reporting
  - Client accounts – sending invoices and monitoring debtors
  - Negotiating financial contracts, e.g. loans
  - Purchase and nominal ledger bookkeeping
  - Preparation of management accounts
  - Payroll and PAYE administration
  - Looking at charges for services and products sold
  - Banking

- **Human resource management:**
  - Recruitment
  - Designing induction programmes
  - Supporting training and development, including booking any approved CPD
  - Performance appraisal systems
  - Updating job descriptions
  - Issuing contracts
  - Dealing with any grievances or disciplinary issues
  - Monitoring any sickness and absence
  - Monitoring holiday leave
  - Keeping up to date with, and implementing, employment legislation
- **Health and safety:**
  - Keeping up to date with, and implementing, any H&S legislation
  - PAT testing
  - Risk assessments
  - Fire assessments
  - COSHH
  - First Aid and completing the accident book as required
  - Notice to contractors
  - Drafting and implementing standards of practice

The way in which offices and wider staff areas are organized and managed can provide an insight into the health of the practice. A disunited and disorganized practice will not perform as well as an organized one, where clinical and non-clinical staff work together well as a team.

KEY POINT

The attitudes and ethics of those who work in the office environments filter through the practice and contribute to the overall morale of the whole team.

Office accommodation

Many offices in veterinary practices use an open working environment approach, often being 'shoehorned' into any available space. In addition, rather than being a successful working environment, the office can become a hub for vets and nurses catching up on phone calls and administration – not to mention the latest gossip. In trying to improve the office environment, the work of the practice, its premises, culture and staff are all important considerations.

Office design

Space

Practical issues in office planning include spatial needs, proximity relations, IT infrastructure and furniture, but also more strategic questions such as effectiveness of the working environment and the environmental impact. In considering office design, a few questions are pertinent:

- What best suits the working processes and culture of the organization?
- Should all employees have their own workstation, or are they going to share desks?
- If sharing a desk, which members of staff should share?
- Which members of staff should share an office?
- Should the office be near reception or away from it?
- What might the future needs be – in five years, or ten years?

Unless designing a practice from scratch or planning an extension, the answer to these questions will often be dictated by the constraints of the building. Generally, groundfloor space is at a premium so offices tend to be located upstairs (Figure 16.1) or, in some cases, in the eaves. Eaves can also be very suitable for archive storage.

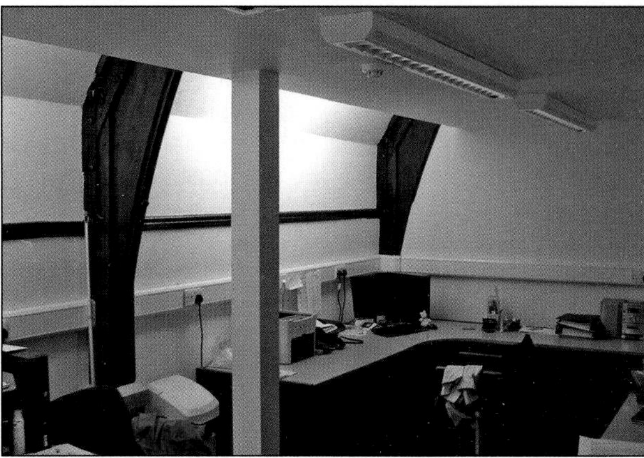

16.1 Offices are often fitted into the upper floors of a practice.

Although the clinical team can use the consultation room for some administrative duties, lack of space can be an issue, a comfortable adjustable chair is required, and clutter in clinical areas becomes unavoidable. Some office space should therefore be allocated to clinical staff (Figure 16.2); they may not necessarily require their own desk but should ideally be provided with a designated administration area. Not every practice will be fortunate enough to have designated workstations for specific functions, individuals or teams or groups of employees. Members of staff often need to share an office and sometimes to share the same desk ('hot desking'; Figure 16.3). This can work well, particularly when staff need to use the office at different times, e.g. part-time

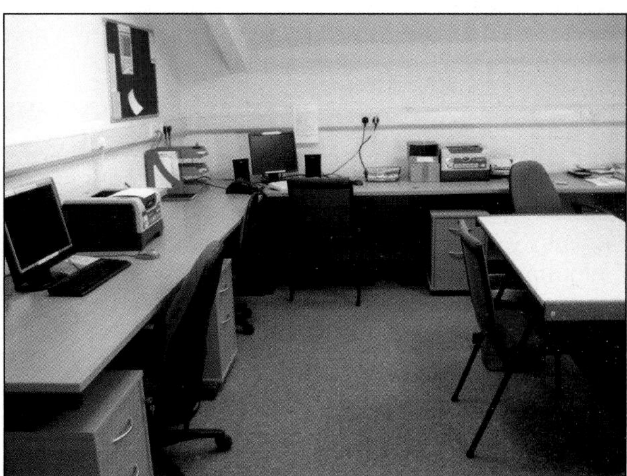

16.2 A dedicated vets office.

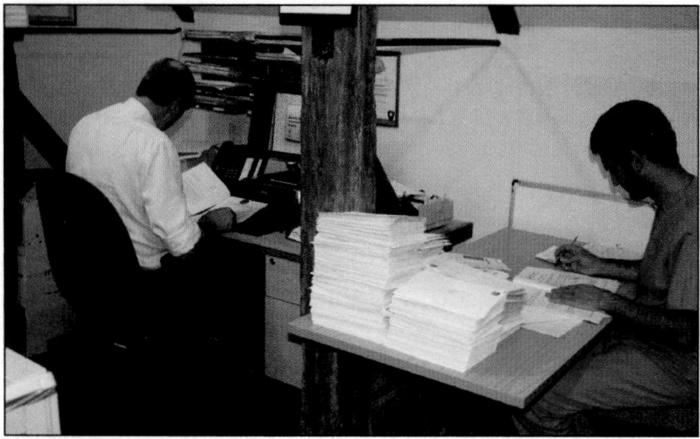

16.3 Hot desking in a quiet corner of the office is appreciated by vets and nurses for essential administrative tasks and for returning telephone calls. Clinicians can keep pending paperwork in personal wall-mounted trays.

workers, vets working different shifts. Hot desks are great in theory but rely on everyone keeping them clean and tidy. In addition, personal preferences regarding workstation set up, computer user settings and log-in details can be an issue. Agreed protocols regarding user etiquette are useful.

Privacy

It is not always expedient – in terms of communication – to have staff members inhabiting their own private offices. Having to get up and go to another room to make a phone call or ask a colleague a quick question is not ideal and can turn a small query into a protracted task. However, in the shared office, although communication may be better there is much more scope for chatter and distraction. Individual offices are an excellent option for silent working, for making a sensitive or confidential phone call, and for private meetings such as discussing a performance issue with an employee.

Managers may have confidential papers on their desks or need to engage in sensitive/private phone calls and meetings, which should not be overheard. For example, the accounts manager will need privacy to deal with the payroll and other sensitive financial details, and different departments are not always at liberty to share all information about staff members. In such scenarios, it would not be practical to keep asking colleagues to leave the office. Too many staff in each office can cause distractions and impede others from working effectively. The correct placing of key staff members can play a major part in efficiency and communication throughout the practice.

KEY POINT

Which staff are to share an office is an important consideration, particularly regarding the need for privacy when it comes to sensitive and confidential information, phone calls or discussions.

Layout and practical considerations

Office space should be adequately designed and properly proportioned. Particularly where space is limited, bespoke units can be commissioned to make otherwise unusable nooks and crannies into places for valuable storage.

Things to keep in mind when setting up or evaluating an office environment include the following:

- **Noise:**
  - In most cases the main noise distractions are: colleagues on the phone; unnecessary telephone lines ringing when incoming lines cannot be regulated; pager systems; and office copiers and printers
  - Noise from clinical areas can be a problem, particularly where offices are above ward or recovery areas. Consideration should be given to the emotional impact this can have on some workers, and effective soundproofing may help.
  - Noise should be kept to a level where it does not cause unreasonable distraction.
- **Office layout:**
  - This should enable efficient working and minimize the time wasted moving around unnecessarily
  - Frequently used equipment and files should be stored within easy reach
  - If possible, employees who work together should be placed close to each other.
- **Temperature, ventilation and humidity:**
  - Due to electronic equipment generating heat, a portable fan or air conditioning may be required
  - Potted plants may help to offset low humidity, as well as adding to the aesthetic appearance.
- **Health and safety:**
  - Equipment should be safely positioned to avoid staff colliding with it
  - Equipment should be positioned to avoid cables crossing pedestrian routes. Where this is not possible, secure purpose-made surface cable covers should be fitted
  - Monitors, desks and chairs should be set up in line with health and safety guidelines relating to a worker's posture and the requirement to provide an adequate desk and comfortable chair (see below)
  - Space is required for recycled and general waste bins. The segregated waste must be removed regularly to minimize fire and trip hazards
  - Mats must be securely fixed without curling edges and work flooring should be kept in a satisfactory clean condition. Where carpet is installed, clear plastic chair mats can be used (Figure 16.4)

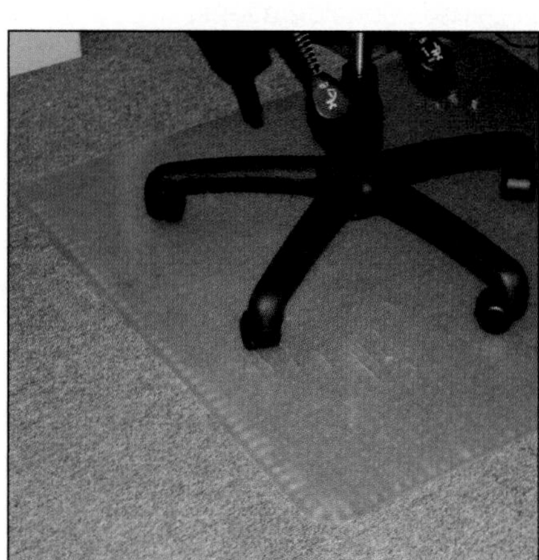

16.4 Clear plastic chair mats facilitate free movement of wheeled chairs and protect the carpet from wear and rucking.

- Office lighting should be bright enough to move around safely and must be adequate for the reading of documents and keyboards. There should be no glare from lights, windows or computer screens. Effective positioning of workstations, blinds and special glare-proof screens might provide solutions
- Opening windows are desirable for fresh air and natural light.

- **Practical considerations:**
  - A large table or desk for collating, printing and preparing mailings is a useful addition
  - There should be sufficient electrical sockets to minimize the use of trailing sockets and multi-way adapters. In new designs, power points coming up from the floor under the desk are useful, and special electrical trunking around the walls offers a flexible solution for electrical and data cables (Figure 16.5)
  - It is useful to have incoming telephone lines and other cables near to the office for ease of access for maintenance and also the computer server, network patch panels and telephone system control unit (see Chapter 4). In larger new builds, these may be situated in a plant room as they generate heat and need to be temperature-controlled
  - If possible, it may be better to situate equipment such as large printers, photocopiers, folding machines and franking machines in a separate room, to reduce noise, heat and fumes (from toner)
  - Consideration should be given as to space for shredders or whether the practice might be better using a confidential waste disposal service.

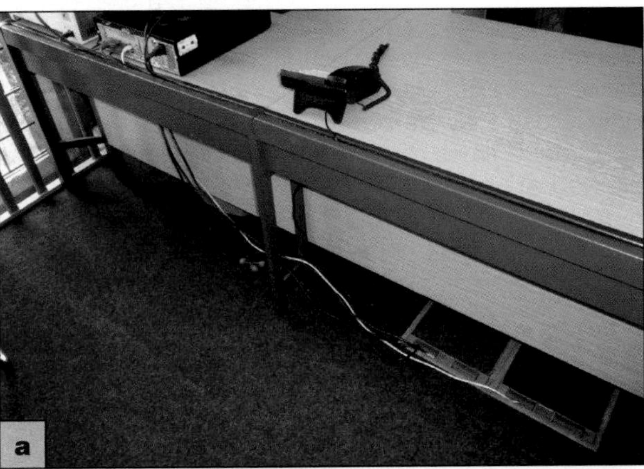

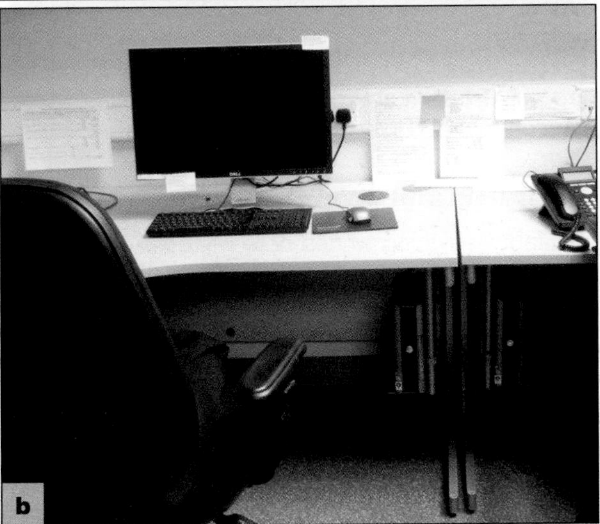

16.5 **(a)** Electrical sockets in floor boxes can be very useful for open-plan offices. **(b)** Clearing PC base units ('boxes') from desks and stowing them neatly can give a less cluttered look.

Future-proofing

Coming up with future-proof solutions that can cope with growth can be tricky; it is advisable to have short-, mid- and long-term plans. Choice of furniture can make a difference to the useable space, and changes can be made economically by judicious choice of units and filing cabinets. Clearing the space and reorganizing seems daunting but is worth it for the long-term benefit achieved.

> **KEY POINT**
>
> Beware of 'temporary solutions': they are often uncomfortable and inadequate set-ups that may not be popular and yet can often end up as permanent.

Workstation design

A workstation should include a standard-height desk, with an adjustable (height and back support) chair on castors (Figure 16.6). An L-shaped or curved desk may be better for using a PC than is a rectangular desk. Adequate space for the IT equipment and paperwork is important.

Training and information

Employers have to provide training, to make sure employees can use their VDU (visual display unit) and workstation safely, and know how to make best use of it to avoid health problems, for example by adjusting the chair. Information should also be provided about VDU health and safety; the *Working with VDUs* booklet available from the Health and Safety Executive is a useful source. Information should also cover more specific details of the steps taken by the employer to comply with the regulations, such as the action taken to reduce risks and the arrangements for taking breaks (see Chapter 22).

Assessing workstations

A VDU workstation checklist is available in a download format from the Health and Safety Executive website (www.hse.gov.uk). Staff and safety representatives should be consulted appropriately and the following considered.

The whole workstation, including equipment, furniture, and the work environment

Employees and safety representatives should be consulted and encouraged to take part in risk assessments. Where risks are identified, the employer must take steps to reduce them and ensure that workstations meet minimum requirements, such as adjustable chairs and suitable lighting. These are set out in The Health and Safety (Display Screen Equipment)

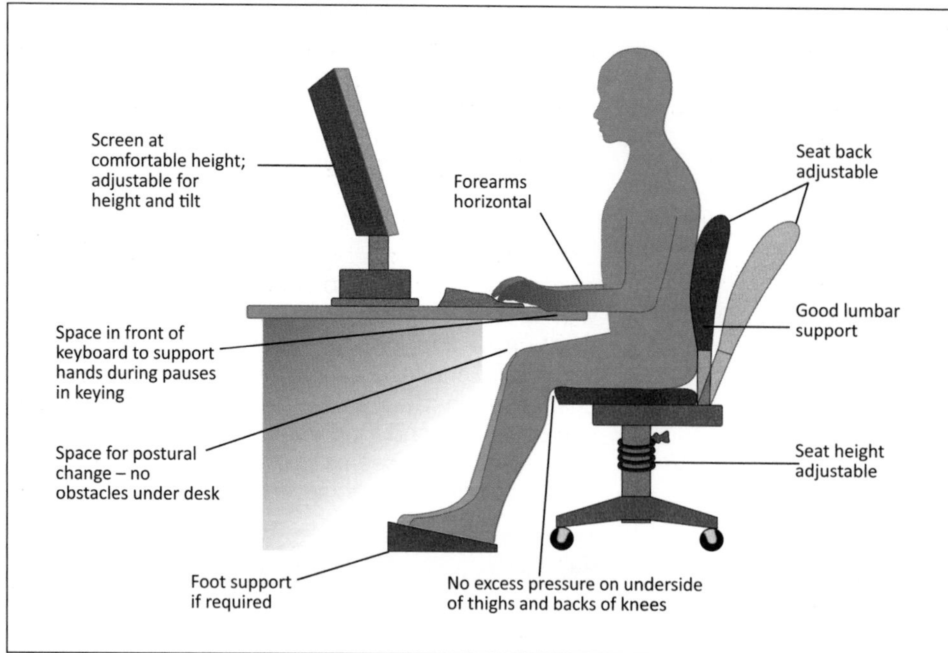

16.6 Elements of a well designed computer workstation.

Regulations 1992, implementing an EC Directive, and came into effect from January 1993 (some small changes were made in 2002). The Regulations require employers to minimize the risks in VDU work by ensuring that workplaces and jobs are well designed. These regulations cover: screens, keyboards, desks, chairs, the work environment and software. All workstations covered by the Regulations now have to comply to the extent necessary for the health and safety of workers. The Regulations apply where staff habitually use VDUs as a significant part of their normal work. Other people, who use VDUs only occasionally, are not covered by the requirements in the Regulations (apart from the workstation requirements). However, their employers still have general duties to protect them under other health and safety at work legislation.

The job being done

Work should be planned so there are breaks or changes of activity. Short, frequent breaks are better than longer, less frequent ones. Ideally the individual should have some discretion over when to take breaks.

Special needs of individual staff

Employees covered by the VDU regulations (see above) can ask their employer to provide and pay for regular eye and eyesight tests, as recommended by an optometrist or doctor. Employers only have to pay for spectacles if special ones (for example, prescribed for the distance at which the screen is viewed) are needed and normal ones cannot be used. Each individual user will need their workstation set up to suit their own preferred position and their physical size. Where appropriate, an individual's choice of chair may be helpful.

Office equipment

Appropriate up-to-date equipment will usually more than justify the expense. Whilst updating a piece of equipment might initially seem costly, the time wastage and frustration of keeping outdated or inefficient equipment in use can be significant.

Computer systems can be used for word processing, spreadsheets, contact database storage and e-mail. E-mail, in particular, can reduce the cost of printing, copying and postage, and is the preferred method of communication for many suppliers, representatives, colleagues and clients. An acceptable user policy (AUP) is strongly recommended to outline the practice's code of conduct in relation to these facilities an example is given at the end of the chapter. Private use may be permitted and may be restricted to certain times or workstations, or may not be allowed at all. This chapter will consider office equipment and computer hardware and peripherals; for details of IT systems and choice of a practice management system, please see Chapter 4.

Any piece of equipment should be tested if possible before purchase to ensure that it is capable of dealing with the typical workload, and consideration should be given as to whether an outside service provider would be preferable. All electrical equipment must be suitable to work in the way intended and physically capable of doing the job. Office IT equipment should be subject to a regular formal visual inspection and a PAT test (if appropriate) by a competent person at recommended intervals (see Chapter 22).

Computer hardware

Inevitably, anything written here will be out of date by the time of publication; therefore, details of current hardware and software options are included for guidance as to the general principles, but must remain general. Advances in computer technology are making smaller and more mobile devices capable of performing the functions of traditional personal computers (PCs), and the computerized veterinary practice will look very different in five years' time. A few principles are important to bear in mind.

Power-hungry main office PCs and servers generally have large outer cases to allow room for maintenance, upgrade and cooling systems (or fans for processors and power supplies). In positioning these units, sufficient space must be allowed for air movement and access for cleaning. Accommodating the necessary wiring for mains supply, network and peripherals is a challenge and is often neglected during design, particularly of clinical areas. Smaller PCs or thin client units and terminals can be used, but wiring to keyboards and mice can still be an issue. Bundles of wires are a safety hazard, a dust trap and look very unsightly. Small PCs are available, which can be attached to the back of TFT (thin film transistor) monitors or can stand upright or lie flat to suit the situation. Laptops and tablet PCs can also be used, but may not cope well with remaining switched on all the time, and laptop fans in particular can be difficult to keep clean.

Computers (and telephones) should be protected by using uninterruptible power supplies, to allow controlled shutdown in the event of power loss, and by using surge protectors. It is best not to install computers in areas that can become dirty, such as where animals are clipped or where there are high moisture levels. Preparation rooms, reception areas and animal wards are the dustiest areas in most practices. If computers in these areas are unavoidable, regular vacuum cleaning around them will prevent dust and hair from building up; keyboard covers should be used to protect against spills and contamination.

All PCs, keyboards and screens, as well as telephones, should be cleaned regularly throughout the day to reduce contamination and spread of infection. They are surprisingly easy to clean. The practice protocol for using disinfectants should be followed. Most business PCs are built for easy access; opening the cases occasionally to clean fans etc. may be straightforward for someone who is competent, and is recommended.

Poorly maintained PC fans and cooling units may be a fire and data loss hazard. Any PC making an unusual noise should be investigated.

TFT screens tend to have reduced life if left on for long periods and so should be turned off when not in use. Computers also refresh computer programmes much more quickly if they are turned off and back on again on a regular basis. However, there are a number of considerations to take into account regarding whether to turn computers off or leave them on, for example, antivirus and operating system software updates and scans. These issues should be discussed with the practice management system (PMS) and hardware supplier(s). Another irritation can be between network users if computers have been left on or turned off unexpectedly – a protocol would be helpful to give guidance to all staff members.

Printers

Locating and selecting printers involves balancing the needs for convenience and immediacy (e.g. for labels in the pharmacy and receipts at reception) with cost, size and printout quality. For larger print runs, particularly if the printer is not designed to print such volumes, it might be cost-effective to outsource after considering the cost of ink, how long the job will occupy the practice's printer, and consequent inconvenience to other staff members.

Many printers are inexpensive to purchase, but running costs can be very high. The quality of a laser printer is usually much better than that of an inkjet printer – but this is usually reflected in the cost of toner. Services are available to refill cartridges and toners to keep costs reduced. Printers can be leased or purchased and there are many offers available regarding maintenance agreements.

The most effective use of a printer is to network it with the PMS so that the printer can be used by several computers, both via the PMS and from standard office programmes. Problems can arise when several people want to print from the same printer at the same time; for example, invoice runs can tie up the printer for some time. It would make sense not to share a printer if there are many different types of paper being used for different tasks.

Outsourcing print runs such as practice leaflets will ultimately look more professional and enhance the image of the practice. Designing documents requires skill and it may not be the best use of staff time, so outsourcing the design work should also be considered. However, if a template document that can be amended is used then it is probably best to produce materials at the practice. Documents can be added to the PMS for use by all staff. Mail merges can be printed from scratch, or on preprinted letterheads, thereby making the best of in-house and outsourced solutions.

Photocopiers

The photocopier must be able to cope with the expected copying workload. When choosing a new machine, the number of copies a minute that it can produce, both in black & white and in colour, should be confirmed in writing. The expected lifespan of the machine must be verified. If the practice decides to lease a photocopier, maintenance charges must be agreed, and the purchasers should be aware of any buyout clauses and minimum usage contracts.

Stand-alone photocopiers should be compared with multifunction networked machines that are capable of printing, copying, scanning and, if required, sending and receiving faxes. A small multifunction machine (Figure 16.7) may be a useful piece of equipment in a compact office. Other features to consider before purchasing a machine are: the need/ability for colour printing, reduction and enlargement; the ability to use A3 paper; and automatic paper handling for multiple sheets, including printing on both sides of the paper. Some machines will also staple and punch, make booklets or fold printed sheets (Figure 16.8). Such convenient machines can be prone to overheating, however, and so a service contract is strongly advised.

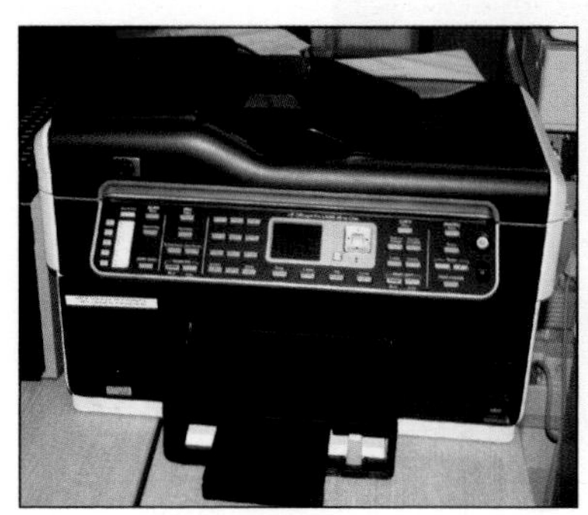

16.7 A small multifunction scanner/printer/fax may be sufficient for personal or light use, and as back-up for a larger machine.

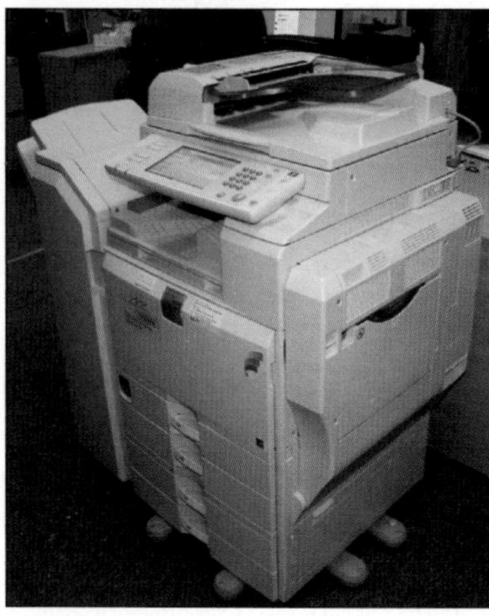

16.8 A large leased networked multi-function printer/scanner/copier on a service contract can be used to: archive patient records electronically; copy and print in colour and black & white; staple; punch; create booklets; and convert documents using OCR.

Fax machine

The practice should evaluate whether paper- or computer-based faxes are most suitable (see Chapter 4). It is possible to use different coloured paper in printer/copying/fax machines so that any faxes are clearly identified. However, it may be more cost-effective and easier to receive and store all faxes electronically.

The cost of toner and print cartridges should also be taken into account when purchasing fax machines, printers and photocopiers. It may be better to purchase a more costly machine in order to reduce the running costs.

Document scanners

The choice of scanner will be influenced by whether scanned items are mostly archived documents, photographic or clinical material (e.g. slides or ECGs), or whether scanning is mostly used for copying and one-off purposes. A multi-sheet feeder and double-sided capability are ideal for archiving; high resolution is essential for photographic or detailed work; and ease of use and optical character recognition (OCR) software may be desirable for other work. If routinely re-typing large volumes of text into the computer, OCR software can save hours of work, by capturing text in a computer file suitable for word processing or other uses. A scanner or scanner/copier that is fast and has a high variable resolution and good software for OCR and saving files in different formats (e.g. .jpg and .pdf) should be chosen (Figure 16.9). If compatible with the PMS, hard-copy lab results, written correspondence, handwritten notes and other useful documentation can be linked to the client records. The PMS supplier should always be consulted before investing in computer peripherals to make sure they are compatible.

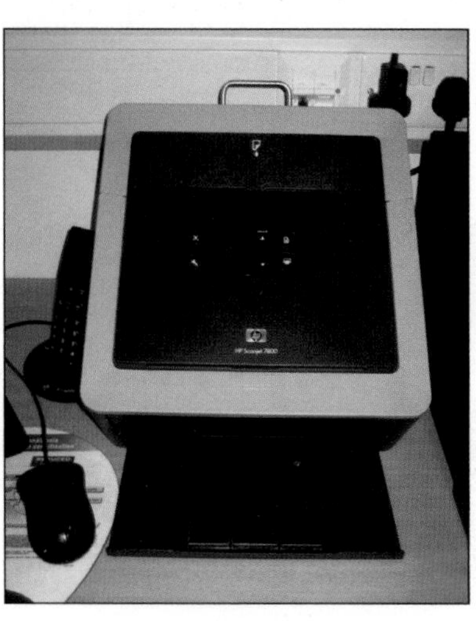

16.9 Auto feed scanner: patient records can be scanned using a stand-alone scanner and attached to individual patient records via the PMS.

Folders and inserters

A variety of machines that fold paper automatically can be leased or purchased. More advanced models can, if required, then insert the document into an envelope and seal it. Such labour-saving devices are extremely useful for practices that frequently send out large mailshots. For smaller practices it may be more cost-effective to outsource the task. Care should be taken regarding the type of paper that can be used with different machines, and a service and maintenance contract should be considered.

Administration

Handling payments

Practices will have individual and specific policies regarding accepted methods of payment, each of which costs different amounts to administer. Many banks charge to deposit cash and cheques, and for changing notes into coins. Card-handling services charge a set fee for each debit card transaction and a percentage of the payment for a credit card transaction. Cash and electronic bank payments are credited to the practice account immediately they are banked; cheque and card transactions may take a few days to 'clear'. Practices may have policies regarding minimum payments accepted on cards or by cheque to allow for the additional costs of the transaction.

Taking payments is a serious responsibility and should never be rushed. Insurance companies will require veterinary practices to have a safe to store money and will specify their terms and conditions. The amount stored should not exceed the amount insured. A safe that takes deposits through a non-return hatch is a good idea and can be fitted into either a wall or floor (Figure 16.10). A policy should be in place as to who has access to the safe, and who takes over responsibility in the event of holiday or sick leave. A night safe service is provided by commercial banks, enabling customers to deposit cash after banking hours, which may reduce the need to keep large sums overnight.

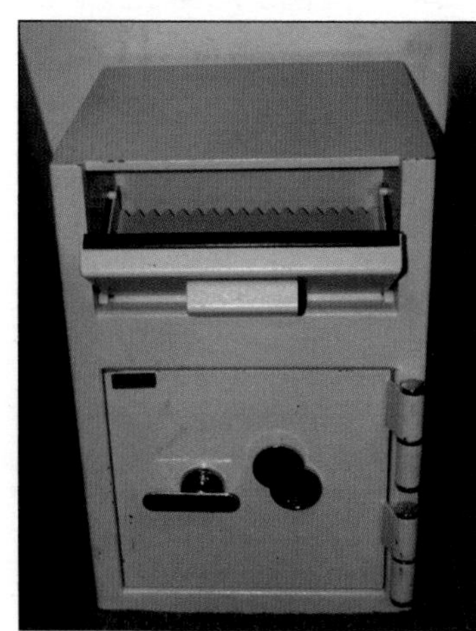

16.10 Floor-standing safe with a deposit drawer. Takings and small items can be deposited into the safe without opening it, by using the deposit drawer. The safe is securely bolted to the floor.

Cash

When taking cash, the amount tendered should be confirmed to the client, particularly if the clinic's till does not have a 'sum tendered' key. Clients may occasionally claim to have tendered a higher sum, and mistakes are less likely if cash changing hands is counted out loud and receipts given. Putting up a notice in the waiting room, suggesting that clients check their change before leaving the clinic, may be helpful. Notes should be checked for authenticity with a special anti-fraud pen.

A secure counter 'cache' adjacent to the till is advisable for increased security (see Chapter 5). If large quantities of bank notes are taken, these should be placed directly into the safe for security reasons.

KEY POINTS

- Staff members unused to handling cash and giving change should practise before taking money in a busy reception area.
- Never let it be known that any amounts of cash are stored on the premises.

Cheques

Cheques are not guaranteed and electronic card payment may be more secure. Banks have been attempting to phase out cheques but at the time of finalizing this chapter, they appear to be here to stay – at least for the foreseeable future. Cheques are still popular for account payments through the post and from businesses, and are still regarded as a contract to pay. Arguably the safest way forward is to take cash, cards and BACS/FPS only – many practices no longer routinely accept cheques.

Credit/debit cards and BACS/FPS payments

Credit and debit card payments may require telephone authorization and it is important to know the procedure for this and what to do if a payment is refused. Some practices allow credit or debit card payment over the telephone; this makes good sense, particularly in cases where a third party may be paying or someone wants to pay in advance. For more information on card handling and security compliance see Chapter 4.

Some practices allow payment direct into their bank account using the BACS/FPS system. In the latter case, the practice's bank details can be included on the invoice.

Selecting a provider

For card transactions, it is important to select the merchant services provider carefully; it is not necessary to use the same bank that provides the main practice account. Shopping around is essential, and the contract should be reviewed regularly, whether or not the practice stays with the same provider. Banks apply different charges depending on a wide range of factors, including the overall value of card transactions and the bank's assessment of exposure to card fraud, and banks will need practice business information in order to set up a card payment system. As credit card and debit card transactions carry different fee rates, tracking the practice's normal value and numbers of each type of transaction is essential for comparing the rates on offer. A small difference in the transaction charge for debit cards can make a large difference if these are the majority of payments, and may offset a higher percentage rate on credit card transactions. Details of charging rates and transaction values and volumes for each payment type should be found on the monthly account statement from the current merchant service provider.

In addition to transaction charges, most providers will charge a monthly card terminal rental fee for the CHIP and PIN unit(s). Choice of provider will also be influenced by the ease of use of the terminals, the connectivity and whether owner-not-present telephone transactions are accepted. Some providers will also offer pre-authorization for large accounts, and other services such as gift cards.

Additional services to consider are a payment service provider (PSP) to process transactions over the Internet. PSP charges can be on a per-month or per-transaction basis. Banks can also ask high-risk businesses for a security bond to cover the costs of unauthorized transactions. Criteria can include the level of online trading, average transaction values and the length of time it takes to fulfil an order.

Although some debit/credit card processors clear all transactions the following day, most processors clear payments two to three days after the customer transaction, with funds available for withdrawal on the working day after they have cleared. Terms and conditions should be checked carefully and the costs of delays in receiving cleared funds calculated in order to compare providers.

The ease of reconciliation is also a significant consideration. Transaction receipts should be reconciled against the end-of-day banking reports for accuracy rather than the X and Z reports produced daily from the terminals. If the terminal is electronically polled by the service provider, a 'poll successful receipt' should be available each morning.

Petty cash

This is a small amount of cash ('cash float') kept separately from the main till to deal with any small items that may have to be purchased during the working day, such as coffee, sugar, etc. It may be kept in a petty cash box, with a book listing any items purchased and in which a running total is recorded. It is essential to keep a precise record, together with all receipts, for any cash used during the day; otherwise time can be wasted wondering why the petty cash float does not balance or whether theft has taken place. A disciplined approach is essential: all staff must always replace cash with receipts and there should be no self-certification. It may also be wise to put in place a limit regarding the amount that can be taken out of petty cash and to set clear access rules. Clear boundaries regarding what the cash can be used for are essential, and formal approval of receipts must be undertaken regularly – are staff permitted to purchase picture frames at £30 for example? Purchases above a certain value should be approved by the practice manager or a partner, and 'IOUs' should be banned. Practices with effective and regular till reconciliation usually find a separate petty cash float unnecessary.

Reconciliation

Reconciliation is the process of balancing up the total payments taken in a period with the amounts recorded as due. By reconciling the totals, errors can be spotted early on, e.g. payments not recorded against the client records. Proper and timely reconciliation is vital to protect the practice against fraud, and to spot errors straight away so that clients' accounts are accurate. Financial recording systems should be checked and audit trails performed regularly. Tight controls regarding cash are essential for a workplace where employees feel part of a well managed trained team, and can help reduce the temptation of theft and/or fraud.

Procedures should be established for recording money transactions, training all staff involved (and recording this training) and, if required, the witnessing of transactions by at least one member of staff

The accounting of monies prior to banking should be completed in a controlled area, either an office or quiet location with the minimum of interruption. Monies waiting to be banked should be retained in a locked container at all times – preferably a safe.

A risk assessment should be in place for staff members taking money to the bank; an example is given at the end of this chapter. It is recommended by some banks that cheques are in one bag and cash in another, so that if challenged the bag with the cheques in can be handed over. The route taken to reach the bank and the timing of the journey should be varied, and cash should not be carried in easily identifiable cash bags. Some larger practices may consider using a security company to collect money and take it to the bank. If anyone is asked to hand over the money, there must be no heroics.

Document (and data) security

Efficient keeping and storage of records is essential for maintaining good communication within the practice. Accurate records aid patient care, protect the practice from legal challenges, and are vital for stock and financial controls (Figure 16.11). Records may be paper-based or electronic, stored in house or on remote servers (cloud-based).

- Client records with contact information
- Supplier records
- Medical records, including ward or hospitalization notes, radiographs, anaesthetic and dental charts, laboratory results, slides, radiographs, digital images and recordings and copies of insurance claim forms
- Personnel records, including salary records, contracts and written statements, recruitment records, application forms and staff reviews or appraisals
- Equipment service records
- Financial records, bank statements, invoices, delivery notes
- Payment records, including electronic payment slips
- Health & Safety records, accident records, risk assessments and Local Rules
- Training records, RCVS CPD record cards, student college reports, centre correspondence, Nursing Progress Logs (electronic and printed hard copies), tutorial records
- Monitoring, e.g. closed circuit television (CCTV) tapes or recording of telephone conversations
- Correspondence

16.11 Examples of records a practice might keep.

Data Protection Act

Practices that keep personal records of staff or clients must comply with the Data Protection Act 1998 (DPA). This requires that anyone holding information about living individuals in electronic format, and in some cases on paper, must follow the eight data protection principles of good information handling (Figure 16.12). The DPA requires that data users, including veterinary practices, must notify the Information Commissioner if they wish to use records for particular purposes. Practices can complete a simple checklist (see www.ico.gov.uk) where full guidance on the Act and need for notification is easy to access. Notification is straightforward. At February 2012, a notification fee of £500 applies to data controllers that have a turnover of £25.9M and 250 or more members of staff, or that are a public authority with 250 or more members of staff. All other data controllers fall into the lower-tier category, paying £35 per annum unless they are exempt. The DPA also gives all individuals certain rights, including the right to see information that is held about them and to have it corrected if it is wrong. Clients may request access to their records under the Act.

Personal information must be:

- Fairly and lawfully processed
- Processed for specific lawful purposes
- Adequate, relevant and not excessive
- Accurate and, where necessary, kept up to date
- Not kept for longer than necessary
- Processed in line with the rights of the individual
- Kept secure
- Not transferred to countries outside the European Economic Area unless there is adequate protection for the information

16.12 The eight data protection principles of good information handling.

Filing

All records should be stored securely and conveniently, using an appropriate filing system. Scanning paper records for electronic storage to reduce volume of archiving and copying, and to ease recall of material should be considered.

The same principles apply to manual and electronic filing. All files should use a standard labelling system, whether in hard copy or electronic format. This will generally include the owner and an animal name, plus a reference number and date.

Non-electronic files should always be returned to the appropriate place after use. A marker can be inserted into the space as the file is removed to aid replacement (Figure 16.13). These markers can also be useful to flag up any files that remain missing.

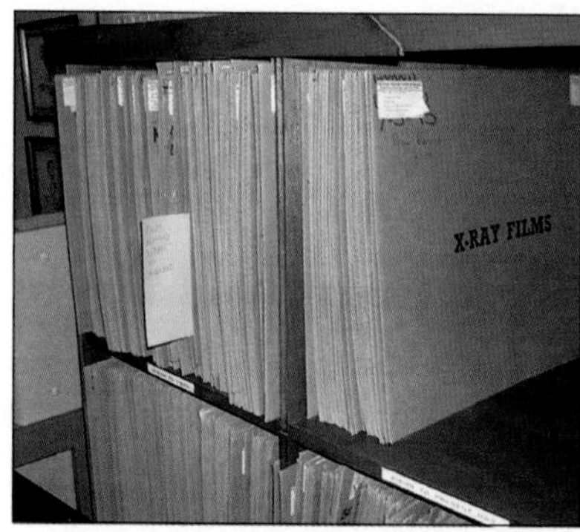

16.13 Leaving a clear marker where a file has been removed alerts others to its absence and facilitates replacement.

Filing systems

Alphabetical: Paper- or card-based client records are usually filed using a system based on surname and house number plus pet name; using a client's individual initials can be problematical where families are owners. Computerized records can be searched using a number of parameters, including pet name, owner name and address, client ID, pet ID, and telephone numbers, and can reduce the drudgery and error of manual filing. Alphabetical filing is not recommended for paper laboratory reports, consent forms, etc., as files are difficult to archive after a period and there is a high chance of misfiling due to manual error.

Chronological: Records such as dental charts, radiographs, ECGs, laboratory reports, hospitalization sheets and consent forms can be filed in date order and cross-referenced to client records. This system is quicker than alphabetical filing, as each new record can just be filed on top of the last one. General filing, particularly where retrieval is less likely to be needed, and archiving old records are also simpler with this system, which saves the continual file expansion required in an alphabetical system.

Numerical: This is a useful way to file purchase ledger invoices for accounts packages, for example. Each invoice will have an individual number (e.g. 12/3465, 12/3466... for 2012). An automatic numbering machine is really useful.

Electronic storage: Laboratory results are now usually e-mailed into the practice and can be attached directly to client computer records. ECG tracings and radiographs can also be stored digitally, and records shared between veterinary surgeons via the Internet. This saves storage space and makes retrieval much faster. As electronic storage increases, however, practices will need to review their back-up systems to include the increasing number and size of files.

Data security

- Records should be kept on *permanent* material, such as good quality paper or other media.
- Non-electronic records should be stored securely, under lock and key if necessary.
- Records may be stolen, and so hard copies should never be left out on reception desks or in other public areas.

Decisions need to be taken regarding which files are suitable for open access by everyone. Secure files with restricted access are required to store: contracts, partners' meeting notes, salary details, financial details, personal development reviews, staff training records, and any other sensitive documents. Access to sensitive documents and records should be reviewed on a regular basis and passwords changed regularly as a security procedure.

Computer records

Magnetic media such as back-up tapes and portable hard drives should be stored in a clean dry place, away from possible sources of radiation and magnetism. Compact discs and DVDs should be kept in protective cases, clearly identified and also stored in a clean dry place. Computer records should be regularly backed up on to storage media, and these back-ups should be verified so that the data are reliable for restoring on to the system should the need arise. It is advisable to have a responsible member of staff in charge of these processes and to store data offsite on a regular basis or in fireproof containers in the practice. A minimum of daily backing up is recommended for medical records and financial information, and weekly for less sensitive records. Many computer networks now include automatic back-up, with duplicate hard drives to take over if one fails; some systems are web-based, with central holding of data. Practices should verify the integrity and security of the data if stored remotely by a third party.

Computers, particularly laptops, are very attractive to casual thieves; locking devices (to fix them down) and alarms are recommended. Computers should never be left in vehicles unless stored in a locked compartment, away from view – many large animal and equine vets now carry mobile devices. Care should also be taken if staff take laptops home that have practice data on them. A robust e-mail and Internet policy is needed (see above).

Information (data) is one of the practice's most valuable possessions and protection with secure passwords is essential so that unauthorized personnel cannot gain access. It is vital for key managers or owners to maintain good password security and access in case of personnel absence or suspected fraud.

Access and ownership of records

RCVS guidance recognizes that clients, who now have access to their own medical records, are likely to seek similar access to their pets' records. In such cases it may be helpful, on the direction of a veterinary surgeon, for a client to be offered sight of the records at the surgery by appointment at a mutually convenient time.

Case records, including radiographs and similar documents, are the property of, and should be retained by, veterinary surgeons, both in the interests of animal welfare and for their own protection. Copies, with a summary history, should be passed on at the request of a colleague taking over a case. Where a client has paid for the radiographs or other reports, the client is legally entitled to them. However, the practice may choose to make it clear that they are charging not for the radiographs themselves but rather for the interpretation and advice. In appropriate circumstances practices may provide copies of radiographs to clients. Practices should consider clarifying their position on ownership of, and access to, diagnostic material in their standard 'Terms of business' document (see Chapter 24).

Disclosure of records may be ordered in disciplinary or court hearings, and the RCVS may request copies of case records as a matter of routine in the course of investigating a complaint.

Confidentiality

All members of the veterinary practice team must maintain the confidentiality of client and practice information at all times, and should never discuss professional or privileged information outside the practice. The RCVS codes of professional conduct for both veterinary surgeons and registered veterinary nurses state that a registered veterinary surgeon or veterinary nurse can be held accountable should practice or client confidentiality prove to have been breached.

Disposal of records

To reduce size and to comply with the DPA, old or unused files should be archived or discarded regularly. There are no legal limits on document storage times, and advice should be sought from the practice's professional advisors, but in general:

- Financial, tax and PAYE records should be kept for 6 years after the financial year end
- Medical records, radiographs, etc. should be kept for at least 6 years in case of legal claims, and longer if deemed necessary by the clinician
- Practice insurance records for employer liability should be kept indefinitely, and it may be prudent to keep health and safety records plus appraisal records of current staff throughout their employment, and as long as is practicable
- Recruitment records, such as application forms and references from unsuccessful candidates, should not be kept for longer than 6 months without permission from the applicant (e.g. to be considered for future vacancies).

KEY POINT

Archived records should be stored securely until destroyed. Garden sheds and outhouses are not suitable; secure storage should be available for paper records.

Practices should ensure secure erasure of data from computers or remote servers. Computers should be disposed of only after permanently erasing any sensitive data and according to local waste regulations. Hard drives may still contain sensitive information, even if 'wiped'. A secure disposal company is recommended, or retention of the hard drives and disposal via a secure data disposal service. Paper records should be destroyed by shredding or burning, or by using a professional confidential waste contractor, which may allow recycling after confidential shredding.

Practice correspondence

Incoming post and faxes

Incoming mail should be opened and handled promptly and efficiently by a nominated person. Letters can be grouped using an agreed system, such as pigeonholes, so that they are passed on to the appropriate persons or departments.

Any private or confidential letters should be passed on un-opened to the addressee. Employees, however, should be discouraged from using the practice address for personal correspondence, so private correspondence would usually only be directed to the practice owners or directors. Some practices may choose to record the date and receipt of all letters and to stamp the date on each letter. Letters (unless private) should not be left unopened; a nominated person should be responsible for opening and dealing with any mail addressed to staff that are absent from work.

Once opened, mail should be responded to as required and without delay. In any situation where the response might be delayed, a brief acknowledgement to the sender that the letter has arrived is essential. This is particularly important regarding letters of complaint, urgent correspondence or for job applicants.

Incoming faxes should be treated in a similar way.

Outgoing post and faxes

The practice should be familiar with local times of postal collections, or have arrangements in place for the mail to be collected direct from the practice. Subject to still being able to send special deliveries and recorded mail, the latter can be a cost-effective option. Nominated trained staff should be responsible for stamping, franking and looking after all post, as items must be weighed and measured in order to be stamped according to current postage rates. A specific place should be designated for outgoing mail.

KEY POINT

Client confidentiality must be maintained for outgoing mail and therefore care should be taken that post is not left on the front desk with client names and addresses exposed. Post on the desk is vulnerable to being stolen.

Stamps and alternatives

Using postage stamps can prove to be expensive but is a convenient method of posting and may suit smaller practices.

Franking is a quick and easy way to manage postage; it can reduce costs and project a professional image. However, as fewer items are now being posted owing to electronic communications, the savings may not be as significant as first expected, particularly for a small practice. Although the actual postage per item is cheaper, the leasing or rental charges of the franking machine must be considered. If a postage meter is used, a specific person should be responsible for topping up postage credit on the meter.

The Royal Mail offers a service for printing postage directly on to envelopes, alongside a personalized logo or message: 'Smart Stamp'. A monthly or annual subscription is payable in addition to the cost of postage. This system can save time when preparing mail with mail merge and multiprint options.

Prepaid envelopes are simple to use, as stamps or a franking machine are not required. There is reduced flexibility, however, and the cost of postage and envelopes, as well as staff time, must be considered when evaluating this method.

Laboratory samples

Most laboratories have a courier collection service for pathological samples but very often lab samples need to be posted (see Chapter 14 for guidance on packaging). It is advisable to have a designated person or department responsible for calling the courier or posting samples. The practice should have a written protocol on the correct packaging and posting of laboratory and pathological samples.

E-mails

It is vital to nominate someone to check the practice e-mail account on a frequent basis throughout the day. Given the 'instant' nature of an e-mail, incoming messages need to be dealt with quickly.

For standard questions (e.g. the cost of vaccinations), standard responses can be devised that can be personalized for each recipient. This can be set up using the 'signature' facility on an e-mail program. Having standardized answers for routine questions means that an approved and consistent response can be issued. While an automated response might be useful in some cases, practice staff must live up to the expectations it creates – if it says that enquiries are dealt with within 48 hours, then this must be the case!

If individual e-mail addresses are not used, e-mails must be forwarded on to the appropriate person and/or department. As well as deciding which staff or which departments in the practice should have direct e-mail access, an agreed standard (e.g. text, wording on the practice's signature) should also be adhered to.

When formulating an e-mail policy, it is worth considering the need for individuals to have their own addresses; this should be balanced against the efficiency of monitoring the accounts, dealing with unsolicited e-mails and spam, and the risk of infected attachments. A strict e-mail policy should be in place (see above), and care should be taken not to forward and reply to e-mails inappropriately. The use of informal language should be discouraged.

Telephone messages

Telephone messages must be delivered to the appropriate person promptly. A telephone message book, duplicate book or a pad of coloured notes can be used so that messages are not lost. Some practice management systems have an internal message feature, where messages are sent directly to the user when he/she logs in, or are displayed until dealt with. Individual voicemail systems allow the caller to be put through so that they can leave their own message. Clear protocols should be in place to ensure that messages are monitored and acted upon within a reasonable timeframe, particularly if people are away from the practice.

When telephoning clients and leaving messages, it may be helpful to use additional lines on the main practice number and to allow the system to transmit the practice number so that clients can identify the caller. These settings can be defined, or can be changed for individual calls using an override number available from the telecom provider, and this may be useful for clients who have phones set not to accept unidentified incoming calls. If using an ex-directory outgoing line, or home number, however, it is useful to withhold the number, as clients often note this down as 'the vet's number' and may use it again.

KEY POINT

Many telephone systems can be set to bar calls to certain telephone numbers, such as premium charged 09 numbers and international calls. A special code can often be used to override this where necessary.

Privacy

It should be made clear within the employee handbook (see Chapter 19) that all post, faxes, e-mails, etc. that arrive at work, even if addressed to an individual employee, are not private and therefore can be opened by the employer. If staff members are on holiday, sick or there is a problem, it may be more appropriate for someone like the practice manager to open and deal with them as required. Use of the practice address for personal correspondence should be firmly discouraged; however, this can be difficult where staff live above the practice or in adjoining accommodation with the same address. A clear protocol should be in place to accommodate this. Where practices permit the delivery of personal items to the practice address, practice policy should state clearly that the staff member's own address must be used for all financial transactions and account details. It is important that no personal shopping is undertaken using the practice name or address for the account holder.

Practice stationery

Stationery quality and a recognizable logo are important factors in creating a good business image (see Chapter 25) and therefore all business stationery should be of the same style and format. Paper weights range from 80 gsm (grams per square metre) for general use to 120 gsm for letters. Card varies from 180 gsm to over 300 gsm. Chosen paper weights must be compatible with the practice printers.

Legal requirements for letterhead stationery

If the owner of the business is a 'sole trader' (see Chapter 24), the business can trade under his/her own name, or a different business name can be chosen. If a business name is chosen that is not the owner's name, the name of the business owner and the business address must be included on all letterheads and order forms.

Businesses that are run by a partnership require letterheads, order forms, receipts and invoices to include the names of all partners and the address of the main office. If there are many partners, however, it is acceptable to state where a list of partners may be found.

If trading as a 'limited company', the letterhead and order form stationery (whether printed or electronic versions) must include:

- The full registered company name
- The company registration number and place of registration
- The company registered address and the address of its place of business, if different.

There is no need to include the names of the directors on the letterhead for a limited company, but if directors are included, all directors must be named.

Most letterheads also include a telephone and fax number, the business's website address and an e-mail address. Where the business is registered for VAT, inclusion of the VAT number is useful if the paper is often used for invoicing.

A clear policy should govern the use of practice-headed stationery (and e-mail accounts), and although not a legal requirement, it would be very advisable to make staff aware that no practice stationery should be used for personal use.

Compliment slips

These are cut-down versions of the letterhead, giving all the basic information (but omitting details such as registered office) on a smaller piece of paper – usually the same width, but one third the depth. Compliment slips can be useful and economical for sending brief messages and cover notes with enclosures.

Invoices

All invoices should clearly state that this is what they are, with the word 'Invoice'. They should also include the following:

- A unique identification number
- The practice name, address and contact information
- The company name or personal name and address of the customer you are invoicing
- A clear description of what is being charged for
- The date the goods or service were provided (supply date)
- The date of the invoice
- The amount(s) being charged
- VAT amount if applicable
- The total amount owed
- Payment/settlement terms and how to pay, e.g. BACS details.

In addition to the above, limited companies and sole traders must by law include the following information on any invoices sent to customers:

- The full company name as it appears on the certificate of incorporation, or the sole trader's name
- Any business name used
- An address where any legal documents can be delivered to using a business name.

Limited companies may include the names of the directors on their invoices. However, if included, this must include the names of all directors.

VAT details: If registered for VAT, whether the business is a limited company or a sole trader, the following information must be included on all invoices:

- A unique and sequential identifying invoice number
- The date the invoice is issued
- The customer's name and address
- The business's name, address and VAT registration number
- Date of supply to the customer
- A description sufficient to identify the supply of goods or services
- The quantity of the goods or services with a unit price – *excluding* VAT
- The rate of VAT per item
- The rate of any cash discount
- The total amount of VAT charged.

A VAT invoice that includes zero-rated or exempt goods or services must:

- Show clearly that there is no VAT payable on those goods or services
- Show the total of those values separately.

If retail sales are made of goods or services for £250 or less, *including* VAT, then when a customer asks for a VAT invoice, a simplified VAT invoice can be issued that only needs to show:

- The seller's name and address
- The seller's VAT registration number
- The time of supply ('tax point')
- A description of the goods or services.

Also, if the supply includes items at differing VAT rates, then for each different VAT rate or item, the simplified VAT invoice must also show:

- The total price including VAT
- The VAT rate applicable to the item.

All transactions should be invoiced, but in practice, invoices are often not printed out or produced formally as payment is often made at the time. The format of receipts should be considered to include the necessary details if this is the case, and itemized receipts must be available for all clients. Most PMS will have editable settings for invoices and receipts.

Business cards

These can be given to clients, suppliers and other contacts, so that they have a record of the practice name and details. Cards can be personalized for individual staff members, adding relevant qualifications as appropriate. Practices may also have specific appointment cards for clients, which can carry appropriate marketing messages.

KEY POINT

A standard card size is preferred so that it will fit into business card holders.

Purchasing stationery

The least expensive option is to print stationery digitally 'on demand'; however, this will lack the quality and image of professionally printed paper.

Order quantity should be decided according to the level of use *versus* the need to update details. The cost of flexibility *versus* print run savings from economies of scale must be weighed up.

Most practices are striving to reduce the amount of paper used within the business and are increasingly using electronic formats to aid this process. However, there is still a need to purchase stationery for the practice, and consolidation of buying these products can reduce costs considerably. The stationery industry is an extremely competitive market and 'shopping around' can prove to be very cost-effective. Having one member of staff in charge of purchasing and keeping the stationery cupboards stocked and tidy can be a very effective form of stock control. Labelling the stationery shelves with maximum and minimum levels can assist with keeping stationery costs under control. A specific stationery cupboard, lockable if desired, can be very useful and many practices find it helpful to keep a hidden 'emergency stock' of commonly used items in case supplies are exhausted unexpectedly and there is a delay in restocking.

Meeting rooms

A meeting room can be an incredibly useful space with many functions, including:

- General staff meetings (Figure 16.14)
- Private meetings when staff members are distressed and need to talk
- Performance reviews and appraisals
- Disciplinary matters
- Interviews
- Meetings with sales representatives
- Meetings with clients.

A telephone line is useful for confidential phone calls and for communication with people within the practice. A flatscreen workstation allows staff to use the room for silent working or to handle particularly discreet matters, away from the main office hub. This is especially handy in the practice that only has an open-plan office.

A busy meeting room may require some kind of booking procedure, so that everyone knows when a meeting is due to take place. As with all communal areas of the practice, protocols should be in place to ensure that the room is kept clean and tidy. If plumbing is available, a small counter top for refreshments and washing up facilities can be useful.

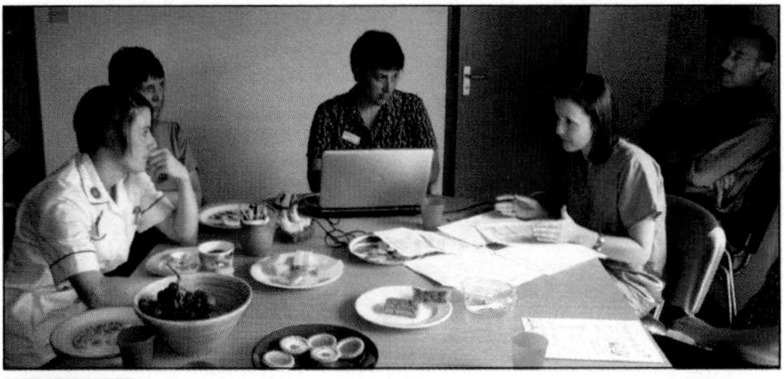

16.14 Making use of the practice meeting room.

Shared areas

Areas such as staffrooms, libraries, the kitchen, cloakrooms and toilets are used by the entire team. Guidelines should be in place to ensure that these areas are well maintained and kept clean and tidy (Figure 16.15), with each person taking a portion of the responsibility. Cleaning schedules or checklists are useful. If washing up tea/coffee mugs becomes an issue, this needs to be addressed: employing an evening cleaner may eliminate the problem; or a practice dishwasher can be an ideal solution. If space is at a premium, named mugs – with a few spares for visitors – and a clear washing up rule will help. Maintaining an adequate supply of cleaning materials is important.

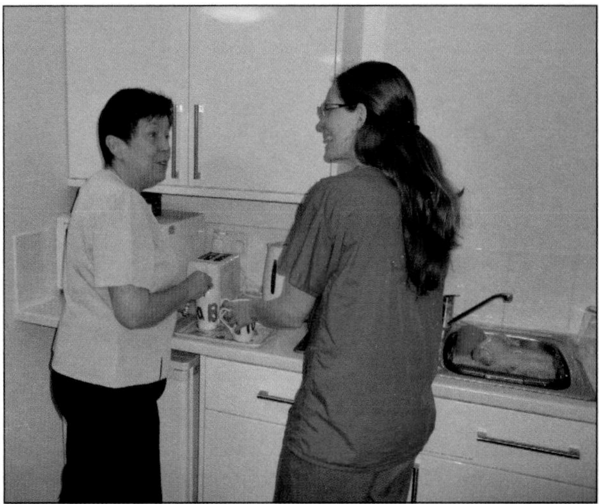

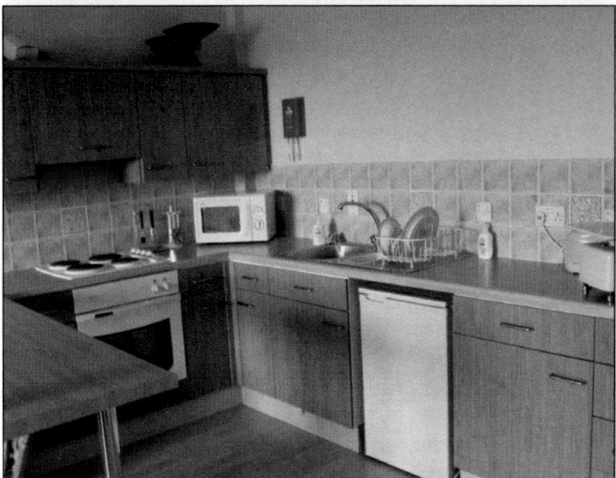

16.15 Staff should have an area where they can relax during breaks. This should be well maintained.

A culture of responsibility and pride should be encouraged. Involving the team in planning and maintaining these areas and deciding what should be provided will help. Employing a cleaner is a financial investment, but may be more cost-effective than using skilled team members to carry out cleaning duties (unless they are not fully utilized). If cleaning out of hours, security and lone worker issues need to be considered.

A fridge of sufficient size for staff to use for packed lunches (Figure 16.16) is always appreciated by the team, but is not mandatory, although perishable food supplied by the practice should be kept safely.

> **KEY POINT**
>
> Staff food must NOT be stored in a fridge used for pharmaceuticals, lab samples or other practice items.

Where cooking facilities are provided, such as a toaster or microwave (and the kettle), appropriate risk assessments should be made and maintenance and

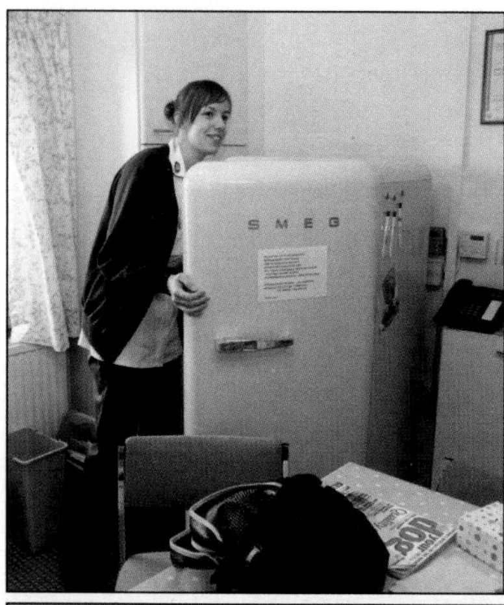

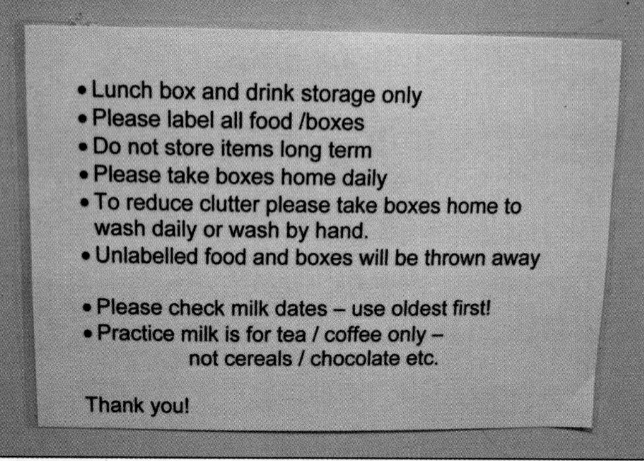

• Lunch box and drink storage only
• Please label all food /boxes
• Do not store items long term
• Please take boxes home daily
• To reduce clutter please take boxes home to wash daily or wash by hand.
• Unlabelled food and boxes will be thrown away
• Please check milk dates – use oldest first!
• Practice milk is for tea / coffee only – not cereals / chocolate etc.
Thank you!

16.16 Although not required by law, providing a fridge large enough to accommodate lunchboxes for staff is always appreciated. A label reminding people of how it should and should not be used is helpful.

testing carried out (see Chapter 3). Provision of a television for staff to watch can cause difficulties – how will it affect the social dynamic of the practice *versus* the need for staff to be able to 'switch off' and relax? Most practices provide a television in overnight and weekend duty accommodation if there is likely to be significant downtime; if provided, a TV licence will need to be purchased.

Space is needed for staff to put their personal belongings into while at work, although long-term and excessive storage should be discouraged. There is no legal obligation to provide secure lockers, although they are recommended.

A clear policy regarding the use and storage of practice telephones and personal mobiles during working hours should be in place (Figures 16.17 and 16.18).

Telephones

- Personal telephone calls should not be made on the practice's telephones or during normal working hours, except in emergencies, without the express permission of the management. Calls should be kept as short as possible and line X should be used to avoid blocking incoming calls.
- All personal calls that appear on the itemized phone bill must be paid for.
- Incoming personal calls should not be taken unless the matter is urgent; any call should be kept brief and the member of staff not distracted from his/her duties.

16.17 An example of a practice policy on telephone use.

Mobiles

- Mobile phones in the workplace can be disruptive, are distracting for other members of staff, cause loss of productive time, and affect concentration and efficiency.
- Mobile phones should be left with your other belongings and answered during a break.

16.18 An example of a practice policy on mobile phone use.

Storage rooms

Storage rooms should be clean, tidy and well organized, with adequate lighting and ventilation. Staff given access to these areas should be made accountable for keeping them tidy and secure. Storage rooms, if placed strategically, can be used as a buffer space for noise reduction in the practice.

For purposes of retrieval, using clearly labelled proper archive boxes for stored files is advisable. Archives should be stacked in a logical manner, clearly marked on the outside with the date, the content and the date for destruction.

KEY POINT

Unnecessary items, such as out-of-date leaflets and obsolete equipment, should not be stored.

Staff accommodation

Overnight duty staff

Emergency Service clinics need a minimum of two people on duty and at least one person awake at all times. It is also mandatory for veterinary hospitals approved by the RCVS Practice Standards Scheme to have staff who are responsible for inpatients staying overnight as part of their duties. Many general practices also choose to provide overnight accommodation for a staff member, whether or not they provide their own out-of-hours services. All members of staff must have working hours that comply with the Working Time Directive (see Chapter 20), and this includes when staff members are staying overnight as part of their duties.

Where there is responsibility for inpatient care, there should be easy access to ward areas. The level of care expected and method of monitoring should be agreed. Patients can also be monitored between formal checks and treatments, using CCTV, a webcam or network camera (Figure 16.19) or via an audio link.

Staff members covering out-of-hours duties should be provided with a list of emergency numbers and must be fully conversant with the phone system and other communication systems. Chapter 7 has more guidance on out-of-hours nursing. Staff on duty should feel comfortable with any security alarm systems. These can be audible alarms or those that ring through to a central control and/or responsible person. Information on security and lone working, including a sample risk assessment, can be found in Chapter 22.

All areas that staff use, including where they sleep and the inpatient wards, must have smoke alarms fitted, and an automatic fire alarm is recommended.

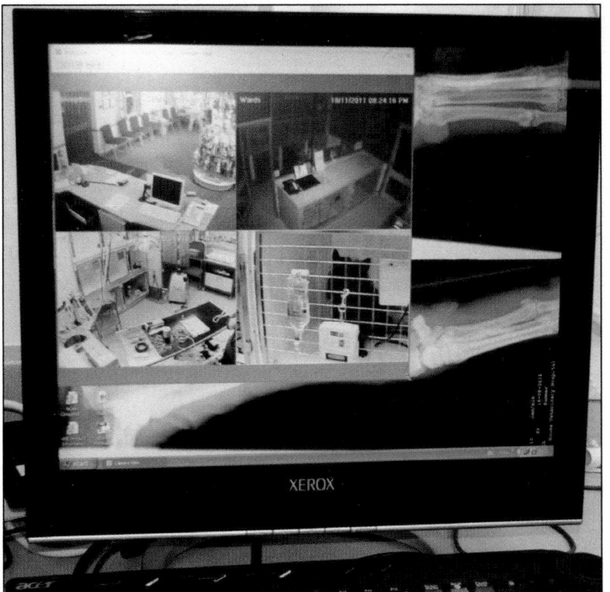

16.19 Particularly when working out of hours, remote monitoring can be useful for observing patients and different areas of the practice.

Responsibility for the tidiness and cleanliness of the on-site overnight staff accommodation (Figure 16.20) should be clear, so staff are aware of what is expected of them including the provision, changing and washing of bed linen. Whilst individuals using overnight facilities should ensure that they keep them tidy and that they clean up any mess made, general cleaning arrangements will need to be in place; the services of a cleaner, who can also wash bed linen and have the room ready for the next duty vet/nurse, may be appropriate. Adequate arrangements for privacy should be ensured if facilities such as showers and toilets are shared, and there should be provision for stowage of personal effects. Adequate kitchen facilities also need to be provided for storing and preparing food and refreshments.

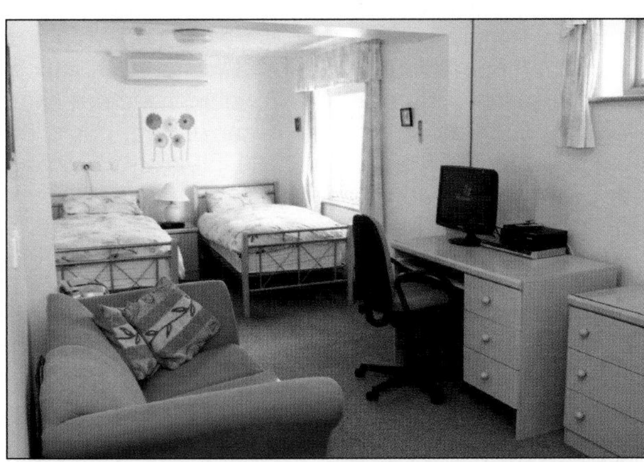

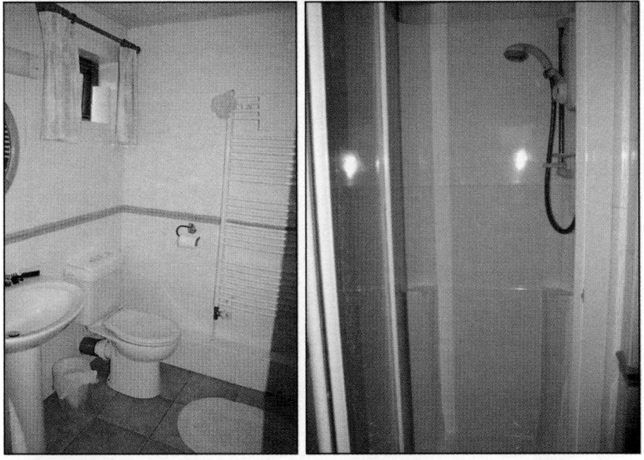

16.20 Duty accommodation should be comfortable and secure with laundered bedding. Two beds allows for clean sheets to be available for consecutive shifts by different individuals. There is a security grille at the bedroom window. Ensuite facilities allow privacy and are secure for lone workers. Easy maintenance is important for duty accommodation: a moulded shower cubicle is easy to clean; shower heads should be descaled regularly in hard-water areas.

KEY POINT

To maintain a professional image at all times, clear guidelines should be in place concerning appropriate dress for out-of-hours care.

Staff living in practice accommodation

Providing staff accommodation can be mutually beneficial to both employee and employer but can prove to be a very complex area. Practice accommodation can be on the premises or away from the practice.

As a landlord, there are a number of legal obligations that must be adhered to, and failing to comply with these could result in prosecution. Regulations vary depending on the type of property. Apart from legal obligations, there are potential taxation issues to consider before the commencement of the tenancy. Professional advice should be sought if the practice is considering renting out accommodation to staff members. Policies should be in place regarding pets in staff accommodation and also a 'No smoking' policy that applies to anyone using the staff accommodation, including visitors. It is vital to have a licence or a tenancy (preferably an 'Assured Shorthold Tenancy') agreement in place.

Agreements

Occupation under licence linked to employment is a type of agreement that gives an employee a licence to occupy premises owned by the practice. It is a short and simple type of commercial agreement that does not form a tenancy. This type of agreement does not create an interest in the property and so the occupant will have to accept that the landlord can enter the property at any time. The agreement can also be drafted to state that the landlord can use the property at the same time as the tenant. The licence to occupy is very popular where a short-term agreement is required and where the property will need to be vacated if the employment ends.

The agreement should specify who is to live there, and set out responsibilities for the payment of insurance, TV licence, utilities and council tax.

Payments and tax implications

Some practices charge the employee rent for use of practice accommodation. This places a value on the accommodation and allows more flexibility for the employee, as they then have the option to move out and rent or buy another property. There is a danger, however, that the practice could be left with unoccupied practice accommodation which may, due to being adjoined to the surgery, be unsuitable to rent out to anyone else. By paying a lower salary, practice accommodation can be offered as part of the package. However, it is not uncommon that, eventually, people's personal circumstances change and they no longer require it. Some staff may expect, or ask for, a salary increase instead. This may not be in the practice's best interest and it is therefore important to ensure that the wording in the contract clearly covers such a scenario.

Employers may be able to obtain a dispensation from HMRC (Her Majesty's Revenue and Customs) for provision of accommodation for veterinary surgeons, provided they can prove they are occupying the premises for the better performance of duties and that it is customary. This means that the accommodation benefit does not have to be declared on the form P11D (see Chapter 24). Other key members of staff, such as nurses, may be able to use the same criteria to obtain a reduction in their tax liability, particularly if the job description specifies duties that must be undertaken from the premises, such as monitoring security.

Rent or licence fees should be set based on advice and the local market rates. Provided there has been agreement from HMRC, rent or fees can be deducted from gross rather than net salary. When the employee moves out of the rented accommodation, this taxation benefit will cease and their salary will be taxed in full, resulting in a slight reduction of their net income.

Security and privacy considerations

Where entrances to practice accommodation and the clinical practice are shared, strict security protocols should be put in place regarding visitors to the practice. For example, visitors will be under the care and direction of a staff member who should ensure that they are accompanied at all times while in the non-public areas of the building. Internal doors to accommodation or staff areas such as offices should be fitted with appropriate security locks to prevent unauthorized access (Figure 16.21).

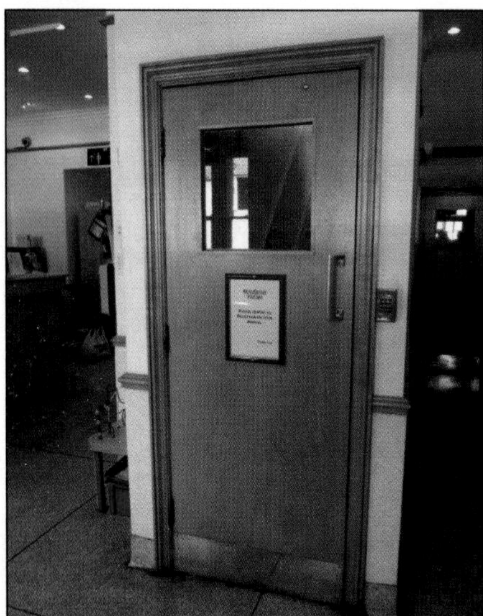

16.21 Internal doors to accommodation or staff areas, including offices, should be fitted with appropriate security locks to prevent unauthorized access.

For all practice accommodation, protocols should also ensure that inpatients, workers and clients are not disturbed, nor the residential member of staff, where possible. Whilst it is reassuring to have a member of staff living on site, clear guidelines should be in place regarding care of the patients, including when the residential member of staff is on duty and when they are not, and the frequency of checks and other duties. Ways to ensure maintaining the tenant's privacy should also be considered and discussed with the tenant before the commencement of the tenancy to avoid any complaints in the future.

Practice vehicles

Many small animal veterinary practices have made the decision not to provide company cars for their employees, as this is generally considered to be no longer tax-efficient for the employee. For the employer, looking after a fleet of cars is very time-consuming, and insurance, repairs, MOTs, accidents and purchases are costly.

Practice ambulance

To conform to UK DVLA regulations (see www.dft.gov.uk), a vehicle designated as a Veterinary Ambulance should be used solely for the purpose of transporting sick and injured animals to and from a place where treatment is given and should be liveried with the words 'Veterinary Ambulance' or 'Animal Ambulance' on both sides (Figure 16.22). A vehicle without such wording, such as an unmarked car or van, could be construed as a private hire vehicle if it is also carrying pet owners, and would need to be licensed as such with the local taxi licensing office. The operation of a Veterinary Ambulance must be overseen by an RCVS-registered veterinary surgeon; the vehicle is then exempt from Vehicle Excise Duty.

The ambulance needs to be kept and maintained in a roadworthy condition and conform to all legal obligations, including a 'No smoking' sign on display. A nominated person must be responsible for the roadworthiness of the vehicle, along with appropriate and adequate insurance. It is also advisable to make one

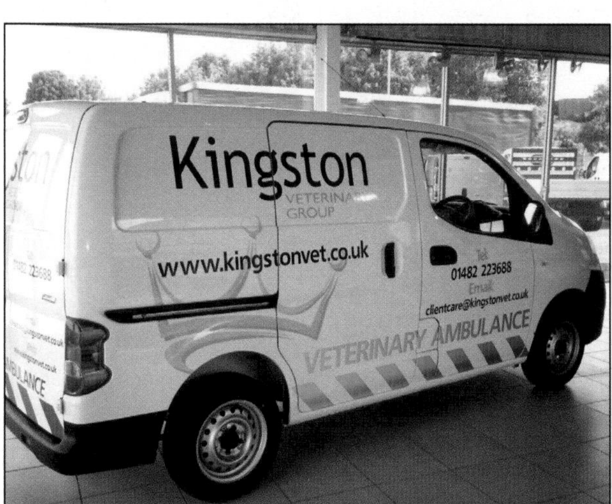

16.22 A well maintained and liveried veterinary ambulance is a great marketing tool, as well as a useful vehicle. © Kingston Veterinary Group

person responsible for the tidiness and cleanliness of the vehicle, bearing in mind the risk for cross-infection from transporting animals.

Many practices choose to use an ambulance as a pool car. Such a vehicle is ideal for using when attending to house calls and for transporting patients between surgeries, and can be branded for advertising purposes (Figure 16.22). The practice will need to have a clear protocol in place as to:

- Who is permitted to drive the vehicle
- What it can be used for
- What restrictions are in place.

Practice cars and car allowances

A clear driving and vehicles policy should be in place and specific elements included in the contract of employment. Examples are given at the end of this chapter.

If staff are given a car allowance, there should be clear guidelines as to what is expected of them (e.g. they may be required to have a vehicle at work in case they need to do a home visit). There must also be clarity as to whether or not travel costs, such as fuel, are included in the allowance paid. Tax implications are covered in Chapter 24.

KEY POINT

If staff are using their own vehicle for work purposes, they will need to ensure that they are appropriately insured and it may be prudent for the practice to request evidence that private cars are covered for business use.

Where a car is provided by the practice for private use, responsibility for its upkeep and maintenance must be clear, as well as any restriction on use and mileage, etc. A list of service dates, MOT dates and all insurance cover details for practice vehicles should ideally be kept at the practice, with responsibility for ensuring renewals of these, plus routine maintenance and repairs, given to a nominated person such as the practice manager. The individual allocated the vehicle should, however, be responsible for reporting any faults or accidents, and for ensuring that cars are kept in a clean and hygienic state with no hazardous materials, drugs or valuables left lying around.

All authorized staff – and anyone else permitted to drive a practice car, e.g. a spouse – will need to provide the practice with a copy of their driving licence and will also need to report any endorsements or penalties. There should be clear written protocols as to who is responsible for paying the excess should an accident/incident occur.

KEY POINT

Annually, every member of staff required to drive for work and any person permitted to drive a practice car should be asked for, and provide copies of, applicable paperwork and certificates, e.g. certificate of insurance, driving licence and MOT, and must report immediately all endorsements and penalties, regardless of whether or not they are incurred during work use.

Any staff claiming mileage must clearly record the purpose of the journey, distance travelled and the date. All expense claims should be submitted promptly within the specified time.

Practice insurance

Practices should ensure that their assets and business activities are adequately insured against adverse events. Insurances will normally be renegotiated and reviewed annually, and competitive quotations should be sought in good time before the renewal date. There are a number of insurance brokers and companies that specialize in the veterinary insurance market, and personal recommendation can be valuable in deciding which to deal with. As well as giving guidance about policy small print, a good broker will also be an invaluable support should the worst happen and a claim be necessary. Many insurers offer monthly premiums with no or minimal credit charges, and this can help cash flow. Whether paying monthly or annually, the total costs – including finance charges – should be compared, along with the excess charged in the event of a claim.

Surgery policies will usually include all or some of the following:

- Premises/buildings insurance – including walls, gates and fences around the building
- Rent – if the event that the building cannot be used due to damage
- Glass – accidental breakage of fixed glass
- Property owner's liability
- Contents – including fixtures, fittings, external signs, drugs and medical stock, telephone installations, computers, cash
- Animals in custody
- Animals in transit
- Employer's liability
- Public liability
- Business interruption
- Fidelity – direct loss of money and/or contents as a result of fraud or dishonesty by staff
- Legal expenses.

It is important to read all current policy and cover documentation carefully at each renewal and to ensure that sums covered are adequate for the practice, taking into consideration any changes in fixed assets (e.g. new equipment), changes in turnover or staffing, and any local factors and risks. The fixed asset register (FAR; see Chapter 24) is useful and is often requested by loss adjusters in the event of a claim; but the practice must be aware of demolition and rebuilding costs, replacement costs for equipment, plant and furnishings, and stock – professional advice is useful. The practice must ensure that the sum insured for the building represents the full cost of rebuilding the property, as this amount may differ from the market value. Claims may be reduced where practices are found to have taken out insufficient cover. It can be useful to video or photograph the practice and its contents regularly to help with a valuation in the event of a claim.

The practice must ensure that all door locks and, if applicable, any alarm systems conform to the requirements of the insurance policy.

Vehicle insurance

Vehicle or fleet insurance should be renegotiated annually and policy cover checked carefully, particularly regarding the excess charged should a claim be submitted. Limiting the number and age of drivers, and using named drivers, can reduce premiums; a low claims history also helps. Where staff are driving their own car for the business, it is important to ensure that their private insurance covers them for business use of that car.

Disaster recovery

Disasters can happen in a veterinary practice as easily as in any other business, and can range from fire or flood to an unexpected power or systems failure. It is vital to have adequate back-up systems and solutions in place to ensure that things run smoothly, paying particular attention to the computer system. The practice should have an emergency procedure that everyone is familiar with.

The practice should have alternative systems in place so that, in the event of a computer failure or power cut, work can continue with minimum disruption (Figure 16.23). Where information needs to be available in hard copy, consideration should be given as to whether a copy of this information should be printed off and kept available and/or stored on a separate PC off site. All information would, of course, have to be updated regularly, and dated to ensure that everyone can see it is the correct version.

- Have hard copies available of:
  - Key forms, such as blank consent forms
  - Price lists for drugs, consumables and procedures
  - Appointment diary
  - Operations list
  - Blank labels for labelling any drugs dispensed
  - A temporary clinical record form, to record all clinical work carried out; if carefully designed, this can be scanned in when systems are back in use
  - Recording form for electronic payments
  - Blank receipts
  - Document containing all the contact numbers of practice contractors and suppliers; a copy should also be kept off-site
- In an emergency, make notes of when clients need to come back, or make provisional appointments. The practice can then call the client back when the crisis is over. This is better than asking the client to phone back
- Set up a clear system to record any payments taken. For example, if the credit card machine is broken, payment may be taken over the phone at a branch surgery. Keep a list of all payments taken and all payments due. Invoices can then be sent out once the system is up and running again

16.23 Office contingency planning.

IT systems

Many veterinary practices strive towards a 'paperless' office. The more reliant a practice is on the computer system, the more acute the problems will be when these systems break down, lose power or have to be disconnected. There are strategies that can be used to avoid 'down time' (e.g. maintaining two live servers for back-up) and practices are advised to investigate and discuss with their IT provider ways to protect their systems (see Chapter 4). Some IT providers now provide a web-based back-up system, which is advantageous. As well as specific reserve capacity for the live system, it is imperative to ensure that computer hardware and software are maintained, up to date and suitable for the tasks required, with adequate and verifiable back-up and reboot systems.

Telephone systems

It is wise to investigate what to do if a power cut should disable the telephone system. Forward planning for this occurrence is essential.

- For telephone systems, power-fail phones should be provided.
- It should be possible to set up 'diverts' at the exchange to mobiles or unaffected landlines in case of faults or other difficulties.
- A battery back-up can be purchased for telephone systems to give a few extra hours of use of the telephone system.

Utilities

It is important to ensure that there is always someone on site, or easily available, to deal with any utilities emergency. It is a good idea to have a plan easily visible, showing how to isolate the electricity supply, gas supply, water and oil or LPG if applicable. Regular practical training on what to do in the event of an emergency, such as leaking, flooding and fire (see Chapter 2) are essential.

Customer service

In order to maintain customer service levels while the practice is without computer/telephone/power systems:

- Where vital maintenance means planned computer down time, staffing levels may need to be higher than usual to cope with less efficient systems
- Appoint one person to be responsible for ensuring that the systems are in place, that paperwork is in sufficient supply, and that everyone knows what they are doing
- Tell the team ahead of time what the expected timescales are, what is to be done and when the system is expected to be back online
- Explain to clients that the computer is down but do not emphasize it as a problem, or blame it for your poor service
- Do apologize if waiting times are increased
- If prices charged or estimated are incorrect because of an error or out-of-date price list, stand by the estimated price if it is less than the actual price. The money lost is small compared to the goodwill lost later from asking the client to pay the difference. Of course, any overpayments will be refunded
- Use the experience of being without the computer to refine your systems, look at the way things are done and streamline client handling.

Acknowledgements

The author and editors gratefully acknowledge the following practices, images of which appear in this chapter: All Creatures Healthcare Ltd; Copeland Veterinary Surgeons; Elands Veterinary Clinic; Goddard Veterinary Group; Mill House Veterinary Surgery and Hospital; Pool House Veterinary Hospital; Willows Veterinary Centre and Referral Service.

Further reading

Health and Safety Executive (2003) *The Law on VDUs: An Easy Guide. Making Sure your Office Complies with the Health and Safety (Display Screen Equipment) Regulations 1992 (as amended in 2002)*. HSE Books. London

McKenna E (2006) *Business Psychology and Organisational Behaviour: A Students Handbook*. Psychology Press, Hove

Stone RJ (2008) *Human Resource Management*. Wiley, Milton, Australia

Stutchfield MS (2008) *Veterinary Practice Management: A Practical Guide*. Saunders Elsevier, London

Examples of practice policies and banking risk assessment ▶

Computer use

To prevent problems with incompatibility and virus infection, you must not install your own programmes on to any Windows or Unix PC (personal computer) in the surgery, nor download programmes from the Internet. If files are brought in on disk, USB stick or other memory card or device, they must be loaded on to a virus-protected PC only and virus-checked before transferring. No programmes or files must be installed in the practice without the express permission of the Partners.

The practice cannot accept liability for corruption or loss of any data held on any PC in the practice, which may be replaced at any time. If you use the network for personal training files, you should keep a regular back-up for your own use. Practice documents, e.g. staff training, manual sheets and area information, must be in appropriately labelled area manual files, and not in personal folders. Important or repeatedly used files should be stored in a properly labelled directory on the network.

Internet and e-mail

Access to the Internet using the practice account is by express permission of the Partners only. Time online should be kept to a minimum, and restricted to surgery business use only, i.e. website maintenance, clinical research, Nursing Progress Log, approved distance learning, practice business and essential business e-mail. You are forbidden to use the Internet at the surgery for non-veterinary purposes, shopping or general surfing. Incoming and outgoing emails are monitored and read by other personnel as part of this policy.

The practice e-mail addresses should not be used for incoming or outgoing personal e-mails. Remember to check for replies regularly and do not delete emails from this interface. E-mails will be archived as appropriate and may be read by other members of the team. The use of the internet to access and/or distribute any kind of offensive material that is not work related will lead to disciplinary action which could result in dismissal.

The identification of the practice or publication of any photographs on any blog or social networking sites is strictly forbidden. In particular, when logging on to and using social networking and video-sharing websites and blogs at any time, including personal use outside the workplace, you must not:

- Publicly identify yourself as working for the practice, make reference to the practice or provide information from which others can ascertain the name of the practice
- Conduct yourself in a way that is detrimental to the practice or brings the practice or your profession into disrepute
- Use your or any work e-mail address when registering on such sites
- Allow your interaction on these websites or blogs to damage working relationships between employees and clients of the practice
- Include personal information about the practice's employees, contractors, suppliers, customers or clients without their express consent (an employee may still be liable even if employees, contractors, suppliers, customers or clients are not expressly named in the websites or blogs as long as the practice reasonably believes they are identifiable)
- Make any derogatory, offensive, discriminatory or defamatory comments about the practice, its employees, contractors, suppliers, customers, clients or patients (an employee may still be liable even if the practice, its employees, contractors, suppliers, customers, clients or patients are not expressly named in the websites or blogs as long as the practice reasonably believes they are identifiable)
- Make any comments about the practice's employees that could constitute unlawful harassment or bullying
- Disclose any trade secrets or confidential information belonging to the practice, its employees, contractors, suppliers, customers or clients or any information which could be used by one or more of the practice's competitors.

If you are discovered contravening these rules, whether inside or outside the workplace, you may face serious disciplinary action under the practice's disciplinary procedure. Depending on the seriousness of the offence, it may amount to gross misconduct and could result in your summary dismissal. Please remember that casual comments made on social networking sites and in e-mails can reach much further than you intend, and are not private. Employees must conduct themselves professionally at all times.

Photographs

Practice cameras are available for clinical use only. Photos taken in the surgery (whether taken with practice or personal cameras) must not be used for any purpose other than that approved by the Partners. Client permission must be sought to use photos for competition entries, VN assessments or marketing purposes, and no pictures may be posted on other websites or networking sites. Photos should be regarded as being part of the clinical record.

If you take photos, please download them yourself as soon as possible. Keep only the photos you need and delete any poor or duplicate ones. Name them, including your initials, and sort into folders as appropriate. Un-named and unidentified photos will be deleted after 3 months. Please delete photos you no longer need to keep for the business, to comply with data protection rules.

An example of a practice policy on computer, camera, Internet and e-mail use.

Driving for work

All vehicle users have a legal and moral duty to reduce as far as reasonably practicable the risks associated with vehicles and driving for work.

If you are driving as part of your work, whether using a practice car or your own, you must:

- Have a current full driving licence
- Report immediately any penalties incurred and involvement in any accidents, regardless of whether driving a practice or other vehicle, for work or personal use
- Ensure you keep up to date with changes to the Highway Code
- Ensure you have the correct class of insurance for the use of a private vehicle on practice business
- Have regular eye tests and ensure that any necessary glasses for driving are worn
- Inform the Partners or immediate supervisor if you think your concentration or driving may be impaired due to fatigue, stress, emotional trauma, pain, reduced mobility, medication or other cause
- If driving long distances (e.g. for CPD), ensure you allow sufficient time for breaks to prevent fatigue and to allow for bad weather, poor road conditions, etc.
- Always drive within speed limits and according to prevailing weather conditions
- Not drink alcohol during working hours or whilst on call if you may need to drive for work
- Not give lifts to unauthorized persons or let others use a practice car without prior consent from the Partners
- Not put yourself or others at risk, e.g. by exceeding the speed limit
- Ensure that vehicles under your charge are well maintained (especially brakes and tyres). Oil and water level and tyre pressures and treads should be checked monthly and every time before a long journey
- Report any suspected mechanical defects to the Partners and do not attempt to drive the vehicle if a defect is suspected
- Keep your vehicle in a clean and hygienic state, with medicines and equipment secure and out of sight, and never left in the vehicle overnight. Vehicles must be locked when unattended
- Not smoke or allow smoking at any time in the vehicle
- Restrain any animals carried to prevent access to the driver
- Always carry appropriate restraint equipment, disinfection and 'sharps' containers
- Always have a functioning mobile phone or supply of change for telephone calls in the event of accident or breakdown
- Never use a mobile phone whilst driving
- Always carry your supplied First Aid kit and insurance policy details (available from the practice administrator)
- Adjust the driver's seat appropriately – headrest 3.8 cm from and level with the bony part at the back of the head; arms loose with elbows bent at around 105 degrees; front of seat higher than back and legs bent 45 degrees to floor; adjustable steering wheel set low to avoid placing stress on shoulders
- When you know you may have to drive, avoid activities that will make or leave you tired, and you should ensure you rest sufficiently in non-working periods.

If you are involved in an accident:

- First ensure your safety and the safety of others involved
- If anyone is injured, call the ambulance and police immediately and cooperate fully
- Never leave the scene of an accident until all parties have been in contact, or if anyone is injured
- Do not drive the car if there is any doubt as to its roadworthiness
- If in a practice vehicle, call the practice if local or your breakdown company if away from home
- Exchange car registration numbers, insurance policy details and name and address and telephone details with anyone else involved in the accident and witnesses
- Do not admit liability
- Make notes at the time of conditions, road layout, how the accident happened, speed, etc. Report all the details to a partner as soon as possible
- If you have a camera with you, photos of the incident and vehicles involved may be helpful.

An example of a practice policy concerning driving for work.

When using your own or a practice car you shall at all times:

a. Duly observe the statutory provisions in force from time to time governing the ownership, driving and use of motor vehicles and in the event of:
   i. your being for any cause disqualified from holding a driving licence or
   ii. your conviction of an offence which in the opinion of the Partners constitutes a serious infringement of the said statutory provisions (the Partners may in their absolute discretion forthwith discharge you from employment without notice)

b. report forthwith to the Partners any accident in which you may become involved

c. in the event of you using a practice car contribute 25% towards motor insurance premiums where the premium has risen as a direct consequence of your driving record

d. take reasonable care to ensure that the car is kept in running order

e. take out insurance cover with the Automobile Association, National Breakdown or other like organization to cover emergency costs and immediate recovery of the vehicle to XXXXXX in the event of breakdown or accident

f. when using the Partners' car, maintain it in a clean and sound condition internally and externally at all times and not fix any accessories or other items which may damage the body or fabric of the car without the express permission of the Partners. Also report any damage to the car however caused and comply with the conditions set out in the separate vehicle agreement

g. in the event of you using your own car with the consent of the Partners in the course of your employment, keep the said car comprehensively insured in particular for use for the purposes of the Partners and so that the Partners shall have a full and complete indemnity in respect of all claims of whatever nature arising out of your ownership of the car and of the its use by yourself, your servants or agents.

Examples of clauses in contracts of employment regarding car use.

Risk Assessment – Banking	Name of Practice/Branch:	Date of assessment:
Issue/factor	**Suggested control measures**	**Action to be taken / N/A**
■ Are frequent banking trips made?	■ Consider storing money on site to reduce the frequency of banking trips. (Check that your storage arrangements and insurance on site are adequate) ■ Consider using a secure collection service	
■ Is the bank a significant distance from the premises?	■ Is there another bank closer to your premises?	
■ Is banking carried out: ▪ on the same day? ▪ at the same time? ▪ using the same route? ▪ or by the same person?	■ Vary the day, time, route and/or person doing the banking	
■ When money is being transported, is it kept out of sight?	■ Keep cash out of sight when being transported	
■ Is the person(s) doing the banking the right person(s)?	■ Avoid using young or immature people	
■ Are the right number of people doing the banking?	■ Provide an escort as required, particularly if there is a large sum of cash (over £..........)	
■ Do people travel on foot to get to the bank?	■ For security, travel by car even if short distances are involved	
■ If travelling by car is there parking at or near the bank?	■ Consider using another person as 'driver' to drop off outside the bank ■ Use a different bank where parking is provided	
■ Does the person doing the banking know what to do if they are attacked or threatened?	■ It must be made clear that they are not expected to put themselves at risk by resisting. They should try to concentrate on observing the attacker to help in the subsequent police investigation	
Please use the space provided below to list any additional factors that have not been consider above:		
Overall assessment of risk (delete as applicable) With current controls in place - High risk Medium risk Low risk		
Manager must sign below to accept the risk assessment and ensure that remedial actions identified are implemented.		
Manager's name:	Signature:	Date:

An example of a risk assessment for banking activities.

Communication

17

Christine Magrath and Geoff Little

Communication affects all members of the practice team. The development of communication skills is not solely the domain of the veterinary surgeon, but also applies to veterinary nurses, receptionists and practice managers.

Good communication is not just about 'being nice' but involves a series of skills that:

- Can be delineated, taught, learned and retained
- Form part of clinical competence
- Need to be updated continually to keep pace with the advances in clinical knowledge
- Can enable individuals to move from knowing what to say to mastering how to communicate the information
- Provide individuals with the tools to improve their communication technique – otherwise experience alone can be the reinforcer of habits and this tends not to discern good from bad.

Communication skills can be categorized into three types (Figure 17.1). These are interdependent and cannot be considered in isolation.

Principles of face-to-face communication

The following principles can be applied when communicating with both clients and colleagues.

Body language

'Actions speak louder than words.' What is actually said accounts for 7% of the message and how the words are said (tonality) accounts for 38% of the message; body language (non-verbal communication) accounts for the remaining 55% of the overall message. Body language is a two-way process and can be either conscious or subconscious. If used effectively, non-verbal communication can enhance and reinforce a verbal message when dealing with clients or colleagues, and being able to 'decode' non-verbal cues is essential to understanding them. Equally, understanding and paying attention to one's own non-verbal skills may prevent misunderstandings and contradictory messages from being relayed. Observation is essential in order to pick up non-verbal cues; however, unless these cues are checked out verbally, it may lead to misinterpretation or in some cases inhibit relationship building.

It is important to think about the following.

- **Proximity to others** – In any interaction it is important that the amount of space between individuals is comfortable; this is particularly pertinent in a professional setting. Many factors can affect this distance, such as prior relationships, age, sex and culture. The use of chairs can alter the dynamics with regard to personal space. More and more veterinary

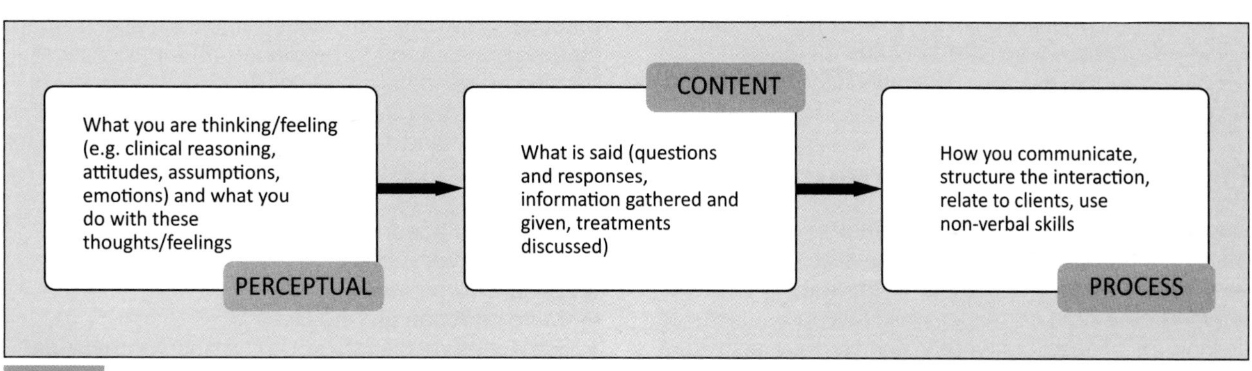

17.1 Categorization of communication skills. These are interdependent and cannot be considered in isolation.

surgeons and veterinary nurses are using chairs in the consulting room, as sitting can be a helpful tool in delivering difficult news to clients. The chairs should not be placed so close together that personal space will be invaded, but sitting too far apart will prevent building feelings of trust and will not encourage discussion. Sitting opposite someone may create feelings of confrontation and increase the defensiveness of anyone feeling insecure. This does not just relate to interactions with clients; interviews and appraisals can also benefit from relaxed or less formal seating, depending on the situation.

- **Body movements** – Many head movements, such as nodding and shaking, can be used to give opposing messages. Nodding often goes hand in hand with listening and conveys interest. However, if it is vigorous, it may signify to the listener that the speaker has made their point or taken up enough time. Shaking the head in most cultures conveys disagreement. Arms may act as defensive barriers when across the body and conversely indicate feelings of openness and security when in open positions, especially combined with open palms.
- **Posture** – Slumped posture can give an impression of disinterest, while a shifting posture may demonstrate unease. A relaxed posture, leaning slightly forward, can help establish rapport by giving the impression of calmness and interest.
- **Eye contact** – Keeping good eye contact with the other person, without staring, indicates genuine interest and empathy.
- **Facial expressions** – These are harder to adjust as facial conformation is often genetically inherited. The basic emotional facial expressions are happiness, sadness, fear, disgust, surprise and anger.
- **Handshaking** – Handshaking can convey a confident, trusting and professional approach. However, if it does not feel comfortable then it may convey disinterest and apathy (see Figure 17.9). In this instance, it may create a more natural approach by not doing it. The common view is that feeble handshakes are a sign of weakness but they can occasionally be due to cultural differences, old people who may be infirm or young people who are unaccustomed to shaking hands.
- **Cultural influences** – Culture can have a significant influence on perceived interpersonal behaviour. An understanding of an individual's preferences and attitude to such things as close contact, informality and forms of address is vital where clients come from a number of different backgrounds, including age, ethnicity, religion and culture.

Use of notes and computers

During a conversation it is important to record information so that key points are not missed; however, it is very easy to lose eye contact when making notes or entering data on a computer while talking to clients or colleagues. Those non-verbal signals may also give the other person the impression that they are not being listened to. Also, cues may be missed and information may be forgotten. The following may be useful to overcome this issue:

- Thorough preparation, to ensure all the information about the client or colleague has been gleaned in advance, may avoid constant reference to notes and computers
- Notes and records could be deliberately postponed until the individual has made their opening statement
- If information must be obtained as a result of new issues coming to light, opportune moments should be waited for before looking at notes
- Listening should be separated from note-reading by signposting an intention to look at the records, or that the procedure is finished. The client or member of staff is then more likely to understand the process
- The lower body should remain facing the other individual. If eye contact is inadvertently lost, it is less damaging if the lower body still faces them
- The client or member of staff should be asked whether they mind if information is entered into the computer during the interaction. It may be less invasive if this information is recorded during summarizing.

Communicating with clients

Whether in a one-off visit or a series of discussions over treatment, communication provides an opportunity to build a valuable relationship with the client.

KEY POINT

Communication with the client extends beyond the consultation process, with many interactions taking place on the telephone or in the reception area.

The consultation

The consultation lies at the heart of almost everything the veterinary team does. Team members other than veterinary surgeons are increasingly conducting consultations, and much of this chapter is therefore devoted to the consultation process. While this process relates to the interaction between clients and practice team members, many of the skills can also be used when communicating with colleagues. There is no doubt that the skills needed for an effective consultation can be applied to many other situations in practice; however, in these other situations more emphasis may need to be placed on a particular skill, depending on the issue at hand.

Improved communication during the consultation process can lead to more effective consultations for both the practice team and the client, including:

- Enhanced accuracy
- Enhanced efficiency
- Enhanced support
- More common ground
- Enhanced relationship building and coordination of patient care
- Reduced conflict and complaints.

These more effective consultations also lead to improved outcomes of care, including:

- Improved client satisfaction, which may generate recommendations and more clients for the practice
- Increased understanding and recall of the case
- Increased concordance and compliance
- Greater satisfaction for the team member.

The structure of the consultation

The format for presenting and recording information (content) is often used as a guide to obtaining and delivering the information (process). Using such a process can prevent some medical information or concerns being elicited. To correct this problem, a veterinary consultation guide has been developed (Radford *et al.*, 2006; Figure 17.2) and is now used at all UK veterinary schools. This offers a repertoire of skills that provide veterinary surgeons and support staff with a detailed process to ensure an effective consultation. At the same time personality is important, and the guide provides individuals with a degree of latitude to develop their own way of putting each skill into practice. On closer examination, the number of skills described in the guide can seem daunting; it is therefore important to be aware that not every skill is needed for every eventuality, although familiarity with each one will help when dealing with difficult or challenging situations.

The guide divides the consultation into six basic stages:

1. Preparation
2. Initiating the consultation
3. Gathering the information
4. Physical examination (including diagnostic procedures)
5. Explaining what has been found and planning the way forward
6. Closing the consultation.

Three constant threads weave their way throughout the consultation model (Figure 17.3):

- Providing a structure to the consultation
- Building the relationship with the client and the patient
- Observation of both client and animal throughout.

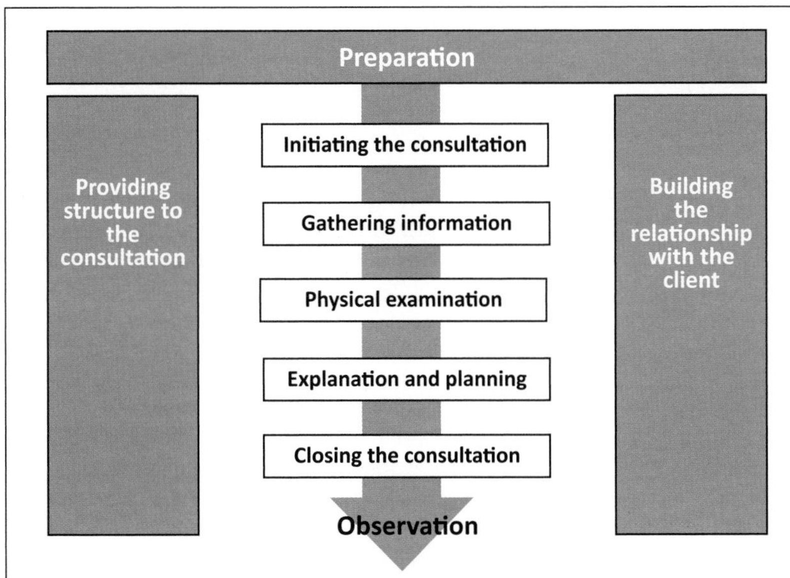

17.2 This guide to the veterinary consultation has been developed based on the medical Calgary–Cambridge Guide and is now used at all UK veterinary schools. (Adapted from Radford *et al.*, 2006)

THE CONSTANT THREADS

PROVIDING STRUCTURE

Signpost and summarize: A signposting statement introduces and draws attention to what is being said next. It is very helpful when introducing the first summary.

Attend to flow: Once an agenda has been set and agreed, the consultation should be carried out in this manner so that the client can see that there is a logical sequence.

Manage time: Balance the time taken over each section of the consultation.

OBSERVATION

BUILDING THE RELATIONSHIP

Appropriate non-verbal communication: Be aware of own facial expression and body posture etc. as well as cues from clients.

Develop rapport: Use empathy to communicate understanding of client's situation, acknowledge client's views, express concern and deal sensitively with difficult topics.

Don't forget the patient: Take time with the patient and acknowledge the relationship between the clent and their pet.

17.3 The three 'constant threads' of a consultation.

Preparation

Without adequate preparation, all other aspects of the consultation can easily be wasted.

KEY POINT

It is essential to be familiar with the clinical notes and to ensure the consultation room is clean, tidy and escape-proof.

Hurrying or becoming distracted can lead to errors at a later stage. It is therefore important to ensure that a previous consultation or personal problems do not impinge on the interaction to hand.

Initiating the consultation

First impressions count. It is essential to start building a good relationship immediately, to encourage trust and make the client feel respected. The factors to consider when initiating the consultation may appear obvious but can often be forgotten, particularly if individuals are following a tight schedule.

- The client and patient should be greeted by name.
- The person carrying out the consultation should then ensure that the client knows who they are (Figure 17.4). Many veterinary surgeons and nurses will often know their clients and patients well and do not need to introduce themselves on every occasion. However, there is sometimes an assumption that, because a client has visited the practice before, they will remember who people are. Not knowing the role or name of the professional can be unsettling for clients, and can even act as a barrier to ensuring that communication is a two-way process.
- Shaking hands can be effective, provided it feels comfortable, but good eye contact and smiling are essential.
- Initially, an open question should be asked in order to invite information from the client and identify the reason for the consultation, e.g. 'How can I help?' 'What's Baxter in for today?' This questioning should take place even if the computer tag or written notes already contain information, as it is possible that the reason for the consultation recorded on the notes is not correct. Also, in follow-up visits veterinary surgeons may assume, erroneously, that the consultation is a direct follow-on from the previous one, thereby preventing new concerns from being brought to the forefront.

The RCVS Practice Standards Scheme stipulates that practices must ensure the public is aware of the identity of individuals involved in the care of their pets. To meet these requirements, the following should be considered:

- Name badges
- Front entrance nameboards and/or consulting room nameplates
- Picture boards
- Staff names and information on websites and newsletters.

In addition to the static media itemized above, personal introductions (to include name and position within the practice team) are paramount.

17.4 Identification of practice staff.

A student elective project at Liverpool Veterinary School suggested that the average time veterinary surgeons and nurses take to interrupt a client is 18 seconds (Gray *et al.*, 2005). A later research project conducted at Nottingham suggested that it took only 13.5 seconds before the client was interrupted (Brightmoore, 2009). Interruption is often due to time constraints and an assumption that the first complaint mentioned is the only one. Interrupting the client at this stage in the consultation may prevent some concerns from being elicited because clients often wish to discuss more than one complaint, and the order in which these problems are presented is often not related to clinical importance. Attentive listening is a very skilled process and the following tips can be useful:

- Do not concentrate on preparing the next question; instead focus on what the client is saying
- Provide the client with enough 'wait time' to complete their story
- Facilitate a response with expressions such as 'hmmm', 'uh huh', 'go on', 'yes', 'I see'
- Pick up on verbal and non-verbal cues. Often the client's ideas, concerns and expectations (ICE) are expressed as non-verbal cues and indirect comments, rather than overt statements. According to medical research, these cues often appear early on in the consultation and will need to be checked out with the client as the consultation progresses
- Ensure the client receives appropriate non-verbal signals, such as good eye contact, direction of gaze, proximity, gestures and vocal cues (tone of voice, speed and volume of speech); otherwise these may contradict verbal messages.

Screening is a technique that encourages, but does not guarantee, the identification of all of the client's problems at an early stage in the consultation before exploring any one of them. This is done by asking further open-ended enquiries instead of assuming that the client has mentioned everything: 'As I understand it Baxter has been coughing for 3 days, off his food since yesterday and appears more tired than usual. Is there anything else you've noticed?'

Screening also provides a method of finding out a client's ideas, concerns and expectations. Making a verbal summary prior to screening helps to facilitate the further responses from the client.

Screening until the client has nothing more to reveal should elicit a number of problems. This is therefore an ideal time to organize thoughts and share them with the client. This 'agenda setting' or structuring of the consultation prevents aimless and unnecessary questioning and allows the client to feel more involved: 'Shall we start with the vomiting and diarrhoea and then tackle the problem with Baxter's ear?'

Gathering information

During the information-gathering component of the consultation, it is important not only to obtain an accurate and complete history of the animal's disease or illness but also to explore the owner's ideas, concerns and expectations.

KEY POINT

It is important that the client should feel valued and listened to.

At this stage, an in-depth analysis of the problems outlined by the client is needed. To ensure that this is done in an effective way, the following skills should be used.

- **A balance of open and closed questions** – Both types of questioning are valuable but starting with an open technique introduces an enquiry without shaping the client's response, e.g. 'Tell me about the cough.' Although a closed questioning technique is important to investigate specific details, it can limit the amount and type of information if used too early in the dialogue. An **open-to-closed cone** (Figure 17.5) therefore tends to be more efficient. More specific but still open questions should straddle the two extremes, e.g. 'What makes the cough better or worse?'
- **Active listening** – This is as important in this part of the consultation as it is at the initiation phase and allows the client to complete statements. Closed questions are often used to interrupt. This causes the individual to follow on with further closed questions and the client becomes a passive contributor. Curtailing the client's responses in this way may force veterinary surgeons into diagnostic reasoning far too early in the consultation.
- **Paraphrasing and repetition** – This should encourage clients to continue their dialogue. Repeating the last few words of a client (echoing) is very effective and encourages clients to continue. Cues should be picked up on continuously. This is likely to shorten the consultation. Comments from the client that are not clear should be clarified. In general these clarifying enquiries tend to be open but they can occasionally be closed, e.g. 'Tell me more about the itching.'
- **Internal summarizing** – This is one of the most important skills at this point in the consultation, as it clearly demonstrates listening and allows the client to confirm or alter the veterinary surgeon's thoughts and understanding. It encourages the client to go further in explaining their problems. There are also certain advantages for the individual gathering the information, as it allows them to check the accuracy of what the client has said and rectify any misconceptions. It also acts as a stimulus for the veterinary surgeon to order their own thought process, recall information at a later stage and help filter the clinical aspects from the client's perspective.
- **Use of easily understood language** – This should be matched to the client's educational level. As the disease and background information is discovered, it is likely that it will be interwoven with the client's ideas, concerns and expectations (ICE). This random gathering of information should then be processed into the biomedical history, background information and the client's ICE for the purpose of recording and presenting a history (Figure 17.6).

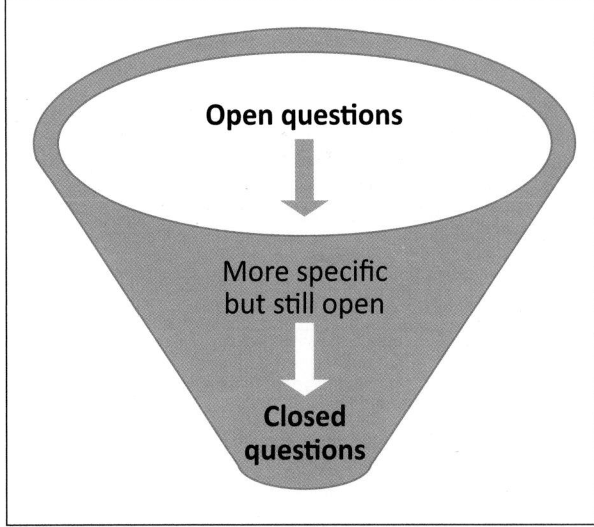

17.5 Open to closed 'cone'. Starting with open questions and moving towards more specific points is an efficient way of eliciting information.

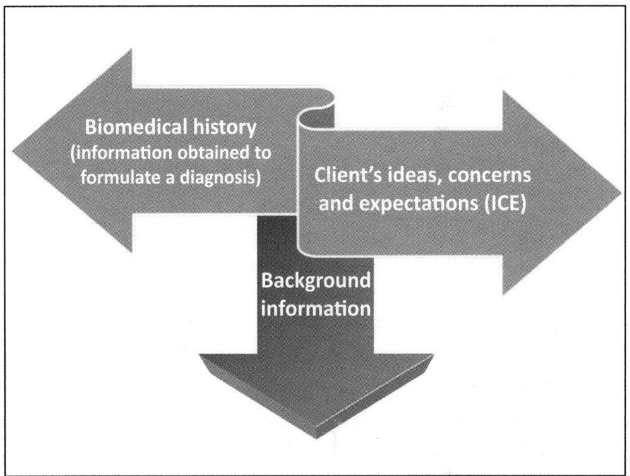

17.6 Grouping of gathered information. Information should be processed into the biomedical history, background information and the client's ideas, concerns and expectations (ICE) for the purpose of recording and presenting a history.

Physical examination

The physical examination is an important part of the consultation process; however, since it is covered in detail in clinical texts, it will not be covered here. It is essential that the examination does not get in the way of the communication process; otherwise clients may feel that they are not being listened to. It is important to check that the client is confident in holding the patient and, as the client may not know what is happening, it is necessary to explain what is going on and outline any procedures that are likely to be uncomfortable for the animal. This also applies to the healthy patient; owners may not be aware that a full health check has taken place during the vaccination procedure, leading clients to believe that they have not had value for money. If the client expresses concern about holding their pet, an offer for a team member to assist should be made.

Explaining and planning

This stage of the consultation should involve the following:

- The client's options should be discussed
- Information should be provided on the procedures or treatments offered
- The client's views should be accepted, although assurance that they understand alternative viewpoints must first be established
- The client's reactions and concerns about treatments and proposed procedures should be elicited
- Perceived benefits and risks should be balanced
- The client should be given an opportunity to ask questions, express doubts and seek clarification.

Investment at this stage in the consultation will pay dividends. Giving information to clients and telling them what to do is not enough; it is essential that they understand and retain details of this aspect of the consultation so that they can make informed decisions about the way forward. The key challenge in giving information is finding out how much detail the client wants, rather than making assumptions, so that the information can be tailored to the client's needs. While many clients would like as much information as possible, there is a minority who would rather have less. The following factors may help to adapt the amount of information that is given to the majority of clients, while being sensitive to the needs of the minority.

- **The client's starting point should be assessed** – The client may be a medical expert or have personal knowledge of the condition, e.g. diabetes: 'Have you any experience of diabetes?', or, 'I don't know how much you know about this condition...'.
- **Information should be recapped in bite-sized pieces followed by a pause** – The client's understanding can then be checked. This process enables the veterinary surgeon to gauge the client's reactions before proceeding. 'Chunking and checking' in this manner also helps the client to recall information accurately and goes a long way to achieving a shared understanding.
- **The explanation should be given at an appropriate time** – Premature reassurance should be avoided. All too often questions arise when veterinary surgeons are gathering information. For example, 'The diarrhoea is making Baxter really poorly. Will he need antibiotics?'. It is tempting to launch into an explanation about antibiotics not being needed in this instance, only to find that as the consultation progresses there is evidence to suggest that there are other clinical signs that may require treating in this manner. It is much better to acknowledge the question: 'That's a good question. Would you mind if we leave it for the time being until I examine Baxter? This way I can put all the information together.' It is useful to prioritize by recognizing that some information may be best provided at a later stage. Organizing the information and 'signposting' it for the client can aid accurate recall and understanding: 'There are three important parts to Baxter's treatment – first we need to keep him off food for the next 24 hours; secondly we need to...'
- **Repetition is a useful skill and can also help recall** – This can be divided into two categories: repetition of important points by the veterinary surgeon; and restatement by the client. Checking the client's understanding in this manner can be a fine balance between being patronizing and being helpful. Tone of voice and paraphrasing are important components. 'I've given you a lot of information about this condition and I'm concerned that I might not have made things clear. It would help me if you could recap on what I've gone through so far, to make sure I haven't missed anything.' Clients need to understand the information as well as being able to recall it. This is more likely to lead to compliance.
- **Categorizing information in order of importance and relating the information to the client's perspective will help to move the client towards a deeper understanding** – 'You mentioned earlier that you thought Baxter might have cancer. I can see why you might think that this is the case but I think it is more likely to be...'.
- **Technical jargon may overwhelm the client** – Many clients will not want to appear stupid and may look as if they understand when the opposite is the case. Hadlow and Pitts (1991) showed that even everyday words can be confusing if used in a medical context. Care should also be exercised with clients who may not be conversant in English, who have learning difficulties or who are illiterate. Four simple steps can help this process:
  - Reduce the use of jargon
  - Explain jargon when it is used
  - Use shorter words
  - Use shorter sentences.
- **Visual techniques paint a thousand words** – Diagrams, wipe boards, models, written information and instructions can help the client's understanding and recall. However, this approach is not a substitute for interaction with the veterinary surgeon and should be used only as part of the overall communication process.

Closing the consultation

Sometimes problems arise at the end of the consultation; these difficulties are often a result of poor communication skills earlier on. This can be very frustrating when there is a tight appointment schedule. However, rushing the client can undo all previous efforts. It is therefore important to consider the following points.

- It is essential that the client knows what is going to happen next, and whether the patient needs to be seen again.
- Encouraging clients to make an appointment with the correct member of the team will help with continuity.
- A 'safety net' should be provided to guarantee that the client knows what to do and who to contact if problems occur or things do not go according to plan.
- The client should be warned of potential, unexpected outcomes.
- If screening has been used at an early stage in the consultation, a final check for 'anything else' should not yield any additional surprises.
- A final summary will help the client to remember the salient facts.
- The client and patient should both be thanked before saying goodbye.

Communicating with colleagues following a consultation

The structured format of a consultation is very effective in bridging the different communication styles within a practice team and, although good communication with clients is paramount, it is essential that there is also clear communication and coordination between managers, veterinary surgeons, veterinary nurses, receptionists, out-of-hours providers and referral centres. Once individuals have extracted information from, or imparted information to, a client they should:

- Record it adequately in a standard format
- Convey it accurately and precisely to other members of the team/other practices
- Impart well defined and accurate instructions.

However, even the most effective communicators can waste their time if they do not have an understanding and appreciation of the contribution that others make towards client and patient care.

Compliance and concordance

Compliance is the extent to which the client carries out agreed actions, such as giving medication to a regimen agreed between the prescriber and the client. Agreement on the regimen is achieved through concordance. **Concordance** involves negotiation between two equal parties, respecting the beliefs and wishes of the client in determining whether, when and how medicines are to be taken. When clients do not administer medications or follow treatment regimens as agreed, they are described as being non-compliant. The relationship between compliance and concordance is illustrated in Figure 17.7.

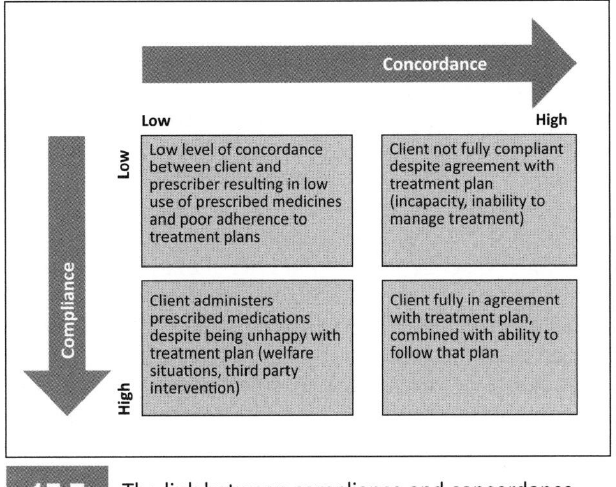

17.7 The link between compliance and concordance.

If the prescriber and client achieve concordance, there is a greater likelihood that the client will make a conscious effort to follow treatment plans. Various steps should be considered:

- Clients should have enough knowledge to participate as partners. This can be achieved by:
  - Relating to the client's ability to understand instructions and their educational level
  - Relating to the health issue at hand and providing realistic expectations of what the medicine or treatment regimen can achieve
  - Providing accurate instructions without the use of jargon in sufficient detail to be meaningful
- Clients should be offered choices rather than directives
- Clients should be encouraged to contribute their ideas and suggestions
- The veterinary surgeon should share his/her thought processes, ideas and dilemmas as appropriate. This encourages clients to share their views and forces the professional to order his/her thinking
- Care should be given to the explanation of risk and side effects.

In the medical profession, 70% of patients wish to be involved and 30% would prefer to leave decisions to their doctor. How much involvement the client would prefer therefore needs to be established:

- Demonstrations and visual material should be provided
- The client's understanding should be checked
- A 'safety net' should be provided in case the treatment plan or administration of medications does not go to plan.

Informed consent

During the veterinary consent process, consideration should be given to:

- The diagnosis or nature of the patient's ailment
- The general nature of the proposed treatment and any other alternatives
- Treatments and the purpose or reason for each treatment
- The risk or dangers involved in the proposed treatments
- The probability or prospects of success with each treatment option
- The prognosis or risk if the client refuses treatment
- The costs of the various treatment options
- The name of the individual who will perform surgery, if not the person obtaining the informed consent
- The location and method of transportation to that location if the treatment is to be administered at another site.

The process of consent is much more than asking a client to sign a written consent form. (Specimen consent forms can be obtained from the RCVS.) Unfortunately, even after signing a consent form, many clients still do not understand basic information about the fees, risks, benefits and alternatives of their proposed treatment options. There are many reasons for this failure of truly informed consent and for the ongoing lack of understanding (Figure 17.8).

A number of studies indicate that by improving consent forms, clients are more likely to read and understand them before signing. However, this is not a guarantee. A properly constructed and clearly formatted consent form is important but not sufficient on

On the client's side
■ Time or stress pressure ■ Feelings of intimidation ■ Learning disabilities ■ Hearing or visual disabilities ■ Limited proficiency at English ■ Poor literacy ■ Poor educational level ■ Perception that the consent form is just a legal procedure
On the provider's side
■ Lack of time from the viewpoint of the veterinary surgeon and other healthcare professionals ■ Overly complex or overly broad written materials ■ Poor explanation of risk ■ Wrong assumptions about client comprehension ■ Poor quality consent forms and lack of associated written material

17.8 Factors that may make it difficult to achieve informed consent.

its own for ensuring that clients read, understand and remember the information presented. A variety of other methods are needed to increase client involvement in the consent process and improve client comprehension of the information presented.

- A consensus should be gained within the practice to make improvements to the procedure.
- The consistency and quality of the written consent form and related written and educational material should be optimized.
- It should be made certain that those presenting the animal are eligible to give consent. The competence of the client to give consent should be assessed.
- The client's prior knowledge should be assessed.
- Differences in educational or literacy levels should be recognized so that help can be given where required.
- All relevant information should be provided to the client and adequate time given to have discussion.
- The information should be given in bite-sized pieces, using clear and simple language. Some jargon cannot be avoided (e.g. chemotherapy) and should be explained in these instances.
- Associated costs should be detailed.
- The risks associated with anaesthetic and surgical procedures should be explained.
- The client should be asked to restate their understanding.
- Individuals should be prepared to repeat components of the explanation if necessary.
- The client's body language should be observed (ideal opportunity to pick up cues if the client is unhappy or doesn't understand the procedure).
- An opportunity for questions should be provided.
- Fact sheets to take home are a useful adjunct.
- The consent form should be used as an outline for discussions.
- Clients should have an opportunity to decline procedures.
- Clients should be given adequate time to read the consent form and consider implications.
- An empathetic approach during the consenting process should be used.
- Phrases such as 'and all other procedures which may be considered necessary' should not be included without some explanation as to what they might include, such as cost, risk and other options.
- A signature should be obtained.
- It is advisable to give the client a copy of the signed agreement.

KEY POINT

At times, veterinary surgeons may consider it inappropriate to insist that clients sign a consent form, e.g. euthanasia of a long-standing patient, emergency First Aid, and euthanasia of a patient that is on the operating table. In such instances it must be recorded in the notes that informed consent has been obtained. It is useful to have another member of staff as a witness. It is also beneficial for the witness to sign the paperwork, or record this independently, for future reference.

Fees

Fees are an emotionally charged topic. Clients may feel guilty that they do not have unlimited resources and so cannot allow treatment to go ahead without considering money. Veterinary surgeons and support staff often have to discuss finance at a time when the client is already emotionally fragile.

Suggested strategies:

- All staff should understand the fee structure and protocols
- Discussions should not be postponed – the situation might get worse
- The client's emotional state should be assessed and then addressed
- If the patient is deemed to be a distraction it may be best for another member of the team to occupy the pet elsewhere
- Technical and financial jargon should be avoided
- The practice should never apologize for the fee or start with the phrase, 'I know it's a great deal of money but...'
- Options should be provided and the subject of cost should be an integral part of explanation and planning
- Signposting can be helpful to alert the client that costs will be discussed, e.g. 'There are three options for treating Baxter's illness, with a range of costs associated with them. I can take you through each one...'
- The client should be encouraged to ask questions
- The client's body language should be observed to see how the information is received
- Information should be backed up in writing and recorded in the clinical notes
- Estimated fees for procedures should be written on the consent form
- A simple explanation of the fees should be given on presentation of the bill and it is important not to be defensive or embarrassed
- Animal welfare should always be considered when discussing fees, and euthanasia may be a valid option.

Estimates

Estimates can be effective but individuals need to recognize that:

- Clients automatically focus on the lower end of the range; this is especially true with verbal estimates
- Linking to a detailed breakdown of individual components will help clients understand the work involved and any uncertainties
- In some instances it can be beneficial to consider an uncertainty factor of 5–10%, to take into account fees exceeding the estimate
- Clients should be contacted as soon as possible if fees look as though they may exceed the estimate. The following may help this process:
  - Ensuring telephone numbers of clients are up to date
  - Explaining why fees will be higher and not proceeding unless the client agrees. These decisions should be recorded in the clinical notes
  - A message should be left to call the practice as soon as possible for clients who are not at home. It is important not to panic the owner in this instance

Further information on fees and estimates can be found in Chapter 24.

Terms and conditions

Whenever a practice deals with a client, there is a contract involved. This is usually verbal and implied rather than written, but is a contract nevertheless. Most businesses publish their terms and conditions – in other words the general and special standards/rules of the agreement. The terms and conditions stipulate the responsibilities that both parties have in this arrangement. They should be freely available to clients and may be published on the practice website, in the brochure, on the reverse side of invoices and in written estimates. For further information on terms and conditions see Chapter 24.

Dealing with difficult situations

The core skills outlined above form the basis of every interaction, including difficult situations. It is only the content of the communication (e.g. what to say when breaking bad news or dealing with anger) and the context of the interaction that changes. The process skills themselves remain the same but may need to be used with greater intention, intensity and awareness. Although the examples given below represent communication with clients, the same skills should be used to overcome communication challenges with colleagues.

Emotions

Emotions that are not addressed will escalate until they are dealt with.

- The emotion should be identified, e.g. sadness, anger, grief.
- The emotion should be reflected back to the client: 'I can clearly see that you are angry'.
- The correct intensity should be indicated. Tone of voice is important.
- A way forward should be mutually agreed: 'I can clearly see that you are angry. Let's see if we can sort this out'.

Anger

Anger in clients is usually obvious but is sometimes expressed in more subtle ways, such as discordant messages between verbal expressions and non-verbal communication. The two common reasons for not dealing with anger are fear of unleashing more anger, and insufficient time.

The following strategies can be applied when dealing with anger.

- Stay calm, as anger feeds anger. It is tempting to take a defensive approach; however, this is likely to exacerbate anger.
- Keep good eye contact.
- Allow the client to express their thoughts and calm down without interruption. Phrases such as, 'I think you should calm down' should not be used.
- Acknowledge the client's right to be angry. 'I understand how you feel' may provoke a response such as 'I don't think you do'. Alternative phrases such as 'I can see why this is frustrating for you' are more appropriate.
- Ask the client to take a seat and then adopt a similar position (mirroring strategy) without an aggressive pose. If the client does not sit down it is still worthwhile taking up this pose – after some time the angry person will often sit. Once seated, it is important to stay seated even if the client gets up – after a while they will often sit down again.
- Pick up on cues, otherwise it is impossible to analyse the root cause of anger and search for hidden agendas. Note that fear may manifest as anger.
- Maintain an empathic stance at all times by acknowledging and indicating to the client that you understand that they are angry ('I can see that you are very annoyed and upset about this'). Try to understand the issues from the angry person's perspective and be sympathetic. Body language should demonstrate interest and concern, and the tone of voice should be appropriate.
- Ensure that you appear comfortable and controlled.
- Use clear, firm, non-emotive language.
- The reason for an angry outburst should be summarized and reflected back.
- Provide the client or staff member with an offer of help or a promise to investigate issues. Avoid giving premature reassurance.
- All individuals should agree a way forward.

Guilt

Guilt can be difficult to identify. In this situation, it may be necessary to interpret statements such as:

- 'Well I didn't know anything about this. I've been away all week'
- 'I wouldn't leave Baxter in this state'
- 'My neighbour has been looking after Baxter while I've been away.'

KEY POINT

It is important to acknowledge any comments and not to judge the client.

Breaking bad news and dealing with grief

Breaking bad news can be difficult, and if not done well it can have devastating and long-lasting repercussions.

- Preparation is paramount, and should involve:
  - Setting aside sufficient uninterrupted time
  - Bringing the client into the practice and sitting them down rather than breaking the news over the phone
  - Being fully up to speed on relevant clinical information.
- The client's starting point should be assessed. This is helpful if dealing with a colleague's client and is also useful in establishing the client's understanding to date. A summary of where things have got to should be given.
- A warning shot should be introduced early in the conversation: 'I'm afraid it looks more serious than we had hoped', 'I'm afraid it's bad news...'.
- Basic information should be given simply and honestly, and important points should be repeated. Too much information should not be given too early; this avoids overwhelming the individual.
- Any emotion shown by the client should be legitimized by listening, as this is an excellent way of demonstrating empathy.
- Body language is vitally important and the listener should demonstrate concern by moving and leaning towards the client while keeping eye contact. Issues surrounding the use of touch are outlined in Figure 17.9.
- Further explanation should relate to the client's perspective.
- The pace of delivery should not be too fast and the client's understanding and feelings should be checked repeatedly.

Touch is a powerful means of conveying concern and empathy. However, touch must be used appropriately, with due regard to the sensitivity of the client and professional codes of conduct. Putting an arm around a distressed client to give comfort or placing a hand on the arm of someone who is having difficulty expressing thoughts and emotions conveys empathy and may help the client to continue. Four key issues are important:

- The client's likely response to being touched should be assessed by picking up cues, such as the way in which they relate their story, their posture and other aspects of their body language
- If you feel uncomfortable about touching a client, it is probably advisable not to do it, as it may then convey anxiety
- Clients from different ethnic, cultural and/or religious backgrounds may interpret body language and physical contact in a very different manner
- Where children are concerned, physical contact could be interpreted as inappropriate.

17.9 Issues surrounding the use of touch.

- Time and space should be given in case the client 'switches off', stops listening and goes into denial. Picking up on this type of shutdown goes hand in hand with reading and responding to cues.
- Emotions should be addressed by accepting and dealing with them; otherwise the client may not be in a position to take on board any further information.
- The client should not be rushed into a decision.
- Support should be offered and a plan identified for what is to happen next.
- It should be noted that everyone grieves differently and this can manifest as anger, depression or guilt.

Handling client complaints

A complaint may be:

- A verbal comment serious enough to demand a direct response
- A letter from a client
- A letter on behalf of the client – probably from a solicitor or the Royal College of Veterinary Surgeons (RCVS).

The practice should have an up-to-date **complaints policy**, with which all members of staff, including locums and new members, should be familiar. When handling a complaint, it is useful to be familiar with the **triple A rule** (Figure 17.10).

- **Acknowledge** – Clients want their feelings and their situation acknowledged. They also want it to be acknowledged that an error has occurred, even if that error was something as simple as a misunderstanding. Effective communicators locked in a difficult conversation learn to acknowledge that that an event has occurred that the client is unhappy about.
- **Apologize** – Ineffective communicators fail to apologize, either because of their egos or because they fail to understand that they can apologize without admitting guilt. Effective communicators learn to apologize for what happened and to apologize for the fact that it happened, without admitting to any personal contribution.
- **Assure** – Complainants want the assurance that their complaint will be fully investigated and that the practice will get back to them with an explanation. In addition, they want the assurance that lessons will be learned and that what they or their pet experienced will not be repeated. Effective communicators learn to give assurances that they will take steps to prevent the problems recurring and outline any steps already taken.

17.10 When something goes wrong from the client's perspective, the 'triple A rule' can be very useful.

The following guidelines are important for initially dealing with a complaint, either in person or by phone:

- Remain calm
- Take the client into a private seated area or transfer the call to a quiet zone
- Thank the client: 'Thank you for bringing the matter to my attention'
- Ask the client to tell the story from the beginning. Once again, listening is important and the client should not be interrupted
- Show empathy by reflecting back the client's emotion. This powerful skill is often forgotten when a complaint is made, as there is tendency to take complaints personally. Avoid phrases such as, 'I know how you feel'

- Pick up on key words
- Take notes. These should be shared with the client to ensure that they agree with the content and identify the specific issues of the complaint. It is sometimes helpful to ask the client to put something in writing
- Demonstrate active listening by summarizing, as this allows the client to alter anything that has been misunderstood or missed
- Say sorry and mean it. An expression of regret will make the client feel heard and understood. It doesn't mean an admission of liability; it is simply an acknowledgement of the upset and not an acknowledgement that what has happened was anyone's fault
- Tell the client which member of the team will deal with the complaint and by when
- Reassure the client that the matter will be dealt with promptly and that they will be kept informed of progress. It is better to get back to clients with an interim report if the investigation looks as though it may take longer than the agreed timescale.

KEY POINT

When a complaint is received in writing, it is important first to send out an immediate, brief letter of acknowledgement. This should inform the client of who is going to deal with the complaint and by when. A full written response should follow as soon as possible.

Once the complaint has been made:

- Record all details of the complaint in a special complaints database or book, separate from the client case notes (complaints can be flagged in the case notes but individuals should avoid recording details)
- Investigate the complaint and record all statements and information in the complaints database
- Ensure that all members of the team involved in the complaint are happy with the proposed response.

The complainant should then be provided with an explanation:

- The key issues that the client is concerned about should be the focus of attention; ask the client in what order they would like them covered
- Use clear language and explain any veterinary jargon
- Never blame other members of staff
- Encourage the client to ask questions throughout
- Check the client's understanding
- Ask the client if the explanation has answered all their concerns
- Inform the client of any changes that have been made as a result of the complaint
- Check whether there is anything else the client would like done
- Once a satisfactory solution has been found, record the way in which the complaint was resolved in the complaints database or book.

When responding to a complaint by letter, the following points should be considered:

- The name and address of the client and the date should be written at the top left hand side
- The opening phrase should address the client by their title and surname, e.g. 'Dear Mrs Smith' (or should address the client by their first name if this is more appropriate for the particular relationship)
- Reference should be made to the last communication with the client, which is probably the acknowledgement letter
- The name and title of the person investigating the complaint should be included
- If the deadline promised in the acknowledgement letter has not been met, an apology for the delay should be given
- The points made in the original letter of complaint should be answered, in the same order if possible
- If clarification is needed, it may be necessary to phone the client first and check what result they are hoping for by making the complaint
- Regret that any upset or inconvenience has arisen should be expressed but liability should not be admitted (liability should only be admitted after consultation with the practice's professional indemnity insurance provider)
- A full explanation of the facts and background to the complaint, including information on relevant staff and policies, should be given
- The language should be clear and easy to understand; any veterinary jargon should be explained
- Any actions that are to be carried out as a result of the complaint and details of who is responsible for these actions should be included
- The telephone number and contact details of the individual who has overall responsibility for handling complaints should be included.

It is prudent to make sure any staff member involved in the complaint has a chance to read the letter and comment. As a final check, the person writing the letter should think about how they would feel if they were the recipient.

The practice's professional indemnity insurer should be informed if the client is still dissatisfied. The client should only be informed of this after the insurer has been contacted.

Encouraging client feedback

In addition to addressing complaints, practices would be well served by encouraging feedback from clients under the two other 'C' headings: **comments** and **compliments**. Compliments and favourable comments are understandably well received by the practice team, with thank you cards and notes often being placed in prominent positions in the practice.

Comment cards

Understanding the client experience is a fundamental aspect of practice growth, and assessing the needs and expectations of clients is part of managing client satisfaction (see Chapter 26). There are several ways to obtain client feedback, e.g. focus groups, client questionnaire mailings. However, it is important to capture a client's experience when it is fresh in their mind, and this is where comment cards can be particularly useful.

Client comment cards should be readily accessible to clients and can be placed anywhere that a client would naturally visit, including the reception area, the waiting room and the consulting room. A comment card collection box should be placed close to where the cards are displayed, in order to facilitate easy card returns.

The management of the client feedback system should be delegated to one member of the practice team. The comment card boxes should be checked on a regular basis, ideally daily, so time is available in which to respond to potential complaints that must be addressed immediately. A database should be created that can be used to track comments, to allow the practice to watch for trends over time that could point to a systemic issue. Issues must be discussed at the appropriate practice meetings and lessons should be learned. Improvements should be incorporated into long-term strategies and business objectives.

Client meetings

If clients are to avail themselves and their pets of the services and products on offer from a practice they need to be told that these services exist and how they will benefit from using them. There are a number of ways in which to convey the message (see Chapter 25), but face-to-face contact is by far the best method. One of the limiting factors for all team members is time, and during a routine consultation it is often not possible for a veterinary surgeon or veterinary nurse to convey all they would like to a client about a particular topic. In addition, the circumstances may prevent the client from taking the message on board, e.g. if the pet is present or if the client is distressed. This is where practice–client meetings can be useful.

When organizing a practice–client meeting, the following should be taken into account:

- What is the objective of the meeting?
- What is the target audience?
- Is the meeting species-driven (e.g. focused on dogs, cats, rabbits, etc.) or clinically driven (e.g. focused on diabetes, senior pets, diet, etc.)?
- Is the meeting an opportunity for new clients to see the practice and meet the team?
- Will the meeting be held in association with a national event? This may help with the promotion.

The use of static media to communicate with clients

Communication can be divided into active and static methods. Active communication involves face-to-face dialogue (in person or over the phone) between team members and clients, whereas static communication depends upon the client seeking out the message. Nothing surpasses active communication, where the message and the style of delivery can be altered depending on the feedback from the client. However, due to time-limiting factors, a practice needs to make use of static communication methods to convey information to large numbers of clients (see also Chapters 5 and 25).

The following static media may be used to educate clients and/or promote services and products:

- Posters, floor displays and interactive displays
- A flat-screen display in the reception area
- Flyers and handouts, which are also useful as memory aids during the consultation process
- Mass mailing (regular mail or e-mail)
- Reminders (e.g. booster reminders)
- Website
- Social media (e.g. Facebook, Twitter, blogs)
- Articles in the public media, such as the local press
- Local radio appearances.

General messages delivered by static media can then be followed up and fine tuned when delivered to individuals via active media in the practice or over the phone.

Social media and websites offer the opportunity to convert a static media message to active communication (see Chapter 25).

Irrespective of which static media are employed to promote services and/or products, face-to-face communication is by far the most powerful and effective method of achieving uptake. It allows the message to be altered to suit the clients, some of whom may respond better to visual rather than verbal messages. Face-to-face communication allows checks to be made, by 'screening', as to whether the client has reservations regarding the proposed course of action, which can then be addressed with reassurances, where appropriate.

Once the client's reservations have been addressed, the necessary steps can be taken to progress matters, e.g. the patient is booked in for surgery.

Communication within the practice

Internal communication networks

Although most practices are small organizations working in small teams out of small premises, internal communication will not necessarily be effective and efficient. A practice must establish an **internal communication network** that meets the needs of the business. Communication must flow in all directions, not just in one, and for this to happen an 'organizational communication structure' (Figure 17.11) must be in place. This should be a published and readily available document that details who is responsible for what in terms of running the practice, and to whom individual team members should direct enquiries, comments, etc. More information on organizational reporting structures can be found in Chapter 19.

The main areas of responsibility should include the following:

- Personnel
- Client base
- Equipment
- Building
- Finance
- Medicines/disposables.

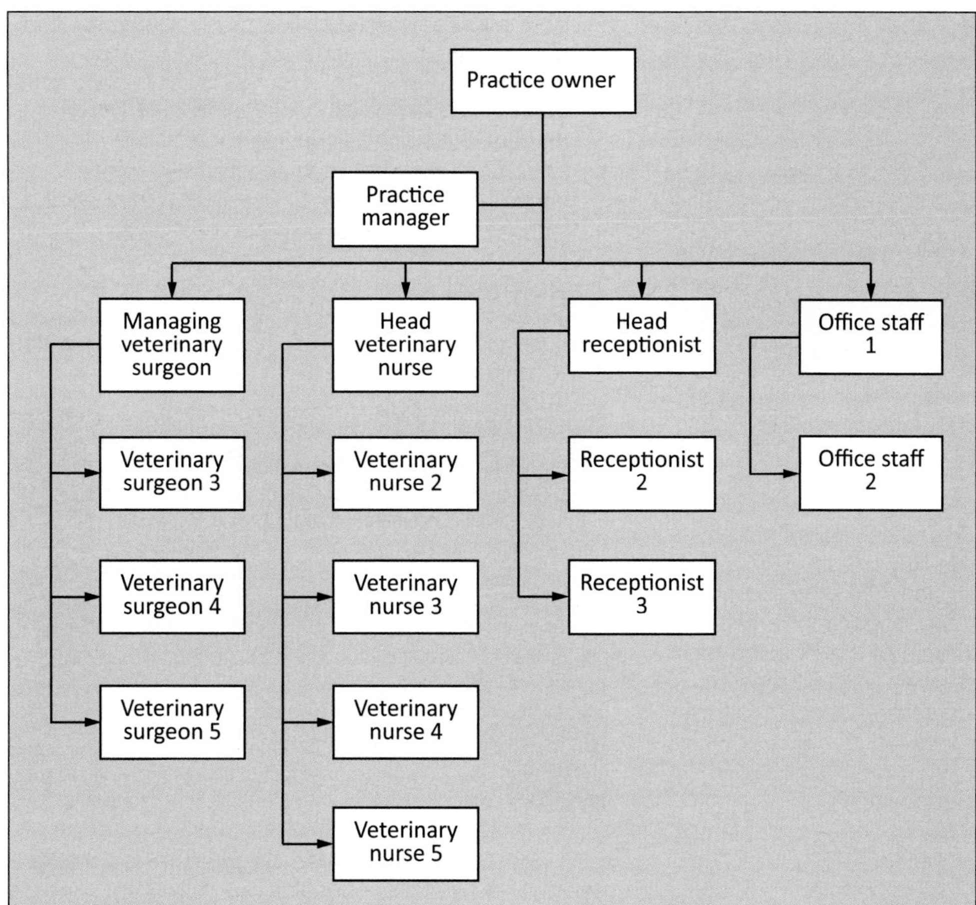

17.11 An example of an organizational communication structure within the practice. This example assumes that the owner is a veterinary surgeon.

Training the team in communication skills

Bringing communication skills training into the practice can:

- Maximize the impact on the whole team
- Reduce communication errors
- Enable practices to look at improving:
  - Consultation techniques
  - The handling of complaints
  - Communication between members of staff.

KEY POINT

Any team is only as strong as its weakest member; all of the good work done by the majority can be undone by the injudicious actions of one individual. In some cases, a weaker member's actions or words can be camouflaged by the rest of the team, but only for so long.

For this reason, communication skills training can benefit all members of the practice team; individuals will begin from different starting positions but even those who have some experience and knowledge can find something to add to their toolbox. It must be accepted that every individual will have their own communication style, and this can be developed with training.

Conventional training methods (didactic teaching, workshops and discussions) can be effective but have limitations where the practice expects individuals to change their behaviour. The acquisition of good communication skills has no ceiling in achievement because of the inherent complexity of the subject. Communication is a series of learned skills that can be taught with the same intensity as clinical and management skills. Figure 17.12 lists some common training methods and their benefits.

Training method	Benefits
Didactic teaching	Stimulating and promotes thinking and understanding of communication but unless supplemented with other teaching methods is unlikely to lead to sustained changes in behaviour when applying communication skills in practice
Trigger tapes, demonstrations, CDs, workshops and discussions	More likely to engage participants but still removed from altering how individuals communicate
Experiential techniques	Can produce an effective and long-lasting change

17.12 Comparison of training methods for developing communication skills.

Experiential techniques

The Veterinary Consultation Guide (see Figure 17.2) provides a comprehensive and manageable delineation of the skills that should be employed during a consultation. In addition to having a knowledge of these skills, whoever is providing the training should have a strategy as to how they will conduct the sessions. Figure 17.13 provides an outline of components that should be considered in order to ensure maximum learning in an environment that doesn't traumatize learners.

Groups	■ Maximum of 10 individuals to one facilitator and one educational role player
Demonstration	■ One learner undertakes a 'consultation' or interaction with a simulated client or simulated colleague ■ Observed by other members of the group and the facilitator
Feedback	■ Learner → group → educational role player → facilitator ■ This order lets the learner rehearse suggestions, allowing multiple opportunities for trial and error

17.13 Components of a training session that should be considered to ensure maximum learning.

Role play

Demonstrating practice scenarios using role play (Figure 17.14) should form a key component of any communication training session. Other members of the group should observe the interaction and a discussion should follow. Members of the practice team can be used as clients. However, enlisting the help of educational role players has several benefits, as they are trained in the following:

- Provision of descriptive feedback:
  - In role in a neutral position
  - In role but still in the emotion
  - Out of role
- The necessary specific skills – They can alter the emotion or direction of the encounter if specific skills are used
- Flexibility – They can change the intensity of the character's emotions if requested by the learner or the facilitator, e.g. the degree of anger or grief
- Ability to rehearse a specific learning point over and over again.

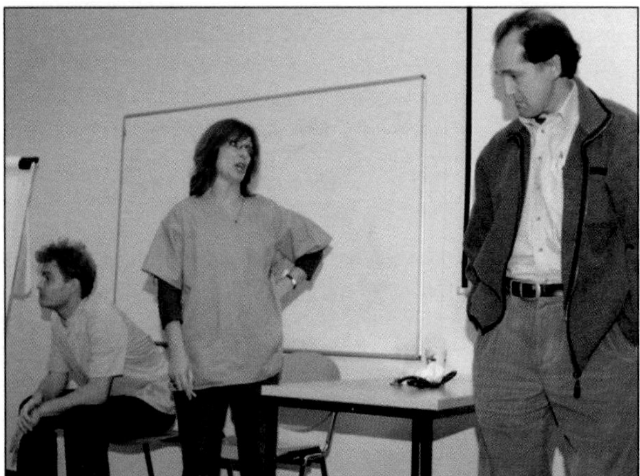

17.14 Experiential training in action: a simulated role play between a senior partner, a nurse and a veterinary graduate.

The facilitator

The role of the facilitator is crucial and it is worth acquiring external training before taking on this role. Facilitators should:

- Ensure all participants engage in feedback
- Ensure participants use descriptive feedback; otherwise the process becomes judgemental and non-constructive. Feedback should be non-judgemental, specific, directed towards behaviour rather than personality, well intentioned, shared and checked with the recipient
- Encourage the learner to use the skills in the Veterinary Consultation Guide so that they can be incorporated into their own personal style.

Use of video

The use of video in role play has its advantages and disadvantages (Figure 17.15).

Advantages
■ More detailed analysis of interaction ■ Learner engaged in role play has an opportunity to look at their performance before feeding back to the group ■ Individuals tend to be less critical about their own performance compared to 'fishbowl' technique
Disadvantages
■ Increased expense: capital outlay for cameras, TV and microphones ■ Additional time needed for training ■ Facilitators need to be familiar with technology

17.15 The advantages and disadvantages of video in role play.

Video cameras can also be used in the practice setting. For example, consultations with clients can be filmed. When using video in this way, the following points should be borne in mind:

- The camera should be placed in an unobtrusive position
- The positioning of the camera should allow a three-quarters body shot of both the client and the member of the practice team
- Permission should be obtained from the client and the member of staff.

Feedback on the success of the encounter can then be given:

- One-to-one
- In small groups
- In small groups plus a role player. The role player can then recreate the encounter, enabling the learner to have a different outcome by trying out different skills.

Practice meetings

KEY POINT

Regular practice meetings play a vital part in good communication, and it is the responsibility of all members of the practice team to ensure that they happen.

Organization of the meeting

- Meetings should be planned ahead and scheduled for a regular day/time/place relatively free from interruptions.

- Even if some practice members cannot attend, meetings should not be cancelled.
- The type and purpose of the meeting (e.g. whole practice or specific group) should be clarified.
- An agenda should be distributed in advance and colleagues should be asked for their input:
  - Action points from previous meetings should be included
  - The last agenda item should be a date for the next meeting.
- Somebody should be asked to take notes (minutes) and record action points during the meeting.

Purpose of the meeting

It is important to establish the purpose of the meeting. This will vary depending on whether it is a general information meeting, a problem-solving meeting or a team training session (Figure 17.16). Different types of meetings have different goals.

A general information meeting should:
■ Inform staff of any upcoming changes at the practice, e.g. new team members, equipment, services, products or procedures ■ Explain any practice decisions that have been made since the previous meeting ■ Set, revise or review goals, policies, guidelines and procedures ■ Review team/practice performance and/or progress toward goals ■ Recognize how each member contributes to the team's goals
A problem-solving meeting should:
■ Identify the problems in advance ■ Discuss the deleterious effects of each problem by analysing them and breaking them down ■ Discuss possible solutions and how they might be put into effect ■ Draw on the whole team's skills and ideas – the more everyone gets involved, the better chance of success
A team training session should:
■ Provide the team with new skills and knowledge ■ Refresh knowledge and understanding of skills and procedures ■ Provide opportunities for staff members or trainers/ representatives from outside the practice to conduct the meeting. DVDs, CDs and journals could also be useful in these situations

17.16 Different types of staff meetings and their purposes.

In the ideal world the entire team would be sent to every relevant CPD meeting, but as this is impossible the next best thing is to have a structure in place to facilitate feedback from those who have attended. Depending on the type of meeting and the content, feedback may include the dissemination of notes or discussion at a practice meeting. Encouraging those who have been on courses to share the information back at the practice is another way of reinforcing the attendee's knowledge whilst at the same time sharing it with the rest of the team.

Guidelines

- The meeting should start at the scheduled time.
- The agenda should be followed.
- Everyone should be encouraged to contribute and listen, and individuals should not be allowed to monopolize the discussion.
- There should be an opportunity to screen for 'anything else' at the end of a discussion.
- The team should reach a consensus.
- Any decisions made and responsibilities assigned should be summarized.
- The meeting should end on time.
- Meeting notes should include any decisions that are made and any agreed action points, with responsibilities assigned and timings outlined.

It is the duty of the chairman to ensure that everybody is included in the discussion. The chairman should consider the following tips in order to encourage participation:

- Prepare well, as discussed above
- Ensure attendees have an interest in the topic that is to be discussed
- Be conscious of the body language of attendees; if necessary, bring an attendee back into the discussion by asking them specifically for their opinion
- Challenge negativity or inappropriate comments
- Ask everybody to write down their comments or suggestions, which can then be displayed and grouped, and may even be photographed as part of the minutes
- Go around the table, asking each person for their opinion
- Use the de Bono hats technique, dividing the meeting up into sections where, for example, only known facts can be tabled, followed by a period when only negative comments can be made, then only positive ones, and so on.

After the meeting:

- Actions should be followed up
- Notes should be distributed to all staff, including those who did not attend
- Someone should be responsible for ensuring decisions/action points have been implemented and they should report on progress at the next meeting
- The meeting/training policy should be reviewed and discussed regularly to assess whether any improvements can be made.

Regular productive meetings in which issues are discussed in an open, no-blame atmosphere, and that result in positive behavioural change and the development of practice protocols are part of good **clinical governance**. This is a stipulation of the RCVS Practice Standards Scheme; for more information, see Chapter 28.

Feedback from the team

There are many good reasons for seeking structured feedback from team members. Feedback may be obtained via a number of channels, including:

- A structured appraisal system (see Chapter 19)
- Regular, frequent, productive practice meetings

- *Ad hoc* feedback through having an 'open door policy'
- Exit interviews, i.e. an interview that is carried out prior to a member of the team leaving the practice
- A staff suggestion scheme.

Staff suggestion scheme

Good ideas, in terms of introducing new services or improvements to existing services, are not the sole prerogative of people in high places. For example, the best person to come up with an idea to improve the kennel area may well be the new recruit working in the area itself. A staff suggestion scheme is one way of encouraging new ideas or improvements from team members.

A meeting should be held to explain what is involved in submitting a suggestion, what feedback can be expected, and any reward system. The scheme itself should provide a mechanism for receiving ideas in writing, with the individual or team providing details of what it is, how it will work, and who it will involve. Above all, the benefits need to be detailed; these can be financial, an enhancement in service to the clients, an improvement in working conditions, or a mixture of all three. Support may be needed to help staff members fill in a complex form.

In return, there must be a commitment from management to get back to that team member with a response within a fixed period of time, such as three weeks. This may be an outright acceptance of the idea, a request for further information or a suggestion of a meeting to move it forward; alternatively, the idea may be declined with a valid reason provided.

A practice may like to consider offering a reward to the individual who comes up with the best suggestion in a given period. Some team members may be reluctant to come forward with their suggestions, fearing their ideas are lightweight and merely offering a reward will not encourage their participation. The message that everybody's contributions are valuable and will be considered must be conveyed. Citing simple examples that have made a significant difference to the practice will help.

An example of a staff suggestion submission form can be found at the end of this chapter. A formal suggestion scheme may not be needed if all staff have ample opportunity to introduce their ideas through day-to-day discussions, informal notes, meetings and feedback sessions, and have their efforts recognized within the team.

Sharing information with the team

Most veterinary practices are small businesses, where it could be assumed that structured internal communications are not required because everybody must know what is going on. However, nothing should ever be assumed. In the absence of a structured communication system, the transfer of information will be by default, osmosis, rumour, etc., and is likely to lead to misinformation, with all the confusion and potential destruction associated with it.

Information can be disseminated in a number of ways, depending on the nature of the information, the target audience, the urgency and the importance. Vehicles used can include:

- Full practice meetings
- Divisional meetings
- Meetings with individuals
- Internal newsletters
- Internal e-mail
- Text messaging.

KEY POINT

One of the definitions of management is 'achieving one's aims through the efforts of others'. The team that understands where the practice is going and why it is being asked to go there is more likely to contribute to the journey.

Every team needs a good leader and every good leader will have a plan that must be communicated and shared with everyone. For more on leadership and business planning see Chapters 18 and 23, respectively.

KEY POINT

People do not like to be changed, but are happy to be involved in bringing about change.

When it comes to shared decision-making and bringing about change in a practice, it is understandable that the practice owners may not want to share all sensitive information, e.g. net profit. However, team members will be aware of certain financial information, e.g. daily turnover, and may well draw incorrect conclusions about the profitability of the business from this information. The revelation that turnover does not equal profit could come as a surprise to some team members, and it may well benefit the business financially to share some figures with the entire team, in a form that is more meaningful to them than standard accounting terminology, for example:

- Percentage of turnover available to the entire team, i.e. the amount of a particular sum received from a client that is available to share between team members (the amount paid less VAT, cost of sales, overheads, etc.)
- The cost of opening the practice for a day
- The financial results of a particular promotion.

Figure 17.17 illustrates the breakdown of a client's bill of £120.

Other information that a practice owner may like to share with the team and that can be published internally can include:

- Graphs of turnover, either as a moving annual total or as a comparison with the figure for last year
- Results of a particular marketing campaign in terms of responses as a percentage
- Number of new clients registered per month
- Level of debt
- Cost of consumables
- Occupancy rate of available appointment slots.

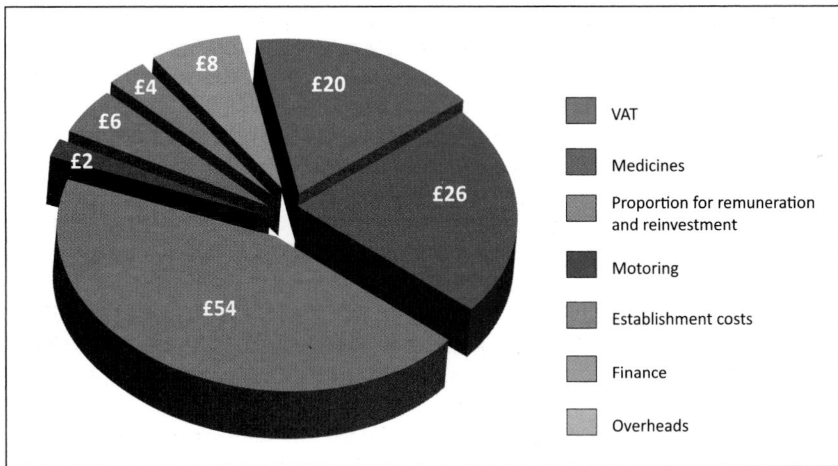

17.17 Illustration of the breakdown of a £120 bill to a client. 'Finance' includes all financial charges including bank charges, interest, depreciation and, in some cases, loan and HP interest.

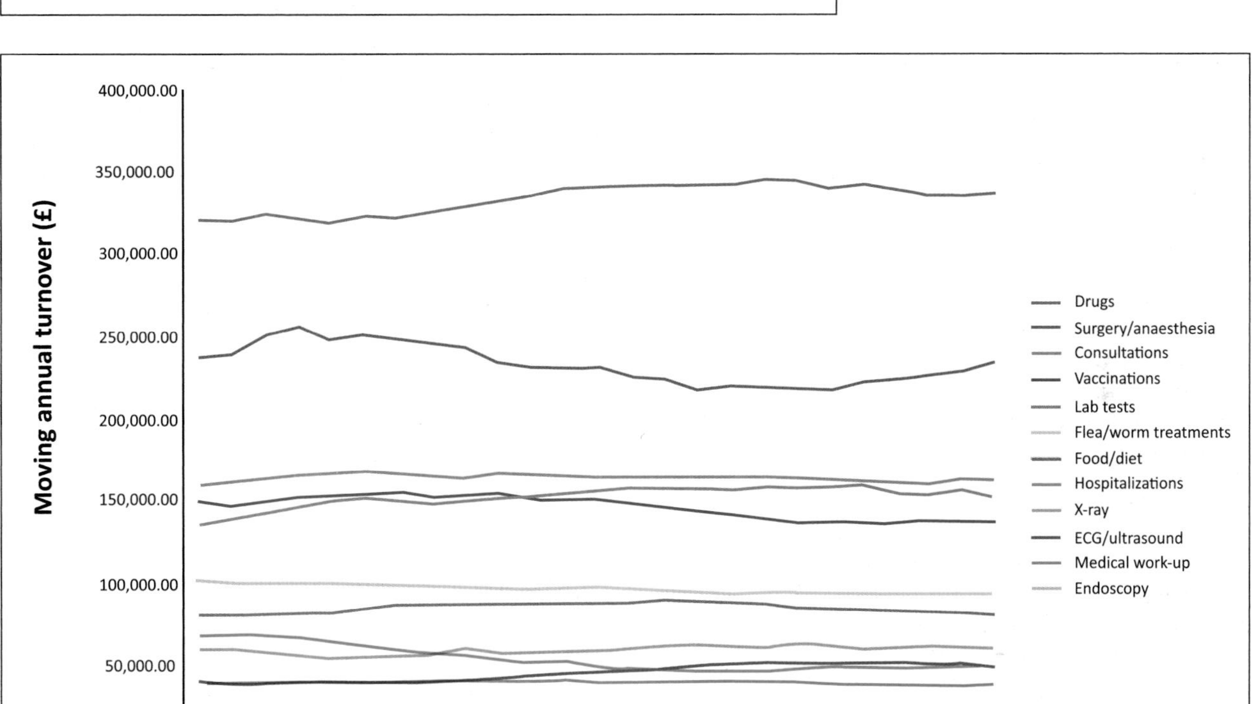

17.18 Moving annual turnover (MAT) can be analysed for a range of categories.

Figure 17.18 gives an example of a graph showing moving annual turnover, split into various income categories. More information on financial reporting is in Chapter 24.

The internal publication of some or all of the above information should form part of a larger picture. In other words, it should be preceded by a full practice meeting to explain the rationale behind sharing the results. This should involve telling staff that every individual is an important link in the chain and can influence results. The sharing of results should be incorporated into the setting of SMART objectives (see Chapter 23), and the team should have an opportunity to celebrate success.

Any business must decide how it will reward success and whether this will involve recognizing individuals or the team as a whole. It must be remembered that an action may be met with a motivational or a demotivational response: making one member of the team ecstatic may result in the alienation of the rest.

Handling complaints from members of staff

Members of staff may wish to make complaints or raise problems or concerns regarding their work, work conditions or relationships with colleagues. Staff members will want their grievances to be addressed, and if possible, resolved. It is in a practice's interest to address any grievances in a timely manner, before any problems develop into major difficulties for all concerned. It is therefore important to have a **grievance policy and procedure** document in place. It may be worthwhile using an external company that specializes in this area to help draw up the required documents. These policies are covered in more detail in Chapter 20. As with all problems, prevention is better than a cure, and hopefully internal complaints and grievances can be averted by having regular meetings to identify commonly occurring niggles and/or complaints, and by putting preventive measures into place.

External communication

When it comes to external communication, a practice needs to take into account all the 'stakeholders' in the business, i.e. all those who have an interest in the practice. This list may include some or all of the following:

- Clients
- Shareholders
- Suppliers
- Professional advisers
- Associated businesses
- Financial backers.

Communicating with suppliers

Manufacturers rely upon the practice, and in particular the practice team, to promote their products to pet owners. Practices, in turn, rely partly on the proceeds from the sale of these products to contribute to the covering of costs.

An individual, not necessarily the 'boss', but somebody who has been suitably trained, should be delegated to be the regular contact with suppliers. Their role is to negotiate on prices and to be the go-between when it comes to disseminating information to the rest of the team. As with all other important meetings, comprehensive notes should be kept, documenting what was agreed in terms of discounts, etc. It is also beneficial to have a member of support staff as a second point of contact, especially when it comes to products that have more of a waiting room presence, and where recording is required, e.g. for free replacement stock or marketing material.

Relying on one individual within the practice to relay all the necessary information to the rest of the team may not always be successful. Practices would be better served, when and where appropriate, to ask company representatives to address the entire practice team, e.g. over lunch or as part of a regular practice meeting.

Negotiating skills

Negotiation is a skill that most people will need to employ, whether dealing with an employer, an employee, a supplier or a customer. Many consider negotiating as an 'all or nothing' exercise; this is far from the case. It should instead be looked upon as a 'win–win' situation.

Customers nowadays are more confident and financially aware and, where possible, will seek to achieve a lower price on products they think they can buy elsewhere. It must be remembered that employees work for the practice and not for the client, and that relationships with existing clients will be undermined if preferential terms are offered to new customers, just to clinch the deal.

When it comes to negotiating with suppliers, the 'game' must be played from the other perspective:

- Do not put yourself in a weak bargaining position by appearing to be desperate to purchase or to have no alternative. The negotiation should take place before a commitment is made to purchase, not afterwards
- Ask the supplier to go first with their opening offer
- The starting offer price you propose should be low. It is not possible to go lower once the opening bid has been named
- Do not give anything away without receiving something in exchange
- If you have to give something away, this should be something that is of high value to the other party but is of lower value to the practice and may not actually cost it that much
- Keep accurate notes. As with all important discussions, it is vital to keep accurate and comprehensive notes that can be referred to if necessary
- Summarize as you go through the negotiation process. Keeping good notes facilitates this process
- Do not be afraid to say no and walk away if the deal cannot be struck.

Communicating with associated businesses

For most general practices, new clients will come from recommendations by existing clients. However, other associated businesses in the community will have influence when it comes to recommending the practice to pet owners. Such businesses include:

- Kennels and catteries
- Groomers
- Pet shops
- Estate agents.

Practices should consider establishing a relationship with such businesses (ensuring they remain within ethical boundaries) to help promote the profession in general and their own practice in particular. Further information can be found in Chapter 27.

Communicating with other professionals

There are a number of 'others' that a practice needs to communicate with on a regular or *ad hoc* basis, including accountants, the bank and professional advisers. With all such encounters, it is important to pre-plan, and also to briefly record the outcome of the meeting if not summarized by the other party in writing. The practice must consider and agree upon what it aims to achieve from such meetings. The objectives must be communicated to the other party and, if costs are involved, an estimate needs to be obtained.

Communicating with other practices

The dynamics of small animal practice have changed in terms of the number of situations in which clients may attend a practice other than their home practice. These situations include:

- Clients that have been referred to colleagues
- Clients who seek a second opinion
- Out-of-hours and emergency cover.

KEY POINT

Communication between colleagues in each of these situations should remain professional at all times (see Chapter 21). Dishonesty, lack of integrity, denigrating others and an unwillingness to discuss difficult issues with colleagues may hamper the progress of cases.

Referrals

When referring clients to a colleague, it is of paramount importance that all information pertaining to that case (e.g. clinical notes and laboratory results) is made available to the referral practice. Information that should be considered includes:

- A comprehensive clinical history
- Supporting material, such as radiographs
- Relevant background history.

This should be sent in good time, together with a referral letter that explains the reason for referral and any other pertinent details about the case. The identity of the referring veterinary surgeon should be clear so that the report and any other queries may be directed to them.

Practices offering a referral service to colleagues should consider providing a **referral pack** for practices to facilitate the process. Ease of use is crucial, and a comprehensive referral pack that provides the practitioner and their clients with as much information as possible and answers the frequently asked questions will greatly encourage the use of the service.

The referral pack should contain the following:

- A list of personnel
- A list of facilities and procedures on offer
- Contact details
- Referral forms (these should also be available online)
- A guide to prices
- Client handouts, which should include:
  - A map and directions
  - Contact details (address, website, phone, fax, etc.)
  - Client-friendly information on the service
  - The protocol regarding communication with the referring veterinary surgeon/practice
  - Terms and conditions.

KEY POINT

Personnel at the referral practice need to be careful when they are dealing with clients that they remain supportive of the referring practice and that they communicate their findings and advice to that practice in a full and timely manner.

References and further reading

Abood SK (2007) Increasing adherence in practice: making your clients partners in care. *Veterinary Clinics of North America: Small Animal Practice* **37**, 151–164

Bark P (2003) Complaints and how to deal with them. *Veterinary Defence Society*. Available at: http://www.bsava.com/LinkClick.aspx?fileticket=QpE2AfZ21h8=&tabid=153

Brightmore H (2009) *Solicitation of agenda and interruption of the opening statement in veterinary consultations: a preliminary study*. BVMedSci dissertation, University of Nottingham

Flemming DD and Scott JF (2004) The informed consent doctrine: what veterinarians should tell their clients. *Journal of the American Veterinary Medical Association* **224**, 1436–1439

Gray CA, Eves RE, Walsh SJ and Wilson CJ (2005) A final year special study module in veterinary communication skills. *AMEE conference abstracts*. Available at www.amee.org

Gray C and Moffett J (2010) *Handbook of Veterinary Communication Skills*. Wiley-Blackwell, Oxford

Hadlow J and Pitts M (1991) The understanding of common terms by doctors, nurses and patients. *Social Science and Medicine* **32**, 193–196

Mossop L and Gray C (2008) Teaching communication skills. *In Practice* **30**, 340–343

Radford A, Stockley P, Silverman J *et al*. (2006) Development, teaching, and evaluation of a consultation structure model for use in veterinary education. *Journal of Veterinary Medical Education* **22**, 38–44

Silverman J, Kurtz SA and Draper J (1996) The Calgary–Cambridge approach to communication skills teaching: agenda led outcome based analysis of the consultation. *Education for General Practice* **7**, 288–299

Silverman J, Kurtz SA and Draper J (2005) *Skills for Communicating with Patients, 2nd edn*. Radcliffe Medical Press, Oxford

Veterinary Defence Society. *The Consultation Process*. VDS

Sample suggestion form ▶

STAFF TEAM SUGGESTION FORM	
Team member's name	**Date**
Concern Please provide details of your suggestion, including how it improves your job, the job of others, benefit to the patients, value to the client and the concern being addressed (e.g. lost time, misuse or wastage of materials, loss of revenue, inefficiency, poor morale).	
Resources required What resources do you think the practice will have to provide in order to support your suggestion? Please provide as much detail as you can under the following headings: Labour Equipment Materials Time Space Money Other (please specify)	
Benefits Please explain what you see as the total benefit to the practice from adopting your suggestion	
Planning Please outline the necessary steps and identify those who are required to accomplish your suggestion: 1 2 3 4 5	
Team member's signature - For management use only	
Supervisor's name	
Receipt date	Response date
Benefits from adopting suggestion Benefits to business Associated costs (financial, time, labour, etc.) Is the suggestion cost-efficient and in keeping with the practice business plan? Priority 1 2 3 4 5 6 (where 1 is low and 6 is high) Action to be taken	
Suggested employee reward Supervisor's name.................... Supervisor's signature....................	

An example of a suggestion form for staff to use.

18

Leadership and self-management

Caroline Jevring-Bäck

Good leadership provides the direction and focus that enables a business to grow and thrive around a stable core of satisfied customers and staff. Poor leadership, on the other hand, creates wasteful inefficiencies, high staff turnover and clients who 'vote with their feet', outcomes which will ultimately drive the practice into the ground.

This chapter will look at a range of issues surrounding leadership, including the critical role it plays in a veterinary practice, and what a leader does when it comes to dealing with change, giving effective and timely feedback, and remaining positive in the face of daily challenges. Topics that will also be reviewed include: the challenges faced by practice leaders in balancing their multi-functional roles; the role and value of a practice manager; and the need for sensible time management to maintain productivity and motivation, and to help prevent and reduce stress. For veterinary surgeons and nurses who are also managers and leaders, continual professional development should include a balance between clinical topics and communication, leadership and management skills.

Do practices need leaders?

Professional and support staff have busy lives, with many conflicting demands on their time and attention. They often become so involved with the minutiae of the present that they lose sight of where they want to go with their professional lives. It is also easy for individuals in the practice to work hard in their own clinical or support areas, or in their own professional career paths, without thinking about how this contributes to the growth and health of the practice business. Pulling together the aims of the individual and those of the business requires focussed leadership.

KEY POINT

Good practice leaders provide the direction and drive to help their staff accomplish more and greater things than they would do on their own. This simultaneously builds a stronger and more productive business.

Leadership and management

The different actions of leaders and managers are summarized in Figure 18.1.

Leader
■ Establishes direction ■ Aligns people ■ Motivates and inspires ■ Produces change and long-term results
Manager
■ Plans and budgets ■ Organizes and staffs ■ Controls and problem-solves ■ Produces predictable short-term results through creating order

18.1 The different actions of a leader *versus* a manager.

In reality, the principals of most practices need to be multi-faceted. They have to be leaders, managers, practice owners and veterinary clinicians; these are different roles, requiring different skills and producing different results.

- A **leader** gets things done through people by giving them purpose, inspiration and a desire to achieve. A leader is *effective*. He/she requires good communication, negotiation, delegation and self-management skills, coupled with a long-term perspective.
- A **manager** creates the environment in which people can be more effective. A manager is *efficient*. A manager's time is more splintered than a leader's, with a greater diversity of problems and situations to deal with in any one day, and the results are more ambiguous and difficult to measure.
- An **owner** is the individual most interested in the practice's profit.
- A **clinician** concentrates on the diagnosis, treatment and management of the consultations, operations and visits booked. His/her day ends with visible signs of progress that can be measured in several different ways, such as the number of clients seen and income generated.

What makes a leader successful?

Much has been invested in trying to pin down what makes a good leader. The behaviours that appear most consistently are:

- **Vision and focus:**
    - Creates and keeps alive a motivating picture of the future
    - Focuses on achieving the most important goals without becoming distracted
    - Really understands what pet-owning clients want and need, and makes sure all business decisions stem from that
    - Is clear in all communication and does a great job of aligning the team around the vision
    - Ties team objectives to the overall business strategies
    - Consistently displays enthusiasm and energy for what is happening
    - Generates excitement about big initiatives
- **Integrity:**
    - Keeps promises and follows through on commitments
    - Gets the planned results
    - Shows genuine concern for colleagues and employees and treats everyone with respect and dignity
    - 'Walks the talk'
    - Consistently has high energy and positive attitude
- **Magnanimity**:
    - Gives credit where credit is due
    - Recognizes the power of the team – does not take all the credit for results
    - Is dedicated to the practice team's growth and development through focused performance coaching
- **Humility:**
    - Shares own strengths and weaknesses with team
    - Learns from mistakes and shares the lessons
- **Openness**:
    - Helps staff understand the 'why' behind major decisions
- **Creativity:**
    - Encourages and supports creative and strategic thinking
    - Challenges ideas respectfully
    - Encourages others to speak up
- **Fairness:**
    - Treats people fairly, if not always equally
- **Assertiveness:**
    - Communicates clearly and well
    - Knows how and when to make decisions that are best for the business as well as the individual
    - Has high standards and holds everyone to them
    - Understands that everyone has a right to their point of view and their own priorities and respects these when negotiating
- **Sense of humour:**
    - Helps maintain team spirit and morale by keeping a realistic perspective on life.

'Emotional intelligence'

Being an effective leader is not simply about *what* the leader does but also *how* they do it. Over and above intellectual intelligence (knowing what to do and getting on with it), a leader also requires emotional intelligence, which is using empathy and social skills to get the best from the people they work with and serve.

Emotional intelligence (or emotional quotient; EQ), is a term made popular by Daniel Goleman in the 1980s. EQ and IQ are not opposing competencies but, rather, separate ones. Using EQ could be compared to writing a letter on the computer: spell-checking can be used to make sure the spelling and grammar are perfect (IQ), but no computer can help select the words and phrasing to express the emotional side of the message (EQ). Everybody uses both and mixes them to a degree, but there is increasing evidence that a balance is needed for real success in life.

KEY POINT

A leader needs both IQ and EQ to be successful.

The competencies that make up EQ are:

- **Knowing one's emotions** – Self-awareness is a cornerstone of EQ. It is about recognizing one's feelings as they happen and is crucial to psychological insight and self-understanding. People who can recognize their feelings are better pilots of their lives than those who are at their mercy
- **Managing emotions** – Self-awareness leads to appropriate management of feelings. People who cannot manage their feelings well and are constantly in a state of distress can have a very negative and energy-draining effect on both themselves and people around them. Those who can manage their feelings quickly bounce back from upsets
- **Emotional self-control** – The ability to stifle impulses and to delay gratification in order to reach a goal underlies every sort of achievement. Focusing emotions in order to achieve a goal enables people to get into a 'flow' state, where outstanding performance is possible. This is the basis of self-motivation
- **Recognizing emotions in others** – Empathy is *the* fundamental people skill. People who are empathetic are more in-tune with the subtle social signals that indicate what others need or want. This makes them better equipped to work in the caring professions, sales, teaching and management
- **Handling relationships** – Social competence is largely about being able to manage emotions in others. This skill set underlies abilities such as popularity, leadership and interpersonal effectiveness.

The importance of EQ in the veterinary business should not be underestimated. Veterinary surgeons have been trained to focus on developing their intellectual intelligence (IQ), with less value placed on EQ.

Competition to get into vet school is fierce and in the past has been judged primarily on the results of intelligence tests such as A levels and other practical achievements. IQ competition continues at university, where huge amounts of information are expected to be assimilated, digested, learnt and regurgitated to pass exams. However, once in practice the rules of the competition change: although IQ remains important, EQ is vital. Being able to get on with fellow team members in practice and relate to pet owners becomes a significant measure of success. The level of EQ in a practice differentiates one practice from another.

KEY POINT

Self-awareness is a cornerstone of EQ, and the ability of a person to get on with their fellow team members in practice and relate to pet owners becomes a significant measure of success.

One of the most important elements of EQ is the ability to show *empathy*. This is striving to see the world through another person's eyes. Offering flexible working hours to a staff member who is trying to juggle full-time work with having a family and studying for a degree, rather than 'forcing' them to work to a rigid schedule, is likely to increase their loyalty to the business. Similarly, a client who feels that they are being properly listened to will be more open to gentle challenges about lifestyle issues and beliefs regarding medication and nutrition that affect the health of their pet.

The possession of good communication skills and the ability to listen also fall under EQ. These skills are very important; enhancing communication skills is not just about psychosocial care but is also about improving physiological outcomes, and can even be a treatment option. In a 1-year prospective study completed by the Headache Study Group of The University of Western Ontario (1986), the best predictor of resolution of headache problems after presenting at family doctors was not diagnosis, intervention, referral or prescriptions, but the patient's perception that they had the opportunity to tell their story and discuss their concerns about their headache fully with their doctor during their first visit.

EQ also has an impact on a person's ability as a leader. Nearly all of the factors that may influence a person's leadership ability (the 'law of the lid', Maxwell (2007)) are linked to EQ, rather than IQ. Information on how EQ competencies contribute to staff and client evaluation of their service experience is given in Chapter 26.

The 'law of the lid' (Maxwell, 2007)

Leadership consultant John Maxwell graphically describes how a person's level of effectiveness influences their leadership ability and how this can set a lid on the development potential of a business. Factors that put a lid on one's success as a leader include:

- **Fear:** of failure, of unwillingness to try new things, of losing face
- **Impatience**: rather than letting people or things take the time they need
- **Denial:** that something wrong has been said or a poor decision has been made ▶
- **Impulsiveness:** linked with erratic, unpredictable behaviour, which is unsettling and does not encourage trust
- **Deceit**: lying or cheating is unacceptable in a leader
- **Jealousy:** a very destructive emotion that does not encourage sharing and growth
- **Anger:** properly managed anger is a powerful tool to set boundaries, but improperly managed it can be terrifying and destructive
- **Lack of confidence:** affects decision-making ability and encourages procrastination
- **Lack of knowledge:** limits choices
- **Lack of understanding:** can create blocks in communication
- **Other people's perception:** especially if this is significantly different from how one sees oneself

The role and function of a leader

A leader has four key activities with distinctly observable actions (Delong *et al.*, 2007):

- Setting the direction
- Gaining commitment to the direction
- Carrying out the necessary actions to keep moving in the agreed direction
- Setting a personal example.

Setting the direction: defining the vision

Businesses need more than short-term goals to succeed. Veterinary surgeons are often focused on specific goals and tasks – managing the next patient, learning a new surgical skill, getting through the day's cases – so they need leaders to express the practice's longer-term objectives and to outline how their work relates to achieving these objectives. Setting the direction or creating the practice vision helps everyone to maintain focus on, and drive towards, the same targets, and reduces false starts and side-tracking. Setting direction is not something a leader decides alone – all practice members should contribute to the process. Creating a vision for the practice is about being clear on the answers to strategic questions. The answers to these questions come from repeated discussions with all staff to get their ideas and contributions. This process creates consensus, buy-in, focus and single-mindedness regarding the organization's direction.

An important aspect of establishing business direction and long-term focus is creating a simple, clear, *written* business plan that is shared, understood and accepted by all practice members. Setting direction also means defining objectives and measuring progress towards targets. This should be on both an overall business level (e.g. setting goals for turnover and profitability), and on an individual level (e.g. setting performance goals for staff). These objectives, however, cannot simply be imposed on the practice team, but should include, for example, regularly sharing financial information about the practice, or managing each individual's performance review cycle. For more information see Chapters 23 and 24.

Gaining commitment to the direction

Ensuring the whole team is working towards the practice's direction is probably the most difficult part of being a leader. Reminding the team frequently of the business focus and goals requires expertise in communication skills (see Chapter 17). Professionals are trained to be independent individualists and often relish working alone; they do not always take kindly to being told what they should be doing and how they should be doing it, but at the same time they expect their leaders to involve them in important processes that affect how they perform their job. The key to getting everyone involved and committed is to engage them in the discussions and thought processes that lead to important decisions about how the business will function. It is also critical to have the right people in the practice team (see later). If this action is missed, or staff have their own agendas that may not be in line with the agenda of the business, then some team members may work against the practice's objectives, showing active or passive resistance.

Gaining commitment to the direction

Just as a football team cannot score well if players are not cooperating to achieve team objectives, so a veterinary practice will not reach its potential if staff members are not fully engaged. Examples of both active and passive resistance are common in daily practice and include:

- Coming late to, not contributing to or not attending practice meetings
- Reluctance to participate in team-building CPD
- Not following agreed policies
- Deliberately not charging correctly
- Deliberately not carrying out reasonable and fair requests when asked.

Over time, these apparently small and individual acts of sabotage will limit change efforts and cripple business development. Unfortunately they are often ignored or 'swept under the mat' because to manage them is uncomfortable. Staff members behave like this for many reasons, ranging from being 'too busy' or not agreeing with the ethos/values of the practice to 'not seeing the need to'. Fundamentally it reflects a lack of understanding about the significance of their individual contribution to the practice and the effect of their behaviours on others. This is the 'rotten apple' syndrome: one rotten apple in a box of fresh apples will slowly and gradually cause them all to rot. A good leader spots and tackles disruptive behaviour promptly and then supports the perpetrator through the discomfort of making the desired changes to their behaviour. (See Chapter 19 for more details about directing behaviours.)

KEY POINT

The behaviour of staff with bad attitude or showing insubordination will ultimately disrupt the whole team. Any such problem must be nipped in the bud quickly, otherwise standards of customer and patient care will be affected, along with respect and courtesy towards colleagues and, over time, practice income and profitability.

Carrying out the necessary actions

A practice will not achieve a competitive difference through doing things reasonably well, most of the time. A good leader makes sure that strategies are in place to create the difference and also that it actually happens. This is often tough because it requires a lot of effort over a prolonged period of time. Typical business strategies in veterinary practice include familiar goals such as 'build client relationships', 'act like team players' and 'provide fulfilling motivating careers'. It is clear that employees want the benefits of these things, knowing what to do, why it should be done and even how it should be done. Yet practice members often do not do what is good for them (and for the business) because they are not prepared to make the effort to change their behaviour. The rewards are far in the future, whereas the disruption, discomfort and discipline needed to get there are immediate.

Strategy and the fat smoker (Maister, 2008)

In his book *Strategy and the Fat Smoker*, David Maister explains why changing behaviours in a business is so difficult by relating it to the need to keep fit. We all know we should not smoke, we should eat less and we should exercise more, but few of us have the self-discipline to do this. 'As human beings', he writes, 'we are not good at delayed gratification. To reach our goals, we must first change our lifestyle and daily habits now. Then we must summon the courage to *keep up* the new habits and not yield to all the old familiar temptations. Then, and only then, will we get the benefits *later*.'

KEY POINT

A good leader makes sure the strategies are in place to create a difference and also that it actually happens.

Setting a personal example

A leader who consistently shows the behaviour they expect from their employees is far more likely to have a successful practice than one who demands one set of behaviours but demonstrates something else. Common examples of unhelpful behaviours include:

- Arriving late and starting consultations late
- Not following protocols, for example:
  - Not booking follow-up appointments
  - Not writing up sufficiently detailed clinical histories
  - Not writing estimates on consent forms
- Charging inconsistently
- Showing favouritism towards an individual
- Exploiting the leadership position by taking time off when they feel like it.

Positive ways in which to work as a leader include:

- Being seen and being actively involved in the daily work
- Taking an individual interest in employees
- Going the extra mile for colleagues and clients

- Following all rules and protocols in the same way that employees are expected to do
- Doing all of this with a positive attitude and good humour.

Employing a practice manager

Shilcock and Stutchfield (2003) define the role of the practice manager as 'enabling the good management of the veterinary practice so that the owner or partners can continue to carry out their clinical functions without the need to devote too much expensive time to management'. This is not the complete story, as an essential role for the owners/partners continues to be leadership, performing the four key activities described earlier.

KEY POINT

Without good leadership from the owners/partners, the practice manager will be not be able to perform his/her job.

The role of practice manager can be undertaken by a veterinary surgeon if they have the inclination and interest for this, and if this is the best use of human resources within the practice. It is important to remember, though, that the skills needed for leading or managing a practice are more than simple common sense. In their role, a manager is just as skilled as a clinical veterinary surgeon.

Management is about coping with complexity in the three primary areas of a business:

- Planning and budgeting
- Organizing and staffing
- Controlling and problem-solving.

Without good management, any business can become chaotic in ways that hinder its health and development. Good management brings a degree of order and consistency to key dimensions such as the quality and profitability of services.

A veterinary surgeon as leader or manager will naturally have insights into the way a practice works, but some practices work very successfully with non-veterinary owners/leaders. Practice managers may come from within the practice and 'grow into' the role, or they may come from outside the profession and therefore bring with them experience from other professions and disciplines.

Increasingly valued are qualified managers who have studied subjects such as business or marketing, or who have achieved the Certificate of Veterinary Practice Management (CVPM).

What does a practice manager do?

Veterinary management in any practice can be broadly divided into six categories:

- Human resources
- Finance and budgeting
- Marketing and sales
- General office management
- Health and safety
- Information technology.

Each of these categories encompasses many different elements, and the skill set a manager requires will depend upon what they are expected to do within the practice. The manager of a medium-sized practice may need to cover all the above, whereas in a larger practice there may be one or more managers responsible for each. In the latter case, this can provide an opportunity for staff development as, for example, nurses move from a clinical role to a managerial support role, or take on more management responsibility in their clinical role.

It is very important that expectations about what the manager is supposed to do are clearly defined and agreed upon. One of the most frustrating situations managers in veterinary practice can find themselves in is when the veterinary owners refuse to truly delegate responsibility to them. Often this can be resolved by having a clear written agreement of responsibilities. Another common frustration for managers is having their role in the practice severely limited to, say, bookkeeping and payroll. This is only one aspect of the myriad things a competent manager must do to ensure a practice runs smoothly and efficiently.

Leading change

Change is a constant in the business world; leading and managing change well is therefore part of the success (or failure) of any business. To lead change in an established practice is a tough challenge. There are already routines, traditions, and ways of doing things which, even if they are not working efficiently, are so deeply ingrained in the practice that they can be difficult to identify, let alone change.

It takes time to define the main problem areas and then to summon the energy needed within the organization to drive through the necessary reforms, by generating a strong will to change and establishing a clear new direction in which to go.

Management supports change by reviewing old and developing new, more efficient routines and processes, and then supporting practice members in learning and implementing them. For example, the leadership in a practice may decide the old labour-intensive system of taking, developing, reviewing and storing radiographs should be replaced by the faster, better quality, space-saving method of using digital radiography.

Leadership creates the focus, enthusiasm and longer-term vision to drive through the change, whilst management is responsible for the practicalities of making it happen, which include helping people learn how to use new machines.

Some employees find change difficult, and in order to ensure success it is important that staff 'buy in' to any proposed changes. To lead change effectively requires a consistent and methodical approach.

The eight-step model for leading change (Kotter, 1996)

1. **Establish urgency.** To create the necessary energy to drive the change process it is vital to establish a sense of urgency. 'Urgency' should not be interpreted as panic, as this is a destructive emotion. Staff should be involved by clearly showing them problem areas, the effect they have on the organization, and how they can personally contribute to making a difference as part of the team.
2. **Form a guiding coalition**. Strong leaders that work well together and inspire their co-workers should be identified at different levels within the practice.
3. **Create a clear description of the future.** A description of what success will look like after the change is necessary in order to guide and shape all decisions. From this description comes agreement on the actions to be taken over the time period that the change will take place. One way of doing this is to express the required change in terms of SMART goals and objectives. SMART stands for stretching, measureable, achievable, results-driven and time-bound. For example, 'By 30 September, three months from now, we will have the new digital radiography system fully up and running. This will include installing the system, training all staff in how to use it, identifying one veterinary surgeon and one veterinary nurse as system specialists, and making information about the new system available for clients on the website.'
4. **Communicate the change.** The change description needs to be kept alive and should be included in meetings and in all internal communications. In addition, practice leaders should model the behaviour they expect from team members to achieve the change.
5. **Empower action.** Systems and methods in the practice that may block or hinder creativity and spontaneity should be reviewed and revised.
6. **Create short-term wins.** It is important to show that change is really happening. Short-term wins should be celebrated to provide incentive for everyone to continue on the new path. In the case above, this could be that half the team has successfully completed their training, or that the first digital radiograph has been taken.
7. **Consolidate.** There is no end point with change or with a change process. Change is continuous and it is therefore important that desirable changes within the organization are consolidated. This is done by, for example, critically reviewing changes and seeing that they function as planned, employing the right people who will contribute to motivating and leading the process forward, and encouraging and rewarding new ideas and more efficient ways of doing things.
8. **Institutionalize change.** The final stage in the change process is institutionalizing it – making it part of the culture so that the organization cannot slip back into 'the good old ways'. This applies both internally for employees, and also externally in how other organizations and clients see the changed ways.

Managing change: working with the change curve

Change can create discomfort and, potentially, chaos which can be disruptive and energy-sapping for all concerned. The change management model offers an understanding of how to be in control when going through the change process. Figure 18.2 illustrates typical emotions and reactions people experience when going through change and how these impact on performance.

Realizing that the emotions experienced are temporary and 'normal' prevents:

- Feelings of being swamped by them
- Getting stuck in negative emotions such as frustration or anxiety
- Being overcome by fear
- Becoming a 'victim'.

Using the change management model empowers proactivity through taking back control and thereby experiencing the change process positively, with a sense of achievement and enhanced self-esteem.

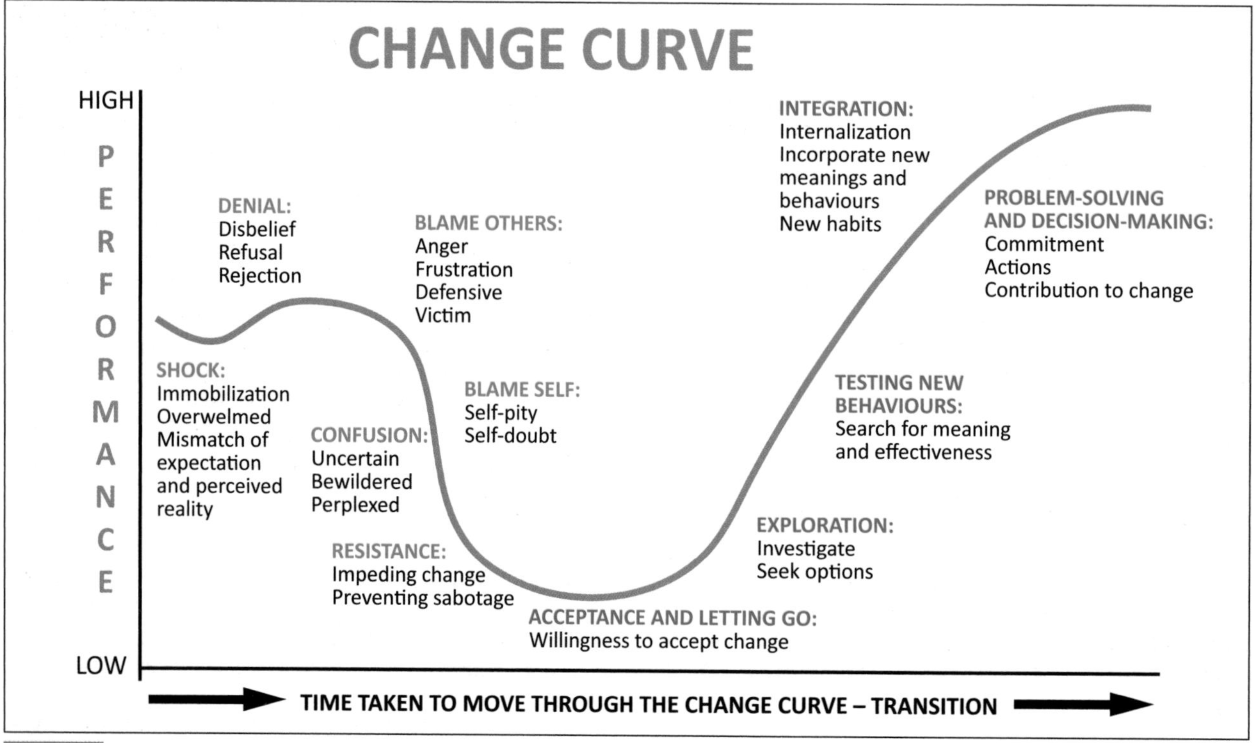

18.2 The emotions involved in change. The initial emotions shown in red are 'negative' and serve to reduce performance. The emotions felt later, shown in green, are 'positive' and lead to enhanced performance.

Change and stress

According to cognitive psychology, human knowledge is organized into mental schemas or habits that guide, to a large extent, everyday behaviour. These habits help people to run their lives smoothly and to manage anxiety and stress. Changing habits is not easy and is often associated with feelings of chaos, discomfort and even stress (Figure 18.3).

KEY POINT

A leader's function is to provide a continued focus on the outcomes and to provide support and encouragement through feedback to achieve the necessary changes.

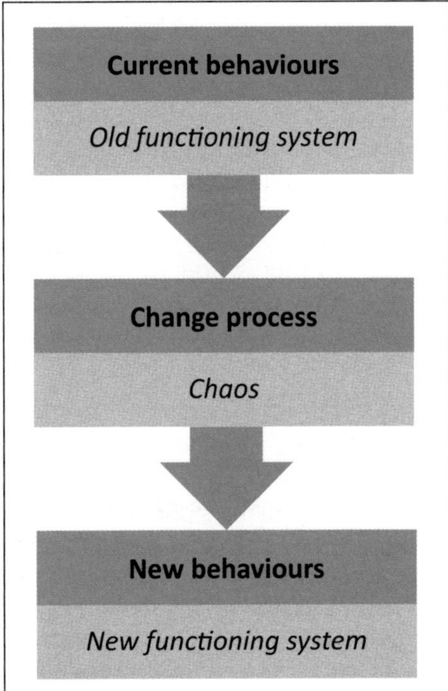

18.3 The change process. The chaos period can be very uncomfortable, as old behaviour patterns are (sometimes reluctantly) abandoned and new ones learnt (sometimes with difficulty).

Getting the right people

As with any professional service firm, a veterinary practice is a people-centred business and its success depends on having happy, productive staff that encourage satisfied clients. It is important to choose the right people to achieve this. Keeping the wrong people in the practice will slow down its development and create dissatisfaction and discomfort for everyone.

Some people are not willing or able to make the changes in their behaviours that are required, even with support and individual coaching. This raises the question of whether or not to keep them, which is not always an easy decision to make and requires careful weighing of the individual's value to the practice against the long-term health of the business.

Removing the wrong people from the practice may happen by itself, in that they may find the changes too uncomfortable and choose to move on. A change of job specification that supports an individual's strengths may be a suitable option, but dismissal is sometimes necessary and appropriate (see Chapter 20). To ensure either of these options is carried out correctly and appropriately requires good performance management and careful documentation of performance records (see Chapter 19).

Having the right people on your bus (Collins, 2001)

The 'right people' are those that are motivated and willing to work together to achieve the business objectives, however challenging these may be. Collins and his team of researchers found that great leaders did not decide where to drive the bus first and then get the people onboard; instead they first got the right people on the bus (and the wrong people off the bus) and then figured out where to drive it. In effect, they worked with three simple concepts.

1. If you begin with 'who' rather than 'what' you can more easily adapt to a changing world. If people join your bus primarily because of where it's going, they can have severe problems adapting if you need to change direction some way down the road. However, if they've joined because of who else is on the bus, they are likely to be far more flexible.
2. With the right people on the bus, the issue of how to motivate and manage people largely disappears. The right people don't need to be tightly managed or fired up; they are self-motivated, with an inner drive to produce the best results and to contribute towards creating something great.
3. If you have the wrong people, it doesn't matter if you decide upon the right direction, because you still won't have a great practice. Great vision without great people is worthless.

The importance of feedback and coaching

KEY POINT

Feedback is the imparting of specific information about specific behaviours to an individual; coaching is about supporting behavioural change.

To be effective and constructive (i.e. helpful to the individual), feedback must be timely, specific and describe the observed behaviours and their effect on the observer (Blanchard *et al.*, 1994). In addition, positive feedback can often be given in a public setting, whereas constructive (negative) feedback should always be given in private. General statements such as 'Good job, Sam' or 'You never do this well, Alex' are not helpful because they are not specific and do not describe the behaviour. The following comments are more helpful:

- 'I'm really impressed with how your surgery skills have come on, Sam. That abdomen yesterday was a mess and you were very careful and thorough in checking it and resecting the right areas of bowel. I think that the dog has got every chance of a good recovery. '
- 'Alex, you haven't cleaned the operating theatre as well as we need you to. I noticed there were still spatters on the walls and floor and you had not

moved the operating table for cleaning. I feel disappointed because we have gone through this several times before, and it is important for everyone that this job is done really thoroughly. Please make sure you pay more attention to detail in the future.'

Using feedback and coaching together

To achieve changes in behaviour three things are required:

- A clear description of the desired new behaviour
- Internal motivation to make the change, which comes from understanding why the change in behaviour is needed
- External supportive actions and encouragement.

The first two involve excellence in communication to paint a vivid picture in people's minds of how the new behaviours will benefit them, which in turn generates excitement and motivation. The last is about coaching to reinforce desired behaviours or modify or eliminate undesirable behaviours. Team members need feedback and coaching to achieve required behavioural changes in many situations from im-proved consultation skills and communication with clients, to managing the installation of a new computerized practice appointment system. Other examples could include introducing improved telephone techniques and handling of telephone calls, converting more enquiries into actual appointments, and changing roles in the practice (e.g. a veterinary nurse becomes head nurse or a veterinary surgeon becomes a new partner).

Coaching for performance is a learnt skill and should be adapted to the needs of the individual who is being coached. Blanchard *et al.* (1994) clearly explains how this works using the situational leadership model (Figure 18.4). The top diagram shows how a leader should vary their level of support (S) depending on the level of skill and development (D) shown by the employee.

Briefly, when learning a new skill or task (D1) the individual initially needs very close supervision and support (S1) – the highly directive behaviour shown in the lower right-hand box. As they gain experience and confidence, this support can gradually be reduced until eventually the individual is fully capable of coping on their own (S4 and D4). To take an example, a new veterinary graduate may require a lot of 'hand holding' and guidance as they perform their first bitch spay, but over time and with more experience they will be able to perform the task well, with minimal input from their coach or mentor. It is important, however, for a leader to appreciate that the level of support required depends on what stage of development the individual is at for a *specific task*; thus, when that graduate performs an orthopaedic procedure for the first time, support and guidance will again be needed.

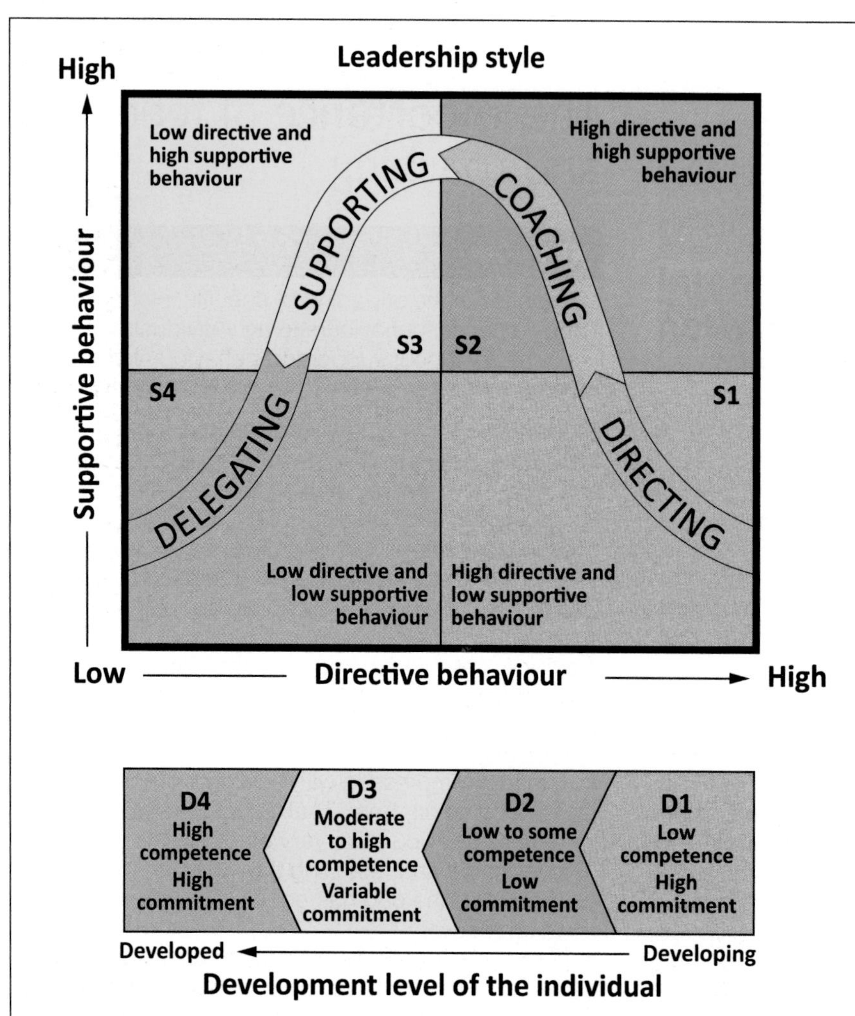

18.4 The situational leadership model (Blanchard *et al.*, 1994). The skill as a leader is to know how much direction and support to give an individual in any situation.

KEY POINT

The skill as a leader is to know how much direction and support to give an individual in any situation, especially as every individual may be at different levels of development for different tasks.

Coaching for correction requires a similar approach, but with the focus on changing observed undesirable behaviour to desirable new behaviour. As already indicated this requires clear feedback about the current behaviour and its effects, and then the creation of a mutually acceptable picture or description of how the new behaviour will look and feel.

To go back to the above example of Alex, who had not cleaned the operating theatre well, coaching questions to ask could include: 'How could you have done this differently?', 'What are you finding difficult or challenging?', 'Is there something you are not clear about?', 'Is there some further help you need?'. Once the description is made, a plan must be agreed as to how to ensure the changes actually happen: perhaps Alex needs to tick off a checklist of duties, or the cleaned theatre could be inspected daily for the next two weeks.

KEY POINT

If a reprimand is delivered it is important for people to understand that they are still valued. People often confuse corrective feedback with a personal attack on them as individuals; it is therefore critical to be very clear that this is about their behaviour. Providing very specific examples of undesirable behaviour and clearer descriptions of desirable behaviour will increase the likelihood that a positive response to change will result.

Coaching for attitude

Where a change in attitude is required, once again very specific feedback about the observed behaviour and its effects are necessary. Many people are genuinely unaware of how their attitude affects others because it reflects their own internal way of viewing the world. Where there is a problem, it is not effective to say 'You have an attitude problem!', but it can make a difference to say 'When you express yourself in that way (using a specific example) it upsets the rest of the team. How do you think you could express yourself more positively?'.

Focused team coaching

Teams have a life of their own, and poor dynamics within a team can render it inefficient and non-productive. Recognizing and managing internal dynamics by coaching for performance is part of good leadership. The team may also need to be divided into sub-teams (such as veterinary surgeon/veterinary nurse teams, the surgery nurse team, the veterinary team as a whole) to coach most effectively. The principles are the same as for individual coaching: clear, precise feedback about performance should be given, working towards an agreed goal or goals.

Self-management and time

Learning to manage time effectively does not require complex analyses and spreadsheets. It does require a critical review of how time is spent and then implementation of some changes that will help improve the use of time. Examples of common time-wasters and time-savers are given in Figure 18.5.

Time-wasters

- Worrying about something and putting it off, so it takes longer to make a decision
- Creating inefficiency by implementing instead of analysing first
- Unanticipated interruptions that do not pay off
- Procrastinating
- Making unrealistic time estimates
- Unnecessary errors (not enough time to do it right, but enough time to do it again)
- Dealing with emergencies
- Poor organization
- Ineffective meetings
- Micro-managing and not delegating
- Doing urgent rather than important tasks
- Poor planning and lack of contingency plans
- Lack of priorities, standards, policies, and procedures

Time-savers

- Manage the decision-making process, not the decisions
- Concentrate on doing only one task at a time
- Establish daily, short-, mid-, and long-term priorities and stick to them
- Handle correspondence quickly with short letters and e-mails where appropriate
- Throw away unneeded things
- Establish personal deadlines and organizational deadlines
- Don't waste other people's time, e.g. with unnecessarily long phone calls to clients
- Ensure all meetings have a purpose and time limit; include only essential people
- Get rid of work that is not really necessary, or due to poor or unwieldy systems
- Maintain accurate calendars and stick to them
- Know when to stop a task, policy, or procedure
- Delegate everything possible and empower subordinates
- Keep things simple
- Set aside time to accomplish high priority tasks
- Set aside time for reflection
- Use checklists and 'to do' lists

18.5 Examples of common time-wasters and time-savers.

Focussing on the big rocks

To identify the important areas of your life, imagine having a glass jar which you aim to fill with big rocks:

- Is the jar full yet? No, then you can pour in some gravel.
- Is the jar full yet? No, then you can add some sand.
- Is the jar full yet? No, then you can pour in some water. Now the jar is full.

Now try and imagine this process in the opposite order. Put the water, sand and gravel in first, i.e., the trivial and less important things that happen in life; the chances are you won't be able to fit the big rocks in the jar.

What does this example show? It shows the necessity for dealing with big rocks first, and this can be applied to time and task management at work as well.

The following steps will aid effective time management.

- **Don't procrastinate; get started** – Often, more time and energy is wasted avoiding doing something than actually needs to be spent on doing it.
- **Get into a routine** – Routines may curb creativity but they also release time and energy. Time should be planned using a day-planning calendar and this calendar should be followed. Larger tasks should be prioritized and completed ahead of smaller ones.
- **Be able to say 'No'** – Saying yes to too many things not only erodes the time needed to spend on one's own activities, it also means living to the priorities of others. Saying no is about learning to set healthy boundaries.
- **Beware of committing to unimportant activities** – Especially when they are far in the future. Although a diary may currently be empty, it will definitely not remain this way and an unimportant activity will remain just that – unimportant.
- **Divide large tasks into a series of small tasks** – By creating small manageable tasks, the entire task will eventually be accomplished. Also, by using a piecemeal approach, it can be more easily fitted into a tight schedule.
- **Accept 'good enough'** – Perfectionism has its place, but for most activities there is not much to be gained from putting extra effort into it. Save perfectionism for the tasks that need it.
- **Deal with it for once and for all** – Often a task is started, then left for a while, then picked up again on a repeating cycle. Either deal with the task right away or plan when to deal with it and stick to the plan.
- **Set start and stop times** – This helps to schedule activities. Challenge the theory, 'work expands to fill the allotted time' by shaving time off deadlines in order to improve efficiency.
- **Plan activities** – Schedule a regular time to plan activities. Allow the time to plan wisely.

References and further reading

Blanchard K, Zigarmi P and Zigarmi D (1994) *Leadership and the one minute manager: Increasing effectiveness through situational leadership*. Harper Collins, London

Buckingham M and Coffman C (2005) *First, Break All the Rules: What the World's Greatest Managers Do Differently*. Simon and Schuster, New York

Collins J (2001) *Good to Great*. Random House Business Books, London

Collins JC and Porras JI (1996) Building your company's vision. *Harvard Business Review*, Sept–Oct, pp. 64–77

Covey SR (1989) *The Seven Habits of Highly Effective People*. Simon and Schuster, New York

Delong TJ, Gabaro JJ and Lees RJ (2007) *When Professionals Have to Lead*. Harvard Business School Press, Boston

Drucker PF (2001) *The Essential Drucker*. Harper Business, New York

Goleman D (1995) *Emotional Intelligence: Why It Can Matter More Than IQ*. Bloomsbury Publishing, London

Goleman D (1999) *Working with Emotional Intelligence*. Bloomsbury Publishing, London

Headache Study Group of The University of Western Ontario (1986) Predictors of outcome in headache patients presenting to family physicians – a one year prospective study. *Headache: The Journal of Head and Face Pain* **26**, 285–294

Kotter JP (1996) *Leading Change*. Harvard Business School Press, Boston

Maister D (2008) *Strategy and the Fat Smoker*. Spangel Press, Boston

Maxwell JC (2007) *The 21 Irrefutable Laws of Leadership*. Thomas Nelson, Nashville

Shilcock M and Sutchfield G (2003) *Veterinary Practice Management: a Practical Guide*. Elsevier Science, Oxford

Wheeler K (2006) Permission to euthanize. *Veterinary Economics* **47**, 88

Self-improvement resource: http://www.i-choose-self-improvement.com

Stress-management tools: http://www.cipd.co.uk/hr-resources/guides/line-management-behaviour-stress-work-line-managers-guidance.aspx

Managing people

19

Maggie Shilcock

Staff are likely to be the practice's biggest ongoing expense. For most practices somewhere in the region of 40% of outgoing costs will be spent on staff salaries and recruitment. However, staff are also the practice's greatest asset. They are the face of the practice and generate the practice's income. It is vital to the success of the practice that staff are well managed so that the practice obtains the maximum return on its 'investment' in them and they gain maximum job satisfaction and opportunities. Poor staff management will result in demotivated, under-performing staff and this will give rise to reduced client numbers and, ultimately, a reduction in income generated.

> **KEY POINT**
>
> Essential to any successful practice is the culture it adopts. That culture should run throughout all the work and operations of the practice and needs to be discussed, agreed and followed by all practice personnel.

The management of a veterinary practice should come within a framework that embraces clear strategies, actions and reviews. Practice planning should consider business, learning and development, people management and leadership strategies. Practice operations should encompass the effectiveness of management, how staff are recognized and rewarded for their work, how staff are involved in the practice and in decision-making and how their learning needs are met. A practice should review its performance continually and look for ways to improve further. By adopting business process management in this way, the practice can become more efficient, more effective and more capable of change, because it is taking its staff along with it at every turn.

Staffing the practice

A veterinary practice should at all times be staffed appropriately to provide for the care and treatment of patients. The number of staff and the skills and qualifications required should be set by the owner of the practice, bearing in mind the volume and nature of the veterinary duties and work to be carried out.

Provision must also be made for staff absence, both for annual holidays and for sickness, so that the practice is not so understaffed that it is unable to provide the required level of service to its clients. This may mean that some staff have to work extra hours when colleagues are absent, or must become multiskilled. Staff absenteeism may also be covered by the use of locum nurses and veterinary surgeons.

As well as covering the normal working day, emergency out-of-hours work must also be covered if it is not outsourced (see Chapter 21). Practices covering their own inpatient and emergency work should consider the number of nurses and veterinary surgeons required to be on duty. The practice must comply with the Working Time Regulations 1998 and the Working Time (Amendment) Regulations 2003. It must also comply with health and safety legislation (e.g. Health and Safety at Work etc. Act 1974), including that relating to lone working (The Management of Health and Safety at Work Regulations 1999 – Working Time Regulations) – see Chapters 20 and 21.

Requirements for 24-hour cover are set out in the RCVS Code of Professional Conduct and Supporting Guidance and in the RCVS Practice Standards Scheme (PSS).

Roles and responsibilities

The veterinary practice team usually includes all or a combination of the following.

Practice owners

The owners of the practice take on the full responsibility for running the business and for the wellbeing of the employees. Their role is to ensure that the practice provides excellent care for clients and their animals, while also keeping the business financially successful. The owner is responsible for complying with all legislation relating to a small business, including employment law (Chapter 20) and health and safety (Chapter 22), and takes the ultimate responsibility for any clinical errors or client complaints.

Practice managers

Practice managers relieve the owners of the basic management of their practice, enabling them to devote more time to their clinical or other roles. However, the role of the practice manager varies considerably, depending not only on the size of the practice, but also on the job description and authority given to them by the practice owner. In some cases the practice manager is a manager in name only and may be carrying out the function of an administrator with no real decision-making responsibilities, while others may be responsible for disciplinary and grievance procedures, staff appraisals and business planning. In smaller practices the practice manager may take responsibility for human resources, health and safety, office management, marketing and financial management, while in larger practices there may be a number of managers, each concentrating on a specific aspect of management.

Veterinary surgeons

The veterinary surgeon's role is to carry out the clinical work of the practice. They are responsible for maintaining the health of clients' animals and for directing and supervising veterinary nurses and clinical support staff.

Nursing staff

Qualified and student veterinary nurses give clinical and surgical support to the veterinary surgeon, as well as providing expert nursing care to hospitalized animals. Many run their own nurse clinics, advising clients on various aspects of pet healthcare. Animal nursing assistants and veterinary care assistants give practical nursing support and animal care under direction. Many nurses also carry out reception duties, particularly in smaller practices.

Reception staff

The receptionist's role is to provide an interface between the client and the practice. They have one of the most varied roles in the practice. They are responsible for answering telephone enquiries, booking appointments and operations, and giving general veterinary advice, as well as promoting the practice and its services to the client. Ensuring clients pay their bills according to the practice's terms and conditions is another key responsibility.

Administrative staff

No medium or large practice can operate without the help of administrative staff, whose role is to ensure that the basic administration of the practice runs smoothly. They are usually responsible for paying practice bills, chasing unpaid client invoices, keeping practice accounts and general record-keeping, IT and secretarial support.

Other support staff

Many practices will employ, often on a part-time basis, other support staff such as cleaners, gardeners and handymen/women.

Organizational structures

Size of practice

Veterinary practices vary in size from the small one-owner practice with perhaps two nurses and a receptionist, to multi-site practices employing large numbers of staff. The organizational structure will vary to suit the size and nature of the practice.

Below are examples of a typical hierarchical structure applied to several different sizes of practice.

Small one-site practices

In the small one-site practice, the owner usually takes responsibility for many of the management tasks, such as planning and development, budgeting, marketing and possibly IT, while delegating some roles to administrative assistants (Figure 19.1). A bookkeeper may be employed, often on a part-time basis, to manage the practice accounts, while other administrative roles, such as payroll, banking, client accounts and personnel, may be the responsibility of an administrative assistant. Health and safety and stock control may form part of a veterinary nurse's role. This will vary somewhat from practice to practice, depending to a large extent on the time and interest the owner has in carrying out management tasks.

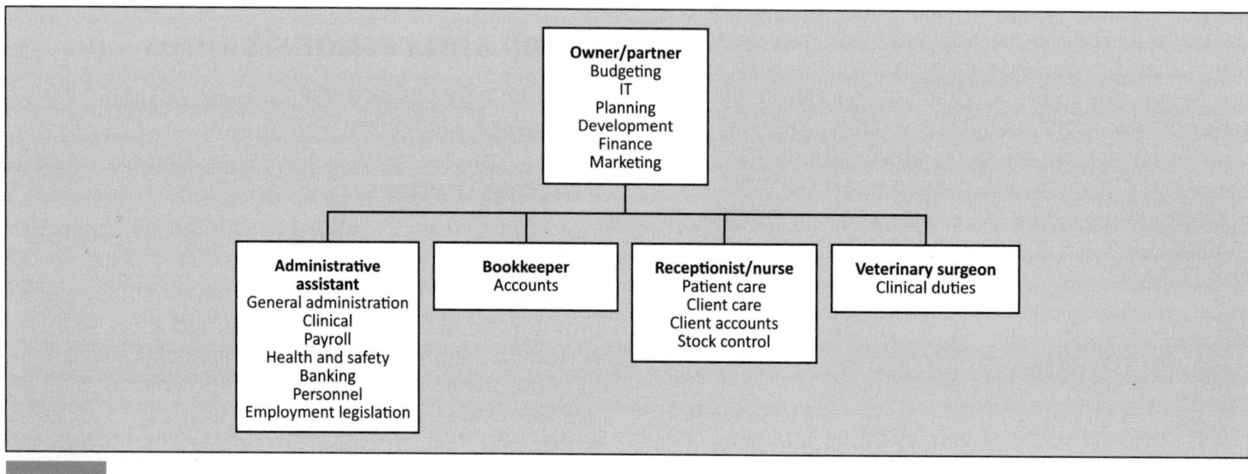

19.1 Typical organizational structure of a small practice.

Larger practices

Larger practices with perhaps a number of owners and assistant veterinary surgeons, and two or three sites, are increasingly likely to have a dedicated managing partner or to employ a practice manager or administrator. The manager is responsible for the daily management of the practice, often delegating a significant number of administrative tasks to other members of the practice (Figure 19.2). In this size of practice there will be greater delegation of roles and separation of tasks. The example shows a practice with a dedicated dispensing team who take responsibility for drug purchase stock control and health and safety with regard to COSHH. However, in other large practices it might be the nursing team that is responsible for stock control and health and safety.

Large multi-site practices

Large multi-site practices (three or more sites) are generally too big to enable management control by a single manager. There may be regional managers responsible for overseeing a number of specific sites and the organizational structure shown in Figure 19.3 is often employed. As the business size grows, the organization becomes more structured and roles become more specific. In a typical large multi-site practice there will be a specific manager for each management area, whilst at each site there is often a 'local manager' responsible for the day-to-day running of the individual practice.

Corporate and joint venture practices

Some corporate practices will organize their practices very much along the lines of the large multi-site practices described above. However, veterinary surgeons/nurses that have invested in joint venture schemes run and manage their practices on a daily basis, while sourcing management skills from the corporate body (Figure 19.4). Joint venture practices are usually small, with one or two veterinary surgeons together with a small number of veterinary nurses and/or receptionists; this is similar to the small one-site practices described above.

Organization

A hierarchical structure is not the only way to organize a practice. Taking a three-vet practice as an example, three different organization structures may be applied.

- **Hierarchical organization:** Figure 19.5 shows a typical top-down organization. Directions are passed from the owner or manager down the lines of command, and authority and responsibility are clearly defined. However, too much bureaucracy and slow communication channels can result and there may be little encouragement of independent thought or ownership of tasks.
- **Flat organization:** Figure 19.6 shows a flat, or horizontal, organizational structure with (in a small practice) no levels of intervening management.

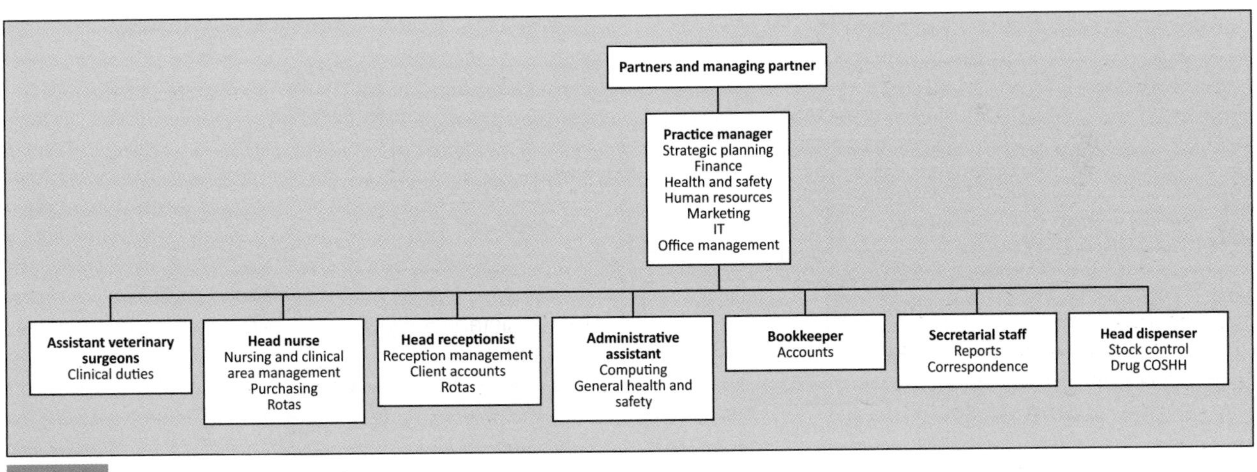

19.2 Typical organizational structure of a large clinic.

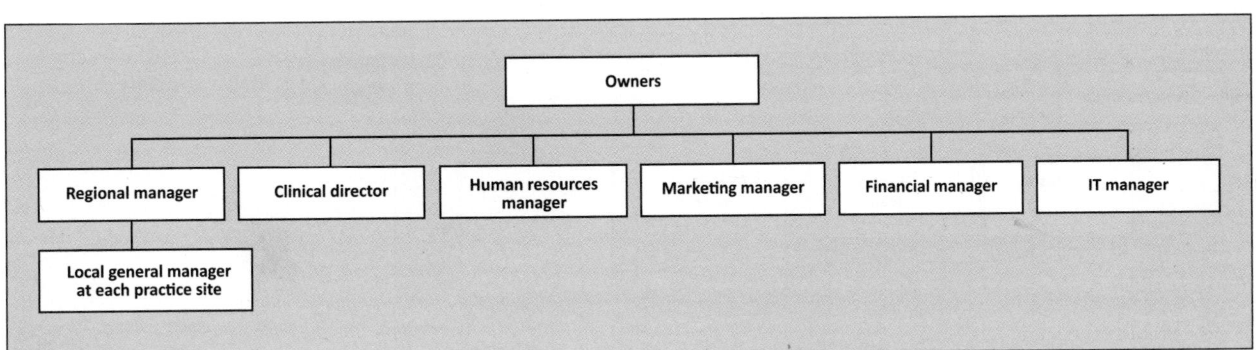

19.3 Typical organizational structure of a large multi-site clinic. In this example the regional manager has a strategic role, working on a par with departmental managers.

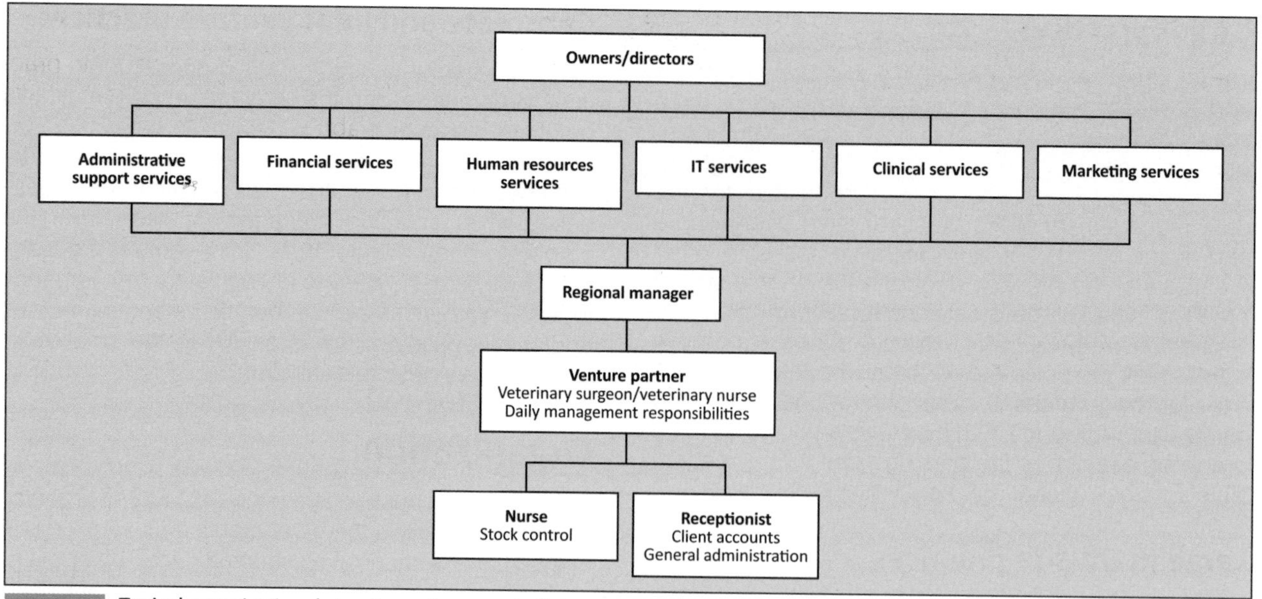

19.4 Typical organizational structure of corporate/joint venture clinics. In this example the regional manager has an implementing role.

Employees will be more productive and motivated, as they are more directly involved in decision-making and there is greater communication between management and employees, who have a very clear picture of the role of the business. However, everyone must communicate and work together effectively.

- **Matrix organization:** Figure 19.7 shows a matrix organizational structure based on a function and product approach, in which those that are skilled in similar areas are placed together to complete certain assignments. This allows the members of the team to share information and work more freely across traditional boundaries. For example, a specific client care initiative can pull members from each team together to complete the project. Members of different teams work together, reducing any 'them and us' culture. Individuals can be chosen to suit project requirements, increasing dynamism. Difficulties can arise, however, if a team has too much independence; projects may be more difficult to manage than if they were more closely monitored. People may also need to learn new skills very quickly.

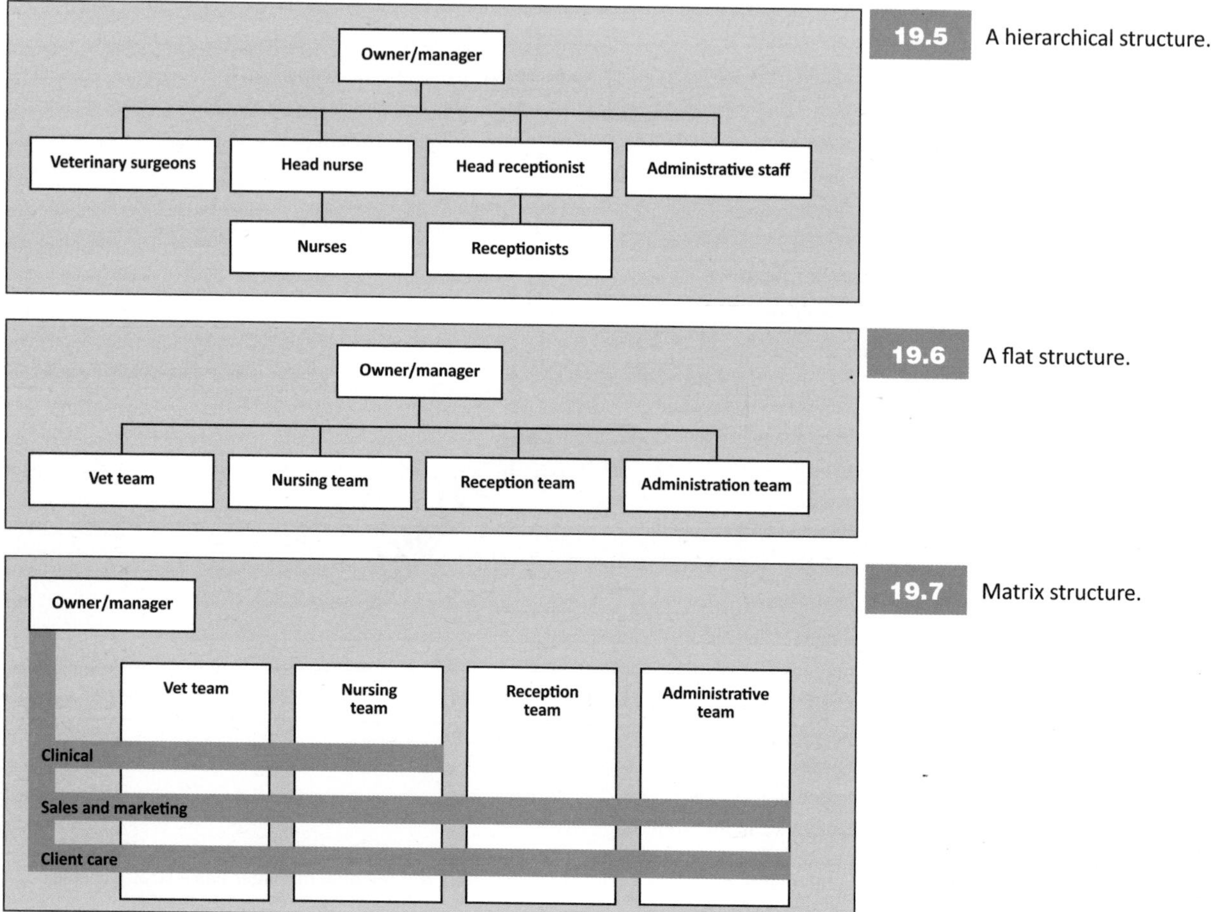

19.5 A hierarchical structure.

19.6 A flat structure.

19.7 Matrix structure.

KEY POINT

The most important people are **customers**, and where they are positioned in the structure will have a major impact on the success of the business.

Customers should have maximum contact with the people and functions of any organization. In the chart in Figure 19.8 the customer interfaces with the functions of the business and the practice staff support those functions in turn, so as to maximize effective customer service. Structures with several layers of the organization between staff and customers are less effective at responsive customer service. Direction is provided by senior management staff, who set up structures, organize management and help ensure the practice is moving in the right direction.

Reporting lines

Clear reporting lines are essential with any organizational structure. Figure 19.9 illustrates the reporting lines for a medium-sized practice with a hierarchical structure where a practice manager is employed. The clinical and the management reporting lines are shown, as these may not coincide for all issues.

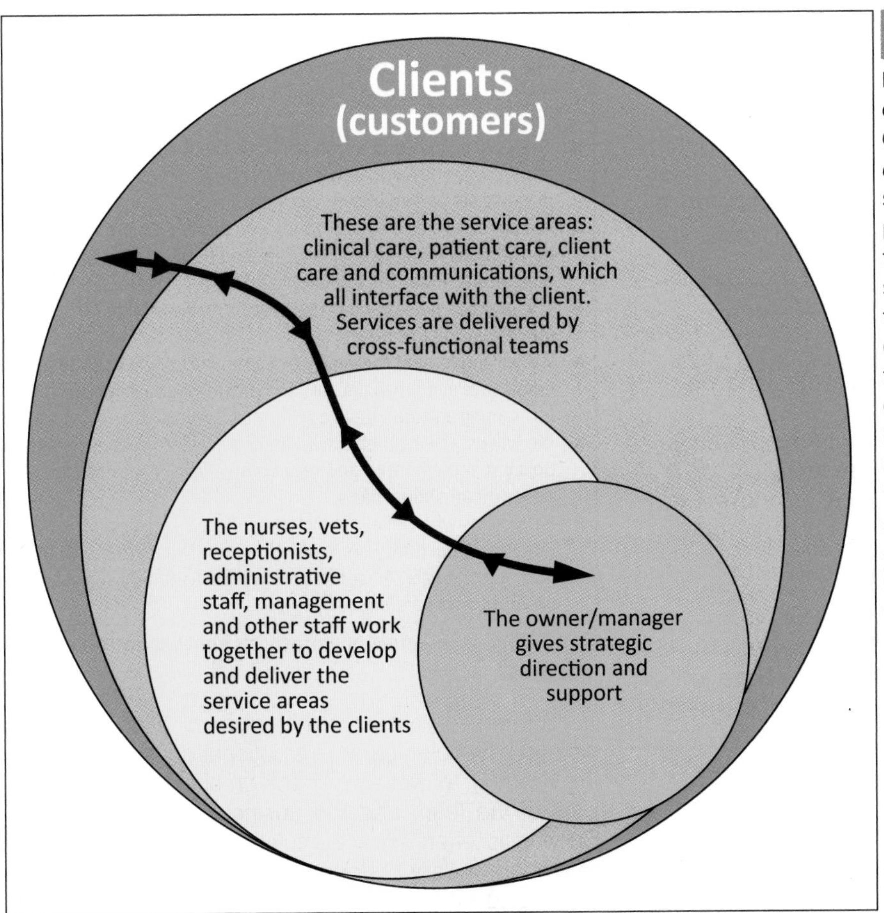

19.8 The customer-focused organizational approach. Individuals in every team interact with clients across the service areas. Cross-functional teams can be created *ad hoc* to develop and deliver new services and improve existing performance. The manager/owner sets the scene and strategic direction, and supports the service teams to deliver the best for each client. Day-to-day direction is from the team itself and from the client. There has to be a cross-team approach – i.e. everyone is responsible for ensuring the client's needs are met, not just in their narrow 'traditional' team area but across the service spectrum. The manager is offset in the chart, as he/she does not hide behind the staff, but interfaces with services and clients as well.

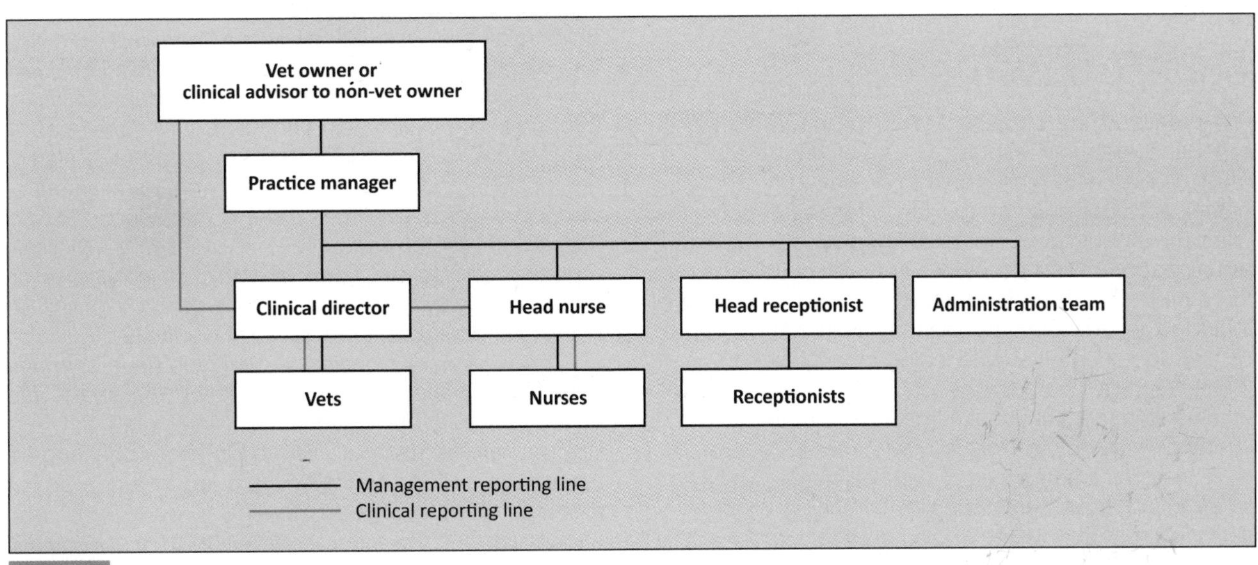

19.9 Reporting lines within the veterinary practice.

Job descriptions

KEY POINT

All staff, however many hours they work, should have a job description describing exactly what their job entails and listing their role, responsibilities and duties. This minimizes misunderstandings between employee and employer.

The job description:

- Should be formally agreed between employer and employee and reviewed regularly, at least annually. A good time for review is at appraisal
- Describes the job within the organizational structure of the practice
- Provides essential information and clarifies employer expectations to potential recruits and the recruiting team.
- Is an important tool for measuring job performance and a useful basis for staff appraisal.

The written job description should contain the following basic information:

- The job title
- The main purpose and responsibilities of the job role
- Lines of authority, specifying who the employee is responsible to and who they are responsible for. It should also include key staff liaison, i.e. those members of staff that the employee will be working with most closely
- Main duties
- Any occasional duties, e.g. covering for others. Adding the phrase 'and any other duties which may reasonably be required' covers the need to ask the employee to carry out occasional tasks that they might not normally expect to do
- Knowledge and skills required to carry out the job
- Any training that may be required.

Examples of job descriptions can be found at the end of this chapter. More information on the recruitment process is given later and in Chapter 20.

Equal opportunities

Full details of the Equality Act 2010 and compliance are dealt with in Chapter 20. A veterinary practice must do all that is reasonable to prevent any discriminatory acts from occurring, and offer equal opportunities to all staff and potential employees. A written equal opportunities policy, which should be given to all members of staff, is essential and should be included in any practice manual, staff handbook or similar document. It should include the following:

- The statement of intent, aims and objectives
- Who the policy applies to
- The commitments the practice will make
- Who will implement the policy
- How the policy will be implemented
- Monitoring and review
- How complaints will be dealt with.

An example of a practice's equal opportunities policy is given in Figure 19.10. Complying with the Equality Act 2010 involves not just the correct paperwork but also adopting a practice culture that embraces equal opportunities. This means that equal opportunity for all staff is a reality for every practice activity and is clear to the staff. Equal opportunities should be discussed at appraisals, considered whenever tasks are delegated or a promotion is considered, and included in training planning to ensure that staff have the necessary skills and understanding to implement the policy in their areas. Specific questions at staff appraisal could bring up the issues, and prompt discussion about equal opportunity in the workplace.

Practice policy on equal opportunities

- The practice aims to be an inclusive organization, where everyone is treated with respect and dignity and there is equal opportunity for all.
- This policy applies to all job applicants, employees, contract workers, agency workers/locums, trainee or work experience placements and volunteer workers.
- We are committed to promoting equality for all, promoting a harmonious working environment and fulfilling our legal obligations under the equality legislation.
- The practice manager has the specific responsibility for implementing this policy.
- We will implement this policy by communicating it in writing to employees and job applicants and providing equal opportunities for training and staff development to all employees.
- We will establish an effective monitoring system to ensure the policy is implemented and review the effectiveness of the policy on an annual basis.
- Employees who believe they have suffered any form of unequal opportunity are entitled to raise the matter with the practice manager. All complaints will be dealt with seriously, promptly and confidentially.

19.10 An example of a practice's equal opportunities policy.

Bullying, harassment and discrimination can have serious psychological and emotional consequences for the victim(s), as well as a knock-on effect on other members of the team and the business, if not addressed. Bullying is often an accumulation of small incidences which individually may appear trivial. These may range from nit-picking, fault-finding, constant criticism, undermining, disparaging patronizing remarks, ostracizing, deliberate isolation and exclusion, humiliating, giving 'the silent treatment' and deliberately expressing doubt over a person's performance or standard of work, through to the victim being shouted at or threatened. It can appear subtle to outsiders. Any member of staff in any position can be subject to bullying, harassment or discrimination at any time, and it is the responsibility of the employer to encourage openness, to facilitate reporting and to deal with all forms of bullying in an appropriate way. An example of a practice policy on bullying and harassment is given in Figure 19.11.

The veterinary practice should also have a written anti-discrimination policy known to all staff, and employers can be responsible if their staff act in a discriminatory manner which is not challenged. Again, the policy should be included in any practice manual, staff handbook or similar document, and should contain the same information as that required for an equal opportunities policy. An example of an anti-discrimination policy is given in Figure 19.12.

Practice policy on bullying and harassment

- We are committed to creating an environment in which individual differences and the contributions of all staff are recognized and valued. This environment should promote dignity and respect to all.
- No form of intimidation, bullying or harassment will be tolerated.
- Training, development and progression opportunities are available to everyone, and employment practices and procedures are regularly reviewed to ensure fairness.

Any action in breach of this policy will be treated seriously and subject to disciplinary procedure, and in serious cases may constitute gross misconduct. If any employee believes they have been treated inconsistently with this policy, or they come across discrimination within their employment, then they should speak to the Partners.

Sexual harassment

- Sexual harassment will not be permitted or condoned, and the Partners and employees all have the right to complain should it ever occur.
- Sexual harassment means unwanted conduct of a sexual nature or other conduct based on sex, affecting the dignity of women and men at work.
- Sexual harassment can include:
  - Unwelcome sexual attention
  - Subjecting an employee to insults or ridicule because of their sex
  - Suggesting that sexual favours may further someone's career or that the refusal of sexual favours may in some way damage their career
  - Over-familiar behaviour, including lewd and suggestive remarks
  - Display of sexually suggestive pictures or other material.
- What is sexual harassment to one person may not amount to sexual harassment to another. If it is unwanted by the recipient then it may amount to sexual harassment.
- It is up to each individual to decide what behaviour is acceptable to them and to decide what is offensive. If an individual decides that behaviour is offensive they must make it clear that they do not accept it. If the behaviour continues then it becomes sexual harassment. A serious incident of harassment may, in itself, constitute harassment.

The Partners will treat any report of sexual harassment seriously. Those complaining will be protected against any form of victimization or retaliation after bringing the complaint. The practice disciplinary procedure will be used, and serious sexual harassment may amount to gross misconduct and could lead then to dismissal.

A formal complaint of sexual harassment is a serious step to take. Any person who has been sexually harassed should therefore, wherever possible, try to tell the person that their behaviour is unacceptable and only formally complain when the behaviour persists. A formal complaint of sexual harassment should be pursued through the process set out in the practice's grievance procedure.

19.11 An example of a practice policy on bullying and harassment.

Practice policy on anti-discrimination

- It is the policy of the practice to maintain a working environment free from all forms of unlawful discrimination.
- The policy applies to all job applicants, employees, contract workers, agency workers/locums, trainee or work experience placements and volunteer workers, and covers discrimination on the following grounds:
  - Race
  - Gender
  - Disability
  - Sexual orientation
  - Age
  - Religion or belief.
- We are committed to fulfilling our legal obligations under the discrimination legislation.
- All staff have the responsibility for implementing this policy.
- We will implement this policy by communicating it in writing to employees and job applicants and providing equal opportunities for training and staff development to all employees. The practice will support staff as needed in the day-to-day implementation of this policy.
- We will establish an effective monitoring system to ensure this policy is implemented, and review the effectiveness of the policy on an annual basis.
- Employees who believe they have suffered any form of discrimination are entitled to raise the matter with the practice manager. All complaints will be dealt with seriously, promptly and confidentially.

19.12 An example of a practice's anti-discrimination policy.

More information on discrimination is given in Chapter 20. Both the Equality and Human Rights Commission (www.equalityhumanrights.com) and the DirectGov website (www.directgov.uk) provide very useful information on equal rights and discrimination.

KEY POINT

Although written policies must always be in place, this is not enough if the culture of the practice is not consistent with them. A culture of equality and anti-discrimination should run through the fabric of all management and employee actions and decisions, and be part of the everyday workings of the practice. Regular discussions of the issues are essential.

Health and wellbeing

Employers have an obligation to ensure the health and wellbeing of their employees while at work. This involves:

- Maintaining healthy relationships between staff
- Building trust between managers and employees
- Having policies and procedures that reward fairly
- Encouraging good communication (see Chapter 17)
- Managing discipline and grievances effectively (see Chapter 20).

Employees need to be involved in decisions that are made about their jobs and how things are done in the workplace, and they need reasonable control over the way they work and should be given the opportunity, where appropriate, for flexible working. Managing change to avoid stress is also crucial.

As with health and safety issues, employees have a responsibility to follow any policies and guidelines their employer has set out in order to provide and maintain health and wellbeing at work.

Providing a completely stress-free environment for staff is probably not possible, and a certain amount of stress is motivating. However, uncontrolled stress is harmful. At appraisal interviews, managers should be mindful of any stress-related concerns, and record and act upon anything that is apparently causing stress to the employee (see Chapter 18). Both ACAS (the Advisory, Conciliation and Arbitration Service; www.acas.org.uk) and the Health and Safety Executive (www.hse.gov.uk) produce excellent guidance notes and advice on preventing and dealing with work-related stress, including a management self-assessment guide.

KEY POINT

It is useful to remember the positive influence that work has on the lives of most employees and that small things can often make a huge difference in the workplace.

Health and wellbeing activities focused in the workplace will have more relevance to employees at work than activities taking place outside work.

The ACAS health, work and wellbeing checklist sets out the six main indicators or standards for health and wellbeing in the workplace:

- **Managers should be trained in people skills.** They should:
  - Be good communicators
  - Be able to deal with emotional employees
  - Understand stress and its causes
- **Employees should feel valued and involved in the organization.** They should:
  - Have control over where and when they do their job
  - Feel that managers listen to them
  - Have support and advice on health and safety issues
  - Be well informed and supported about change
- **Managers should be able to use appropriate health services to tackle absence and help people get back to work.** They should:
  - Use health professionals when necessary to help employees return to work
  - Tackle bullying and harassment at work
  - Make reasonable adjustments to accommodate disabled employees
- **Managers should promote an attendance culture.** They should:
  - Promote return to work discussions following sickness absence
  - Recognize the importance of rehabilitation following long-term sickness
  - Focus on positive aspects of employees' abilities
- **Jobs should be flexible and well designed.** Employees should:
  - Be given the opportunity to discuss flexible working
  - Be given the opportunity to put forward ideas about how their jobs could be improved
  - Receive suitable training and skill development
- **Managers should know how to manage common health problems such as mental health and musculoskeletal disorders.** They should:
  - Know key facts about important health issues, such as depression, back pain, drugs and alcohol.

Managers should explain policy implementation to employees and know the law on discrimination and victimization (see Chapter 20). More details on health and wellbeing standards can be found in the ACAS advisory booklet *Health Work and Wellbeing* and at the Investors in People website (www.investorsinpeople.co.uk). See Chapter 18 for more information on self-management and stress.

The practice manual and staff handbook

Providing employees with an agreed framework within which to operate is a vital part of a healthy and productive workplace. From the employee's perspective, understanding why they must do certain things in certain ways is key to job satisfaction and self-esteem. A written practice manual is a key tool with which to achieve both of these objectives.

The **staff handbook** should contain employment policies, practice rules, the main health and safety policy document and commonly referred to information such as common clinical protocols (e.g. vaccination). A copy of the staff handbook is usually (but not always) given to every staff member and is a useful reference, particularly for new members of staff. It is normally a pocket-sized affair. As a minimum, it should contain any supplementary information referred to in the employment contract or written statement. This would usually include the disciplinary and grievance policy, and sickness and absence policy.

The **practice manual**, on the other hand, normally refers to a comprehensive collection of written policies, procedures and protocols, and information necessary for the effective and correct running of the practice.

- **Practice policies** are the principles or rules that must be followed in order to achieve required outcomes or to comply with regulations, and the manual should set out in simple terms its policies on subjects such as health and safety, equal opportunities, discrimination, dress, behaviour, drink and drugs, and CPD, and its procedures for booking holidays, completing absence forms, etc.
- **Procedures** are specified sets of actions that need to be carried out in order to achieve the desired needs of the practice, and the manual might include information on cashing up, answering the telephone, fees and the charging policy.

- **Protocols** are the guidelines or rules agreed by the team, which should be followed by all staff in the same way, and the manual should include protocols on subjects such as worming and flea advice, investigation of common problems, nurse clinics, handling of certain situations, etc.

The manual should be respected and used as a basis for everyday working. To retain the respect of staff, it should be followed by everyone and kept updated as things change. Every member of staff should have access to a copy (preferably one each) and should have read or been taught its contents. It is important to discuss the contents of the manual at the induction of a new employee, rather than relying upon the employee to read it. It is also good practice for the employee to sign a statement to confirm that they are fully aware of and understand the contents. This can be done at the induction appraisal (see later).

The manual can take the form of a booklet, a loose-leaf folder or a computer resource, whichever is easiest to use and most appropriate for the practice. Specific information must be easy to find, with a clear listing of sections and their contents, and possibly also an index. Provision for updating should be considered when deciding on the format. Keeping staff informed of any updates is essential. Staff memos or e-mails may be sufficient for minor updates or, in the case of a loose-leaf format, a replacement page can be issued to all staff. For more major changes, staff meetings and consultations may be in order.

Every practice will have its own priorities, but the information below is suggested.

Section 1: General

- Introduction – What the manual is for and what it contains.
- Mission statement – This is usually a simple statement about what the practice is trying to achieve. Mission statements are discussed later in this chapter and in Chapter 23.

Section 2: Practice structure

- Practice history – Simple details of how long the practice has existed and how it has developed.
- Practice premises – Details of the premises, including any branch surgeries, maps, telephone numbers, etc.
- The work of the practice – Species treated and special organizations who are clients.
- The practice structure – An explanation of the organizational structure of the practice (see above) and a list of personnel and their titles and roles in the practice.
- Practice hours – Details of opening hours and emergency provision.

Section 3: Personnel and administration

- Employment policies.
- Training and development – The CPD policy (Figure 19.13).
- New staff induction – An explanation of the induction programme all new staff will follow in the first few days of their appointment. (Induction of new staff is dealt with in detail later in this chapter.)
- Holidays and holiday booking procedures.
- Absence from work – Details of the practice regulations regarding absence through sickness, absence through official reasons such as jury service, absence on compassionate grounds and absence for family responsibilities, who to report to and by when if there is a need to be absent from work.
- Dress and appearance – An explanation of how staff are expected to look and dress (Figure 19.14).
- Behaviour – An explanation of how staff are expected to behave, including the practice's policy on drink and drugs (Figure 19.15).

Practice policy on CPD

- We actively encourage the personal development of all staff and the acquisition of new skills relevant to the position they hold.
- We require all professional staff to complete at least the minimum CPD required by the RCVS Code of Professional Conduct.
- Maintaining clinical and non-clinical skills and staying up to date with new knowledge and techniques is the responsibility of each employee.
- We expect each employee to maintain an up-to-date CPD record.

In order to support staff, the practice will also:

- Help to identify training and development priorities for each team and individual within the practice
- Provide relevant training in house or through external providers
- Keep records of the training provided to staff
- Monitor and evaluate the efficiency and effectiveness of all training and development carried out
- Review training and development needs annually.

19.13 An example of a practice CPD policy.

Practice policy on personal hygiene and appearance

The appearance of all staff is considered by the practice to be extremely important in terms of meeting clients' expectations. Staff are expected to appear neat, clean and tidy with appropriate dress for the post they hold, as detailed below.

- All staff members are identified by name badges or embroidered uniform and are expected to wear this identification at all times.
- Hair must always be clean and tidy. Long hair must be worn off the face and tied back during theatre procedures.
- Moustaches and beards must be kept neat and trim.
- Fingernails must always be kept short and clean. Coloured nail varnish is not allowed.
- Jewellery may be worn but only stud earrings, wedding rings and watches. No other jewellery is acceptable.
- Makeup, if worn, should be tasteful and in keeping with a professional image.
- Uniform and clothing must be regularly laundered, in good repair and ironed.
- Shoes must be clean and polished.
- The wearing of non-practice badges is only permitted with the consent of the practice manager.

19.14 An example of a personal hygiene and appearance policy. Additional biosecurity measures, such as bare below the elbow and no hand or wrist jewellery, may be necessary depending on the job role.

Practice policy on behaviour

- Staff are expected to conduct themselves in an appropriate and professional manner at all times. Any behaviour that reflects badly on the practice or the profession must be avoided.
- Staff must avoid giving offence to a client or potential client. Staff should never argue with, or be rude or offensive to, a client.
- Chewing gum at work is not permitted.
- The illegal use of prohibited substances at any time, but specifically on practice premises, is incompatible with employment by the practice. If misuse is discovered, offending staff may be dismissed without further warning.
- Smoking will not be permitted anywhere on the premises, including the grounds.
- Alcohol consumption during work or duty hours is not permitted.
- Honesty is expected in all aspects of a member of staff's work.

19.15 An example of a practice behaviour policy.

- Personal communications at work – A statement outlining the practice rules on use of personal mobiles at work, the personal use of the practice telephones and the personal use of the practice computers for e-mails and the Internet (see Chapters 4 and 16).
- Security – Practice procedures for staff personal safety, such as panic buttons and lone working (see Chapter 22). Rules about dealing with cash, computer discs, alarms, etc. (see Chapter 16).
- Use of practice vehicles and private cars – Rules for the use of the practice vehicles and what to do if staff have an accident when driving a practice vehicle, car parking rules on the practice premises, and the driving for work policy (see Chapter 16).
- Staff pets – The practice policy for the treatment of staff pets should be explained, along with any staff discounts allowed. The practice's policy regarding staff pets at work should also be in writing.
- Disciplinary procedure – An explanation should be given of the steps in the disciplinary procedure followed by the practice (see Chapter 20). Examples should be given of what is considered unsatisfactory conduct, misconduct and gross misconduct, and the possible consequences.
- Grievance procedure – An explanation should be given of the steps in the grievance procedure that is followed by the practice (see Chapter 20).
- Appraisals – An explanation of the purpose of appraisals and how they are carried out in the practice. Appraisals are discussed later in this chapter.
- Equal opportunities policy – See earlier.
- Anti-discrimination policy – See earlier.
- Confidentiality – A statement about the confidentiality of practice and client records. Staff may be required to sign a confidentiality agreement (Figure 19.16).

KEY POINT

Clear guidance on confidentiality is essential for all staff, including temporary staff and visitors such as work experience students. Requiring a signature on the policy will highlight the importance of the issue.

This agreement is between:

Practice name

and

Staff member

- The business of *practice name* is confidential. You agree that you will not use, divulge or communicate to any person, firm or organization (and in the course of your business) any of the trade secrets or other confidential, technical or commercial information of the practice relating to the business, organization, accounts, analysis or other affairs of the practice and partners which you may have received or obtained while working for the practice. This includes any information relating to the trading position of the practice, including in particular names of clients or customers and any document or item marked as confidential. This restriction will continue to apply after the termination of your employment but will cease to apply to any information which may come into the public domain through disclosure by the partners.
- Client records must be treated as confidential at all times and no information about a client or their pets may be divulged to anyone not in the employment of *practice name* or on the Internet or any social networking site.

Signed .... (staff member)

Date ....

19.16 An example of a confidentiality agreement.

Section 4: Client care

- Client care standards – A statement on how staff are expected to behave towards and communicate with the general public. This should include standards expected for answering the telephone, making appointments, recognizing emergencies, booking operations, and advising on veterinary products and practice services (see Chapters 5 and 27).
- Complaints handling – A statement about how the practice client complaints procedure operates, explaining how the complaint is received, recorded and dealt with and how the results are communicated to the client (see Chapter 17).

Section 5: Health and safety

The full practice health and safety policy should be included here. Health and safety is dealt with in Chapter 22.

Recruitment

Staff need to understand that by delivering practice services and benefits and satisfying customers, they are delivering what the practice has promised and thereby reinforcing the brand. It is they who ultimately create a successful or unsuccessful practice and, although recruiting a new member of staff involves a considerable amount of time, effort and money, it is well worth it if the right person is appointed.

Identifying the role

KEY POINT

Before planning any recruitment advertisement, it is essential to be clear about exactly what the practice is looking for in a new employee.

The following questions should be considered.

What will the person do?

It is vital to be absolutely clear about what the job entails. Is it the same job that the previous occupant has just left, or does it need to be changed? Is there a need to add extra duties, change the emphasis of the job, or give the role more responsibility? This is the time to make changes to the job description if required.

What kind of person is required?

It is important to have a good idea of the kind of person needed and the skills they should have. A profile should be drawn up, listing essential and desirable qualifications, experience, communication skills, client care skills, personality, the need to be able to drive a vehicle, and so on (Figure 19.17).

Skills required

- Educational standard/qualifications
- Work experience
- Generic or general skills required
- Specialist skills required
- Computer and IT skills
- Communication and people skills
- Ability to work as a team member

Personal profile

- Personality
- Flexibility
- Travelling time from home to work that is acceptable
- Driving licence
- Date available to start work

19.17 Issues to consider for a personal skills profile. This will vary in level of detail according to the job role and the expected range of applicants for the position.

What is being offered?

The practice should think about the salary package it is prepared to offer, the hours of work, rotas, night duty, working conditions and the training and CPD to be provided, and what benefits will be given. Is there a private healthcare scheme, accommodation, car allowance, pension scheme, CPD allowance or staff discount? These are all things the potential candidates will want to know.

Advertising the post

Where a post is advertised depends very much on the job. Support staff posts would normally be advertised in the local press, while veterinary surgeon and veterinary nursing posts would usually be advertised nationally, almost always in veterinary journals but increasingly on appropriate websites. Most veterinary posts are advertised for up to 4 weeks, while local advertising for support staff may be on a week-by-week basis.

Having established the job specification, an advertisement will need to be designed that will attract the right candidates (Figure 19.18). The kind of person required and the experience they need should be indicated, to avoid wasting both the practice's and the applicant's time. Care should be taken to avoid any wording that could be interpreted as misleading or discriminatory. More information on job advertising compliance is given in Chapter 20.

- Practice logo and/or name
- The job title or eye-catching headline
- Brief resumé of what the practice does
- Details of the job (responsibilities, duties, hours, etc.)
- The skills, abilities, sort of person required
- The benefits that go with the post
- Ways to apply (application form, application letter and/or CV)
- Contact details for further information (if appropriate)
- Closing date
- Any additional relevant accreditations, e.g. Investors in People, Positive about Disabled People

19.18 Items to be included in a job advertisement. It should be borne in mind that every job advert is also a practice advert.

KEY POINT

A job advertisement is an opportunity to market the practice, as is the whole of the recruitment process. It is a chance to show applicants how good the practice is and how good an employer it is. However, it is important not to oversell the job.

Some adverts ask for CVs, whereas others indicate that job application forms should be requested. CVs are difficult to compare fairly and come in a variety of formats, while application forms ask the same questions of all candidates. Generally, the use of application forms is a fairer and more straightforward selection method. A job application form allows the interviewer to probe more deeply into the candidate's experience and suitability, and perhaps makes it easier to choose a shortlist of interviewees, as gaps in experience and training should be easier to spot. Application forms and CVs should not be mixed when selecting. It is also helpful when defending a claim for discrimination if the practice can show that everyone has completed the same job application form. A closing date for the job application must always be given, and the post should also be advertised internally so that all current employees have the opportunity to apply for it. An example of a job application form can be found at the end of this chapter.

References

It is standard practice to ask potential employees to provide details of referees on their CV or application form. Current or former employers, however, are under no legal obligation to provide a reference. If a reference is given, there are no rules to say how comprehensive it must be.

Many organizations, including veterinary practices, have a policy when contacted for references concerning ex-employees, and this is strongly recommended. It is very important that the policy names those members of staff who are authorized to give official practice references. and this must be known by all staff. The permission of the leaver is essential. If employees ask other members of staff for references it must be clear that: these are personal; they do not represent the practice; and they are not on practice headed paper. All members of staff should be clear about the possible consequences of inaccurate or misleading references.

Some organizations will simply not provide references; others will verify the dates of employment, position title and salary only. This policy avoids any possibility of being sued by a former employee who may claim he/she was defamed by the organization. Many employers, however, are only too happy to help by offering a meaningful reference for a good ex-employee.

A referee has a duty to take reasonable care not to give misleading information about the employee, so it is quite possible that a current or previous employer may not disclose that an employee has performed at an unacceptably low level or has been dismissed for a reason that would cast doubt on his/her suitability for future employment. It is always worth asking for, and following up, references and it is worth asking permission to contact any of the previous employers – not just the previous one. In order to give a meaningful reference, it is helpful if the referee is given some details of the proposed job role and a list of the information the prospective employer is looking for. This will usually include the question 'Would you re-employ the candidate?' If an employer is provided with a poor reference from a candidate's previous employer, the offer of employment can be withdrawn. References should always be treated confidentially by the manager and interviewing team, and should be filed with the other interview paperwork.

An example of a reference request form can be found at the end of this chapter.

Pre-employment health checks

Information on pre-employment health checks can be found in Chapter 20.

Selecting for interview

Matching the applicant's CV or application form to the job description and personal profile requirements can be a difficult task. Instinct can play a part in selection and that 'feeling' about an application can often be the correct one.

In addition to checking the applicant's qualifications, the way any supporting letter/e-mail is set out should be considered, along with its neatness (the handwriting if it is handwritten), and the grammar, as well as the content and reasons given for wanting the job. The application should be studied carefully, looking out for gaps in employment, checking that experience is relevant, and looking for indications given of future ambitions. Hobbies, interests, etc., should be looked at, and whether the candidate sounds like the sort of person who would fit in with existing staff or into the locality should be considered. Any recommendations that may have been given (and who they are from) should also be considered.

The applications should then be divided into three groups:

A. Yes – Interview
B. Possible – Only interview after group A interviews
C. No – Do not interview.

All members of the interview panel should carry out the above procedure, independently if possible. Group C applicants should be informed immediately that they have not been selected for interview.

The interview

Good interviewing has three phases: pre-interview planning, conducting the interview and post-interview assessment. An interview checklist should be drawn up to make sure that each phase has been carefully considered.

- **Who will interview the candidates?** Ideally, candidates should be interviewed by the person who will be their immediate supervisor and the practice manager or managing partner. It is unwise to have too many people interviewing as this can be intimidating.
- **Where will the interviews take place?** Interviews should take place in a quiet room away from the hustle and bustle of the practice and where there will be no interruptions. Staff should also be informed that interviewing is taking place.
- **When will the interviews take place?** Interviews should be timetabled so that all of the interviewers are free. If possible, they should take place over a short period of time so that all the candidates are fresh in the interviewers' memories. It is also sensible to consider how far the candidate will have to travel to get to the practice when scheduling their interview (e.g. the interview for the candidate that lives 200 miles away should not be scheduled for 9 am).
- **What questions will be asked? Who will ask each of the questions?** This should be discussed and agreed between interviewers beforehand.
- **How long will the interviews be?** At least 30–45 minutes should be allowed for each interview. More time may be needed for more senior positions, second interviews and for writing up and discussions between interviews.
- **Who will show the candidates around the practice?** The candidate should be shown around the practice; this may be before they are interviewed, or possibly mid-interview. This places the interview in a better context and enables candidates to ask questions about what they have seen. It is often a good idea to ask one of the candidate's potential colleagues to give the practice tour. The candidate will be able to identify with this member of staff and the member of staff can assess how the candidate might fit in with other members of the team.
- **How will the interviews be assessed?**
- **Will there be second interviews?** These can be cancelled later if there is one outstanding candidate.
- **What records need to be kept?**

KEY POINT

The interviewer should not take phone calls during an interview and all mobile phones should be switched off.

The practice is also trying to sell the job to the candidate. The benefits of working with the practice should be outlined, ensuring that the expectations of the candidate are matched by what they see. It would be disappointing if the best candidate turned down the job because they had not been given the right impression of the practice.

KEY POINT

Candidates invited to the practice for an interview should be asked to bring identification, proof of qualifications, original certificates, etc., once the practice has checked the RCVS registers or VN list, as applicable.

Interview candidates should be given enough notice, as the best candidates may well be in a job where they will be reluctant to inconvenience their current employer with short-notice leave. It is often a good idea to contact potential candidates for reception-based jobs by telephone to offer them an interview, just to hear how they sound on the other end of the telephone. Is this the voice the practice wants its clients to hear? Candidates must be told how long the process will take on the day, so they can plan work absence and travel.

The structure of the interview

There is a logical order to an interview, which, if followed, enables a smooth progress from greeting to farewell.

1. The candidate should be welcomed using their name. This is polite and indicates friendliness.
2. The candidate should be introduced to the interviewers and their role in the practice explained.
3. The candidate should be invited to sit down, indicating where they should sit. They should not be placed in front of a row of interviewers. The seating arrangements should be as informal and comfortable as possible.
4. The candidate should be put at ease, e.g. by asking them what their journey was like or if they know the area. This helps to break the ice and makes the candidate feel a little more comfortable.
5. The interview procedure should be explained, making sure the candidate understands how the interview will be conducted and how long it will be.
6. The candidate should be allowed to introduce themselves; this also helps them to relax. They should be asked to talk about themselves and their career to date.
7. The interview questions should then be asked as arranged beforehand with colleagues, but members of the interview panel should always be prepared to alter or abandon questions if necessary, especially if a 'new line of enquiry' arises. The interview questions should be designed to obtain as much information as possible about the candidate, their ability, experience and personality.

   Open questions should be asked to reveal what a person has actually done or experienced, by enabling them to talk about events or situations rather than giving short yes or no answers – e.g. 'Tell me about the last time...', 'Tell me about the last complaint you had to deal with,' 'Describe the last difficult case you had to operate on,' 'What did you find most (or least) motivating in your last job?' Open questions can be followed by probing questions if the answer given is not satisfactory, but closed questions should be avoided unless necessary for clarification. The secret is to get the candidate to talk to the interviewers. The more they talk, the more the panel will find out and the better they will be able to judge the candidate's suitability

   Behavioural and situational questions should also be asked. These look for specific examples of past behaviour that show that the candidate has the required abilities for the role. Behavioural questions require the candidate to describe how they have performed a number of different duties based on their past experience. This allows the interviewer to find out about the candidate's past behaviour, how they carried out tasks, and the situations or circumstances that they have dealt with, i.e. *what they did*. Situational questions require the candidate to describe how they would deal with a particular hypothetical scenario, i.e. *what they would do.*

   Examples of interview questions for vets, nurses and receptionists are shown in Figures 19.19 to 19.21. Discriminatory questions must not be asked, e.g. relating to age, sex, marital status, religion, ethnic background or such family matters as child care arrangements (see Chapter 20).

   Notes should be made. It can be a good idea to have a fresh sheet of questions for each candidate so that notes can be made directly against the question, remembering to identify the applicant on each sheet.
8. The candidate should always be given time for questions at the end of the interview.
9. Interviewers should ensure they have references and permission to follow them up.
10. The next stage of the process should then be explained to the candidate (e.g. whether there will be second interviews). The candidate should be told how (and when) a decision will be reached and the job offer will be made (e.g. by letter or telephone). They should also be told how to claim expenses if this is the practice policy.
11. The candidate should be thanked for coming. Politeness and friendliness should be maintained to the closing of the interview. The candidate should be left with a good impression of the practice.
12. Time should be taken once the candidate has left to complete any candidate assessment forms while impressions are still fresh in the interviewers' minds.

Receptionist

- What attracted you to apply for this post?
- Why do you want to leave your present post?
- What were the things you liked most and least about your last job?
- How does this job fit in with your long-term career objectives?
- What motivates you?
- What situations do you find difficult or uncomfortable?
- There are happy and sad occasions involved in working in a veterinary practice. How do you think you would cope with the sad things?
- What qualities do you possess that make you a good receptionist?
- What do you think clients are looking for from the receptionist?
- What differences have you found between working alone and working in a group of people?
- Can you think of any mistakes you have made in your current job and what you learnt from them?
- Can you think of an example of having to work with someone who was difficult to get along with and how you handled this situation?
- Veterinary practices provide more services and sell more products than they used to. What sales and marketing skills do you have and how would you feel about promoting new products and services?
- Give some examples of changes or improvements you have made in your current/previous role.
- What experience do you have of dealing with difficult or awkward clients?
- What would your current employer say were your strengths and weaknesses?

19.19 Some example interview questions for a receptionist.

Veterinary surgeon

- What attracted you to apply for this post?
- How does this job fit in with your long-term career objectives?
- We are able to provide increasingly more sophisticated treatment for pets but at a financial cost to the client. Where do we draw the line?
- What did you enjoy most about working for your last practice?
- Describe your ideal employer.
- What last made you angry at work and what form did your anger take?
- What qualities do you possess that make you a good vet?
- What do you see as the main aims of a veterinary practice?
- What other interests or specialties do you have?
- What have you contributed to team working at your current practice?
- Tell me about a good decision you recently made at work.
- Tell me about a recent problem you faced at work and how you resolved it.
- How do you think new clients can be attracted to the practice?
- What do you see as the role of veterinary support staff?
- What do you see as your main strengths, both in and outside work?
- How important is the client care aspect of your work in relation to your animal care role?
- What is the most difficult veterinary situation you have found yourself in?
- Give some examples of changes or improvements you have made in your current/previous role.
- Where do you see the veterinary surgeon's role with regard to discussing costs with clients?
- What are your views on promoting products and services in the consulting room?

19.20 Some example interview questions for a veterinary surgeon.

Veterinary nurse

- What attracted you to apply for this post?
- How does this job fit in with your long-term career objectives?
- What do you see as the major role of the veterinary nurse?
- What qualities should a good veterinary nurse possess?
- What motivates you?
- Do you have any areas of special interest that you would like to develop?
- What qualities do you possess that make you the right person for this post?
- What experience do you have of dealing with difficult or awkward clients?
- What do you see as your main strengths, both at and outside of work?
- What have you contributed to teamworking at your current practice?
- Have you ever experienced problems with information that has only been offered verbally? How did you resolve these?
- Can you give an example of a mistake you recently made at work and how you resolved it?
- Give some examples of changes or improvements you have made in your current/previous role.
- What are your views on promoting products and services in the consulting room?
- How important is the client care aspect of your work in relation to your animal care role?

19.21 Some example interview questions for a veterinary nurse.

Candidate assessment

The assessment form for each candidate is used to make an overall judgement of the suitability of the candidate and to clarify what the interviewers think about each applicant (Figure 19.22). The form can be used to score their suitability or just to make comments against each skill requirement. If a scoring system is used, the interviewers must agree on a consensus rating for each selection criteria, work independently when allocating scores for each candidate, and then discuss scores before making the final decision. At the end of all the interviews, these assessments can be compared in order to help choose the right person for the job.

When making the final choice, interviewers must:

- Be as confident as possible that this is the right person for the job. If in doubt, they should not appoint the candidate
- Not take second best, however tempting this may be. They should re-advertise instead
- Listen to staff; they are the ones who have to work with the new employee. If they have reservations about a candidate, their reasons should be listened to. If current employees have not bought into the recruiting choice, they may not be supportive to the new employee.

Very careful records should be kept of the interview. These should include:

- The original personal skills profile (see Figure 19.17)
- The questions asked (see Figures 19.19 to 19.21)
- The candidate assessment form (see Figure 19.22)
- Any other relevant material.

Skills/qualities	Score 1–4	Comments	Other information
Personality			
Appearance/dress/manner			
Flexibility			
Education/qualifications			
Communication skills			
Specialist skills			
Client care skills			
Ability to work as a team member			
Fitting in with staff			
Computer skills			
Common sense and initiative			
General comments			

19.22 An example of a candidate assessment form. Rating: 1, does not meet expectations; 2, meets expectation; 3, exceeds expectations; 4, outstanding candidate.

Records and feedback

The record of the successful candidate will be of use during employee appraisals. The records of all candidates should be kept for at least 6 months, in case any of the unsuccessful candidates question the decision that was made, suggest some form of discrimination has taken place, or ask for feedback as to why they were not offered the post. It is important to make this feedback very clear and to be able to justify the selection decision objectively. The manager should be ultimately responsible for giving this feedback if it is requested, based on notes taken at the interview and discussions between the interviewers. As candidates may ask to see notes from the interview, nothing should be recorded that could be interpreted as discriminatory or could appear trivial or unprofessional.

Most requests for feedback, however, are made by keen candidates who want to know how to improve their application next time. Below are a few tips for giving feedback to candidates:

- Feedback should only be given if a candidate wishes to receive it
- The candidate should be asked what he/she thought went well and what did not go so well
- Positive points should then be confirmed/shared
- Any negative points suggested by the candidate that were also picked up on by the interview panel should be acknowledged
- Only one or two negative points should be offered to the candidate; the most significant issues should be concentrated on
- The focus of the discussion should be on information that would help the candidate to prepare effectively for selection on another occasion.

Communication with applicants

All letters of application must be replied to promptly, thanking the applicant for their interest in the practice. This is only polite, and if not done can leave a very bad image of the practice. A standard letter can be used for applicants that have not been invited for interview, as the reply is simply a formality. This is becoming increasingly time-consuming due to the number of unsuitable applications via internet agencies. Enquiries and applications received by e-mail should also receive a standard polite e-mail response. For those applicants that were interviewed, a personalized letter should be sent.

Candidate acceptance

The letter offering the job to the successful candidate should include the following information:

- The formal offer of the job, subject to any references (if appropriate)
- The contract of employment or written statement
- The proposed start date
- A statement regarding any existing holidays the person may be taking
- Uniform/dress details
- Reporting for work details – where and to whom
- A contact name for information before employment starts
- A request for written confirmation of acceptance of the post and deadline for response.

Once references have been obtained and the job offer formally accepted, there is only one final step to take, and that is to inform existing employees of the appointment. Brief details of the new employee should be given, as well as the date they will be starting, and any impact on the team should be outlined. Introducing the new team member to the workplace is covered later in this chapter.

KEY POINT

Many practices invite all candidates that have been shortlisted to come in for a half day, to spend time with the team and meet everyone. A second interview can then be carried out at the end of the visit.

Shared values

Everyone working in a veterinary practice must share the same values, aims and objectives if there is to be a successful working partnership. This involves all staff agreeing and having input into the concepts shown below.

The practice vision

The practice vision must encompass the goals of the team as well as those of the owners. The vision should include the activities of the practice, the size of the practice, including the number of sites or branches, the number of clients, the staffing, the style of medicine practised, and the veterinary and client care provided. The vision may be for the next 5 years or may be for longer, and it will vary from practice to practice according to how the owners see their business developing (see Chapter 23).

Practice values

Values can be defined as a person's set of beliefs, which influence how they wish to run their life. They provide the code by which that person works – for a practice owner this includes the things they find acceptable and unacceptable when running the business.

Led by the owner, the team should set the values that the practice will work to. These values must be owner-driven, modelled and disseminated to all staff and committed to by everyone in the practice. This will create the culture of the practice and can form the basis for recruiting for attitude and training in the skills required by the practice.

Without values it can be difficult to plan the future development of the practice, and even more difficult to ensure that staff are providing the kind of service the practice would like for its clients. If staff do not share or understand the practice values, they will work to their own, which may be quite different. Without values it is very easy to give mixed messages, not only to staff but also to clients.

KEY POINT

Underlying all that is done in the practice should be the values that all staff work to. The practice may have set aims and objectives for the next 5 or 10 years and have goals it wishes to achieve. The values for the business must fit in with these aims, objectives and goals.

It is important to set values regarding:

- The practice – The values for organizational standards and the running of the practice and its services
- Clients – The values for the care of clients and the service provided for them
- Pets – The values for the care of pets in the practice
- Medical and scientific – The values for the standards of veterinary care provided
- Staff – The values that are held towards staff and how they are treated
- Community – The values held by the practice towards the local community
- Family and self – The practice must be run in such a way that these important personal values are accommodated.

Recruiting the right person is crucial, but sometimes mistakes are made because however well an interview is planned and carried out, it can at times be difficult to establish an individual's true values and attitudes. It is therefore inevitable that there will be times when the owner or manager will have to deal with staff or situations where the practice values are not being upheld. For example, there may be a situation where a veterinary surgeon views animals differently, due to cultural differences, and is unable to understand why a client is treating their pet like they would their child. This needs to be dealt with quickly before the client becomes upset or alienated. The manager or owner will need to explain the human–animal bond in detail to the veterinary surgeon, making sure he/she fully understands and from then on handles clients in the appropriate manner.

Similarly, if someone is found to have a problem taking instructions from a senior member of staff or shows a lack of respect for colleagues, the matter needs to be addressed immediately by the manager or owner. The culture of the practice and the required behaviour should be carefully explained to the individual and their behaviour monitored sympathetically and assessed on a frequent basis until it falls in line with practice expectations.

Practice culture

The culture of the practice affects the whole working environment and the attitude of staff to their duties, their employer(s) and the clients, as well as having a direct bearing on stress-related illness in the workplace. How the practice deals with the demands that may be placed on an employee by their job and the control they have over it, employee relationships at work, the management of change and the support and training an employee receives, defines the nature of the practice culture. This topic is dealt with in more detail later in this chapter.

Practice and personal goals

Personal goals need to be in line with those of the practice. For example:

- If the personal goal of the owner is to spend more time with his/her children this year, then a practice goal to expand the business, which will involve more time working in the practice, will not be realistic
- If a potential member of staff states at interview that they wish to concentrate on a particular avenue of medicine and perhaps gain a certificate, but the practice goals do not include expanding the service in this area, this person may not be suitable for the job.

Practice mission statement

The mission statement is a short, formal, written statement of the purpose of the practice (see

Chapter 23). It provides the framework within which the practice operates.

The statement should be simple, easy to remember and known by all staff. For example: 'To provide the highest standards of care and expertise to our clients and their animals', or even simpler, 'To excel at everything we do'. The mission statement can be used and reflected in other documents, such as job descriptions, and should be regularly reviewed by the team.

Empowering staff

> **KEY POINT**
>
> Practice owners/managers must trust their staff and the decisions they make in order for them to feel empowered.

Owners/managers must also support staff when things do not go well. Empowerment encompasses many areas of staff management. It is implicit in staff consultation, delegation, teamwork and staff development, and should be part of the practice culture.

For staff to give their best they need to feel that they have a stake in the success of the practice. Forcing staff to stick to rigid rules can leave them feeling helpless and frustrated in situations where, with a little flexibility, problems could have been solved or client care issues or complaints sorted out successfully. Not allowing staff to make any decisions can lead to unnecessary stress, demotivation and lack of productivity, and can seriously affect the health and wellbeing of staff. It is important to share information with staff so they have the necessary background to make the right decisions – i.e. they understand the impact their decisions will have on the business.

Empowering staff to think and behave as individuals gives them 'permission' to take action in situations that cannot be overcome by simply following the general rules. This gives staff ownership and control of their job, and more pleasure and satisfaction in carrying it out. An example would be the head veterinary nurse who, in the practice manager's absence, cancels a locum veterinary surgeon as their services were no longer required, thus saving the practice money.

Receptionists are responsible for booking appointments. If they are to be empowered with this task they need to have real involvement in the structure of the appointment system and the freedom to move appointments if the surgery is too busy. They need to know that any suggestions they make for change or improvements in the appointment system will be seriously considered and discussed. They also need to know that owners or managers will truly consult them about how to run this important aspect of the practice and be committed to allowing and trusting them to make decisions.

Managers who feel that their staff do not have the skills, enthusiasm or desire for empowerment, or who may have tried to encourage this but have not succeeded, should first look at their own behaviour and management skills, followed by a serious consideration of the current skill level of their staff; this should highlight some of the hurdles that need removing.

> **KEY POINT**
>
> It is then the manager's job to investigate the issues and correct them by effective performance management.

Staff motivation

Motivation involves creating an environment – both working and emotional – in which staff do things because they want to. It is the manager or team leader's job to motivate staff and help them develop a 'can do' rather than a 'can't do' attitude. Motivation comes from the top, and a highly motivated manager will inspire their staff. Lack of motivation in a manager is very likely to produce a similar attitude in their staff. This is explored further in Chapter 18. Motivated and de-motivated staff will behave differently:

- **Motivated staff:**
  - Happier, positive attitude
  - Energetic and enthusiastic
  - Cooperative
  - More productive
  - Work better as a team
  - More committed
  - Motivate others
- **De-motivated staff:**
  - Poor or negative attitude, apathy
  - Poor work
  - Poor timekeeping; absenteeism
  - Lack of cooperation
  - Exaggerate difficulties
  - Poor client care
  - Poor promotion of services and products
  - Low productivity
  - De-motivate others.

It can be a useful exercise for owners, managers and team leaders to take a little time to consider what their image is and how the rest of the practice sees them, by asking themselves the following questions:

- Do I look forward to going to work each day?
- Do I enjoy my job?
- Am I enthusiastic about the work the practice does?
- Do I show my enthusiasm?
- What do my staff see?

The answers should be self-explanatory in terms of how much motivation exists.

Showing motivation comes in many guises. It is not just a happy face; it is also being visible and accessible to staff. Staff need to see their manager or team leader in their workplace and feel that they are also part of the practice team. They need to feel able to go and see them if they have problems and to know that they will be listened to.

Nothing is more de-motivating than people feeling that they are unable to talk to their manager or that, if they do, nothing will happen and their ideas or problems will be ignored. This situation also seriously hampers the empowerment process. People often moan about things but can find it difficult to talk to the management team about them. Staff may feel that their ideas and suggestions are not listened to by management and therefore give up putting forward their suggestions for improvements. Quite apart from de-motivating staff, this can also mean that potentially good ideas from the people working close to the ground are lost. Listening to and, in particular, asking for staff opinions and suggestions makes staff feel cared for, and this in itself is very motivating for many employees. The manager may not be able to act on all suggestions or solve all the problems but if they listen and explain why a 'great idea' is actually difficult to put into operation, at least the member of staff will know that the time has been taken to consider it.

Different things motivate different people and it is not always easy to determine what these factors are. Staff appraisals can be a great help in finding out what motivates someone, what their aspirations are and where they want to go within the practice. Regular consultation and discussions are also key to success.

For most staff there are two types of motivation:

- **Intrinsic motivation** comes from rewards inherent to the job itself and, for many working in veterinary practice, this is simply the love of animals. One is said to be intrinsically motivated when engaging in an activity 'with no apparent reward except for the activity itself'
- **Extrinsic motivation** comes from outside. Money is perhaps the most obvious example, but recognition, encouragement, praise and promotion are also good examples. These rewards provide satisfaction and pleasure that the task itself may not provide.

Because of the nature of the work in a veterinary practice, it is likely that staff will be intrinsically motivated. This should make the job of motivating staff a lot easier and should allow managers and team leaders to concentrate on some of the external factors that help to create a motivational environment.

Employees have some basic needs when it comes to carrying out their role:

- To know what is expected of them in terms of role, results and responsibilities
- To be allowed to do their job
- To know how well they are doing
- To receive guidance, training and support
- To be rewarded in accordance with their contribution
- To receive praise and thanks where it is due.

One of the easiest ways to de-motivate staff is to fail in this last employee need by not giving praise, thanks or recognition.

Praise is also the easiest and least expensive way to motivate.

KEY POINT

Praising or thanking an employee for something they have done well, especially if this is done in front of their team mates, can be highly motivating.

Maintaining a motivational environment is an ongoing management responsibility but on a day-to-day basis there are some simple practical steps to support motivation.

- Staff should be made to feel valued. Success should be made easier than failure and a no-blame culture of approval should be established, rather than one of criticism. For example, if a member of staff has made a mistake it is fair to point out the consequences but it is important to concentrate on ways to avoid this happening again.
- Opportunities for development should be provided. Targets should be set, training provided, and all of the skills possessed by staff should be used.
- Achievements should be recognized by giving praise and thanks when due.
- Staff should be set challenges, e.g. objectives should be set and opportunities for greater responsibility should be provided by encouraging ideas and building on people's strengths.
- Belief in staff should be expressed by delegating and empowering appropriately.
- Care should be shown by listening and displaying interest, but letting staff get on with the job at hand.

Motivation tools can be as simple as giving an employee a name badge or personal business card or stocking a pet product recommended by a member of staff, or can be as complex as training, delegating or mentoring a member of staff to take on more responsibility. The important thing is to know which it should be, by treating staff as individuals and finding out what really motivates them.

Teams and teamwork

Good teamwork is essential for good service to clients and a happy atmosphere within the practice. It involves members of the team treating each other as they would wish to be treated. For example, it is important that veterinary surgeons do not leave syringes out on the side for the veterinary nurse to clear up when there is a bin to hand; this will be seen as lazy and disrespectful as well as poor safety practice. In the same way, respect must be shown to the client (e.g. not keeping them waiting by starting consults late) and the patient treated with dignity.

KEY POINT

Good teamwork is about respect. It is about respecting each other and each other's roles, including the client.

Analysing team members and working out who is the 'challenger', 'doer' 'thinker', etc., can be very helpful in enabling understanding of why certain colleagues do or don't work well together. It can also improve success in recruitment by seeing how someone new will fit into the team. However, the reality in most veterinary practices is that there is a group of people who, more by circumstance than planning, must work together to create results. The luxury of being able to move a 'problem' team member in order to create a more harmonious team is rare. This being the case, it helps to have fairly clear guidelines about how the people in the group need to work together.

Aims and beliefs

It is fundamental for team members to understand the aims of the practice. If staff are unsure about what the practice is trying to achieve, it is unlikely that they are going to be working towards the vision the owner has. Probably the second most important aspect of good teamwork is that everyone truly believes in what they and the practice does. Staff must believe that the practice provides a caring service that gives clients value for money.

A culture of care

The members of the team need to care about each other. This simply means supporting each other when there are problems and sharing the bad as well as the good times and the failures as well as the successes of the veterinary day. Team members need to be generous enough to support each other in times of failure or stress while taking pleasure in combined success.

Good communication

This is where so many teams fall apart. It is essential to have good lines of communication within the team (Figure 19.23) and it is worth remembering that usually the larger the team the more difficult this becomes. It does not matter what system is used to communicate, the important thing is that it happens (see Chapter 17). People must not feel left out because they work part-time or work at another branch for part of the week, and afternoon staff must know what the morning staff have been dealing with. Daily communication systems regarding rotas, operations, telephone messages and clients must work. Poor communication means poor working procedures and poor client care and leads to poorer working relationships among staff.

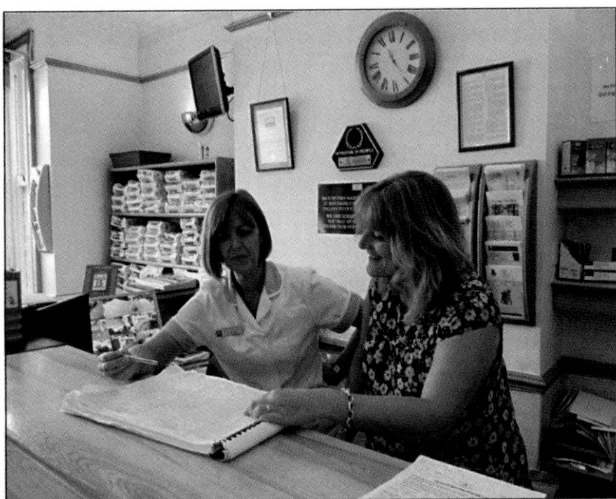

19.23 A member of the management team discusses rotas with the head receptionist. Good communication within and between teams is essential.

Contribution

In a good team, everyone should be able and willing to contribute. It is important for members to be able to say what they think and make suggestions without fear of being put down or rebuffed or upsetting anyone. Not all ideas are good, but they do deserve to be heard, and any good team leader will make sure that they respond to all ideas put forward, whether they are good or bad. A good team is one in which contribution is actively encouraged; this helps to bind the members and makes them feel that they really are working as a team.

Protocols

Teamwork is about working together in the same way for the same outcome. For this to happen smoothly, protocols/rules/procedures are necessary. These should be set, and should avoid conflicting messages from different members of staff. This enables staff to hand over to others knowing that their work will be continued in the same way, and fewer uncertainties, misunderstandings or conflicts between team members will result. Staff members need to understand their individual role and their role within the team, where they stand and to whom they report.

Good leadership

The acid test of the good leader is the extent to which they can select their style to suit the circumstances they find themselves in, how well they can adapt to a variety of situations and how good their ability is to get people willingly to perform to a level they did not believe they were capable of.

Although good leadership is influenced by the individual's personality, a good leader also needs to have a set of qualities that make people want to 'follow' them and work with them.

> **KEY POINT**
>
> Good leaders have respect for the people in their team. It is essential that a leader works to create a positive and cheerful workplace.

If a leader has a negative attitude, it is hard to expect staff to be otherwise. A good leader must be highly motivated and make sure that their staff see this at all times. Providing support is an important part of the leader's role. Supportive leaders listen to their team members, praise them when praise is deserved and seek their ideas (see Chapter 18).

Team dynamics

Team dynamics are the unseen forces that operate within the team between the different members. These dynamics can have a strong influence on how a team behaves or performs. Team dynamics are complicated; teams may have ups and downs, working well and then perhaps not so well for a while. Changes in team members can have a strong effect until the group relationships are sorted. Change within the practice, especially if it is not well handled, can also have an adverse effect on how well a team works together.

Recognizing and managing team dynamics

The forces that influence team behaviour should be recognized.

- **Personality** – Teams should embrace members with different personalities, strengths and weaknesses, but sometimes these differences cause problems, which need to be addressed before they get out of hand. Understanding how different people communicate and adapting one's own style in order to relate better to them can have a major positive impact.
- **Team roles** – Teams are about working together; if roles clash or members misunderstand each other's roles, problems arise.
- **Communication** – Poor communication always causes difficulties among any group of people.
- **Organizational culture** – A poor culture within the organization or the team (e.g. a culture of blame or criticism) can lead to dissatisfaction and de-motivation. This can quickly spread to all team members.
- **Processes and procedures** – If the way the team works and the procedures it has to follow are inadequate, it will not be long before members become dissatisfied.

Any one of the above forces can cause upset in the team, but problems are usually due to a combination of factors, and it is up to the person leading the team to identify where the problems are and to remove them. Teams are not static: the dynamics of the team cycle with time.

Running successful meetings

Good teamwork and successful teams are based to a huge extent on good communication. Good internal communication is vital and the larger the practice is, the more important it becomes. Meetings play a very important role in internal communication and relationships between practice teams, as well as in the consultation process. However, they are only successful if organized and conducted in an efficient and effective manner (see Chapter 17). Poorly organized meetings with no outcomes are a waste of everybody's time and can be very de-motivating.

Staff consultation

Staff consultation involves taking account of and listening to the views of employees. It is something that should take place before making either minor or major decisions that will affect them. Staff consultation is valuable, and is also a great motivator, helping employees to feel 'part of the practice' and to feel that their opinions, views and ideas are listened to and count.

For example, the decision to install a new computer system in a practice can be taken with or without consultation. Where there is no consultation, staff will be told the following:

- A new computer system will be installed in the practice next month
- This is how it will be installed and this is how it will operate
- This is what staff need to do to prepare.

Where there is a consultation, the decision will be discussed with staff.

- Staff are told the problem/issue: the computer system needs upgrading as the current one is too slow and out of date.
- Staff are asked for their input regarding what they would require from a new system.
- An agreement is reached as to how things will proceed and how systems will be changed with the least amount of disruption and stress.
- Staff explore how the decided plan can be put into action.

Successful consultation requires that there is a free exchange of ideas and views on any issue that affects the interests of the employees and of the practice. This does not mean that the employees' views always have to be acted upon or accepted, as there may be very good practical or financial reasons why their suggestions may not be able to be put into practice. However, the employer must consider all employee suggestions and opinions and, if they are rejected, explain why this is. The worst-case scenario is to have consultation but no feedback; this is highly de-motivating.

There is no one best way to carry out staff consultation, but underpinning the whole procedure is the requirement for every member of staff to have had the opportunity to 'have their say'. If the practice team has bought into the ideas and procedures agreed, then the practice will run more smoothly because everyone will be pulling in the same direction. Consultation can take a number of different forms:

- **Staff meetings** – Full staff meetings are not easy to arrange in veterinary practices but they provide the ideal opportunity for the employer to discuss with all their staff the possibility of changes in the practice. It is also a chance for staff to talk directly with employers or managers about their own ideas or where they think working systems could be improved. However, this is less practical for large practices as the more people present, the less most will say
- **Team meetings** – These can be used to gather information from the vet, nurse or reception team members, which can then be passed on up the system by the team representative, e.g. at a team leaders' meeting. Management responses to the suggestions would then be passed back to the team members by the team representative at the next team meeting. Team meetings are also useful for problem-solving in specific areas, while *ad hoc* groups can be formed for particular projects
- **Brainstorming** – This can be a very effective method of staff consultation, especially if there is a major issue to discuss, or there are going to be big changes in the practice, e.g. the introduction of a new admissions and discharge procedure. At this meeting everyone can put forward their ideas, however extreme, and all are considered later, discussed and then accepted or rejected until a consensus has been reached.

The employer has a legal duty to consult their employees over health and safety matters (see Chapter 22). This involves not just making sure that they have read health and safety information but that they have an opportunity to discuss how the practice health and safety procedures are put into place and make suggestions for change and/or improvements.

Staff training and development

Practices spend time, effort and money on training staff and developing their skills; both the staff members and the practice have the potential to benefit greatly from this. The practice should make use of the full skill set of its trained staff; it is de-motivating for staff if they are held back from putting into practice the skills and knowledge that they have acquired.

KEY POINT

Training in itself is motivating, and external training offers the opportunity for team members to benchmark themselves and their skills and to meet colleagues from other practices or people from outside the industry.

People need to be given a chance to shine and show just what they can achieve. Even for those that have been working in the practice for a long time, including the owner, training and self-development is a continuous process. The practice should aim to develop a training culture in which all staff know that training and continuous improvement is a normal ongoing activity. Without fully trained staff no veterinary practice can reach its full potential.

Managers and supervisors will need to adopt different training styles according to the skills and knowledge shown by their employees. Different individuals learn in different ways, so taking a blanket approach for training all staff will have more limited success. Particular consideration should be given to individual learning styles; that is, whether people prefer to learn by seeing, listening, reading or actually practising the task. Usually a combination of all three is used, and the trainer should adapt their one-to-one style to the individual.

Staff training and development can be divided into three stages:

1. Induction training
2. Initial job skills training
3. Ongoing training and development.

Induction training of new staff

It is vital that new employees get off to a good start; those first few days can make a lot of difference to their comfort, confidence and enthusiasm. Starting a new job is both exciting and frightening, and every employee, particularly when new or in a new role, needs support and encouragement. The start day and time must be considered carefully – a busy Monday morning may not be the best time.

All staff should be briefed before the new employee arrives so that they know who the new staff member will be and what it is they will be doing. The induction process should be planned for the new employee, who should be given all the details in advance of their arrival so they know what to expect. A timetable should be drawn up that provides details of what they will be doing, when they will be doing it and who will be involved. The first day, week and month should be considered. The manager/owner must ensure that the members of staff involved have set aside time for the induction and that there is cover provided for them.

The new employee should have been told what time to arrive on their first day, where to park (if applicable), where to go and who they will be meeting. Normally this would be the practice manager, the staff member responsible for personnel or possibly a team leader.

An important part of this initial induction is handing over and explaining the often considerable amount of paperwork involved in taking on a new employee. It can be useful to have a checklist (Figure 19.24) to

Item	Date completed and signature
Before the new employee starts: ■ Provide contract of employment/written statement ■ Issue dress policy ■ Order uniform and PPE ■ Order badges ■ Label locker ■ Arrange personal space and equipment ■ Prepare copy of staff manual ■ Induction paperwork ■ Inform team	
Job description	
Contract of employment	
Identification and evidence of eligibility to work in UK (see Chapter 20)	
P45	
Salary payment details	
Organization chart, lines of responsibility and report	
Rota	
Details of next of kin	
Doctor's telephone number	
Car documentation/driving licence	
Uniform/protective clothing	
Locker keys	
Fire procedure	
First Aid arrangements, accident book	
Disciplinary and grievance policies	
Health & safety policy and regulations	
Practice/departmental manual	
Staff manual	
Training programme – agreed and issued	

19.24 An example of an induction checklist for a new employee.

provide a reminder of what the new recruit requires, as well as the information needed from them. This paperwork will vary depending upon the practice but, with the exception of the job description and salary payment details, most of the information should be in the practice manual, which can be explained and given to the new employee at the start of their induction process. If possible it is a good idea for the new employee to visit the practice a week or two before starting in order to try on uniforms for size, to check spellings of names for badges, etc. and to have dress codes explained so that the employee can come prepared and properly attired. Once this part of the induction is complete, the rest of the induction timetable can be set in motion.

The first day should be devoted to meeting staff, reading and going through protocols, work shadowing, an overview of the computer system, and perhaps a visit to any other sites. At the end of the day it can be useful to have a de-briefing meeting with the practice manager or their equivalent. Whatever is in the timetable, the new employee should not be given difficult or lengthy work to do; this first day should ideally be kept for induction, observation and learning. However, if appropriate, involving the new member of staff in some work and asking for input into discussions can help add variety to the day and make them feel useful. It is a very good idea to allocate a team colleague to the new employee, to give the starter the lowdown on things such as tea and coffee arrangements, staff rooms, cloakrooms, and the 'do's and don'ts' of the practice in an informal way. They can also offer to accompany the starter during lunch and other breaks.

During the employee's first week, a timetable of induction training and work activities can be implemented, with the aim that by the end of the week they have a very clear idea of the organization of the practice, know who does what, and have spent some time shadowing other members of staff. Daily debriefing of the new starter and their team colleague will be useful for offering positive feedback and making adjustments to the induction process.

KEY POINT

A good induction programme is designed to help guide the new member of staff gently into their new job and make them feel comfortable, confident and enthusiastic in their role.

Induction training programme

Initial induction programmes may last for one or two days, or for up to two weeks, depending on how they have been designed and what is appropriate for the practice and the new employee. For positions where a high level of training is required, such as with a new veterinary graduate, student nurse or office junior, initial induction will be followed by ongoing job training that may last a year or more (see below). The aim of the induction programme is to familiarize the new employee with all the work of the practice and enable them to place it in context with their own specific job. The longer induction programmes will combine observation of other areas in the practice with practical work in the employee's specific area, so that they are learning their own job as well as observing those of others. It can be useful to have an observation checklist to ensure that the observation has taken place; however, it is important to remember that observation is not training, and care must be taken that the two are not confused. Examples of observation and training checklists for new receptionists, veterinary nurses and veterinary surgeons are provided in Figures 19.25 to 19.27.

Skill/task	Demonstrated	Trainee happy that they are competent	Supervising staff member confirms competence	Date
Using computer to administer client records				
Booking appointments				
Answering the telephone and taking telephone messages				
Working knowledge of office equipment, its use and maintenance				
Working knowledge of practice policies and procedures				
Working knowledge of new products, medicines and services				
Advising clients on pet healthcare				
Advising on and selling pet products				
Dealing with client account queries				
Awareness of and compliance with practice health and safety regulations				
Cashing up				
Dealing with client complaints and problems				
Puppy party bookings				
Handling euthanasia appointments				
Other				

19.25 An example of a receptionist induction training plan.

Observation	Trainee	Trainer	Comments	Date
Reception				
Administration				
Dispensary				
Laboratory				
Consulting room				
Nurses' clinics				
Puppy parties				
Other				

19.26 An example of a veterinary nurse induction training observation checklist.

Observation	Trainee	Trainer	Comments	Date
Reception				
Administration				
Admissions				
Discharges				
Recovery				
Dispensary				
Laboratory				
Nurses' clinics				
Puppy parties				
Other				

19.27 An example of a veterinary surgeon induction training observation checklist.

It is important for everyone to consider the individual's learning style and pace in working through induction training, and to reassure the learner that repetition of training is often needed before some skills are mastered. Having a protocol for the induction of new employees will ensure that all the necessary steps in the process are followed. An example of a protocol for new employee induction is given in Figure 19.28.

Staff induction protocol
■ Provide new member of staff prior to their employment start date with information regarding their induction programme. ■ Inform all staff of appointment of new staff member and their start date. ■ Design day one induction programme. ■ Design induction/observation program for employee. ■ Appoint appropriate member of staff to be 'the friend/support' of the new employee during first few days. ■ On arrival of new staff member, using documentation checklist to ensure all documentation has been supplied by both practice and employee. ■ After day one put into operation the induction/observation programme. ■ Monitor progress of employee using induction appraisal system.

19.28 An example of a protocol for new staff induction. An example of an induction checklist for a receptionist is given in Chapter 5.

Monitoring induction training programmes

The success of the induction programme and how the new employee is getting on with both their work and their colleagues should be monitored. The best way is to carry out induction appraisals after 1, 3 and 6 months or as required according to progress. These give the employees an opportunity to discuss any problems and the manager/team leader a chance to discuss the employee's progress and plan future action. Induction appraisals are discussed later in this chapter.

Induction for existing staff

Induction does not just apply to new staff. Newly promoted staff may find themselves in exactly the same position as a new recruit. They may now be working at a different branch of the practice with new colleagues, or their job and routines will have changed and they may need to familiarize themselves with new procedures and protocols and changed relationships with co-workers. Induction for these members of staff should follow similar lines to those for new employees, with an induction checklist being drawn up as well as a timetable for settling in to the new job. The same applies to those returning from extended leave (e.g. sick or maternity leave).

KEY POINT

It is good practice when someone is away on extended leave to make a note of all equipment, stock and procedure changes as they happen, and to add these to the induction checklist, in order to bring the returning staff member back up to speed as quickly as possible.

Initial job skills training

New employees, or those who have been promoted to a new post within the practice, need specific job training to enable them to carry out their designated role.

This specific job training should be carefully planned, identifying the skills that need to be taught. Scheduled time should be set aside for training the employee and for the employee to carry out personal study. Consideration should be given as to whether all the training can be carried out within the practice or whether external courses or trainers will be required. However the training is to be delivered, it is important to have a timetable drawn up, setting out what training is required and when. A training skills checklist will help to assess progress, should list the skill areas required, and should be completed by both trainee and trainer as the training progresses. The checklist will help encourage the trainee to direct their own learning, as they can see what has been delivered and what there is still to do. It also facilitates the involvement of other team members, who can see easily where the trainee has got to and what still needs to be covered. The employee can start working on the checklist during the induction period. It is worth noting that each business will have its own training needs, so external training checklists may not fully meet the practice's requirements. For example, although the current veterinary nursing training programme includes a skills checklist (the Nursing Progress Log), this may not cover all of the same areas in the same timescale that the practice needs for a practice nurse, so should not be relied upon as the only training structure for an employed student nurse.

If training is being provided within the practice, the employee should have the opportunity to learn by theory, observation and then practice. So, for example, teaching computer skills might involve:

- **Theory** – The employee being told about the system, reading about or being given basic notes about the use of the computer
- **Observation** – The employee watching another member of staff using the computer
- **Practice** – The employee 'having a go' themselves, usually under supervision.

It is important to understand that people have different learning styles; when designing the employee's training, the four main learning styles should be considered.

- **Activist** – Those who want to 'have a go' and have 'hands-on experience' right from the start. These people will benefit from a very practical training programme.
- **Theorist** – Those who want to learn about a new skill first. These people will benefit from theory and observation training before putting their knowledge into practice.
- **Reflector** – Those who are cautious and methodical. These people will benefit from an observation-based programme.
- **Pragmatist** – These are the planners who learn, design and then test out their skills. These people will learn best from a theory-based training programme.

Identifying training needs

Before any training programme can be set up, the training and development needs of staff need to be identified. There are a variety of ways to do this:

- **Brainstorming** – Involves gathering together all the staff for whom training is to be designed and giving everyone an opportunity to make suggestions on the skills and training required, as these both need to be connected
- **Questionnaires** – Involves sending a questionnaire to all staff, asking them to identify areas where they consider they need new skills or knowledge and require training
- **Interviews** – Involves interviewing staff individually to discuss their training needs
- **Observation** – The manager's own observation, or that of the heads of departments, team leaders, etc., are valuable in assessing the training requirements of staff
- **Appraisals** – If the practice carries out annual appraisals, training and development needs will be discussed at these meetings.

Practice staff may require new skills and learning due to:

- Changes in practice procedures
- The introduction of new equipment or techniques
- The provision of new services
- Advances in knowledge or technology.

Training may be needed in order to decide whether to offer a new service or purchase new equipment, e.g. before considering purchase of an ultrasound machine or digital radiography unit.

KEY POINT

Ongoing cross-training is invaluable for ensuring that team members can cover for each other during busy times or periods of absence.

Designing the training programme

Having established training needs, the delivery method must be decided. One of the best ways to design the programme is to draw up training plans. These may be for everyone in the practice, whole teams within the practice, such as receptionists or nursing staff, or can be designed for each individual member of staff. In all cases, the following issues must be considered.

- **Training required** – Training needs should be established.
- **Training delivery** – This will depend on the learning abilities of the staff, the logistics of staff working and the number of staff that need to be trained. The most effective way to train should be chosen; this may, in some cases, be a lunchtime seminar, or it may be an external course. How the individual staff members prefer to learn should also be considered (see earlier).
- **Who trains** – Training may be: carried out in house by experienced members of the team or delivered by outside trainers in the form of external courses or distance/Internet/ DVD training.
- **When to train** – Whenever possible, training should take place during working hours and lunchtimes. Distance and private learning is very much up to the individual, but it would be reasonable to allow some of the employees' working time to be given over to this type of learning if it is structured.
- **Where to train** – Some practices will have a dedicated meeting or training room, which is ideal for in-house staff training. If this is not the case, it may be better for training to take place away from the practice in a quieter environment with no distractions. The reception area can be used out of hours.
- **Training targets** – Target dates for the completion and evaluation of the training must exist. Staff need something to aim for and a deadline to meet.
- **Training costs** – Training and development must be budgeted for. Decisions will have to be made about affordability and the return on investment made in training provision. This includes whether, for example, two short courses for two different members of staff are better value than one longer, more expensive course for a single member.
- **Training outcomes** – These should be set at the planning stage and expectations should be clear. If the desired outcome is not considered, assessing the success of the training will not be possible.

KEY POINT

Training is not an end in itself – it should lead to enhanced performance.

An example of a practice training programme is provided in Figure 19.29.

Individual training plans

It is a good idea to give each member of staff their own training plan (Figure 19.30). This gives them a clear idea of what training there will be, how it will be organized, and what will be expected of them at the end of the training (e.g. what skills and knowledge they will have gained and what they will be able to do that they could not do before). It is also useful during an appraisal to have the training plan to refer to and discuss.

Monitoring and reviewing training

It is important to monitor the training provided so that its success can be measured. Discussing training at appraisals will provide one way of doing this, as will the completion of training evaluation forms (Figure 19.31) by employees. At the end of any training period, employees should be asked to complete an evaluation form which asks some or all of the following questions:

- What did you expect to learn from the training?
- How did it meet up to your expectations?
- If it did not meet your expectations, how could it be improved? What do you still need to learn?
- How has the training helped you to carry out your job better? What can you now do?

Assessing staff training needs, developing training plans, monitoring progress and reviewing performance forms an ongoing cycle which helps ensure that standards and service quality are maintained and improved.

Training required	Delivery	Trainer	Time of training	Venue	Completion target date	Employees to be trained	Required training outcomes	Cost
Use of new computer system	Group and individual training	Clinic IT manager	14–15 March 20XX	Main clinic	24 March 20XX	All	Complete competency in use of computer records	Some overtime payments: approx. £.....

19.29 An example of a practice training programme, with one item entered.

Name				Job title		
Skills required	**Training to be provided**	**Date and time of training**	**Venue**	**Training completed**	**Trainer comments**	**Trainee comments**

19.30 An example of an individual training plan.

Name .... Training	Job title .... Specify type of training, e.g. course, talk, handouts, meeting ....
Length of training	
Date of training	
Location	
Trainer	
Cost (including travel and accommodation)	
What did you hope to gain from attending this training?	
What did you actually gain from attending this training?	
How could the training have been improved?	
How has the training helped you to carry out your job better?	
Please asses the usefulness of the training on a scale of 1 to 3: 1. No help 2. Helpful 3. Very helpful	
Please assess the delivery of the training on a scale of 1 to 3: 1. Poor 2. Good 3. Very good	
General comments on the training, e.g. did you feel it was value for money?	

19.31 An example of an employee training evaluation form. Employees should fill out the form within a few days of completing any training.

Putting training to work

An action plan should be discussed and agreed with the employee (Figure 19.32). It should be split into two parts:

- What the employee will do differently or start to do as a result of what they have learned
- What will be done differently in the practice and what support the employee will need in order to achieve the above.

KEY POINT

Training will remain a passive process without an action plan.

Evaluating training

It is not enough just to provide training and hope that it has worked. All training should be evaluated. There are several ways to evaluate what staff training has achieved, what its limitations might be and how it can be improved.

- **Employee performance** – The impact the training has had on the employee's performance should be reviewed. The best way to do this is as part of a regular appraisal process.
- **Business performance** – This is a more tangible evaluation, which looks at performance indicators such as sales.

Personal objective	How this will be achieved	Help/support required	Achieve by date
Practice objective	**How this will be achieved**	**Resources needed**	**Achieve by date**

19.32 Once the employee has completed a training evaluation form (see Figure 19.31) they should complete an action plan showing how they are going to use the skills they have acquired. The action plan should include both personal aims and action points for the practice or other team members as a result of the training.

- **Qualitative performance** – This considers improvement in the quality of, for example, teamwork or client satisfaction.
- **Employee feedback** (see above) – This should cover whether employees thought the training was relevant to their job and their level of expertise, what they thought about the training methods used, what worked and did not work, and what could be improved. A training evaluation form is a useful aid (see Figure 19.31).

An evaluation of training will enable employers to find out how well it is working and to identify any aspects that need to be improved or changed.

For the training organizer and the employee, this evaluation is really part of a reflective process (described below) that asks:

- Have the training objectives been achieved from both the practice's and the individual's points of view?
- Is more training needed and, if so, what?
- Is a different method of training needed?
- Are training times appropriate?
- Did all the staff have a reasonable access to training?
- Are the training resources sufficient?
- Has the training been good value for money, and kept within budget?

The training programme can be changed at any time if it will benefit staff or the practice. Any programme must be flexible. Staff members change and the skills required change, as do the available methods of training, and it is important to achieve the best mix. If this means altering the training programme, then this should be done. What worked well 10 years ago will not necessarily work well today. Availability and delivery of training can be limiting factors, and arrangements may have to be changed to suit the provision and availability of expertise within the practice.

Recording training and CPD

Staff should be given **CPD record cards** to record training and progress. These are not only a good way for them to keep accurate records of their training hours but are also useful at the appraisal interview when training needs and outcomes are discussed. An example of a CPD record card is provided in Figure 19.33. RCVS record cards (downloadable from www.rcvs.org.uk) are recommended for veterinary surgeons and registered veterinary nurses, and may be requested by the RCVS for monitoring purposes at any time.

For veterinary surgeons and registered veterinary nurses, maintaining adequate CPD for the role they have in practice is their own responsibility, as is the completion of the record card, although in practical terms practices will share this with an agreed level of financial and time support in most cases. To maintain standards, practices should require submission of all CPD record cards at the end of each year and retain

Name .... Job title ....

Training record from .... to ....

Date	Course/CPD	Venue	Length/time spent	Evaluation

19.33 An example of a CPD training record.

a copy on file for RCVS Practice Standards Scheme inspections. Scrutinization of CPD records is strongly recommended for all recruits, including temporary and locum staff, as part of the selection process. The RCVS has comprehensive guidelines on CPD, and the obligation to keep up to date in active areas of work, as decided appropriate by the individual. More information can be found about this at www.rcvs.org.uk. Where less than the recommended minimum CPD has been undertaken, an action plan must be put in place.

At the time of writing there is no official RCVS accreditation of CPD *per se*. Certificated hours etc. offered by training providers are their own assessments, and training should be evaluated by the recipient according to their previously defined needs and outcomes achieved.

KEY POINT

For veterinary surgeons and registered veterinary nurses, maintaining adequate CPD records is their own, and not the practice's, responsibility, as is the completion of the record card. To maintain standards, practices should require submission of all CPD record cards at the end of each year and should retain a copy on file for PSS inspections.

Reflective learning

Part of the learning process for anyone who has had new training or has had to use new skills should be to reflect on what they have learnt and how it has helped them. This reflection enables the learner to see a clear link between the effort they have put into the learning and the benefits they have achieved. Put simply, reflection means asking the following questions:

- What was I trying to achieve?
- What should have happened?
- What actually happened?
- What went well and why?
- What didn't go so well and why?
- How did it affect me?
- How did it affect others?
- What were the consequences?
- What could be done differently next time?
- What else can I learn from this?
- What personal learning/skill/knowledge development needs have I identified?

Reflective practice has many benefits for everyone in the team: it helps to improve performance and allows everyone in the team to take an objective look at what they do, and think positively about it.

Coaching and mentoring

There is much confusion between the terms coaching and mentoring, particularly as they are often used interchangeably. Coaching is a tool for supporting personal development, while mentoring provides for the transmission of skills and knowledge. A good training programme will involve both of these activities, and both should be seen as part of the practice culture.

Coaching

Coaching is a two-way process, where the member of staff or trainee develops skills and achieves desired competencies through regular assessment, guidance, practical help and, very importantly, feedback, with the aim of improving their personal performance (see Chapter 18). Coaching can be used for a number of purposes, including:

- Performance coaching – Aimed at enhancing an individual's performance in their current role
- Skills coaching – Concentrates on the core skills the individual needs to perform their role
- Life or career coaching – Helps an individual look at the bigger picture and their own life and career goals and achieve their personal aims.

Coaching is not simply training or teaching an individual how to do a job, it is a continuous process, developing the individual and their own ability to improve their skills and performance. For example, a head veterinary nurse may provide coaching for a student veterinary nurse. The head nurse will need to know enough about the person and their work to be able to offer helpful guidance and support. He/she will help to develop plans and set goals and targets for improving or developing the trainee's skills and will then spend time reviewing the results and providing advice or help where there are any difficulties. One of the important roles of a coach is to provide feedback to the trainee and suggestions and guidance for the way forward.

Coaching is appropriate for any member of staff who has received training but still needs a little extra support, help and motivation to carry out their role to the standards required.

Mentoring

Mentoring provides support and encouragement to staff to help them manage their own learning, develop their skills and improve their performance. It is, in essence, a partnership between two people (the mentor and the mentee) and is a relationship based upon mutual trust and respect. In the case of veterinary practice, the mentor may be a practice owner guiding a new graduate veterinary surgeon through their first years in practice, or a head veterinary nurse providing mentorship for a student nurse who is working their way through their training. Mentors often rely upon having had similar experiences in order to establish an empathy with the mentee and an understanding of their issues. The mentor should help the mentee to believe in themselves and boost their confidence. A mentor should ask questions and challenge, while providing guidance and encouragement.

Counselling

It is sometimes difficult to distinguish clearly between coaching and counselling. The key distinction is that coaching in the workplace is for individuals who are psychologically well. If a manager or owner is able to identify any staff member who is distressed by personal, social or work issues they should offer to arrange for specialist counselling or other support.

Managing staff performance

Managing and analysing staff performance, providing appropriate training and helping staff to develop skills are vital to the success of the veterinary practice.

> **KEY POINT**
>
> Staff performance can be split into two areas:
>
> - **Ability** – This is the individual's skills and knowledge. If they are considered lacking, appropriate training needs to be arranged
> - **Willingness and motivation** – In effect, this is the individual's attitude to work and their work colleagues.

Clearly, any deficiencies that have a negative effect on an employee's performance, and/or on the performances of their colleagues, need to be addressed immediately. A lack of ability can be addressed by extra and appropriate training and mentoring. Poor attitude and behaviour of a staff member can be difficult to deal with, however, and will require a one-to-one discussion, which looks at:

- The problem, i.e. the attitude or behaviour
- Any underlying reasons or explanations for it
- The effect this is having on others, e.g. colleagues, the business and clients
- The consequences of this effect on themselves
- How to address the problem – i.e. what the manager and the staff member can do to change attitude and behaviour
- Designing an action plan that deals with the problem.

A very simple example would be a receptionist who always arrives late yet leaves 5 or 10 minutes early. This situation, if left, will cause resentment among the other staff and possibly lead to 'copycat' behaviour. The problem, once identified, needs to be dealt with straight away. The member of staff should be asked to attend a meeting with their supervisor, who should:

- Explain what the problem is – i.e. arriving late and leaving early
- Find out the reason for the behaviour – in this example it could be due to a variety of reasons, e.g. family problems, problems with other staff or health, or lack of motivation
- Explain the effect this is having – i.e. it causes disruption for other staff because they are shorthanded. This in turn looks inefficient to clients
- Explain the consequences – i.e. other staff feel annoyed and resentful, and clients see an inefficient reception service
- Design an action plan that addresses whatever the problem is. This is a plan that sets out the actions required from the receptionist and from the practice. The team leader and receptionist should agree to meet at regular intervals to discuss how the plan is working. The action may be to insist on better timekeeping, or an alternative solution could be agreed, e.g. a change in working hours.

The performance appraisal or development review

A long-term view should also be adopted in order to manage staff performance. One of the most important ways to achieve this is through regular development reviews or appraisals. The performance appraisal is a very effective means of ensuring that managers and their staff meet regularly to discuss past and present performance issues, to identify training and development needs and to agree what future action is appropriate on both sides. Appraisals are very useful management tools. They can improve communications and the quality of working life for employees and make them feel more valued by the organization.

The appraisal should assess an employee's performance, look at past achievements and agree objectives for the future. As well as increasing staff motivation and commitment, it should build on the employee's strengths and help resolve any weaknesses. However, a poorly managed appraisal is worse than no appraisal.

> **KEY POINT**
>
> Appraisals should not be linked to pay. The appraisal should only be used as a tool for developing a staff member's skills and abilities. Linking pay to the outcome of the appraisal will alter the whole character of the interview.

Performance appraisals should not be used for any disciplinary issues. These should be dealt with on a separate occasion and at the time. The appraisal should always be a positive meeting. Even if issues are identified that show an employee needs to improve standards, the discussion must be looking to how they can improve rather than how bad their performance might have been in the past. There should be no surprises at an appraisal; no issues should be brought up suddenly by the manager without warning. The appraisal consolidates everything that has happened and draws up plans for the future.

Who should be appraised?

All members of the practice should be appraised, including the partners and owners of the practice. This avoids the 'them and us' scenario, where junior staff are appraised by seniors who themselves are not appraised.

Who appraises?

Traditionally in veterinary practice employees are appraised by their immediate manager. This is based on the assumption that those who delegate the work and monitor performance are best placed to appraise performance. In the case of a small practice this may mean that most of the appraisals are carried out by one person, i.e. the manager or senior partner. In larger practices, head veterinary nurses and head receptionists appraise their staff and, in turn, are appraised by the practice manager. Figure 19.34 shows a typical appraisal hierarchy.

An alternative to the traditional appraisal is the 360-degree appraisal or feedback, where appraisal

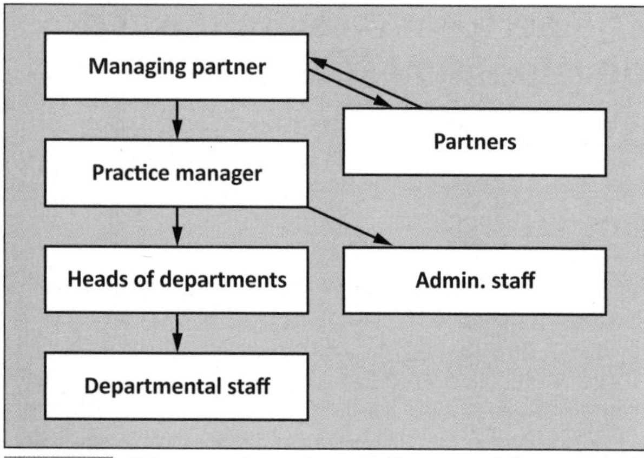

19.34 Who appraises whom. In the case of the appraisal of the partners, it is best for each partner to be appraised by all the others

feedback is given by subordinates, peers and supervisors. This type of appraisal is typically carried out using a written feedback form, which describes the individual's job skills, abilities, attitude, behaviour, etc. The appraisee also assesses themselves, using the same feedback form.

There can also be upwards feedback, where managers and/or partners are given feedback by the rest of the staff on an anonymous basis. This is often carried out by an external organization to ensure anonymity.

A practice must consider carefully whether the culture in the organization would support this kind of appraisal system, and full consultation must take place before introducing it. Objectivity is paramount, and training in appraisal technique is essential before 360-degree feedback is given by the team.

The timing of appraisals

Appraisal should be a continuous process and, once begun, should take place on a regular basis. This should be at least every 6 months but, ideally, a short one-to-one quarterly meeting is advised. In some instances, appraisals will need to be more frequent; e.g. induction appraisals for new employees, one of which may be a probationary appraisal if a probationary period has been agreed.

Appraisal success

Successful appraisals are based on:

- The commitment of the owners to supporting and encouraging appraisal of all staff, including themselves
- Communication with staff about appraisals, initially when they are being set up for the first time and then continuously where appraisal information needs to be disseminated
- Good training of all those who will be carrying out appraisal interviews. A badly conducted interview can set back an employee's progress and be very de-motivating
- Simplicity in terms of appraisal paperwork. There is no need for long and complex forms to be completed
- Effective monitoring. This is achieved by employee feedback and productivity, effective teamwork and both employee and appraiser reflection, to assess if the scheme is working well or needs modification.

Appraisal paperwork

Written records of appraisals should always be kept. This enables previous appraisals and decisions to be looked at, as well as providing evidence of ongoing agreed training. The paperwork gives the history of the employee's development in the practice; it can be used to assess their suitability for promotion, as well as (in the worst scenario) to assess the need for any disciplinary procedure. The essential paperwork is listed below.

- **The job description** – The employee's performance will be based on how well they are carrying out the responsibilities and tasks in their job description. This should be agreed at each appraisal.
- **The personal skills profile** – This is the profile drawn up when the employee was interviewed and sets out the skills and individual requirements required for the job (see Figure 19.17). It will provide a very useful guide when completing the employee's appraisal form.
- **The self-appraisal form** – This is the form the employee completes before the appraisal interview. It asks questions about their achievements, difficulties, skills and training (Figure 19.35). The completed form is handed to the appraiser a few days before the appraisal so that they can study it and prepare comments.

- What do you feel have been your major achievements at work in the last 12 months?
- How well do you feel you have achieved the objectives set at your last appraisal? (if applicable)
- Do you feel that you fully understand your role in the practice? Is your job description accurate?
- List any difficulties or frustrations you have in carrying out your work.
- Do you feel that there is anything that the practice can do to alleviate or remove these difficulties?
- What parts of your job do you:
  - Do best?
  - Do less well?
  - Fail to enjoy?

  (Please give reasons for your answers)
- Have you any skills, aptitudes or knowledge not fully utilized in your job? If so what are they and how could they be used?
- Are there any areas where you would like more support from your immediate supervisor?
- What support do you receive from your fellow workers and what help and support have you given your colleagues since the last appraisal?
- Do you have any difficulties with personal relationships in the practice? If you do, how could the practice help you?
- Are there any ways in which the practice could provide you with more support?
- Do you feel that you are always well informed about changes that are made to the way you work and the practice operates?
- What additional training have you received in the last 12 months and what difference has it made? What are you doing now that you didn't do before?
- Do you feel that you have received all the training promised at the last appraisal? (if applicable)
- What training, support or help do you think would enable you to do your job better?
- How would you like to see your job and role in the practice developing over the next 12 months?
- What work goals/ambitions do you have for the next 12 months?
- Please list any other comments, questions or suggestions here which you would like to discuss at the appraisal interview.

19.35 An example of a list of questions that may be included in an employee self-appraisal form.

- **The performance appraisal form** – This is the form the appraiser completes. It is used to assess the performance of the employee (Figure 19.36). There are many ways of assessing performance but, increasingly, the use of a comments-based form is being accepted as the most useful method. The appraisal form can be given to the employee a few days before the appraisal so that they can study it and prepare comments.
- **The personal and training action plan** – The training action plan (Figure 19.37) is drawn up as a result of the appraisal interview discussions. It sets out the training for the employee, agreed by the employee and appraiser for the next 12 months. The action plan should be discussed at intervals throughout the year to ensure the training is progressing, and is brought to the next year's appraisal for discussion. It will usually be helpful to note down a practice or manager's action plans as well, as this is a good opportunity to get ideas to improve resources, systems and relationships.

The appraisal interview

At least an hour should be set aside for the appraisal interview. It should be held somewhere quiet and should not be interrupted. As with any interview, seating arrangements should be comfortable and the appraiser should aim to create a relaxed atmosphere.

The appraiser should explain the purpose and scope of the interview and ensure that there is a constructive and positive discussion. The employee's job should be discussed in terms of its objectives and demands, and the comments made by the employee and appraiser on the appraisal forms discussed. Any future objectives (and how these will be achieved) should be discussed and agreed.

The appraiser must not promise help or training that cannot be delivered, and only realistic goals should be agreed. At the end of the appraisal the appraiser should summarize the discussion and the plans or training agreed and explain that a summary of the interview, or a copy of notes made, will be given to the appraisee.

Name .... Job title ....
Appraiser .... Date ....

Performance	Comments
Quality of work	
Practical and technical skills	
Job knowledge	
Organization and efficiency	
Productivity	
Degree of motivation	
Communication skills – oral and written	
Cooperation and work with colleagues	
Degree of support given to fellow employees	
Maintaining a positive attitude	
Use of initiative	
Client care skills	
Attendance and punctuality	
Achievement of objectives set at last appraisal (if applicable)	
Any other comments	

19.36 An example of an annual performance appraisal preparation assessment framework. If scores are desired, the following might be used: 1, improvement essential; 2, improvement desired; 3, performs to level expected of the job; 4, consistently gives outstanding performance with added value.

Name .... Date ....

Objective	Training or help needed	Action to be taken	By whom	Achieve by (date)

19.37 An example of a post-appraisal action plan. The appraisal should bring up actions for the individual, for the supervisor and for the practice.

KEY POINT

It is good practice for both parties to sign the appraisal summary and action plan and for both parties also to record a comment.

The manager should monitor the progress of the objectives agreed at each appraisal, checking that they are being achieved and that any agreed training is being carried out. The appraisal process can be summarized as follows:

1. Inform employee in writing of date of appraisal and how the appraisal will be managed.
2. Provide employee with the employee self-appraisal form to complete and return by a set date.
3. Appraiser completes employee appraisal form (the employee could complete this for themselves as well).
4. Appraisal forms are exchanged.
5. Appraisal takes place, content of the forms is discussed and the action plan is agreed.
6. Employee is informed in writing of appraisal discussions and decisions (or appraisal notes are shared) and any training and development plans are agreed.
7. Both parties record their comments and sign the document
8. Monitor and review action plan on a regular basis.

Induction appraisals

These appraisals follow the same structure and routine as a normal appraisal but are held 1, 3 and 6 months after a new employee has been recruited. The aim of the appraisal is to ensure that the new member of staff in their early days and weeks with the practice is progressing well and has no problems or difficulties. It is important that there is a formal opportunity for the employee to talk about their job with their line manager or team leader early in their employment so that any problems are sorted out at an early stage. It also helps with confidence boosting if the employee can be told that they are doing a good job. Questions that might be included in an induction appraisal form are shown in Figure 19.38.

Performance-related pay

Performance-related pay schemes link pay to a measure of individual or group performance. Such schemes have advantages, e.g. the staff get a 'cut' of practice income and are therefore rewarded for generating additional work, staying late, etc. Any such financial rewards are usually motivational. Importantly, the practice pricing policy will have a significant effect on behaviour when it comes to all bonus schemes.

There can be unintended consequences, however, such as extra work being done for the wrong reasons, e.g. cases not referred when they should be or products being sold when not needed. Where rewards are based on individual achievement, such schemes can be very effective for the 'workaholic' but do not always encourage teamwork and can sometimes result in resentment, particularly if work is not always shared out appropriately. Generally, the best bonus schemes are those that are equally shared by all staff and are applied *pro rata* for part-time staff. This reinforces teamwork and shows that everyone is valued and that no one person's role is more important than another. If the receptionist does not book the appointment when the call is taken, the veterinary surgeon cannot do the work, therefore both should equally share in the bonus that consultation generates. Work that is not directly income-generating, such as staff development, is also recognized this way.

- Is the job what you expected – does it vary from the job description discussed at interview? If so, in what ways?
- In which areas do you feel insecure, or lack knowledge necessary to perform tasks?
- In which areas do you feel confident, or feel you have received good training?
- How useful is the staff handbook?
  - Who's who?
  - Employment policies section?
  - Health and safety policy?
  - COSHH risk assessments?
  - Practice rules?
  - Clinical protocols?
  - Pricing and charging policy?
- What suggestions do you have for improving our induction training?
- Have health and safety issues been discussed with you adequately?
  - Please confirm by signing here that you have read and understand the practice rules and health and safety rules:

    ....
  - Any queries arising?
- How easy do you find other members of staff to work with?
- Are you having any problems with your relationships with other members of staff? Are you getting enough support/help when you need it?
- What do you most enjoy about the job?
- What do you least enjoy?
- How do you think you best contribute to the aims of the practice?
- Do you feel you have adequate opportunities to discuss your progress, and your position in the practice, with your supervisors?
- Are there any areas you would like to become more involved in, or where we are not using your skills to the best advantage?
- Have you any other comments or suggestions at this time?

19.38 An example of a list of questions that might be included in an induction appraisal checklist.

Some schemes are based on the whole salary being performance-related; this can greatly benefit the hard worker and leaves no room for those who wish to coast along on a guaranteed annual salary. It also eliminates the need for regular salary reviews. Other schemes operate on the basis of staff receiving a set salary plus a performance-related bonus.

Any performance-related pay scheme needs to be worked out carefully to suit each individual practice. It is important to be clear which criteria are to be used to measure performance, e.g. growth in turnover (excluding VAT) or increased profit. If schemes are based on turnover, the percentage that is to be paid must be carefully calculated as costs will not have been removed at this stage. If a scheme is based on profit, care must be taken regarding the influence of management decisions on spending that could significantly reduce that profit. The owner or management team needs to be in a position to make decisions regarding investment and spending without protests from staff, so gross profit or profit before investment or certain spending categories could be used. Some practices may prefer to keep things simple, with a performance-related pay scheme based on turnover.

In order to calculate bonus payments, the practice will need to decide which time periods they will base figures on (e.g. growth in turnover compared to the same period for the previous year), how long each scheme will run for (e.g. renewed annually), how often the bonus is to be paid (e.g. quarterly) and whether or not any deficits are carried forward. The last point is important: in the case of an annual scheme with quarterly payments, if turnover is down in the first 9 months of the year and deficits are not carried over, should practice income increase significantly in quarter 4, a large bonus could be paid out when, over the 12-month period, the practice has actually remained static and no extra income has been generated overall. It should be borne in mind that if this scheme is applied year on year, the ability for staff to continue to influence growth will slowly diminish as the market becomes saturated.

In practices with multiple branches, it is usually better to treat each branch as a separate entity; however, if staff rotate between branches then branch figures can be included in with the main surgery's figures.

KEY POINT

Bonus schemes are very exclusive to a practice, the way it operates and the staff it employs. Managers should be aware of the advantages, disadvantages and unintended consequences of such schemes, apply any scheme to the needs of the individual practice and keep the whole scheme and its results under review. It is useful to bear in mind that money is rarely the sole motivator of performance, particularly where complex work is involved.

It is advisable to seek professional advice on the mechanism, payment structure and contractual implications of any proposed practice- or personal-performance-related pay scheme.

Handling performance problems

Dealing with poor performance should be carried out with empathy and understanding. Although the appraisal is an excellent opportunity to discuss performance issues, poor performance should never be discussed for the first time at an appraisal. Just as thanks and praise must be given at the time and whenever appropriate, so must constructive criticism. Issues must never be saved up for appraisals or the appraisal system will fail.

If a member of staff is under-performing, the team leader or line manager needs to arrange an informal meeting with them to discuss any concerns and how they may be resolved. Identifying and dealing with poor performance depends on the presence of clear expectations for performance in the first place. The approach to performance should be a positive one with the assumption that everyone comes to work to do a good job. The manager may need to go through a problem-solving process to try to find the root cause of the problems. These could be, for example:

- A lack of understanding of what was expected
- An unwillingness to follow the ethos of the practice
- A lack of training to do the job correctly
- A system breakdown or inappropriate approach to the issue or task
- A lack of aptitude for the job which may be approached by changing the job expectation
- A problem originating outside of work.

An action plan should be agreed and targets set for improvement, necessary support/training should be agreed and provided and the whole process should be monitored.

It may be that the problems cannot easily be solved and, despite supportive training and encouragement, improvement does not occur. In this case, dismissal may become the only option (see Chapter 20). Wherever possible, however, if the wrong person is in the job, it is best to part on amicable terms and with the employee leaving voluntarily, having understood their own limitations and that of the job. The possibility of changing the job role to suit the individual's strengths should always be considered but may not be possible, particularly in smaller practices.

The correct handling of poor performance is vitally important. If things go wrong and there is no amicable parting between employee and employer, the consequences could be a constructive dismissal claim with accusations of bullying, harassment or even discrimination (see Chapter 20); if issues have not been fully and formally addressed at work and at appraisal, this may be difficult to defend, particularly if the employee produces evidence of an unblemished appraisal record.

Managing absenteeism and sickness

Absenteeism and sickness can be very expensive to any business, not just in monetary terms but also in reduced staff morale. Practices should have very clear guidelines and policies regarding staff absence and sickness. These should be included in any practice manual.

The main reasons why employees take time off work are:

- Holiday
- Short-term sickness
- Long-term sickness
- Authorized absence, e.g. maternity leave, parental leave, emergency leave, agreed compassionate leave, jury duty
- Unauthorized absence.

Absence due to ill health is normal for all businesses. However, excessive time off work for this reason needs to be addressed. One of the ways to measure staff absenteeism is to use the Bradford Factor or Formula. Bradford scores are a way of identifying individuals with serious absence and patterns of absence worthy of further investigation. How the Bradford Factor is calculated is shown in Figure 19.39.

B = S x S x D

B = Bradford points score
S = the number of occasions of absence in the last 52 weeks
D = the total number of days of absence in the last 52 weeks

Examples:

- 1 instance of absence with a duration of 10 days (1 x 1 x 10) = 10 points
- 3 instances of absence; one of 1, one of 3 and one of 6 days (3 x 3 x 10) = 90 points
- 5 instances of absence; each of 2 days (5 x 5 x 10) = 250 points
- 10 instances of absence; each of 1 day (10 x 10 x 10) = 1000 points

19.39 How to calculate the Bradford Factor, used to monitor absenteeism.

Frequent or high levels of sickness and absenteeism can be an indication that the culture of the practice is poor. Low staff morale and de-motivation as well as poor health and safety practices can all lead to higher than normal staff absence. Having good health and wellbeing standards (see earlier) will certainly help to keep staff absence at a minimum, but it is still necessary to have a sickness and absence policy in place. A sickness and absence (including holiday) policy should contain the information given in Figure 19.40.

A practice's sick pay policy can affect staff attitudes to taking sick leave. Statutory sick pay is paid to employees who are unable to work for at least 4 calendar days because of sickness. It is paid by the employer for up to a maximum of 28 weeks to all employees who satisfy the conditions for payment.

Practices should set their own discretionary sick pay agreements, e.g. they may make a discretionary sick pay payment to an employee for the first 3 days of illness or they may pay discretionary sick pay for a certain number of days per year. Such discretionary sick pay is open to abuse by employees and if a practice does provide this type of sick pay they should monitor employee illness/absence rates carefully. The practice can do this by employing and acting upon the Bradford Factor and making sure that any employees with high Bradford scores are interviewed to pick up/identify not just sickness but also unhappiness, personal problems and possible malingering. A return-to-work interview should apply to everyone, however long they have been off sick. It is important to encourage an attendance culture and make appropriate adjustments so that people can come back to work if they are able, even if they are not fully fit. For example, seated or part-time work can be offered to injured staff members who are otherwise feeling well. The manager should ensure that staff who have been off work because of an infectious disease are (as far as they can ascertain) free from infection before they return. Good attendance should be celebrated, being careful not to fall foul of disability discriminatory legislation.

The legal aspects of drawing up a sickness and absence policy are dealt with in Chapter 20, and more information about handling sickness and absence can be found on the ACAS website (www.acas.org.uk).

Holiday

- The holiday year – when the 12-month period runs from and to
- Holiday entitlements
- Booking holidays – who they should be made through, forms to complete, notice to be given, how decisions are made if more than one person requests the same holiday period, etc
- Carry-over holiday (if applicable)
- Christmas and bank holiday rotas

Illness

- How the member of staff should notify the practice if they are ill, or going to be late for work or absent for other reasons, e.g. by what time in the morning they should inform the practice and who they should inform
- When they should submit a medical statement from their doctor or self-certify their illness
- Statutory (and any contractual) sick pay arrangements
- Health insurance arrangements (if applicable)
- Possible procedures for using the employer's own doctor/medical advisor if there is a long-term illness
- The need to attend a return-to-work interview if these are held by the practice
- Consequences of not complying with the policy, e.g. what disciplinary measures may be taken

Official absence from work

- Antenatal appointments
- Jury service
- Maternity/paternity leave
- Parental leave
- Emergency time off for dependants – this is usually unpaid leave of absence

19.40 Items to be included in a practice policy for holiday, illness and official absence from work.

Handling long-term illness

When an employee is sick for a long period of time, they may feel isolated from work and worry about losing skills. Regular telephone calls or contact, appropriate to the situation, will help to keep the employee in the loop, keep stress levels at a minimum and motivate them to return to work. The secret is to keep in touch, understand the employee's problems and worries, and determine the exact nature of their illness and the estimated time they expect to take before returning to work.

Return-to-work interviews

The aim of the interview is to welcome the employee back, establish why the employee has been absent, check that they are well enough to be working again and whether, in the short term, they need any special accommodations to help them back into their job. It is also an opportunity to find out if there are or were any underlying problems causing the illness that are work-related and, if so, what can be done about them (Figure 19.41).

As with any other interview, the return-to-work interview should be held in private. The person conducting the interview should:

- Explain the reason for the interview – i.e. so that problem areas can be identified and appropriate support provided
- Ask about the reasons for the employee's absence
- Ask whether the employee consulted a doctor
- Try to establish the underlying cause of the absence without asking intrusive questions
- Check that the employee is well enough to return to work
- Check any discrepancies between the original reasons for absence and the reason given at the interview
- Review, check and ensure that the employee has correctly completed and signed their self-certification form
- Discuss and agree any support needed if recovery is ongoing.

For employees on long-term or maternity leave it is good practice to agree how to keep in touch beforehand (e.g. by e-mail, post or telephone). The practice must decide whether it is going to send details of ongoing training sessions to these employees, and whether they are welcome to attend discussions and training. Vacancies, team changes and other things happening in the practice that the rest of the staff would be informed about must all be communicated. In the case of maternity leave, the practice may have 'keep in touch days' when the employee attends the practice for an update on issues that affect them and their role in the team, or participates in the working day.

Handling grievance and disciplinary issues

The mechanism for handling grievance and disciplinary issues is dealt with in Chapter 20, but it is worth saying a few words here about how to avoid potential problems.

If a practice has a good communication system in place between line manager/team leader and staff there is less likelihood of grievances occurring. In many cases it is poor communications and misunderstandings that lead to disharmony among staff and unhappiness or upset with the practice. There needs to be an effective way of communicating information to staff and an equally good system of encouraging them to communicate back. Genuine grievances need to be addressed as soon as possible and all staff should be made aware of the grievance procedure by providing this information in the practice manual. The quicker a problem or grievance is dealt with, the less disruption there will be to the smooth running of the practice and to staff morale, and the less likely is an Employment Tribunal.

The same applies to dealing with disciplinary issues. What constitutes unacceptable behaviour should be explained in the practice/staff manual, as should the disciplinary process that will be carried out if an employee is considered to have breached any disciplinary rules.

KEY POINT

As with grievances, discipline should be dealt with as soon as possible. The longer the problem is left, the more difficult it will be to resolve.

Name of employee	Job title ....
Name of interviewer	Date and time of interview ....
Date of first day of absence	
Date of return to work	
Total days absent	
Reason given for absence	
Was correct notification of absence given?	
Was a doctor consulted or a hospital attended?	
Were any work factors connected with the absence?	
If work factors were connected with the absence what were they and what action has been agreed to support the employee?	
Interview discussion notes: Any accommodations needed to facilitate return to work/phased return?	
Signature of interviewer	
Signature of employee	

19.41 An example of a format for a return-to-work interview.

Exit interviews

Exit interviews are interviews conducted with departing employees, just before they leave. The aim of the exit interview, apart from confirming the reasons for the person's departure, is to find out useful information about the practice, which may be used to alter and improve aspects of the working environment, culture, processes and systems and management.

The interview is a unique chance to survey and analyse the opinions of departing employees, who will often be more forthcoming, constructive and objective than staff still in their jobs. From the point of view of the employee who is leaving, it is an opportunity to give some constructive feedback and for them to leave on a positive note. This is also important from the point of view of the existing staff, who will see the exit interview as a sign of a positive practice culture. A practice that cares about staff's reasons for leaving and is prepared, in some instances, to accept criticism and act upon constructive suggestions made by the leaver, is a listening employer. The exit interview helps to support good and effective people management in the practice.

Exit interviews are best conducted face to face because this enables better communication and understanding, although sometimes an employee may prefer to give their feedback in a questionnaire form. The exit interview should be organized in the same way as any other, with careful planning and attention to the need for time and privacy. Examples of exit interview questions are given in Figure 19.42.

It is also useful to have a leaver's checklist of items borrowed/used by the leaving employee (e.g. uniforms, badges, keys, equipment, books) to ensure that all items are left at the practice. Having a forwarding address is advisable for redirected mail and it is important to have reviewed the confidentiality clause.

Losing someone from the team and saying goodbye can be difficult. If good management practices are in place, however, there should be no regrets or surprises, and the leaver should be going on good terms, with a wealth of excellent experience and good times behind them. Recruiting to fill their shoes is an opportunity for the team, just as their new job or lifestyle is an opportunity for the leaver. The challenge should be embraced and the practice should look forward.

- What is your main reason for leaving?
- Are there any other reasons for your leaving?
- Is there anything that the practice could have done to avoid the situation that has influenced you to leave?
- What specific suggestions have you for how we could have managed this situation better?
- What has been good/enjoyable/satisfying for you during your time with the practice?
- Is there anything that has been frustrating/difficult/upsetting for you during your time with the practice?
- What could you have done better if you had been given opportunity?
- Were there any extra responsibilities that you would have liked?
- Could the practice have helped you to make fuller use of your capabilities and potential?
- What training would you have liked or needed that you did not receive, and what effect would this have had?
- How good do you think the communication is within the practice?
- What improvements do you think the practice could make to customer service?
- How would you describe the culture or 'feel' of the practice?
- What improvements could be made to the induction training you received?
- Do you think that you received enough helpful feedback about how you were performing your role in the practice?
- How well do you think the appraisal system worked for you?
- How do you think the practice could have improved your job motivation?
- Were there times when you felt stressed in your job and, if there were, how could the practice have helped to reduce that stress?

19.42 Sample exit interview questions.

Acknowledgements

The author and editors gratefully acknowledge Goddard Veterinary Group for the image in Figure 19.23.

Further reading

Advisory, Conciliation and Arbitration Service. *Health, Work and Wellbeing*. (available from www.acas.org.uk)

Bower J, Gripper J, Gripper P and Gunn D (2001) *Veterinary Practice Management, 3rd edn*. Blackwell Science, Oxford

Moreau P and Napp RC (2010) *Essentials of Veterinary Practice: An Introduction to the Science of Practice Management*. Henston Veterinary Publications, Peterborough

Shilcock M and Stutchfield G (2008) *Veterinary Practice Management: A Practical Guide, 2nd edn*. Saunders Elsevier, Oxford

Examples of job descriptions and forms ▶

Clinical Partner (Veterinary Surgeon)

Main purpose of the job:
To formulate and monitor practice clinical and business policy, together with the Managing Partner. To work together with the Managing Partner in business and financial planning, marketing, and maintaining the practice business, premises and contents. To select staff and appraise senior staff. To work as a veterinary surgeon.

Lines of authority:
Joint responsibility with Managing Partner for all staff.

Key staff liaison:
Partners and heads of sections.

Main duties:
- Setting and reviewing clinical policies in consultation with the veterinary team
- Coaching and instructing assistant veterinary surgeons and students in practical techniques and practice procedures, and encouraging them to keep up to date and maintain adequate CPD
- Instructing support staff re nursing procedures and general care of each patient; supervising nursing staff where appropriate. Training nurses according to the practice training schedules, both in practical and theory areas for the VN Diploma and further qualifications, and in equipment use and health and safety in the practice
- Directing the nursing staff towards achieving and maintaining the practice aims, and maintaining the high standards of the practice facilities and resources
- Holding local training sessions for colleagues in referral discipline, and other professional involvement
- Clinical diagnosis, treatment and care of animals both in the surgery and at other locations, following practice policy. Provision, on an equally shared basis with the other full-time and part-time vets, of the 24-hour emergency service
- Liaison with owners and ensuring good client communications are maintained at all times
- Seeing referral cases in .... disciplines as accepted and according to practice policy – including preparing referral written reports, follow-up telephone calls and liaison with referring practices
- Maintenance of accurate and complete computerized and manual medical records
- Charging for and recording all work done; taking and recording accurately all cash payments where required
- Ensuring that pet insurance claims and related correspondence are accurate and are dealt with in a timely manner
- Advising and educating clients on pet healthcare; answering telephone and general queries
- Participation in marketing initiatives, staff and management meetings and client meetings
- Radiation Protection Supervisor: responsible for ensuring the health and safety of all employees in the designated area and for liaison with the RPA.

Knowledge and skills required:
- Sound business knowledge and skills
- Good communication and coaching skills
- Personnel skills
- Clinical skills
- Specialist or recognized certificate level qualifications and recognition in relevant discipline for referrals
- Up-to-date veterinary clinical knowledge in all areas.

Training that may be required:
- Attendance at relevant clinical specialist conferences; speaking or writing in area of special interest; further reading in referral discipline and non-veterinary journals
- Training in coaching and leadership skills, interpersonal communications.

Some examples of job role descriptions. (continues) ▶

Managing Partner

Main purpose of the job:
To take overall responsibility for the business of the veterinary practice, ensuring that financially the practice is sound, with adequate generated profit, and that strategic plans are in place and implemented. To take ultimate responsibility for all personnel issues, training policy, and development of staff and the practice as a whole. If applicable, to carry out clinical veterinary surgeon duties, as described in Clinical Partner and Veterinary Surgeon job descriptions.

Lines of authority:
Responsible for all staff via the management team.

Key staff liaison:
Partners, veterinary surgeons, heads of sections.

Main duties

Responsibility for (via delegation):

- Credit control
- Production of accurate monthly management accounts and reporting these to practice teams
- Budgeting, cost control and income analysis
- Accurate and regular bank and cash reconciliation
- Liaison with accountant at year end
- Purchase of assets and setting buying policy
- Production of Practice Annual Report and its presentation
- Recruitment and staffing
- Maintaining IiP and Health and Wellbeing standards
- Staff appraisal
- Salary setting and review
- Staff manual and Health & Safety policy
- Organizing training and evaluation
- Standards of production of in-house publicity and educational material
- Marketing
- Maintaining premises in good order
- Monitoring and maintaining high standards of customer service and patient care
- Chairing weekly vets meetings and ensuring they are recorded accurately
- Chairing practice meetings.

Knowledge and skills required:

- Sound business experience
- Clear leadership qualities and excellent delegation skills
- Good communication skills
- Financial analysis skills
- Planning skills
- Personnel skills
- Problem-solving skills
- Marketing skills, creativity.

Training that may be required:

- Attendance at relevant management and veterinary courses/events
- Maintaining up-to-date knowledge of veterinary clinical issues and current business performance and benchmarking.

(continued) Some examples of job role descriptions. (continues) ▶

Associate Veterinary Surgeon

Main purpose of the job:

To provide high quality veterinary services to clients and their animals. To continuously develop personal clinical skills, to achieve practice goals and to communicate effectively with clients and the team.

Lines of authority:

Responsible to the partners.

Key staff liaison:

Veterinary surgeons, Practice Manager and Head Nurse.

Main duties:

- Consultations
- Surgical operations
- House visits
- Investigative procedures
- Care of hospitalized patients
- To present a caring, professional attitude to clients, patients and other staff members
- To abide by the rules set out in the RCVS Code of Professional Conduct
- To communicate effectively with colleagues in order to ensure continuity in care of patients
- To communicate promptly and effectively with clients regarding progress of hospitalized patients and reporting of laboratory results
- To regularly undertake CPD in order to maintain and increase veterinary skills and knowledge
- To make use of internal or external referral services as appropriate, and seek the advice or assistance of colleagues when needed
- To train and develop staff members to enable them to carry out their role
- To follow practice protocols
- Any other duties that may be required.

Knowledge and skills required:

- Clinical and surgical skills
- Client care skills
- Communication and personal organizational skills.

Training that may be required:

Attendance at any relevant training that is considered necessary for carrying out the role of Associate Veterinary Surgeon at the practice.

Veterinary Nurse

Main purpose of the job:

To act as a veterinary nurse in the clinic nursing services team to provide high quality surgical, nursing and animal care skills to the veterinary team. To provide excellent client care to all owners.

Lines of authority:

Responsible to the Head Nurse.

Key staff liaison:

Veterinary surgeons and the Head Nurse.

Main duties:

- To provide nursing support to the veterinary team
- To provide animal nursing for hospitalized animals
- To act as a consulting room nurse when required
- To dispense animal medicines
- To maintain clinic hygiene standards
- To sterilize surgical equipment
- To assist in radiography
- To provide pre- and postoperative animal care.

Knowledge and skills required:

- Currently registered or listed veterinary nurse
- A sound knowledge of practice protocols
- At least RCVS minimum required CPD
- Good client care skills
- Competency in the use of the clinic computer and word processing systems
- Up-to-date knowledge of the clinic services and products.

Training that may be required:

- Attendance at any relevant in-house training sessions
- Attendance at any appropriate external training courses which will enhance skills and personal development.

(continued) Some examples of job role descriptions. (continues)

Practice Manager

Main purpose of the job:

To facilitate and manage the day-to-day business of the practice and to implement the owners' vision for taking the business forward.

Lines of authority:

Responsible to the partners.
Responsible for veterinary surgeons (non-clinical) and for nursing and administrative staff.

Key staff liaison:

Partners and heads of sections.

Main duties:

- To promote and grow both the first opinion and referral sides of the business
- To expand the business and develop branches in the local area
- Personnel management
- Recruiting and interviewing
- Staff training
- Staff appraisals
- Discipline and grievance procedures
- To ensure good communication within the business
- Financial planning
- Monitoring practice financial accounts
- Generation and presentation of financial and management reports
- Overseeing financial accounts
- Managing cash flow
- Debt control
- To liaise with practice accountants and solicitors
- Overall responsibility for drug purchase and stock control
- Practice insurance
- Car and equipment leasing, fleet management
- Equipment purchase
- Computer hardware and software management
- Overall responsibility for implementing legislative requirements relating to the business, in particular health and safety and employment requirements
- Development of new practice services
- Marketing
- Public relations and media liaison
- Client complaints
- Overseeing of building maintenance and any other duties which may reasonably be required.

Knowledge and skills required:

- Previous business experience
- Sound knowledge of accounting procedures
- Personnel skills
- IT skills
- Marketing experience
- Good communication skills.

Training that may be required:

Attendance at relevant management training course/events.

(continued) Some examples of job role descriptions. (continues)

Nursing Assistant

Main purpose of the job:
To assist the nursing and veterinary teams with basic animal care and nursing.

Lines of authority:
Responsible to the Head Nurse.

Key staff liaison:
Veterinary surgeons and the Head Nurse.

Main duties:
- Assisting the veterinary surgeon or nurse
- Holding patients for blood samples and non-surgical treatments
- Feeding patients under instruction
- Maintaining a clean and hygienic environment
- Washing and drying bedding
- Processing blood samples.

Knowledge and skills required:
- A sound knowledge of practice protocols
- Animal knowledge and handling skills
- Familiarity with commonly used veterinary terms and drugs
- Good client care skills
- Competency in the use of the clinic computer and word processing systems
- Up-to-date knowledge of the clinic services and products.

Training that may be required:
- Attendance at any relevant in-house training sessions and appropriate external training courses.

Receptionist

Main purpose of the job:
To provide a friendly, efficient and effective reception service to our clients.

Lines of authority:
Responsible to the Head Receptionist.

Key staff liaison:
Head Receptionist.

Main duties:
- Booking appointments
- Answering the telephone and taking phone messages
- Using computer to administer client records
- Working knowledge of office equipment, its use and maintenance
- Advising clients on pet healthcare
- Working knowledge of new products, medicines and services
- Advising on and selling pet products
- Dealing with client queries and problems
- Dealing with client account queries
- Cashing up
- Supporting bereaved clients
- Stocking shelves in waiting room
- Booster reminder administration
- Faxing, photocopying and filing
- General cleanliness and tidiness of surgery
- Awareness of and compliance with practice health and safety regulations.

Knowledge and skills required:
- A sound knowledge of practice policies and protocols
- Good client care skills
- Competency in the use of the practice computer and word processing systems
- Up to date knowledge of practice services and products
- Sound knowledge of common veterinary terms
- Sound knowledge of commonly used veterinary drugs
- Sound knowledge of common veterinary treatments and operations
- Basic knowledge of cat, dog and rabbit anatomy and physiology
- Basic knowledge of common microorganisms
- Basic knowledge of common parasites
- Ability to give immediate animal First Aid advice to clients.

Training that may be required:
Full initial training will be provided. All staff are expected to attend appropriate staff training and development courses.

(continued) Some examples of job role descriptions. (continues)

Administrative Assistant

Main purpose of the job:
To provide administrative and secretarial support to the Practice Manager. To provide a friendly, efficient and professional service to clients.

Lines of authority:
Responsible to the Practice Manager.

Key staff liaison:
Partners and the Practice Manager.

Main duties:

- To type and process various documents, presentations, reports and electronic documents
- To create reports using spreadsheets
- To set up and maintain filing systems
- To be responsible for stationery purchase and stationery stock control
- To implement and adhere to stated policies and procedures relating to health and safety
- To maintain staff leave and sickness records
- To maintain debtors' records and deal with overdue accounts.

Knowledge and skills required to carry out the job:

- A sound knowledge of practice protocols
- Good organizational skills
- Good client care and communication skills
- Competency in the use of the clinic computer and word processing systems
- Up-to-date knowledge of the clinic services and products.

Training that may be required:

- Attendance at any relevant in-house training sessions
- Attendance at any appropriate external training courses which will enhance skills and personal development.

Cleaner

Responsible to:
Practice Manager.

Responsible for:

General duties

- To ensure high standards, by offering a service of quality and efficiency, administered with total integrity in a helpful, cheerful and friendly manner.
- To take proper care of all surgery equipment, including correct cleaning of equipment, and to report any items in need of maintenance or repair.
- To ensure that work is carried out in an economical manner and that all wastage is kept to a minimum, particularly with regard to consumable items.
- To carry out general and specific cleaning duties, helping to ensure that all areas of the premises are maintained in a neat, clean, tidy and presentable state.
- To carry out the specific weekly duties relating to the offices, stairs, staff toilets, staff room (including the refrigerator) and training room (including training room toilet). Duties include cleaning, vacuuming, wiping any linoleum floors, emptying the bins and replacing bin liners, cleaning out the refrigerator, bleaching any work surfaces, wiping over any sinks, changing towels and restocking.
- To maintain a safe working environment for all staff by observing and implementing all health and safety regulations and requirements.
- To ensure that the Practice Manager is notified of any relevant personnel/management issues that may arise.
- To foster an excellent level of communication between all staff.
- To assist in implementing any new practice protocols or standards of performance in conjunction with the Practice Manager or Principal, and to put forward any suggestions for further improvements and refinements.
- To carry out any other reasonable task or any duties, which fall within your capabilities, as requested by the Practice Manager or Principal.

Professional duties

- To observe and conform with the RCVS code of ethics in accordance to how it relates to lay staff.
- To ensure a smart and professional appearance and to conduct a professional manner at all times.

(continued) Some examples of job role descriptions.

Job application form

Please complete the following application form and return to the Practice Manager by ....
If there is further information you wish to add please attach a separate sheet to the application form.

Post advertised: ....

Where did you hear about this post? ....

Personal details

Name: ....

Address: ....

....

....

Telephone: .... (daytime) Telephone: .... (evening) Telephone: .... (mobile)

E-mail: .... Fax: ....

Do you have a current British driving licence? ....

Please state the number of endorsement points on this licence: ....

Are there any restrictions regarding your right to work in the UK? If yes, please provide details. ....

....

....

Do you have any criminal convictions? If yes, please provide details ....

....

Education

School dates: ....

Please give NVQ, GCSE and A-Levels, and grades achieved:

....

....

....

University/college dates: ....

Name of institution: ....

Address: ....

....

....

Please give degrees/qualifications achieved:

....

....

Other further education dates: ....

Name of institution: ....

Address: ....

....

....

Please give details and qualifications obtained:

.... Dates ....

.... Dates ....

Professional membership and qualifications

Please give full details:

....

....

....

....

....

An example of a job application form. (continues)

CPD

Please give details of any training and development courses which support your application.

....

....

....

Work experience and employment

Present employment

Employer: ....

Position: ....

Please describe the work you do and your responsibilities:

....

....

Length of time in this post:

From: .... To: ....

Starting salary: .... Leaving salary: ....

Reason for leaving: ....

....

Previous employment

Employer: ....

Position: ....

Please describe the work you did and your responsibilities:

....

....

Length of time in this post:

From: .... To: ....

Starting salary: .... Leaving salary: ....

Reason for leaving: ....

....

Previous employment

Employer: ....

Position: ....

Please describe the work you did and your responsibilities:

....

....

Length of time in this post:

From: .... To: ....

Starting salary: .... Leaving salary: ....

Reason for leaving: ....

....

Your application

Please tell us why you are applying for this position:

....

....

....

....

Please describe your skills and experience which are relevant to the position applied for:

....

....

....

(continued) An example of a job application form. (continues) ▶

Please tell us why you feel you are the best candidate for this post:

....

....

....

Interests and activities

Please describe your interests and activities outside work:

....

....

Interview assistance

We are an equal opportunities employer and need to be aware of any adjustments we may need to make to assist you at interview. Please specify below:

....

....

Referees

Please give the names and contact details of referees for each job above:

....

....

....

Please give the name and contact details of a personal referee who is not a present or past employer:

....

....

Do you give the practice permission to approach referees if you are short-listed for the position?

....

When would you be available to start employment? ....

I confirm that the information I have given on this form is accurate to the best of my knowledge and belief.

Signature: .... Date:...

(continued) An example of a job application form

Reference request form

The person below has applied for employment with *practice name* and has supplied your name as a referee in support of their application.

Name of applicant:..

Post applied for:..

Name of referee:...

Position: ....

Name of organization: ....

In what capacity do you know the applicant? ....

....

To be completed by current or previous employer:

Capacity in which person was employed: ....

....

Dates of employment: From .... to ....

Main duties: ....

....

....

Number of days of absence due to sickness/injury in the last 2 years: ....

How long have you known the applicant?...

To be completed by all referees

Please rate the applicant on the following by placing a tick in the appropriate box.

Trait/skill	Excellent	Good	Adequate	Poor
Honesty				
Punctuality				
Motivation				
Flexibility				
Reliability				
Communication				

Additional information to be completed by all referees

A job description and personal specifications are supplied.
Please comment on the applicant's suitability for the post with reference to the job description:

....

....

....

....

Do you have any other relevant comments to make regarding the applicant?

....

....

....

....

Would you re-employ the applicant if applicable? Yes No (please circle)

The details supplied are to the best of my knowledge correct.

Signature: .... Date:...

Thank you for taking the time to complete this form. Please return it to ....

An example of a reference request form

Practical employment law in the United Kingdom

20

Margaret Keane

Employment law is complex and wide-ranging, changing frequently and permeating every part of the relationship between an employer and an employee, from recruitment to leaving employment.

It is important to have an understanding of the terms 'reasonableness' and 'reasonable' in the context of employment law. Whenever a decision is taken to resolve an employment dispute, reasonableness should always be considered. At a tribunal the question asked is, 'Did the employer act reasonably or did the employee?'. If a party is judged to have acted unreasonably, the complaint is more likely to be upheld.

The words 'reasonable' and 'reasonably' can be interpreted by different people in different ways: what is reasonable behaviour for one person may be seen as outrageous by another. The root of these words is reason, which means being rational. Therefore, in the context of employment law, did the parties act in a rational way without being prejudiced or influenced by emotions like anger? Employment law is based on rational behaviour by employees and employers.

The approach of this chapter is to look at the different life stages of an employee (Figure 20.1) and explain which legislation employers should be aware of when dealing with different situations.

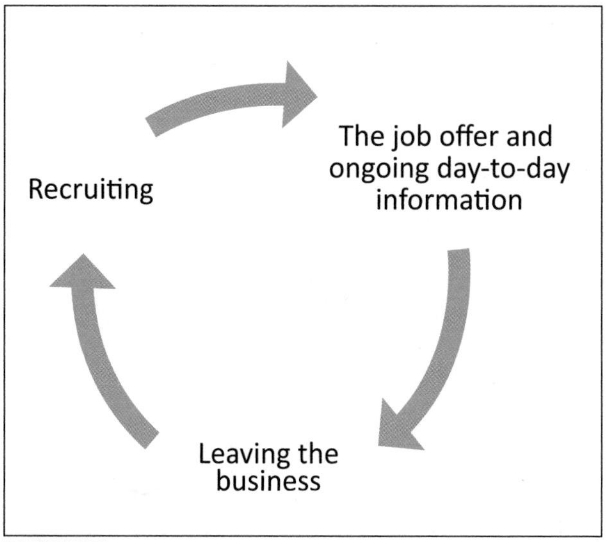

This chapter provides guidance on employment law at the time of writing for the United Kingdom generally. There are some minor differences for Scotland and Northern Ireland. **This is not legal advice** and so readers are strongly advised to seek independent legal advice for any employment law issues with reference to their national law. Many professional organizations such as the BVA may have access to telephone legal helplines as a member benefit. As for searches on the Internet for any subject, readers must ensure that the sites are up to date.

More information about recruitment and selection procedures and staff management can be found in Chapter 19.

Recruiting

The job offer and ongoing day-to-day information

Leaving the business

20.1 The life cycle of an employee.

Recruitment

Attracting and short-listing candidates

Once the decision has been taken to recruit a new employee, the usual starting point is writing a job description or reviewing an established one. Under the RVCS Practice Standards Scheme it is a requirement to provide employees with a written job description, although there is no legal obligation to do so. The role/job description is useful information for applicants. It should be specific enough to identify the job role but general enough to enable changes within the context of a contract of employment.

The usual way a business attracts candidates is by advertising the role both internally and externally. It is not unlawful for an employer just to advertise internally; however, some organizations in the public sector are required to apply open competition rules when recruiting.

An advertisement could be deemed to be unlawful if the wording could be interpreted as discouraging applicants from a particular group. For example, to advertise for a man or a woman or to state a preference for candidates from a certain racial or religious group is unlawful unless it is an occupation requirement (see later).

Discrimination

The aim of the Equality Act 2010 was to bring together all of the different pieces of discrimination legislation. This piece of legislation affects all areas of the relationship between an employer and employee.

Candidates for a job are protected against discrimination throughout the recruitment process on the following grounds:

- Sex
- Race
- Disability
- Sexual orientation
- Age
- Religion and belief
- Marriage and civil partnership
- Pregnancy and maternity
- Gender reassignment.

These are the protected characteristics as stated in the Equality Act 2010.

If at any time during the recruitment process a candidate believes they have been subjected to discrimination, they may bring a claim against the potential employer to an employment tribunal.

Types of discrimination

There are four types of discrimination:

- Direct discrimination (including perceptive and associative discrimination)
- Indirect discrimination
- Victimization
- Harassment.

Direct discrimination: This would occur if an applicant could show that they had been treated less favourably than another applicant on one of the prohibited grounds. The other applicant would be known as the 'comparator'. The comparator must be someone whose circumstances are the same or not materially different.

In cases where there are no comparators, e.g. where there was only one applicant for the job and they allege discrimination, the law will allow a hypothetical comparison to be drawn. The applicant would have to show that they were treated less favourably than someone older or younger, of the opposite sex or of a different race, religion or sexual orientation would have been treated in the same or similar circumstances.

In the Equality Act 2010, the terms perceptive and associative discrimination are defined as follows:

- **Perceptive discrimination** – When a person is discriminated against because it is perceived that they have a particular protected characteristic, such as they are perceived to be of a certain age. This is unlawful even if the individual is not of the perceived age
- **Associative discrimination** – When an individual discriminates against someone because they associate them with someone with a particular protected characteristic.

Indirect discrimination: Indirect discrimination occurs where a policy, act or decision is applied to everybody, but that policy, act or decision has a disproportionate impact on people with a protected characteristic. Indirect discrimination has been extended to cover disability discrimination and gender reassignment. An example would be requiring that employees must be 6 feet tall, as this would disproportionately disadvantage women. Indirect discrimination can be justified if the employer can show that the policy, act or decision represented a proportionate means of achieving a legitimate aim.

Victimization: The law protects individuals from discrimination on the protected characteristics and it also precludes an employer from victimizing an employee or a job applicant if they have made a 'protected act' or the employer believes that the employee has done, or may do a 'protected act.' Protected acts include bringing proceedings under discrimination law or making an allegation of discrimination. They also include giving evidence in respect to a claim of discrimination, in someone else's complaint of discrimination. For example, if decisions were taken not to shortlist a candidate or not to offer employment because they had appeared at an employment tribunal to give evidence in respect of a claim of discrimination, this would be victimization. The candidate would have to show that their treatment was caused by their involvement in a previous complaint of discrimination.

Harassment: The general definition of harassment is unwanted conduct related to a relevant protected characteristic, which has the purpose or effect of either violating an individual's dignity or creating an intimidating, hostile, degrading, humiliating or offensive environment for that individual. Harassment may also arise where an individual engages in unwanted conduct of a sexual nature and that conduct has the purpose or effect as described above, or where because of an employee's rejection of, or submission to, that unwanted conduct they are treated unfavourably. This could happen in the interview stage of recruitment, for example if the interviewer made sexist or racist remarks or made demeaning or degrading observations about candidates' religious beliefs.

Exceptions: occupational requirements

This is a very limiting exception and would be for specific circumstances where an employer could set out to recruit a man or a woman, someone from a racial group, someone of a particular religion, sexual orientation or someone who possesses a characteristic related to age. It has to be shown that some aspect of the job creates a genuine need for the job to be carried out by a person from a specific group. These regulations might apply to modelling or acting jobs. Within a veterinary practice it would be difficult to state that any role would need to be performed by a person from a specific group.

Positive action and positive discrimination

Positive action happens where members of an under-represented or disadvantaged group are encouraged to apply and are prioritized. An example of this would be when the police force advertised for members from minority ethnic communities. The Equality Act

2010 contains provision for lawful positive action, which is designed to apply where persons who share a protected characteristic suffer a disadvantage connected to that characteristic, have particular needs, or are disproportionately under-represented.

Compensation

A claim for discrimination gives rise to awards for injury to feelings as well as loss of earnings compensation. The level of compensation will depend on the seriousness of the complaint and there is no upper limit. At the time of writing, the injury to feeling award can be from £600 for a one-off incident up to £30,000 for a campaign of harassment. Compensation payments under all discrimination legislation are calculated on the basis of what is just and equitable for the employee to receive. Discrimination cases can make newspaper headlines, such as in 2008 when a top female City lawyer won £13.4 million in compensation. This would have been calculated by an amount for injury to feelings and a claim for loss of earnings. The purpose of the award is to put the employee back into the position they would have been in had the discrimination not occurred.

Job advertising compliance

When advertising for a role the following should be checked:

- The wording used in the advert should not be sexist, e.g. 'taxi man'
- Any pictures of teams should not create a stereotypical image, e.g. contain only white people
- The wording must not be ambiguous or open to misinterpretation
- The job requirements are stated appropriately and are correct for the job
- The advertisement does not imply that the role is not suitable for a disabled person
- Age limits or ageist terms (e.g. 'young vet') must be avoided.

Advertising in this context includes all forms of advertising, both internal and external, and includes all types of media.

Recruitment agencies

The Conduct of Employment Agencies and Employment Business (Amendment) Regulations 2010 exist to establish the rules that govern how a recruitment agency works with its clients and the candidates they wish to place, either temporarily or permanently.

The Employment Practices Data Protection Code issued by the Information Commissioner is a formal guide that helps recruitment agencies and employers to comply with the Data Protection Act. The Code in itself is not legally binding, but failure to comply with its guidance can be taken into account by a court or employment tribunal.

Application forms and short-listing

Applications forms should be designed so that they only ask relevant questions. It is acceptable to ask questions that relate to gender, date of birth, marital status, address, nationality, age and disability, but this information must only be used for monitoring purposes. Some companies split the application into two forms and the part that contains the monitoring information is not seen by the person who is responsible for short-listing. In a small business this might not be a possibility and so whoever is responsible for short-listing must ensure that job applicants are treated fairly and equally, regardless of their personal circumstances (i.e. gender, age, religion, sexual orientation, marital status, disability, maternity issues or gender reassignment).

Any questions asked prior to short-listing in relation to disability should be purely for determining whether reasonable adjustments might need to be made for a disabled person to attend the interview. Once the job has been offered, questionnaires such as pre-employment health questionnaires can then be used but, again, the information is used to ascertain whether any reasonable adjustments are required to assist the new employee on a day-to-day basis at work. For example, a person who is diabetic may need extra breaks to administer their medication and check sugar levels.

KEY POINT

Pre-employment health questionnaires should not be part of the recruitment process and should only be requested once a job offer has been made. The information contained in them should not be used to judge the ability of an applicant to do a job.

It is good practice to monitor recruitment processes in order to promote equality.

Data protection

Under the Data Protection Act, employers should not collect information that is classed as 'sensitive' unless the individual has consented and the use of the information is for monitoring.

Questions asked on an application form should be either relevant to determining the suitability of an individual to perform the role or for general administration purposes. Any questions relating to trade union membership or activities should not be included as, if an employer refused to employ a person because they were a member of a union, this would be unlawful.

Interviewing

Questioning

When preparing for interviews, an employer should decide beforehand what questions to ask.

A list of key job-related questions should be prepared (see Chapter 19), with the intention of asking such questions (in the same order and in the same way) of every candidate for the post under review, to help ensure consistency and fairness in interviewing. There will also be a need to ask questions that are specific to each candidate.

The interviewer should look for features of each application that:

- Require clarification
- Require verification
- Have experience expressed in vague terms
- Have information or time periods missing.

The Equality Act 2010 applies during the interviewing process. Questions are discriminatory if they:

- Show an intention to discriminate on any of the prohibited grounds listed earlier
- Indicate a biased view on the interviewer's part for any of the prohibited reasons
- Put the applicant at a disadvantage on any of the prohibited grounds, e.g. a question asked of a Muslim applicant as to how much time off he or she would require for prayer would discriminate on the grounds of religion
- Are derogatory on any of the above grounds, e.g. a comment made about a female applicant's family commitments conflicting with work requirements could be construed as sex discrimination.

The purposes of an interview are to find out whether the applicant can do the job and, for the applicant, to ascertain whether the role is going to meet with their expectations. Questions must be asked about the capability of the applicant while at the same time not asking questions which could be potentially discriminatory.

Questions to avoid

Questioning on the following areas could be regarded as discriminatory.

Questions about place of birth, ethnicity and religion

- Where were you born?
- What is your native language?
- Do you observe religious holidays that may not be national holidays?

Employers do need to ensure that employees have the correct paperwork to work in the UK and can ask for specific proof (see below). Employers cannot, however, ask about the place of birth or personal history of an applicant. If during an interview, questions are asked regarding someone's place of birth, it could be interpreted that the company was asking this because it was going to base its decision on the grounds of nationality, race or religious preference or background.

Questions about marital status, children and sexual preferences

- Are you married?
- Are you gay?
- Do you plan to start a family soon?

If an employer asks about marital status it can be perceived that they would prefer either to employ a married person because they are thought of as being more stable, or to employ a single person without children because it could be assumed that they would have more time to devote to the job. Enquiring about a person's personal sexual preferences is strictly a no-go area.

Questions about age

- How old are you?

If there is a minimum age for a person to carry out a role, e.g. bar staff must be at least 18 years of age, then an employer can ascertain this fact (see above).

Questions about disability and illness

- Do you have a disability or chronic illness?

Asking direct questions to a person about a disability, whether or not it would affect their ability to do the job, could be grounds for disability discrimination.

If a role needs a certain level of fitness (e.g. a scaffolder) then, once the job has been offered, a company could say it was conditional on passing a medical as this attribute is imperative to the role.

Other questions to avoid

In most cases, a potential employee or current employee's activities outside of work are not the business of the company, e.g. their alcohol consumption or whether they smoke. However, a company can set out the policy for using these kinds of substances within the working environment. These policies should be set out in the staff handbook.

If it is a requirement of the job, employers are entitled to run a CRB (Criminal Records Bureau) check prior to the interview. However, information obtained from this check should never form part of the interview process.

Direct questions regarding an applicant's membership of organizations can only be asked if there are concerns about time commitments and how that would affect the ability to do the job. Not employing someone on the grounds that they were a member of a trade union would be illegal (see later).

Checking eligibility to work in the UK

KEY POINT

Employers are responsible for making reasonable checks to ensure that their employees are legally entitled to work in the UK.

To do this, the employer can ask the applicant to provide appropriate evidence. Under the Immigration, Asylum and Nationality Act 2006 it is illegal to employ someone who does not have the right to work in the UK. The Home Office has produced two lists, known as List A and List B (Figure 20.2). The employer should ask all potential employees to show them either one document from List A or two of the documents in the combinations specified in List B. Only original documents should be accepted.

- Documents in List A indicate that the holder is entitled to live and work in the UK without restriction. Checking a document included in this list will provide a statutory defence and will mean there is no need to check further documents from List B.

List A

- A United Kingdom passport describing the holder as a British citizen or as a citizen of the United Kingdom and Colonies having the right of abode in the United Kingdom; or:
- A passport containing a certificate of entitlement issued by or on behalf of the Government of the United Kingdom, certifying that the holder has the right of abode in the United Kingdom; or:
- A passport or national identity card, issued by a State which is a party to the European Economic Area Agreement or any other agreement forming part of the Communities Treaties which confers rights of entry to or residence in the United Kingdom, which describes the holder as a national of a State which is a party to that Agreement; or:
- A United Kingdom residence permit issued to a national of a State which is a party to the European Economic Area Agreement or any other agreement forming part of the Communities Treaties which confers rights of entry to or residence in the United Kingdom; or:
- A passport or other travel document or a residence document issued by the Home Office which is endorsed to show that the holder has a current right of residence in the United Kingdom as the family member of a named national of a State which is a party to the European Economic Area Agreement or any other agreement forming part of the Communities Treaties which confers rights of entry to or residence in the United Kingdom, and who is resident in the United Kingdom; or:
- A passport or other travel document endorsed to show that the holder is exempt from immigration control, has indefinite leave to enter, or remain in, the United Kingdom or has no time limit on his/her stay; or:
- A passport or other travel document endorsed to show that the holder has current leave to enter, or remain, in the United Kingdom and is permitted to take the employment in question, provided that it does not require the issue of a work permit; or:
- A Registration Card which indicates that the holder is entitled to take employment in the United Kingdom.

List B

First combination

A. A document issued by a previous employer, Inland Revenue, the Department for Work and Pensions, Job Centre Plus, the Employment Service, the Training and Employment Agency (Northern Ireland) or the Northern Ireland Social Security Agency, which contains the National Insurance number of the person named in the document; AND ONE OF THE FOLLOWING DOCUMENTS FROM (B TO H):
B. A birth certificate issued in the United Kingdom, the Channel Islands, the Isle of Man or Ireland which specifies the names of the holder's parents.
C. A birth certificate issued in the Channel Islands, the Isle of Man or Ireland.
D. A certificate of registration or naturalization as a British citizen.
E. A letter issued by the Home Office, to the holder, which indicates that the person named in it has been granted Indefinite Leave to Enter or Remain in the United Kingdom.
F. An Immigration Status Document issued by the Home Office, to the holder, endorsed with a United Kingdom Residence, which indicates that the holder has been granted Indefinite Leave to Enter or Remain in the United Kingdom.
G. A letter issued by the Home Office, to the holder, which indicates that the person named in it has subsisting leave to enter or remain in the United Kingdom and is entitled to take the employment in question in the United Kingdom.
H. An Immigration Status Document issued by the Home Office, to the holder, endorsed with a United Kingdom Residence Permit, which indicates that the holder has been granted Limited Leave to Enter or Remain in the United Kingdom and is entitled to take the employment in question in the United Kingdom.

Second combination

A. A work permit or other approval to take employment issued by Work Permits UK; and EITHER:
B. A passport or other travel document endorsed to show that the holder has current Leave to Enter or Remain in the United Kingdom and is permitted to take the work permit employment in question;
OR:
C. A letter issued by the Home Office to the holder, confirming the same.

20.2 It is essential to check that all new employees are eligible to work in the UK. The Home Office has produced two lists: List A and List B. Employers must ask all potential employees to provide either one document from List A or two documents, in the combinations specified, from List B. Only original documents should be accepted.

- Documents on List B indicate that the individual may work in the UK but with restrictions, normally in respect of the length of time the holder may continue working. List B covers *combinations* of documents. Both documents in the combination list must be seen in order to have a defence. It will not provide a defence to see one document from one combination and one from another. If the family name or other personal details on the two documents do not match, further proof must be produced of the reason for this – in the form of a marriage certificate, divorce document, deed poll, adoption certificate or statutory declaration.

KEY POINT

Employers should always take copies of original documents and keep them for the duration of employment and 2 years after the employee's departure from the business.

Although it is not a legal requirement to conduct the document check or to retain copies of the documents, employers will, by doing so, have a statutory defence against liability for civil penalties in the event that the person turns out not to have the right to work in the UK. The fine for employing a person who does not have the necessary permission to work in the UK is in the region of £10,000.

UK immigration scheme

Currently the UK has in operation a five-tier immigration scheme. As part of this scheme, there is a Shortage Occupation list. Up until 2011, this list included veterinary surgeons. This meant that if an employer wished to employ a veterinary surgeon from overseas, they could do so without having first to fulfil the Resident Labour Market test by advertising the vacancy in the UK. However, from 2012 employers will have to satisfy the requirements of the Resident Labour Market, as it has been decided that statistically there is no longer a shortage of vets within the UK; employers may still recruit from the EU without doing this. The UK Shortage Occupation list is revised annually.

Tier two of the scheme replaced the work permit scheme in 2008. When looking to recruit from abroad, an employer should check the current information available from the UK Border Agency (www.ukba.homeoffice.gov.uk).

The job offer and ongoing day-to-day issues

KEY POINT

Job offers are usually conditional on passing the probation period and receiving suitable references. This should be stated in any offer letter sent to the new employee.

In theory, the employer could sue for breach of contract if the potential employee changed their mind once they had accepted a job offer and had not given at least the amount of notice required in the contract or offer letter. This rarely happens due to the cost of suing someone for breach of contract and because the financial loss is limited to the notice period, which is usually 1 week.

Where an employer withdraws the job offer, there could be cases where the potential employee could claim for breach of contract. This would not be the case if the job were withdrawn because the candidate did not meet one of the conditions set, e.g. not providing satisfactory references or not passing a medical. A potential employee could sue for breach of contract; again this could be limited to the amount of the notice period set in the offer letter. If the job has been withdrawn for reasons of unlawful discrimination then the potential employee could make a claim against the company.

Contracts of employment

The contract of employment should form the basis of the relationship between the employer and the employee, as it gives information about starting at, working at and leaving the company.

A contract of employment, like any other contract, is an agreement between two parties – in this case an employer and an employee. For a contract to exist there needs to have been an offer and an acceptance. In employment terms the employer agrees to pay an employee if they work for them. A contract can be in writing or oral, or a combination of the two. Contracts of employment are individual to the employee.

A full written contract gives an extra layer of certainty to employer and employee alike. Whereas a statutory written statement of employment is simply evidence of what has been agreed, a written contract contains the terms themselves.

It is a legal requirement for employees to have received from their employer within the first 8 weeks of employment a written statement containing the main terms and conditions of their employment. These terms are the administrative clauses; the contract of employment includes these plus other terms, including other express terms and implied terms (see below).

KEY POINT

It is best practice for contracts of employment to be signed prior to a person starting in the business.

The statement must contain the following:

- The names of the employer and the employee
- The place of work
- The job title
- The date upon which employment began
- The date of any period of continuous service
- The wage or salary, including how it is calculated and the frequency of payment (e.g. monthly)
- Information relating to hours of work
- Entitlement to holidays, including public and bank holidays, and details of pay when on holiday
- Terms and conditions in relation to sick pay
- Pension scheme details and a note stating whether there is a contracting-out certificate in force under the Pension Schemes Act 1993
- Notice period that the employee has to give and their entitlement if the contract is terminated by the employer
- If it is a fixed-term contract, how long the employment will last
- If it is a temporary contract, how long the employment is expected to last
- Any collective agreements that are applicable
- Details if the employee needs to work outside the UK.

Also included should be notes of where other required documents can be found, e.g. the discipline and grievance policy.

Discipline and grievance procedures are generally non-contractual. They are usually based on the Advisory, Conciliation and Arbitration Service (ACAS) codes of conduct. A failure to follow the codes does not in itself make a person or organization liable to proceedings. However, an employment tribunal will take the code into account when considering relevant cases.

If the discipline and grievance policy were to be made contractual, an employer could then be liable to be sued for breach of contract if they did not follow the policy when dismissing an employee.

The information can be given to the employee (as per regulations) before or during the 2-month period from the beginning of employment. If the employment ends within the 2 months, at least the names of the parties, start date, period of continuous service, details of salary payment, hours of work, holiday entitlement, job title and place of work must be given.

An example of a written statement of employment is provided at the end of this chapter.

Types of contractual terms

Contained within a contract of employment will be express terms and implied terms.

Express terms

Express terms are always the principal terms unless a term contravenes a statutory right. For example, if a contract stated that an employee was not entitled to maternity rights, this term would be null and void as it would take away a right under statute law. Statute law is written law (as opposed to oral or customary law) set down by legislature.

Within the workplace various documents can be used to establish an employee's express terms, e.g. the staff handbook, which may contain contractual policies and procedures, notices, work rules and collective agreements.

Implied terms

Implied terms are not usually written down anywhere, but are understood to exist if there is nothing clearly agreed between the employer and employee about a particular matter. Many issues may be covered by an implied term, e.g. turning up to work on time.

Terms that are necessary to make the contract work

Terms can also be implied because they are necessary to make the contract work. The most important of these is the 'duty of mutual trust and confidence'. This means that the employer and the employee need to rely on each other to be honest and respectful. For example, the employer should trust the employee not to destroy company property, and the employee should trust their employer not to bully them.

Terms that are obvious or assumed

Some terms are not included either because they are so obvious that it is not felt necessary to write them down, or because it will be assumed that such a term exists. An example of this might be where a contract provides for sick pay without saying how long it will be paid, as it will be assumed that it is not intended to be paid forever.

If there is a breakdown in an employment relationship due to a contractual dispute, e.g. an employer promised to pay overtime at double time but only paid at single rate, the employee could consider making a claim. It would then be down to the tribunal to decide what the intention was at the time of the promise.

KEY POINT

Important terms should be written down in a contract so that there can be no misunderstandings.

Terms implied by custom and practice

These are specific to an employer or type of work. They are arrangements that have never been clearly agreed but over time have become part of the contract e.g where it is the norm to give employees a Christmas bonus every year, or where the business closes early on particular days. In employment law terms, when a custom becomes part of a contract will depend on the circumstances. If a company practice has become a part of a contract then an employer must stick to it and cannot normally change it without the employee's agreement.

Collective agreements

Collective agreements are agreements between trade unions and the employer. It is important to establish the status of these agreements for the employees. An employee may be bound by a union-negotiated collective agreement even if he/she is not a member of the union, provided the agreement is expressly incorporated. The agreement must be brought to the attention of the employee and not just be in the wording of the contract.

Variations of contracts of employment

Employment contracts are binding on both the employer and the employee; it is therefore unlawful for an employer to change an existing employee's contract of employment without agreement. If an employer is going to impose a change using flexibility clauses contained in the contract, it is always advisable to consult with the employee on these changes. Negotiation and agreement to alleviate misunderstandings is advised. It is important not to give the opportunity for employees to believe that the implied term of trust and confidence has been breached. If the change is minor or administrative then these changes would be permitted.

Varying the contract of employment with consent

For any changes an employer wishes to make, an employee's written agreement should be obtained after a period of consultation as appropriate. Changes should be communicated verbally and in writing and should be stated as a proposal, i.e. communication should include why the change is important and should give the employee the opportunity to consider the change and put forward their views. If it is agreed, the employee's acceptance should be obtained in writing and the change can then be incorporated into their contract. Contractual changes that are beneficial to the employee, such as increases in salary or annual leave, are not expected to cause problems but should still be recorded in writing.

KEY POINT

For any changes an employer wishes to make to the contract of employment, an employee's written agreement should be obtained after a period of consultation as appropriate.

Varying the contract of employment without consent

If an employee does not accept the proposed change even after a period of negotiation, the employer could offer an incentive to encourage acceptance. This incentive could take the form of a salary increase or a one-off bonus, or the employer might consider amending the proposal so that it is acceptable to the employee.

If this is not a possibility, the employer may consider imposing the change (which could risk difficulties surrounding breaches in contract) or terminating the employee's current contract of employment and then offering to re-engage them on new terms and conditions. If an employer imposes the terms unilaterally, the employee can continue to work under the new terms and not make the employer aware of their objections. After a period of time (usually months) it could be deemed that they have accepted the change and therefore, the change could be made to their contract of employment. This can be a risky strategy and can cause problems if the change is fundamental and employees were not made aware of it.

In some cases employees will work under the new terms but under protest. This still puts the employer in breach of contract and a claim could be put against them for this breach.

If an employee resigns as a result of the breach and they have been employed for more than 1 year (or 2 years if employed on or after 6th April 2012) they could claim constructive unfair dismissal before an employment tribunal. It is worth remembering that there is no limit on the time that an employee can continue to work under protest and retain the option of resigning and claiming constructive dismissal at a later date.

KEY POINT

An employer should not assume that an employee has accepted a change just because he/she has not specifically objected.

Dismissals and re-engagement

If an employer plans to dismiss an employee and re-engage them on new terms and conditions, it must be for sound business reasons. If, after consultation, the employee does not agree with the new terms and conditions under any circumstances, the employer may decide to give the employee notice that their current contract of employment will be terminated and then offer them re-engagement on the new terms and conditions of employment. The amount of notice must be the employee's contractual notice period or the statutory minimum notice period (whichever is the longer).

Terminating the current contract of employment with due notice can be deemed as not a breach of contract; however, the termination still constitutes dismissal and hence can still be unfair dismissal. This can be the case even where an employee has accepted the new terms and conditions of re-engagement, whether under protest or not.

If dismissing and re-engaging an employee on new terms and conditions, the employer must be prepared to carry out a full consultation procedure and consultation must be meaningful.

KEY POINT

It is always recommended to seek up-to-date professional advice if making major changes to employees' terms and conditions.

Employment status

Within UK employment law there are three categories of employment status:

- Employee
- Worker
- Self-employed.

Each category has different legal rights, e.g. an employee is entitled to a considerably greater level of statutory and common law protection than a worker or a self-employed person. Likewise, a worker benefits from certain employment law rights that a self-employed person does not have.

Employees

An employee is engaged under a contract of employment. The contract of employment can be in writing and/or verbal with implied and express terms plus custom and practice (see earlier). Employees have the full protection of employment law. Some employment rights are earned by employees once they have worked continuously for 1 or 2 years. For example, the right to claim unfair dismissal requires 1 year's service (except in the case of discrimination claims) if employed before 5th April 2012, and 2 years' continuous service if employed after 6th April 2012. The right to a statutory redundancy payment requires 2 years' continuous service.

An employee has the right to:

- Be issued with written particulars of employment (the written statement of employment, or contract)
- Not be unfairly dismissed
- Receive statutory redundancy pay on redundancy
- Receive notice of termination of employment
- Receive guarantee payments in respect of lay-off and short-time working
- Receive itemized pay statements
- Receive statutory sick pay
- Take maternity, paternity and/or adoption leave and receive statutory maternity, paternity and/or adoption pay (as appropriate)
- Take parental leave and time off for family emergencies
- Request flexible working arrangements if they meet the prevailing criteria
- Not receive less favourable treatment on account of working under a fixed-term contract
- Have protection of their employment upon the transfer of the business under The Transfer of Undertakings (Protection of Employment) Regulations 2006 (Figure 20.3).

As well as full-time staff, employees include part-time staff, temporary/fixed-term staff, casual/seasonal workers and zero hours/bank workers.

Part-time staff

The Part-time Workers (Prevention of Less Favourable Treatment) Regulations 2000 give part-time staff parity of treatment with full-time staff. Therefore, a part-time worker should not be treated any less

TUPE is the acronym for these regulations. The purpose of these regulations is to protect employees if a business is sold. This, in effect, transfers the employee's current terms and conditions over to the new employer (the purchaser), along with any liabilities associated with them.
TUPE can apply in the following examples:

- Selling or buying part or all of a business as a going concern
- Outsourcing or making a 'service provision change', e.g. where a business contracts an outside company to provide a service or if the service transfers from one contractor to another or the service is brought back in house
- Taking over the lease of a premises and operating the same business from the new premises.

When dealing with issues of transferring a business, it is advisable to obtain up-to-date legal advice.

20.3 The Transfer of Undertakings (Protection of Employment) Regulations 2006.

favourably on a *pro rata* basis than comparable full-time employees doing the 'same or broadly similar work'. The Regulations state that part-time workers should have 'equal treatment', not only in contractual terms and conditions of employment, but also in the way they are treated.

Guidance from the UK Department for Business, Innovation and Skills (BIS) states that the Regulations give part-time workers the right:

- To receive the same hourly rate as comparable full-time staff
- Not to be excluded from training simply because they work part-time
- To receive the same entitlements to annual leave, sick pay, family leave and access to occupational pensions as their full-time colleagues, on a *pro rata* basis, where appropriate
- Not to be treated any less favourably than comparable full-time employees with respect to redundancy selection.

Temporary and fixed-term staff

A temporary employee can be employed on a fixed-term contract or on a casual basis. A fixed-term contract has a specific end date. If a contract terminates when an event occurs at some indeterminate date, e.g. the funding for a project is exhausted, this is not a fixed-term contract but rather a limited-term contract. This type of contract intends the employment not to be indefinite.

A notice clause can be lawfully inserted into a fixed-term contract; this gives the employer flexibility if the employee's performance or conduct has been unsatisfactory but has not been so serious as to invoke summary dismissal. This notice clause could be used effectively in conjunction with a probation clause.

The Fixed-term Employees (Prevention of Less Favourable Treatment) Regulations 2002 protect these employees from being treated less favourably than comparable permanent employees. Fixed-term employees are entitled to be informed of any permanent vacancy at their place of work. After a 4-year period a series of one or more fixed-term contracts is converted to a permanent contract.

Zero hours or bank workers

These contracts are used for individuals who agree to be on standby, e.g. in case of staff shortages. It is important that mutuality of obligation is avoided in these situations; therefore, no payment is forthcoming when no work is available. Also the employer is not obliged to give work and the individual can refuse work. There can be cases where a core number of hours are set. A time notice clause can also be included to give employees a reasonable amount of time before they are called into work. Zero hours staff can build up continuous employment, e.g. 2 days per week, provided their employment has been governed by a contract of employment for all or part of each week during any particular period.

Workers

A worker is someone engaged in the business who is not an employee (though may be self-employed) but is so integrated into an organization that they deserve some basic protection at work. This can include some people who are referred to as 'casuals', or casual workers.

The rights that would be afforded to workers are as follows:

- To receive paid annual leave
- Working time limited to a maximum number of hours per week as per the Working Time Directive
- To have rest breaks
- To be paid not less than the national minimum wage
- To not have unlawful deductions made from wages
- To not receive less favourable treatment on account of working part-time
- To be protected from discrimination because of age, disability, gender reassignment, marriage and civil partnership, pregnancy and maternity, race (including colour, nationality and ethnic or national origins), religion or belief, sex or sexual orientation
- To receive equal pay and conditions for equal work.

Casual workers

True casual workers are hired on a one-off short-term basis, or in an *ad hoc* way without any pattern of employment. There should be no obligation on the employer to provide work and no obligation on the casual worker to accept work. This term is mutuality of obligation. If a casual worker is to remain casual, no pattern of work should be established.

Seasonal work is a form of casual employment and can be a type of a fixed-term contract. The contracts need careful monitoring and wording to ensure that long-term contractual commitments that were not intended are not acquired inadvertently.

Self-employed persons

Self-employed contractors or locums usually work under 'contracts for services', are independent and are in business on their own account. For an employment relationship to exist, the employer is obliged to provide work for the employee, to decide when and how the work is carried out and to pay for the work. A self-employed person is obliged to perform the work; however, the contract for services should contain a substitution clause, which allows the self-employed person to send a substitute to perform the contracted work if they wish. The practice is permitted to specify the criteria of the substitute, e.g. within a veterinary locum agreement it would state that the substitute must be a member of the Royal College of Veterinary Surgeons. In practice, if a locum cannot provide a substitute, the practice will usually find its own cover.

KEY POINT

For an employment relationship to exist, the employer must have control over when and how the work is carried out and by whom.

People who are self-employed cannot be paid through the payroll. By the very nature of self-employment this person is in business in their own right and is responsible for their own tax and national insurance, whether as a limited company or sole trader. It is preferable to contract a self-employed person who works through a limited company, as if they are investigated by HM Revenue and Customs they will usually investigate the limited company of the self-employed person rather than the engager, which in this case would be the veterinary practice.

Self-employed persons are not employees but in some cases could be classed as workers. If a disagreement arises about a self-employed person, an employment tribunal will look at this on a case-by-case basis. The tribunal will take into account a range of factors to decide whether a person is an employee or self-employed (Figure 20.4). They will also take the written agreement into consideration, as well as enquiring how this agreement worked on a daily basis. However, the terms of the written agreement will not be determinative and if the working arrangements differ from the terms of the written agreement tribunals will generally give greater weight to the actual working arrangements.

It is worth remembering that tax and employment law are separate entities, and that some people engaged in the business could be classed in one way for tax purposes and another for employment law purposes, although this is rare. Full details of employment from a tax point of view can be found at the HM Revenue and Customs website (www.hmrc.gov.uk).

Statutory rights

Rights at work will depend on the employee's:

- Statutory rights
- Contract of employment.

A contract of employment cannot take away statutory rights which are law. For example, if a contract of employment states that the entitlement is for 15 days of paid holiday per year when, by law, all full-time employees are entitled to 28 days of paid holiday per year, this part of the contract is void and does not apply. The right received under law (to 28 days holiday in this case) applies instead. If the contract gives greater rights than under law, e.g. it states 6 weeks paid holiday per year, then the contract applies.

Factor	Employee	Self-employed
Is the worker contracted to provide the work personally?	Yes	No. Can send along a substitute if unable or unwilling to do the work personally
Does the worker work exclusively for the other party?	Yes	No. Can do work under two or more contracts with different parties at the same time
Does the worker work as part of the other's business?	Yes, an integral part of their employer's business, working within the core of the business	No. Works as and when required
Does the worker provide their own equipment?	Employer provides all tools, machinery and equipment required	Most often provides own tools and equipment
Does the worker provide their own support staff?	Employer provides all required support staff	Provides own support staff as required and pays them directly at own expense
Is the worker responsible for own profit and loss?	Not able to increase profits over and above wage received	Ability to enhance profit by maximising efficiency. Puts errors right at own cost
Tax, NI and VAT arrangements	All dealt with by employer. Subject to PAYE rules	Produces own accounts and paid on invoice
Is the arrangement designed purely to achieve tax advantages and/or to avoid employment legislation?	If yes, it is likely to fail and the worker will be regarded as an employee	
Does the worker receive paid holidays, sick pay and/or a company pension scheme and do they receive regular wages?	Yes (note: workers are also entitled to receive paid annual leave)	No
Is the worker subject to disciplinary action in the event of misconduct or poor work performance?	Yes	No

20.4 The multiple factor test. This list is not exhaustive.

Statutory rights are legal rights based on laws passed by Parliament. Nearly all workers, regardless of the number of hours per week they work, have certain legal rights. A part-time or fixed-term worker is entitled to the same contractual rights (*pro rata*) as a comparable full-time worker. There are some workers who are not entitled to certain statutory rights. Sometimes an employee only gains a right when they have been employed by their employer for a certain length of time.

When dealing with statutory rights it is advisable to check the prevailing rights at the time.

Payment

An employee has the right to:

- A written statement of terms of employment within 2 months of starting work
- An itemized pay slip from day 1 of employment
- Be paid at least the national minimum wage from day 1 of employment
- Not have illegal deductions made from pay from day 1 of employment
- Paid holiday. Full-time employees are entitled to at least 28 days a year. Part-time employees are entitled to a *pro rata* amount.

Trade union activities

An employee has the right to:

- Join a trade union, and should not be refused a job, dismissed, harassed or selected for redundancy because they are a member of or wish to join a trade union
- Not join a trade union if they wish, and should not be refused a job, dismissed, harassed or selected for redundancy because they refused to join.

An employee who is a member of a trade union has the right to:

- Take part in trade union activities, e.g. recruiting members, collecting subscriptions and attending meetings
- Be accompanied by a trade union representative to a disciplinary or grievance hearing
- Take time off for trade union duties and activities from the day they start work. If an employee takes part in official industrial action and is dismissed as a result, this will be an automatically unfair dismissal. Trade union activities must take place either outside the employee's normal working hours or at a time agreed with the employer. An employee has no right to be paid for this time off work unless their contract allows for this.

Time off work

An employee has the right to:

- Paid time off to look for work if being made redundant. This usually only applies for employees with 2 years' service, but good practice would include all employees that are being made redundant
- Time off for study or training for 16–17 year olds from day 1 of employment
- Paid time off for antenatal care from day 1 of employment
- Paid maternity/paternity leave. Amount of payment will depend on prevailing regulations
- Ask for flexible working to care for children or adult dependants. It is the duty of the employer to consider this
- Paid adoption leave. Amount of payment will depend on prevailing regulations
- Take unpaid parental leave for both men and women if they have 1 year's service
- Reasonable time off to look after dependants in an emergency from day 1 of employment, usually unpaid
- Under health and safety law, work a maximum 48-hour working week from day 1 of employment (see later)
- Under health and safety law, weekly and daily rest breaks. This applies from the day the employee starts work. There are special rules for night workers (see later).

Most employees have a right to take time off work, although not necessarily with pay, for the following:

- To participate in trade union activities (see above)
- To perform 'public duties', for example, being a Justice of the Peace (JP), local authority councillor or school governor
- To attend to unexpected problems with dependants, e.g. where childminding arrangements break down. A dependant includes anyone who reasonably relies on the employee.

Lay-offs and short-time working

If the employer has no work for the employee to do they may put them on short-time working or lay them off, provided that this is in their contract.

If employees are laid off, they will not usually get paid. Short-time working means receiving only part of the normal wage. If employees are laid off or put on short-time working, they may be entitled to a payment from the employer, called a 'guarantee payment'. In some cases, lay-offs or short-time working may be offered as an alternative to redundancy. However, some employees may be able to claim a redundancy payment if laid off or put on short-time working.

Sickness

Many employees will be entitled to statutory sick pay if they are off work due to sickness. In addition, some employees may receive occupational sick pay from their employer but this will depend on their contract of employment.

Health and safety

All employers have a statutory duty to take care of the health and safety of all their employees. For example, employers must provide First Aid equipment, protective clothing and adequate means of escape in case of fire, and they must also ensure that all machinery is safe (see Chapter 22).

Harassment and discrimination

Discrimination is the unfair or prejudiced treatment of one person or a group of people. Employees have the right not to be discriminated against on grounds such as:

- Age
- Disability
- Pregnancy or maternity leave
- Race
- Religion or belief
- Sex
- Sexual orientation
- Gender identity.

A form of unlawful discrimination may occur where a female worker is paid less than a male worker for doing the same or similar work.

'Whistle blowing' at work

There is some protection for workers who are concerned about malpractice at work and who publicly disclose information about their employer's activities. This is called 'whistle blowing'. The information disclosed must relate to:

- A criminal offence
- A failure to comply with a legal obligation
- A miscarriage of justice
- A health and safety issue
- Damage to the environment
- An attempt to cover up any of the above.

Surveillance at work

Employers have the right to monitor their employees' communications, provided they have warned them first that they are doing this. Employers can monitor, for example:

- Postal communications
- Telephone calls
- Faxes
- E-mails
- Internet use.

In some circumstances, an employer can also monitor what their employees are doing by using CCTV.

Monitoring and surveillance is only permitted by law if:

- The monitoring is relevant to the employer's business
- The telecommunications system is provided for use partly or wholly in connection with the employer's business
- The employer has made all reasonable efforts to inform users that their communications will be intercepted.

Ideally, an employer should have a code of conduct or policy about surveillance. If it has been agreed with the employees, it will form part of the contract of employment and can be the basis for disciplinary action or a grievance.

Working Time (Amendment) Regulations 2003

The Working Time Regulations are linked to health and safety legislation. Employers must keep proper records of hours worked per week for all employees working days and nights, including the times during which rest breaks are taken if compensatory rest periods are implemented, plus work patterns and annual leave.

The Working Time Regulations apply to everyone apart from self-employed persons, as they are free to work for different clients and customers.

48-hour week

Adult workers (aged 18 and over) cannot be forced to work more than 48 hours per week on average. Working time includes:

- Travelling time, where this is part of the job
- Working lunches
- Job-related training days.

Working time does not include travel between the home and place of work, lunch breaks or day release courses.

KEY POINT

On-call time is not working time if the individual is not restricted to their place of work and is free to pursue leisure activities. On-call time would be working time if the individual were required to be at their place of work, even if they were provided with residential accommodation at their place of work.

The average working time is normally calculated over a 17-week reference period, although this can be longer in some situations (e.g. seasonal work), and can be agreed for periods of 26 or 52 weeks, usually by a collective or workforce agreement.

Adult workers (over the age of 18) can sign an 'opt out' agreement but this must be in writing and be signed by individual workers. These agreements can be cancelled by the individual by giving written notice (length of time to be agreed when signing the opt out agreement). An individual cannot be forced to sign an opt out agreement and it would be unfair to dismiss or subject them to a detriment for refusing to sign an opt out agreement or for cancelling one that has been signed.

Night workers

A night worker is someone who normally works at least 3 hours of their working time between 11 pm and 6 am. The night period can be varied by agreement between employers and employees/workers, but the designated period must be at least 7 hours long and span the hours from midnight to 5 am.

Practices that employ workers for night work (or shift work) should carry out appropriate risk assessments. Under Working Time Regulations, employers are required to ensure that workers are fit for night work and must offer a free health assessment to all night workers on a regular basis as well as to anyone who is about to start working nights. Specialist advice should be sought regarding devising and assessing the results of health assessments.

A night worker cannot opt out of the night work limit. A night worker has a right to a limit of an average of 8 hours' work in each 24-hour period. Employers must take reasonable steps to ensure that night workers do not work more than 8 hours in a 24-hour period. Where a night worker's work involves special hazards or heavy physical or mental strain, there is an absolute limit of 8 hours on the worker's working time each day; this is not an average. Nightly worked time is worked out over a 17-week period; however, again this can be extended by agreement (see Chapter 22 for information on lone workers).

The practice should periodically review the effectiveness of any shift-working arrangements.

Rest periods and in-work rest breaks

Adult workers (over the age of 18) are entitled to:

- 11 hours of uninterrupted rest between each working day
- 1 whole day off per week (can be averaged over a 2-week period)
- If a worker is required to work a shift of more than 6 hours, they are entitled to take a rest break of at least 20 continuous uninterrupted minutes at some point during that shift.

Workers under the age of 18 are entitled to:

- 12 hours of rest between each working day
- 2 days off per week (cannot be averaged over a 2-week period)
- Rest breaks of 30 continuous uninterrupted minutes if required to work over 4.5 hours continuously.

There is no requirement in the regulations for rest breaks to be paid; however, payment may well have been promised as a matter of contract.

Young workers and the time limits

Young persons are defined as those over the minimum school-leaving age but under the age of 18. Young workers cannot normally work for more than 8 hours per day, totalling 40 hours per week. These hours cannot be averaged out over the 17-week or more reference period and there is no opt out available. If a young worker works for more than one employer, the total number of hours worked should be spread among the employers. Young workers may work longer hours where this is necessary to maintain the continuity of service or production, or in response to a surge in demand for a service or product; however, the employer must always ensure that there is no adult available to perform the task and that the young person's training needs are not adversely affected.

Young workers can be asked to work at night if there are no adults available to perform the task. Young workers are allowed a period of compensatory rest and need to be supervised adequately where it is necessary for their protection.

The Working Time Directive is enforceable by the Health and Safety Executive, with failure to comply being an offence.

Annual leave

All workers are entitled to a minimum of 28 days' paid annual leave, including bank holidays and public holidays for full-time staff. Part-time workers receive an equivalent amount calculated on a *pro rata* basis. Details on how to calculate holiday entitlement and pay can be found at www.acas.org.uk.

Discipline and grievances

There will be times when some employees are not behaving or performing their role to the employer's satisfaction or there may be events that cause the employee to feel aggrieved. In most cases these situations can be resolved informally. In others a more formal approach is required, resulting in the disciplinary or grievance procedure being implemented; this must be followed correctly and fairly.

The ACAS Code of Practice on Discipline and Grievance Procedures states what a fair procedure should involve. The code is not law, but the failure of an employer to follow its provisions could render a dismissal unfair. In addition, if either party has unreasonably failed to comply with any of the provisions of the Code, the tribunal has the discretion to adjust any award by up to 25% (depending on which party was at fault). However, the tribunal will only make an increase or a reduction to any award if it considers it to be just and equitable.

Disciplinary action

In general, disciplinary procedures are there to assist and improve conduct and performance of employees and not as a means of imposing sanctions. Prior to starting a formal procedure, an employer should consider dealing with the situation informally through discussions with the employee and performance appraisal (see Chapter 19).

ACAS recommends three formal stages for disciplinary matters other than gross misconduct:

1. Written warning
2. Final written warning
3. Dismissal.

A fair disciplinary procedure will go through the following stages:

- Ensure any allegations have been thoroughly and properly investigated to establish the facts of the case
- Consider whether informal action is appropriate
- Provide the employee with full details of the allegations made
- Allow the employee to be accompanied at the disciplinary hearing. The employee is allowed to be accompanied at the meeting (and at any appeal meeting) by a fellow employee, a trade union representative or an official employed by a trade union

- Hold a disciplinary hearing to discuss the problem and give the employee an opportunity to explain their side of the story
- Ensure the hearing is conducted in good faith, having regard for the principles of natural justice
- Provide for an appropriate disciplinary sanction
- Provide employees with an opportunity to appeal
- Adhere to the employee's contract of employment.

A copy of the ACAS codes and booklets can be found at www.acas.org.uk.

Special cases

Where disciplinary action is being considered against an employee who is a trade union representative, the normal disciplinary procedure should be followed. Depending on the circumstances, however, it is advisable to discuss the matter at an early stage with an official employed by the union, after obtaining the employee's agreement.

If an employee is charged with, or convicted of, a criminal offence outside work, this is not normally in itself reason for disciplinary action. Consideration needs to be given to any effect the charge or conviction might have on the employee's suitability to do their job and on their relationship with their employer, work colleagues and customers.

Gross misconduct

Offences of gross misconduct usually warrant summary dismissal for a first offence, i.e. dismissal without notice. However, 'summary' is not synonymous with 'instant' and incidents of gross misconduct will still need to be investigated and dealt with as part of a formal disciplinary procedure. It is still important to establish the facts before taking any action. A short period of suspension on pay may be helpful or necessary, although it should only be imposed after careful consideration, should not represent any form of disciplinary sanction, should be for as brief a period as possible and should be kept under regular review.

Again, there should be a disciplinary hearing before deciding whether to take action. The principles of fairness apply as much to cases of gross misconduct as they do to ordinary cases of misconduct or poor performance.

Acts that constitute gross misconduct are those resulting in an extremely serious breach of contractual terms and will be for businesses to decide in the light of particular circumstances. Disciplinary rules should give examples of acts of gross misconduct and these may vary according to the nature of the business. Gross misconduct offences might include:

- Theft, fraud, unauthorized possession of company property, deliberate falsification of records or any other form of dishonesty
- Physical violence
- Serious bullying or harassment
- Deliberate damage to the employer's property
- Extremely serious insubordination
- Gross negligence
- Bringing the employer into serious disrepute
- Serious incapacity through an excess of alcohol or drugs.

The above is intended as a guide only and is not a definitive list.

Grievances

Grievances are problems or complaints raised by employees in relation to aspects of their work. Grievance procedures should be used to deal with grievances fairly, consistently and expeditiously. Grievances may be raised by employees for the following reasons:

- Disputes over terms and conditions of employment
- Health and safety concerns
- New imposed working practices
- Problems with the working environment
- Work relationships
- Bullying and harassment.

The ACAS Code of Practice on Disciplinary and Grievance Procedures sets out the following general principles for dealing with grievances:

- Issues should be raised and dealt with promptly and the parties should not unreasonably delay meetings and decisions
- Employers should act consistently
- Any necessary investigations should be carried out to establish the facts
- Employers should allow employees to be accompanied at any formal grievance meeting
- Employees should be allowed to appeal against any formal decision made.

The following five steps are recommended:

1. The employee should report the nature of the grievance, usually to their supervisor or line manager.
2. A meeting should be held with the employee to discuss the grievance.
3. The employee should be allowed to be accompanied at the meeting (and at any appeal meeting) by a fellow employee, a trade union representative or an official employed by a trade union.
4. Appropriate action should be decided upon, if any is required, to resolve the grievance, and the decision should be communicated to the employee in writing without unreasonable delay. The employee should be informed that they can appeal if they are not content with the action taken.
5. The employee should communicate the grounds for their appeal without unreasonable delay and in writing. Appeals should also be heard without unreasonable delay and at a time and place notified to the employee in advance. The appeal should be dealt with impartially and wherever possible by a manager who has not previously been involved in the case. The outcome of the appeal should be communicated to the employee in writing without unreasonable delay.

Wherever possible, a grievance should be dealt with before the employee leaves employment.

Special cases

Grievances regarding bullying, discrimination, harassment and whistle blowing are highly sensitive issues. Larger organizations often have separate grievance procedures, which are more detailed, for dealing with these issues. The normal grievance procedure should be used if no others are issued but care should be taken to deal with grievances as sensitively and confidentially as possible.

> **KEY POINT**
>
> Where an employee raises a grievance during a disciplinary process, the disciplinary process may be suspended temporarily in order to deal with the grievance. However, where the two issues are related, it may be appropriate to deal with them concurrently.

Finally, the provisions of the ACAS Code do not apply to collective grievances raised on behalf of two or more employees by a recognized trade union representative or other appropriate workplace representative; those grievances should be handled in accordance with the employer's collective grievance process.

Leaving the business

Resignation

In employment there is a contract between the two parties (the employer and the employee), with a 'get out' clause known as the notice period. In most cases employees will resign for normal reasons, such as moving away from the area, better job prospects or different hours.

A resignation should be a clear statement (preferably in writing) from the employee, stating their intention to leave. Employees threatening to leave and informing the employer that they are looking for another job have not necessarily resigned.

If an employee resigns verbally, it is advisable to confirm the resignation in writing so there can be no misunderstanding at a later stage. If an employee wishes to retract their notice, this can only be done if the employer agrees. If an employee resigns during a 'heat of the moment' conversation, it advisable to give them a cooling-off period followed by the opportunity to discuss the problem and look at ways in which the situation might be resolved.

The leaving date would normally be at the end of the notice period. In some cases an employee may request to leave earlier and give less notice; it would be for the employer to agree to this and the salary would be paid to the last day of the revised notice period. If an employee does not work their notice period then they are not paid for this time and the employer could sue for breach of contract. Any compensation would, however, be limited to the financial loss to the employer of the notice period and therefore would not be worth the legal fees.

If an employee resigns and the employer wishes them to leave before the end of the notice period, then the notice period would have to be paid in full. Contracts of employment may contain a clause whereby an employee is put on 'gardening leave'. This gives the employer the right to allow the employee to leave early but not to join their new employer until the leave has expired. During the period of gardening leave the employee is still employed.

For clarity, a clause can be inserted in the contract of employment to state that if an employee who is leaving has taken more holidays than accrued, the overpayment of these will be deducted from the final salary payment. Likewise if an employee has not taken all holidays accrued, then a payment for outstanding holidays is made.

The employee does not have the right to receive their final salary on their last day unless it is the normal pay day. Holiday pay should be given up to the last/termination date, even in the cases of a gross misconduct dismissal, and a form P45 issued. This is a record of pay in the current tax year along with total amounts deducted for tax and National Insurance.

Where an employee feels that they have been made to resign in response to a fundamental breach of contract on the part of their employer, they could consider taking their employer to a tribunal for constructive unfair dismissal (see later). For this to happen the problem should have been raised as a grievance and an employment tribunal can refuse to hear a constructive dismissal claim or reduce the amount of compensation if the grievance has not been raised.

> **KEY POINT**
>
> It is advisable for the employer to request that an employee confirms their resignation in writing.

Notice and dismissal

Employees have the right to:

- Notice of dismissal, provided the employee has worked for the employer for at least 1 month
- Written reasons for dismissal from the employer, providing the employee has worked for the employer for 1 year. Women who are pregnant or on maternity leave are entitled to written reasons without having to have worked for any particular length of time
- Claim compensation if unfairly dismissed. Up until 5th April 2012, an employee will have to have worked for 1 year to be able to claim unfair dismissal. From 6th April 2012, the length of service required to take an employer to a tribunal to claim unfair dismissal will be 2 years. This will be applicable to those employed on or after 6th April 2012
- Claim redundancy pay if made redundant. In most cases the employee must have worked for 2 years to be able to claim redundancy pay
- Not to suffer detriment or dismissal for 'blowing the whistle' on a matter of public concern (malpractice) at the workplace (see later). This entitlement is from day 1 of employment.

Most employees have a legal right to a period of notice if their employer dismisses them. Many employees will have extra rights to notice under their contract of employment. There will always be a contract of employment, even if there is nothing written down. When it comes to dismissal, even if the law or the contract of employment does not give an employee the right to a minimum amount of notice, they are still entitled to 'reasonable' notice. In most circumstances, if the employer wishes to dismiss an employee they must follow a proper dismissal and disciplinary procedure.

The law does not give the following employees the right to a minimum period of notice:

- Those employed for less than 1 month by their employer
- Crown servants
- Seamen employed under a crew agreement on a ship registered in the UK
- Employees who have been dismissed for gross misconduct.

The law gives all other employees the right to a statutory minimum amount of notice. This period of notice is:

- 1 week for employees that have worked for their employer for longer than 1 month but less than 2 years
- Or 2 weeks if the employee has worked for their employer for 2 whole years
- Plus 1 extra week for each further whole year's employment at the date the notice period expires, up to a maximum of 12 weeks' notice in total.

Contractual notice

The contract of employment may state more notice than the statutory minimum. However, employees can never receive less than the statutory minimum period of notice, regardless of what their contract states.

If the contract does not specify a period of notice, in most cases the notice period will be the statutory amount. However, this would depend on the employee's status and the normal practice within the business.

> **KEY POINT**
>
> Where there is no express term stated in the contract, the statutory minimum notice from an employee to an employer is one week, regardless of status or length of service.

Entitlement to pay in the notice period

If normal working hours are worked during the notice period, then employees are entitled to be paid their normal salary. Payment will be due as stated in the contract of employment if an employee is unable to work during the notice period because:

- They are given no work to do, even though they are willing to work
- They are on holiday
- They are off work due to sickness or injury.

Payment in lieu of notice

An employee is entitled to receive pay in lieu of notice if they are dismissed without being given a notice period. The term **severance pay** can be used. The only exception to this is if the employee was dismissed due to gross misconduct. The amount of pay in lieu of notice will depend upon the amount of notice to which the employee is entitled.

Redundancy

Redundancy is a form of dismissal. An employer may make an employee redundant for one of the following reasons:

- Where the business closes
- Where a particular workplace closes
- Where there is a reduced requirement for employees to carry out work of a particular kind.

A redundancy situation must follow one of the above reasons and not be contrived so to remove an employee who, for example, is not performing their role to the standard required. Redundancy needs to be genuine.

Once an employee reaches 2 years' service they will be entitled to a statutory redundancy payment, which is a tax-free lump sum and is calculated according to age, length of service and gross weekly wage. The gross weekly wage can be capped at the statutory minimum of £430 (as of 1st February 2012) as long as there is no provision within the contract, either express or implied, for an enhanced redundancy payment.

For a redundancy to be found unfair it is usually because a fair procedure was not followed. A fair procedure would involve holding meaningful consultation, a fair selection procedure, and considering whether there is any other suitable alternative employment available within the company or, in some circumstances, associated companies.

Consultation

Consultation must take place with individual employees, irrespective of the number of proposed redundancies. This consultation should not just inform the employee of the decision to make them redundant, but should also explain the reason for the redundancy and then give the employee the option to suggest alternatives. The number of actual consultation meetings will depend on the circumstances. To preserve employment in cost-cutting exercises, it has been known for employees to take pay cuts.

Where employees have been put at risk of redundancy and are being consulted, they have the right to reasonable time off to attend interviews and register with agencies.

Where more than 20 employees are made redundant, the law imposes far-reaching obligations on employers to notify both recognized trade unions and the Department for Business, Innovation and Skills of forthcoming collective redundancies and to consult with representatives. The regulations guiding collective consultation periods set the minimum amount of time for consultation to be:

- At least 30 days before the first dismissal takes effect where 20–99 redundancies are proposed at one establishment within a 90-day period
- At least 90 days before the first dismissal takes effect where 100 or more redundancies are proposed at one establishment within a 90-day period.

The dismissal is considered to have taken effect when the contract of employment is terminated. If employers are considering making more than 20 employees redundant it is sensible to source current advice on collective redundancy.

Fair selection

In considering a fair selection procedure, this will depend on how many redundancies will be made and what types of role are proposed for redundancy. A fair selection procedure would be required if an organization had, for example, a team of five employees performing the same role and the requirement for the future was four. The five employees would be the pool for selection. Selection criteria must be applied to choose one person out of the five.

The criteria must be objective and reasonable and therefore measurable. If a level of skill is required it must be considered how this will be measured so that employees are being assessed fairly. Vague and/or subjective criteria, such as quality of work, would be hard to assess if there were no documentation, such as a discipline record, to verify a low score.

Where fair selection is not relevant (e.g. where everyone in a particular department is being made redundant, or where there is only one person in a unique job role being made redundant), it is still important that the reason for redundancy is fair. For individuals, the role in the organization must be unique, not just the job title.

Consideration for alternative employment

During the consultation period, a discussion between the employer and employee needs to take place regarding the possibility of suitable alternative employment. All alternatives should be explored, including roles that may be assumed to be unacceptable due to their terms and conditions. An employee can accept a new role on a 4-week trial. If, after this 4-week period, the role is not an acceptable alternative, the employee can still be made redundant. If an employer considers it to be suitable and it is believed that the employee is being unreasonable in not accepting it, the employer could refuse to pay a redundancy payment and the employee would need to claim the payment through the tribunal system.

Where there are no other vacancies, the employee must be informed.

At all stages of a redundancy process, all conversations should be documented and confirmed in writing to the affected employees. At the consultation stage it is not a statutory requirement for the employee to be accompanied but good practice would be to allow an employee to be accompanied by either a fellow employee or a trade union official.

An opportunity to appeal

Offering an appeal for a redundancy situation is not a statutory requirement; however, it allows the employer to demonstrate that they acted fairly in the redundancy process.

An employee is likely to appeal against the redundancy decision if they are not satisfied with it, e.g. because they believe the redundancy is not genuine, because they feel they have been unfairly selected or because they think consultation was inadequate. If this is the case, the employer would have a chance to review the process and if the employee were still not accepting the decision, they could consider taking the employer to a tribunal for unfair dismissal (see below).

For up-to-date information about how to handle redundancies, ACAS produces a Redundancy Handling Booklet (see www.acas.org.uk).

Dismissal

If an employee is dismissed, the employer must have a fair reason to do so and must follow a fair procedure. The ACAS Code of Practice on Discipline and Grievance Procedures must also be adhered to when dismissing an employee for reasons of poor performance and misconduct (however, the ACAS Code specifically states that it does not apply to dismissals by reason of redundancy or the non-renewal of a fixed-term contract).

Fair reasons for dismissal

There are five fair reasons to dismiss an employee:

- **Conduct** – including gross misconduct
- **Capability** – the employee is not able to perform their job due to capability, including illness
- **Redundancy** – a fair selection procedure must be in place and the employer has a duty to consult with the affected employees
- **A statutory restriction** – e.g. dismissing a veterinary surgeon who had been removed from the register by the Royal College of Veterinary Surgeons
- **Another substantial reason** – this applies to situations where there is a reason to dismiss that does not fall into the above categories, e.g. imprisonment, or unreasonably refusing to accept a company reorganization that changes the terms and conditions of employment.

KEY POINT

Wrongful dismissal and unfair dismissal are different:

- Wrongful dismissal is a contractual claim
- Unfair dismissal is a statutory claim.

Unfair dismissal

If an employee is dismissed for a reason not given in the above list, this could be considered unfair.

Making a claim to a tribunal

If an employee feels that they have been dismissed unfairly they may decide to make a claim of unfair dismissal at a tribunal. Full details of the rules regarding employment tribunals can be found at www.justice.gov.uk.

When deciding whether to take the case to an employment tribunal, the following points must be considered.

Who has the right to make a claim for unfair dismissal? Self-employed people cannot claim unfair dismissal. This is why it is important to understand the employment status of people engaged in the business.

In general terms, up until 5th April 2012 an employee will have to have worked for 1 year to be able to claim unfair dismissal. From 6th April 2012 the length of service required to take an employer to a tribunal to claim unfair dismissal will be 2 years. This will be applicable to those employed on or after the 6th April 2012. Employees who were employed before the 6th April 2012 will still have the right to claim unfair dismissal with 1 year's service.

Has a dismissal taken place?

Dismissal is where:

- The employee's employment has been terminated with or without notice
- A fixed-term contract has come to an end and is not being renewed
- The employee has been made redundant
- After a strike or a lockout, the employer refuses to let the employees return to work
- The employee was made to resign – i.e. constructive dismissal (see below)
- A woman returning from maternity leave is not allowed to return to work
- An employee is laid off or put on short-time working when the contract of employment does not allow for it.

Dismissal is not:

- A resignation without pressure from the employer
- A suspension on full pay during a disciplinary procedure
- When a contract is frustrated (i.e. if circumstances change so that the contract can no longer be fulfilled, for example if an employee is sent to prison for a substantial period of time – although this will depend on the reason for the prison sentence)
- A resignation in the heat of the moment.

Has the employee been discriminated against? If an employee has been dismissed because of age, disability, gender reassignment, marriage/civil partnership, pregnancy/maternity, race, religion or belief, sex or sexuality then a claim for discrimination can be made. The employee does not need 1 year's service to make a claim.

Is the reason for dismissal automatically unfair? There are a number of circumstances in which a dismissal could be deemed automatically unfair. The following non-exhaustive list details some of those circumstances. An employment tribunal will automatically decide that a dismissal is unfair if:

- The employee was dismissed for reasons connected with pregnancy or maternity leave
- The employee was dismissed for reasons connected with an application for flexible working
- The employee was dismissed for a reason related to their part-time or fixed-term status
- The employee was dismissed when trying to enforce a statutory right
- The employee was dismissed for invoking the health and safety law
- The employee was dismissed because he/she was a trade union member, had taken part in trade union activities or had acted as another employee's representative at a statutory meeting, e.g. a disciplinary meeting
- The employee was dismissed in connection with exercising the right to be accompanied to a disciplinary or grievance hearing
- The employee was dismissed for 'blowing the whistle'.

One year's service is not required to make a claim for the above reasons.

If the reason for dismissal was not automatically unfair, did the employer act unreasonably in dismissing the employee? For an employee to claim unfair dismissal they must, subject to certain exceptions, have completed at least 2 years' service if employed on or after 6th April 2012 (and at least 1 year's service where employed before 6th April 2012). The employer will have to demonstrate that it had a potentially fair reason for the dismissal (see above). If it cannot demonstrate a potentially fair reason the dismissal will be unfair. If the employer can show that, on the balance of probabilities, it had a potentially fair reason for the dismissal, it is then for the tribunal to consider whether the employer acted reasonably in coming to the conclusion to dismiss. The tribunal will apply an objective test and will consider whether the employer's decision fell within a band of reasonable responses open to a reasonable employer in the circumstances. The tribunal will, as part of that consideration, take into account the procedure followed by the employer in coming to the conclusion to dismiss.

When must a claim be made? If an employee believes they were dismissed unfairly they must make a complaint to an employment tribunal within 3 months of the date of dismissal, which is defined as:

- The date on which the notice period ends if notice is given
- The date an employee is dismissed without notice (not the date that that the employee would have worked until had they worked a notice period)
- If paid in lieu of notice, the last actual day worked
- The end date of a fixed-term contract.

Compensation

If the employment tribunal decides that dismissal was unfair, it can order the employer to pay compensation. This is normally made up of a basic award and a compensatory award.

- The basic award will depend on the age of the ex-employee and their length of service. The maximum number of years is 20 and the maximum weekly pay is £430 (as of 1st February 2012). The maximum basic award is £12,900.
- The compensatory award is for the loss of earnings and can include loss of pension rights. The maximum for this type of compensation is £72,300 (as of 1st February 2012).

There is no cap on awards for discrimination cases.

Reinstatement

Reinstatement would need to be negotiated with the employer; usually tribunals do not and cannot force re-employment.

The ACAS Arbitration Scheme and mediation

The ACAS Arbitration Scheme is for straightforward unfair dismissal cases. The Scheme is quicker and more informal than a tribunal hearing but, by using it, the right to go to tribunal is waived. There is also no right of appeal.

Mediation within the workplace will become more prevalent over the next few years, as the government is encouraging the system.

Constructive dismissal

Constructive dismissal is a form of dismissal whereby the employee resigns promptly in response to a fundamental breach of contract on the part of the employer. An employee would need to prove that:

- The employer had committed a serious breach of the contract of employment and it caused the employee to feel that they were forced to resign
- The employee has not accepted the breach or the change or has not done anything to suggest that they have accepted the breach or a change in employment conditions.

The employee's reason for leaving their role must be a serious fundamental breach of contract. For example:

- A serious breach of the contract (e.g. not paying the employee or suddenly demoting them for no reason)
- Forcing an employee to accept unreasonable changes to their terms and conditions of employment without their agreement (e.g. relocation without informing the employee)
- Bullying, harassment or violence against the employee by work colleagues and no action taken when reported
- Employees made to work under dangerous conditions.

A breach of contract can be one serious incident or a series of incidents; it would depend on the circumstances. If an employee feels they are being made to resign they should try to resolve the situation internally by raising a grievance. In some cases mediation could be applied.

If an employee resigns and makes a claim against the employer for constructive dismissal it could be for unfair or wrongful dismissal. How the claim is constructed will determine whether it is for unfair or wrongful dismissal.

Wrongful dismissal

Wrongful dismissal refers to a contractual claim by an employee where there has been a breach of the oral or written terms of an employment contract by an employer, which led to a dismissal. This could be either an actual dismissal by the employer or constructive dismissal claimed by the employee. There is no qualifying period of employment, so a claim can be brought within the first year of service if need be. An example of wrongful dismissal would be not giving an employee the correct length of contractual or statutory notice.

Where an employer has dismissed an employee for gross misconduct (which is, in most cases, a breach of contract), the employee is dismissed immediately and, if stated in the contract, will not be entitled to notice pay.

If the employee has the required length of service and alleges that the decision to dismiss them was unfair because, for example, the correct procedure was not followed, they would then have a claim for unfair dismissal *and* a claim for wrongful dismissal. This is because the decision not to pay them for their notice period, which is contractual, relied on the fact they were dismissed but this may not have been a fair dismissal.

In wrongful dismissal cases, damages are based on salary and benefits for the notice period, while under unfair dismissal the concept is based on a basic award and a compensatory award derived from ongoing and future loss.

The future

In April 2011 there were approximately 150 different pieces of legislation related to employing people. There has been a commitment from the UK government to cut back on red tape in all areas of business. One of the main current proposals is to reform the way tribunals work in order to encourage early settlement of disputes and to reduce costs.

Planned implementations include the following:

- Claims to go to ACAS for conciliation first, before the tribunal sees them, to encourage the use of internal mediation
- A pilot scheme will be started at the end of 2012 to encourage and explain the benefits of using mediation to settle disagreements before they reach the tribunal stage
- Claimant deposits and fees, and the ability to award increased costs to deter vexatious claims
- Penalties of up to £5000 will be introduced for employers who lose tribunal cases but this will not be automatic; judges will have discretion to impose a penalty where the employer's breach of employment rights has aggravating features, such as negligence or malice.

Employment law changes throughout the year, with different case law going through; legislation is implemented twice a year, in April and October. Public consultation is in place to find out what businesses think of the regulations and what should be changed to encourage employers to take on more employees without the associated risks.

Useful websites

- Advisory Conciliation and Arbitration Service: www.acas.org.uk (code of practice on discipline and grievance; *Discipline and Grievances at Work: the ACAS Guide*; calculating holiday entitlement)
- Business link: www.businesslink.gov.uk
- Her Majesty's Revenue and Customs: www.hmrc.gov.uk: (information for the self-employed)
- Ministry of Justice: www.justice.gov.uk (tribunals)
- UK Border Agency: www.ukba.homeoffice.gov.uk (eligibility to work legally in the UK)

Example of T&C statement ▶

STATEMENT OF TERMS AND CONDITIONS OF EMPLOYMENT IN ACCORDANCE WITH SECTION 1 EMPLOYMENT RIGHTS ACT 1996

This agreement is between

NAME AND ADDRESS OF THE COMPANY

and

NAME AND ADDRESS OF THE EMPLOYEE

It is agreed that the employer will employ the Employee and the Employee will work for the Employer on the following terms and conditions:

1. Job title
Your position is that of *JOB TITLE*

You may from time to time be required to carry out such other reasonable duties as the Company may decide should be necessary to meet the needs of the business, without additional remuneration.

2. Commencement and continuity of employment
Your employment with the Company began on *date*
Your continuous employment, taking into account any service with [insert names of any previous employers for which service counts towards continuity] with *NAME OF COMPANY* began on *DATE*

NEED TO STATE THE TYPE OF CONTRACT (FIXED-TERM, TEMPORARY, ETC.)

3. Hours of work
Your normal working hours per week are *HOURS* with a statutory rest/lunch break of *XXX* minutes per day, which is *PAID/UNPAID.*

You may be required to work such further hours as may be necessary to fulfil your duties and/or the needs of the business. Wherever possible, the responsible manager will give the employee reasonable notice of any additional hours.

You agree that your average weekly working hours may be in excess of those prescribed by law ('the Waiver'). The Waiver will remain in force indefinitely but you may give the Company not less than three months notice in writing of your intention to terminate the Waiver.

For part-time employees, entitlement to holidays, sick pay and all other benefits is *pro rata* based on the hours worked compared to those worked by a full time employee. Full time hours for this purpose are 40 hours per week.

4. Place of work
Your normal place of work will be *** premises; the Employer reserves the right to change this to any place within the group.

5. Payment
DETAILS ABOUT WHEN BEING PAID AND HOW THE PAY IS TO BE CALCULATED, OVERTIME REQUIREMENTS OR TIME IN LIEU

6. Pension
CONTRIBUTIONS IF ANY OR A STAKEHOLDERS' SCHEME
A contracting-out certificate is (not) in force in respect of your employment.

7. Holiday entitlement
You will receive *XXX* weeks' paid holiday during each complete year of service which includes Statutory Bank and Public holidays (*pro rata* for part-time staff).

Your entitlement in the first year of service will be *XXX.*

The holiday year runs from *DATES.*

(Where the holiday year is 1st April to 31st March: Because Easter dates vary from year to year the April to March period may include two Easter holidays. To compensate for this we will allow you to carry forward 2 days from one year to the next.)

Holiday must be taken and unused holiday entitlement cannot be carried forward to the following year.

Holiday must be taken at a time convenient to the Company and no more than *XXX* working days may be taken at any one time.

Holiday will accrue, but may not be taken, during the first month of employment.

8. Sick pay
If you are ill and unfit for work, you must personally contact your line manager as early as possible on the first day and certainly by *DATE* and comply with the absence policy.

If you are ill for fewer than 7 consecutive days (including weekends) you must complete a self certification form. For longer periods of illness a Doctor's certificate must be supplied and additional ones sent to cover the whole period of sickness.

Statutory Sick Pay is paid to employees in accordance with the Statutory Sick Pay Regulations and Company Sick pay will include any Statutory Sick Pay due. Company Sick pay is paid at the absolute discretion of the Company.

An example of a statement of terms and conditions of employment. (continues) ▶

After the probationary period and subject to the correct notification, Company Sick Pay may be paid at the Company's absolute discretion.

9. Notice period

The first 3 months of your employment will be a probationary period during which either party may terminate the contract by giving 1 week's written notice.

Following the probationary period, you are required to provide the Company with written notice of your intention to terminate your employment.

Following the probationary period, and up to 2 years' continuous employment, the Company will provide you with 1 week's notice. Thereafter, the notice period the Company must give will increase by 1 week per complete year of service, to a maximum of 12 weeks.

If written notice is given by you or by the Company to terminate your employment, the Company may, notwithstanding any other terms of these terms and conditions, and at its absolute discretion, require you to:

Continue to perform such duties as the Company may direct or to perform no duties during the period of your notice provided always that it shall continue to pay you your salary and provide all contractual benefits to which you are entitled during such notice period.

Accept a payment of salary in lieu of notice and your employment shall terminate immediately but without prejudice to any other claim the Company or you may have against the other.

The Company has the right to terminate your contract of employment without notice in the event of serious misconduct or some other fundamental breach of contract on your part.

10. Discipline and grievance

The Company want to resolve issues speedily, ensuring fair and consistent treatment for all employees. The Disciplinary and Grievance Procedure is attached; this does not form part of your contract of employment.

11. Collective agreements

There are no collective agreements applicable to your employment.

12. Working outside the United Kingdom

There is no requirement for working outside the United Kingdom.

This contract is subject to:

- Receipt of two references in terms acceptable to the Company;
- You being contractually free to join the Company on the day of commencement;
- That you are not subject to any contractual term that would be breached by you commencing work with us;
- That on commencement date you supply relevant documents to the Company proving your legal right to work in the Country.

For and on behalf of:

Signed..

Dated ....

I acknowledge receipt of these written particulars of employment.

Signed..

Dated ....

(continued) An example of a statement of terms and conditions of employment.

The professional context

21

Bob Moore

This chapter looks at a range of issues relating to the status of being a member of a self-regulating profession. The influences impacting on the veterinary profession include primary, secondary and tertiary legislation, approved codes of conduct, codes of conduct and best practice protocols. For veterinary surgeons in the UK, these will include legislation affecting every member of society and, in addition, that applying specifically to members of the Royal College of Veterinary Surgeons (RCVS).

The trust of the public in the veterinary profession relies on the public's assurance and confidence that the veterinary profession behaves in a totally professional manner, with personal wishes and desires subservient to the requirements of professional behaviour. International readers should refer to their own competent authority and the legislative framework in place in their own country and/or state.

Being a veterinary surgeon involves being a member of a profession (or being a professional). This description carries with it benefits and responsibilities. The following is a non-exhaustive list of characteristics that identify a person as a member of a profession:

- **Integrity** in exercising professional judgement
- **Trust** – professional relationships with clients, based upon trust
- **Ethics** – a commitment to abide by a code of ethics
- **A licence to practise** and a wide range of alternative job opportunities
- **A qualification and title**, as indicated by letters after one's name
- **Betterment of society** – ability to contribute to the betterment of society
- **Membership** of the governing body (i.e. MRCVS).

KEY POINT

Accessibility, accountability and transparency are core requirements expected of every self-regulating profession.

The Royal College of Veterinary Surgeons

The RCVS is the regulatory authority for the veterinary profession and derives its authority from the Veterinary Surgeons Act 1966 (VSA). With an overall aim to protect the public interest and to safeguard animal health and welfare, it has three main functions:

- To maintain a Register of Members
- To monitor the standard of undergraduate education
- To regulate the profession (through the disciplinary process).

The RCVS also has a role as a Royal College, as which it awards certificates and diplomas, and administers veterinary nursing qualifications.

The RCVS Code of Professional Conduct

The Code of Professional Conduct (the Code), formerly known and published as the RCVS Guide to Professional Conduct, is written and updated regularly by the RCVS. The Code addresses the behaviour of veterinary surgeons and their relationships with the public, staff and colleagues. It does not directly address matters of best practice in running the business or of providing a service to clients and their animals. The Code sets out veterinary surgeons' professional responsibilities, and supporting guidance provides further advice on the proper standards of professional practice. On occasions, the professional responsibilities in the Code may conflict with each other and veterinary surgeons may be presented with a dilemma. In such situations, veterinary surgeons have a responsibility to balance the responsibilities, having regard first to animal welfare.

At the outset, the Code says: *'Rights and responsibilities go hand in hand. For this reason on admission to membership of the Royal College of Veterinary Surgeons, and in exchange for the right to practise veterinary surgery in the United Kingdom, every veterinary surgeon makes the following declaration: "I PROMISE AND SOLEMNLY DECLARE that I will pursue the work of my profession with integrity and accept my responsibilities to the public, my clients, the profession and the Royal College of Veterinary Surgeons and that ABOVE ALL my constant endeavour will be to ensure the health and welfare of animals committed to my care".'* These promises acknowledge the obligation of every veterinary surgeon to observe the provisions of the current RCVS Code of Professional Conduct, and in so doing make animal welfare their overriding consideration at all times.

KEY POINT

At the time of writing the Code of Professional Conduct is due to replace the former RCVS Guide to Professional Conduct. Although the exact wording of the oath is changing, the principles of the oath remain. To date, the RCVS guidance has been in the form of:

- The Guide to Professional Conduct
- The Annexes to the Guide
- Advice Notes issued by the RCVS from time to time.

Throughout this chapter, references are made to:

- The Code of Professional Conduct
- Supporting Guidance.

These replace the three sets of documents used previously.

The Code is the benchmark for judging whether the actions or behaviour of a veterinary surgeon fall within acceptable limits. It is not possible within practical limits to mention in the Code every conceivable situation in which a veterinary surgeon might find him/herself, but the provisions of the Code are such that the principles are clear for making a judgement. The Supporting Guidance amplifies the Code and provides examples of situations. Current guidance can be found at www.rcvs.org.uk, and veterinary surgeons in the UK should be familiar with this and any updates made from time to time. It is also advisable for managers and support staff to be familiar with sections of the Code and Supporting Guidance relevant to their roles in practice.

The RCVS has included a Health Protocol within the Supporting Guidance. This provides that a veterinary surgeon with any health issues that affect his/her capacity to perform – with the safety and welfare of animals adversely affected – will have the matter dealt with compassionately rather than with the full force of the disciplinary process. There is a requirement that the veterinary surgeon agrees to undertake some therapy and to provide the RCVS with regular progress reports. This enables colleagues to request help from the RCVS for a colleague they have concerns about, without automatically invoking disciplinary sanctions on them.

The Advisory Committee of the RCVS writes and maintains the Code and Supporting Guidance, and deals with topics that have been raised by veterinary surgeons or members of the public and that the College feels require more detailed explanation. As well as communicating by post, the RCVS offers a regular e-mail update service for members, to alert them to RCVS news, changes and new publications. As RCVS news is generally sent only to veterinary surgeons and veterinary nurses, managers and other support staff may wish to keep themselves up to date by regularly visiting the RCVS website or by ensuring that RCVS publications and mailings sent to members or nurses are circulated appropriately within the practice.

The RCVS Code of Professional Conduct for Veterinary Nurses

The RCVS recognizes training programmes for those wishing to qualify as a veterinary nurse. On 1st September 2007 the non-statutory register for veterinary nurses opened, following a voluntary decision by the Veterinary Nurse Council to create a Register of Veterinary Nurses. Previously, veterinary nurses' names were entered on a non-statutory 'List' and they were referred to as listed VNs. All veterinary nurses listed since 1st January 2003 were automatically transferred to the Register, and other listed VNs were invited to transfer. Registered veterinary nurses can use the post-nominal RVN (listed nurses use VN). RVNs are subject to the Code of Professional Conduct for Veterinary Nurses, together with Supporting Guidance similar to that for veterinary surgeons. RVNs thus have professional responsibility and accountability.

KEY POINTS

- Only registered or listed veterinary nurses may use the post-nominal RVN or VN, respectively.
- Only registered or listed veterinary nurses may work under the exemptions set out in Schedule 3 of the Veterinary Surgeons Act (VSA, see later).
- Previously qualified nurses who have not maintained their listing nor transferred to the register should not use the post-nominal VN and are not permitted to work under Schedule 3 of the VSA.
- It is also worth noting that under current VN Diploma training arrangements, only RVNs may be clinical coaches for student nurses.

The RCVS disciplinary process

Veterinary surgeons

The RCVS is given the responsibility of regulating the veterinary profession under the Veterinary Surgeons Act 1966 (VSA). The Act specifies that the RCVS shall have a Preliminary Investigation Committee (PIC) and a Disciplinary Committee (DC). At the time of writing Defra (Department for Environment, Food and Rural Affairs) is proposing to seek a Legislative Reform Order that will effectively separate the two statutory committees (PIC and DC) from RCVS Council. In modern judiciary thought, it is preferable to have total separation between the 'law makers' and anyone judging those accused of failing to comply with the law. More detailed information will be available as the process progresses. It is unlikely that the actual process of dealing with complaints will alter significantly from the current arrangements.

- The Preliminary Investigation Committee is composed of six veterinary surgeons, three lay observers (appointed by RCVS Council) and some of the legally qualified permanent members of staff present when the committee meets. Only the veterinary surgeons have the right to vote on any case.
- The Disciplinary Committee is composed of twelve members of RCVS Council, not all of whom are veterinary surgeons; some are Privy Council or university appointees who may be laypeople.

The RCVS has a duty to investigate every complaint made against a veterinary surgeon. When a complaint is received, it is assessed by an RCVS lawyer, usually with advice from a veterinary surgeon on the PIC. If it is found that there may be a case to answer, the respondent is asked to provide his/her side of the story. If not, the case is closed at that point. When the respondent has replied, the case is considered by a veterinary surgeon on the PIC and a lay observer who sits with the PIC. Again, if it is agreed that there may be a case to answer, the case is referred to a full meeting of the PIC. If not, the case is closed at this stage.

The referred cases are considered by a full meeting of the PIC, which has a number of options in dealing with the complaint:

- The case may be closed
- It might be that aside from giving suitable advice to the veterinary surgeon there is no need to pursue the case further
- If more information is required the case is deferred to the next meeting while it is collected
- If the case is not considered likely to result in a finding of guilty of serious professional misconduct, but there is concern that further instances of the same type might occur, the PIC can opt to hold the case open so that if further complaints should be received, the current case can be included in any considerations
- The case may be considered sufficiently serious for referral to the DC.

Disciplinary hearings are effectively court hearings, with an adversarial process. The standard of evidence has to be 'so as to be certain', equivalent to that required in a criminal court. The RCVS and the respondent usually have legal representation and the proceedings are overseen by a legal assessor, who is usually a Queen's Counsel (QC).

The sanctions the DC can impose are:

- A warning
- A deferred sentence
- A suspension of registration
- Removal of the respondent's name from the Register.

The RCVS has a target timescale for each stage of the investigation. It is important that witnesses and respondents reply to enquiries from the RCVS promptly. If a respondent wilfully delays their response to the RCVS, that in itself may be considered as professional misconduct.

Registered veterinary nurses

Registered veterinary nurses (RVNs) also have, since 1st April 2011, their own disciplinary process, which mirrors that of veterinary surgeons. Only RVNs are subject to the process; listed veterinary nurses (those who qualified before 2003, who remain on the List but have not voluntarily entered the VN Register) are not subject to the disciplinary process.

Other professional bodies and organizations

The British Veterinary Association

The BVA is a professional association that represents the interests of its members, who are largely veterinary surgeons. It is important to recognize the difference between the roles of the BVA and the RCVS. As explained above, the RCVS is the *regulator* of the profession and has no remit to represent its members; it more properly protects the public against the few instances of professional misconduct by veterinary surgeons. In contrast, the BVA represents its members (e.g. in lobbying parliament and others), and provides a range of services (e.g. insurance and legal advice) for the benefit of its members, as well as negotiating fees for certain activities.

The BVA consists of its membership across the UK. It has a number of divisions, with special interests in particular aspects of veterinary medicine. The British Small Animal Veterinary Association (BSAVA), BCVA (cattle) and BEVA (equine) are the largest of the species divisions. The Society of Practising Veterinary Surgeons (SPVS) is an example of a non-species division; its interests are the business of veterinary practice, management topics and financial issues. Full details of the BVA's structure and various divisions can be found at www.bva.co.uk.

The British Small Animal Veterinary Association

The BSAVA is a membership association specifically for companion animal vets and nurses. It provides a forum for the discussion of issues of importance to veterinary surgeons and nurses in small animal practice and submits evidence on their behalf to the BVA and RCVS as well as to government departments. It also liaises with other veterinary professionals through regular meetings and represents member interests internationally through various european and world small animal veterinary organizations. On behalf of its members, the BSAVA encourages veterinary surgeons and nurses to develop their professional skills through CPD courses, postgraduate certificates and the biggest annual small animal conference in the world. It publishes information on a diversity of small animal topics, including the prestigious BSAVA Manuals and the *Journal of Small Animal Practice,* in a range of traditional and electronic formats. Through its charity, Petsavers, BSAVA funds clinical investigations into the diseases of companion animals. More details are available at www.bsava.com.

The Veterinary Defence Society

The VDS is a mutual insurance company run by experienced veterinary surgeons on behalf of the veterinary profession. Its function is to provide professional indemnity insurance for veterinary surgeons against possible claims by owners for negligence in respect of animals treated. The VDS will, in most circumstances, extend its insurance cover to non-veterinary surgeon members of a veterinary practice who are working under the direction of the employing veterinary practice.

The VDS provides support for insured veterinary surgeons by providing legal representation should events progress to a court hearing. This applies to civil courts where claims for negligence are heard, or allegations of professional misconduct before the Disciplinary Committee of the RCVS. Registered veterinary nurses must take out an additional personal policy if they wish to be insured by the VDS for support in the event of allegations to the RCVS of professional misconduct.

There are a number of other commercial companies who will provide professional indemnity insurance cover for veterinary surgeons. Charges will vary and the veterinary surgeon should consider the way in which the indemnity insurer chooses to handle claims against a veterinary surgeon. Some are more ready to pay compensation and avoid a lengthy battle, whilst others will choose to defend the veterinary surgeon against what it perceives to be an unjustified accusation of negligence on the part of the veterinary surgeon. It is up to each individual veterinary surgeon to decide how he/she can best meet the requirement of the Code to provide professional indemnity insurance (PII) cover for him/herself.

British Veterinary Union in Unite (BVU)

The BVU was formed in 2011 and is led by a professional advisory committee of veterinary surgeon employees and employers and veterinary nurses. It is based in the health sector of the trade union Unite. The BVU has objectives to ensure and enhance the welfare of vets and nurses as personnel, to safeguard and promote the welfare of vets and nurses as professionals, and to set up and operate proactive welfare programmes for vets and nurses. Membership is open to veterinary surgeons, veterinary nurses, students and support staff working in and with the veterinary profession. Further details can be found at www.unitetheunion.org.

The Veterinary Practice Management Association

The VPMA is an association for those with an interest in the management of the business of running a veterinary practice, and is also affiliated to the BVA. Membership is open to veterinary surgeons, practice managers and anyone with an interest in such management issues. The VPMA has a Code of Conduct with which its members are required to comply (Figure 21.1).

I pledge that I will:

- Maintain and promote the profession of veterinary practice management;
- Seek every possible opportunity to enhance my personal experience, skill and expertise in the profession of veterinary practice management;
- Seek and maintain an equitable, professional and co-operative relationship with fellow members of the Veterinary Practice Management Association and with my colleagues in my business and professional life;
- Fulfil my obligations and responsibilities to the best of my ability to enable my employer and colleagues to deliver the highest possible standards of service to our clients and their animals within the guidelines set down in the current RCVS Guide to Professional Conduct; [a]
- Pursue my profession in veterinary practice management with honesty, integrity and industry, placing the emphasis of my efforts on the highest possible standards of service to my employer(s);
- Ensure the confidentiality of any information relating to the business or personal affairs of my employer(s) and the clinical or other details of their clients and patients, except as may be required or compelled by appropriate law or other regulation;
- Protect any of my employer's property under my control and acknowledge that all information gathered, maintained or produced within the practice is the exclusive property of the practice owner(s) and will not be reproduced, shared or distributed outside the practice without the owner's consent.

21.1 The VPMA Code of Conduct. [a] From 2012 The RCVS Code of Professional Conduct.

The British Veterinary Nursing Association

The BVNA is the only national representative body for veterinary nurses. It advises and represents veterinary nursing interests and supports veterinary nurses and practice staff with legal advice and support. Associate membership is available for people other than nurses. It publishes a monthly journal, the *Veterinary Nursing Journal*, and runs regional meetings, CPD and an annual congress. Further details can be found at www.bvna.org.uk.

The Veterinary Medicines Directorate

The VMD is an agency of Defra and is responsible for legislation affecting all veterinary medicinal products (VMPs) (see Chapter 15). It writes the Veterinary Medicines Regulations (VMRs) and updates these annually. It also provides Guidance Notes to assist in understanding the VMRs. Suspect Adverse Reactions (SARs) should be reported to the VMD on the appropriate forms, which can be downloaded at www.vmd.defra.gov.uk. The regulations governing the importation of VMPs, the licensing, manufacture, classification and supply of VMPs all come within the jurisdiction of the VMD.

The registration of practice premises is required under the VMRs, and the VMD has a cadre of inspectors who carry out inspections for those practices not registered under the RCVS Practice Standards Scheme (PSS). The RCVS maintains the register of practice premises for the Secretary of State and PSS members are registered on the basis of their PSS membership.

Animal Medicines Training Regulatory Authority

AMTRA is the independent regulatory body whose task it is to ensure that the prescription and supply of POM-VPS animal medicines in the UK is undertaken in a responsible manner by AMTRA-qualified persons. Under the Veterinary Medicines Regulations, AMTRA is the body appointed by the Secretary of State to keep a register of Suitably Qualified Persons (SQPs), who are a category of professionally qualified animal health advisors who are entitled to prescribe and/or supply POM-VPS medicines. Full details of the qualifications necessary and the responsibilities for SQPs, together with their code of conduct, can be found at www.amtra.org.uk.

Key legislation and regulations

The Veterinary Surgeons Act 1966

All legislation governing the veterinary profession is designed to meet the requirements of animal welfare and to protect the public interest by ensuring a high level of education and training, combined with personal and professional integrity. The VSA provides the authority for the RCVS to regulate the veterinary profession. The VSA does not set the standards directly but allows the RCVS to set standards of education, professional behaviour and regulation.

The Act states that subject to certain provisions, no individual shall practise, or hold him/herself out as practising or as being prepared to practise, veterinary surgery unless he/she is registered in the Register of Veterinary Surgeons or the Supplementary Veterinary Register. The Act makes clear the requirements for registration, including the registrable degrees from EU states, and recognizes the RCVS as the Competent Authority. It sets out the composition of the council of the RCVS and its disciplinary process and procedures. It also restricts the practice of veterinary surgery by unqualified persons, and allows exceptions (in Schedule 3) to this for veterinary students and certain other categories, subject to prescribed conditions.

Veterinary nurses and Schedule 3

The VSA recognizes the special position held by veterinary nurses. Schedule 3 to the VSA allows anyone to give First Aid in an emergency for the purpose of saving life and relieving suffering. The owner of an animal, or a member of the owner's household or employee of the owner, may also provide minor medical treatment. Owners of farm stock or their employees may carry out a limited range of minor procedures to farm animals, such as castration of lambs and disbudding of calves; other legislation covers ages at which these can be done, and anaesthesia requirements.

The exemptions to the Act that apply to veterinary nurses are shown in Figure 21.2. In this context 'veterinary nurse' means a listed or registered veterinary nurse. The exception does not apply to nurses whose names are not on the List or Register.

Practices should check that all veterinary nurses carrying out Schedule 3 procedures, including minor treatments, are currently registered or listed and should verify their identification. In addition to their badge, both carry cards which must be in date (Figure 21.3).

Applying to listed or registered veterinary nurses

Any medical treatment or any minor surgery (not involving entry into a body cavity) to any animal by a veterinary nurse if the following conditions are complied with:

- The animal is, for the time being, under the care of a registered veterinary surgeon or veterinary practitioner and the medical treatment or minor surgery is carried out by the veterinary nurse at his/her direction
- The registered veterinary surgeon or veterinary practitioner is the employer or is acting on behalf of the employer of the veterinary nurse
- The registered veterinary surgeon or veterinary practitioner directing the medical treatment or minor surgery is satisfied that the veterinary nurse is qualified to carry out the treatment or surgery

For a student veterinary nurse

Any medical treatment or any minor surgery (not involving entry into a body cavity) to any animal by a student veterinary nurse if the following conditions are complied with:

- The animal is, for the time being, under the care of a registered veterinary surgeon or veterinary practitioner and the medical treatment or minor surgery is carried out by the student veterinary nurse at his/her direction and in the course of the student veterinary nurse's training
- The treatment or surgery is supervised by a registered veterinary surgeon, veterinary practitioner or veterinary nurse and, in the case of surgery, the supervision is direct, continuous and personal
- The registered veterinary surgeon or veterinary practitioner is the employer or is acting on behalf of the employer of the student veterinary nurse

Activities specifically excluded from being done by veterinary nurses

- The castration of a male animal being: a horse, pony, ass or mule; a bull, boar or goat which has reached the age of 2 months; a ram which has reached the age of 3 months; or a cat or dog
- The spaying of a cat or dog
- The removal (otherwise than in an emergency for the purpose of saving life or relieving pain or suffering) of any part of the antlers of a deer before the velvet of the antlers is frayed and the greater part of it has been shed
- The desnooding of a turkey which has reached the age of 21 days
- The removal of the combs of any poultry which have reached the age of 72 hours
- The cutting of the toes of a domestic fowl or turkey which has reached the age of 72 hours
- The performance of a vasectomy or the carrying out of electroejaculation on any animal or bird kept for the production of food, wool, skin or fur or for use in the farming of land
- The removal of the supernumerary teats of a calf which has reached the age of 3 months
- The dehorning or disbudding of a sheep or goat, except the trimming of the insensitive tip of an ingrowing horn which, if left untreated, could cause pain or distress

21.2 Exemptions from restrictions on practice of veterinary surgery: treatment and operations that may be given or carried out by unqualified persons. Adapted from Schedule 3 of the Veterinary Surgeons Act 1966.

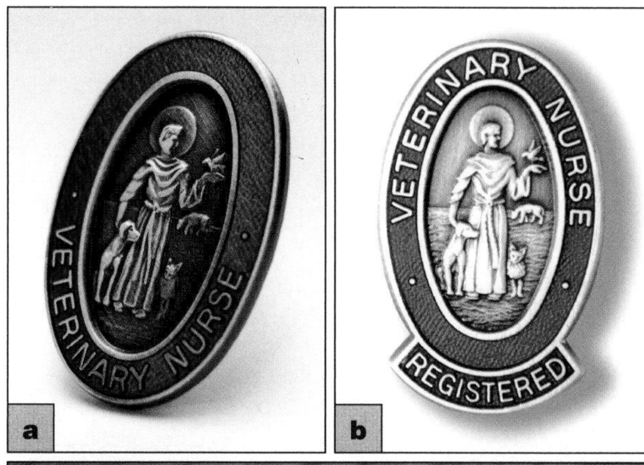

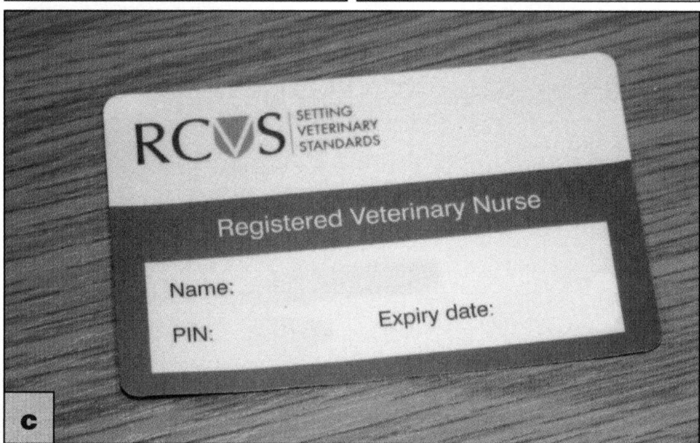

21.3 **(a)** Veterinary nurse badge awarded to all qualified VNs until the end of 2011. **(b)** Registered veterinary nurse badge awarded to RVNs from 2012. **(c)** An example of a card issued annually to Registered VNs; Listed VNs carry a pale purple card. (a,b © RCVS)

Delegating to a veterinary nurse

There are two levels of responsibility to be considered when deciding whether a veterinary nurse should carry out a procedure:

- The directing veterinary surgeon must be confident in the competence of the veterinary nurse or student veterinary nurse to perform the task satisfactorily and without danger to the animal or its welfare
- The veterinary nurse or student veterinary nurse must be satisfied of their own competence or confidence to carry out the procedure without danger to the animal or its welfare.

If either party is not entirely happy with the above provision, then the process of delegation to a veterinary nurse should be reviewed. A young or inexperienced veterinary nurse or student veterinary nurse may find it difficult to express their concerns. It is the duty of the supervising veterinary surgeon to be sensitive to the concerns of their staff and to encourage nurses to be realistic in assessing their own abilities. If a veterinary surgeon has worries about the competence of a veterinary nurse in their practice, they should discuss the matter with other colleagues (including nurses) in the practice, with a view to helping the veterinary nurse achieve competence. Veterinary nurses should recognize that it is not a right to carry out Schedule 3 procedures. Further information regarding delegation to veterinary nurses is set out in the Supporting Guidance to the RCVS Code of Professional Conduct.

It would be prudent for a veterinary practice to record and keep documentation relating to the assessment of the training and competence of veterinary nurses. Inspection or challenge by any competent authority (such as RCVS Practice Standards Scheme inspectors) would be easily satisfied by such record-keeping, and colleagues would have a ready reference for training and competence completed by staff members.

The Animal Welfare Act

The Animal Welfare Act 2006 replaces earlier legislation and brings animal welfare issues together in one place. It places an onus on the owner of the animal to ensure the welfare of their animals (Figure 21.4). Section 18 of the Act sets out all the conditions and situations where a veterinary surgeon can act in assisting 'an officer or constable' in arriving at a decision if an animal may be judged 'to be in distress' and may need to be euthanased (see www.legislation.gov.uk).

Duty of person responsible for animal to ensure welfare:

(1) A person commits an offence if he does not take such steps as are reasonable in all the circumstances to ensure that the needs of an animal for which he is responsible are met to the extent required by good practice.
(2) For the purposes of this Act, an animal's needs shall be taken to include:
  (a) its need for a suitable environment,
  (b) its need for a suitable diet,
  (c) its need to be able to exhibit normal behaviour patterns,
  (d) any need it has to be housed with, or apart from, other animals, and
  (e) its need to be protected from pain, suffering, injury and disease.

21.4 An extract from the Animal Welfare Act 2006.

Other legislation

A significant amount of government legislation impacts on all businesses, whatever their nature may be. It is the responsibility of the practice owners and management to ensure that all relevant legislation is complied with. Important areas are noted below, though this is by no means an exhaustive list.

- **Health and safety** is an all-embracing section of legislation, with significant sanctions for non-compliance. Its range and ramifications will affect every veterinary practice. It covers Control of Substances Hazardous to Health (COSHH) regulations, radiation regulations, personal protective equipment, use of VDUs, fire safety, RIDDOR and much more. See Chapter 22 for more information.
- **Employment legislation** is a major subject in its own right, and is covered in Chapter 20.
- **Anti-discrimination legislation** now covers every conceivable aspect of potential discrimination; see Chapters 19 and 20.
- **Financial regulations** and advice on HM Revenue and Customs matters, etc., can be found in Chapter 24.

- **The Bribery Act 2010:** This was introduced to prevent bribery by companies or individuals. In summary, it is not acceptable to give, to promise to give or to offer a payment, gift or hospitality with the expectation or hope that a business advantage will be received, or to reward a business advantage already given, or to accept a payment, gift or hospitality from a third party if it is known or suspected that this is offered or provided with the expectation that that party will receive a business advantage. Any payment or gift to a public official or other person to secure or accelerate the prompt or proper performance of a routine government procedure or process, otherwise known as a 'facilitation payment', is also strictly prohibited. Facilitation payments are not commonly paid in the UK but they are common in some other jurisdictions. A company may have a written policy (Figure 21.5).

Practice Policy on Gifts

The giving of business gifts to clients, customers, contractors and suppliers is not prohibited provided the following requirements are met:

- The gift is not made with the intention of influencing a third party to obtain or retain business or a business advantage, or to reward the provision or retention of business or a business advantage
- It complies with local laws
- It is given in the company's name, not in the giver's personal name
- It does not include cash or a cash equivalent (such as gift vouchers)
- It is of an appropriate and reasonable type and value and given at an appropriate time
- It is given openly, not secretly
- It is approved in advance by a director of the company.

21.5 An example of a practice's anti-bribery policy.

Animal welfare

Every veterinary surgeon registered in the UK makes a declaration on admission to membership of the RCVS that he/she will ensure the welfare of animals committed to his/her care. This is fundamental to the professional standards of all veterinary surgeons.

Veterinary surgeons may meet a situation where they consider that there are welfare issues with animals presented to them, or which are coincidentally observed during a consultation. Small animal and farm animal practitioners may from time to time encounter situations that they feel compromise the welfare of animals on their clients' premises. The veterinary surgeon should try to resolve the issue directly with the client by giving suitable advice, and assisting the owner if it is a matter of ignorance or incompetence on the owner's part. Such advice may not always be welcome and the veterinary surgeon should approach the situation with tact and diplomacy.

KEY POINT

Advice from a partner or senior member of the practice should always be sought by inexperienced veterinary surgeons.

There will, inevitably, be occasions when a veterinary surgeon feels that more direct action may be required. They may feel that the owner should face prosecution or some sort of sanction for actions concerning welfare of animals. The veterinary surgeon immediately faces the problem of client confidentiality in revealing information gained by virtue of their position as the consulting veterinary surgeon. It is essential that the matter is discussed with colleagues in the practice and, moreover, it is advisable to seek advice from the Professional Conduct Department of the RCVS, who are experienced in dealing with such matters.

Veterinary surgeons should be particularly careful that they never put themselves in the position of appearing to breach any welfare code in dealing with any animal – their own or those of their clients. All veterinary surgeons in practice will recognize the need for firm handling of difficult patients, for the safety of themselves, the animals, and the owners or staff assisting in the handling process. However, there can be a fine line between firm handling and over-enthusiastic restraint. Owners may not be used to seeing animals handled at all and may misunderstand what is being done, or may fail to realize the need for the actions taken by the veterinary surgeon or their staff. Suitably warning the owner, explaining what is going to happen, or removing the animal to a separate room can usually avoid owner complaints with regard to mistreatment of pets.

Patient's wellbeing

The Code states that veterinary surgeons must make animal health and welfare their first consideration when attending to animals, providing veterinary care that is appropriate and adequate. They should keep within their own area of competence and refer cases responsibly.

It is important that animal owners are given the opportunity to be involved in the selection of the treatment their animal receives. RCVS guidance is that having reached a provisional diagnosis taking into account the animal's age, the extent of any injuries or disease and the likely quality of life after treatment, veterinary surgeons should make a full and realistic assessment of the prognosis and the options for treatment or euthanasia and communicate this to the client. Veterinary surgeons and nurses should seek to ensure that what both they and clients are saying is heard and understood on both sides, and encourage clients to take a full part in any discussion. Chapter 17 gives more detail on the consultation process and communicating with owners.

Clients should be made aware of the cost of providing care for inpatients. In some instances it may be appropriate for an experienced owner to provide nursing care at home. Before leaving an animal at a practice, the owner, keeper or carer should be made aware of the level of supervision that will be provided to the animal, particularly the level of supervision during an overnight stay. Different levels of care are required, depending on a wide range of factors. Where the owner cannot afford private treatment and may be eligible for charitable assistance, veterinary surgeons should redirect the animal for further treatment to a charity where possible, supplying full details of the case in the proper manner.

The welfare of animals committed to the care of veterinary surgeons is fundamental to their professional behaviour. Pain relief is now sophisticated and available for most species. With judicious use of the prescribing cascade (see Chapter 15), pain relief should be available for all species. Whilst there is no specific advice given by the RCVS about preventive healthcare, this remains an important part of the service veterinary surgeons will provide for their patients.

Euthanasia

The subject of euthanasia is dealt with in the RCVS Supporting Guidance (Figure 21.6). Issues that may arise include:

- The owner may find the decision difficult and will need reassurance
- Communication is paramount (what is likely to happen?)
- Judging the optimum time to discuss the disposal of the body may be difficult
- Does the owner wish to be present, or remain in a side room?
- The amount of restraint required will vary and should be appropriate
- Support staff may be required to restrain animals
- Explaining to owners that old or sick animals may have poor circulation, and the possible outcomes that may ensue
- Considering sedation and explaining why this may be needed
- In cases where the procedure does not go according to plan, providing owners with a detailed explanation and support.

Euthanasia and the owner's wishes

Euthanasia is not, in law, an act of veterinary surgery, and may be carried out by anyone provided that it is carried out humanely. No veterinary surgeon is obliged to kill a healthy animal unless required to do so under statutory powers as part of their conditions of employment. Veterinary surgeons do, however, have the privilege of being able to relieve an animal's suffering in this way in appropriate cases.

From time to time veterinary surgeons may face difficulties. For example, an owner may want to have a perfectly healthy or treatable animal destroyed, or an owner may wish to keep an animal alive in circumstances where euthanasia would be the kindest course of action. The veterinary surgeon's primary obligation is to relieve the suffering of an animal but account must be taken not only of the animal's condition but also the owner's wishes and circumstances. To refuse an owner's request for euthanasia may add to the owner's distress and could be deleterious to the welfare of the animal. Where, in all conscience, a veterinary surgeon cannot accede to a client's request for euthanasia he or she should recognise the extreme sensitivity of the situation and make sympathetic efforts to direct the client to alternative sources of advice.

Where a veterinary surgeon is concerned about an owner's refusal to consent to euthanasia, the veterinary surgeon can only advise their client and act in accordance with their professional judgement. Where a veterinary surgeon is concerned that an animal's welfare is compromised because of an owner's refusal to allow euthanasia, a veterinary surgeon may take steps to resolve the situation, for example an initial step could be to seek another veterinary opinion for the client, potentially by telephone.

21.6 RCVS Supporting Guidance on euthanasia. (continues) ▶

Euthanasia and the owner's wishes

The Animal Welfare Act 2006 (which applies in England and Wales), the Animal Health and Welfare (Scotland) Act 2006 and the Welfare of Animals (Northern Ireland) Act 2011 contain provisions to safeguard the welfare of animals. For animals in distress, there are no provisions in these Acts which specifically authorize a veterinary surgeon to destroy an animal. Powers to destroy an animal or arrange for its destruction are conferred on an inspector (who may be appointed by the local authority) or a police constable. A veterinary surgeon may be asked to certify the condition of the animal is such that it should in its own interests be destroyed. An inspector or constable may act without a veterinary certificate if there is no reasonable alternative to destruction and the need for action is such that it is not reasonably practical to wait for a veterinary surgeon.

A person with responsibility for an animal may commit an offence if an act, or failure to act, causes an animal to suffer unnecessarily. An owner is always responsible for their animal, but a veterinary surgeon is likely to be responsible for the animal when it is an inpatient at the practice. If, in the opinion of the veterinary surgeon, the animal's condition is such that it should, in its own interests, be destroyed without delay, the veterinary surgeon may need to act without the owner's consent and should make a full record of all the circumstances supporting the decision in case of subsequent challenge. Generally there should be discussions with the owner of the animal before such a decision, which should be endorsed by a veterinary surgeon not directly involved in the case until that time.

21.6 (continued) RCVS Supporting Guidance on euthanasia.

Tail docking

The Animal Welfare Act 2006 prohibits the removal of any part of a dog's tail for other than medical reasons. The Act then makes exceptions: the veterinary surgeon may remove part of a dog's tail before the dog is 5 days old if the vet is presented with specific evidence that the dog is to be used as a working dog in relation to law enforcement, the armed forces, emergency rescue, pest control or the lawful shooting of animals, and is of a type of dog that may be docked. In Scotland there are no exceptions. In Wales the types of dog allowed to be docked are more closely defined.

Under the Animal Welfare Act it is an offence to cause unnecessary suffering to any animal; in the section dealing with mutilations, besides specifically banning tail docking, the Act states that it is an offence to *carry out a procedure which involves interference with the sensitive tissues or bone structure of the animal.* This will preclude procedures such as ear cropping and claw removal, unless done for valid medical reasons. The BVA publishes a detailed guide (for the UK) on docking and the processes advised should a docked dog be presented without a certificate; members can access this at www.bva.co.uk.

Animal breeding

Veterinary surgeons have a professional interest in breeding animals, especially where extremes of conformation lead to difficulties either for the dam giving birth (e.g. fetal oversize or conformation of head) or for the animal during its lifetime. The problem may be one of conformation affecting the animal's ability to lead a normal life, or a predisposition to disease processes developing in later life. Patrick Bateson's 2010 *Independent Inquiry into Dog Breeding* made reference to these topics and encouraged the veterinary profession to be active in promoting responsible breeding of companion animals. Veterinary surgeons have a responsibility to advise breeders if they consider it appropriate.

The Kennel Club is amending its procedures for registration of dogs. Owners now have to agree when signing the application form that they are giving veterinary surgeons authority to report to the Kennel Club any operations to alter conformation, and any caesarean sections. This will resolve any confidentiality problems associated with revealing specific details about a client's animal or any treatment administered.

If a veterinary surgeon recognizes any defect affecting the welfare of the animal in question it is their responsibility to give advice to the owner of the animal. They should recognize that if the animal is registered with the Kennel Club then they already have permission to divulge information relating to surgery, either to alter conformation or for caesarean sections.

It is not compulsory for a veterinary surgeon to report any defects or alterations (provided they are not illegal!), but it will help to improve the breeding of dogs if reporting is approached responsibly.

Strays

Every practice will be familiar with the scenario: a concerned and conscientious member of the public presents an animal at the practice that is obviously in need of veterinary attention. The member of the public frequently does not wish to 'adopt' the animal or to take on the potential expense of any treatment that might be required. They merely feel they have acted responsibly in bringing an injured or sick animal to the right place for attention. They wish to leave the animal at the practice. What should the veterinary practice do? Who is going to give consent for any treatment?

There is a series of issues for the practice to consider:

- Is the animal microchipped?
- Is there a need for emergency relief of pain or suffering?
- Is euthanasia required if the condition is severe?
- Can the owner be traced?
- Who pays, and should an animal charity be approached?

Any stray presented at the practice should be scanned for a microchip (Figure 21.7). If a microchip is identified, the practice should then take all reasonable steps to contact the database holder and trace the owner. Consent can then be sought and the matter of fees discussed before any treatment is initiated. The Preliminary Investigation Committee of the RCVS (PIC) has been called upon to issue advice to a veterinary surgeon who euthanased a stray cat without first checking for a microchip (which was present) and whose owner subsequently complained that they were not contacted prior to the cat being euthanased.

Emergency treatment for the relief of pain and suffering should not be withheld solely on the basis of non-payment. The treatment need be no more than the minimum required to relieve pain or suffering. If the client is not eligible for charitable assistance, euthanasia may have to be considered on economic grounds.

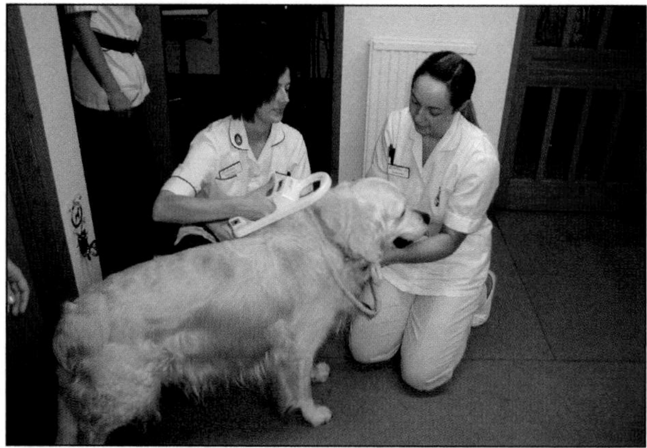

21.7 All strays presented at the practice should be scanned for a microchip. As scanners vary in sensitivity, choosing a good quality scanner that can detect a range of chips is vital.

In some instances euthanasia may be the correct clinical choice in the judgement of the attending veterinary surgeon. In the absence of an owner or person able to give consent, the veterinary surgeon should, if possible, seek the opinion of a colleague before carrying out the procedure. In all cases, whether acting alone or with a second opinion, the veterinary surgeon should record in writing the reasons leading him/her to arrive at that judgement.

Invariably, when an owner cannot be traced and the animal is healthy or makes a good recovery, practice staff will want to re-home the animal. The practice should make every effort to find the owner by searching for a microchip, advertising locally and contacting local police and animal charities to enquire whether a lost animal has been reported. Provided the new owners are aware of the situation, the practice is then at liberty to re-home the stray. If re-homing is not an option and if there is no charity able to take the stray and the practice has made reasonable efforts to find the owner, then euthanasia may be the only option. The time period before euthanasia is carried out will depend on the circumstances, available space, type of animal and its condition at the time.

Wildlife

There is no specific guidance provided by the RCVS on treatment of wildlife by veterinary surgeons, but the Code's requirements to not unreasonably refuse First Aid and to facilitate the provision of pain relief continue to apply.

Members of the public or laypeople will always want to 'do something' but under the VSA they are limited to administering First Aid. Veterinary nurses will be better trained to administer First Aid but are still limited in what they can do. Access to veterinary medicines will be limited and veterinary surgeons should always be wary of leaving veterinary medicines with laypeople for administration to wildlife, particularly POM-Vs.

The question of fees for such treatment will always be raised. Some animal charities will provide payment for treatment of wildlife and local arrangements can be established. If a veterinary surgeon is requested by an animal charity or the police to attend at a wildlife incident, the requesting authority should be expected to bear a reasonable charge for the service provided. The RSPCA has a policy regarding animals and birds brought to their wildlife centres of only providing treatment if the animal will ultimately be able to be returned to the wild.

Almost all local areas will have either a branch of a national animal charity or a locally based group. Life in practice can be much easier if the practice establishes and maintains a good relationship with their local animal charity, as sources of funding for treatment can be established in advance. Involvement of the practice with their local 'open day' or the local charity with the practice open day can promote cooperation.

Animal abuse

If a veterinary surgeon suspects animal abuse, as a result of examining an animal, it should be considered whether the circumstances are sufficiently serious to justify breaching the usual obligations of client confidentiality. If appropriate, the veterinary surgeon should attempt to discuss his/her concerns with the client, but if this is not possible or appropriate, the relevant authorities (e.g. RSPCA, SSPCA (Scotland), USPCA (Northern Ireland)) should be contacted to report alleged cruelty to an animal. The veterinary surgeon would in this case make a judgement that the public interest in protecting an animal overrides the professional obligation to maintain client confidentiality. In general, confidentiality should only be breached where there is direct evidence (i.e. not hearsay or third-party evidence) that an animal has suffered abuse or neglect.

Child abuse and domestic violence

RCVS guidance indicates that a veterinary surgeon reporting suspected animal abuse to the relevant authority should consider whether a child might be at risk. A situation may also arise where a child may be considered at risk in the absence of any animal abuse. The NSPCC leaflet *Understanding the Links: Child Abuse, Animal Abuse and Family Violence – Information for Professionals* provides further information (see www.nspcc.org.uk).

Continuity of care and case handover

KEY POINT

Once an animal has been accepted as an inpatient for treatment by a veterinary surgeon or practice, responsibility for the animal remains with that veterinary surgeon or practice until another veterinary surgeon or practice accepts the responsibility.

Primary practices and out-of-hours emergency service providers must provide uninterrupted treatment of an inpatient if it is not fit to be moved. Where an animal needs continuous inpatient care, a veterinary surgeon should not leave the animal until appropriate care is provided by a suitably qualified colleague (e.g. an MRCVS, or a listed, registered or student veterinary nurse). It is up to the veterinary surgeon dealing with the particular case to decide on the level of care required.

Transport

It is recognized that critically ill animals will sometimes need to be moved in order to receive appropriate treatment, and primary practices should have appropriate transport and transfer arrangements in place. This may necessitate trained staff travelling with the animal. When considering the transfer of critically ill animals, veterinary surgeons should consider the long-term care that may be required and avoid, so far as possible, the need for such animals to travel more than necessary. Where it is necessary and appropriate to transfer an animal between the primary practice and an out-of-hours emergency service provider, the responsibility is that of the veterinary practices involved, *not the client*. Normally, the practice from which the animal is transferred is responsible for the transfer or arranging the transfer.

KEY POINT

The transfer of a critically ill animal between practices should be in the animal's best interests, not for the convenience of the practices involved.

Out-of-hours cover

The Code of Professional Conduct currently requires anyone in practice 'to take steps to provide 24-hour emergency First Aid and pain relief to animals according to their skills and the specific situation'. It is important to differentiate between a 24-hour service (open for all business 24 hours) and emergency 24-hour cover (emergency First Aid provided). Out-of-hours cover may be provided by the practice itself, in cooperation with local practices, or by using the services of a dedicated out-of-hours clinic. In every instance the practice must make details of the emergency service available to its clients, with information about location, distances, and possible fees to be charged. This can be through practice newsletters, information on accounts rendered, notices in the waiting room, vaccination reminders, terms of business notices, or 'mailshots' (bulk mail advertising).

Dedicated emergency clinics are required to meet all the same standards as normal practices. The area requiring particular attention is the responsibility for continuity of care provision. When premises are shared between normal-hour clinics and emergency clinics, arrangements must be in place to deal with animals that cannot be moved after admission during overnight hours.

Referral

Veterinary surgeons should facilitate a client's request for a referral or second opinion. A referral may be for a diagnosis, procedure and/or possible treatment, after which the case is returned to the referring veterinary surgeon; a second opinion is only for the purpose of seeking the views of another veterinary surgeon.

In recent years there has been an increase in the number of referral practices offering specialist services to first-opinion practices. All arrangements must be made for the benefit of the patient and its owner. This will require both parties to have in place a protocol dealing with transfer of patients, records and advice.

- **The first-opinion practice** must ensure that the referral practice has all the necessary information prior to the patient being transferred.
- **The referral practice** must ensure that the owner and the first-opinion practice are provided with full details about treatment programmes and how follow-up or emergencies arising with the case are to be managed. This may be achieved by the veterinary surgeon at the referral centre providing the owner with written instructions for ongoing treatment and follow-up consultations with the first-opinion practice. The referral centre veterinary surgeon should, *before the date of any check-up required at the first-opinion practice*, telephone the first-opinion veterinary surgeon or, preferably, send a written report of what has been done and any ongoing medication or treatment recommended.

KEY POINT

First-opinion and referral practices should have clear protocols in place to ensure that all relevant information and case records are passed to and from the veterinary surgeons involved, both before and after the case is seen, and that clear follow-up guidelines are communicated.

Client transfer

If a client chooses to transfer the care of their pet to another veterinary practice, the original practice must not obstruct them in making the move. It is acceptable to ask them for the reasons, explaining that it may help to avoid similar problems in the future. The clinical records of the animal involved must be provided to the new veterinary practice. This is particularly important when an animal is undergoing treatment; details of diagnosis and treatment protocols are required before a new veterinary surgeon can take over the case. Only those records pertaining to the pet while it was owned by the current owner have to be supplied. The new practice should contact the previous practice to inform them of the change in arrangements.

Access to clinical records

Under the rules of the Data Protection Act 1998, the owners of an animal may request a copy of their animal's clinical notes and the practice is under an obligation to provide a copy, for which it may make a reasonable charge. The notes should only cover that period during which the animal has been the property of the current owner.

KEY POINT

All practice staff members should ensure that their entries on the records are appropriate, professional, accurate and easy to understand.

The impact of ethics on staff, clients and colleagues

Mental health and wellbeing

The veterinary profession has the unfortunate distinction of having the highest suicide rate of any profession in the UK. The precise reasons behind this statistic are unclear but, whatever they are, it is important that every graduate takes care to protect their own mental health and that of their colleagues. Information on The Veterinary Surgeons' Health Support Programme (VSHSP) can be found at www.rcvs.org.uk. Help and support is also given by Vetlife (www.vetlife.org.uk).

In practices where out-of-hours cover is provided by that practice, care must be taken to comply with the Working Time Regulations (see Chapter 20). Adequate rest times and the maximum working hours per week must be monitored so that individuals are not exposed to unnecessary stress.

At times, the practice of veterinary surgery can be a very stressful occupation. It is the responsibility of every member of the practice, whether a veterinary surgeon or not, to learn how to manage stress. Ways of de-stressing will vary between individuals but everyone should recognize the need to take personal responsibility for their own wellbeing (see also Chapter 18). The managers of the practice should bear these matters in mind when arranging the work rotas for the practice; e.g. some flexibility may be required to ensure that an individual can organize to be a member of a local activity group on a regular weeknight. At the same time, managers should ensure that one individual is not always scheduled to be on duty at a 'bad' or unfavourable time. For example, Friday evenings/nights should be shared among everyone, as should weekend duties, unless individuals prefer to work such duties for their own work–life balance.

Every member of staff should be alert to potential problems in the team. One regrettable feature of any large group working together is bullying or harassment. This can take many forms and can be exceedingly destructive for the targeted individual. If those that observe bullying are not able to deal with it themselves they should seek advice from senior members of the practice or from the Professional Conduct Department of the RCVS. A bullying and harassment policy should be in place and followed by all staff. Chapter 18 includes more guidance on stress management.

'Whistle blowing'

Veterinary surgeons and veterinary nurses may consider that they have witnessed inappropriate conduct in the workplace, on the part of a professional colleague or the practice as a whole. Inappropriate conduct may include a breach of the RCVS Codes of Professional Conduct for veterinary surgeons and veterinary nurses or unethical behaviour, e.g. false certification, care of an animal which falls far short of the expected standards, or practising under the influence of drugs or alcohol. Individual members of the practice may see other activities that they find unsettling or recognize as wrong on any number of levels.

The advice of a senior colleague should first be sought. If a veterinary nurse becomes concerned about the competence of a veterinary surgeon, they should discuss these concerns with another veterinary surgeon in the practice or, if this is impractical, seek advice from the Professional Conduct Department of the RCVS. It is vital that issues such as these are approached sensitively and through the appropriate practice channels in the first instance. There are also Vet Health helplines, which can offer assistance and advice informally. Only when other channels have been exhausted should whistle blowing be considered.

Before alerting any statutory body, the whistle blower should have first-hand evidence, should consider the effect that whistle blowing might have on the staff involved, and must be prepared to lose anonymity. RCVS guidance on 'whistle blowing' can be found in Figure 21.8 and at www.rcvs.org.uk. Further information can be found at: www.bva.co.uk; www.bvna.org.uk; www.rspca.org.uk; www.acas.org.uk (Advisory, Conciliation and Arbitration Service); www.citizensadvice.org.uk; www.hse.gov.uk (Health and Safety Executive); www.pcaw.co.uk (Public Concern at Work); and www.lawsociety.org.uk and in Chapter 20.

Relationships with the community

Many practices will work, either alone or in collaboration with local charities, to provide help for disadvantaged groups of petowners, or for strays brought in by members of the public when no owner can be traced. The practice activities can take many forms, from having a collection tin on the front desk to holding a full-day fundraising event. Such activities will create a positive link with the local community and practice clients but should at all times be professional in execution and it should be made abundantly clear that the funds are not to swell the profits of the practice.

Relationships with colleagues

Communication within the practice can sometimes be overlooked, resulting in unfortunate outcomes. It is essential to have a system of information exchange for all members of staff (see Chapter 17). It is particularly important to ensure the continuation of a programme of treatment initiated by a colleague in the practice. Changes should be introduced only after discussing the reasons with colleagues. It can appear to clients that the practice is disorganized if treatment is changed for no apparent reason.

The Code also requires all RCVS members and veterinary nurses to treat colleagues with respect and not disparage them in front of clients or the public. Disagreements should be resolved in private, if necessary seeking advice from other colleagues or advisors.

Certification

One of the criteria for being a professional is that the individual has the trust of his/her clients. This is particularly so in the case of certification. Veterinary surgeons are called on to provide certification on a wide range of issues, including pre-purchase examination of horses and freedom from disease and

Reporting inappropriate conduct

- The first consideration in reporting inappropriate conduct is for the veterinary surgeon or veterinary nurse to consider resolving the matter internally, discussing it with the senior veterinary surgeon of the practice.
- Veterinary surgeons and veterinary nurses who have concerns about the competence of a colleague are encouraged to discuss the matter with the senior veterinary surgeon of the practice. If the matter cannot be resolved by such an approach, any concerns should be brought to the attention of the RCVS Professional Conduct Department.
- A veterinary surgeon or veterinary nurse may consider that the matter of inappropriate conduct is particularly serious or may involve senior members of the organization. The matter may also have been reported internally but remains unresolved. In these circumstances, veterinary surgeons and veterinary nurses should consider bringing the issue to the attention of the RCVS Professional Conduct Department.

Resolving the matter

- A veterinary surgeon or veterinary nurse reporting inappropriate conduct internally will need to observe any internal protocol for whistle blowing, and resolution will be dealt with by the employer.
- If the matter has been brought to the attention of the RCVS Professional Conduct Department it is likely that the veterinary surgeon or veterinary nurse will be asked to submit a formal complaint. (The RCVS complaints procedure can be viewed at www.rcvs.org.uk.) If the matter involves allegations of illegal conduct or inappropriate action that come within the jurisdiction of another regulator or authority, then the RCVS Professional Conduct Department may advise that the matter also be brought to the attention of the relevant body, for example the police.
- It is important for veterinary surgeons and veterinary nurses to acknowledge that the RCVS may be unable fully to investigate anonymous complaints.
- Certain whistle blowing is protected under The Public Interest Disclosure Act 1998, which seeks to protect employees from detrimental treatment by employers if they blow the whistle. Veterinary surgeons and veterinary nurses should consider obtaining independent legal advice if they may qualify for protection under the Act, and for further guidance on how their employment may be affected. It may also be beneficial to consider whether membership of a trade union or similar organization would be of assistance, or whether relevant legal cover is provided by, for example, any household insurance policy.
- Whistle blowing may be carried out whether the Act applies or not.

Client confidentiality

- Veterinary surgeons and veterinary nurses must also be aware of their duty to keep client information confidential. If reporting inappropriate conduct involves the disclosure of client information, the veterinary surgeon or veterinary nurse must disclose information only for public interest or animal welfare reasons.

21.8 RCVS Supportive Guidance on 'whistle blowing'. (Courtesy of RCVS Professional Conduct Department, February 2012)

export certificates for live animals and animal products. Veterinary surgeons are asked to provide these certificates because they can be relied on to be truthful and diligent in providing the certification. Detailed guidance on certification is contained within the Supporting Guidance.

KEY POINT

The RCVS puts great emphasis on the integrity of certification, and the Disciplinary Committee has consistently given the severest sanction to veterinary surgeons found guilty of false certification.

Official veterinarians

Official veterinarians (OVs) are private practice veterinary surgeons who are licensed by Defra to perform work on behalf of an EU member state. The work performed by OVs is normally of a statutory nature (i.e. is required by law). In small animal practice, it includes signing export and import certificates, and pet passports under the Pet Travel Scheme.

Informing clients of withdrawal of service

There are occasional times when the trust and respect between a client and a practice breaks down and a continuing business relationship is untenable. The reasons leading up to the breakdown can be varied; bad debts leading to court action, or abusive behaviour towards staff members are among the commonest.

If the decision is made to withdraw services from a client, the practice should do so in writing. The letter should inform the client of the practice's intention to withdraw services from a specified date. The date should be sufficiently far in the future to enable the client to make alternative arrangements for veterinary services. In most instances this would be about 2 weeks. There is no need to give any reason for withdrawing services. Everyone in the practice must be aware of the date of withdrawal of services and must comply with the intention not to provide service.

In instances where there are no other practices in the area (e.g. remote areas or islands) and it would adversely affect animal welfare to withdraw services, the practice can impose conditions under which it will provide veterinary care. These conditions can be firmly applied and can be suitably severe where needed. Provided the conditions are made clear in advance of veterinary care being needed, they may include a requirement for some payment in advance of supply.

Practice and professional insurance

There are three types of insurance that practices *must* carry:

- **Employers' liability insurance:** Legislation requires all employers to have in place insurance to cover their employees against harm or damage at their place of employment. This is to meet the cost of compensation for employees' injuries or illness, whether caused on or off site (Employers' Liability (Compulsory Insurance) Act 1969)
- **Public liability insurance (third-party):** This protects the practice against claims for compensation by anyone who might allege that they were harmed as a result of the practice's negligence. It is voluntary under national legislation but is a requirement under the RCVS Practice Standards Scheme
- **Professional indemnity insurance:** PII (or equivalent arrangements) to cover all the professional activities of the practice is a requirement of the Code. It protects the individuals and the practice against claims for negligence in the provision or execution of professional work.

In addition, property insurance and fire insurance are examples of those considered prudent to have in place.

Money matters

Fees

The RCVS has no power under the VSA or any other legislation to set or adjudicate on fees charged by veterinary surgeons. It recognizes the right for veterinary surgeons to make a charge for services and goods supplied and will only take issue where such charges may be judged to be so extreme as to amount to possible professional misconduct. It does require veterinary surgeons to ensure that the treatment offered is for the benefit of the animal and not solely to increase the bill to the client.

Businesses working together to set fees for services might be guilty of violating anti-competition rules.

The person responsible for the veterinary fees is the person presenting the animal and requesting treatment. This may not be the legal owner of the animal. It could apply to any member of the public presenting an animal (such as a stray) at the surgery. However, in that instance most practices would adopt a pragmatic approach and would not ask a member of the public acting in a responsible manner and with a genuine concern for animal welfare to pay for the proposed veterinary care.

It is perfectly acceptable for practices to pursue bad debts through normal business arrangements. Chronic bad debts may be one reason for a practice to withdraw services from a client. Although veterinary surgeons do have a right in law to hold an animal until outstanding fees are paid, the RCVS believes that it is not in the interests of the animal so to do, and it can lead to the practice incurring additional costs which may not be recoverable. This right should therefore only be exercised in extreme cases and after discussion with the RCVS.

The RCVS cannot make an order for fees to be refunded if a client claims the veterinary surgeon has been negligent in treating an animal. Such claims are a civil matter and the Code requires all veterinary surgeons to have PII in place to cover such situations (see earlier).

Pet insurance

An increasing number of pet owners are insuring their animals against veterinary fees. This has a number of benefits for the owner, their pet(s) and their veterinary surgeon. For example, it means that procedures and operations that would otherwise be prohibitively expensive can be carried out.

Pet insurance companies offer a number of policy types to suit differing needs. Options include an annual policy, life cover, and varying maximum amounts that can be claimed in a specified timeframe. Veterinary practices can display literature provided by insurance companies, for example in the waiting area, to provide clients with the relevant information.

KEY POINTS

- A veterinary practice that is neither authorized by the Financial Services Authority (FSA) nor an Appointed Representative of a particular insurance company can only encourage clients to take care in selecting a policy that suits their particular requirements. Specific advice cannot be given regarding any specific insurer or policy. The practice is, however, permitted to display and hand out insurance policy leaflets.
- A practice that is an Appointed Representative of a particular insurer is able to give specific advice about that insurer's policies. Staff must have regular training and assessment, which is provided by the insurer. However, staff are still not permitted to give advice on alternative policies.
- Full advice on all policies can only be given if a practice is FSA-authorized.

Following treatment it is necessary for claim forms to be completed for the insurance company. Invariably, because of the technical nature of the replies required, it falls to the veterinary surgeon to ensure that these forms are completed accurately, although administration is often delegated to a senior staff member. It is not unreasonable for a veterinary practice to make a charge for the time taken to complete insurance claim forms, but this is not usually claimable under the policy. Any additional or administrative charges should be shown separately. In cases where the bill is sent direct to the insurance company, a copy should be sent to the client. RCVS Supporting Guidance states that pet insurance schemes rely on the integrity of the veterinary surgeon, who has a responsibility to both the client and the insurance company, and any material fact that might cause the company to increase the premium or to decline a claim must be disclosed.

Misunderstandings between veterinary surgeons and clients about the amount of insurance cover available can lead to disputes. This is particularly relevant when an animal is referred for treatment. For example, if the first-opinion practice carries out investigations or treatment that exhaust the majority of the insured sum, there may be insufficient funds available for the referral centre to provide the treatment within the remaining insured amount. Equally, if a referral practice exhausts the insured sum, there may be nothing left to cover follow-up by the original practice. Both practices should keep in mind such issues when a case is likely to be referred.

KEY POINT

It is important that veterinary practices are aware that they must charge for services supplied for an insured animal at the same level as for non-insured animals.

Business and practice core values

Every business needs to be financially sound in order to continue in business and, as a result, will have a set of principles that govern how it functions, even if these are not written down. In a veterinary practice or business, these principles, or core values, will need to reflect not only the financial basis of trading (see Chapter 24), but also the ethical, health and welfare needs of the animals undergoing treatment, and their owners.

The five principles of practice set out in the Code of Professional Conduct are:

- Professional competence
- Honesty and integrity
- Independence and impartiality
- Client confidentiality and trust
- Professional accountability.

The core business values of a veterinary practice must comply with these ethical considerations and allow those employed in the practice to comply with the provisions of the Code. Practice core values are discussed further in Chapters 19, 23 and 25.

Ethics *versus* sustainability of practice: social responsibility

It could be postulated that being an ethical practice might adversely affect profitability and make life difficult for the practice to function effectively. However, maintaining ethical standards can improve the standing and success of a business in the local community.

Ethical standards have an impact on employees, customers, suppliers, the local community and the environment. It is important that the practice carries out more than the basic requirements with regard to its employees. Gaining a reputation as a good employer will make it easier to attract and retain employees. This will apply to both professional staff and support staff. The details of exactly what is involved will vary according to the type and location of the practice. Pay rates, annual reviews, appraisals, overtime, sharing rotas equitably, social events, rewards, working conditions, provision of uniform, and payment of membership fees for professional associations and CPD might be part of the consideration.

The customers of the practice will expect to be treated well. Practice brochures and similar material should be written in clear and understandable English. The practice should be truthful at all times and restrictive phrases in small print avoided.

KEY POINT

Practice staff should all be honest and open and, on the rare occasion that a complaint is received, it should be dealt with promptly, fairly and the complainant given a chance to meet face to face with the practice owners. Complainants to the RCVS often quote the lack of a reasonable response from the practice owners as the reason for sending their complaint on to the RCVS.

Suppliers might appear to have little to do with the social responsibility of the practice; however, the practice should ensure that suppliers demonstrate social responsibility as well. Their impact on the environment and the local community will have a bearing on how the practice might be viewed in the community.

The impact of the practice on the environment will be evident to all onlookers. Waste disposal is covered by legislation and has to be complied with (see Chapter 3) but the wider picture also applies. Development of premises that are sympathetic with the local environment, and the responsible use of motor vehicles, will have a positive impact on the impression of the practice in the community. The involvement of the practice in the local community provides enormous opportunity for securing a positive benefit for the practice. The opportunities are wide-ranging and include writing articles for the local press, supporting local charity events, giving talks at local schools and social clubs, and holding practice open days.

References and further reading

Bateson P (2010) *Independent Inquiry into Dog Breeding.* London: Dogs Trust (see www.ourdogs.co.uk)

Royal College of Veterinary Surgeons (2012) *RCVS Code of Professional Conduct and Supporting Guidance for Veterinary Nurses.* (available at www.rcvs.org.uk)

Royal College of Veterinary Surgeons (2012) *RCVS Code of Professional Conduct and Supporting Guidance for Veterinary Surgeons.* (available at www.rcvs.org.uk)

Walsh L and Ravetz G (2011) Managing employees with mental ill health. *In Practice* **33**, 228–230

Principles of health and safety

22

Mark Enright and Alison Clark

For some, the many acts and regulations pertaining to health and safety (H&S) are simply bureaucratic 'red tape' that puts too great a burden on small and medium-sized enterprises, and hinders them in their efforts to get on with the business of doing business. This is despite the fact that H&S legislation since 1992 has been based on risk assessment and self-regulation ('*you think about* and *you decide* how best to keep *your employees* healthy and safe'), the previous style of legislation having been seen as reactive rather than proactive, too prescriptive, drawn up with big businesses in mind and therefore unnecessarily burdensome for small businesses.

In October 2010 Lord Young published his review of 'health and safety and the compensation culture', entitled *Common Sense; Common Safety.* He made several recommendations for simplifying H&S administration and for helping small businesses to do simple risk assessments. Following this, the Department for Work and Pensions published plans entitled *Good Health and Safety, Good for Everyone*, for further major reform. In March 2011 the government established an independent review of H&S legislation; the report *Reclaiming Health and Safety for All: An Independent Review of Health and Safety Regulation* was published in November 2011 (see www.dwp.gov.uk). It aims to reduce regulatory requirements on business where they do not lead to improved H&S outcomes, and to remove pressures on business to go beyond what the regulations require, enabling them to reclaim ownership of H&S management.

At the time of writing, these proposals are being considered and reviewed, with a plan to phase them in and amend the relevant regulations by the middle of 2012. In response to the report, the Health and Safety Executive (HSE) produced a guide entitled *Health and Safety Made Simple: The Basics for Your Business* (see www.hse.gov.uk). The claim is that the amended regulations will make it easier for a business to comply with the law and to manage H&S. Some welcome this 'new thinking', whilst others are concerned about the risk of 'dumbing down'.

According to the HSE, 70% of accidents are preventable if businesses adopt good systems of H&S management.

KEY POINTS

- To comply with the Health and Safety at Work etc. Act 1974 (HASAWA) and the Management of Health and Safety at Work Regulations 1999 (MHSWR) the employer must be aware of, and must appropriately address, all H&S legislation that applies to their business.
- How H&S will be managed in the business constitutes the Health and Safety Policy. If the business has five or more employees, this policy must be set out in a written policy document. The H&S policy must be reviewed at least annually, or more frequently if there are significant changes to personnel, premises, plant or procedures.

Health and Safety Policy Statement and Management Arrangements

The written Health and Safety Policy should show that the employer is aware of its obligations under all applicable H&S acts and regulations and has considered all relevant issues. It must include a Statement of General Health and Safety Policy and must specify who is responsible for what, i.e. the arrangements (see below) to ensure that risks to the H&S of employees, clients, contractors, visitors, etc., are kept as low as is reasonably practicable. It should also give instruction to employees regarding their general responsibilities and refer them to specific policies, rules, procedures and risk assessments regarding specific issues. A template Health and Safety Policy document that covers many of the relevant issues is available to BSAVA members at www.bsava.com. The HSE also provides a template on their website; this is useful to refer to but is less specific. Some examples of policy statements are given at the end of this chapter.

The lines of responsibility regarding H&S issues in the practice (i.e. who will do what, when and how) constitute the Health and Safety Management

Arrangements. By law, the practice must have such management arrangements in place and must make them known to employees. The simplest way to do this is to display pages similar to the examples at the end of this chapter.

KEY POINT

Copies of the Health and Safety Policy Statement and Management Arrangements should be prominently displayed at each surgery or issued to all staff.

It must be clear to all staff where to access the full policy document and other essential H&S information. An approach adopted by many practices is to keep all relevant documentation – such as specific policy statements, risk assessments, Local Rules, standard operating procedures, safety data, records, etc. – in a Practice Health & Safety Manual, to which all staff have access. In addition to this, it is a good idea to reproduce the key pieces of H&S information and instructions in a Practice Health & Safety Handbook or Mini-Manual, which can be issued to all staff and which can refer to more detailed information where appropriate.

KEY POINT

Ultimate responsibility for ensuring that H&S is managed effectively rests with the employer. However, if he or she is not on site for all or much of the time, or there is a group of practices, it is advisable to appoint one or more senior members of staff to oversee and manage H&S issues on their behalf.

Assigning responsibilities

Safety officers

The key roles, which carry a significant degree of responsibility, are Practice Safety Officer (PSO) and Fire Officer (FO). Each branch surgery may have its own PSO and FO, or one PSO/FO may cover more than one location. If there are five or more employees it is recommended that some Area Safety Officers (ASOs) are also appointed to carry out most of the day-to-day H&S duties and to ease the burden on the PSO and FO. H&S issues will be managed more effectively if staff know that they are all involved and have specific responsibilities.

Before appointing specific individuals and entering their names in the policy document, there are four points that must be addressed and confirmed:

- Individuals understand their responsibilities and are prepared to accept them
- Employer and employee are confident of their competence to carry out the duties
- Individuals will be given the necessary time, training and assistance to do the job
- There is no confusion regarding who is responsible for what, and no areas/issues are left out.

Practice Safety Officer and Fire Officer

If employees are expected to take on significant H&S responsibilities, such as PSO and FO, they must be fully prepared and understand their responsibilities, and should not take these on lightly. They have a right to say 'No'. Individuals can be held personally liable if incidents occur as a result of poor H&S management or a failure to discharge their responsibilities effectively.

The FO is responsible for all aspects of fire and emergency procedures, including carrying out an assessment of the fire risks in the practice (a legal requirement); see Chapter 2 for more on fire safety policy and procedures.

Area Safety Officers

The duties of an ASO are no more than would be expected of a manager or supervisor in any workplace, so it could be stipulated that being an ASO is an integral part of the job for say, the head nurse or head receptionist. However, because the duties and responsibilities of an ASO may be new to proposed appointees, it is important to ensure that they are fully prepared and comfortable with the role before appointment. This is for the employer's benefit as much as the employee's, since the employer is ultimately responsible if anything should go wrong and must therefore be confident in the competence of the appointed ASOs. The appointed ASOs are unlikely to do the job properly if they are anxious, overworked or uninterested.

It is important that employees know what is being asked and expected of them before they accept the roles. For example, it is quite common to assign one ASO to 'staff/client areas' and another to 'clinical areas', which is fine, as long as it does not lead to confusion as to who is responsible for outside areas (yard, storage sheds, etc.), drug room, and whether the consulting rooms are staff/client or clinical areas.

Health and Safety Coordinator

Practices with more than two full-time surgeries are advised to appoint a Health and Safety Coordinator (HSC), to be responsible for chasing up and issuing reminders to the relevant people at each surgery to ensure and confirm that the H&S policies and management procedures are being fully implemented and that the necessary records are being kept. The HSC should also issue reports to the employers, directors, partners and PSOs on how things are going overall and in relation to each surgery. The identity of the HSC should be clear in the policy document.

Competent Person

Employers must, by law, appoint a CP to help with the management of H&S and to comply with their obligations. An employer can appoint themselves to be the Competent Person (CP); however, if they do not have the 'necessary skills, knowledge and experience', they must instead appoint a member of staff (if appropriate) or a specialist Health and Safety Advisor (HSA). If appointing an external advisor, it is important to ensure that they can produce evidence of relevant training and knowledge and of any formal qualifications required.

The Occupational Safety and Health Consultants Register (OSHCR) is now open to the public (www.oshcr.org). This is a register of consultants who can offer general advice to UK businesses to help them manage H&S risks. All those consultants on the register will belong to a participating professional body and will have met set standards. The minimum standard for consultants to join the register has been set at a degree level qualification, at least 2 years' experience and active engagement in a continuing professional development scheme. All consultants who join the register are bound by their professional body/bodies' code of conduct and are committed to providing sensible and proportionate advice. The aim of the register is to help businesses find advice on managing their general health and safety risks.

KEY POINT

The name of the appointed Competent Person, along with a description of their role, should be included in the Health and Safety Policy document.

First Aid personnel

To comply with The Health and Safety (First Aid) Regulations 1981, the practice must provide adequate and appropriate equipment, facilities and personnel to ensure that its employees receive immediate attention if they are injured or taken ill at work. Although not specifically mentioned in the First Aid regulations, under other regulations (e.g. MHSWR), and as common sense dictates, employers must also consider their 'duty of care' regarding First Aid provision for non-employees (e.g. clients, visitors, contractors, etc.). What constitutes 'adequate and appropriate' will vary from practice to practice and therefore an assessment of First Aid needs should be carried out. The issue of adequate and appropriate 'First Aid provision' is discussed in more detail later. With regard to H&S management arrangements, the minimum requirement is to appoint a person to take charge of First Aid arrangements. The roles of this appointed person (AP) include: looking after the First Aid box; and, if required, calling the emergency services. The HSE website includes a self-assessment for employees to help decision-making for First Aid provision, and useful guidance on the regulations. Before designating any First Aiders (FAs) and/or APs it must first be confirmed that nominated staff are prepared to be responsible for First Aid; as employees they are not obliged to accept the role. Full and clear details must be given as to what the role as FA or AP will entail with regard to administering First Aid. If the practice is close to a medical centre or a hospital, it might be stipulated that they are simply to call the doctor or an ambulance, or escort the casualty to the surgery or A&E department.

- Appointed persons are not First Aiders and should not attempt to give First Aid for which they have not been trained.
- A First Aider is someone who has undertaken training and has a qualification that is HSE-approved. It is very unlikely that any action would be taken against an FA who was using the First Aid training they have received, but an FA should never go beyond their training when attending to someone.

Risk assessments

To comply with MHSWR, risk assessments must be carried out to determine exactly:

- What risks exist in the practice
- What the levels of those risks are
- What would be considered reasonably practicable in terms of how low those risks should be
- What the practice should be doing to attain and maintain such levels or to lower them.

Practices should carry out risk assessments for *all areas and activities* to comply with MHSWR. There are also some H&S regulations that require 'specific' risk assessments to be conducted, such as the Control of Substances Hazardous to Health (Amendment) Regulations 2004 (COSHH). Details of the acts and regulations that apply when carrying out a risk assessment are given in Figure 22.1 and the issues to be considered are shown in Figure 22.2.

Reference number for Figure 22.2	Acts and regulations
1	**Management of Health and Safety at Work Regulations 1999** Require employers to carry out risk assessments, make arrangements to implement necessary measures, appoint competent people and arrange for appropriate information and training
2	**Workplace (Health, Safety and Welfare) Regulations 1992** Cover a range of health, safety and welfare issues including ventilation, heating, lighting, work space, etc.
3	**Health and Safety (Display Screen Equipment) Regulations 1992** Set out requirements for risk assessment of work with visual display units (VDUs)
4	**Personal Protective Equipment at Work Regulations 1992** Require employers to provide appropriate protective clothing and equipment for employees
5	**Provision and Use of Work Equipment Regulations 1998** Equipment for use at work, including machinery, must be safe and appropriately serviced/tested
6	**Manual Handling Operations Regulations 1992** Cover the need to assess risks associated with moving objects by hand or bodily force

22.1 Acts and regulations that apply to carrying out a risk assessment. (continues)

Reference number for Figure 22.2	Acts and regulations
7	**Health and Safety (First Aid) Regulations 1981** Cover requirements for First Aid personnel, equipment and facilities
8	**Health and Safety Information for Employees (Amendment) Regulations 2009** Require employers to display a poster telling employees what they need to know about H&S
9	**Employers' Liability (Compulsory Insurance) Act 1969** Requires employers to take out insurance against accidents and ill health to their employees
10	**Reporting of Injuries, Diseases and Dangerous Occurrences Regulations 1995** Require employers to report certain occupational injuries, diseases and dangerous occurrences
11	**Control of Noise at Work Regulations 2005** Require employers to assess risks and take action to protect employees from hearing damage
12	**Electricity at Work Regulations 1989** People in control of electrical systems must ensure all systems are safe and maintained in safe condition
13	**Control of Substances Hazardous to Health (Amendment) Regulations 2004** Require employers to assess the risks from hazardous substances and take appropriate precautions
15	**Construction (Design and Management) Amendment) Regulations 2000** Cover safe systems of work on construction sites. Applies to planning new build and refurbishments
16	**Gas Safety (Installation and Use) Regulations 1998** Safe installation, maintenance, use of gas systems/appliances in domestic and business premises
17	**Environmental Protection Act 1990** Hazardous waste and pollution control legislation
18	**Equality Act 2010** Discrimination, bullying, harassment. Prohibits use of pre-employment health questionnaires
19	**Misuse of Drugs Act 1971 and Misuse of Drugs Regulations 2001 as amended** Covers controlled drugs
20	**Regulatory Reform (Fire Safety) Order 2005** 'Responsible person' to carry out fire risk assessment and implement a fire management plan
21	**Road Safety Act 2006** Employers and employees must recognize legal and moral duties regarding driving for work
22	**Collection and Disposal of Waste Regulations 1988** Covers disposal of clinical waste
23	**Control of Asbestos at Work Regulations 2006** Requires building owners and other parties with legal responsibility to 'manage' asbestos
24	**Control of Pollution (Oil Storage) Regulations 2001** Covers oil storage (e.g. central heating oil tanks)
25	**Controlled Waste Regulations 1992** Covers disposal of clinical waste
26	**Hazardous Waste (England and Wales) Regulations 2005** Covers disposal of hazardous waste
27	**Health and Safety (Consultation With Employees) Regulations 1996** Requires employers to consult with their employees on all issues/proposals that affect their health and safety
28	**Health and Safety (Miscellaneous Amendments) Regulations 2002** Amends First Aid, personal protective equipment, work equipment, signs and signals, HASAW regulations
29	**Health and Safety (Safety Signs and Signals) Regulations 1996** All health and safety signs and signals (e.g. regarding hazards, safety, fire and First Aid) must meet specific criteria
30	**Health and Safety (Training for Employment) Regulations 1990** Specifically with regard to training for young people (e.g. work experience)
31	**Ionising Radiations Regulations 1999** Covers any work with ionizing radiation
32	**Lifting Operations and Lifting Equipment Regulations 1998** Requires all lifting equipment (e.g. slings, hoists, lifts) to be regularly inspected and tested
33	**Pressure Systems Safety Regulations 2000** Autoclaves and pressure vessels over 250 bar litres must have 'written scheme of examination'
34	**Smoke-Free (Premises and Enforcement) Regulations 2007** No smoking in any enclosed premises or shared work vehicles. Must display a 'no smoking' sign

22.1 (continued) Acts and regulations that apply to carrying out a risk assessment. (continues)

Reference number for Figure 22.2	Acts and regulations
35	**Water Supply (Water Fittings) Regulations 1999** Must have appropriate back-flow devices on washing machines and X-ray developers
36	**Social Security (Claims and Payments) Amendment Regulations 2011** Must have an accident book if more than 10 employees
37	**Work at Height Regulations 2005** Specify the hierarchy of controls that must be adopted for any work at height
38	**Working Time (Amendment) Regulations 2003** Specify maximum working hours and minimum time off for employees, including persons under 18
39	**Carriage of Dangerous Goods and Use of Transportable Pressure Equipment Regulations 2007** Covers the use and transport (e.g. in practice vehicles) of gas cylinders

22.1 (continued) Acts and regulations that apply to carrying out a risk assessment.

Issues to be specifically addressed and/or considered in risk assessments	Applicable health and safety legislation (see Figure 22.1)
Building and modifications	1, 15
Design/layout/materials (access, traffic routes, doors, windows, heating/lighting/ventilation, washing/rest/toilet /eating/changing facilities, drinking water, slips/trips)	1, 2
Security measures (protection against break-ins)	1, 2
Disabled access/use	1, 18, 28
Fire, First Aid, hazard and safety signage	1, 29
Consultation with employees	1, 27
H&S law poster	8
H&S training (induction, basic, specific, revision)	1, 30
Stress, bullying, harassment, discrimination	1, 18
Alcohol and drugs	1
Smoking in premises (and work vehicles)	1, 34
Working time	1, 38
New and expectant mothers	1, 2, 6, 13, 31
Young persons, work experience	1, 30, 38
Personal safety and security (including lone working)	1
Contractors	1
Work equipment	1, 5, 28
Lifting equipment (e.g. use in hydrotherapy)	1, 5, 32
Electrical safety	1, 12
Autoclaves (and dental compressors possibly)	1, 5, 12, 33
Gas supply and installation (e.g. central heating)	1, 16
Oil storage (e.g. central heating boiler)	1, 24
Washing machines (back-flow device)	1, 5, 12, 35
X-ray developers (back-flow device)	1, 5, 12, 13, 35
Practice vehicles, driving for work	1, 5, 21
Use of mobile phones	1, 5, 21
Display screen equipment	1, 3, 5, 12, 28
Personal protective equipment (PPE)	1, 4, 13, 28
Working at height	1, 37
Use of ladders and stepladders	1, 37
Manual handling	1, 6, 28
Clearing snow and ice	1, 2
Noise	1, 11
Hazardous substances (COSHH)	1, 13
Cleaning and disinfection	1, 2, 13
Legionella (water supplies and air conditioning)	1, 2, 35
Latex	1, 4, 13
Asbestos management	1, 23
Anaesthetic gases and vapours	1, 5, 13
Anaesthetic monitoring	1, 2, 13
Medicinal and veterinary products	1, 13, 19
Cytotoxic drugs	1, 7, 13, 19
Medical gas cylinders and pipelines	1, 5, 6, 13, 39
Liquid nitrogen	1, 5, 13
Lasers	1, 5
Ionizing radiation (X-rays, radioisotopes)	1, 31
Handling of animals	1, 6, 13
Isolation, barrier nursing	1, 13
Post-mortem examinations	1, 5, 13
Pathological specimens by post	1, 2, 13
Biosecurity policy and procedures	1, 2, 13
Disposal of waste	1, 2, 6, 13, 17, 22, 25, 26
Laboratory/lab area, procedures (Local Rules)	1, 2, 13, 17, 22, 25, 26
Accident/incident recording and review	1, 36
Accident/incident reporting (RIDDOR)	1, 10
First Aid personnel, facilities and information	1, 7, 29, 28, 30
Fire risk assessment	1, 20
Fire procedures, training and information	1, 20, 29, 30
Safety data (regarding equipment, drugs, microbial agents, chemicals)	1, 5, 13, 32

22.2 Issues to be considered when carrying out risk assessments in practice, with relevant legislation (for an explanation of the numbering please see Figure 22.1).

In addition to the many H&S acts, orders and regulations listed in Figure 22.1, there are official Approved Codes of Practice, guidance notes and information leaflets on the HSE website about many of the specific issues that apply to veterinary practice (e.g. gas cylinders, *Legionella*, cytotoxic drugs, asbestos, First Aid, H&S management, benchmarking), which are a useful reference for queries and clarification. There are also additional resources such as self-assessments for First Aid provision and tools for stress management, which provide questionnaires and checklists to help with consultation and formulating policy and Local Rules.

To clarify the HSE terminology and the legal position:

- Acts and Orders – are 'enabling' and 'must do' legislation. Regulations are made 'under' them
- Regulations – are 'must do' legislation
- Approved Codes of Practice (ACoPs) – give recommendations on what should be done, and how; but they do not have to be followed if you can *prove* you do better
- Guidance – is simply guidance, and comes in two forms:
  - How to comply with the Acts and Regulations
  - Examples of 'best practice' (similar to an ACoP)
- Information – is informative but has no legal standing.

The HSE advises employers to follow 'the five steps to risk assessment'. The HSE guide to the five steps can be downloaded from www.hse.gov.uk and example documents are easy to download and use. 'The five steps to risk assessment' is also available as a display poster for the practice. The first three steps constitute the actual risk assessment.

These details may make the process of risk assessment seem complicated and time-consuming. However, rather like driving a car, it can be difficult to describe and explain but is easy to do once mastered, though always requiring due care and attention. The main purpose of risk assessment is to identify the most significant risks and to address those first. Risk assessment is a skill with which all members of staff should be familiar. In veterinary practice, situations can occur daily where immediate assessment of risk is required, e.g. a visit to an unknown client, or handling a dog of questionable temperament.

Step 1: Identify the hazards in the workplace

A hazard is anything that has the potential to cause harm to a person. There are six types:

- Physical hazards (e.g. noise, electricity, X-rays)
- Biological hazards (e.g. viruses, bacteria, fungi, parasites)
- Chemical hazards (e.g. cleaning agents, anaesthetic agents, drugs, latex)
- Mechanical hazards (e.g. animals (bites, scratches), vehicles, work equipment)
- Ergonomic hazards (e.g. narrow corridors, cramped workspaces, high shelves)
- Psychosocial hazards (e.g. workload, office politics, bullying, stressful situations).

Step 2: Decide who might be harmed by them and how

Who

The people who might be harmed are those who might be 'exposed' to the hazards identified, either as a consequence of their work or of their presence and actions in an area where the hazard is. It is important to appreciate, therefore, that in addition to employees of the practice, clients, visitors, contractors and members of the public may also potentially be exposed to some of the hazards.

How

How a person might be harmed depends on the nature of the hazard. For example, if a person is exposed to a cleaning agent that is caustic, they could suffer skin burns; but if a cleaning agent is harmful rather than caustic, they could develop occupational dermatitis over time. A knowledge of the harm each hazard could cause is essential in order to determine how people might be harmed.

Step 3: Evaluate the risks and decide on appropriate control measures

Risk evaluation

Risk is a term that reflects both the likelihood of harm occurring and the severity of the harm (i.e. how many people might be harmed and how badly).

Risk = Likelihood × Severity

To assess risk, in addition to identifying who may be potentially exposed (see Step 2), due consideration must also be given as to whether any people may be *particularly vulnerable* to the hazards identified (given the nature of the hazard). This might include young people, new and expectant mothers, or those with specific allergies or sensitivities. In each case the degree of injury or ill health they could suffer as a result of exposure to the hazard(s) must be considered. For example:

- An experienced veterinary nurse handling a fractious and injured dog could be at some risk of being bitten, but the risk to a young work experience student is much higher – a bite may be very likely
- Cleaning out a hospitalized rabbit may present little risk to most members of the nursing team, but for one nurse with a severe allergy to rabbit fur it could bring on an anaphylactic reaction, necessitating emergency treatment.

For an identified risk, consideration must then be given as to whether enough is currently being done to control it adequately or whether action is required to eliminate or reduce it further.

It is useful to conduct risk assessments in relation to the six Ps of veterinary practice:

- **Premises:** the practice and other premises where staff may work, including any shared premises

- **Plant:** air conditioning, heating, ventilation, computer systems, all work equipment
- **Procedures:** how people do what they do (i.e. the tasks and activities in the practice)
- **Products:** hazardous substances used (by whom, when, where and how)
- **Pets:** different types and temperaments, handling (who, where, how)
- **People:** staff, clients, visitors, contractors, persons on shared sites.

Premises

When it comes to identifying hazards in the premises, the advice often given is to 'walk around the workplace and look at *what could reasonably be expected* to cause harm'. However, a person needs to know what they are looking for or they will almost certainly miss important things. In addition to the duty to assess risks under MHSWR, there is a duty under the Workplace (Health Safety and Welfare) Regulations 1992 (HSWR) to ensure that the workplace is 'safe and suitable' and meets the defined minimum standards in terms of comfort, space, heating, lighting, ventilation, sanitary conveniences, vision panels, safety glass, cleanliness, and freedom from 'unnecessary' hazards (e.g. inherently slippery floors and trip hazards that could or should have been designed out). It is therefore a much better idea to walk around the premises with a pre-written checklist of the issues to consider, and the types of hazards to be looking out for. It is important to inspect all the practice premises, inside and out, including garages, sheds, workshops, car parks and grounds.

An example of a checklist is given at the end of this chapter. This is not a comprehensive list and it should be revised as other known or new hazards are identified. Each practice should develop its own detailed list. A checklist can be used both as a memory jogger and as a means to document the inspection and risk assessments. In the case of the example shown, if the answer to any question on the list is 'No' it is likely that it presents a risk and that action will need to be taken to eliminate or reduce it. This should be indicated on the checklist and brief details either written on the back or on a separate record.

Plant

Some practices have installations and equipment that can genuinely be considered as 'plant' and some may even have a plant room. However, in the context in which it is used here, 'plant' is just another term for work equipment.

Hazards to consider include:

- Those associated with location, position and condition of the equipment:
  - Is it in the way?
  - Is it unstable?
  - Does it have damaged or sharp edges?
- Those associated with its use.

Some 'safety-critical' items of work equipment, e.g. X-ray machines, autoclaves, lifting equipment, must – to comply with specific regulations – be regularly inspected, serviced, tested and certified as safe to use. Therefore, if any such equipment has not been inspected and tested in accordance with its appropriate schedule, it must be considered a hazard. It is useful to have a comprehensive checklist of all items of work equipment in the practice that need to be formally inspected, tested and certified safe (how, when and by whom), ideally one that can serve as a risk assessment record as well.

Procedures

There are duties imposed by specific regulations to ensure that risks associated with several specific issues are assessed (e.g. COSHH, manual handling, display screen use). However, under MHSWR there is a general duty on practices to assess the risks associated with all aspects of their business – which can include such things as cleaning the stairs, changing a light bulb (see Figure 22.8) or cutting a hedge. These examples are procedures for which veterinary practices have been told (by a Health and Safety Inspector) that they should have carried out risk assessments. In each case, accidents had occurred because no one had considered what could have happened, and what could/should have been done to prevent it. In each case, the employer was deemed to be at fault and the employee claimed and won compensation. These examples serve as reminders that it is not just the veterinary aspect that practices have to think about – every activity must be considered.

> **KEY POINT**
>
> It is not realistic to expect the employer personally to carry out a risk assessment of every procedure. However, the employer must ensure that every procedure is assessed.

The way to address this issue is to instruct employees to conduct their own assessment if there is not already one available for them to refer to. The person who carries out the procedure is often the best person to carry out the risk assessment. This does not mean that all responsibility can be, or is, passed to the employee, but it does make the point that they carry some responsibility for their own safety and that the employer can, and does, expect them to give due thought to the safe way to do their job (Figure 22.3). It must therefore be a formal instruction and should be accompanied by information on, and training in, how to identify hazards and carry out a risk assessment.

The practice Health and Safety Policy document, together with Local Rules and Health & Safety Handbook (or alternatives) should provide staff with information on the types of hazards to be aware of and the sorts of controls necessary to reduce risks. In essence, the process of risk assessment is simply a stop and think exercise. Employees should be instructed that before performing *any* activity they must ask themselves the following questions:

- Do I fully understand what it is I've got to do and how to do it?
- Do I know what hazards the activity might expose me to?
- Do I know what harm those hazards could cause – and how?

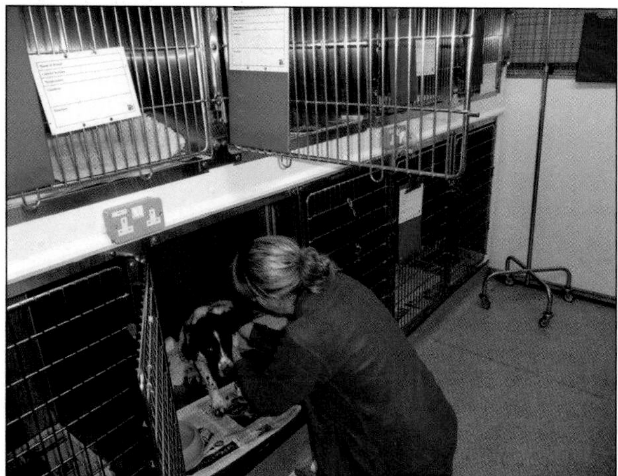

22.3 Employees should understand that it is their responsibility to give due thought to the safe way to do their job. This may include, for example, ensuring that upper cage doors are not left open as shown in this photograph. Everyone should be alert at all times to anything in the workplace that might increase risk to themselves or others.

- Are there sufficient precautions in place (training, facilities, equipment, systems)?
- Is it safe for me (and those around me) if I continue?

It should be made clear that if the employee cannot answer 'Yes' to all of the above questions they should not continue until they can acquire whatever training, information, safety data, equipment or assistance they need. This is primarily to prevent accidents occurring due to basic oversights. For example: the bucket should not be behind the operator when working backwards down the stairs; the employee must be familiar with the instructions for the hedge trimmer – which clearly state that the power must be turned off before freeing the blades. It also reduces the likelihood of anyone being able to claim, 'I didn't know; no one ever told me'. To assist in training, and to emphasize the need for employees to think about the work they do – and how they do it, practices should consider displaying the HSE's poster *Five Steps to Risk Assessment.*

> **KEY POINT**
>
> If an employee requires assistance to carry out a risk assessment or assurance that their assessment is sufficient, a Competent Person must be available to provide it. If an assessment cannot be carried out, the employee should be instructed not to undertake the specific procedure.

For many procedures it will not be necessary to record the risk assessment. However, for some procedures the risk assessment will be significant and it is important to keep written records once completed. Such procedures would include: working at height (Figure 22.4), e.g. to access the loft; cutting the hedge; and pressure-washing cars; as well as veterinary activities such as performing a dental procedure or administering an injection to an inpatient. The list is endless but it does not take long to compile a record and once done it is there for anyone to refer to.

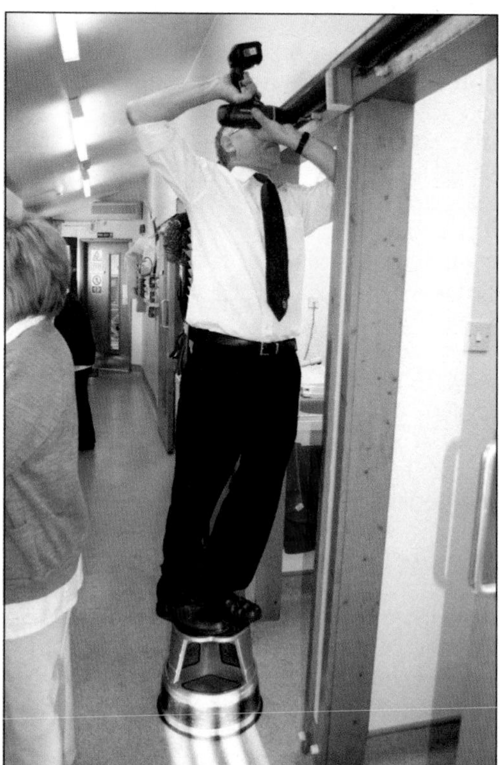

22.4 Routine maintenance can often involve working at height, even if ladders are not needed. A quick repair job such as shown here (tightening a screw in a door mechanism) can represent significant risks in a busy area, particularly when animals are being moved. Risk assessments should be completed and appropriate control measures in place to minimize risk during these procedures. There are several possible hazards in this picture to consider.

> **KEY POINT**
>
> The practice should keep a list of all specific procedures for which there is a formal record and should periodically review all records and revise the assessments as necessary.

Products

These are the items and substances used or stored in the practice, such as cleaning agents, dog leads, pet food, boxed files, and waste – basically, anything not classed as 'work equipment'. It is not uncommon for practices to assume that most of these items and substances are non-hazardous or of low risk, but this is not necessarily true. Serious consideration must be given as to how they are stored, displayed and handled (i.e. where, how, who uses them, who has access to them). For example: a case of cat food or a big bag of dog food may present significant manual handling risks; an air freshener spray in the toilet may seem sensible enough, until a client's child sprays it in their eyes.

An employer has a legal duty under the COSHH Regulations specifically to assess the risks associated with the way hazardous substances, such as cleaning agents, radiograph developing chemicals (see Chapter 13), gases and anaesthetic agents (see Chapters 2 and 8) and medicinal products (see Chapter 15) are handled, used and stored. In general, substances can be grouped into classes of hazard (Figure 22.5) and

Symbol and classification	Precautions
Toxic	Wear PPE, including eye protection Rinse immediately if in contact with skin or eyes Dispose of safely
Explosive	Use only as directed Keep tightly closed, cool and in a well ventilated area Keep away from heat or ignition Dispose of safely
Flammable	Keep away from heat or ignition Keep container tightly closed away from sunlight Do not breathe vapours
Oxidizing	Use only as directed Keep tightly closed, cool and in a well ventilated area Keep away from heat or ignition Dispose of safely
Corrosive	Wear PPE, including eye protection Rinse immediately if in contact with skin or eyes Dispose of safely
Harmful	Avoid contact with skin and eyes Do not inhale vapour, dust or spray Rinse immediately if in contact with skin or eyes
Dangerous for the environment	Dispose of safely – do not empty into drains or water sources The container must also be disposed of safely

22.5 'Dangerous substances' – common health hazards.

then risks assessed following examination of the datasheet and any associated manufacturer guidance. The aim is to produce a COSHH risk assessment that is logical and easy to understand by all the staff that may come into contact with the substances, so that they know what to do should there be, for example, a spillage, an accidental self-injection, or a chemical splashed into an eye.

For each group of products, a general procedure can be drawn up, but hazardous items need to be dealt with individually. Where detailed information is necessary (e.g. volatile anaesthetics, cytotoxic drugs, oil-based vaccines, hazardous chemicals), there should be clear guidelines on where to find the information quickly and what to do. This information can be kept in a file or online, where Summaries of Product Characteristics (SPCs) (see Chapter 15) are now easy to find. Hazardous substances can also be, or contain, biological agents such as bacteria or viruses (see biosecurity advice in Chapters 6, 7 and 8).

The general guidance is the same as for any risk:

- Remove the hazard altogether (e.g. do not treat cases with toxic chemotherapeutic agents on the premises, but refer them elsewhere)
- Replace the hazard with something less hazardous (e.g. use less harmful cleaning agents)
- Restrict access to the hazard (e.g. restrict access to a patient with suspected *Salmonella* infection in the isolation ward)
- Reduce exposure to the hazard (e.g. wash hands after use; wear gloves when handling).

Pets

Bites and scratches should not be considered as 'part of the job', as the HSE considers that most could, and should, be prevented. This also applies to back injuries that are the result of poor manual handling, and to the diseases that staff and clients contract due to a lack of awareness of zoonoses and the need for good hygiene practice.

The designs of some practices dictate that patients may have to walk, or be transported, up or down steps, and this can present risks for staff, owners and pets. Pets should be restrained in the car park and waiting room, but frequently are not.

Noise can create stress, and can be a safety hazard at work, interfering with communication, acting as a distraction and making warnings harder to hear. Depending on how loud a noise is and how long an employee is exposed to it, if the noise is intrusive then ways of controlling, reducing and monitoring it should be investigated. For example, it may be best for all involved, including the patient, for a dog to be taken outside rather than to sit barking continuously in the waiting room.

People

The hazards that people themselves present and whether they are a risk to themselves and/or others must be considered. Examples that highlight this issue include:

- Abusive clients (e.g. physical abuse/injury, verbal abuse/stress)
- Contractors (e.g. a builder could drop a brick on someone)
- Drink and drugs (e.g. someone with their own problem can cause problems for others)
- Young people (e.g. immaturity and lack of awareness could put themselves and others at risk)
- Pranksters (e.g. what may seem like a joke to them might backfire).

When completing a risk assessment and considering a person's susceptibility to one or more hazards, in the absence of specific information it has to be assumed that all are equally and particularly susceptible, because it cannot be known whether someone is pregnant or has osteoporosis, a bad back, a weak heart, haemophilia or other susceptibilities. The worst-case scenario for severity of harm has to be assumed (i.e. severe) and risk can only be reduced by reducing the *likelihood* of an event occurring.

For particularly susceptible employees where more is known of their personal situation, the practice can take appropriate actions to eliminate or reduce their exposure. For example, if a member of staff has a chronic back problem, measures can be put in place to ensure that the risk of a manual handling injury is minimized, such as by removing, replacing, restricting or reducing their manual handling activities (Figure 22.6).

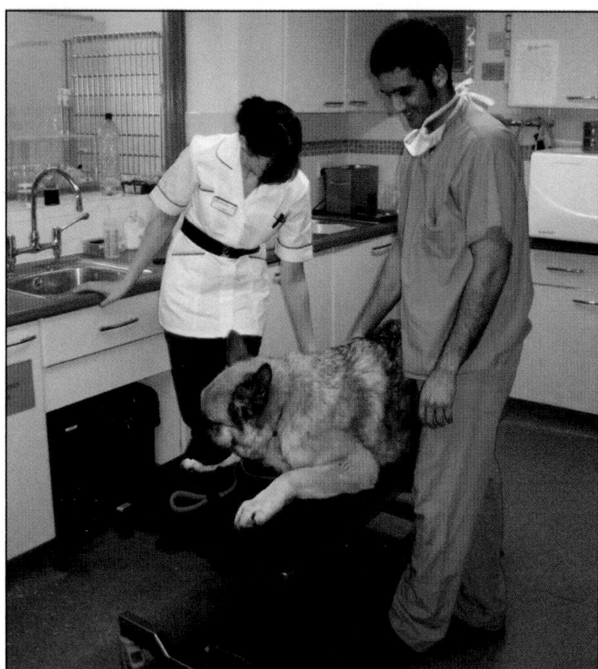

22.6 An electrically operated lifting table will help reduce risks associated with manual handling of large patients.

Risk assessments should be carried out on an individual basis as frequently as necessary. A useful aid, as with all risk assessments, would be a checklist of the hazards and risks to discuss, ideally cross-referenced to a list of conditions that could predispose a person to being at greater or particular risk from those hazards.

Although not compulsory, it is a good idea to conduct a basic health surveillance of all members of staff; *confidential* records should be kept of all illnesses and absences, including reasons. These should be reviewed periodically to look for trends associated with specific tasks or hazardous substances. Adverse reactions or poor working practice can then be assessed and redressed if necessary. Because of the nature of the hazards present in veterinary practice, and the growing trend in personal injury claims and litigation, a health check and health surveillance system is good practice. As a minimum, practices should carry out monitoring of anaesthetic gas exposure (volatile agent and nitrous oxide) and radiation exposure from X-rays (see Chapters 8 and 13). This can be regular sampling or continual monitoring, according to the findings of the risk assessments.

Health and wellbeing and stress management are important factors for the people in the practice team; see Chapter 19 for further guidance on this subject.

With regard to contractors, the practice needs to identify clearly all aspects of the work to be carried out and then consider the H&S implications of the job to be done. The practice must satisfy itself that any contractor used is competent. It is important for contractors to know what is expected of them, to have the practice's H&S arrangements explained to them and to be shown any procedures. They should understand the practice's Health and Safety Policy Statement and agree to act in accordance with it; a written signature to confirm this is prudent. A risk assessment should be completed jointly by the practice and the contractor, and both parties should inform each other of any relevant and specific information such as risks, relevant H&S procedures, and any instructions or training requirements. The practice should provide management and supervision to ensure the safety of all involved, and should keep a list of approved contractors.

Deciding on appropriate control measures

By law, employers must do everything *reasonably practicable* to protect their employees and workers from harm. A control measure would not be reasonably practicable if the cost and inconvenience of implementing it outweighed the benefits in terms of risk reduction. For example, switching to digital radiography just to prevent exposure to film-developing chemicals would not be a reasonably practicable thing to do.

When deciding on appropriate control measures and acceptable levels of risk in the practice, the procedures adopted and standards achieved by other similar veterinary practices must be considered. If they are achieving lower levels of exposure and risk, or if they adopt more effective control measures, for example by having an extractor fan in the darkroom, it would be difficult for a practice to justify that it was not reasonably practicable for them to do the same.

In acknowledgement of the need for businesses to compare themselves with others in their sector, and to improve H&S standards in small businesses generally, the HSE advise benchmarking. In other words, businesses should not and do not have to: live in ignorance; go it alone; or re-invent the wheel. Where there is a recognized sector-specific *benchmark* H&S management system, it makes sense (business and common) to adopt it.

Ideally, any hazard should be removed altogether, but if this is not practical (e.g. there is no alternative), control measures should be implemented. These may be physical controls, which are directed against the hazard itself, and/or personal controls, which apply to the people who might be exposed.

Physical controls are usually the most effective, and MHSWR require employers to consider and implement them according to the following hierarchy:

1. Remove the hazard altogether (e.g. go digital and avoid using radiographic film-developing chemicals).
2. Replace the hazard with something less hazardous (e.g. use less harmful film-developing chemicals).
3. Restrict access to the hazard (e.g. only designated persons may enter the darkroom or handle the chemicals).
4. Reduce exposure to the hazard (e.g. fit an extractor fan in the darkroom).

In addition, personal controls are required in most cases:

- Training (e.g. training in safe film processing)
- Instruction (e.g. written SOP for film processing)
- Information (e.g. provision of developer and fixer product safety data)
- Supervision (e.g. of new employees, employees developing films for the first time)

- Welfare facilities (e.g. First Aid and washing facilities for removal of contamination)
- Personal protective equipment (e.g. disposable apron, disposable gloves, eye protection).

Ideally, personal protective equipment (PPE) should only be used as a control measure if there is no other way to prevent exposure to a hazard. However, realistically some types of PPE (e.g. gloves; aprons) are essential in veterinary practice.

In addition to the controls described above, safety signs also have an important part to play with regard to controlling risks. To comply with the *Health and Safety (Signs and Signals) Regulations 1996* the approved colour coding of safety signs (Figure 22.7) is as follows:

- Blue: Mandatory (i.e. MUST do something – e.g. 'fire door – keep shut')
- Red: Prohibition (i.e. MUST NOT do something – e.g. 'no unauthorized entry')
- Yellow: Warning (i.e. HAZARD – e.g. 'wet floor')
- Green: Safety (i.e. SAFE CONDITION – e.g. 'First Aid box'; 'fire exit route').

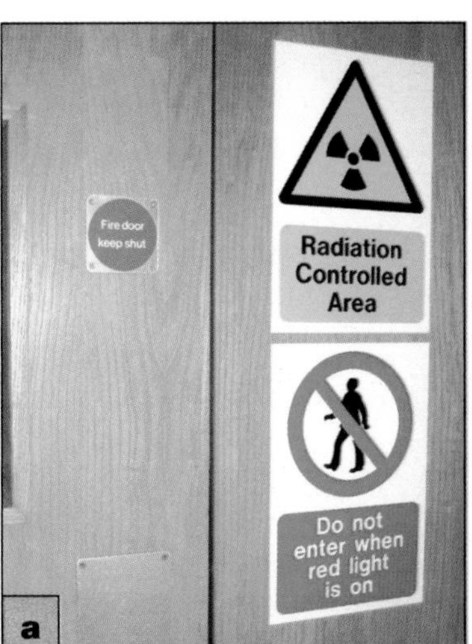

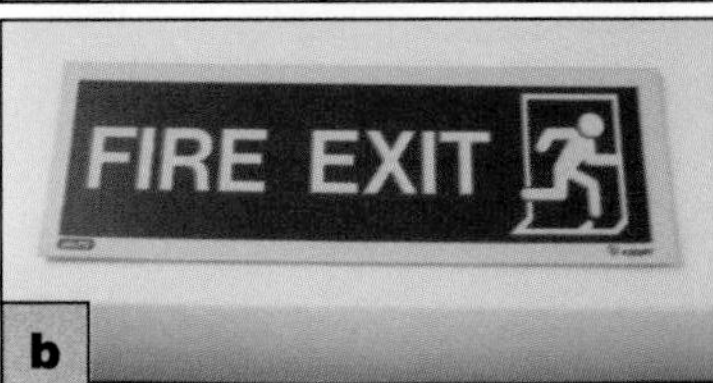

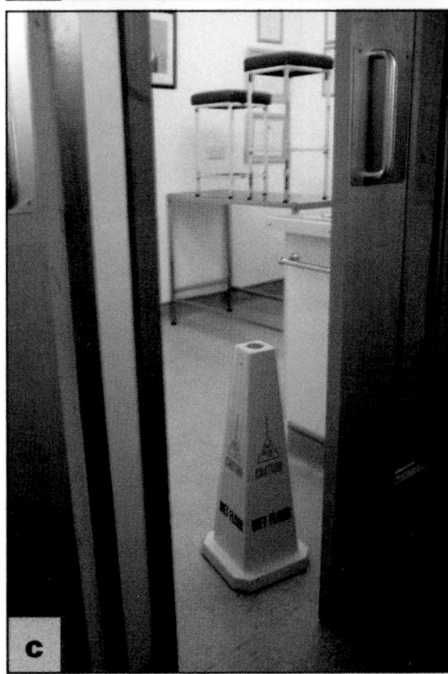

22.7 **(a, b)** A variety of safety signs, showing the approved colour coding. **(c)** A wet floor sign deters people from entering a risky environment (i.e. an area/room with a wet floor), or alerts them to the additional slip risk if crossing the floor is unavoidable.

It is compulsory to display some safety signs (e.g. 'radiation controlled area', 'fire exit', 'smoking is not allowed on the premises') and it is advisable to display others (e.g. 'First Aid box', 'not drinking water', 'fire assembly point').

KEY POINT

Safety signs should not be seen as a quick fix. Risk assessment should determine whether or not there is a better way to control risks. For example, in some cases drying a floor rather than displaying a wet floor sign might be a more 'reasonably practicable' way of reducing the risk of slips; i.e. eliminate the hazard rather than warn people of it.

Step 4: Record findings and implement them

- If the practice has five or more employees the significant findings of risk assessments must be recorded.
- Where there are fewer than five employees, although not required by the regulations, it is still advised that the main points of the risk assessments are recorded as this may be helpful in the case of any legal or civil action brought following an incident.
- In all cases, risk assessments must be carried out, whether recorded or not, and any significant findings must be brought to the attention of employees.

Risk assessments need not be onerous. The HSE advises when writing down records to 'keep it simple', e.g. 'Tripping over rubbish: bins provided, staff instructed, weekly housekeeping checks'. In many cases combined 'assessment checklists' can address several issues on one record. However, oversimplification may fail to identify risks that could cause harm. There is no right or wrong answer as to what is significant. Only the employer or worker, with their knowledge of the practice layout, staff and procedures, can really make such a judgement.

Figure 22.8 shows a record of a risk assessment for changing a light bulb/tube. It is an extreme example but actually each of the hazards identified could apply and should therefore be subject to 'appropriate controls'. The record also shows that it would be difficult and time-consuming to state control measures for each of the hazards (such as electricity/shock) if the practice does not have specific policies and Local Rules that address the 'general' risks associated with each of them. If it is known that the electrical system and light fittings are in good order, because the policy is to have them regularly inspected and tested, and it is known that this has been done, then there is a far lower likelihood that the bulb changer will get electrocuted. However, given knowledge of the practice, the actual risk assessment might be: 'Blown and broken bulbs/tubes only ever changed by Dave, who is a qualified electrical engineer and fitter. Minimal risk'.

Figure 22.9 shows a risk assessment for slips and trips in the practice.

<table>
<tr><td colspan="2">Risk Assessment No......</td></tr>
<tr><td>Procedure:</td><td>Changing a light bulb/fluorescent tube.</td></tr>
<tr><td>Description:</td><td>Replacing a blown or broken light bulb/fluorescent tube in a ceiling or wall fitting, desk lamp, theatre light, etc.</td></tr>
<tr><td>Location:</td><td>Various locations inside and outside the practice buildings.</td></tr>
<tr><td>Frequency/ duration:</td><td>Occasional short periods.</td></tr>
<tr><td>Nature of hazards:</td><td>▪ Electricity: electric shock, burns.
▪ Broken glass: cuts, fragments in eyes, toxic (fluorescent tubes).
▪ Hot bulb/fitting: burns.

If the procedure involves work at height:

▪ Falls: injury to person or others
▪ Falling objects: injury to others.

Possibly (depending on location):

▪ Hazardous substances, e.g. X-ray chemical fumes in the dark room, infectious agents in the laboratory.</td></tr>
<tr><td>Who might be affected:</td><td>The person carrying out the procedure, and persons (e.g. staff, clients) who are in or may enter the location when the procedure is taking place.</td></tr>
<tr><td>Control measures required:</td><td>▪ The procedure must only be carried out by persons who have received specific instruction and training (verbal or written).
▪ Do not carry out the procedure if alone on the premises (assistance must be available in event of accident – e.g. shock).
▪ The light/lamp must be switched off. If unsure (e.g. pull cord switch) the electrical supply to the light/lamp must be switched off at the mains, or the relevant fuse removed. Follow the electrical safety guidance in the health and safety manual.
▪ The bulb should be allowed to cool before removal.
▪ Bulbs/tubes must be handled in accordance with manufacturer instructions (e.g. use gloves or tissue when handling halogen bulbs, to reduce the risk of oil from the skin causing the bulb to shatter when it gets hot).
▪ Appropriate protective clothing must be worn as necessary, e.g. wear gloves to remove broken bulbs/tubes, and eye shield/goggles if there is potential for bulb/tube to shatter or for glass to fall into eyes (e.g. if removing a broken bulb/tube from above head height).
▪ Ensure persons in the location are not likely to be exposed to glass fragments (including if the bulb/ tube is dropped).
▪ If the procedure involves work at height, those involved must follow the guidance in the health and safety manual regarding: work at height; use of ladders and stepladders; work equipment.
▪ Persons carrying out this procedure must be familiar with the relevant Area COSHH Assessment (as documented in the health and safety manual) and must adhere to/implement the necessary control measures as specified on the record.
▪ Bulbs, glass and fluorescent tubes (hazardous waste) must be disposed of according to the disposal of waste guidance.</td></tr>
<tr><td>Risk (high, moderate or low) if all controls are implemented:</td><td>Low.</td></tr>
<tr><td>Actions required:</td><td>Ensure all control measures are implemented.</td></tr>
<tr><td>When:</td><td>On each occasion.</td></tr>
<tr><td>Responsible persons</td><td>Area Safety Officers and person engaged in the procedure.</td></tr>
<tr><td>Date for next assessment/ review:</td><td>12 months from today.</td></tr>
<tr><td>Signed:</td><td></td></tr>
<tr><td>Date:</td><td></td></tr>
</table>

22.8 An example of a risk assessment for changing a light bulb/tube.

Risk Assessment No......	
Procedure:	Slips, trips and falls.
Description:	Slips, trips and falls within the practice.
Location:	
Frequency and duration:	
Nature of hazards:	Physical injury from slips, trips and falls, including fractures, sprains, strains, cuts, abrasions, bruises, etc., which could be caused by the following: ▪ Wet floors ▪ Cluttered areas and corridors ▪ Loose cables/wires ▪ Loose carpet/flooring/mats ▪ Poor lighting ▪ Changes of level in flooring ▪ Unsuitable footwear.
Who might be affected:	Staff, clients and visitors.
Control measures required:	▪ Clean up any spills immediately. Ensure appropriate signage is displayed when floor is wet. Arrange an alternative route if possible. ▪ Keep all areas free from clutter at all times. Deliveries must not be left on the floors. ▪ Position equipment to ensure that cables do not cross pedestrian routes. Use cable covers/ties and fix securely to surfaces. ▪ Provide warning signs/tape and sufficient lighting to indicate steps or changes in level of floor. ▪ Improve or reposition lighting. ▪ Ensure appropriate footwear (correct type of sole) is worn by all practice staff. ▪ See the Premises Inspection Checklist in the H&S Manual.
Risk (high, moderate or low) if all controls are implemented:	Low.
Actions required:	Ensure that the control measures are implemented.
When:	At all times.
Responsible persons:	Area Safety Officers and staff involved.
Date for assessment review:	
Signed:	
Date:	

22.9 An example of a risk assessment for slips and trips in the practice.

The most important point of risk assessment is to put into practice the controls that have been determined are necessary. In the case of the light bulb, this could be to implement appropriate management systems and Local Rules, or to appoint a 'Dave'. Employers are not expected to do everything at once. If the practice can implement some quick and simple changes to improve things straight away, it should. Otherwise, it should prioritize and tackle the significant risks first. Continual changes, even if they are small, may then be required to achieve continued improvement.

Step 5: Review assessments and update if necessary

All things change: premises, plant, procedures, products, pets and people. If the changes are significant (e.g. first parrot patient diagnosed with psittacosis), assessments should be reviewed. Even if there have been no changes, it makes good sense (and in some cases is a legal requirement) to review assessments at least annually. A review of accident records, or simply thinking about an issue or a staff suggestion, may indicate that further improvements are necessary. All records should have a review date on them and the people responsible for them should have a reminder system in place. H&S should be managed – not left to chance.

Lone working

The five steps to risk assessment may need to be followed in the case of staff working alone. Lone working is not limited to out-of-hours duties but can include other scenarios such as being alone at reception or when out on visits. Protocols and standard operating procedures (SOPs) can never completely cover every eventuality, and staff members should be empowered sufficiently to make their own risk assessment of each case. However, for specific lone working scenarios such as out-of-hours, SOPs should be in place regarding basics such as door security, e.g. Don't admit owners without prior arrangement when there is only a lone worker on the premises – always wait until another member of staff arrives to open the front door. Thought should be given to how to deal with a life-threatening veterinary emergency that is presented unexpectedly.

It is advisable to avoid having staff working alone in the practice unless absolutely necessary. There are a number of issues to take into consideration and some simple safety mechanisms that can be put in place in order to reduce the risk. An example of a risk assessment to be completed for a lone worker is given in Figure 22.10.

Considerations

- Will the lone worker be using equipment and, if so, can this be handled safely by one person?
- Will the lone worker be required to lift or move objects too large for one person?
- Are there any chemicals or substances which might pose a risk to the lone worker?
- Is the lone worker pregnant or suffering from a medical condition that could increase the risk of working alone?
- Is there a risk of violence against the lone worker?
- Is the lone worker new to the job or inexperienced?
- Back-up and security must be available for lone workers out on call, e.g. equine vets, house calls.

Risk Assessment No.....		
Activity	**Hazard**	**Control measure**
Low risk		
Reception Office-based Cleaning Attending to inpatients Clearing up theatre	Illness	If known illness then consideration should be given to restricting working alone as appropriate.
	Fire	Follow standard fire procedure and evacuate to assembly point.
	Intruder	Out of hours the building must be kept secure at all times. Contact police if anything suspicious is seen or heard.
Staff entering/leaving premises	Assault	There must be adequate lighting, e.g. outside light or street lamp. The main reception entrance may be used if staff prefer. Cars can be parked near entrance.
Walking dogs	Intruder	Door must be kept locked whilst walking patients. There must be adequate lighting outside.
	Stress	Double lead must be used to reduce risk of patients escaping and avoid stress for staff involved.
Persons entering the practice	Assault	Authorized persons may enter the practice during normal opening hours but are not permitted in any areas other than reception. All entrances apart from the main entrance must be kept locked. The main entrance can be locked if there is a cause for concern.
Use of equipment	Injury	Do not use unfamiliar equipment if alone.
House calls	Assault	Plan the route in advance and take a map. Ensure colleagues know when and where you are going and have the client's full details. Any daytime visits to new clients must be accompanied, as must *all night visits*. It may be prudent to carry a basic First Aid kit if there is a foreseeable risk of injury.
	Illness	If known illness then consideration should be given to restricting working alone as appropriate.
Medium risk		
Handling aggressive/difficult to handle/nervous/very strong patients	Injury	Work not to be undertaken alone.
Controlled drugs	Abuse	Staff are not permitted to access the controlled drugs cupboard when lone working. Controlled drugs may be administered by a lone worker but the dose will need to have been dispensed in another location other than the controlled drug cupboard.
Persons entering the practice	Assault	Staff are not permitted to allow persons into the practice out of hours if they are alone, unless they know the person and prior arrangements have been agreed.
High risk		
Unplanned events, including accidents and emergencies	Injury	Follow emergency procedures and call for assistance as required. A First Aid kit must be available on site.
Signed:		
Date:		

22.10 An example of a risk assessment for lone working.

- How are aggressive, large or difficult patients to be handled?
- What access will there be to controlled drugs?

KEY POINT

Everyone in a client consultation is, in essence, working alone, so these issues do not just apply to out-of-hours or remote working.

Reducing the risks

- Ensure that clients are aware of the practice out-of-hours safety arrangements (Figure 22.11).
- Ensure that every lone worker has received appropriate safety and job training, and is able to perform their own risk assessment for every task or call.
- Ensure all appropriate entrances into the practice have been shut and secured.
- Consider using a service that offers lone worker monitoring checks.
- Ensure that the building is adequately alarmed.
- Install panic buttons within the practice (can be linked to a police station or monitoring service).
- Provide a personal alarm that alerts a responsible person.
- Provide an emergency telephone.
- Provide contact details for appropriate colleagues.
- Ensure that there is a 'panic-room' within the building (i.e. a secure room which can be locked from the inside and from which a telephone call can be made).
- Ensure that there are clear written rules on tasks the lone worker may and may not carry out.
- Consider providing formal training for difficult situations – this can help greatly in preventing panic when faced with an unusual situation.
- Ensure that the lone worker understands that risks should not be taken and that if they are worried about a potential intruder the police should be called without hesitation (ensure police know there is a lone worker on the premises).
- Install a video intercom so that any callers to the practice can be seen and questioned before being admitted.
- Maintain a list of expected visitors, and ensure that unexpected visitors are treated with caution; record all activity, for example telephone calls and consultations with clients and other staff.

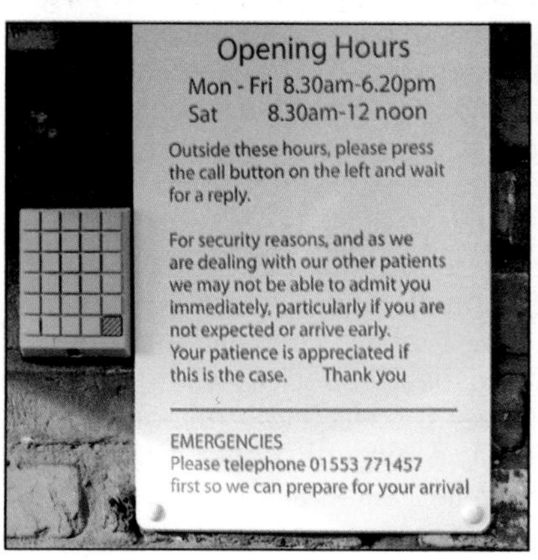

Opening Hours
Mon - Fri 8.30am-6.20pm
Sat 8.30am-12 noon
Outside these hours, please press the call button on the left and wait for a reply.
For security reasons, and as we are dealing with our other patients we may not be able to admit you immediately, particularly if you are not expected or arrive early.
Your patience is appreciated if this is the case. Thank you
EMERGENCIES
Please telephone 01553 771457 first so we can prepare for your arrival

22.11 Making clear to clients the practice out-of-hours safety arrangements will reduce frustration and help lone workers to feel safe.

Staff consultation

As well as informing all personnel of the practice's Health and Safety Policy, Management Arrangements and risk assessment findings, as required under HASAWA and MHSWR, the employer must consult employees on all matters and proposed changes that may have implications for their health and safety. The requirement is set out in the Health and Safety (Consultation with Employees) Regulations 1996. Areas to consider include:

- Changes to working practices (e.g. out-of-hours duties, new methodologies)
- New equipment, new technologies (e.g. MRI, new laboratory tests, new display screens)
- Different products/substances to be used (e.g. cleaning agents, anaesthetic agents)
- Appointing or changing H&S personnel (e.g. Competent Person, consultant)
- How the practice will provide H&S information (e.g. results of assessments)
- Planned H&S training (for specific individuals or for all staff).

Consultation procedure

Consultation is a two-way process. There must be specific arrangements in place for raising issues and proposals with employees *and* for allowing them time to consider them, to raise any concerns they may have, and to have their views taken into account and fully considered before any changes are implemented. This can be on an individual or group basis, or via a Representative of Employee Safety (RES). Employees have the right to choose how they wish to be consulted and so must be asked what arrangements they would prefer. If they opt for an RES, they must nominate someone and that person must be asked if they are willing to take on the role. The employer cannot decide who the RES will be. Anyone who is appointed to the role must be given sufficient training to enable them to carry out their duties, which include:

- Distributing information from employer to staff, and relaying staff opinions back
- Raising any H&S suggestions or concerns staff may have
- Representing the staff in consultations with Health and Safety Inspectors.

For many practices, appropriate consultation arrangements could simply be, and usually are:

- An open-door policy
- Informal discussions on safety issues through the working day
- Regular practice meetings, with H&S a specific topic always on the agenda.

The policy document should specify the practice arrangements for consultation, and appropriate records should be kept of the issues discussed and of any follow-up actions. It is important that consultation with employees takes place *before* anything that may affect or concern them is done. Through effective consultation, the practice will be ensuring that the health, safety and welfare of staff are given a high priority. The practice will run more effectively and safely as a result and, by giving staff the opportunity to discuss H&S issues, they may well suggest safer, cheaper and more practical approaches to manage H&S and reduce risks.

Informing staff

To comply with the law, employers must provide all employees with sufficient information, instruction and training to enable them to work safely and without risks to their health. To emphasize the priority given to H&S and to effective consultation, with regard to information and instruction, it is essential that someone goes through it with the employee, either individually or as a group, and explains how it applies to individuals and to the practice as a whole, rather than simply telling everyone to read the Policy document and sign the declaration.

The points to be discussed should include:

- The practice's overall Health and Safety Policy and who is responsible for what
- The hazards to which people in the practice might be exposed
- Findings of risk assessments, and measures in place to minimize risks
- Accident, fire and emergency procedures
- First Aid facilities and procedures
- Specific policies, Local Rules, work instructions, SOPs
- Where to find operating instructions and product and equipment safety data
- How individuals can find information of relevance to themselves
- Who to ask for advice
- How to report H&S concerns and problems
- H&S training.

This should not be done all at once, but issues should be introduced and explained, and full training given over a prolonged induction period, with regular checks on understanding and performance.

Health and Safety Law poster

To comply with the Health and Safety Information for Employees (Amendment) Regulations 2009 the practice must display a copy of the approved Health and Safety Law poster, or provide each member of staff with a copy of the equivalent pocket card. The poster must be displayed in a location where employees can easily read it. A new version of the poster was introduced in 2009 (Figure 22.12). However the old 1999 version and equivalent leaflet is valid until 5 April 2014. After that date only the new versions must be used. The Health and Safety Law poster is available from most safety suppliers and from HSE Books. The poster outlines H&S laws and states in clear terms what employers must do for their employees and what they, in turn, must do to help. It also has space to record the names and details of any Representatives of Employee Safety (RESs) or other H&S contacts, but this is not compulsory. Unfortunately, the new poster contains some information and guidance that is out of date.

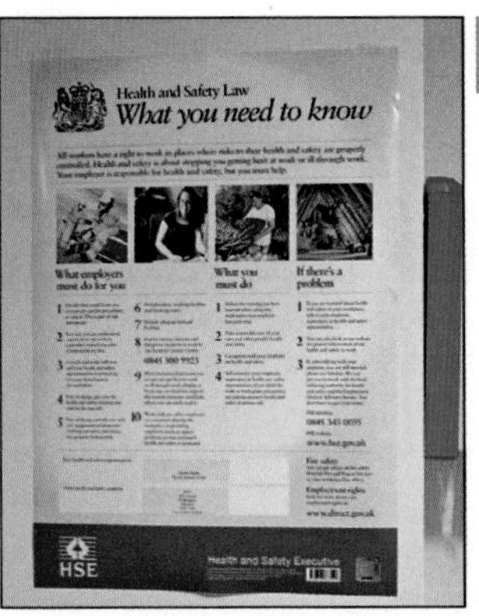

22.12 Health and safety poster on display.

KEY POINT

The HSE Infoline referred to on the poster, for employees to obtain advice, is no longer in service. Information is available via the website www.hse.gov.uk. Reports made under RIDDOR (see below), with the exception of fatalities and major incidents and injuries, should no longer be made via the Incident Contact Centre telephone number on the poster but via the website www.hse.gov.uk/riddor.

Training

Determining and meeting the training needs of staff is a critical issue, and one that must be discussed with them. All H&S information, instruction and training provided needs to be relevant to the individual and in a format that is easy to understand.

Consideration should be given with regard to who needs to know what, and when and how best to provide training. For example: a receptionist probably does not need to know about the hazards and risks associated with a hydrotherapy unit (except perhaps the wet floor) or to be given training in how to lift a big dog on to an operating table; a head nurse will need to know both, but referring him/her to a generic risk assessment attached to a list of chemical safety datasheets and sending him/her on a manual handling course run by someone from the construction industry would not be appropriate.

As with so many issues, a checklist is a good place to start. The employer and employees should make a list of topics for which specific training is or might be necessary. The list of topics in Figure 22.2 could be used as a start, as almost everything on the list is likely to be relevant to one or more people in the practice. This should form the basis of an induction plan for new employees. There will be some other general issues and many specific tasks with H&S implications that are not on the list (e.g. regarding MRI; transporting healthcare waste and gas cylinders between surgeries).

In many cases it is simple enough, and perfectly acceptable, to provide appropriate training in house. An experienced member of staff showing an inexperienced one how to do something safely, then observing them doing it, and then both agreeing competence to 'go it alone' constitutes training. However, for some issues, especially with regard to employees who have specific H&S responsibilities (e.g. PSO, FO, RES), it may be better for them to attend an appropriate external training course. Training needs are summarized in Figure 22.13.

Type of training	Who requires this training?	What should the training involve?	When should the training take place?
Induction	New employees; returners from extended leave, e.g. maternity leave, sabbatical; and locum staff	Health and safety policy; employer and employee responsibility; importance of understanding one's own limitations; who to ask for guidance; accident, First Aid, fire procedures	As soon as possible after starting work
General	All employees	Health and safety policy; accident, First Aid and fire procedures; Local Rules	Whenever changes are made following review or new regulations
Specific	All relevant employees	Specific tasks	When employees start new tasks
Specialist	Employees with specific health and safety, First Aid or fire safety responsibility	Fire marshall; specific technical training or management of health and safety qualifications	As required or on promotion
Refresher (CPD)	All	All areas of health and safety	As necessary, to update on latest regulations and advice and to maintain standards and confidence

22.13 Training needs should be considered for each member of staff and at each stage of their employment or when things change.

By law, the employer is obliged to provide all necessary H&S training free of charge to employees. Training must be provided within working hours, or employees must be given paid time off to compensate. It is essential that appropriate staff training records are kept (a checklist would be useful) and that training needs are continually assessed and refresher training provided to keep people up to date and to prevent standards slipping, which could result in greater risks arising.

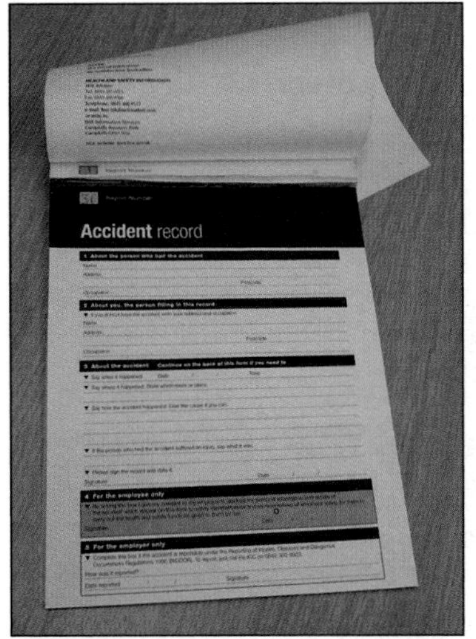

22.14 Practices are recommended to use the HSE-approved Accident Book B1 510, which allows employers to comply with legal requirements to record work-related accidents and the requirement to keep personal details in confidence, whilst enabling information to be available for accident investigation and prevention purposes.

Accident recording and investigation

Veterinary practices are potentially hazardous workplaces. Injuries such as cuts, 'needle sticks', bites and scratches often occur. Chemicals in the eyes, self-injection, burns, electric shock, fractures and deep wounds occur less often but are certainly not unheard of. Stressed staff, squeamish or aggressive clients, inquisitive (or naughty) children, clumsy workmen and various other scenarios can and do occur in practice. All contribute to the potential for a variety of injuries to occur to staff, clients and visitors.

Reporting accidents

- To comply with The Social Security (Claims and Payments) Amendment Regulations 2011, a practice with 10 or more employees must keep an Accident Book.
- For those with fewer than 10 employees this is not compulsory, but it is good practice and it is recommended.

The Accident Book must be one that complies with the Data Protection Act 1998. Practices are therefore recommended to use the HSE-approved Accident Book B1 510, which allows employers to comply with legal requirements to record work-related accidents and the requirement to keep personal details in confidence, whilst enabling information to be available for accident investigation and prevention purposes (Figure 22.14). Completed pages are numbered and removed, to be filed confidentially. The HSE Accident Book also contains advice and guidance on the Reporting of Injuries, Diseases and Dangerous Occurrences Regulations 1995 (RIDDOR), under which an employer must report and keep a record of certain injuries, incidents and cases of work-related disease, even if they have fewer than 10 employees.

Reportable injuries

The following must be reported without delay to the HSE's Incident Contact Centre (ICC) by telephone (number currently 0845 3009923):

- Death of an employee, member of the public, or self-employed person working on practice premises
- Any injury that results in a member of the public being taken to hospital
- Major injury to an employee or self-employed person working on the premises, for example:

- Fracture, other than to fingers, thumbs and toes
- Amputation
- Dislocation of the shoulder, hip, knee or spine
- Loss of sight (temporary or permanent)
- Chemical or hot metal burn to the eye or any penetrating injury to the eye
- Injury resulting from an electric shock or electrical burn leading to unconsciousness, or requiring resuscitation or admittance to hospital for more than 24 hours
- Any other injury leading to hypothermia, heat-induced illness or unconsciousness, or requiring resuscitation, or requiring admittance to hospital for more than 24 hours
- Unconsciousness caused by asphyxia or exposure to a harmful substance or biological agent
- Acute illness requiring medical treatment, or loss of consciousness arising from absorption of any substance by inhalation, ingestion or through the skin
- Acute illness requiring medical treatment where there is reason to believe that this resulted from exposure to a biological agent or its toxins or infected material.

Any injury not included above which results in the injured person being off work for a specific number of days (includes weekends but not the day of the injury) must be reported via the HSE's RIDDOR website using form F2508. There is also a deadline by which the injury must be reported.

Reportable diseases

If the practice receives notification from a doctor that a member of the staff is suffering a reportable work-related disease, this must be reported via HSE's RIDDOR website using form F2508A.

Reportable dangerous occurrences

Incidents that could have caused a fatality or major injury but did not must be reported immediately via HSE's RIDDOR website, using form F2508. For example:

- Collapse, overturning or failure of load-bearing parts of lifts and lifting equipment
- Explosion, collapse or bursting of any closed vessel or associated pipe work
- Plant or equipment coming into contact with overhead power lines
- Electrical short-circuit or overload causing fire or explosion.

The HSE's approved Accident Book and their RIDDOR website both include comprehensive lists of what constitute major injuries, reportable diseases and dangerous occurrences.

KEY POINT

Although the legal requirement to investigate accidents and incidents applies to those that are reportable under RIDDOR, it is very useful – and good practice – to investigate all accidents and, ideally, all near misses.

Bird's triangle (Bird and Germain, 1986) (Figure 22.15) shows that for every major accident that occurs there are many more that result in minor injury or property damage, and considerably more near misses or 'accidents waiting to happen'.

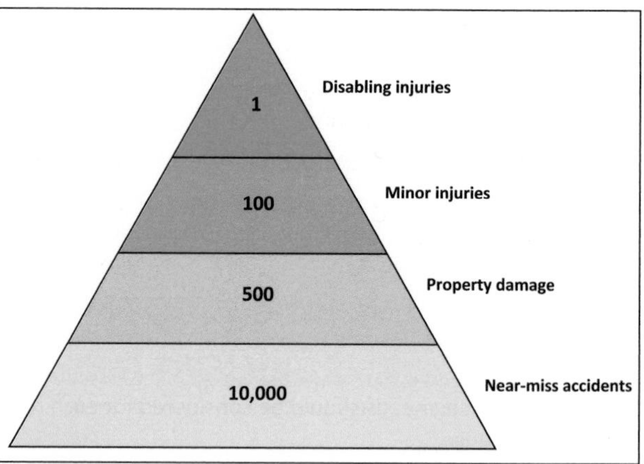

22.15 Bird's triangle (Bird and Germain, 1986), showing the relative frequency of different categories of accident.

For full up-to-date information on what must be reported, how and when under RIDDOR, consult the HSE's RIDDOR website: www.hse.gov.uk/riddor.

Most common accidents in veterinary practice

Of the major and 'over 3 days' accidents reported under RIDDOR by veterinary practices (not just small animal practices) the statistics provided by the HSE are:

- 47% involved animals (bites (Figure 22.16), scratches, kicks, butting, crushing)
- 17% manual handling injuries
- 17% slips, trips and falls
- 10% struck (by clients or other staff members)
- 9% other (e.g. electric shock, burns, chemicals).

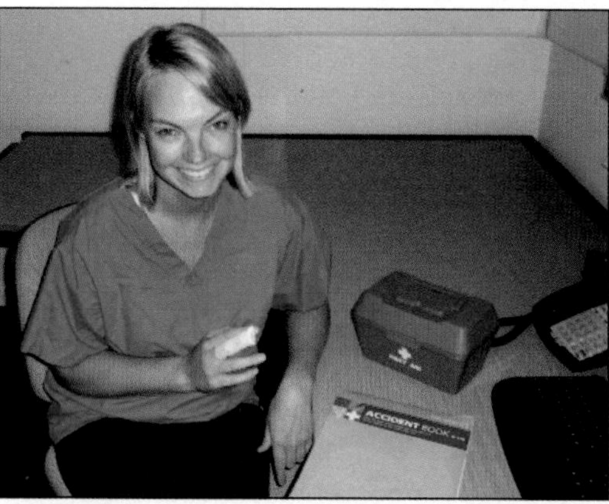

22.16 Cat bites can be serious and any staff bitten should seek medical attention, ensuring that the wound is washed and dressed and that appropriate antibiotics are prescribed if required. The Accident Book should be completed.

For minor accidents, i.e. those not reported to the HSE, the order is similar but manual handling injuries (e.g. bad backs) are significantly higher and 'needle-stick' injuries (which do not feature as a category on the HSE statistics) far outnumber slips, trips and falls (unpublished data collected by Salus QP).

Investigation

Ideally, a practice should have a defined investigation procedure, with responsibility for implementing it as-signed to a senior member of the practice. An essential component of an effective investigation system is the keeping of detailed records:

- Date and time of the accident/incident
- Area in which it happened
- Type of work being done, and equipment in use
- Details of person(s) involved
- Nature of the accident/incident, i.e. what happened
- Nature of injuries or damage sustained
- First Aid/actions taken at the scene at the time
- Eye-witness accounts
- Probable cause of the accident/incident
- Any immediate measures taken to prevent recurrence.

The purpose of investigation is to establish the cause of the accident or incident rather than to establish blame. Only when the cause is known can it be decided what, if anything, could and should be done to reduce the likelihood of recurrence.

It is important to record all incidents, even the minor ones. 'Needle sticks' and small cuts and scratches may seem trivial, and a slight trip at the top of the stairs may be simply shrugged off. But next time that scratch could turn nasty and that trip could lead to a fall. Major accidents very often have the same causes as minor ones.

As well as recording any on-the-spot actions, although not a legal requirement (in most cases), practices are strongly advised to review their accident records annually, in order to determine what steps, if any, could and should be taken to reduce the number of accidents in future. Figure 22.17 shows an example of a record form that could be used to document reviews. It also gives guidance on the points to consider, such as: repeats of the same accident; accidents of a similar nature; accidents associated with one area, one activity, or one member of staff; and whether accidents are due to the equipment (unsafe or unsuitable), the surroundings (poor lighting, insufficient space), or poor working practice (negligence, insufficient training, pressure of work).

KEY POINT

For practices that have more than one surgery, or are part of a group, it is good practice carry out an overall accident review and to compare accident rates and types between sites and between groups of employees, such as experienced *versus* less experienced.

ACCIDENTS AND INCIDENTS REVIEW

It is the policy of the practice that ALL accidents (major and minor), **near misses** (no injury, but could have been) and **dangerous or potentially dangerous occurrences** are recorded in the Accident Book, together with details of the incident, including some or all of the following:

- **Who** was involved (name, age, sex, job description)
- **What** they were doing
- **What** was involved (e.g. property, equipment)
- **What** injury, illness or damage was sustained
- **When** it happened
- **Where** it happened
- **How** it happened.

Accidents and incidents are investigated at the time and the records are reviewed annually as a whole, in order to detect any underlying causes and to determine what actions, if any, could and should be taken to reduce the number of accidents and incidents in future.

Use the grid below to categorize the accidents and incidents in terms of their associations and causes; each accident or incident may have more than one of each. You can rule lines and put more than one number in each box if you wish to categorize the accidents and incidents, e.g. two trips on the same step and two shocks from the kettle could be recorded in 2a) as 2 and 2 or 4, in each case with 2 in 5a) and 2 in 4a).

Date of current review:.................................
Date of previous review:.................................
Review carried out by:.................................

Number of accidents/incidents in current 12-month period:..............
Number of accidents/incidents in previous 12-month period:..............

1. Accidents and incidents associated with:	2. Total number	Number of accidents and incidents caused by poor:			
		3. Working practices	4. Equipment	5. Surroundings	6. Other
a) Same accident/incident (e.g. trip on same step)					
b) Similar accidents/incidents					
c) Same area					
d) Same activity					
e) Same individual					
f) Similar groups of individuals or team members					
g) Other					

Give further comments on the causes (e.g. whether poor working practice is due to negligence, lack of training, pressure of work; is the equipment unsafe or unsuitable; the surroundings too cramped or dark or lacking facilities; etc.).

Comment on any other causes and state whether accident/incident stats have improved, worsened or stayed the same as the previous period (i.e. in nature/number).

Continued on the back? YES/NO

If specific actions are required tick here ❑ Please give details on the back or attach an additional sheet.

22.17 An example of an accident records review form.

First Aid facilities and procedures

As discussed above, to comply with The Health and Safety (First Aid) Regulations 1981 a practice must appoint sufficient and appropriate First Aid personnel. The practice must also provide First Aid equipment and facilities 'appropriate for the circumstances in the workplace' – but there are no hard and fast rules. To determine what is appropriate, the employer will need to carry out a risk assessment and be prepared to defend it if necessary.

Requirements for First Aid provision should not be based solely on the number of staff present. Split sites, work rotas, the hazards present, and availability of professional assistance must be taken into account. Provision should be considered for all times that workers are present. Practices also have a 'duty of care' to provide adequate facilities for clients and visitors invited to the premises. Although under the regulations there is no legal duty to provide First Aid for non-employees, the HSE strongly recommends that they are included in First Aid provision. Practices must therefore consider students, seminars, open days, puppy parties, etc.

First Aid box

At least one suitably stocked First Aid box should be readily available, situated near to hand-washing facilities that are maintained to a high standard of hygiene, in a place that is always accessible, preferably hazard-free and, ideally, where a casualty (staff or client) can sit down to be treated if necessary. The staff kitchen or rest room (if one exists) is often the best place. A First Aid box must also be provided for each practice vehicle.

There is no standard list of items to be included in the First Aid box, although there is a suggested minimum:

- Leaflet giving general guidance on First Aid
- 20 individually wrapped sterile plasters of assorted sizes
- 2 sterile eye pads
- 4 individually wrapped triangular bandages
- 6 safety pins
- 6 medium-sized, individually wrapped, sterile unmedicated wound dressings
- 2 large, individually wrapped, sterile unmedicated wound dressings
- 1 pair of disposable gloves.

The contents of the First Aid box should be listed on the lid. Items can be ticked off as they are used and the designated person can easily check the contents/expiry dates. Boxes should be checked regularly (according to usage); the primary FA or AP should put reminders in their diary. Tablets or medicines should not be kept in the First Aid box.

First Aid boxes should be clearly identified with a white cross on a green background (Figure 22.18). If risk assessment indicates that a First Aid room is necessary, a notice should indicate who the FAs are and how to contact them.

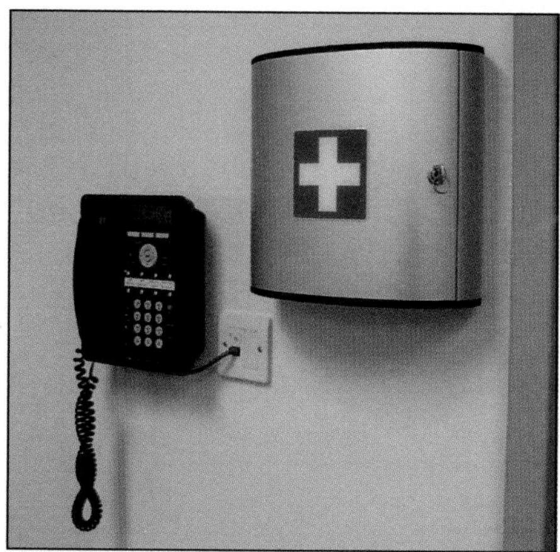

22.18 A First Aid box, in this case affixed to a wall, should be identified by a white cross on a green background.

KEY POINT

Staff should be aware of who the First Aiders, emergency First Aiders or appointed persons are. There should be no doubt as to who is to take charge of an incident.

Employees who travel regularly or work elsewhere

Employers are responsible for meeting the First Aid needs of their employees working away from the main site. The assessment of First Aid needs should determine:

- Whether those who travel long distances or are continually mobile should carry a personal First Aid box
- Whether employees should be issued with personal communicators/mobile phones.

Eye washing

In areas where drugs, chemicals, animals or clinical materials are handled, there is the potential for eyes to be splashed with hazardous substances. In such an event the most important First Aid is prompt and thorough irrigation of the eyes with sterile buffered saline or water from a clean tap. Eyewash bottles (Figure 22.19) or sinks (ideally with flexible rubber

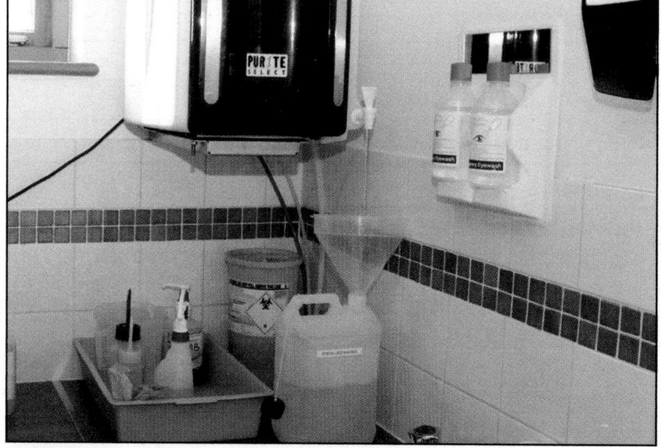

22.19 Eyewash bottles should be readily available for immediate emergency flushing of eyes.

hoses on the taps) should be readily available in all such areas. The practice must decide whether current arrangements provide adequate facility for eye washing, i.e. whether enough sinks are available, always accessible, clean and easy to use, or whether additional sinks and/or eyewash bottles should be provided.

Although there are no rules on this, and it is for each individual practice to decide for itself, it is good practice as a minimum to keep a large sterile eyewash bottle with each First Aid box. Indeed, having sterile eyewash bottles in all clinical areas is the cleanest and safest option.

The Approved Code of Practice (ACoP) to the First Aid Regulations recommends that employers display First Aid posters, particularly if they do not have a fully qualified FA on site all of the time.

Electrical appliances

Electrical equipment should be checked visually, at least annually, to spot early signs of damage or deterioration. Additional regular inspections may be required where a risk assessment indicates this is necessary. Equipment that is used in a harsh environment should be checked and/or tested more frequently than equipment that is less likely to become damaged or unsafe. It is good practice to:

- Assess how often equipment being used for work purposes should be checked and/or tested
- Write down the findings
- Ensure checks and tests are carried out and results recorded.

All electrical installations must be inspected and tested by a person who is competent to do so. A Competent Person should advise the frequency of both visual inspection and a test, e.g. portable appliance test (PAT). Guidance is available on the HSE website and an example of an electrical testing policy for an office or low risk environment is given in Figure 22.20. PAT testing must be carried out by someone who is trained and competent. Equipment should be labelled with the date of inspection. Failed equipment must not be used and repaired equipment must be retested before use.

All staff should be trained to spot common visible faults and problems with electrical equipment and wiring at point of use so that a responsible person can be alerted to any problems (Figure 22.21).

KEY POINT

Staff concerned about the safety of electrical equipment should stop it from being used and ask a Competent Person to undertake a more thorough check.

Category of equipment	User check	Formal visual inspection	Combined inspection and testing
Battery-operated: (<20 volts)	No	No	No
Extra low voltage: (<50 volts AC), e.g. telephone equipment, low voltage desk lights	No	No	No
Information technology, e.g. desktop computers, VDU screens	Yes	Yes – every 2 years	Power supply leads every 2 years. If equipment is double-insulated then it does not require testing. If it is not double-insulated, test every 5 years
Laptops	Yes	Yes – annually	Power supply leads, annually
Equipment that is **not** handheld and rarely moved, e.g. photocopiers, fax machines	No	Yes – every 2 years	No if double insulated; every 4 years if not double insulated
Double-insulated equipment, whether handheld or not	Yes	Yes – every 2 years	No. For double-insulated equipment, breakdown is almost always caused by physical damage, which should be identified by visual inspections
Double-insulated equipment that is handheld, e.g. some floor cleaners	Yes	Yes – every 6 months to one year	No
Earthed equipment (class 1), e.g. electric kettles	Yes	Yes – every 6 months to 1 year	Yes – every 1 to 2 years if not in a high risk environment and not subject to abuse. Combined inspection and testing will be required more frequently if in a high risk environment/subject to abuse
Extension cables, leads (for mains voltage equipment)	Yes	Yes – annually	Yes – every 2 years
Cables, leads and plugs connected to the above	At the same frequency as the equipment		

22.20 This example of a practice electrical testing policy for low-risk and office areas indicates the results of that practice's risk assessment and shows the testing plan, which should be regularly reviewed. Testing frequency may need to be increased in higher risk environments. Experience of operating the system over a period of time is used, together with information on any faults found, to review the frequency of formal visual inspection and combined inspection/testing.

Checklist for inspecting electrical equipment	
1. Switch off and unplug the equipment before you start any checks	
2. Check that the plug is correctly wired (but only if you are competent to do so)	
3. Ensure the fuse is correctly rated by checking the equipment rating plate or instruction book	
4. Check that the plug is not damaged and that the cable is properly secured, with no internal wires visible	
5. Check the electrical cable is not damaged and has not been repaired with insulating tape or an unsuitable connector. Damaged cable should be replaced with a new cable by a competent person	
6. Check that the outer cover of the equipment is not damaged in a way that will give rise to electrical or mechanical hazards	
7. Check for burn marks or staining that suggests the equipment is overheating	
8. Position any trailing wires so that they are not a trip hazard and are less likely to get damaged	

22.21 An example of a simple checklist to help staff spot potential problems with electrical equipment. Many faults with work equipment can be found during a simple visual inspection. If anyone is concerned about the safety of the equipment they should stop it from being used and ask a competent person to undertake a more thorough check.

Gas appliances

To comply with the Gas Safety (Installation and Use) Regulations 1998 the practice must ensure the safe installation and maintenance of gas appliances (see Chapter 2). Whenever a gas appliance is installed in the workplace or maintenance work is carried out on existing gas appliances or fittings, the person carrying out the work must be competent to work on the type of equipment concerned. At present, such persons can prove this by appearing on the Gas Safe Register.

Employers, self-employed persons and anyone responsible for business premises must not allow a gas appliance to be used if they suspect that it may be dangerous. To help reduce the risks presented by use of gas in the workplace it is essential to:

- Have new gas equipment supplied and fitted by a Gas Safe Register engineer
- Have all gas appliances serviced regularly by a Gas Safe Register engineer, in line with the manufacturer's instructions
- Keep the areas around external flue outlets clear of vegetation, etc. to make sure that combustion gases can be effectively removed
- Ensure there is an adequate airflow around gas appliances.

Specific duties of landlords

If staff accommodation is provided, the owner or person with responsibility for the accommodation must:

- Ensure that gas appliances and flues are maintained in a safe condition
- Ensure that annual safety checks are carried out by an appropriately qualified Gas Safe Register engineer
- Retain records of these checks for at least 2 years and issue them to tenants within 28 days of the checks being carried out.

Carbon monoxide

Carbon monoxide is an odourless and invisible gas that can kill within hours if inhaled. It is produced when methane, propane, liquefied petroleum gas (LPG) and other gases burn incompletely because of poor appliance maintenance or lack of ventilation. Although not a legal requirement, for extra safety practices may wish to install a carbon monoxide detector and alarm system anywhere gas is burned, particularly in any staff accommodation or sleeping areas. The landlord must make sure that the alarm meets safety standards BS 7860 or BS EN 50291, has a BSI Kitemark and is sited in line with the manufacturer's guidance. It is important to ensure that the detector is tested regularly.

KEY POINT

Carbon monoxide detectors are safety devices and are not a substitute for basic safety precautions, staff awareness and regular maintenance by an appropriately qualified engineer.

Acknowledgements

The authors would like to thank Salus QP (a division of VetsNow Ltd), from which some of the examples have been adapted. The authors and editors are grateful to the following practices, images of which appear in this chapter: Elands Veterinary Clinic; Mill House Veterinary Surgery and Hospital; Willows Veterinary Centre and Referral Service.

References and further reading

Bird FE and Germain GL (1986) *Loss Control Management: Practical Loss Control Leadership*. Det Norske Veritas, USA

BSAVA: Health & Safety resource available for members at www.bsava.com

Health and Safety Executive (2006) *Electric Shock: First Aid Procedures*. HSE Books (other advice and H&S Law poster available at www.hse.gov.uk)

Suzy Lamplugh Trust: training and useful handbooks for staff and lone workers available at www.suzylamplugh.org

Examples of Health and Safety Policy documents ▶

General Health and Safety Policy Statement

The Health and Safety at Work etc. Act 1974 (HASAWA)

To comply with the **HASAWA** (and all subordinate legislation) *The Practice* must do all that is 'reasonably practicable' to ensure the health, safety and welfare of all employees, trainees, students, clients, contractors and visitors – and all others who may be affected by their actions (volunteers, unpaid helpers, members of the public, other employers/persons with whom they share business premises, etc.).
To ensure compliance *The Practice* will implement an overall health and safety policy, and specific policies on all specific health and safety regulations/issues that directly apply to the business.

***The Practice* undertakes to ensure that all personnel will receive appropriate information and training to ensure that they:**

- Are aware of the hazards at 'the workplace' (e.g. at The Practice or on client premises)
- Are familiar with all relevant safety rules, procedures and codes of practice
- Know where and how to access all necessary safety information, advice and guidance
- Know where to find and how to use First Aid and firefighting equipment
- Are familiar with the procedures for reporting accidents and for reporting or raising other health and safety issues.

***The Practice* also undertakes to ensure that:**

- Staff/trainees/students will be supervised until fully trained and assessed as competent
- Machinery, equipment and safety devices are regularly inspected and maintained and are safe and suitable to use
- The workplace is safe and suitable in terms of comfort, space, heating, lighting, ventilation, cleanliness and freedom from unnecessary hazards
- All hazards are identified and the associated risks are assessed, and that all risks will be removed or reduced to as low as is reasonably practicable
- Working practices are regularly reviewed to improve health and safety
- Accidents and incidents are investigated and appropriate actions taken to prevent recurrence
- Individual members of staff/trainees/students will not be expected to perform tasks that may present risks to them specifically due to their age, sex or health status
- An ongoing health surveillance scheme is in operation; that the records are regularly reviewed to check for possible links between working practice and ill health; and that any such links are investigated and appropriate actions taken
- **'Named individuals'** will be appointed as **Practice Safety Officers** and designated as the **'responsible persons'** for managing health and safety at their specific Practices and for ensuring the implementation of all health and safety policies.

See also the poster 'Health and Safety Law' displayed ....

This health and safety policy will be reviewed annually or sooner if/as necessary.

Signed: (employer).......... Date:..........

Signed: (Practice Safety Officer).......... Date:..........

An example of a General Health and Safety Policy Statement.

Health And Safety Policy: General Duties of All Personnel

The Health and Safety at Work etc. Act 1974 (HASAWA)

It is the duty of ALL personnel:

- To take reasonable care for their own health and safety and the health and safety of other persons who may be affected by their acts or omissions at work
- To co-operate with their employer and safety officers so far as is necessary to enable them to comply with any duties or requirements imposed on them under health and safety legislation
- Not to intentionally or recklessly interfere with, or misuse, anything provided in the interest of health, safety or welfare.

Detailed in *The Practice's* **HEALTH AND SAFETY MANUAL** are **specific policies, Local Rules and procedures** – i.e. the Codes of Practice (COPs) – which must be followed by **ALL** personnel.

All personnel must sign the declaration in the manual to indicate that they have read and understand them.

The key points of the practice's **H&S policy** are:

- All personnel will receive formal instruction and training in the relevant health and safety aspects pertaining to them. Written records of this training will be retained
- All personnel must not perform any tasks for which they have not received formal instruction or training detailing the health and safety procedures and precautions involved
- All personnel must not perform any task or handle any equipment or hazardous substance if they know that the required health and safety procedures and precautions cannot be complied with
- All personnel must approach their manager or the relevant safety officer (or their deputy) if/when they need authorization, training, advice or health and safety information or equipment for specific purposes.

All personnel should be familiar with H&S aspects of each task carried out and know what safety precautions must be taken. Each individual must take responsibility for doing their own risk assessment every time and seek help and advice if there is any doubt regarding the safety of themselves or others.

An example of a practice Health and Safety Policy Statement: general duties of all personnel.

Health and Safety Policy: Health and Safety Management Arrangements

The Management of Health and Safety at Work Regulations 1999 (MHSWR)

The overall policy of *The Practice* with respect to all matters concerned with health, safety and welfare has been drawn up/ agreed by...('the employer') in consultation with the practice team. The persons with specific responsibilities for ensuring that appropriate details of the policy are specified and fully implemented at The Practice are the:

1. **Practice Safety Officer**... who, under the direction of and in liaison with the employer or practice manager.., undertakes to:

- Ensure the implementation of all practice H&S policies
- Keep up-to-date with H&S legislation and associated practice policies (as directed)
- Ensure ALL staff who work at the practice receive appropriate H&S instruction and training
- Keep ALL staff aware of the high priority given by the practice to health and safety: advise and remind staff of their **general** responsibilities to themselves and those around them; advise and remind the **Fire Officer, Area Safety Officers** and **First Aiders**, of their **specific** responsibilities
- Advise/liaise with those responsible for the design and construction of new buildings and modifications to existing buildings, to assist them to ensure all necessary and appropriate safety features and procedures are included in all designs and work programmes
- Ensure provision of First Aid personnel, materials and procedures appropriate for the practice
- Compile and review data concerning accidents, incidents and staff health issues and ensure that all are recorded, reported and investigated in accordance with practice and legislative procedures.

The Practice Safety Officer will also, directly or by delegation to the following area safety officers:

AREA SAFETY OFFICERS:	Responsible for (specific areas)
....	....
....	....
....	....
....	....

undertake to:

- Disseminate information on specific safety matters within specific areas
- Advise on and check procedures to ensure the safety of work within specific areas
- Ensure that new employees are fully aware of specific safety policies and standards if/as they apply to arrangements and procedures for specific areas
- Ensure all relevant employees are made aware of any special or new hazards about to be introduced into specific areas
- Ensure that all accidents, incidents and staff health issues associated with specific areas are reported promptly in accordance with the procedures of The Practice
- Carry out or arrange for the necessary safety inspections, checks and assessments, and the recording of the results on appropriate record forms, as required for specific areas – i.e. as specified in the Local Rules and Codes of Practice section of the practice health and safety manual.

2. **Practice FIRE OFFICER**..who, under the direction and on behalf of the person with ultimate responsibility for the building..undertakes to:

- Ensure that a fire risk assessment has been carried out and is reviewed as necessary
- Ensure that the firefighting equipment and the automatic fire alarm system (if installed) is examined and serviced by approved contractors at appropriate intervals (at least annually)
- Ensure that any/all fire detection and alarm systems installed are tested weekly in house
- Ensure that sufficient legally compliant fire safety signage is displayed
- Ensure all fire exits and escape routes are regularly checked and kept free of obstructions
- Ensure all staff receive appropriate training in the use of emergency firefighting equipment
- Ensure that sufficient and appropriate fire drills are carried out
- Ensure that all architect's drawings for proposed alterations/extensions to the premises are submitted to the appropriate planning/fire authorities for approval; and maintain liaison with outside inspectors (e.g. from the fire service and insurance companies) and ensure that their recommendations/stipulations are fully considered/ implemented
- Provide advice to staff and contractors, etc. on any topic related to the fire precautions
- Maintain a record of all fires (and near incidents) and the steps taken to ascertain their cause.

continues

An example of a practice Health and Safety Policy: Management Arrangements. (continues) ▶

Health and Safety Policy: Health and Safety Management Arrangements *continued*

3. H&S COORDINATOR.. who, in consultation with

4. H&S 'COMPETENT PERSON'.. undertakes to:

- Serve as the source of 'competent advice' to enable the practice to appropriately and effectively manage health and safety
- Ensure the Practice Safety Officer, Area Manager and Fire Officer are kept up-to-date with H&S legislation; maintain a log of when specific health and safety inspections and risk assessments are to be carried out or reviewed, and issue reminders to relevant persons in the practice
- Ensure the practice H&S manual is reviewed/revised as necessary to address all new/amended legislation, and that up-to-date health and safety records are maintained.

		Level of FA training:
5. FIRST AIDERS	(1)	....
	(2)	....
and/or		
APPOINTED PERSONS	(1)	....
	(2)	....

who undertake to:

- Regularly check the contents of all First Aid boxes and eye wash bottles (to comply with HSE/RCVS approved contents/standards) and re-stock or renew as necessary
- Keep up-to-date with accepted First Aid practices (appropriate to their role as FA or AP)
- Carry out or witness all initial First Aid treatments, **and/or** take charge in an emergency – i.e. administer emergency First Aid **and/or** call for an ambulance or medical assistance
- Never go beyond their level of training regarding provision of First Aid treatment or advice
- Ensure all accidents are recorded/reported in accordance with the practice procedures.

(continued) An example of a practice Health and Safety Policy: Management Arrangements.

Requirement	YES	NO/?
Physical conditions		
1. Are all areas inside and out (including doorways, stairways, walkways, car parks, etc.) free from:		
▪ Obstructions?		
▪ Loose/trailing cables (i.e. that may present trip and/or electrical hazards)?		
▪ Other slip/trip/fall hazards (wet/uneven/moss-covered floors/paths/steps; raised/loose tiles/paving/drain covers; damaged/loose flooring/carpet; potholes; shallow/unmarked steps; loose/non-existent handrails; items/papers left/stored on stairs, etc.)?		
▪ Risk of collision with structures or objects (obscured pillars, low beams, filing cabinet drawers, cupboard doors, etc.)?		
▪ Risk of falling objects (top-heavy filing cabinets, unstable/poorly stacked racks/shelves, loose roof tiles, unprotected low lights, etc.)?		
▪ Unstable/insecure fixtures/fittings/structures (walls, fences, roofs, pipes, floors, scaffolding, equipment mounts/brackets, etc.)?		
2. Are all hazards and safety features signed as necessary (and do signs comply with The Health and Safety (Safety Signs and Signals) Regulations 1996, if/as necessary)?		
3. Are all 'non-work' areas adequately lit (e.g. stairways, store rooms, entrances, exits, outside walkways)?		
4. Are pedestrians (staff/clients) adequately protected from vehicles (e.g. in drives, car parks, delivery areas)?		
5. Are all traffic routes appropriately signed and free from blind spots or equipped with safety mirrors?		
6. Do service engineers/maintenance workers have easy/safe access to areas and equipment as/when needed?		
7. Is all work equipment, etc. safely supported by the furniture, floor or stand, etc. on which it sits?		
8. Are all items of furniture, fixtures, racks, shelves, etc. stable such that they cannot give way or topple over?		
9. Are all items of equipment/furniture free from broken or loose parts, sharp/rough edges, protruding keys, etc.?		
10. Are all items in store easily and safely accessible – especially those needed frequently?		
11. Are heavier items that have to be manually handled stored at waist height (or on the floor if a trolley can/must be used)?		
12. Are appropriate, safety-checked steps or ladders available for work above head height (e.g. storing/retrieving, fitting bulbs)?		
13. Are all hazardous substances (drugs, chemicals, gases, paints, etc.) clearly labelled and kept safely/securely at all times?		
14. Are all safety-critical machines/appliances (X-ray, anaesthetic, lifting, electrical, heating, etc.) appropriately serviced?		
15. Has the electrical system (wiring, RCDs, fuses, earth bonds, etc.) been checked and passed/certified within the last 5 years?		
16. Are all sockets/switches in good order, in appropriate/safe places and/or protected (e.g. from rain, leaks, splashes)?		
17. Is the rule of one plug per socket being adhered to?		
The Workplace (Health, Safety and Welfare) Regulations 1992 **In all work areas:**		
23. Is the temperature within The Workplace (Health, Safety and Welfare) Regulations 1992 guideline limits all year (i.e. not so hot or cold that it affects concentration)?		
24. Is the fresh air ventilation sufficient all year (not too humid/stuffy or high CO_2 to cause headaches, lethargy, flu-like symptoms)?		
25. Is lighting, space, layout, equipment acceptable according to The Workplace (Health, Safety and Welfare) Regulations 1992 (such that tasks can be performed safely and comfortably)?		
26. Is the noise in each area below The Control of Noise at Work Regulations 2005 action and nuisance levels (not too loud, distracting or wearing)?		
27. Are washing and sanitary facilities sufficient and appropriate, clean and well appointed (i.e. as required under The Workplace (Health, Safety and Welfare) Regulations 1992)?		
28. Are eating/rest areas sufficient and appropriate, and kept clean and tidy?		
29. Do all doors open freely and easily?		
30. Do all doors that need them have safety vision panels?		
31. Is any full length glass conspicuously marked so as to make it apparent?		
32. Are any wide, tall or low level windows made of safety glass or covered with anti-shatter film?		
33. Can all windows (that will/need to be) be opened/closed easily/safely, with no broken or damaged fittings or glass?		

An example of a checklist that can be used for assessing potential hazards related to premises. (continues) ▶

Hygiene and housekeeping		
34. Are all areas, floors, work surfaces, etc. kept clean and tidy and free from litter and other waste (especially clinical waste)?		
35. Are there appropriate bins for all categories of waste, and are they used correctly and emptied regularly?		
36. Are appropriate spillage kits available for dealing with spills of hazardous substances (e.g. X-ray chemicals, lab reagents)?		
37. Are heaters, air conditioning vents, passive anaesthetic scavenging outlets, etc. kept free of obstructions?		
38. Are coats, bags, personal possessions stowed safely and away from work areas (i.e. secure and unobstructive)?		
39. Is used protective clothing/soiled bedding, etc. kept away from clean clothing/bedding and clean surfaces?		
40. Are good hygiene practices adopted for food/drink, animals/drugs/chemicals, clothes and handwashing?		
Public areas and access/egress		
41. Are all entrances/exits free from obstructions and slip/trip hazards (e.g. loose/damaged doormats)?		
42. Are suitable facilities/provisions available/made for disabled access and use of sanitary facilities?		
43. Are toilets that are used by clients kept free of hazardous chemicals and maintained to high standards of hygiene?		
44. Are members of the public prevented from unauthorized/unsupervised access to hazardous substances?		
45. Are the premises adequately protected against intruders/break-ins (e.g. alarm, barred windows, manned 24 hours)?		
46. Are staff adequately protected from risk of assault by clients/intruders (e.g. by barriers, panic buttons, personal alarms)?		
Accident and First Aid facilities and procedures		
47. Is an accident book compliant with the Data Protection Act 1998 provided and readily available?		
48. Are adequate First Aid boxes and eyewash facilities provided, in appropriate places, clearly signed and unobstructed?		
49. Have First Aid boxes and eyewash facilities been checked/re-stocked in accordance with relevant schedules?		
50. Are First Aid action and information notices prominently displayed or available, and do they give clear up-to-date instruction/information?		

Inspection carried out by:............................ **Record appraised/confirmed by:**............................

Date:............................

Next inspection due:............................

(continued) An example of a checklist that can be used for assessing potential hazards related to premises.

Strategic and business planning

23

Pippa Reffold

All veterinary practices should consider themselves to be businesses. In simple terms, a practice offers a product or a service to meet a customer need. The aim of this chapter is to give all veterinary practices, no matter what size, a workable guide to strategic and business planning. Strategy and planning should not be viewed as theoretical enigmas, but as essential tools for survival and growth.

What is strategy?

In simple terms, strategy is the long-term intent of a practice or business, which can be visualized by a team. It encompasses the following elements:

- **Visionary ideas** – Where does the practice want to be?
- **Competitive advantage** – How will the practice differentiate itself in the market?
- **Objectives** – How is the practice going to get there?

Revitalizing, growing or starting up a business will require some important decisions to be made in order to achieve goals and targets. By developing and then implementing a realistic strategy, the long-term business potential will be maximized.

> **KEY POINTS**
>
> A strategic plan is different from a business plan:
>
> - A **strategic plan** focuses on the *mid- to long-term* goals of a business and the *broad strategies* needed to achieve them
> - A **business plan** focuses on the *short- to mid-term* goals of a business and how it will achieve them.

Devising the strategic plan

Devising a workable strategic plan should be a critical consideration for any business or practice. Time must be set aside for this and the right people must be involved in the process. A realistic and achievable timescale should be set.

Who to involve

In order to help eliminate bias, the plan should ideally be devised by more than one person. Involving the team, accountant, advisors, suppliers and clients should be considered. Involving somebody who will play 'devil's advocate' is also recommended, as they will really test the strategy.

> **KEY POINT**
>
> Managers should be prepared to delegate some elements of the planning to other people and to enlist external support where necessary in order to stay on top of the process.

The process

There is no set way to run the process whereby the strategic plan is devised. However, it is important to ensure that everyone knows how they will be involved and when meetings will be held. One person should facilitate all meetings. Individuals and teams may be given investigation projects, which they work on independently and then bring back to the meetings.

In order to develop a good strategic plan, two steps must first be taken:

1. Preparation – including the use of models to assess the current situation and explore the direction the business should be taking.
2. Competitive strategy – to be decided on by the business.

A timescale should be set for this process and meeting dates should be entered into the diary – two to three months should be adequate for the formulation of most strategic plans.

Preparation for developing the strategic plan

When developing a strategic plan, intensive research and analysis will need to be undertaken. This is as appropriate for a start-up or growing practice as for one that needs revitalizing. Good preparation will ensure a well thought-through and, more importantly, achievable strategy.

In order to work out the best strategic plan, time should be spent thinking about the current situation. It may be worthwhile to engage a specialist consultant or advisor to help with this process. Owners and managers become very close to the business and therefore do not always have a realistic perspective of the situation. Guidance from an impartial person can be very enlightening.

Models to assess the business

Strategic planning is not an exact science but is a process that allows choices to be made based on assessment and identification. It is therefore crucial that ample time is allocated to the use of appropriate models, so as to provide a strong foundation of knowledge upon which the business can map its future. Three models are commonly used to help businesses assess their strategic direction:

- STEEPLE
- SWOT
- Porter's five forces.

To enable these models to be used effectively, the difference between the internal and external environment must first be understood. In simple terms:

- The **internal environment** is the practice itself
- The **external environment** covers all areas affecting the internal environment that the practice does not have direct influence or total control over, e.g. government legislation and social trends.

An awareness of external changes and trends is necessary to ensure that the internal environment, which is controlled, meets the business needs of the practice. Informed decisions can then be taken within the internal environment to gain a competitive edge.

STEEPLE

The strategy should enable the business to meet the market need, whether current or future; the strategy will therefore be based on assumptions of the current and future external environment. These assumptions are made using an understanding of the key areas that can influence the environment. That is where the STEEPLE model comes in.

An extension of the much used PESTEL analysis, the STEEPLE analysis considers **s**ocial, **t**echnological, **e**conomic, **e**nvironmental, **p**olitical, **l**egal and **e**thical factors that affect the market and the wider environment. The external environment is comprised of these and all general external uncontrollable forces and pressures that indirectly influence and affect the practice. This analysis is useful when considering the wider impacts that the external environment has on the business. Each of the potential external factors should be explored, considering anything that is happening that could present a possible threat or opportunity. It is important to be specific with regard to the level of risk or benefit to the business. Grading the level as high, medium or low risk could be helpful. It can also be useful to map out the factors that are identified, e.g. on a flip chart. It is important to be prepared to investigate some of the findings more thoroughly. Findings should be written up and distributed to all those involved. Quite often when using this type of model certain areas are clearly identified (they may 'jump out of the page') and these may form the basis of the strategy.

Social factors

These will include the demographic and cultural aspects of the external environment. These factors will affect customer needs and the size of the potential market. Areas to consider include:

- Health
- Human and specific animal population growth rates
- Popular pets and animals
- Age profile of humans and animals
- Age distribution
- Working profiles
- Values and culture
- Lifestyles
- Attitudes to work and culture
- 'Green' environmental issues
- Education
- Demographic changes
- Distribution of income
- Attitude to pets.

Technological factors

Technology can define a differentiating factor; it can influence capital expenditure and outsourcing decisions. Areas to consider include:

- Latest research and development activities and trends
- Rate of technological change and cost
- Government and regional (e.g. European Union) investment policies
- New research incentives
- New patents and products
- Incentives and support to invest in new patents and products
- Speed of change and adoption of new technologies
- Level of expenditure on research and development (R&D) by rivals
- Developments in unrelated industries that could be adapted for use in the veterinary industry.

Economic factors

Economic factors will affect the purchasing power of potential customers, as well as the cost of expenditure and supplies. Areas to consider include:

- Local, national and global economic growth
- Interest rates
- Exchange rates
- Inflation rates
- Total gross domestic product (GDP) per head, consumer expenditure and disposable income
- Currency fluctuations
- Investment trends
- Cyclicality
- Unemployment
- Energy, transport, communication and raw materials costs.

Environmental factors

These will affect decisions regarding market placement, physical location and product or service choice. Areas to consider include:

- 'Green' issues
- Government environmental policies
- Environmental regulations
- Renewable energy
- Waste and its disposal
- Veterinary environmental trends
- Cultural perception
- Environmental trends
- Animals in the environment.

Political factors

These define formal and informal rules within which the practice must operate. Areas to consider include:

- Trade restrictions
- Political stability
- Government ownership and attitude to monopolies and competition
- Relationships between government and committees, regulatory bodies and trade associations
- Trade restrictions and tariffs
- Local authorities
- Specific regulations within the sector.

Legal factors

These will define the formal rules that the practice must abide by or be prepared to influence. Areas to consider include:

- Current and future legislative changes
- Regulatory guidelines (e.g. RCVS)
- Health and safety laws
- Veterinary medicines legislation
- Medical laws
- Competition law
- Employment law
- Animal welfare legislation
- Drugs or working practices becoming illegal
- Legislation relating to drugs for competition animals
- Legislation relating to animals for food, e.g. withdrawal times
- Other relevant national legislation (e.g. Dangerous Dogs Act 1991 and proposed changes for control of dogs).

Ethical factors

These factors are the ethical or moral issues that currently or potentially affect the veterinary industry and market (see Chapter 21). Areas to consider include:

- Interactions with other professionals
- Euthanasia policies
- Where an animal is kept
- What conditions animals are kept in
- Domestic pets *versus* wildlife
- Cleaning principles
- Feeding principles
- Administration of drugs
- Medical intervention
- Guidance and advice
- Involvement of RSPCA/the law
- Knowledge of owners.

SWOT

SWOT is the acronym for **s**trengths, **w**eaknesses, **o**pportunities and **t**hreats. It is probably the most commonly known analysis and is useful for a number of reasons:

- It is a good mechanism for assessing a business's capabilities and resources in comparison to the external environment
- It is an excellent way to identify the overall strategic position and direction of the business in its environment
- It can be used to assess a business, a proposition or an idea, and can therefore be used when assessing diversification of the business
- It is very simple to use
- It can be used for businesses of all sizes
- It will normally throw up significant issues that would otherwise have remained hidden.

The SWOT analysis is normally presented as a grid with four sections, one for each of the SWOT headings. When embarking on a SWOT analysis it is important to be clear on what is being assessed. In the case of a strategic plan, the practice is being assessed against the external environment.

Figure 23.1 gives an idea of what to consider when preparing a SWOT document and, although not an exhaustive list, it demonstrates some of the core areas that should be discussed and included in the document.

Figure 23.2 is an example of a completed SWOT analysis. The action plan from this would contain the following points:

- Define core competency – e.g. do surgeons offer the best service for existing clients? If not how can these be improved?
- Investigate who the target clients are
- Investigate where target clients are located
- Consider outsourcing marketing
- Consider further CPD in business development and leadership skills for the practice principal
- Look at options to gain financial investment.

Once the SWOT analysis is complete, the findings can be used to create action points. The best way to work out the action plan is by segment:

- Strengths – maintain, build and leverage the practice
- Weaknesses – remedy or exit
- Opportunities – prioritize and optimize
- Threats – counter.

KEY POINT

It is useful to complete the STEEPLE analysis before carrying out the SWOT analysis. This will help to identify external factors prior to considering the internal factors of the SWOT (strengths and weaknesses). There is an overlap between the two models: STEEPLE provokes consideration of the external environment and SWOT allows the practice to map itself within that environment.

Strengths (internal)	Weaknesses (internal)
■ Advantages of service/product ■ Capabilities ■ Competitive advantages ■ USPs (unique selling points) ■ Resources, assets, people ■ Experience, knowledge, data ■ Financial reserves, likely returns ■ Marketing – customer base, distribution, awareness ■ Innovation ■ Customer service and loyalty ■ Location ■ Price, value, quality ■ Accreditations, qualifications, certifications ■ Processes, systems, IT, communications ■ Cultural and behavioural issues ■ Management cover, succession ■ Values ■ Employees' skills ■ Speed of decision-making ■ Implementation skills	■ Disadvantages of service/product ■ Gaps in capabilities ■ Lack of competitive strength ■ Reputation, presence and customer base? ■ Customer loyalty ■ Financials ■ Vulnerabilities ■ Pressures ■ Cash flow ■ Continuity ■ Supply robustness ■ Effects on core activities, distraction ■ Reliability of data ■ Planning ability ■ Morale, commitment, leadership ■ Accreditations, etc. ■ Processes and systems, etc. ■ Management cover, succession ■ Speed of decision-making ■ Implementation skills
Opportunities (external)	**Threats (external)**
■ Market developments ■ Competitors' vulnerabilities ■ Industry or lifestyle trends ■ Technology development and innovation ■ Global influences ■ New markets ■ Niche target markets ■ Geographical, export, import ■ New USPs ■ New product or service ■ Business and product development ■ Information and research ■ Economic environment ■ Partnerships, agencies, distribution ■ Economy ■ Seasonal, weather ■ Fashion influences	■ Political effects ■ Legislative effects ■ Environmental effects ■ IT developments ■ Competitor intentions – various ■ Market demand ■ New technologies, services, ideas ■ Partners ■ Reliance on customer base ■ Threats to internal capabilities ■ Obstacles faced ■ Insurmountable weaknesses ■ Loss of key staff ■ Threats to financial backing ■ Economy – home, abroad ■ Seasonality, weather effects ■ Financial markets and lending ■ Health scares ■ Demographics

23.1 Areas to consider in a practice's SWOT analysis. In this process, one of the objectives should be to turn weaknesses into strengths and threats into opportunities. It is important to remember that strengths and weaknesses relate to the internal environment (i.e. the practice) and opportunities and threats relate to the external environment.

Strengths	Weaknesses
■ Only practice to offer in-house surgery for a variety of domestic animals ■ Experienced team ■ Domestic animals ■ 25 years established ■ Own premises ■ Team involved in lectures and demonstrations ■ Experts in our field ■ Repeat business and referrals ■ Currently financially sound ■ Owner managed ■ Excellent IT processes	■ Clients need to travel a long distance ■ Reliant on experienced team ■ Long-term finance draining ■ Owner managed ■ Lack of succession ■ Customer base reducing ■ Lack of marketing skills ■ Lack of management experience in business to encourage growth ■ Aftercare service
Opportunities	**Threats**
■ Expansion ■ Referrals from other practices and colleges ■ Franchise ■ New location(s) ■ Marketing ■ Add-on products and services ■ Work with universities and colleges ■ Succession ■ Leadership development	■ Economic climate ■ New practices in area ■ Loss of key employees ■ Retirement of owner ■ Lack of lending by institutions ■ Not enough money for new ideas ■ Changes in local authority and government ■ Decline in disposable income

23.2 An example of a SWOT analysis.

Porter's five forces

The last tool to consider is 'Porter's five forces' (Figure 23.3). Michael Porter provides a framework that models an industry as being influenced by five forces (Porter, 1979). This is an excellent tool with which to develop an edge over competitors. It is similar to STEEPLE in that it facilitates the understanding of the environment within which the practice operates. It is, however, more specific to each individual business and the direct influences of competitors, suppliers and clients. The risks and opportunities that arise in each of the market forces must be considered when using this model, along with their potential impacts on the practice.

The five forces are:

- Supplier power
- Barriers to entry
- Rivalry
- Threat of substitutes
- Buyer power.

Completion of the five forces exercise should throw up some key strategic objectives. The business may be vulnerable because it relies on just one supplier for the majority of its products. It could be that the practice is located in an area in which its services are in over-supply. The practice may find that it has no identity or differentiation in the market so customers may choose to go elsewhere. As with STEEPLE and SWOT, some key action points can be fed into the strategic planning process through this model.

Supplier power

How easy is it for the practice's suppliers to find alternative buyers for their product or service? How much can the practice's suppliers push up prices (e.g. if the practice has only one supplier, or if the supplier is the only company to make the product)?

These factors will have a significant impact on the costs and profitability of the practice. These factors also apply to drug manufacturers that sell to wholesalers as well as to wholesalers that sell to veterinary practices. For example, some products that were classified as POM-V prescription-only medicines have changed their legal category and can now be sold in other outlets such as pet shops. This has been good for suppliers in providing alternative buyers for their products, and potentially increasing their sales, but has not been good for veterinary practices.

Supplier power is also relevant when considering a specific drug for which there is just one manufacturer with a veterinary authorization. While there are no alternatives the price will remain high. The situation will change, however, if a new product or human generic drug becomes authorized for veterinary use.

Barriers to entry

How difficult is it for potential competitors to enter the practice's market? If more businesses compete in the market, it makes it difficult to retain market share and maintain price levels to the customer. The corporate joint venture partnership model is encouraging more veterinary surgeons to set up small practices with one or two veterinary surgeons, resulting in overall

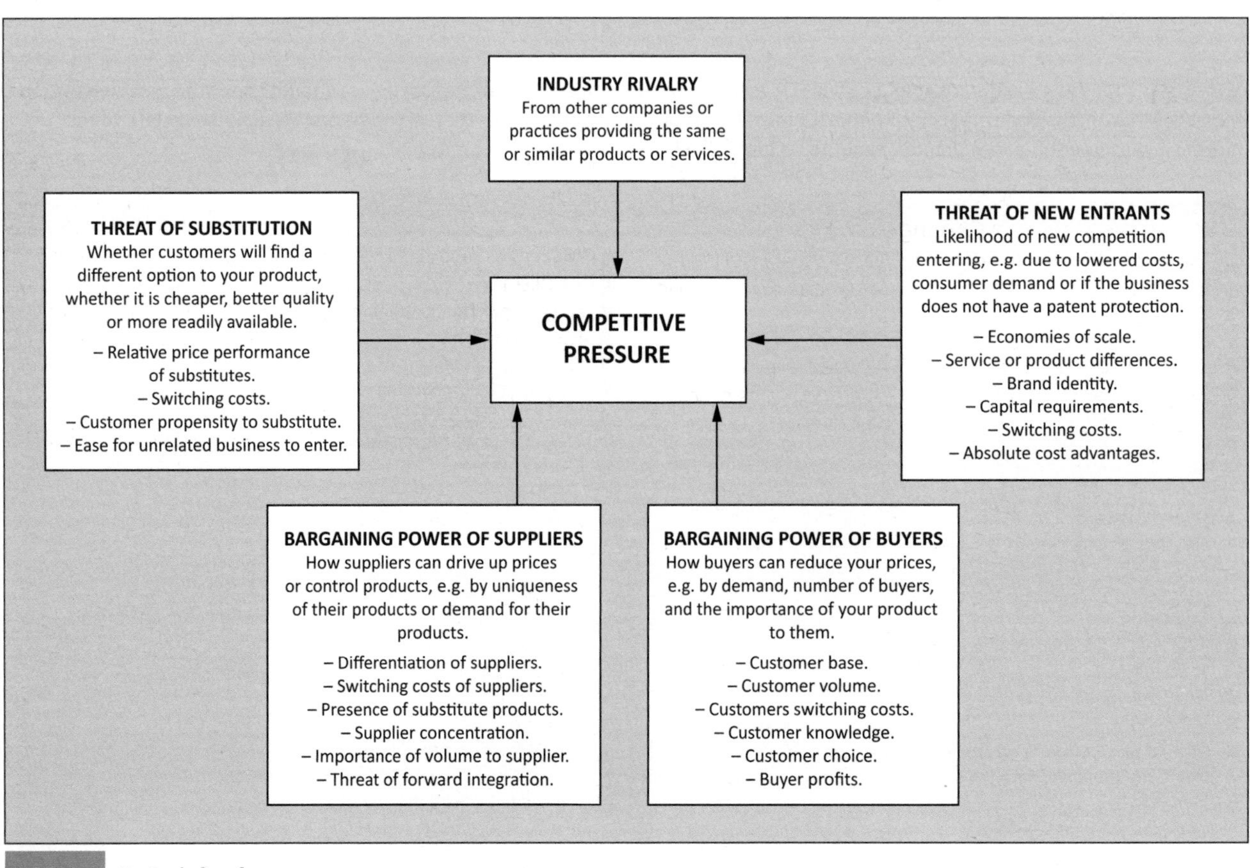

INDUSTRY RIVALRY
From other companies or practices providing the same or similar products or services.
THREAT OF SUBSTITUTION
Whether customers will find a different option to your product, whether it is cheaper, better quality or more readily available.
– Relative price performance of substitutes.
– Switching costs.
– Customer propensity to substitute.
– Ease for unrelated business to enter.
COMPETITIVE PRESSURE
THREAT OF NEW ENTRANTS
Likelihood of new competition entering, e.g. due to lowered costs, consumer demand or if the business does not have a patent protection.
– Economies of scale.
– Service or product differences.
– Brand identity.
– Capital requirements.
– Switching costs.
– Absolute cost advantages.
BARGAINING POWER OF SUPPLIERS
How suppliers can drive up prices or control products, e.g. by uniqueness of their products or demand for their products.
– Differentiation of suppliers.
– Switching costs of suppliers.
– Presence of substitute products.
– Supplier concentration.
– Importance of volume to supplier.
– Threat of forward integration.
BARGAINING POWER OF BUYERS
How buyers can reduce your prices, e.g. by demand, number of buyers, and the importance of your product to them.
– Customer base.
– Customer volume.
– Customers switching costs.
– Customer knowledge.
– Customer choice.
– Buyer profits.

23.3 Porter's five forces.

increased numbers of practices. Competition is not only from other veterinary practices, but may also come from the Internet, charities, pet shops or retailers.

> **KEY POINT**
>
> What is unique about the practice's offering that will prevent others from entering the market?

Rivalry

How many other companies or practices are providing the same or similar products or services? This depends on the number and relative strengths of the businesses within the market and the ease with which customers can switch between them. More importantly, what can be done to prevent this?

Threat of substitutes

Is there a possibility that the products or services the practice is offering will no longer be required? Could an alternative be offered by someone else (e.g. a major retailer/pet shop offering veterinary services)? Clients are now searching the Internet for advice, paraprofessionals offer their services and there are an increasing number of part-time courses on subjects such as canine massage, physical therapy, behavioural therapy and hydrotherapy.

Buyer power

How easy is it for buyers to find alternative vendors for products? The higher the bargaining power of customers, the more this puts a downward pressure on prices and revenue. For example, clients are increasingly choosing to buy on the Internet rather than from the practice.

Other issues to consider

Strategic tools such as STEEPLE, SWOT and Porter's five forces may lead to the discovery that fundamental changes are needed in order for the business to survive and grow. These changes must feature in the strategic plan; to ensure that the plan will be successful, some of the following areas may need to be challenged.

- **The role of the owner:** Many owners make excellent leaders and managers; some focus on this aspect and employ someone else to do the routine clinical work, allowing them more time for the development of the strategic plan. However, where owners do not have management skills in abundance, it may be more appropriate for them to concentrate on the clinical area and allow someone else with the necessary knowledge, skills and experience to run the business. Not everyone makes a good leader or manager, and the owner may have to make a conscious decision to step back and, more importantly, to allow another person to take over if required.
- **The location:** The assessment process may indicate that the practice is not located in the best position to target its chosen clientèle. In order to gain market share and better skilled employees, the practice may need to move. As discussed later, care must be taken when opening new branches; the location must be correct for the practice's core competency – cost or differentiation (see Chapter 1).
- **Ownership structure:** The more a business grows, the more sophisticated it needs to be regarding finance, processes and procedures. In order to achieve this, new skills and additional finance may need to be brought in. Financial investment could be through giving up shares, accepting investment or borrowing from the bank, and will very much depend on the needs of the business.

Choosing a competitive strategy

It is difficult to be successful if the practice is trying to be all things to all people (i.e. being the cost leader and yet differentiated, and serving both the mass and niche markets). The practice must define its competitive strategy so that it can determine its marketing strategy (see Chapter 25). In particular it must understand market needs and then offer its service or product; the practice's core competencies must be considered in relation to the market in which it competes. Within a practice there may be a multitude of competencies, e.g. specialist veterinary skills, customer care, accounting skills, technical equipment expertise. These must be matched with the needs of the market, which must therefore be understood. There is no point having a highly specialized veterinary practice with state-of-the-art equipment if the client does not recognize this, does not need it, or cannot afford it. This is not just a poorly thought-out strategy; it may affect the sustainability of the practice.

Leading on differentiation or cost

In order to gain competitive success, the practice will need to know what its core focus is: cost or differentiation. The choices a practice makes will enable it to lead on one or the other. To be somewhere in the middle of the two can be very dangerous, particularly if the client cannot identify either. This does not prevent a practice from appearing to be leading on cost, e.g. cheap vaccines, but in fact being more expensive for other services.

In order for the business to consider its future, it must develop a competitive edge. Generic competitive strategies, as devised by Michael Porter, are summarized in Figure 23.4. According to Porter (1980), in order to define the strategy a choice will

	Low cost	Higher cost
Broad	Overall cost leadership, e.g. vaccination clinic or charity	Differentiation, e.g. developed general practice with range of services through different branches
Narrow	Cost focus, e.g. 'cheap and cheerful' single practice	Differentiation focus, e.g. referral practice

23.4 Generic competitive strategies (Porter, 1980).

have to be made as to whether the practice wishes to compete to achieve a narrow or broad target. In the case of a veterinary practice, this will normally depend on the number of sites it operates from.

Cost leadership

If the strategic direction is based on competing on cost, then the practice must lead its competitors on price. In order to do this all practice costs must be low and sustainable. This is called cost leadership.

If a practice chooses to provide a low-cost option for clients and the intention is to remain a one-practice organization, this strategy will be within the narrow target low-cost segment of Figure 23.4. The strategic drivers will be to monitor the competition and to keep prices below those of competitors whilst keeping overheads low. This strategy is vulnerable as the practice could fail or, at the very least, just break even if a client base is not generated quickly or if competitors continually drop their prices.

If, however, a practice decides to offer a 'cheap and cheerful' service at multiple sites, it will be the low-cost option for clients but will have more than one practice or outlet and so will fall within the broad target low-cost segment of Figure 23.4. The strategic drivers will be the same as for the above example but the practice will aim for a wider market. Offerings will have to be more general within the domestic animal sector, as the practice will not be able to afford costly equipment to specialize. All practice sites will have to be based within the cheapest rentable or affordable areas in order to maintain the cost base and be located close to target clients (i.e. price-conscious families and individuals). The practice will not be attempting to offer all types of service to everyone, but will focus on one segment of the market. It will be clean and modern with no room for anything else. It should be seen as convenient and cost-effective. For example, many charities offer a reduced 'no nonsense' veterinary service to people who re-home their animals.

Differentiation leadership

When a practice differentiates itself as opposed to copying the competition, it will normally aim to ensure that the veterinary offering is better than the competitors' offerings. This will usually allow the practice to charge more for products and services. If the value of the differentiation is not recognized by the client, however, the practice will lose out as it will have to cut its prices to get more business and yet carry higher internal costs.

Whether differentiation is to a broad or narrow target (see Figure 23.4), the practice will need to concentrate on offering a unique service that competitors cannot easily copy. For example, possessing the latest technical equipment within the small animal sector, which competitors cannot easily replicate, will differentiate the practice within its sector. It will be able to charge more for its services due to the lack of competition and the higher cost of the technical equipment and specialist skills. In order to retain the competitive advantage, it will need to differentiate itself from competitors constantly. The costs and skills required to run the practice will be higher. The most important thing to establish when considering this strategy is whether there is a market for the service. A multi-site practice should tread cautiously when expanding by acquiring new practices, as these may not have the same differentiating skills. Care should also be taken with regard to differentiating when opening new branches; it is important to research the geographical area in which the practice intends to open its new business outlet. The local market may not need or even recognize the differentiated service offered.

Diversification

Diversification is an option that a practice can consider in order to offer a different service to clients and thus make more profit. Diversification is not always as easy as it may at first appear, and the idea may be best assessed as if it is a separate business. Ideas can be tested using analyses such as STEEPLE, SWOT and Porter's five forces (see above). Just because the practice has a strong customer base, it does not always mean there is a market for the new idea or that the practice has the internal skills to implement a diversification.

An example of diversification is a practice that may want to offer dog grooming. The strengths might be that it would be convenient for clients and there is a demand for the service; the weakness could be space limitations. The opportunity might be to sell more over-the-counter products such as brushes and shampoos; the threat could be from a new dog grooming business that has opened in the next town. The practice would need to consider whether any members of staff have sufficient dog grooming experience and skills and, if not, whether someone with the required skills could be recruited.

Whatever the diversification idea may be, it is important to go through the whole process of planning again, methodically, setting key performance indicators (KPIs) and/or objectives. An implementation plan should be set in place and progress monitored.

Putting the strategic plan together

Encompassing the conclusions of the preparation stage and the chosen competitive strategy, the strategic plan should now be devised. It is the owner of the business who, having involved all the team in discussions, will ultimately need to decide on the strategic plan. A realistic vision and mission statement need to be written down. The practice vision must be compelling and inspiring, as it will need to motivate those involved in order to turn it into reality.

The vision and mission statements may be only a paragraph long but have to answer the following questions fully and clearly:

- What is the business?
- What is the market?
- What is the potential of the business?
- What are the forecast profits?
- What money is needed?

A clear set of objectives, responsibilities and budgets should then be set against this strategic intent.

Implementing a strategic plan

To implement a strategic plan, the goals and timescales required should be defined meticulously. The implementation of a strategic plan can be thought of as crossing a river using a series of stepping stones: each stone is critical to ensure completion of the journey and each one has to be completed in sequence. At this stage it may be necessary to involve more people who understand the workings of the business. Those who work in the practice on a day-to-day basis will have a very good idea as to whether something is going to work or not. Another option is to use an external advisor or consultant to monitor and review progress with the team; they will do this dispassionately and ensure that everyone is held accountable.

Each area of the business must be assigned goals, responsibilities and deadlines. For example, if the goal is to increase the number of vaccinations in dogs, cats and rabbits, current numbers should be identified and increased to a realistic level over an agreed timeframe (Figure 23.5). For each goal one person should be held accountable.

Patient type	Now	Quarter 1	Quarter 2	Quarter 3	Quarter 4
Dogs	30	50	60	70	90
Cats	25	35	50	65	80
Rabbits	15	20	25	35	40

23.5 In order to increase the number of vaccinations for dogs, cats and rabbits, current numbers should be identified and realistic targets set over an agreed timeframe.

KEY POINT

All objectives must be SMART:

- **S**tretching
- **M**easureable
- **A**chievable
- **R**esults-driven
- **T**ime-bound.

Reviewing and monitoring how objectives are being met and implemented is absolutely crucial, with any amendments being made as necessary. The use of key performance indicators (KPIs; Figure 23.6) should be considered. These define the key objectives that indicate how well the business is doing. KPI targets are normally set against revenue, profit, customer service, new clients, client retention, overhead costs, new market penetration and employees' objectives.

KEY POINT

Only the KPIs most appropriate to the chosen strategy should be selected. There should not be too many KPIs, otherwise more time will be spent monitoring than implementing.

The business plan

In order for the business to flourish and grow, it is imperative that a business has a manager/owner that is prepared to put time and effort into devising a business plan. The manager/owner must be clear as to whether the business is being reactive to the market or proactive – in other words, is it just 'fighting the fires' or is it wanting to steer itself to growth?

The following should be borne in mind when devising a business plan:

- It can be put together:
  - On an annual basis
  - Over a 3-year period with a 5- to 10-year strategic plan
  - Or combined according to preference
- It does not need to be any more that five to ten pages long; a brilliant plan that fills lots of paper and is left on a shelf to gather dust is not helpful
- It should be a working document that defines the practice's direction
- It must be easily accessible to all those who need to implement the vision
- It should be a reminder of practice strategy, and should also serve to remind everyone what has to be done, by whom and by when
- It should ensure support in the right places and secure finance
- It should provide a blueprint to run the business
- It should be achievable
- It should allow the business to be steered through the good and the harder times.

KEY POINT

The business plan must be completely consistent with the strategic plan in order for implementation to succeed.

KPI	Now	Quarter 1	Quarter 2	Quarter 3	Quarter 4	Annualized
Turnover	£250k	+ £15k	+£15k	+£20k	+£20k	£320k
Profitability	£2.5k	+ £5k	+£5k	+£10k	+£10k	£32.5k
Overheads	£200k	–£2.5k	–£2.5k	–£5k	–£5k	–£15k
New clients	20	10	10	10	10	40
Customer complaints	10	2	1	1	1	5

23.6 An example of the KPI targets set by a veterinary practice.

What benefits can a business plan provide?

- A clear and concise business plan will draw a clear picture of the business objectives.
- It will facilitate the identification of the key driving forces required to make the business thrive.
- It will allow all staff to concentrate on the core requirements of the business and therefore drop other time-wasting tasks or responsibilities.
- Very importantly, it will provide an up-to-date understanding of the state of the industry that the business operates within.

All stakeholders (i.e. shareholders, owners, directors, partners, staff, suppliers and clients) need to have a clear perspective as to where they fit into the business. It is important that the business embraces all stakeholders as part of its long-term plan and considers the impact that each may be able to have on the business as a whole. A plan that celebrates their inclusion will enable any potential investor, partner or bank to see clearly whether the business is suitable for them to invest their time and/or money in.

Lastly, planning provides the opportunity to give a chronology of events and financial milestones against which actual results can be compared. It will allow alternative actions (contingency plans) to be considered if an objective is falling short of the original requirements.

What should be included in the business plan?

The elements of a business plan are listed in Figure 23.7. This type of business plan is used for driving the business forward from day to day; a different type of plan will be needed for submitting to a bank or investor when financing or refinancing a business.

- Executive summary
- The business
- The team
- Business environment
- Sales and marketing plan
- Operations
- Finance
- Risk

23.7 Elements of the business plan.

Executive summary

The executive summary should be written last, as its purpose is to summarize the business plan. Although this is the last page to be written, it is the opening page of the plan. The executive summary should be concise and need only fill half an A4 page. It will often be read by people unfamiliar with the business, so technical jargon should be avoided.

KEY POINT

The executive summary may be the only page of the business plan that is read.

The executive summary highlights the most important points of the business and should summarize the six key areas:

- The business's product or service and its advantages (strategic intent)
- Its opportunity in the market (strategic intent)
- Its management team (core skill)
- Its track record to date (how the business started)
- Financial projections (could be KPIs)
- Any funding or ownership details (strategic intent).

The business

The background to the business should be explained, including:

- The amount of time that has been spent on developing the business idea in its present form
- The work that has been carried out to date
- Any relevant experience the owner has or the business has used.

The product or service the business is offering should then be explained. It should:

- Stand out from others (cost or differentiation)
- Define what customers will gain through buying the business's product or service
- Explain how the business will be developed to meet customers' changing needs in the future. Any disadvantages or weak points should also be explained (SWOT). This will inspire confidence.

Finally, the key features in the industry (STEEPLE and Porter's five forces) should be explained.

The team

This section should address the following questions:

- Who is in the team and what does the structure chart look like?
- What are the reporting lines and who are the senior members?
- What roles and specific skills does the team possess and where do they need to develop?
- Which skills will the team need to possess in the future, and how many staff will be required to support any changes and developments?

This section should include any outside stakeholders that have an impact on the business, e.g. the bank, auditors, key consultants and investors.

Business environment

This section should include where the business started, what stage it is at, the size of the industry and the business's position within that industry environment. The following questions should be answered:

- What are the long-term views of the industry? How will the trends affect the business?
- Does the business have any legal patent, trademarks or copyrights that protect it? If so, are they up to date and valid?

- Who are the business's clients and what is the demographic breakdown of their profile? (Published demographic data are available.)

Sales and marketing plan

This should focus on the segments of the market that the business proposes to target, indicating how large each market may be and whether it is growing or declining. Important trends should be illustrated, along with the reasons behind them. This section should address why clients come to the business. What benefits do they enjoy? Is it the value for money, friendly reliable service, new technologies, or after-care support? It should also define the clients that the practice wants to attract, and outline the required numbers of these clients. Too many clients may weaken the benefits of the practice; this may therefore be an opportunity to expand by acquisition or by physically enlarging the premises, or both.

Lastly, the marketing materials that will be needed to attract and, most importantly, maintain the client base should be considered, remembering that it can cost up to ten times as much to attract a new client as to maintain a current one. Consideration should be given to the required marketing activity, e.g. public relations support, advertising, promotional literature, website and social networking (see Chapter 25). The following questions should be considered:

- How will the practice sell its existing or new products and services?
- How will the practice be positioned in the marketplace? Price, quality and after-sales?
- Will sales activity be face to face (e.g. in a consultation), by phone, website or through an agent (e.g. via referral practices)?
- Will a new product or service start in one practice and then expand to any branch surgeries?
- What will be the profit contributions? Sales forecasts are very often over-estimated. Useful check points include:
  - How soon can the practice start selling its services or product?
  - How big is the target market? (e.g. a new product for rabbits may not sell in the same quantity as one for dogs)
  - Is there potential for repeat business?

Operations

These are the facilities the business will need to have in order to deliver the product or service.

- Which premises will the practice operate from and will this be owned or rented?
- Who will be the suppliers and what should be expected of them regarding support, discounts, staff training, etc.?
- What equipment will be needed to support the practice, including that for surgery, offices and home visits (mobile equipment)?
- Which industry and professional bodies will the business belong to and which guidelines will it follow?

Finance

- Will the business be self-funded or does it need investors? How will financial resources be managed?
- What are the business's financial projections, investments and, most importantly, cash flow projections? Profit and loss, balance sheets and cash flow spreadsheets should be included in this section (see Chapter 24).
- Who will manage the financial aspects of the business and who will audit them?

Risk

This is a very valuable 'what if' section:

- What will the business do if the number of competitors increases?
- What if a key employee leaves?
- What if the business falls into financial difficulties?
- What are the risks specific to the veterinary industry?
- What if demand for all or some of the practice's services or products diminishes?
- What if technology moves on?

Devising the business plan

The following steps should be taken when devising the business plan:

- Decide when the process is going to start, and set a realistic completion date
- Involve key members of the team and stakeholders (as previously discussed) and an external person if appropriate
- Decide from the start what the purpose of this plan is and who will be using it
- Assign sections to others and give them deadlines to complete, if necessary/appropriate
- Take some time to investigate and research the sections to make sure that value is added to the plan
- Always make sure that SMART objectives and milestones are set for the business, and make sure these are reviewed. This is fundamental to a successful plan.

Once all of the above has been carried out, the information should be collated and the first draft of the plan completed. The draft should be read carefully and any grammatical, tactical or spelling mistakes corrected. At this stage, someone impartial could be asked to read the content to make sure it flows and is understandable. All final adjustments should be made and the executive summary should then be written.

Implementing the business plan

- The plan or a section of the plan should be communicated to all members of the team. They will be responsible for the implementation of the plan, which could lead it to succeed or fail.

- Quarterly or monthly meetings should be arranged with the team at which the progress of the business plan is reviewed. At these meetings it will be important to consider any changes required to the plan due to unforeseen circumstances or if some of the risk factors have occurred or altered.
- If the business is looking for investment, any good investor or bank will ask for a formal review with the owner and the team on a regular basis. They will want to see where their money is being spent and when they can expect to get a return.

KEY POINT

A business plan should be work in progress as the practice continuously evolves.

References

Porter ME (1979) How Competitive Forces Shape Strategy. *Harvard Business Review*. March/April 1979.

Porter ME (1980) *Competitive Strategy: Techniques for Analyzing Industries and Competitors*. Macmillan, New York

Finance

24

Andy Moore

Finances are fundamentally important to every practice, no matter how large or small. Profit is essential for the survival of the business. The systems, reporting and analysis will vary substantially between practices, and a firm grasp of the basic principles and broad concepts is needed for anyone involved in ownership or management of a veterinary practice. When it comes to staff, finance is a subject of discussion that was historically considered to be taboo; in the past, any performance information was confined to owners and managers. This approach ignores the very real impact practice staff can have on the performance and profits of the practice, and has become outdated. Communication and feedback of appropriate information relating to practice performance and finances should be part and parcel of practice life and the overall management of the practice. The financial principles and concepts contained in this chapter are universal. Points relating to taxation are specific to the UK tax system and legislation. Non-UK resident readers should seek advice specific to their location.

KEY POINT

To produce numbers that summarize what has happened and then do nothing risks the practice doing no more than recording its demise. The value of numbers lies in the action that is taken based on what they show; this is always the difficult part of management.

All references to taxes (direct or indirect) within this chapter relate to the UK tax system and rates.

The basics of practice finance

A sound understanding of the basic terminology of practice finance (Figure 24.1), definitions and calculations of key percentages is required for interpreting and understanding the numbers.

Term	Definition
Cost of sales	The cost incurred in a period, net of VAT, of all goods purchased for re-sale and any other direct costs incurred in order to achieve the turnover generated in that period. The cost figure is adjusted for the value of any items in stock at the start and end of the period, i.e. it is only the value of goods consumed or sold that is recognized as a cost in the period. Within veterinary practices, it is common for labour costs to be excluded from this figure initially and considered separately for analysis and benchmarking purposes. If they are included here as a personal preference then it will only be professional salaries that are included.
Cost-plus pricing	One method used to determine the selling price of an item. It is calculated on the cost price of an item, to which a percentage mark-up is then added. The cost price is normally taken as the list price of the item purchased but can also include an amount for a proportion of the variable costs incurred in the business.
Current assets	The value of current assets is the value of all assets that are reasonably expected to be converted into cash within 1 year in the normal course of business. Current assets include cash, current bank accounts, the value of debtors, stock held for resale, prepaid expenses and any other assets that can easily be converted to cash.
Current liabilities	The value of current liabilities is the value of all creditors who are owed money by the business, together with any other liabilities or obligations due for payment within 1 year. They include any short-term debt (e.g. bank overdraft), creditors, accrued expenses and any other short-term liability.

24.1 Definitions of some of the terms used in this chapter. (continues)

Term	Definition
Fixed costs	Expenses that do not vary with the level of income or activity of the business. An example would be rent that remains fixed at the level agreed, regardless of whether no fees are generated or substantial fees are generated.
Gross profit (gross margin)	Calculated by deducting the cost of sales for the period from the turnover generated in the same period.
Gross profit percentage	The gross profit for the period in monetary terms divided by the turnover for the same period, expressed as a percentage (i.e. multiplied by 100).
Mark-up	The amount added to the cost price of medicines and other purchased items for resale to arrive at the selling price. The mark-up is added so as to generate a surplus over costs to pay for wages and overhead costs and generate a profit.
Net profit	The amount remaining after all trading expenses incurred in a period have been deducted from the total turnover generated in the same period.
Overheads	The ongoing expenses of running a business other than the costs of sales (direct costs). For analysis purposes, they are normally grouped into: establishment costs, administration costs, financial costs and depreciation (see Figure 24.2). Labour costs may be considered separately or included under costs of sales or under overheads, depending on the accounts structure.
Stock	The value of all items held for resale. The value shown should be the cost of purchase net of all discounts and rebates received relating to the purchases.
Turnover	The total value of work undertaken and goods sold in a period, net of (i.e. without) VAT (see below). The figure is the value of the work undertaken and goods sold, regardless of whether they have been paid for by the client.
Value added tax (VAT)	Tax paid on all taxable supplies made by VAT-registered business and on all taxable goods sold by a VAT-registered business.
Variable costs	Expenses that change according to the level of activity of the business. Examples would include postage costs, telephone charges and some labour costs.
Working capital	The funding that a business uses in its day-to-day trading operations. It is calculated as the current assets of a business less its current liabilities.

24.1 (continued) Definitions of some of the terms used in this chapter.

Turnover

It is crucial to appreciate that all figures should be considered net of VAT. At the current rate of 20% VAT (April 2012), of every £1.20 received by the practice, 20p never belongs to it.

Net	100p
VAT	20p
Gross	120p

- To get net from gross, divide gross by 1.2
- To get gross from net, multiply net by 1.2

Each £1 of turnover (net of VAT) received by the practice will be made up of two types of income:

- **Professional fee income** incurs the direct cost of the labour needed to generate that income; this may be either employed labour or proprietorial labour (that of the owners)
- **Medicine and retail sales** incur the direct costs of drug purchases, to which a mark-up is applied to arrive at the selling price. There is some labour cost incurred in achieving these sales but it should not be material in terms of the marginal staffing requirement and is commonly ignored for analysis purposes.

Within first-opinion small animal practice, the ratio of fee income to medicine income (fee to drug ratio) will usually range between 60:40 and 70:30. Total vaccine sales are included within the fee income figure for this key performance indicator (KPI).

Turnover monitoring can be of use as a quick and easy headline figure for communication with staff. A rolling annual figure is best used so as to adjust for seasonality of workload and provide a very quick, easily digested indicator. Turnover provides an easily monitored figure for staff to focus on and encourages them to drive the practice forward. For more on communicating practice performance to staff see Chapter 17.

Mark-up and gross profit

These terms are easiest to understand using an example.

Drugs purchased for	£100
Mark-up applied	50%
Selling price of drugs	£150
Turnover (drugs sales)	£150
Costs of drugs purchased	£100
Gross profit	£50

The gross profit % is then calculated as:

(gross profit ÷ turnover) x 100 = (£50 ÷ £150) x 100 = 33.33%

At a 50% mark-up, the gross profit is 33.33%

Discounting

If a discount is given to a client of, say, 10% on an invoice of £150 (excluding VAT), many people simply believe that £15 has been given away and that has little impact. However, if the position is considered:

	After discount	Before discount
Turnover (discounted) (£150 less 10%)	£135	£150
Costs of drugs purchased	£100	£100
Gross profit	£35	£50

Gross profit before discount (£50) – gross profit after discount (£35) = £15 lost

(£15 ÷ £50) x 100 = 30% lost profit

In terms of gross profit given away, the loss is £15 out of a gross profit of £50. This means that 30% of the gross profit has been given away for a 10% discount to the client. Discounting must be treated with caution!

Cost-plus pricing

Historically, veterinary practices have adopted cost-plus pricing, as defined in Figure 24.1. This has worked in broad terms but needs to be reviewed for specific products to ensure that profits are not given away.

This is best considered with an example. Drug 1 has traditionally been used. The purchase cost is £5 per unit and mark-up (MU) is 100%, giving a sales price of £10 per unit. In the year, the practice sells 250 units. The position is then:

Scenario 1	
Selling price	£5 + 100% MU = £10
Sales (units)	250
Sales income	250 x £10 = £2,500
Unit cost	£5
Cost of sales	250 x £5 = £1250
Gross profit	£2,500 - £1,250 = £1,250

Following a review, the practice locates a cheaper alternative with a purchase cost of £2.50 per unit. If the same cost-plus approach is used, the figures then become:

Scenario 2	
Selling price	£2.50 + 100% MU = £5
Sales (units)	250
Sales income	250 x £5 = £1,250
Unit cost	£2.50
Cost of sales	250 x £2.50 = £625
Gross profit	£1,250 - £625 = £625

By improving the buying position, the practice has reduced turnover by £1,250 and has reduced profits by £625. If no price pressure existed from clients, the practice could have retained the higher selling price and benefited from increased profits:

Scenario 3	
Selling price	£10
Sales (units)	250
Sales income	250 x £10 = £2,500
Unit cost	£2.50
Cost of sales	250 x £2.50 = £625
Gross profit	£2,500 – £625 = £1,875

A further alternative to consider is one in which drug 1 can be sourced more cheaply but the selling price is set so as to maintain profits, passing on a price reduction to the client.

Margin per unit required:	
Gross profit as per Scenario 1	£1,250
Units to sell	250
Gross profit per unit required	(£1,250 ÷ 250) = £5
Buying price per unit	£2.50
Add gross profit per unit	£5.00
Selling price per unit	£7.50

The results then become:

Scenario 4	
Selling price	£7.50
Sales (units)	250
Sales income	250 x £7.50 = £1,875
Unit cost	£2.50
Cost of sales	250 x £2.50 = £625
Gross profit	£1875 – 625 = £1250

The effect is that the practice maintains profits and the client pays less. This may be an option for chronic medications in the face of price pressure or competition.

To summarize the scenarios:

Scenario	***1***	***2***	***3***	***4***
Sales income	£2,500	£1,250	£2,500	£1,875
Cost of sales	£1,250	£625	£625	£625
Gross profit	£1,250	£625	£1,875	£1,250
Mark-up	100%	100%	400%	200%
Gross profit	50%	50%	75%	66.67%

So, if better buying is possible, cost-plus pricing may need specific review by product to vary the mark-up according to market conditions. Every practice and practice owner will have a different view on this but a conscious decision must be taken.

Gross profit

The gross profit for a veterinary practice is calculated as shown below. The items included within cost of sales are for illustration and are not intended to be exhaustive.

	£	£
Turnover:		
Fees		70,000
Drugs		30,000
		100,000
Cost of sales:		
Drugs used	20,000	
Lab fees (external)	2,000	
Lab consumables (internal)	1,000	
Cremation fees and waste disposal	1,000	
Surgical and other consumables	1,000	
Pharmaceutical rebates	(2,000)	
		(23,000)
Gross profit (GP)		77,000

GP % = (£77,000 ÷ £100,000) x 100 = 77%
Fee to drug ratio =
(£70,000 ÷ £100,000):(£30,000 ÷ £100,000) = 70:30

The gross profit is calculated before taking account of any labour costs or other costs of running the practice. It gives an indication as to:

- **The pricing structure of the practice** – Practices vary considerably with respect to the mark-up applied to drugs and the charge they make for professional fees, e.g. within consulting charges and surgical theatre time
- **How that pricing structure is applied by the practice staff** – On occasions staff will not apply the price structure set, either consciously (override of clinical system pricing) or subconsciously (free-of-charge consultations or underestimation of surgical time, for example). In this situation, the GP% will drop
- **The nature of work undertaken** – The mix of fee income relative to drug income will be affected by the type of practice (first-opinion or referral), the nature of any referral specialism, the level of work-up of cases, client compliance, client finances, the type of client base and the current economic climate.

It is from the gross profit generated that all other costs have to be met, such as:

- The costs of staffing the practice
- The costs of running the facilities
- All other overhead expenses (Figure 24.2)
- The cash required for funding equipment and other capital expenditure
- A reward for the proprietor's clinical time, skills and expertise
- A reward for the proprietor's management time, skills and expertise
- A return for the proprietor's investment of funds
- A return for the risk taken by the proprietors.

Gross profit therefore plays a pivotal role in the success (or survival) of a practice. Many people focus on turnover; however, conversion of turnover to gross profit and then to net profit is of far greater (and fundamental) importance.

Establishment

- Rent
- Rates and water
- Premises insurance
- Light and heat
- Repairs and maintenance

Administration

- Telephone
- Printing, postage and stationery
- Advertising and practice development costs
- Computer costs
- Sundry expenses and cleaning
- Motor expenses and travelling
- Equipment leasing
- Subscriptions
- Professional indemnity insurance

Financial

- Bank interest
- Bank loan interest
- Hire purchase interest
- Bank charges
- Bad and doubtful debts
- Credit card charges
- Accountancy and bookkeeping
- Legal and professional fees

Depreciation

24.2 Overhead expenses are the ongoing costs of running a business other than the costs of sales and are normally grouped for analysis purposes.

Net profit

At its simplest, net profit is the invoiced turnover (net of VAT) less the expenses incurred (net of VAT) in order to achieve that turnover.

The net profit is stated after all staff costs and costs of running the practice have been deducted. The cash in the bank account of the practice does not necessarily reflect the net profit the practice generates. This is a fundamental concept to grasp. The net profit is calculated by reference to work invoiced, regardless of when paid, and the expenditure incurred to generate that turnover, regardless of when or how the expenditure is paid. The production of accounts to arrive at the net profit involves numerous accounting adjustments, as discussed below.

Cash flow

Cash flow is, in essence, the money coming into and going out of the practice: cash, cheques, FPS (faster payment service), BACS, debit cards and credit cards. If everything goes through a single bank account then it is the bank balance that reflects the practice cash flow.

The old adage of 'cash (flow) is king' holds a great deal of truth, particularly in recessionary or volatile economic times. Management of the practice to protect cash flow and ensure it is healthy (and positive) is fundamental. This is considered in detail later.

Tax

To quote Benjamin Franklin, 'in this world nothing can be said to be certain except death and taxes'. The main taxes to be aware of are discussed in broad terms below.

Value Added Tax (VAT)

A business is compelled to register for VAT when the turnover of the business exceeds the VAT registration limit in any 12-month period. Alternatively, a business may choose voluntarily to register for VAT. At the time of writing (April 2012), the VAT registration limit is £77,000.

- **Output VAT** is charged on all taxable supplies made by a VAT-registered business. Certain supplies to registered charities can be exempt and thus supplied with no VAT charged.
- **Input VAT** is paid on all taxable purchases made by a VAT-registered business.

The practice is acting as an unpaid VAT collector and is required to pay over to HM Revenue and Customs (HMRC) the difference between output VAT charged (collected) by the practice and input VAT suffered by the practice. There are a number of adjustments made to the payments in a situation where there is any private use of vehicles, rental income received and private use on any other expenses incurred.

The frequency with which the difference has to be paid can be monthly, quarterly or annually; a quarterly return period is the most commonly used. The quarterly return details certain financial information about the trade of the practice. Penalties may be imposed if there is repeated late submission of returns, and interest will normally be charged on late payments.

HMRC will visit businesses to ensure they are making correct returns. Some businesses will never have an inspection; some will have inspections frequently. To a large extent, inspections are a random selection process, although certain anomalies in returns or persistent late submission may well encourage a visit.

Pay As You Earn (PAYE) and National Insurance Contributions (NIC)

All employers are obliged to set up payroll schemes with HMRC, no matter how few employees they have (see later for more information on payroll). The employer is obliged to deduct tax at source from each employee, as determined by a notice of coding (issued to the employee and copied to the employer by HMRC) that is then applied to the HMRC payroll tables or input into a proprietary payroll software package.

The employer also has to deduct employees' NIC from the employee and to pay employer's NIC on the gross wage. Reports are required to be submitted to HMRC and to employees from time to time. An example, with figures for illustration only, is given below.

Gross salary	£1,000
Employer's NIC	£55
Employee's NIC	£45
PAYE	£80
Paid to employee:	
Gross salary	£1,000
Less PAYE	(£80)
Employee's NIC	(£45)
Net pay	£875
Paid to HMRC:	
PAYE	£80
Employee's NIC	£45
Employer's NIC	£55
	£180
Gross cost to practice:	
Gross salary	£1,000
Employer's NIC	£55
	£1,055

The deductions are paid over to HMRC monthly (or quarterly for small employers). The employer also has to pay National Insurance (Class 1a NI) on the value of any benefit provided to employees. This is currently charged at 13.8% of the value of the benefit provided and is paid to HMRC in one lump sum annually.

Income tax

Individuals must pay income tax (and NIC) on earnings less allowable expenses on a tax-year basis (i.e. between 6th April and the following 5th April). Income tax is paid by individuals on their total income, regardless of whether this comes from a partnership, limited liability partnership (LLP), property rental, dividend income or salary. In a partnership, the partners pay income tax and NIC on their share of the profits made each year, regardless of how much they withdraw from, or introduce to, the business.

Corporation tax

Corporation tax is paid by a limited company on the profits generated by the company in each accounting year.

Trading structures

It should be noted that, regardless of trading structure or ownership structure, the financial principles remain. It is only the accounting, taxation and legal treatment of the entities that differ.

Within veterinary practice, the most common trading and ownership structures are:

- Sole trader
- Partnership
- Limited liability partnership
- Limited company.

Another structure increasingly appearing in the veterinary profession is the joint venture (JV), either with corporate JV partners or with other independent practices. Detailed consideration of this type of structure is beyond the scope of this chapter but all financial principles remain unchanged.

The trading structure and ownership structure are one and the same. If a practice trades as a partnership it is owned by the partners; if it trades as a company it is owned by the shareholders. The key points relating to the legal and accounting issues of the different trading structures are set out below in summary form. The most appropriate structure for any practice depends on a multitude of factors. Selection of the appropriate structure or structures is beyond the scope of this chapter and a matter where specific specialist professional advice must be taken.

Sole trader

- A sole trader is not a separate legal entity.
- A sole trader is a trading name for the individual owner.
- A sole trader is one individual.
- The individual owner will be responsible for running the business and owns the profits that it makes.
- The liability of the individual owner is unlimited in respect of business debts and liabilities.
- Annual accounts have no statutory format.
- Accounts do not need to be filed on any public record and are compiled to give the owner a picture of the business performance and to facilitate the completion of a tax return.
- Profits generated are taxed on the individual owner as they arise, regardless of how much that individual introduces to or withdraws from the business.

Partnership

- A partnership is not a separate legal entity.
- It is registered with HMRC and is issued a unique tax reference number.
- It is owned by the partners.
- A partnership must comprise two or more partners.
- The partners normally share in both the responsibilities of running the business and the profits that it makes.
- It is also possible for limited companies to be partners.
- A partnership agreement should be drawn up to govern how the rights and responsibilities of partners are defined and divided, as well as how profits should be allocated.
- The liability of the partners is unlimited, joint and several in respect of partnership debts and liabilities.
- Annual accounts have no statutory format.
- Accounts do not need to be filed on any public record and are simply compiled to give the partners a picture of the business performance and to facilitate the completion of tax returns.
- Profits generated are taxed on the individual partners as they arise, regardless of how much a partner withdraws from the partnership.

Limited liability partnership

- A limited liability partnership (LLP) is a separate legal entity from its members.
- An LLP is formed at Companies House and has a unique identification number at Companies House.
- On formation, a certificate of incorporation is produced by Companies House – in effect, the LLP's birth certificate.
- It is owned by its members. In effect they are the same as partners.
- An LLP must have at least two members, and at least two must be 'designated' members.
- The members of an LLP normally share in both the responsibilities of running the business and the profits that it makes.
- It is also possible for limited companies to be members of an LLP.
- Designated members have responsibilities in addition to those of ordinary members in relation to ensuring that the LLP meets various legal obligations, including: making sure that the annual accounts and returns are properly signed and delivered to Companies House; and being responsible for appointing auditors if necessary. Designated members are legally accountable if they fail to carry out their duties properly.
- A members' agreement should be drawn up to govern how the rights and responsibilities of members are defined and divided, as well as how profits should be allocated.
- The liability of the members is limited to the amount of capital they have invested, provided that there has been no fraud or intentional wrongdoing.
- Annual accounts are prepared in a statutory format in accordance with UK Accounting Standards and other accounting requirements relating specifically to LLPs.
- Accounts are required to be filed at Companies House (and are placed on the public record), generally within 9 months of the year end.
- Small LLPs (those with a turnover of less than £6.5 million) can take advantage of the option to submit abbreviated accounts. The abbreviated accounts are, in effect, a foreshortened balance sheet with brief associated notes. Anyone viewing these would have very limited information as to the financial position of the practice and no information relating to profitability.
- Profits generated are taxed on the members in the same way as a partnership, i.e. as they arise.

Limited company

- A limited company is a separate legal entity.
- Companies are formed at Companies House. On incorporation, a company is given a unique company number and the Certificate of Incorporation is issued – in effect, the company's birth certificate.
- The company has directors who are responsible for the running of the company. All limited companies must have at least one director.
- The company is owned by its shareholders.
- The directors and shareholders do not need to be the same individuals but can be the same (and often are in smaller companies).

- Directors usually receive a salary for the work undertaken on behalf of the company. This is subject to PAYE and National Insurance in the same way as for any other employee.
- If the company is profitable, dividends can be paid to the shareholders as a return for their investment in the company. Dividends received by an individual are subject to income tax but are not currently liable to National Insurance.
- Directors have certain legal responsibilities as set out in the Companies Act 2006, the details of which can be obtained from the Companies House website (www.companieshouse.gov.uk).
- Directors are required to act in a way that is most likely to promote the success of the company for the benefit of the shareholders.
- Directors also have many business and legal responsibilities for ensuring the success of their company, in areas such as health and safety, employment law and tax.
- The liability of the shareholders is limited to the value of the capital they have invested (i.e. shares and retained profit). In some cases this may also extend to personal guarantees given to, for instance, banks to secure finance.
- Annual accounts are prepared in a statutory format in accordance with UK Accounting Standards.
- Accounts are required to be filed at Companies House (and are placed on the public record), generally within 9 months of the year end. Small companies (turnover less than £6.5 million) can take advantage of the option to file abbreviated accounts, i.e. foreshortened balance sheet and restricted notes, revealing limited information to external parties.
- Profits generated by the company are currently subject to corporation tax of: 20% (small companies rate) on profits up to £300,000; 27.5% (marginal rate) on profits between £300,001 and £1.5 million; and 26% (main rate) thereafter. (The rates are scheduled to reduce over the course of the next 3 years, currently set to become 20% small companies rate and 23% main rate (24% marginal rate) effective from 1st April 2014.)
- Payment of the tax liability is due 9 months and 1 day after the year end of the company (where taxable profits are less than £1.5 million per annum).

Practice financial software

All practices will have some form of financial systems in place.

The practice management system

The practice management system (PMS) is also considered in detail in Chapter 4. The financial module of the PMS will provide detailed analysis of the turnover generated by the practice. Reports can be produced to analyse the split of income between fee income and medicine sales, the work type undertaken, the work undertaken by each member of staff, etc. The range of reports, flexibility and the ease of extracting information for financial and staff management should be one of the key factors when selecting a PMS.

Whilst many practice management systems can potentially integrate with accounting software, in practice the most efficient accounting and recording method tends to be a straightforward manual summary entry (from the PMS) within the accounting software. This avoids the duplication of holding the data in two locations and saves the time, effort and frustrations of data mapping between clinical and accounting software. Any analysis of turnover is then normally produced from the PMS, rather than from the accounting software. Commonly, the PMS will be used to record and manage the sales ledger (invoices to and payments received from clients). The PMS will be used to generate sales invoices and issue statements to chase up debtors (clients who owe money to the practice). The PMS should be capable of maintaining stock control records and producing stock valuation reports. To produce accurate figures requires strict discipline to be in place; this often proves problematic in practice.

The accounting software

There are a number of software packages on the market and also software designers who will construct bespoke packages if required. The accounting software is used to process purchase ledger payments (payments to suppliers), bank payments and cash payments, and to produce quarterly VAT returns for the practice. It also is used to record the turnover and draw together the figures so as to produce accounts (management and draft financials) for the practice. In most cases it will be used to generate monthly, quarterly and annual accounts information, as referred to below. Within some packages the facility exists to import (or input) the practice's financial budgets so as to facilitate easy reporting of actual results against budgets; this feature is often ignored but is very useful.

Financial information available to practices

Profit and loss account

The profit and loss account summarizes the turnover generated by the practice (net of VAT for a specific period of time) (Figure 24.3). From that turnover, the direct costs of generating that turnover are deducted, leaving the gross profit. The remaining expenditure incurred in generating that income is then shown, also net of VAT. The resultant figure is the net profit for the practice.

It is worth noting that a figure is included for depreciation. Depreciation is normally calculated by the accountant, and is designed to reflect the wearing out of the assets.

When an item of equipment is purchased, such as a digital X-ray machine, this cost is shown in the balance sheet (see below) as an asset, and is not shown in the profit and loss account. The cost of that equipment is then written off against profit by way of a depreciation charge over a period of time as the

	Current year £	Current year £	Previous year £	Previous year £
Sales				
Fees		700,000		600,000
Drugs		300,000		285,000
		1,000,000		885,000
Cost of sales				
Opening stock	80,000		70,000	
Purchases	220,000		185,000	
Lab and specialist fees	30,000		28,000	
Waste disposal and cremation	10,000		9,000	
Referral fees	10,000		9,000	
Rebates received	(20,000)		(2,000)	
Closing stock	(100,000)		(80,000)	
		(230,000)		(219,000)
Gross profit		770,000		666,000
Expenses				
Labour	300,000		270,000	
Establishment	40,000		38,000	
Administration	70,000		65,000	
Financial	50,000		48,000	
Depreciation	34,250		25,000	
		(494,250)		(446,000)
Trading profit		275,750		220,000
Other income				
Interest receivable	100		100	
Miscellaneous income	1,000		800	
Rent receivable	20,000		20,000	
		21,100		20,900
Net profit		**296,850**		**240,900**

24.3 An example of a profit and loss account.

X-ray machine is used. In effect, the depreciation charge should be building a cash reserve from profits to facilitate the replacement of the asset when, ultimately, it is worn out. This can be a difficult concept, but one that is important for a number of reasons. It particularly becomes an issue where practices are managed on a 'cash basis', i.e. if there is cash in the bank, extra drawings are taken without realizing that part of the cash is to replace equipment.

Fixed assets

A fixed assets register (FAR) is illustrated in Figure 24.4. Practices can maintain their FAR in house, although it is normally left to the accountant to prepare and maintain it.

An FAR can easily be set up in a spreadsheet. The minimum information to be recorded is:

- Date of purchase
- Description of asset
- Purchase cost (net of VAT).

Ideally, it should also record:

- Serial number of asset (useful record for insurance purposes if required)
- Other details for identification purposes.

For accounts purposes it should then also contain:

- Depreciation charge to date brought forward
- Depreciation charged in the period
- Depreciation charge to date carried forward.

There is no hard and fast rule as to which purchases should go into fixed assets (be capitalized) and what should be written off to the profit and loss account as repairs and renewals. Each item of expenditure must be considered individually.

Small items under a certain monetary value would normally be classed as 'repairs'. The monetary limit will often be determined by the size of the practice and what is considered material. For example, a small start-up practice may view £100 as material and show all items costing over £100 as fixed assets, whereas a larger practice may view an individual item limit of £500 as more appropriate.

Replacing part of a larger asset will normally be a repair, regardless of cost; e.g. a new engine in a car is a repair; a replacement camera for an endoscope is a repair.

A number of small items grouped to form a larger asset would normally be capitalized; e.g. when buying computer parts to build a new computer, all parts purchased would be capitalized.

A new asset of continuing use to the practice, not intended for resale, would be capitalized, e.g. a new endoscope or digital X-ray machine.

Special rules exist for 'fungible' assets: these are groups of smaller items such as the initial equipping of a surgery with surgical equipment or the initial forming of a clinical reference library. The initial purchases are capitalized but subsequent updating and replacements are treated as repairs.

Description	Cost				Depreciation				NBV this year	NBV last year	Disposal proceeds	Profit/loss on disposal
	Brought forward	Additions	Disposals	Carried forward	Brought forward	Charge	Disposals	Carried forward				
Land and buildings:												
Property 1	750,000	–	–	750,000	–	–	–	–	750,000	750,000	–	–
Property 2	500,000			500,000	–	–	–	–	500,000	500,000	–	–
	1,250,000	–	–	1,250,000	–	–	–	–	1,250,000	1,250,000	–	–
Vehicles:												
Vehicle 1	20,000	–	–	20,000	6,000	3,500	–	9,500	10,500	14,000	–	–
Vehicle 2	15,000	–	–	15,000	5,000	2,500	–	7,500	7,500	10,000	–	–
Vehicle 3	25,000	–	–	25,000	6,000	4,750	–	10,750	14,250	19,000	–	–
Vehicle 4	–	30,000	–	30,000	–	7,500	–	7,500	22,500	–	–	–
	60,000	30,000	–	90,000	17,000	18,250	–	35,250	54,750	43,000	–	–
Equipment:												
Scanner	10,000	–	(10,000)	–	8,000	–	(8,000)	–	–	2,000	2,000	–
X-ray	50,000	–	–	50,000	25,000	5,000	–	30,000	20,000	25,000	–	–
Computers	50,000	–	–	50,000	20,000	6,000	–	26,000	24,000	30,000	–	–
Endoscope	–	5,000	–	5,000	–	2,000	–	2,000	3,000	–	–	–
Scanner	–	15,000	–	15,000	–	3,000	–	3,000	12,000	–	–	–
	110,000	20,000	(10,000)	120,000	53,000	16,000	(8,000)	61,000	59,000	57,000	2,000	–
	1,420,000	**50,000**	**(10,000)**	**1,460,000**	**70,000**	**34,250**	**(8,000)**	**96,250**	**1,363,750**	**1,350,000**	**2,000**	–

24.4 An example of a fixed assets register. NBV = net book value.

Depreciation

As noted above, the basic principle of depreciation is to reflect the wearing out of an asset as it is used to generate income for the practice. An example of this would be a blood analyser machine, which may wear out over a 4-year period. The calculation to arrive at the depreciation charge is, at its simplest:

Asset purchase cost	£10,000
Assumed sale value in 4 years	£2,000
	£8,000
Useful life of asset	4 years
Depreciation charge per year	£8,000 ÷ 4 = £2,000 per annum

Alternatively, a straightforward reducing balance method can be used.

	25%	**20%**
Cost	£10,000	£10,000
Year 1 depreciation	(£2,500)	(£2,000)
WDV c/f	£7,500	£8,000
Year 2 depreciation	(£1,875)	(£1,600)
WDV c/f	£5,625	£6,400

(WDV = written-down value; c/f = carried forward)

There are more involved depreciation methods, e.g. the 'sum of the digits' method, where the depreciation charge is loaded into the earlier years when the reduction in value of the asset is higher than in the later years. However, in veterinary practice very few would use this approach.

The balance sheet

The balance sheet (Figure 24.5) provides a snapshot of the assets and liabilities of the practice at a point in time. It will record the tangible assets, and the value shown will be the written-down value of the equipment and other assets within the practice. This figure is not designed to be a market value, but simply records the historical cost less any depreciation charged during the life of each asset. Intangible assets within a veterinary practice will commonly be goodwill.

Goodwill

Special consideration must be given to the subject of goodwill. At its simplest, goodwill is the difference between the total value of a business that someone is prepared to pay, as compared to the underlying net value of the assets in that business. A goodwill value arises from the ability of the business to generate returns for the owners in excess of what they could generate for their time in the market place (i.e. working as an employee). In effect, it is buying future profits. Taking a straightforward example:

- An owner of a business could earn £40,000 salary for the clinical work they undertake in their practice
- The practice generates £100,000 per annum total profit for them
- The business is generating £100,000 minus £40,000 = £60,000 of 'super profits' each year. The goodwill value is often calculated as a multiple of the super profits
- Many factors influence the value of goodwill, but ultimately the fundamental issue is the level of additional income the purchaser will receive in excess of a normal return.

	Current Year £	Current Year £	Previous Year £	Previous Year £
Fixed assets				
Tangible fixed assets:				
Property		1,250,000		1,250,000
Equipment		113,750		100,000
Goodwill		100,000		100,000
Investments		1,000		1,000
		1,464,750		1,451,000
Current assets				
Stock	100,000		80,000	
Debtors and prepayments	210,000		200,000	
Cash at bank and in hand	50,000		10,000	
	360,000		290,000	
Current liabilities				
Creditors and accruals	170,000		120,000	
Loans due within 1 year	60,000		60,000	
	230,000		180,000	
Net current assets		130,000		110,000
		1,594,750		1,561,000
Long-term liabilities				
Loans due after 1 year		(540,000)		(600,000)
		1,054,750		**961,000**
Financed by:				
Capital accounts		**1,054,750**		**961,000**

24.5 An example of a practice's balance sheet.

Within the veterinary profession, there are a number of generally accepted valuation methods and it is beyond the scope of this chapter to consider each of these. Within veterinary practices, individual valuation models are often adopted by a practice, which function adequately for its particular circumstances. In all of the valuation methods, there is no exact formula. Every method relies on some form of adjustment, practice factor, multiplier or other element of judgement. Ultimately, an individual purchaser must judge the value to them, based on the likely returns they will achieve and their perceived risk profile of the practice being purchased.

For any prospective purchaser, the goodwill payback period is commonly used to help consider the proposal and whether the value put forward represents a fair value. The goodwill payback period (in outline) considers, notionally, how long it would take to repay the entirety of the goodwill investment by applying the total additional returns obtained (after costs of finance) to repaying that goodwill investment. An example is given below.

Goodwill element of purchase price	£100,000
Additional income (pre-tax) per annum	£40,000
Finance costs of buy-in (per annum)	(£10,000)
Post finance costs increase in earnings	£30,000
Tax and NI on additional earnings	(£12,600)
After tax increase in earning	£17,400
Payback period £100,000 ÷ £17,400 = 5.75 years	

It should be stressed that the above is a very simplified discussion of goodwill within veterinary practices and it is essential that specialist professional advice is sought before reaching any conclusions. Furthermore, if any external bank finance is required to purchase goodwill, the banks will normally require an independent external professional opinion on the valuation of goodwill prior to offering finance.

The question is sometimes posed as to why some practices do not value goodwill whereas others do. In practical terms, every practice will have a goodwill value of some sort attaching to it, assuming that it is sufficiently profitable. The individual practice may choose not to recognize any goodwill value on its balance sheet and may choose not to pay a goodwill value to outgoing owners nor require incoming owners to purchase goodwill. That does not mean the goodwill does not exist or is valueless; it simply means that they choose to not recognize it.

Again, a straightforward example illustrates the point: Consider a partnership with three partners, where no partner replacements can be found when two of the partners retire, and the partnership agreement states that goodwill is not recognized in the accounts and no payment will be made to the outgoing partners for goodwill. When there is a sole owner of the practice, that owner may decide to offer the practice for sale on the open market. At that stage, assuming a reasonable level of profitability, there would be a goodwill value attaching to that practice which they would realize on sale. In this scenario, the practice has always had a goodwill value throughout its life, but the arrangement between the partners was that goodwill was not recognized.

The reason for goodwill disappearing from balance sheets stems from the 1970s and 1980s. At that stage, many of the other professions began writing out goodwill from their balance sheets as it was becoming increasingly difficult to attract incoming partners where the buy-in costs were substantial. Ultimately, that came from reducing levels of profitability and a very high level of finance costs due to high interest rates at the time.

A number of other mechanisms were designed to replace goodwill, e.g. the lock-step method and the super profit earn-out method. In each of these the senior partners would receive an enhanced profit share and the junior partners would gradually work up to the higher profit shares over a period of time, without having had to buy goodwill on their admission.

Annuities have also been used to replace the goodwill valuation, whereby an outgoing partner would receive some form of annuity from the practice after retirement effectively to compensate them for the absence of a goodwill payout. Annuities are a complex area and, in general, veterinary practices are not actuaries and the build-up of a number of annuities has caused financial angst to a number of practices; they are therefore not recommended but are not uncommon within not only the veterinary profession but other professions too.

Stock

This is the net value of stock on the shelves. The value should be stated for in-date items net of wholesaler discount and net of any pharmaceutical company rebates relating to that item. In practical terms, the net valuation tends to be calculated by taking the list price of the stock on the shelves and deducting an average discount. The average discount is calculated as follows:

Wholesaler discount	12%
Average rebates	11%
	23%

Average rebates in turn are calculated as:

Total rebates received in the year, say, £15,000 ÷ total drugs purchases of £136,000 = 11% average rebate

Debtors

This is the amount owed to the practice by clients in respect of work undertaken and invoiced but not yet paid for. When any work is undertaken for a client and an invoice is generated on the PMS, that work is recognized in the accounts as having been completed; where work has been undertaken but not yet invoiced, technically that should be valued as 'work in progress' (although that very rarely happens within the veterinary profession). Work is recognized in the accounts when invoiced. Until the invoice is paid, it is recorded as a debt in the practice accounts. This is the amount due to the practice recorded in the PMS. When a client pays all or part of that invoice, the amount outstanding reduces and hence the debtor balance also reduces.

Bank and cash

These are the combined cash and bank balances as at the balance sheet date.

Creditors

These are amounts that the practice owes to suppliers.

Loans

These are long-term loans that the practice has a liability to repay at some point in the future, commonly to one of the major banks.

Prepayments and accruals

These are accounting adjustments in respect of goods or services used at the balance sheet date which have not yet been paid for (accruals) or paid for at the balance sheet date but not yet used (prepayments). Examples would be telephone line rentals paid in advance (prepayments) and electricity used in the period but not yet billed to the practice (accruals).

As mentioned above, there are certain times when the practice will have received or paid out cash where those items do not impact directly on the profit and loss account. Furthermore, there will be certain areas where an invoice has been issued and recognized in the profit and loss account but the invoice has not been paid by the end of the period. The cash movement schedule (Figure 24.6) seeks to reconcile the profit to the movement in the cash within the practice, allowing for these types of issues; such schedules are normally prepared by the external accountant.

Practice budgets

In the past, it has been relatively uncommon for veterinary practices to produce annual budgets. However, the current economic climate, the current lending climate and the increased competition between practices, along with practices becoming more financially developed, have all contributed to the increasing use of annual budgets. Rather than using the budgets as a tick box exercise to satisfy banking requirements, practices should use them to:

- Review practice development plans
- Consider the capital expenditure plans for the coming year
- Review practice performance
- Review the proprietors' aspirations for the practice and themselves
- Review staffing needs, potential salary reviews and training plans.

All of these are then reflected within the projected financial position for the coming year. Budgets should also be used as a mechanism to review expenditure programmes and to attempt to set budgets for each individual item of expenditure, such as targeted staffing requirements, the marketing budget, advertising budget, etc.

The practice budgets will normally include a projected profit and loss account, balance sheet and cash flow forecast. Commonly, budgets are used when agreeing the funding requirements for the practice for the coming year and securing the appropriate overdraft facility with the practice bank, but they also present a huge opportunity to undertake an annual review.

KEY POINT

Annual budgets present a real opportunity for forward planning, reflecting on what has been done well and done badly, and taking charge of the direction of the practice.

	£	£
Profit for the year		296,850
Add		
Depreciation	34,250	
Sale of equipment	2,000	
		36,250
Net cash profit		333,100
Less		
Capital expenditure	50,000	
Loan repayments	60,000	
Drawings	203,100	
		(313,100)
Cash generated		20,000
Movement in working capital		
Increase in stock	20,000	
Increase in debtors and prepayments	10,000	
Increase in trade creditors and accruals	(50,000)	
		(20,000)
Movement in overdraft		
Bank balance this year	50,000	
Bank balance last year	10,000	
		40,000
		20,000

24.6 An example summary of cash movement.

Many practices do not produce budgets, as the initial hurdle of setting up the templates for the first time can be off-putting. Normally, a few hours of input from the practice's external accountant will enable the required templates to be put in place and, once established, these can be used year after year. An example of an annual practice budget is shown at the end of this chapter and some important items are explained below.

- **Turnover and cost of sales –** The starting point of a budget is normally the turnover achieved in each month of the previous year. These figures should then be uplifted by an amount for inflation or, alternatively, the amount of any known or projected price increases to be applied during the year. Cost of sales should automatically follow turnover, assuming that the gross profit percentage will remain relatively constant. Any large fluctuations in projected GP% should be investigated.
- **Labour costs** – These will normally be one of the largest expenses for a veterinary practice and time should be spent considering staffing levels, rates of pay, projected salary increases, additional staffing needs, and so on. A spreadsheet can be used to undertake a sensitivity analysis, whereby expenses can be flexed to consider the likely impact on profits before reaching a final decision. A spreadsheet for each class of employee is useful and should be used to record their gross salary and total employment costs. This would include employer's NIC, projected CPD costs, projected job-related accommodation costs, professional subscriptions, and any other costs related to employment of the individuals. Broadly, the groups of employees will be veterinary surgeons, veterinary nurses, reception staff and administration staff.
- **Other overheads** – In general, establishment costs, administration costs, financial costs and depreciation should be relatively fixed costs, i.e. they are not correlated directly with the level of turnover generated by the practice. For each of these items, the opportunity should be taken to plan the capital expenditure for the coming year, any repairs and redecorations required, any changes in utilities, etc. At the budgeting stage, the likely costs can be flexed to consider the impact of changes before reaching a decision for the coming year.

Practice accounts

The profit and loss account and balance sheet together are normally referred to as the practice accounts. In general, there are two types of accounts produced:

- Financial accounts
- Management accounts.

The financial accounts tend to be used for tax purposes and are produced annually. Historically, accountants have tended to produce the financial accounts and use them to do nothing more than establish tax liabilities. In effect, it is a cost of being in business. Since financial accounts are used to agree the tax liabilities, it is fundamental to ensure that they are correct and compliant with HMRC legislation.

Management accounts are used, as the name suggests, for management of the practice. Given that they do not need to be as accurate as financial accounts, management accounts need to show the position sufficiently accurately to give a reasonable indication of performance. The distinction between financial accounts and management accounts and accuracy of the figures relates to the detailed work that needs to be undertaken by the external accountant in order to produce financial accounts that are adequate for tax purposes. To undertake all of those adjustments on a monthly or quarterly basis would be excessively time-consuming and costly.

> **KEY POINT**
>
> In the past, practices would generally produce accounts to record what happened previously as a historical exercise. It was a retrospective thing and often left until the last minute, driven by tax-reporting deadlines. It is far better to use the figures to allow forward planning, to save tax, to make changes within the practice and to learn from the past.

- **Financial accounts** tend to be produced annually, although they can be produced at any time if required, e.g. if there is a change in partners part way through an accounting year.
- **Management accounts** tend to be produced quarterly (or monthly). Considering the financial performance of the practice in detail at any shorter interval risks being inefficient in terms of time expended, given the fluctuations occurring through timing of expenditure alone.

In certain situations, monthly management accounts are entirely appropriate and necessary; it should be straightforward to produce monthly management accounts, assuming the accounting systems are accurate and reconciled. However, the question must be asked as to what is gained from looking at full accounts in detail on a monthly basis given that most costs, other than drugs, consumables and labour, are relatively fixed (or at least should be). Care has to be taken so as to avoid 'micro-managing' the practice. It is far better to monitor certain key performance indicators (KPIs) and certain rolling 12-month figures on a monthly basis to keep track of overall performance without utilizing vast amounts of administrative and proprietorial time. The figures need to be simple, concise and digestible.

> **KEY POINT**
>
> With all financial information, the real value is derived from what action is taken in respect of that information. Inherently, that is the far more complex area to consider.

Working capital management and practice funding

The working capital of a practice is, in essence, the more liquid assets and liabilities. The liquidity of assets and liabilities refers to the speed at which they could be converted into cash (i.e. the more quickly they can be converted into cash, the more liquid the assets are considered to be). Specifically, liquid assets and liabilities are: the value of stock on the shelves; the amounts owed to the practice by clients; and the amounts owed by the practice to suppliers. The working capital requirement links directly to practice funding, which is the amount of finance required for the practice to operate from day to day.

Practice funding may be short or long term:

- **Short-term funding** will tend to be provided by way of an overdraft. Short-term increases in funding may be required for increased stock levels, an extension in the level of debtors or some such change
- **Long-term funding** tends to be provided by way of either long-term loans (from the banks) or amounts invested by the proprietors. The level of the long-term (fixed capital) funding is normally taken to be the value of the fixed assets and goodwill, less any long-term loans taken by the practice as a starting point.

There is no right or wrong level of funding, as it is individual to every practice and personal circumstance. It does, however, need to take into account the likely capital expenditure for the following year when it is reviewed annually. If the long-term funding is set at the wrong level, the overall costs of funding will increase due to the need to operate with an annually renewable overdraft facility. In general, it is better to be slightly over-funded on the long-term fixed capital funding as this leads to a more cost-effective funding solution in terms of charges.

Working capital management will be affected by the type of practice (first-opinion or referral) and the type of work undertaken, the level of direct insurance claims and the proprietorial attitude to funding. In some practices, the proprietors wish to extract all funds possible from the practice and run the practice by relying entirely on external finance. In other scenarios, the proprietors wish to retain all profits within the practice and operate with minimal reliance on external funding. Ultimately, there is no right or wrong answer but simply one of personal preference, taking into consideration the availability of external finance in the market.

Conveniently, working capital management can be broken into its component parts: stock control; debt control; and creditor control. Combined, the subject is effectively one of cash flow management.

Stock control

Purchasing stock means that practice finances are tied up in drugs on the shelves, rather than being cash in the bank. Ultimately, if the drugs purchased do not go out of date and are eventually sold, the only issue is one of tying up cash for a period of time and, therefore, it is a cost of funds issue. Keeping £10,000 of stock on the shelves with funds costing, say, 6% per annum will cost the practice £600 per annum of pre-tax profits (£348 after higher rate tax and NI relief for a partnership).

Practices will often look to arrange a bulk purchasing discount; this allows them to buy at preferential rates but they have to pay for a greater value of the product upfront. Every practice has a different viewpoint on this and it has to be considered for each individual case, as the deals are always different. In addition to consideration of the cost of funds, there is often also a consideration of space in storing the bulk orders. Furthermore, the bulk deals often come just before a product switch by the manufacturers or new product release by a competitor, which increases the risk of the practice holding stock that cannot be sold, or cannot be sold at the current price.

As an aside, with bulk purchases it is always worth considering the timing of the placement of the order within the credit cycle from the wholesaler. A bulk order placed on the first day of the purchasing month will often afford a 6-week credit period, allowing time for the drugs to be sold and cash received before the purchase is paid for. This can provide a useful way of managing working capital.

In general, there is a risk that practices may carry more stock than is necessary, in particular considering the prevalence of next-day deliveries from wholesalers. Some practices are happy to run with a smaller range of drugs on the shelves, giving the clinicians less choice and running the risk that clients cannot have what they want immediately. Others will stock multiple ranges of drugs. In reality, this becomes an issue of protocol-setting by the proprietors and managers of the practice. See Chapter 15 for more information on stock control.

KEY POINT

Ultimately, individual practice protocol on stock control is a very personal matter. The loss of a good client or a good member of staff due to lack of availability of products when required or a restriction in clinical freedom through a restricted drugs selection can far outweigh the costs of the extra stock on the shelves. However, a line must be drawn somewhere and this has to be considered on an individual basis.

Debt control

Debt control is a difficult area. Within first-opinion small animal practice, the business should be considered as one of retail. Within that definition, clients should pay at the time of treatment with limited exceptions (e.g. emotionally difficult situations, approved accounts such as charities or kennels or pre-approved insurance cases). In general, first-opinion small animal practice should run on a debt period of roughly 8 to 10 days, excluding direct insurance claims. The debt period is commonly calculated as follows:

Value of debt outstanding ÷ total amount invoiced in month x 28 = debtor days

Or

Value of debt outstanding ÷ total amount invoiced in year x 365 = debtor days

In referral practice, the situation is considerably different given the preponderance of insurance work, which results in inevitable delays in payment. Benchmarking is therefore inherently difficult as far as expected debtor days are concerned.

It is essential that **terms and conditions** are clearly defined when any client joins the practice and that those terms and conditions are enforced. Even if terms and conditions were not in place in the past, they should be put in place now for existing clients at their next visit. They could, for example, be pre-printed on the reverse of invoices. Alternatively, a copy could be handed to each client at their next visit. Whilst there is no legal requirement to provide terms and conditions to clients of a practice, it is undoubtedly best practice and can save disagreements at a later stage. It will also give the practice greater ability to be able to charge interest and late payment fees on any amounts that are not paid within credit terms. An example of terms and conditions can be found at the end of this chapter.

The whole debt control process should be run efficiently and effectively. Ideally, it should be run autonomously within the administration and management team and without requiring input from veterinary surgeons. It is generally preferable for the professional fee-earners to be one step removed from the debt control and late payment procedures; the professional delivering the clinical care and advice in a caring profession could encounter a conflict if they then had to pursue late payment of fees. It is better if the debt recovery procedure is undertaken by someone within the practice who is removed from the clinical care but is able to call in the veterinary surgeon to assist as and when appropriate. Furthermore, efficient running of a practice dictates that the fee-earning professionals do just that (i.e. generate fees) and so should not become embroiled in administrative tasks, which should be undertaken by administrative staff.

Booking of work

It is important that work is booked (i.e. priced or written up on the computer) and invoiced on a timely basis. Late bookings undoubtedly contribute to increased difficulties with debt collection. Extending the period between the work being carried out and clients being expected to pay is detrimental to cash flow. With a few exceptions, it is in a practice's best interest to ask for payment at the time of treatment or on collection of any drugs or goods purchased.

Where procedures are priced up promptly and treatment given to hospitalized patients is recorded daily, missed bookings due to chargeable items and services being forgotten or missed off are less likely. Missed and inaccurate bookings result in a decreased turnover and ultimately impact upon the profit of the practice. The practice should look to share some financial figures with staff in order that the whole team understands the importance of this.

Credit terms

Credit terms could be as follows:

- Small animal – payment at time of treatment
- Small animal credit account holder – 14 or 30 days from date of invoice.

The terms should be clearly displayed in reception and issued to clients in writing. Some clients, particularly if new to the practice, may need the policy explaining to them politely but firmly and whilst this initially may present a challenge, it is essential to enforce all terms and conditions.

Frequency of invoicing

Small animal customers with no account (which should be the norm) should be invoiced at the time work is carried out and payment obtained before the client leaves the premises. On occasions where clients do not pay they should either be given an invoice to take with them or, if this does not happen for any reason, an invoice should be posted out that day and a note made on the record. The only exceptions to this are for euthanasia, where a few days may be left before sending the invoice (certainly after the condolence card has been sent) or where it has been agreed that an insurance company will pay the practice directly. For direct insurance claims, any charges for this service, the excess and anything not covered by the insurance should be paid for at time of treatment.

Where 14- or 30-day credit terms are in force, an invoice run should be prepared weekly or, at the least, fortnightly to shorten the period from the work being carried out to monies being collected.

Credit control

Trade suppliers can provide a useful form of practice finance. Most suppliers will give a 30-day credit period, which can be used if desired. Some practices choose to pay suppliers by return, as it is perceived to give a better working relationship. However, this becomes a decision based on the availability of other finances and the ethos of the practice owners. Consideration must also be given to any early settlement discounts that are available and this will need to be taken into account with the cash flow requirements of the practice. In new start-up situations, wholesalers may give deferred payment terms during the first three months. This is dealt with on an individual basis and is subject to status.

Set out below are suggested credit control procedures for the two groups of debt (non-account and 14- or 30-day credit terms). For credit control to be successful, clients should be told that the procedures are automated to streamline the debt collection process and improve efficiency for the practice. A process should be in place such that it cannot be overruled by individual members of the team.

On the rare occasions where there are specific reasons that a client is not going to pay at the time of treatment, the practice should have a protocol and this must be followed. There should also be a protocol in place for occasions when payment is expected and the client then indicates that they are not intending to pay. For example, it may be that if the client is at the front desk and cannot pay, the receptionist asks for assistance from the practice manager who, as long as there are no safety concerns, can then take the client into a more private area to discuss payment issues. If different payment terms are agreed, the client should be informed as to why they are being permitted to be treated as an exception, and credit control should be notified to ensure that appropriate revised debt collection procedures are adopted on that debt. Clear notes should be made for future reference, which should be separate from clinical notes.

Clients must be informed of any late payment fees and interest charged by the practice. This information can also be printed on invoices and should be included in the practice's terms and conditions.

The practice should have a clear protocol setting out who is allowed to agree and authorize non-standard payment terms and credit notes. It is important that all staff, including veterinary surgeons, have support regarding all aspects of clients being unwilling or unable to pay.

KEY POINT

In order for debtors to be identifiable if there is a need to take further action, the client's initials and full address are required. It is good practice to ensure that full client details are always recorded on the PMS and that all details are kept updated.

Non-credit accounts

The information below gives an example of a non-credit accounts policy; the process may vary from practice to practice but should be along these lines.

- Where a client does not pay at the time, they should either be sent away with an invoice or an invoice should be posted to them that day.
- After 7 days, a statement should be sent marking the amount as overdue and requesting immediate payment and re-stating the practice's right to charge interest and late payment fees if the account is not settled. This may also be followed up with a phone call.
- After 14 days, a further statement should be sent and this should be followed up with a phone call.
- After 21 days, a letter should be sent advising the client that if payment is not received within 7 days then the matter will be passed to solicitors or a debt collection agency. At this stage, a late payment fee may be applied (e.g. £15 to £25, plus VAT).
- After 28 days, rather than giving notice of legal proceedings, a solicitors' letter might be sent as a first course of action. This approach can be relatively successful at a fairly low cost.
- If after another 14 days there has been no success with the solicitors' letter, then court proceedings against the client may well be instigated. At this stage, it is important to consider how far to pursue the debt, taking into account the level of the debt and the client's personal financial position.
- The stage at which treatment is withdrawn (other than emergency care) should be considered, and the client should be notified that they should seek an alternative veterinary service provider.

14- or 30-day credit terms

Again, the credit control procedure for these clients should be automated as far as possible. Where payment is not received within the 14- or 30-day terms, the procedure should be as follows:

- After 14 or 30 days, a statement should be sent to the client, clearly showing the debt as overdue and stating that payment is expected by return.
- If not paid within a further 7 days, a further statement should be sent, along with a letter stating that the invoice is now overdue and immediate payment is expected. At this time, a late payment fee of £15 to £25 (plus VAT) may be added to the account.
- After a further 7 days, a final reminder should be sent and followed up by a phone call indicating that debt collection procedures will commence if not paid within 7 days.
- After a further 7 days, the debt should be chased by phone and this should be followed up with a letter saying that the debt will be passed to solicitors if payment is not received within 7 days.
- After a further 7 days, a solicitor's letter should be sent to the client and further administration fees added to the client's account.
- If after a further 14 days the debt remains outstanding, the decision needs to be taken whether to initiate legal proceedings or pass the debt to a debt collection agency.

Again, the course of action will depend on the level of debt and the client's personal financial position.

Many practices are now handling their own bad debts and completing the small claims court process themselves via the Internet. Clients receiving a signed copy of all the paperwork 7 days before the court paperwork is due to be sent tend to be more inclined to settle their outstanding account before proceedings are actually issued.

New client procedures

Before new clients are given credit terms (or, ideally, before they are approved as clients), it is strongly recommended that certain checks are carried out to confirm their identity and address and also to identify any historical credit issues. The easiest and most straightforward way to do this is to obtain a credit reference. It is relatively inexpensive to do this and it should help reduce the number of debt issues experienced with new clients.

Insurance

In addition to general debt control, there is a need to review how direct insurance claims are administered. The practice should have clear criteria for offering this service, e.g. there may have to be a minimum amount claimed, there may be certain insurance companies that the practice will not deal with and direct claims may only be agreed for claims on procedures rather than ongoing conditions.

One option may be to put additional onus on the client by obtaining agreement, in advance, that after a period of, say, 6 weeks, if an insurance claim has not been settled, the debt will revert to the client and they will need to pursue the claim themselves. The client should also be made aware that it is their responsibility to pay for anything not covered by the insurance company. It is prudent for the client to sign to say that they have understood and agree to this.

If this course of action is taken, then a pre-authorized credit card swipe could be used in order to secure a form of payment. This would need to be approached with a certain amount of discretion and each case would need to be reviewed on an individual basis. This can be useful on the basis that, although it is assumed that insurance claims will be paid at some point, in fact, the claim could either have been rejected or the funds paid directly to the client.

Direct claims have an impact on cash flow and there is an increased risk that the practice may not receive full payment. Some practices therefore charge a fee for this service and others take a minimum payment of £100 to £150 before treatment as a guarantee. This is particularly useful when the client is not sure of the excess sum on the policy as any excesses and costs known not to be covered should be paid for at the time.

Cash and banking control

Within veterinary practice, there is a reasonably high level of cash received and it is not uncommon to encounter cases of misappropriation of practice funds by staff and others. Robust control systems must therefore be established and enforced.

Specifically, daily cash reconciliations should be carried out and control must be exercised in respect of which members of staff are able to make any adjustments to client balances outstanding on the PMS. It is also advisable to have an individual undertaking the reconciliations who is not involved with the collection of cash and delivering of cash to the bank. Involvement of more than one individual in the cash and banking control process is essential to provide a second check on the figures.

Daily banking is good practice and should take place as a matter of course. If insufficient cash is being received during the course of the day to warrant daily banking then banking may take place less frequently, although consideration must be given to the level of insurance cover if there are material cash balances left on the premises overnight.

The PMS is fundamentally important in the banking control process. Controls are normally available to prevent any editing of financial information within the PMS, but this control is often left open to provide flexibility for the correction of mistakes. This also provides an ideal opportunity for manipulation of figures and presents a real risk of misappropriation of funds. Whilst it is more cumbersome and, at times, frustrating for the editing of financial figures to be restricted to specified authorized individuals, this is preferable to funds being misappropriated. There is also an issue as far as HMRC are concerned if financial data can be amended retrospectively. The risk is that amendments would alter figures that have been entered on to VAT returns and thus give an incomplete audit trail, which is one aspect that HMRC will consider should an inspection take place. Where possible, the editing of clinical text and typographical errors could be permitted with attendant audit trail, but financial transactions should be non-editable.

Payroll

One of the unenviable administrative burdens of running any business is the need to handle the payroll for all employees. It is a monthly task, where any inaccuracy in processing will directly impact on that employee's finances – a subject very close to their hearts. The options are broadly: to use proprietary payroll software to process the payroll in house; or to outsource to a payroll processing bureau (of which there are many). Although there are still some instances of weekly paid employees, this should be discouraged and payroll should be run monthly.

The requirements are such that a payroll scheme must be registered with HMRC, even for a sole employee. A simple call to the HMRC helpline (currently 08456 070 143) will set the wheels in motion and all paperwork will be dispatched to set up the scheme. Alternatively, full information and guidance is given at www.hmrc.gov.uk.

Payroll is assumed to be straightforward but is, in fact, complex. HMRC have very good helplines:

- For those that have been an employer for more than 3 years: 08457 143 143
- For those that have been an employer for less than 3 years: 08456 070 143
- National minimum wage helpline: 08456 000 678.

However, payroll is an area for which advice can yield savings through planning and pre-empting problems that may arise through the incorrect application of the legislation.

Once the scheme is established, the next point to address is how to process and manage the payroll for the practice. Whether the scheme is to be processed internally or outsourced, a decision has to be made as to:

- What the processing date each month will be
- What the cut-off date for overtime and salary adjustments will be (i.e. will it include overtime and extra hours monthly in arrears?)
- What the pay day each month will be.

Once the internal logistics have been established, the method of processing can be considered.

In-house processing

There are a number of payroll packages on the market. HMRC has its own (free to use) software for use where employees number nine or fewer, which handles basic payrolls adequately.

Outsourcing

It is hard to understand why businesses choose to process their payroll internally when payroll services can be bought in so cost-effectively. Many of the largest businesses in the UK outsource their payroll function as they cannot achieve the economies of scale of payroll bureaus. Outsourcing alleviates the need to buy software (which must be updated annually), saves on management time and can, if managed correctly, save costs. The bureau will also remind the practice of all filing and payment deadlines and help with (or deal with) all returns required.

Statutory obligations

Employers have an obligation to pay statutory payments in certain circumstances, e.g. for maternity leave, sickness or redundancy. It is beyond the scope of this chapter to consider these aspects in detail but further guidance can be found at www.hmrc.gov.uk/employers. In most situations, specific professional advice should be sought. National minimum wage (NMW) legislation applies in most situations and again, specific advice should be sought as there are circumstances where benefits and training costs can be factored into the salary for NMW purposes. More information on statutory rights is given in Chapter 20.

The PAYE calendar

The PAYE year runs to 5th April annually. The deadlines applicable are given in Figure 24.7.

- Monthly payments for PAYE and NIC must be made by the **19th** of each month (by cheque) or by the **22nd** of each month (by electronic transfer). These deductions are withheld from employees and belong to HMRC. The practice is acting as an unpaid tax collector. Non-payment by the employer of PAYE and NIC deductions is dealt with firmly by HMRC and should be avoided
- Final payment of PAYE and NIC due for the year to 5th April must reach the Accounts Office by **19th April** (cheque) or **22nd April** (electronic)
- Form P35, the Employer's Annual Return, must be submitted online to HMRC by **19th May**. Failure to submit will result in a penalty being charged
- Forms P60 for the year to 5th April must be distributed to all employees in the employment of the practice as at 5th April by **31st May**
- Forms P11D declaring benefits supplied to directors and/or employees must be submitted to HMRC by 6th July and copies distributed to employees. Items constituting a benefit include (not exhaustive):
  - Car and car fuel
  - Van and van fuel (if private use other than incidental)
  - Interest-free or low interest loans
  - Medical insurance
  - Payments made on behalf of employees (e.g. settling their personal expenses and/or bills)
  - Telephone landlines (in some circumstances)
- Payment for Class 1A NIC due on benefits must reach the Accounts Office by **19th July** (cheque) or **22nd July** (electronic).

24.7 PAYE deadlines.

Improving practice profitability and efficiency

Generating an adequate level of profit and working efficiently is fundamentally important to allow:

- Remuneration of staff
- Reinvestment in the practice, in terms of equipment, staff development and practice development
- The proprietors' provision for their retirement
- Flexibility on succession planning for the practice
- A better work/life balance.

Generating an adequate profit within veterinary practice should be achievable, providing the practice is run efficiently and assuming there is a critical mass of turnover. As to the definition of adequate profit, this will vary from practice to practice and from owner to owner; it is a very personal judgement.

Fee setting

It is of fundamental importance that the practice establishes a simple and straightforward pricing structure, which is communicated to all staff. That pricing structure should be primarily based on the individual practice's cost structure and then referenced to what the market will pay. The fee-setting process is complex, although historically practices have tended towards one of two approaches: looking at what everyone else is charging locally (either geographically local or in the specific referral specialist area) and adjusting prices relative to others; or looking at what the practice is currently charging and adding a percentage across the board to allow for inflation. With the evolution of the profession, the development of the pet insurance market, increased competition generally and the changes in medicines pricing, either of these approaches is fraught with risk.

Practices will often set out a pricing structure, but the financial results achieved by the practice do not reflect it. A common issue is staff not charging correctly for the work that has been carried out. Staff may be giving conscious or subconscious discounts, or they may be charging incorrectly because they are too busy, or have a lack of confidence or understanding. Incorrect charging may also be due to the practice having unclear policies, poor systems or an unrealistic pricing structure. It is of paramount importance that appropriate coaching is given to staff so that they understand the practice's requirements and expectations.

Medicines pricing

The traditional blanket cost-plus pricing is, to an extent, outdated. Internet pharmacies have brought price pressure to bear akin to that experienced within the farm animal sector several years ago. This is driving long-term prescribed medicine prices down. As to whether this will suppress the entire market or just the 'price shopper' clients remains to be seen. As far as other medicines are concerned, a value pricing approach appears to be emerging, i.e. what will the client pay to fix the problem? Many practices use specific pricing and mark-up by product, with the cost-plus approach being used as the backstop position.

Professional fees

To set fees in a way that is technically correct for the practice:

- All staff must maintain detailed accurate timesheets for a full year, recording how each member of staff divides their time between activities such as consultations, minor procedures, surgery under general anaesthetic, nurse clinics, administrative paperwork, etc. Gathering this information is often the first stumbling block for practices

- Accurate costings are required for all items in the practice; this is normally an easier piece of information to obtain, although it is inherently difficult to be entirely accurate
- The practice needs to have accurate square footages of all areas of the practice; this is normally easily identified
- The practice needs to identify the fee revenue generators. Broadly, these would be:
  - Consultations – veterinary surgeons, nurses
  - Minor surgery
  - Surgery under general anaesthetic
  - Hospitalization.

With all this information to hand, fees can be set by looking to recover costs and generate suitable profits based on the use of man hours. Ultimately, the costs of running the practice, together with profits required, must come from what is charged for time spent by staff and from the margin generated from drug sales. In reality, most practices will arrive at the fees they charge by undertaking a review process partly based on their own cost structure, partly based on what the market can carry, and partly based on what the local competition is charging. The weighting that each of these factors has on the ultimate pricing decision depends on the individual practice.

The process might involve:

- Mystery shopping local competition
- Considering what is currently charged by the practice
- Considering the current results and profits achieved by the practice
- Considering the number of fee complaints received from clients
- Considering the rate of inflation.

Fees are then reviewed, often by a set percentage, either annually, half-yearly or quarterly. This is a less than scientific process but is one that has worked for many practices over the years and continues to be widely used now.

Estimates

In general, fee complaints from clients will occur where inaccurate or inappropriate estimates have been given in respect of the treatment required. It is therefore of fundamental importance that a clear estimating procedure is set out and applied on every occasion. Absence of a procedure that works will almost always result in fee complaints. It is important to understand the distinction between a quotation and an estimate.

- **A quotation** is a fixed price offer that cannot be changed once accepted by the client. The price quoted holds even if the practice has to carry out much more work than expected. If a quotation is being given then it must define precisely what is covered and what is not covered and specify that variations outside of this work will be subject to additional charges.
- **An estimate** is an educated guess at what a procedure or item of work may cost, but is not binding. To take account of possible unforeseen development complications, either a best estimate should be given or estimates based on various circumstances, preferably including the worst-case scenario, should be provided.

Most PMSs can carry out estimating procedures; and incorporation of the estimate on the consent form for inpatient work is best practice. Clear communication with the client is of fundamental importance and that in turn must be defined and set out by the proprietors and managers of the practice.

KEY POINT

It cannot be over-emphasized that communication with all practice staff regarding practice finances is fundamentally important to the overall success of the practice. Coaching and mentoring of staff is crucial for achieving good results.

Benchmarking and profit maximization

Within veterinary practice, the two largest costs will always be the drugs bill and the wages bill. Commonly, the drugs bill might amount to 20–25% of turnover and the wages bill, including a notional salary for proprietorial input, might represent 35–40% of turnover for non-hospital status first-opinion practices. Therefore, the starting point for profit maximization must always be to consider whether these two areas are running as efficiently as possible.

Drug purchasing

A large practice will inherently have better buying power and should therefore achieve a better margin. However, for smaller practices, similar buying power can be achieved by using the services of a buying group. A number of these operate within the UK, each with their own terms & conditions and membership criteria.

Labour costs

In respect of labour costs, efficient working is of great importance. At the outset, defining what is included within labour costs for a practice is key. This will include:

- Gross salary
- Employer's NIC
- CPD costs
- Professional subscriptions
- Any benefits in kind provided (car, employer's pension contributions, job-related accommodation, mobile phones, practice computer, etc.)
- Staff uniforms
- Staff Christmas party and social events throughout the year
- Training and development costs.

Veterinary surgeons generate the lion's share of the income for the practice, and their performance can be benchmarked by considering fee turnover per MRCVS and total turnover per MRCVS. Total turnover per MRCVS in practice may range from £200,000 to £350,000 per full-time equivalent (FTE) MRCVS in first-opinion practice. This indicator is total practice turnover divided by FTE MRCVS in the practice, i.e. it apportions the over-the-counter and other income across the MRCVS numbers. The range in turnover per MRCVS is considerable and will depend on a variety of factors, including work/life balance, type of client base, types of work undertaken and the demographics of the clients of a practice.

Labour costs can also be benchmarked as a percentage of turnover to identify the efficiencies of labour utilization: 35–40% for non-hospital status is common, with up to 42% for a hospital status practice running at less than full capacity.

Most other practice costs will be relatively fixed. For example, the cost of the property will be fixed and should not fluctuate materially month on month. The practice therefore needs to consider whether it is running at sufficient critical mass of turnover, so as to maximize the use of those assets and minimize the fixed costs as a percentage of turnover.

Variable costs will fluctuate with the level of turnover. In this area, practices should generally be looking to ensure they are getting value for money. Examples of variable costs are telephone charges, marketing and advertising, postage and stationery – in essence, any cost that fluctuates with the level of income as distinct from fixed costs, which do not fluctuate. For example, rent paid for the practice property will remain the same regardless of level of work undertaken. Utility cost reviews can yield some savings but the numbers involved do not tend to be substantial.

Practice investment decisions

Before any investment is made, a cost–benefit analysis should be undertaken to assess the financial implications of the purchase to ensure that, at the very least, the asset will generate a contribution towards practice overheads and, ultimately, profit. In addition to this standalone analysis, consideration will also need to be given to the impact on the existing practice of making that investment. For example, opening a new branch may, if not managed correctly, have a detrimental effect on the profitability of existing branches; it is therefore important to ensure that consideration has been given to the impact of the investment decision and steps taken to address this.

As well as considering the potential negative implications, consideration should be given to the positive impact on the rest of the practice of any investment. For example, a new piece of diagnostic equipment may allow further work to be undertaken in house rather than referred, and this could generate additional income streams and provide additional motivation and self-esteem to existing staff.

Figure 24.8 sets out the template for undertaking a cost–benefit analysis for the purchase of a new piece of equipment. To undertake a cost–benefit analysis, the following steps must be taken:

1. Identify the cost of the investment.
2. Identify the likely useful economic life of that item.
3. Make a 'best guess' of the number of times that item of equipment will be used each year.
4. Establish the income that will be generated from each use of the equipment.
5. Identify the cost of funds used in acquiring the item of equipment.
6. Identify the labour costs incurred in undertaking each procedure.
7. Identify the annual maintenance and running costs for the new equipment.
8. Identify any other incurred costs, e.g. marketing, advertising, training, gaining experience in the use of the equipment.

With the above identified, it is then possible to calculate the time it will take for the equipment cost to be recovered (the payback period). Provided this is less than the estimated useful life, purchasing the equipment should generate additional profit for the practice.

There are two main ways to assess the payback period (see Figure 24.8). The first of these is to look at the contribution to the fixed costs of the practice generated by the equipment. The contribution is the marginal income after direct costs have been deducted. To establish this, a contribution per procedure is calculated by taking the anticipated income less the variable costs. This can then be used to establish an annual contribution and the payback period calculated in this way, taking into account projected number of uses per annum and then considering the contribution in context of the capital investment. Provided the contribution pays back the investment in less than the anticipated usual economic life, this will generate some additional profit for the practice. However, this may be to the detriment of net profit margin. This method would tend to be used only for relatively small investment decisions, and also where there are no alternative investments.

A more robust approach is to calculate the payback period after allowing for a contribution to practice overheads and allowing for the practice to generate its target profit percentage. This method will be more suitable for larger investment decisions, for example the opening of a new branch or the installation of a substantial new piece of equipment.

In any cost–benefit analysis there will always be certain variables, with the main items being the level of income generation per use and the number of uses. The less certain the above variables are, the shorter the payback period required so as to allow for any variability within these.

Once a cost–benefit analysis has been completed and the decision to invest has been made, consideration must then be given to:

- The funding method most appropriate, e.g. long-term lending, HP, lease purchase
- The structure of the investment or purchase, e.g. equipment may be bought outright or leased
- The tax implications of the investment or purchase (method and timing).

These points normally require the input of the external accountant to establish the most appropriate option for the practice.

Summary	
Cost of new asset	£25,000
Useful Economic Life of new asset	6–7 years
Estimate usage of asset	150 times per annum
Cost of funds to purchase asset	6%
Labour costs involved	One veterinary surgeon and one veterinary nurse
Annual estimated maintenance costs	£2,000 per annum
Profit per use	
Time taken for procedure	20 minutes
Charge	85.00
Vet cost	(8.33)
Nurse cost (see Note 1)	(4.14)
Maintenance and consumables [a]	(13.33)
Finance costs (at 6%)	(10.00)
Contribution generated	49.20
Less: overhead absorption at 15%	(12.75)
Less: required profit at 25%	(21.25)
Contribution to cover equipment replacement	15.20
Total number of scans	150
Annual position	**£**
Turnover	12,750.00
Variable costs	(5,370.00)
Overheads and profit	(5,100.00)
Contribution to cover equipment replacement	2,280.00
Payback period	
Payback period – Turnover: How long will it take for the turnover generated to repay the initial cost, ignoring other costs?	1.96 years
Payback period – Contribution: How long will it take for the contribution (turnover less direct costs) to repay the initial cost?	3.39 years
Payback period – Allowance for profit: How long will it take to repay the initial cost allowing for all costs and target profit element?	10.96 years

Note 1: Salary costs [b]

	Vet	Nurse
Annual salary	37,500.00	19,000.00
Employer's NI	4,386.00	1,833.00
Allowance for CPD, insurance and subs	2,500.00	1,250.00
	44,386.00	22,083.00
Total available days	222	222
Daily cost	199.94	99.47
Cost for 20 minutes (based on 8-hour day)	8.33	4.14

24.8 Practice investment decisions: example cost–benefit analysis. [a] Assumes space available to use the equipment within existing premises and no installation costs. [b] Salary costs are for illustrative purposes only.

Using external accountants

How a practice uses its external accountants will very much depend on the specific requirements of the practice, the level of involvement they want from their accountants and the degree of specialist knowledge the accountant has of the veterinary profession. Consideration must also be given to the financial knowledge and business acumen of the practice owners and managers, as this will directly affect the type of relationship the practice has with its accountant and the type of service required.

Historically, external accountants have provided a basic compliance-led service, preparing the annual accounts and tax return forms with little involvement in practice development or the more proactive planning work and tax mitigation work that adds tremendous value for any practice. As the veterinary marketplace becomes more competitive and economic pressures increase, the historic service becomes of limited value but it does depend on what the practice wants and needs.

Many industries and professions are moving towards the use of accountants who are specialists in their field, and the veterinary profession is no different. Veterinary specialist accountants understand the issues facing the profession, the terminology of the profession and should be able to give advice on benchmarking, practice development, profit maximization, and so on. A major factor may be whether the accountant is able to provide detailed benchmarking services from their own client base and whether that client base is of sufficient size to make the results meaningful.

Using a specialist accountant can add significant value to the practice and can make managing the practice easier. The external accountant should be in a position to provide meaningful financial information, benchmarking analysis against up-to-date practice-specific data and national trends.

In addition, the external accountants can be used to provide practical advice on:

- Specialist accounting systems
- Cash flow and drawings projections
- Management accounting
- Restructuring, including incorporation
- Succession planning
- Partnership agreements
- Tax efficiency of borrowing
- Outsourced finance and payroll function
- Tax planning and compliance
- Retirement advice and planning
- Practice acquisitions, sales and mergers.

Ultimately, the role of external accountants for any veterinary practice is to provide a level of service and strategic advice, to enable the practice to maximize profits, minimize tax liabilities and work towards the practice's strategic aims as part of the practice's management team. The key issue is to discuss what the accountant can offer, agree what the practice and owners need and want and then work towards that over time.

Further reading

Bower J, Gripper J, Gripper P and Gunn D (2001) *Veterinary Practice Management, 3rd edn.* Blackwell Science, Oxford

Drury C (2006) *Cost and Management Accounting: An Introduction.* Thomson Learning, London

Impey D and Montague N (2008) *Running a Limited Company, 6th edn.* Jordan Publishing, Bristol

Moore A (2000) SIPPs – an alternative means of practice property purchase. *In Practice* **22**, 218–221

Moore A (2002) Finding the best route to driving a practice car. *In Practice* **24**, 604–610

Moore A (2003) Making it all add up – choosing and using an accountant. *In Practice* **25**, 285–288

Moore A (2004) Trading structures for veterinary practices. *In Practice* **26**, 394–396

Moore A (2010) Getting involved in a joint venture. *In Practice* **32**, 315–316

Wood F and Sangster A (2008) *Business Accounting, 11th edn.* (2 vols) Pearson Education, Essex

Examples of budgets and T&C 

	Jan	Feb	Mar	Apr	May	Jun	Jul	Aug	Sep	Oct	Nov	Dec	TOTAL
	£	£	£	£	£	£	£	£	£	£	£	£	£
Receipts:													
Income	12,000	12,000	12,000	12,000	12,000	12,000	12,000	12,000	12,000	12,000	12,000	12,000	144,000
Interest received	1	1	1	1	1	1	1	1	1	1	1	1	12
Miscellaneous income	10	10	10	10	10	10	10	10	10	10	10	10	120
Rent received	150	150	150	150	150	150	150	150	150	150	150	150	1,800
Total receipts	12,161	12,161	12,161	12,161	12,161	12,161	12,161	12,161	12,161	12,161	12,161	12,161	145,932
Payments:													
Cost of sales	2,640	2,640	2,640	2,640	2,640	2,640	2,640	2,640	2,640	2,640	2,640	2,640	31,680
Labour costs	2,800	2,800	2,800	2,800	2,800	2,800	2,800	2,800	2,800	2,800	2,800	2,800	33,600
Establishment	440	440	440	440	440	440	440	440	440	440	440	440	5,280
Administration	720	720	720	720	720	720	720	720	720	720	720	720	8,640
Financial	400	400	400	400	400	400	400	400	400	400	400	400	4,800
Loan repayments	150	150	150	150	150	150	150	150	150	150	150	150	1,800
Equipment additions	1,200	–	1,200	1,200	–	–	–	–	–	1,200	–	–	4,800
HP repayments	100	100	100	100	100	100	100	100	100	100	100	100	1,200
VAT payments	2,000	–	–	3,800	–	–	4,000	–	–	4,200	–	–	14,000
Tax payments	2,000	–	–	–	–	–	2,000	–	–	–	–	–	4,000
Drawings	750	750	750	750	750	750	750	750	750	750	750	750	9,000
Total payments	13,200	8,000	9,200	13,000	8,000	8,000	14,000	8,000	8,000	13,400	8,000	8,000	118,800
Net cashflow	(1,039)	4,161	2,961	(839)	4,161	4,161	(2,161)	4,161	4,161	(1,239)	4,161	4,161	26,810
Opening bank balance	3,000	1,961	6,122	9,083	8,244	12,405	16,566	14,405	18,566	22,727	21,488	25,649	3,000
Closing bank balance	1,961	6,122	9,083	8,244	12,405	16,566	14,405	18,566	22,727	21,488	25,649	29,810	29,810

Sample budgets – Cashflow.

	Jan	Feb	Mar	Apr	May	Jun	Jul	Aug	Sep	Oct	Nov	Dec	TOTAL
	£	£	£	£	£	£	£	£	£	£	£	£	£
Income	10,000	10,000	10,000	10,000	10,000	10,000	10,000	10,000	10,000	10,000	10,000	10,000	120,000
Cost of sales													
Opening stock	10,000	10,000	10,000	10,000	10,000	10,000	10,000	10,000	10,000	10,000	10,000	10,000	120,000
Purchases	1,800	1,800	1,800	1,800	1,800	1,800	1,800	1,800	1,800	1,800	1,800	1,800	21,600
Lab and specialist fees	300	300	300	300	300	300	300	300	300	300	300	300	3,600
Waste disposal and cremation	100	100	100	100	100	100	100	100	100	100	100	100	1,200
Closing stock	(10,000)	(10,000)	(10,000)	(10,000)	(10,000)	(10,000)	(10,000)	(10,000)	(10,000)	(10,000)	(10,000)	(10,000)	(120,000)
	2,200	2,200	2,200	2,200	2,200	2,200	2,200	2,200	2,200	2,200	2,200	2,200	26,400
GP	***7,800***	***7,800***	***7,800***	***7,800***	***7,800***	***7,800***	***7,800***	***7,800***	***7,800***	***7,800***	***7,800***	***7,800***	***93,600***
	78.00%	***78.00%***	***78.00%***	***78.00%***	***78.00%***	***78.00%***	***78.00%***	***78.00%***	***78.00%***	***78.00%***	***78.00%***	***78.00%***	***78.00%***
Overheads													
Labour costs	2,800	2,800	2,800	2,800	2,800	2,800	2,800	2,800	2,800	2,800	2,800	2,800	33,600
Establishment	400	400	400	400	400	400	400	400	400	400	400	400	4,800
Administration	600	600	600	600	600	600	600	600	600	600	600	600	7,200
Financial	400	400	400	400	400	400	400	400	400	400	400	400	4,800
Depreciation	150	150	150	150	150	150	150	150	150	150	150	150	1,800
	4,350	4,350	4,350	4,350	4,350	4,350	4,350	4,350	4,350	4,350	4,350	4,350	52,200
Net trading profit	3,450	3,450	3,450	3,450	3,450	3,450	3,450	3,450	3,450	3,450	3,450	3,450	41,400
Interest received	1	1	1	1	1	1	1	1	1	1	1	1	12
Miscellaneous income	10	10	10	10	10	10	10	10	10	10	10	10	120
Rent received	150	150	150	150	150	150	150	150	150	150	150	150	1,800
Net profit	3,611	3,611	3,611	3,611	3,611	3,611	3,611	3,611	3,611	3,611	3,611	3,611	43,332

Sample budgets – Profit and Loss account.

	Jan	Feb	Mar	Apr	May	Jun	Jul	Aug	Sep	Oct	Nov	Dec
	£	£	£	£	£	£	£	£	£	£	£	£
Fixed assets	100,850	100,700	101,550	102,400	102,250	102,100	101,950	101,800	101,650	102,500	102,350	102,200
Current assets												
Debtors	12,000	12,000	12,000	12,000	12,000	12,000	12,000	12,000	12,000	12,000	12,000	12,000
Stock	10,000	10,000	10,000	10,000	10,000	10,000	10,000	10,000	10,000	10,000	10,000	10,000
Cash at bank	1,961	6,122	9,083	8,244	12,405	16,566	14,405	18,566	22,727	21,488	25,649	29,810
	23,961	28,122	31,083	30,244	34,405	38,566	36,405	40,566	44,727	43,488	47,649	51,810
Current liabilities												
Creditors	5,000	5,000	5,000	5,000	5,000	5,000	5,000	5,000	5,000	5,000	5,000	5,000
VAT liability	1,200	2,600	3,800	1,200	2,600	4,000	1,400	2,800	4,200	1,200	2,600	4,000
HP liability	5,000	4,900	4,800	4,700	4,600	4,500	4,400	4,300	4,200	4,100	4,000	3,900
	11,200	12,500	13,600	10,900	12,200	13,500	10,800	12,100	13,400	10,300	11,600	12,900
Long-term loans												
Bank loan	(35,850)	(35,700)	(35,550)	(35,400)	(35,250)	(35,100)	(34,950)	(34,800)	(34,650)	(34,500)	(34,350)	(34,200)
	77,761	80,622	83,483	86,344	89,205	92,066	92,605	95,466	98,327	101,188	104,049	106,910
Financed by												
Capital accounts	77,761	80,622	83,483	86,344	89,205	92,066	92,605	95,466	98,327	101,188	104,049	106,910

Sample budgets – Balance sheet.

Terms and Conditions

1. Fees

1.1 VAT is charged at the prevailing rate on all fees, diets and drugs.

1.2 Charges are determined according to the drugs, materials, consumables and diets used, together with the type of work undertaken and time required.

1.3 You will receive a detailed fee note for every consultation, surgical procedure or transaction with us.

1.3 Our fee list is available on request.

2. Methods of payment

2.1 Accounts are due for settlement at the end of consultation, on the discharge of your pet or upon collection of drugs/diets.

2.2 You may settle your account using the following:

- Cash
- Cheque or BACS/FPS
- Credit/Debit Card – Switch, Solo, Mastercard, Visa, Delta (not Amex)

2.3 Accounts are only available by prior agreement.

3. Estimate of treatment costs

3.1 We will happily provide a written estimate as to the probable costs of a course of treatment.

3.2 Please bear in mind that any estimate given can only be approximate. A pet's illness may not follow a conventional course and your pet's welfare is our primary concern.

4. Settlement terms

4.1 Should an account not be settled within 14 days , a reminder will be sent with an additional fee in respect of administrative costs incurred.

4.2 Interest will be added to overdue accounts at the rate of 8% over base lending rate.

4.3 Should it be necessary for further reminders to be sent, further charges will be incurred.

4.4 After due notice to you the client, overdue accounts will be referred to our debt collection agency or solicitors and further charges will be levied in respect of costs incurred in collecting the debt, such as:

- Production of reports
- Calls
- Home visits, etc.
- Court fees.

4.5 Any cheque returned by our bank as unpaid, any credit card payment not honoured and any cash tendered that is found to be counterfeit will result in the account being restored to the original sum, with further charges being added in respect of bank charges and administrative costs, together with interest on the principal sum.

5. Inability to pay

5.1 If for any reason you are unable to settle your account as specified, we ask you to discuss the matter as soon as possible with a member of staff.

5.2 Please note that installments or part payments of accounts may only be sanctioned with the express written permission of the Practice Principal, or the Practice Manager.

6. Pet health insurance

6.1 We strongly support the principle of insuring your pet against unexpected illness or accidents. Please ask for details about insurance from any member of staff.

6.2 Please note that it is your responsibility to settle our account and then reclaim the fees from your insurance company.

6.3 We do not conduct any treatment or procedure subject to the costs being covered by your insurance company.

7. Complaints and standards

7.1 We hope you never feel the need to complain about the standards of our service. However, if you feel that there is something you wish to complain about, please direct your comments in the first instance to the Practice Manager.

8. Ownership of records

8.1 Case records and similar documents are the property of, and shall be retained by the practice.

8.2 Copies with a summary of the history will be passed, on request, to another veterinary surgeon taking over the case.

9. Ownership of radiographs and similar records

9.1 The care given to your animal may involve making some specific investigations, for example taking radiographs or performing ultrasound scans.

9.2 Even though we make a charge for carrying out these investigations and interpreting the results, ownership of the resulting record, for example a radiograph, remains the property of the practice.

10. Out-of-hours service

10.1 The practice operates an out-of-hours service for emergencies.

10.2 The out-of-hours service can be accessed by telephoning any branch and the call will be diverted to a telephonist, who can contact the duty veterinary surgeon as necessary.

10.3 Out-of-hours small animal emergency cases are seen at a nominated branch, which varies depending on the veterinary surgeon on duty.

10.4 You will be expected to transport your animal to the nominated surgery for treatment, which may not be the usual branch your animal attends.

Example of terms and conditions of business. Some aspects of the terms may not be relevant to all clients. (continues) ▶

11. Variations in terms of trading

11.1 No addition or variation of these conditions will bind the practice unless it is specifically agreed in writing and signed by one of the practice principals.

11.2 No agent or person employed by, or under contract with the practice has the authority to alter or vary these conditions in any way.

12. Applicable law

12.1 These terms are governed by, and constructed in accordance with, English law. The Courts of England will have exclusive jurisdiction in relation to any claim, dispute or difference concerning these terms and any matter arising from it. Each party irrevocably waives any right it may have to object to any action being brought in these courts, to claim that the action has been bought in an inappropriate forum, or to claim that those courts do not have jurisdiction.

12.2 If any provision in these standard terms of business, or its application, is found to be invalid, illegal or otherwise unenforceable in any respect, the validity, legality or enforceability of any other provision shall not in any way be affected or impaired.

13. Data Protection Act

13.1 We may obtain, use, process and disclose personal data about you in order that we may discharge our duties as your veterinary surgeon under these standard terms of business, and for other related purposes including updating and enhancing client records, analysis for management purposes and statutory returns, crime prevention and legal and regulatory compliance. You have a right of access, under data protection legislation, to the personal data that we hold about you. We confirm that when processing data on your behalf we will comply with the provisions of the Data Protection Act 1998. For the purposes of the Data Protection Act 1998, the Data Controller in relation to personal data supplied about you is the Practice Manager.

(continued) Example of terms and conditions of business. Some aspects of the terms may not be relevant to all clients.

Principles of marketing

25

Helen Kington, Marion Chapman, Carole Clarke and Susan Beesley

Marketing is defined by the Chartered Institute of Marketing as 'The management process involved in identifying, anticipating and satisfying customer requirements profitably'. Marketing therefore is not just about promotion, brochures, advertising and special offers. It is about people – both customers and the people in the practice. It is about emotions, loyalty, listening, learning and sharing knowledge. It is about what happens every day in every transaction and interaction, not just how the practice projects itself externally, and it draws on much of what is discussed in all the other chapters in this Manual.

Professional service businesses deal in knowledge, and veterinary surgeons and veterinary nurses value highly their knowledge and skills, which are fundamental to the jobs they are doing. This must, however, always be balanced with the client or customer relationship. Clients tend to take a practice team's knowledge and skills for granted and so place more value on their experience and how their needs are met, rather than the qualifications and specific skills of the clinician or nurse; Chapter 27 discusses this core concept in detail.

Many firms recognize the importance of marketing, and employ marketing specialists with market research departments and product development sections. They study the trends, invent new materials, devise better processes and try to keep one step ahead of their competitors. Most veterinary practices do not have professional marketing departments, but understanding the basics of marketing is fundamental to success.

Coordinated marketing activities will start to build a successful corporate image, which fosters the idea of brand loyalty. This chapter will discuss in detail the importance of positioning and branding, segmentation and targeting, customer retention strategies and the offerings, which are much more than just the services and products offered by the practice.

The theory of marketing

There are four main aspects of marketing, sometimes referred to as the 'marketing mix'. The theory of marketing involves modifying the marketing mix variables of product, price, promotion and place. These are relevant to all business, and are called the 4 Ps of marketing (Figure 25.1). The extended marketing mix (also known as the 7Ps) includes a further three variables – people, processes and physical evidence. By mixing and modifying all these variables, the practice can build a marketing strategy tailored to the needs and requirements of its clients.

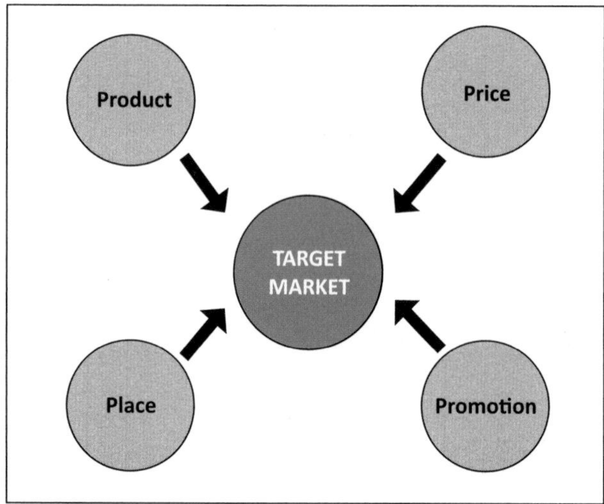

25.1 The 4 Ps of the marketing mix.

Product/Service

Product is a generic term that, for marketing purposes, can also include any services provided. Services differ from products or goods sold as they are:

- Intangible – cannot be seen, touched or displayed. The customer has nothing physical to show as a result of the purchase
- Inseparable – production and consumption of a service cannot be separated. Services cannot be produced and then stored but are produced on demand in the presence of the client. This can create problems with demand levels, such as on a busy day at the practice when several emergencies come in
- Heterogeneous – the quality of the service delivered is often dependent on the quality of the personnel involved, in the same way as when

visiting a hairdressing salon, a client's haircut will differ slightly according to each stylist. It is therefore very important in any service industry (including veterinary practices) that the level of service delivered is consistent, regardless of who delivers the service.

In order to help overcome these issues, businesses can use a promotional strategy to differentiate their services, such as establishing brand loyalty.

Price

Every product/service has its own demand curve, which relates sales volume to selling price. Generally, this shows that the lower the price, the greater is the quantity sold. The sensitivity of demand to price changes is called 'price elasticity'. If demand increases more than proportionately when a product price is reduced, then the demand is elastic. If it does not, it is inelastic.

Quality products should not be underpriced. Indeed, the appeal may be diminished. A practice must quickly get a feel for how sales volume is affected by price changes and this is where monitoring key performance indicators (KPIs) can help to assess the effect that price may have on sales.

Promotion

This involves communication with current and potential customers via advertising, promotions, direct mail, events, etc.

Place

This concerns how to make products and services available to the target audience, e.g. opening hours, location. Place also refers to the channels of distribution and method of delivery used to reach the marketplace.

People

This aspect is particularly important when the offering is a service. Good staff can offer added value to delivery of a service.

Processes

Practice processes are key to customer appeal and retention (see Chapters 26 and 27). Where services are difficult to access, or opportunities missed because of poor systems, clients will go elsewhere. Customer focus is key, and processes must be refined with the customer in mind, rather than concentrating on or prioritizing the needs and interests of the practice staff.

Physical evidence

It is important to remember that the presentation and packaging is a crucial element in customers' buying decisions. In veterinary practice, this relates to the appearance of the premises, signage, the style of the reception, the furniture and seating, the consulting rooms, etc., and to the clinical offerings and how these are bundled together.

Marketing strategy and the SCORPIO model

Marketing strategy is the process by which an organization aligns itself with the market it has decided to serve. In this way marketing strategy translates the business's objectives and strategy into marketing activities. It is the process by which the practice engages with its staff and how they then focus activities on the clients' current and future needs.

The SCORPIO model (Fifield, 2007, 2008; Figure 25.2) includes the various elements of the marketing strategy and illustrates a useful approach to the issues practices should consider. At the centre is the customer, or client, without whom there would be no practice or service business. The customer must drive practice activity.

KEY POINT

Understanding what the customer wants or needs is central to the marketing effort, and adapting to changes in customer requirements is key to success.

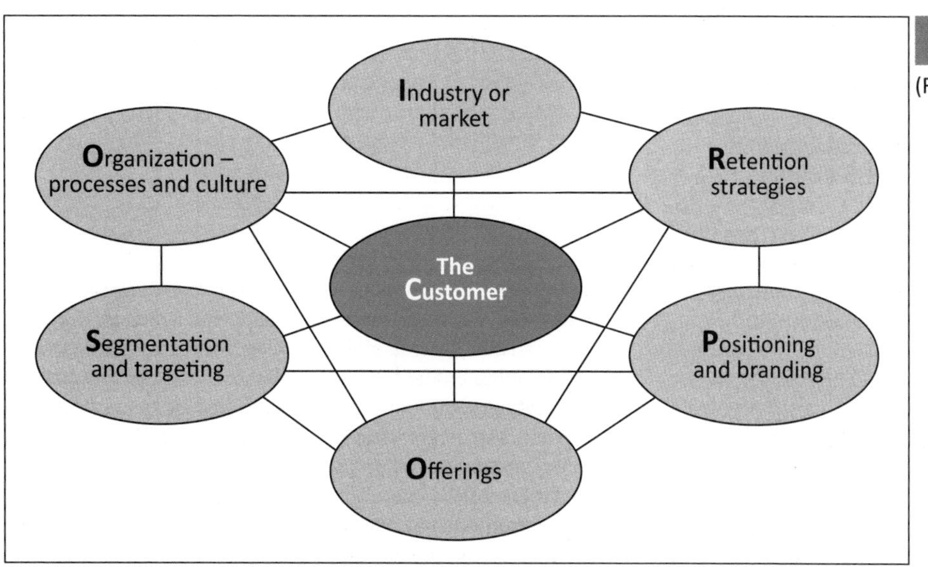

25.2 The SCORPIO model of market strategy (Fifield, 2008).

Industry or market

It is important to be clear about what the practice does, and where it wants to go (see Chapter 23). In the SCORPIO model this is represented by 'Industry or market', and is also referred to as the **marketing orientation** of the practice. Three orientations can be described.

- **Product/service-oriented** organizations concentrate on the products and services they offer. Such businesses believe that the demand for their product or service is obvious and therefore they do not take into account the needs of the customer/client.
- **Sales-oriented** organizations focus on maximizing sales through sales techniques and a sales force.
- **Market-oriented** organizations focus on the needs of the customer, and all business activities will be coordinated around the customer. Practices that are truly market-oriented take a longer term view of business.

KEY POINT

The difference between selling and marketing is that selling focuses on the needs of the seller, whereas marketing focuses on the needs of the buyer (whilst making money in the process).

If it is felt that the marketing is not working, it may be because of the following factors:

- Inadequate market research: practices must be familiar with the needs of current and potential clients to plan a worthwhile marketing strategy
- Inadequate client profiling: asking questions of customers can be a key step to improving and expanding customer service
- Off-the-shelf marketing programmes: any standard plan will fail unless it is customized to a fit a practice's goals, values, operating principles and personnel
- One-shot sale mentality: a narrow focus on 'getting money' rather than 'getting the client back' can undermine marketing efforts
- Lack of incentives: unless practices allow members of staff to engage in practice development during working hours, the commitment to the idea will be minimal and consequently the results disappointing
- Lack of sales skills: any practice development programme that does not assess skills and provide group and individual sales training will fail
- Lack of personal accountability: all employees and partners must be accountable, not only for their own duties but also for upholding, and delivering implied promises relating to, the mission statement and the practice vision.

If the practice does not understand what clients need or want, then the success of any marketing activities will be limited. In order to succeed in the long term, there have to be ongoing and coordinated activities to ensure that the practice understands its clients and caters for their needs better than the competition would.

Organization – processes and culture

Central to all marketing activity is the culture of the organization, which reflects the attitudes and beliefs of all the personnel. Management systems and processes need to be supported by consistency in staff attitude and by everyone believing in the core goals of the practice.

The 7S McKinsey Model (Figure 25.3) can be used in a wide variety of situations; for example:

- To analyse and improve the performance of a business
- To examine the likely effects of future changes within a business
- To align departments and processes during a merger or acquisition or during any changes
- To determine how best to implement a proposed strategy.

The 7S model can be used to help analyse the practice's current situation, and a proposed future situation (where the practice wants to be) and to identify gaps and inconsistencies between them.

- **Strategy**, **structure** and **systems** are known as the 'hard' elements. These are easier to define or identify, and management can directly influence them. They include organization charts and reporting lines, formal processes and IT systems.
- **Shared values**, **skills**, **style** and **staff** are known as the 'soft' elements. They can be more difficult to describe and are more influenced by culture.

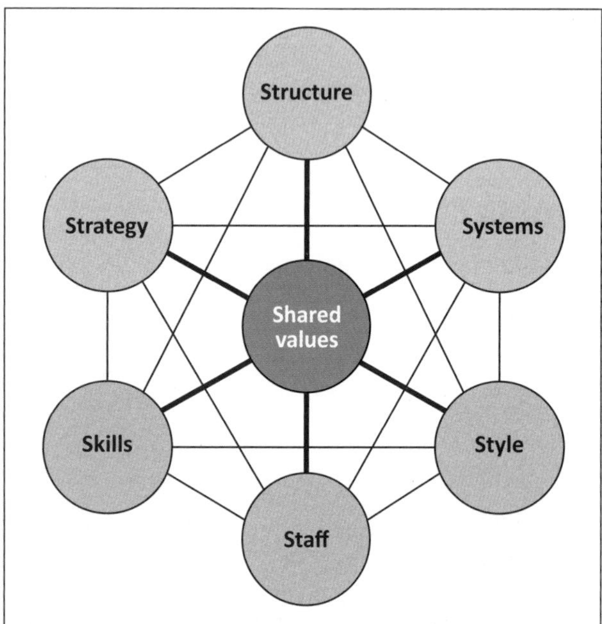

25.3 The 7S McKinsey Model. The interdependency of the seven elements means that a change in one of them can affect all the others. Placing 'Shared values' in the middle of the model emphasizes that these values are central to the development of all the other critical elements. The company's structure, strategy, systems, style, staff and skills all stem from why the organization was originally created, and what it stands for. The original vision of the company was formed from the values of the Principal. If the values change, so do all the other elements.

Each element will need to be compared against the other six elements in the matrix. Having a framework will help to ensure that the right questions are asked. Examples of questions that may arise are listed below.

- Are the practice's shared values consistent with its structure, strategy and systems?
- Is the style of management in line with practice values?
- Do the attitude and actions of the team reflect practice values? For example, are they dedicated and caring?
- Are there gaps in required competencies?
- Are there any gaps in the skills of staff, including the management team and the practice principal?
- Do the current employees/team members have the ability to do the job?

Discussing some of the seven elements and identifying gaps might be done as a team brainstorming session. It is far easier to implement changes if the team has, for example, looked at the systems that are currently in place and concluded that they are no longer appropriate and no longer ensure the best possible client care or patient care as per the values of the practice.

The 7S model can be applied to almost any organizational or team effectiveness issue. If something within the practice or team is not working, there will be inconsistency between some of the elements identified by this classic model. By analysing and determining the ultimate state for each of the factors, inconsistencies will be revealed. Once identified, they can be addressed and resolved. Only when the internal elements are realigned can the practice and the team move forward.

The knowledge-based business

As knowledge-based businesses, practices that manage and use knowledge effectively will have an advantage. The following areas are useful to consider.

- **Internal awareness:** The business's ability to assess its own core competencies and abilities.
- **Internal responsiveness:** The business's capacity to change and respond to new market challenges and customer needs – how it uses the knowledge and skills of its staff to effect change and drive the practice forward to keep up with changes in demand.
- **External awareness:** This is about understanding changes in the marketplace, what is going on elsewhere in the sector, and how customers perceive what the practice currently offers. It may use surveys and market research. Responding to the challenges, however, requires the internal responsiveness described above.
- **External responsiveness:** This is the ability of the business to respond to challenges and changes in the external and economic environment.

In a knowledge-based business, individuals and teams may be able to move and adapt quickly and this will give them a competitive advantage over less responsive businesses that may be slow to adapt. This means setting broad goals and guidelines and managing effectively, so that individuals have the knowledge and skills to realign themselves and adapt quickly to external pressures. In a fast-moving market, the speed of flow of knowledge will have a significant effect on the adaptability and success of the practice, as long as team members are empowered to use it (see Chapter 18).

Positioning and branding

Positioning is the outcome of a process by which a business or practice decides how it wishes to be perceived by its customers. Rather than being about products and services specifically, it is about how customers perceive a service or the practice as a whole, and the aim should be to develop clarity and simplicity in communications, so that customers associate clear concepts with the particular business offering. Positioning can also be decided by the customers themselves, and may be different from that intended by the practice.

Differentiation

A differentiated market position is one that is clearly different from other competitors; e.g. a practice might offer 'keyhole' surgery, 24-hour hospitalization or an in-house grooming service. However, differentiation is not just about different products and services; it is often about a different approach, e.g. a more customer-friendly welcome, tea and coffee in reception, a more personal telephone answering style, more comfortable seating, or a more caring manner. Differentiation may also be about quick and efficient service for busy commuters, or a relaxed style for those with more time to chat. However the practice is differentiated, there are usually one or more USPs (unique selling points or propositions). The USPs should be well defined and should be included in the marketing effort, so that clients and potential clients are aware of them. Each one of a number of differentiated practices in one area can stand out from its competitors and can still be profitable with a lower volume of sales but at higher prices. Customers choose a particular practice for a number of different reasons, and the skill in positioning is understanding what these are or are likely to be, and then working consistently to meet expectations every time (see Chapter 27).

Commodity marketing

In commodity marketing, competition is based upon price alone, with little differentiation. The trend with 'commoditization' is that prices are driven lower and lower, generally at the expense of profit, quality and service (Figure 25.4); there is usually only one clear winner in the marketplace – the one with sufficient volume of sales to succeed. When mass marketing techniques are used, it is more difficult to cater for individuals, and customers' needs may not be satisfied. The other danger is that once the market becomes saturated, demand for a product or service will fall and a new focus will be required.

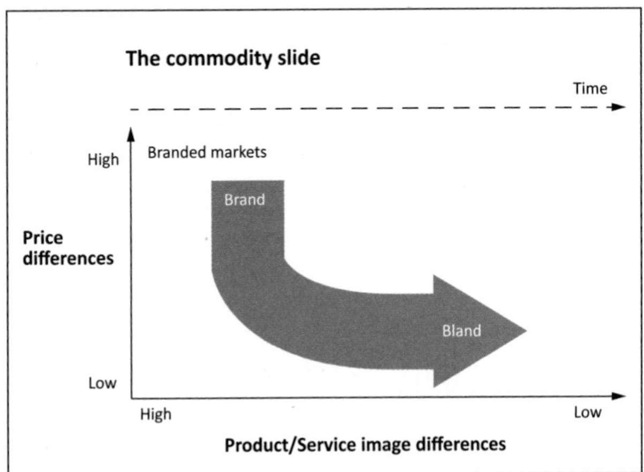

25.4 The commodity slide (after Fifield). Differentiated services that are branded can be highly priced. Commodity products or services that are not branded tend to be low priced. Where clients cannot see any added value or differences between the products or services offered by different practices, they may make a choice just on price.

In veterinary practice it is becoming common for some products and services to become more 'commoditized'. In this instance, the cheaper services, such as vaccination or microchipping, become 'loss leaders' (a product/service sold at a low price to attract clients in and then encourage other more profitable sales). However, the clients attracted in by these may not remain loyal to the practice. Although it is possible to combine some differentiation with low pricing, generally this will be at a more basic 'hygiene' level rather than in more complex services and offerings. As clients' perceptions of service and value for money change, particularly during times of economic uncertainty, it is becoming much more usual for them to use more than one practice for different services, choosing from a menu of commoditized and differentiated offerings. For example, a dog may receive routine vaccinations and be neutered in one clinic but be taken to a full-service veterinary practice or hospital when it is ill. For differentiated practices, the decision on whether to stay in the commodity market for certain items must be driven by overall net profit, which will be influenced by the additional level of differentiated sales; it may not be financially viable for a veterinary hospital to carry out cut-price neutering. The growth of referral services has further differentiated the market, and clients are much more used to shopping around now than they were 20 years ago.

Brands

Where there is clear differentiation (and more than one winner!) these are termed branded markets. Brands are not just about logos, advertising and memorable jingles. Brands are product and service offerings that are recognizable, and consistent. Successful brands are trusted, different in an easy-to-understand way, and relevant to customers' lives and experiences.

In building a clearly recognizable and successful brand, it is important to know, therefore, what customers' wants, needs, aspirations and feelings are. Market research can help with this, and client surveys are invaluable in helping gather evidence to define what it is that clients value about the service they receive (see Chapter 27). As well as identifying areas for growth and innovation, practices should also look at declining or non-profitable areas and consider whether these do still represent customer value. If they do, then restructuring may be required, rather than dropping the service.

An exercise

1. List a few well known brands and the values or 'personality' they represent.
2. List a few product types (e.g. cars, flea treatments, airlines, vacuum cleaners), and list three common brands for each.
3. Note what differentiates each brand from the other and try to work out the positioning for each brand.

It should be clearer now where emotions come into play, and although advertising and promotion play a large part in the development and prominence of some brands, service and experience generally is a major factor in their success. Promotion cannot prop up a poor product or service for long. It is also worth thinking about the effect of time on the success of these brands – some may be new, others long established. How have the older players maintained their position? Or have they changed it? Brands can never stand still, they must adapt to changing attitudes and needs; however, most established brands will retain a recognizable form or theme through any change.

Branding in veterinary practice

Product branding is very relevant to over-the-counter sales and to commonly purchased items, such as flea and worm control. Where a manufacturer supports a valued brand with good quality advertising, sales can grow and margins can be maintained. However, it is the practice branding that will have the biggest influence when it comes to ongoing success. The successful brand is a trusted choice for the customer.

To think of it a different way, the practice's brand is its flagpole. This is very visible and clear, and clients will hang on to it (Figure 25.5). The strength of the brand acts as a glue on that flagpole: the stronger the brand, the less likely clients will be to migrate to a different practice. To be strong, the flagpole (services, products and practice staff) must be reliable, performing as expected all the time.

Maintaining and renewing customer loyalty is the secret to a successful brand and a healthy net profit. Doing more work on a product or service does not necessarily enhance the brand (strengthen the 'glue'), however; it is important to work on how customers feel about the brand (see Chapter 27). A successful practice will be regarded by its clients not just as somewhere necessary to visit when they have a problem, but as a positive partner in the care of their pet. Visits should be anticipated eagerly, not dreaded. Customers that are passionate about the brand are reluctant to move away from it. Small changes can maintain performance, loyalty and the positive relationship.

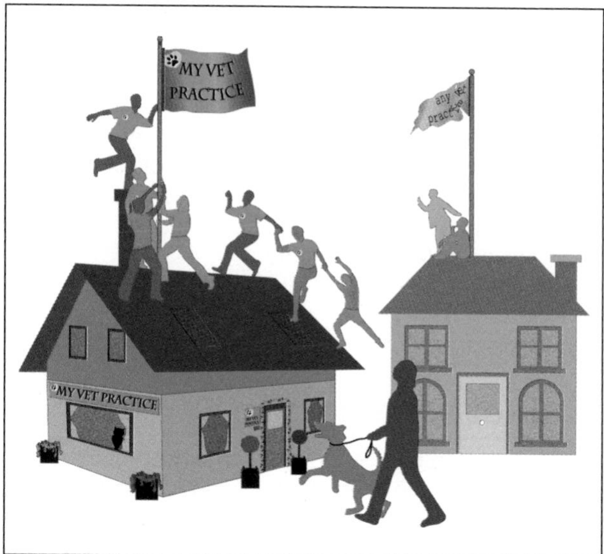

25.5 Hanging on to the flagpole: the stronger the brand 'glue' that holds clients to the flagpole, the more loyal they will be. If there is no brand 'glue', customer drift will be a reality.

Developing and maintaining a successful brand

The practice should be clearly positioned so that clients know what is on offer and that it is relevant to them. Most importantly, this must be clearly communicated and must be consistent. Factors that contribute to a clear brand image include:

- A clear set of goals and/or mission statement
- Clear culture and beliefs of the team
- Name of the practice, and recognizable logo
- Position and appearance of the premises
- Level and style of customer service
- Quality of the customer experience from arrival to departure, and follow-up
- Word-of-mouth communication – talking about the experience
- Being clearly different from competitors in the client's perception
- Consistency in image projection (Figure 25.6)
- Visibility in the marketplace – advertising and community activity
- Social responsibility and ethical behaviour.

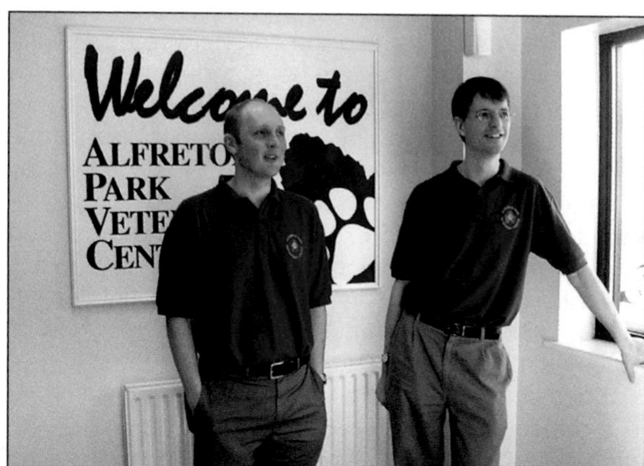

25.6 A consistent brand image can include extensive and prominent use of the practice logo and colours, and can be extended to staff clothing.

Many of these aspects are discussed elsewhere in this Manual, but a few will be expanded upon here. It is useful to think about what the brand would look like if it were a person: What sort of person would it be? Do the practice, the logo and strap line (short advertising message) match this?

Being clearly different in the client's perception

Being clearly different means being clear about what the practice offers that clients value – repeatedly stating what differentiates the practice from others, in clear terms and without jargon. The message(s) should not change too frequently or this will dilute the brand. This is an important consideration when planning advertising materials and practice brochures.

> **KEY POINT**
>
> A consistent message should be conveyed across all types of media.

Being consistent in the client's perception

A consistent message is of no value if it does not reflect reality. The practice must be consistent in all areas and in everything it does. Clients will expect the same level of care and attention from every member of staff every time they visit.

Image projection

As well as strap lines and written copy, the name of the practice and its logo must be considered.

- **Practice name:**
  - Is the practice name well known, and what does it stand for in the client's and community's eyes?
  - Would people immediately think of the name and link it with the USP(s) offered by the practice?
  - Do the staff feel proud to work under this banner?
- **Logo:** It is not essential to have a specific logo, but a well designed logo is useful for immediate brand recognition and as shorthand on any marketing and communication materials, such as badges, uniforms, letterheads and advertisements.
  - Is the logo consistent with the practice's position in the marketplace?
  - Is it modern?
  - Does it project the values of the practice and reflect the name of the practice?
  - Does it indicate location? (Can be useful if the practice is not very visible in the environment)
  - Does it look professional? (This is where a good graphic designer is essential)
  - Is it easy to produce in black and white, in two colours (one colour plus black) and in full colour?
  - Does it look good large and small?
  - Is it unique or could it be easily confused with other well known logos?
  - Does it work in electronic media and paper-based media?
  - Are colours consistent with other materials, and with the practice position?
  - Is the logo being used everywhere it could be?

Matching the projected image with the reality of practice positioning is vital for brand success. If the practice is offering high-quality veterinary medicine in a professional style, do the logo, staff uniform, shoes, décor and business cards also project the same image? Without a clear marketing strategy and understanding of client perceptions of an individual practice, it can be difficult to design a logo that will adequately support the brand. Where a new logo or practice name is being considered, great care must be taken not to lose the brand associations with the existing ones, and some linkage is often advisable. There are many examples of organizations that have changed their names and branding only to have to change back again further down the line.

Maintaining a brand means keeping a close rein on all external communications so that they reflect the brand guidelines. The guidelines should include new media communications, so that everything the practice publishes or writes is consistent with the planned image.

Brand guidelines should include:

- How and when to use the logo
- The correct font (typeface) and size to use for letters, brochures, etc. (using templates for layout)
- How colour should be used, including guidelines for monochrome.

KEY POINT

A professional image can be destroyed instantly in the eyes of a client if poorly spelt or punctuated letters are sent, if handwriting is not neat and legible, or if inaccurate information is given. The small things really matter; ideally, one or two people in the practice should have the responsibility of ensuring that all new communications follow the guidelines, and that communications are subject to some form of quality control.

Brands in the community

Visibility in the community is an important aspect of branding, and the brand image will be enhanced by activities that demonstrate environmental and social responsibility. Practices that spend time with schools, youth groups and charities will project a positive image and encourage the community to engage with them. Environmentally friendly policies, sponsorship and prudent purchasing can all help show the community how caring the business is. Getting staff personally involved in local projects and on committees is invaluable for networking, and professional networks in the community should not be ignored.

Why do brands work?

It is clear that customers like brands. Brands make buying decisions easier and take the decision-making away from price alone. Customers like to feel part of the brand and can be enthusiastic about 'spreading the word'. This is exactly what a successful veterinary practice should be aiming for in order to maintain a good flow of new clients and patients. Brands can offer the buyer security and help reduce the risk of purchasing, as the offering should be familiar and predictable and quality generally assured. This is particularly important when customers want to use a new product or service – if they are familiar with the brand (the veterinary practice), trust is already in place. Brands can also be aspirational – people like to feel they are buying the best, or doing the best for their pet. A trusted brand will be something to aim for – the best quality a client can afford.

Segmentation and targeting

Market segments

The market can be divided or 'segmented' into subsets of clients that can then be targeted using a distinct marketing mix. For example, the product or price may vary depending on the segment targeted. The customer profiling concept is a compromise between mass marketing (one size fits all) and individual bespoke offers, and is the foundation for the development of a customer-driven marketing strategy. For the customer, segmentation provides not only an increased choice of products and services, but also a range that should more closely match their needs. For the organization, marketing and sales activities can be more focused, resulting in more sales, reduced costs and higher profitability.

There are numerous options and approaches to categorizing/segmenting customers:

- **Geographical factors:** the market is divided into locations and regions, according to where the customer lives, e.g. neighbourhoods or postcodes
- **Demographic factors:** characteristics of a population such as age, gender, occupation, income, marital status
- **Geodemographic factors:** a combination of geographical and demographic segmentation – the demographic characteristics of particular regions
- **Psychological factors:** customers can be divided on the basis of lifestyle, opinions, interests, values
- **Behavioural factors:** the consumer's relationship with the product; this approach divides customers according to usage rates, brand loyalty, readiness to buy.

It is interesting to note the link between segmentation and branding; they are not stand-alone issues.

Segments that have been mainly divided demographically (e.g. by client age or gender) are simple classifications. Segments that have been divided by emotional factors, such as motivation or loyalty, represent true segmentation and are more strategic and long term. It may be more productive to send out a promotion to loyal clients who have actively recommended the practice than to send it it, for example, to all female clients of a certain age.

Care should be taken not to assume that everyone in a subset has the same characteristics. Poor segmentation, analysis or choice of variables within the marketing mix can lead to failure. Over segmentation can lead to market fragmentation, resulting in client confusion due to the variety of choices available.

Overall, a company cannot cater for all segments within their marketplace. As with any business, a practice will need to analyse the market, including competitor strategies, and identify and then consider which segments it can cater for and are a viable target, and which to avoid. In order to do this, it will need to carry out:

- Qualitative market research – to establish customer attitudes and what factors are driving behaviour in the target market
- Quantitative research – to look at demographics, product usage and purchasing behaviour.

The more that is known about clients' needs and wants, the more closely a business will be able to match the services required and to meet client expectations. Recognizing the needs, characteristics or behaviours of clients enables marketing to be targeted.

Target marketing

Target marketing recognizes the diversity of customers and does not try to please them all by offering the same one product or service. There are three broad approaches to targeting.

- **Undifferentiated** strategy: this is the least demanding approach, with a single marketing mix or offer served to more than one segment. Whilst keeping costs low, this mass marketing approach will not accommodate the needs of all customers.
- **Differentiated** strategy: this involves the business developing a different marketing mix for each segment. This is a more challenging approach that can dilute effort and resources but is useful in a very competitive marketplace.
- **Concentrated** strategy: this focuses on delivering only a specialist offering to one specific segment for which a premium price may be charged. There is only one marketing mix to manage and resources are concentrated; however, if the 'niche' segment fails to respond as anticipated, there is no fallback position.

When a target market is divided up into relevant segments to allow a tailored offering to be developed, to be successful each segment must be:

- Distinctive: each segment must be significantly different from any other to ensure a sufficiently well tailored marketing mix that will attract and retain customers
- Commercially viable: if there is a gap in the market, is it an opportunity or is it too small to be commercially viable?
- Accessible: the business must be able to deliver its goods and services and its promotional message to the customer
- Defensible: the business must take into account whether or not it can develop a strong enough differential advantage to defend itself against its competitors.

Once a practice has decided which segment of the market to target, in order to be successful it will need to penetrate the chosen segment and gain a greater share of it.

Retention strategies

All businesses need both to acquire new customers and to keep existing ones. Customers should be regarded as the most important asset to the organization, and it is important that all staff understand and acknowledge the lifetime value of each client. Whilst registering new clients is one important aspect, looking after and keeping profitable existing clients is crucial. It is important to acknowledge that the more investment that is made in acquiring a new client (e.g. advertising, promotions, special offers, discounts, puppy/kitten packages), the longer they need to remain as clients in order for this investment to be paid back.

Clients will stay with a practice if:

- They perceive they are getting value for money
- Their needs and wants are satisfied
- They cannot get a better offering from a competitor
- Communication is good and clients are aware of what the practice offers and what is different or unique about the offering.

Ideally, the practice will be moving beyond a straightforward business transaction and will be looking at establishing a relationship with the customer. A relationship is a two-way process; this therefore involves asking the customer what they want out of the relationship. The needs and wants of customers will change over time and for some, the practice will not want to, or will not be able to, accommodate their new requirements. The practice needs to maintain its market positioning and cannot cater for everyone. If a client naturally moves into other segments which may be better served by a competitor, then it may be best that they leave.

According to the 80:20 rule, the top 20% of clients provide 80% of turnover. The importance of customer care for these top clients cannot be underestimated (see Chapters 26 and 27), whilst some clients that are not bringing in the money and do not create a profit for the business may need to be reviewed. The top 20% of clients will change over time and may be made up of those with older pets (these often visit the surgery more frequently), pets with ongoing chronic conditions or pets who have required expensive surgery. A good practice management system should allow easy access to such data. It may also, for example, be useful to know who the top 20% of referrers are, as these will ensure maintenance of the client base.

It is important that, as well as new client acquisitions, the number of defecting clients and their reasons for moving are also monitored and recorded. Trends need to be identified and the reasons behind the trends need to be understood:

- Is there a new practice in the area?
- Is a competitor running any special offers?
- Has the practice changed its offering and not got the marketing mix correct?
- Does the practice need to update its offering?

Satisfied clients can still defect. The practice therefore needs to take the process one step further and ensure their clients keep coming back (they are loyal) and keep returning because they want to (they are committed). To help ensure loyalty is maximized and not compromised, a number of factors need to be considered, including competitor offers, the value proposition (see below), changing customer needs and wants, or any changes within the practice which may have caused a decline in loyalty (e.g. a change in veterinary staff can cause clients to defect).

Should a long-term bonded client change practice, it can be extremely beneficial and enlightening for someone from the practice to phone them to ask why, and to request some constructive feedback. Most clients are very obliging, open and honest, and practices may be surprised to find out that it is not always about price.

KEY POINT

It is important that all staff understand and acknowledge the lifetime value of each client. Whilst registering new clients is one important aspect, looking after and keeping profitable existing clients is crucial.

Offerings

The offering is not just about the product or service: it is about the process of how to meet the needs of the customer, i.e. the thinking, planning and implementing involved. It is the link between differentiation and value.

A product is an item that can be sold to clients. A service is something that is provided; by adding in and including the seller's expertise, value is then added to the transaction. It is best to think that clients visiting the practice are not buying specific goods, treatment and services but rather are looking for solutions to problems. They will attach a value to the service that is provided, depending on the benefit it offers in solving the problem. Clients therefore purchase 'value'.

KEY POINT

Practices that offer more value tend to be able to charge more, ultimately generating more income and profit for the business.

Value

Value represents different things to different clients; it is therefore difficult to quantify. Value should not be linked just to price, as this is just one aspect.

The product benefit or solution to a problem that the customer purchases is another component of value, as are effort and risk. A business can increase benefits by differentiating its services, increasing client convenience and reducing perceived risks. Clients will see a greater value in purchases that offer less effort and are more convenient, e.g. many clients will favour a long-acting injection or a spot-on drug to tablets, despite a higher cost. Clients also have perceived risks when purchasing products or services. The lower the perceived risk, the greater the value. For example, many clients will favour a specific surgeon to carry out a procedure, as they perceive the risk of something going wrong to be reduced. Offering guarantees and warranties, or free trials, may be beneficial. The most effective way of reducing a client's perceived risk, however, is to offer something they believe in and trust that represents reassurance – a brand.

The best value does not necessarily mean the cheapest price. Clients compare the perceived values from different practices against the prices charged. Smart clients want value for money and will pay as long as the service is perceived to offer them what they want and therefore to be of value.

The value proposition

The USP, also known as a 'value proposition', is a business's offer and promise of what it is going to deliver to a customer, and the benefits the customer is assured of receiving in exchange for payment. It is a combination of product, service, pricing and delivery system. In order to ensure a successful offering a business will need to:

- Know its target market (see above)
- Understand the needs and problems of its customers (via market research)
- Understand what is driving these needs, wants and purchasing behaviour
- Create and maintain a profitable market position and brand, and focus all marketing activities
- Ensure differentiated products or services
- Communicate the value and benefits of the offering to customers.

It is vital that clients prefer an offering over that of a competitor; clients will use the services of the practice they believe offers them best value.

Product life cycle

The product life cycle concept reflects the theory that products and services have a life and that they grow, mature and eventually die (Figure 25.7). Marketing support for each product will vary according to what stage the product is at, and elements of the marketing mix will vary at different stages in the product life cycle. This model can be applied to a product, service, product category or brand, and can be used to develop

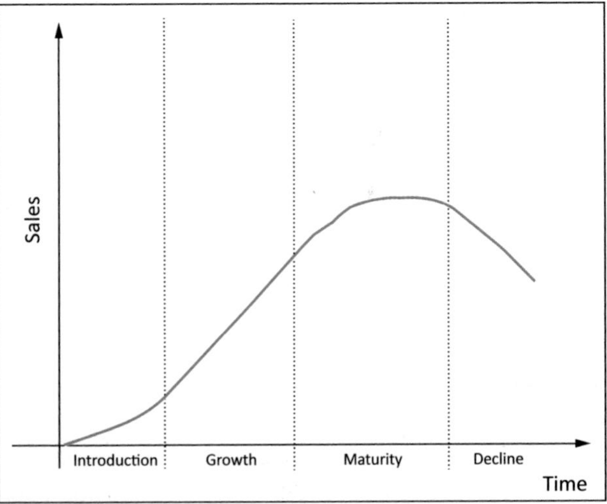

25.7 The product life cycle.

and manage the offerings part of the marketing strategy. For example, bringing forward the demand for a product or service during the growth stage may not increase the whole market but may increase overall market share: a practice promoting a new surgical procedure can create a demand and be ahead of its competitors, and hence increase market share. It can be argued that products and services do not have to 'die' and that, as long as the offer is still valued and profitable, the maturity stage should be extended. For more mature products and services, subsequent growth is still possible. Growth can be stimulated by modifying the product to increase its value, as currently seen in the mobile phone market, and by marketing different benefits for the same product, or suggesting different uses, to a wider range of clients. The product life cycle is a guide, providing useful indications of marketing problems and issues that may arise.

Product portfolio

Many factors need to be taken into account and evaluated when it comes to the product portfolio; these include product performance, demand, market share, potential product growth, and repeat sales.

Implementation

The implementation process consists of the marketing mix being applied to the value proposition. The 4Ps, product, price, promotion and place, are therefore aligned to the customers' (the target market) needs and wants.

Ansoff marketing matrix

In order for a business to grow, a strategy to introduce, develop, extend or modify the range of products sold or services offered can be used. The Ansoff matrix (Figure 25.8) looks at four combinations of product–market options:

- **Market penetration:** This is where a business aims to increase sales volumes in current markets. This can be achieved by better segmentation and increasing marketing effort and by encouraging existing customers to buy more through advertising, publicity, special promotions (e.g. vaccination amnesty or worming reminders)

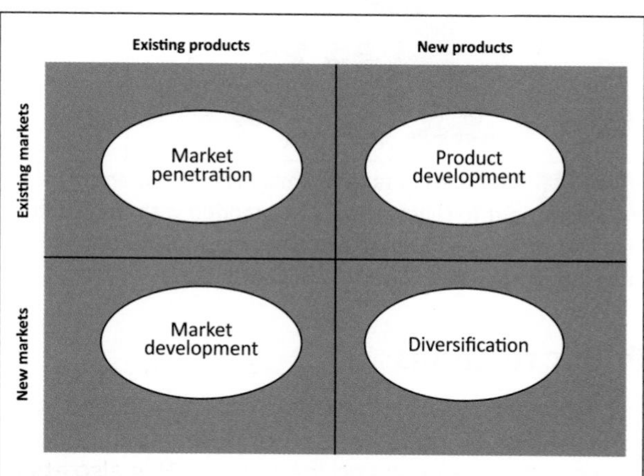

25.8 The Ansoff matrix: a model to help businesses decide on their product and market growth strategy.

- **Market development:** This involves introducing current products to new markets (e.g. different regions) or new market segments (e.g. offering services available at the practice, such as acupuncture or hydrotherapy, to other practices and their clients). There is a clear need for market research when adopting this strategy
- **Product development:** This involves selling new or improved products into existing markets, e.g. spot-on wormer, laparoscopic bitch spay
- **Diversification:** Entering new products into new markets is a higher-risk strategy, e.g. dog grooming, cat boarding, behaviour classes.

Promotion

Promotion is one of the 4Ps of the marketing mix (see earlier); the promotional mix is the combination of marketing and communication strategies. The practice must look at the way it makes the market aware of, and how it communicates, its services and the benefits to both existing and potential clients. This includes looking at other factors, such as packaging and branding as well as practice literature.

KEY POINT

Communication is an integral and vital aspect of the promotional mix.

The promotional mix

The promotional mix includes a number of tools.

Sales promotions

These are short-term inducements to encourage purchases and increase sales. Sales promotions can be used tactically to:

- Launch new products
- Stimulate interest from new consumers
- Move old stock
- Encourage increased product uptake and/or repeat purchases from existing consumers
- Counteract competitor activity.

Examples include:

- Special offers
- Coupons
- Free samples
- Discounts
- Free gifts
- Competitions
- Short-term price offers
- Combination pack offers.

It is vital to know who the customers are and how to reach them. Customer data will enable current customers to be profiled and help target them correctly. If key performance indicators (KPIs) are used as a management tool, these can also highlight areas where special offers can be run in order to improve take-up of certain services. These should then be measured to see whether the promotion has worked (Figure 25.9).

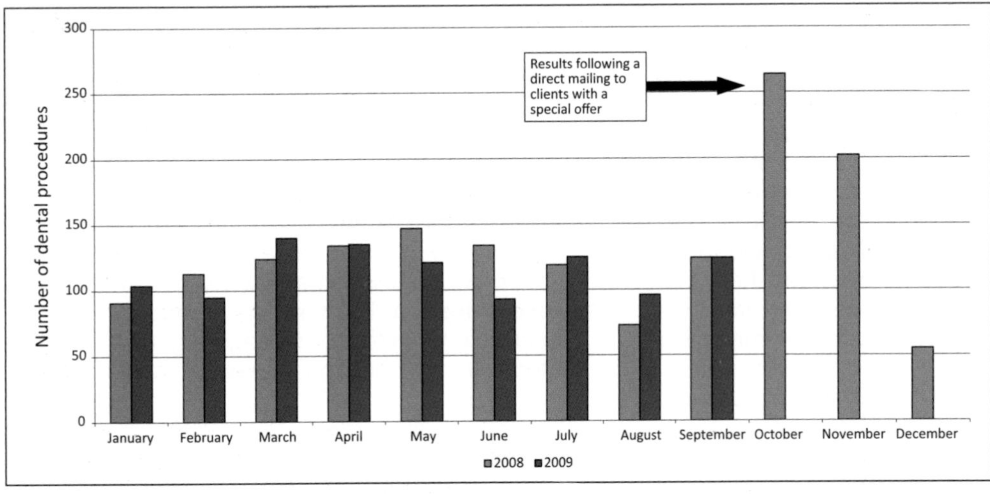

25.9 This graph illustrates an increase in dental procedures following a marketing promotion.

> **KEY POINT**
>
> Take care not to make the mistake of thinking increased sales means an increase in profits. Marketing performance must be judged on profit rather than purely on sales volume.

Advertising

Advertising creates awareness and an interest in the product or service and in the organization. It is paid-for mass communication and therefore is often non-personal. It can reach a large audience at low cost but the audience may include people who are not the appropriate target market and will never become clients, e.g. the non-pet-owning public.

Personal selling

Personal selling is very effective, as it uses face-to-face communication between staff and clients, allowing a tailored approach according to the needs of the individual client. Technical advice can be given and the sale secured and closed.

Direct marketing

- Direct marketing may take the form of mailshots to select client and patient groups about specific health issues, procedures and treatments (Figure 25.10), using the database of a practice management system.
- Most practice management systems now have the ability to e-mail clients. This is a cost-effective way to communicate a promotion.
- SMS texting is also available through many practice management systems, and most clients will have a mobile phone. What can be included in a text message is limited, however, so the wording has to be simple and to the point. This tool is very useful for clinical reminders such as for vaccinations.
- Well designed posters and displays in the reception area are also useful to promote a product (see Chapter 5). Several commercial companies offer design and printing of promotional materials, so it is possible to display well designed professional-looking material at minimum cost.
- A regularly and professionally produced newsletter can be: left in reception; put up on the website to be downloaded; e-mailed; and/or sent out with invoices. This is a great tool for keeping in contact with clients and updating them with practice news and events as well as promotional offers. Interesting case histories can be included to promote services.
- Joint ventures and working with other local businesses, such as breeders, catteries, dog groomers, kennels, training centres and feed merchants, can be mutually beneficial when it comes to promotion and recommendations.

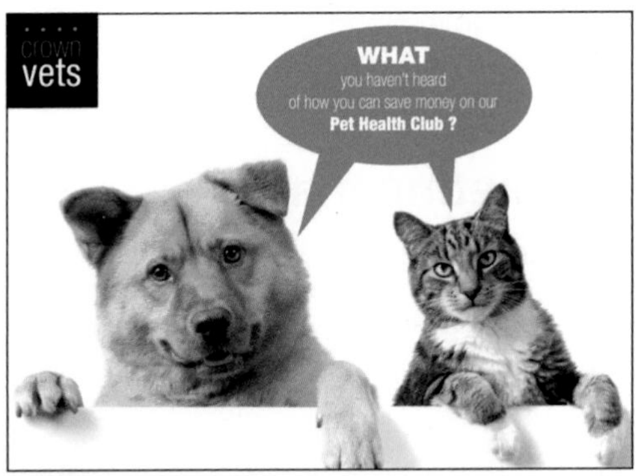
crown vets
WHAT
you haven't heard
of how you can save money on our
Pet Health Club ?

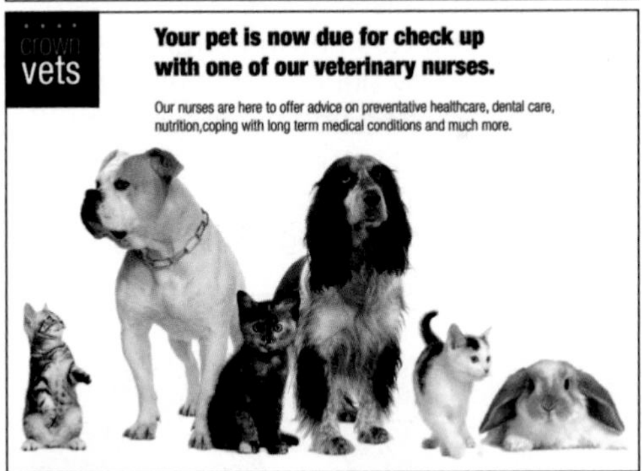
crown vets
Your pet is now due for check up with one of our veterinary nurses.
Our nurses are here to offer advice on preventative healthcare, dental care, nutrition,coping with long term medical conditions and much more.

25.10 Examples of targeted mailings. All material sent out to clients should be branded with the practice logo and should be of suitable quality to complement the image of the practice. (Courtesy of Crown Vets)

Public relations

Public relations (PR) involves the planned and sustained effort to communicate and promote goodwill between the business and the public. PR is also about educating and informing customers and is seen as a long-term commitment. Where information appears in the media, editorial material is seen as more credible than paid-for advertising space, although the business may not have total control over what is eventually printed or over the timing of any press releases.

Press releases

A press release about the practice must be a story that: is relevant to the publication; contains new information; is factual; and is of interest to the readers. The story can be about the business, a new product, people (clients or staff) or patients. The first paragraph must contain key elements and any vital information about the story to catch the editor's eye. If writing a story for a local paper, it should start with the name of the practice and where it is located, so the editor is instantly made aware that the practice is in the catchment area for the paper's readers. Editors are more likely to print a story that does not overtly promote the practice, which has an intriguing headline, and which is written in plain English with no long medical terms. It should also be well presented (1.5 or double line spacing so that editors can make notes). Full and correct practice contact details must be submitted. A good photograph can increase chances of publication, along with short, relevant and meaningful quotes.

Marketing literature

Practice literature is an important tool for communicating with clients; when done well it can help build a strong and professional brand. Examples of marketing literature that can be produced by the practice include:

- Welcome letter
- Opening hours
- All about the practice
- Terms and conditions
- Any promotional offers
- Staff details
- Neutering guidelines
- Flea and worming guidelines
- Vaccination guidelines
- Details on health clubs.

When designing marketing literature, it is helpful to use the AIDA format:

- **A**ttention: something eye-catching for the customer
- **I**nterest: mention some features of the product or service
- **D**esire: explain to the customer the benefits
- **A**ction: tell the customer how and where to contact you.

Using new media

Traditional advertising is losing its influence on consumers and there is a growing trend, backed by statistical evidence, of consumers making purchasing decisions from Internet research and referrals. Consumers are more inclined to believe feedback from like-minded peers than corporate-style marketing dispensed via traditional direct mail and advertising. Since veterinary practices around the world talk repeatedly about building trust with their clients, it would make good business sense to harness the Internet to build on this and incorporate it into the practice marketing mix. People with access to a computer with an Internet connection are much more likely to use a search engine than a printed directory when they are looking for a veterinary practice.

New media marketing uses traditional forms of media (e.g. images, written and spoken words) and publishes content on computer-enabled devices or the Internet, enabling interactive user feedback, creative participation and community formation. Developing an online community allows customers to congregate and, in a best-case scenario, extol the virtues of the brand. Sir Timothy John Berners-Lee, creator of the World Wide Web in 1989, has said, 'The ultimate goal of the web is to support and improve on our existence in the world...to develop trust across the miles and trust around the corner...the web is more a social creator than a technical one. I designed it for the social effect – to help people work together'.

> **KEY POINT**
>
> New media marketing is about people, relationship building and being social – this is the new way of doing business.

The practice website

It is not difficult to set up a website quickly and easily. With the popularity of easy-access publishing platforms it is now possible for anyone to set up their own website and integrate social networks (Figure 25.11). Alternatively, practices can choose from a number of 'ready to go' websites especially designed for the veterinary market. The first thing that the practice will need

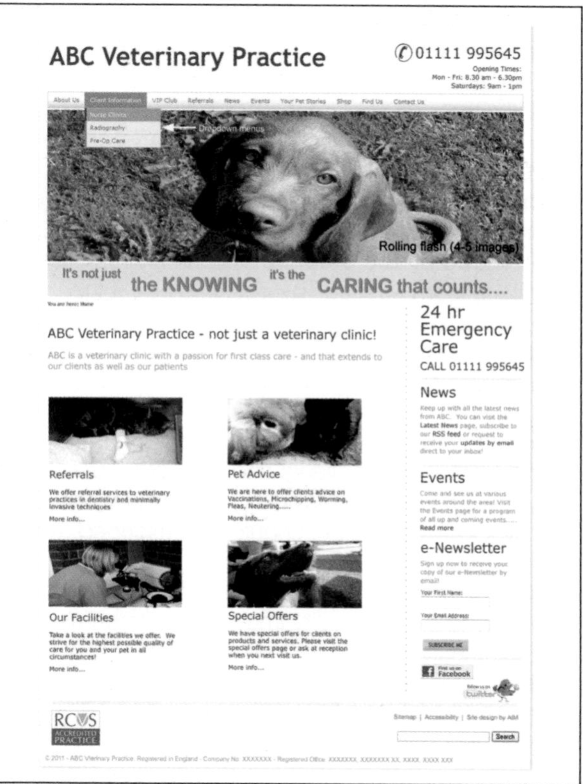

25.11 An example of a practice website homepage. (Courtesy of aimweb.co.uk)

is a 'domain name'; this is the address that people use to find a business online (e.g. yourvetpractice.com or yourvetpractice.co.uk, depending on the practice's location in the world). A degree of creativity is required where there are practices with the same or a similar name or where the name is long or difficult to spell. The website is the practice 'storefront' and the practice should put as much into its virtual storefront as it would to the front window/reception display at its physical premises. The website needs to attract customers and keep them coming back for more.

KEY POINT

The website should be easy to use. Visitors should be able to learn as much as possible about the practice in a short space of time and should be able to find exactly what they are looking for within three clicks of the mouse.

Design

Whether someone in the practice puts the website together or a designer is hired, there are some key points to consider, and care should be taken to see things from the customer's point of view. Looking at the practice website from the visitor's perspective, the practice should ask themselves the following questions.

- **Where do the visitor's eyes go first?** It is important to ensure that the first image seen is something interesting enough to keep the visitor on the site. Colourful images and videos work well.
- **Does the visitor know straight away what the website is about?** There is a limited time to get the practice message across. Are there too many distractions? The practice phone number should be prominently displayed.
- **Is the important information 'above the fold'?** This means that the visitor does not have to scroll down the page to find the practice's unique selling proposition (USP) because it is clearly spelled out as soon as they arrive at the website.
- **Can the visitor find out easily what the benefits are to them of the products and services provided by the practice?** A visitor should be able to learn as much as possible about the practice in a short space of time. The information should be about the benefits of the practice products and services, and not the features. For example, visitors should be informed that the practice has a big car park (the feature) that will make life easy for clients and less stressful for pets (valued benefit). If promoting a particular product, the benefits to the pet should be described rather than the product.
- **Are the colours and images aesthetically pleasing?** High-quality images should be used and time taken to coordinate colours.
- **Do the menu items clearly tell the visitor where they will be taken?** Site design and usability are important considerations. Menus should be carefully planned and there should always be an 'About us' and a 'Contact us' page that visitors can find easily to get in touch with the practice. If the navigation is well designed, a visitor should be able to find exactly what they are looking for within three clicks of the mouse.
- **Does the visitor feel personally connected?** Visitors who feel personally connected with the practice will be more likely to stay on the website and/or become a customer. A conversational style should be used when detailing products and services – it is far more effective than 'brochure speak'. This is why social media always use the word 'you'.
- **Is there a 'webform'?** A webform on a web page is a way of collecting data automatically, using specialized software in order to capture leads from website visitors (see later). It should be visible and should offer a good incentive to encourage the visitor to give the requested information.
- **Is there multimedia content?** Multimedia content (e.g. video, audio, animation, images and, importantly, interactivity) is an excellent way to add character and interest to a website. For example, videos, podcasts and tutorials allow the practice to present its message to its visitors in a human way that appeals to them, rather than the formal approach that many businesses still use.
- **Are there links to social media?** Social media allow the practice to communicate with its customers and potential customers and allow them to communicate with each other. Links to a practice 'blog' and to Facebook, Twitter and other social media accounts should be included. It should be easy for everyone to find the practice on social media. Potential clients who do not fill out a webform may still choose to 'follow' the practice in some fashion.

Traffic generation

A good website must be designed in such a way that it can generate and maximize traffic flowing through it and ultimately attract potential clients to the practice. A few simple steps can encourage visitors to a website. The more that is put into traffic generation, the better the chances of converting visitors to clients. This includes search engine optimization (SEO), local search listings, Google AdWords and Facebook Ads, for example.

The design and wording of the website should maximize the practice's exposure in searches. For those familiar with the keywords that relate to the practice, 'pay per click' advertising can be very effective, but it can also be very expensive. It is therefore far better to ensure that the site fits all the guidelines as far as the main search engines (Google, Yahoo and Bing) are concerned, and that it is developed ethically within these guidelines to ensure maximum exposure within the indexes using no 'black hat' tactics. Black hat tactics are search engine optimization techniques that are used to try to get higher rankings in an unethical manner (e.g. invisible text methods where keywords are hidden in the hope of attracting more search engine 'spiders'). Such tactics will provide short-term gains in terms of rankings but, if they are discovered, the business runs the risk of being penalized by search engines and even removed from their listings.

KEY POINT

Traditional methods of marketing – printed newsletters and brochures, leaflets, posters, etc. – can be used to bring clients online. To achieve this, the practice website must be clearly displayed and existing clients and prospective clients should be guided to the website.

Using social media

Social media is an umbrella term that defines the various activities that integrate technology, social interaction, and the construction of words and pictures. Over 75% of consumers use social media in some form or another (e.g. Facebook, Twitter, YouTube) to learn about products and services. The practice cannot afford to miss out on the action. One of the most cited reasons for practices not getting involved with social media is that it is felt that they would be exposing certain weaknesses to the marketplace by allowing individuals, or even competitors, to post critical comments. However, responding with honest and transparent answers designed around solving the issue at hand mitigates any potential risks and actually establishes and strengthens the practice brand. Clients are likely already to be 'talking' about the practice but because it is not a part of the conversation the practice may not even know about it.

KEY POINT

It is important to understand that businesses should not sell their products and services on social media sites; this should be done by other means, such as the website. Using social media is about the practice becoming part of a 'community'. It is important to concentrate on getting the practice name out there, and building likeability and expertise.

There is plenty of pet-related content generated within the practice that can be published on blogs or in ezine articles, or turned into videos. The practice can also subscribe to sites that provide a digest of information either daily, weekly or monthly that can be used and commented upon. Services are available that will keep all bookmarked blogs and websites in one place for the user to revisit, and alerts can be set up to find anything published on a particular subject.

The person responsible for social media marketing for the practice should be trustworthy, and ready and able (and empowered) to 'speak' on behalf of the practice. A senior administrator or senior nurse would be an ideal choice. Clear guidelines should be laid out. Many businesses use an imaginary 'persona' to represent the practice on social media so that if the employee leaves the relationship the practice has built up with its clients through the 'spokesperson' is not damaged.

Social media marketing is no different to any other type of marketing in that it needs to be planned and incorporated into the marketing mix so that it becomes a part of the whole. Getting started in social media is not as daunting as it may seem and there are a few simple things the practice can do to get noticed in the online community.

Blogs

The word 'blog' originates from the term web log and is a tool for businesses of all sizes to publish content on the Internet. It is a way to become a respected provider of knowledge in the veterinary industry. Blogs are easy to create and maintain and a 'webmaster' does not need to be consulted. Figure 25.12 lists some examples of websites that may be helpful. Figure 25.13 shows an imaginary blog put together by the author [SB] using free software.

A name for the blog that is either the practice name or reflects the theme of the practice should be chosen. It needs to be inviting to readers. Once the blog has been set up it is time to start creating content. This could be stories, promotions, topics of interest – anything that is relevant to the practice's target audience. There should never be any shortage of content in a veterinary practice.

Blog programs	Automation
Wordpress.com Wordpress.org Blogger.com Blog.com	Socialoomph.com Hootsuite.com MarketMeSuite.com

25.12 Examples of websites that may be helpful when creating content for social media.

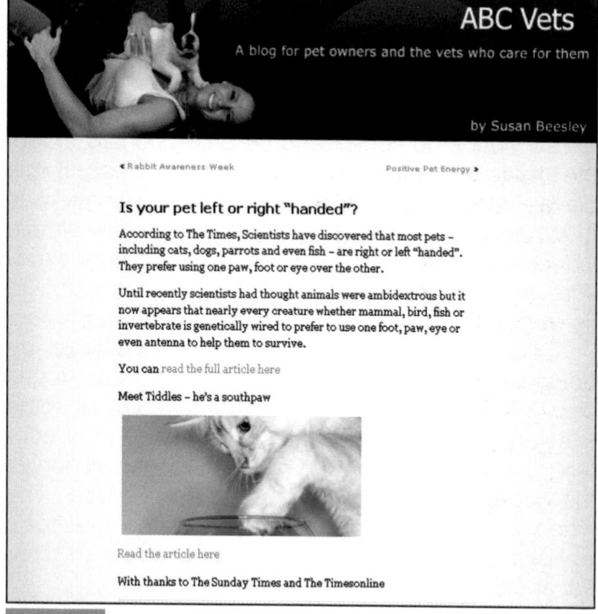

25.13 An example of a blog posting.

KEY POINTS

- Blog readers should be encouraged to interact with the practice by being asked questions and being asked for feedback and comments, and these should always be responded to. People like to be noticed!
- The practice should contribute regularly to its blog (at least once a week). This will ensure that content is fresh and that visitors keep coming back. It should be kept consistent and enjoyable for the audience.
- Content should be providing information, not selling.

Facebook, Twitter and LinkedIn

Social media options such as Facebook, Twitter and LinkedIn will help to increase brand exposure and allow the practice to communicate with existing customers and potential new customers. These are all free, easy to set up and widely used. Once the accounts have been set up, it is a matter of posting content and making sure that any responses or messages from customers are replied to quickly. Services are available that enable the practice to consolidate its social media dashboard, schedule updates ahead of time and even monitor conversations about its brand.

Article marketing

Article marketing, if done correctly, is an easy and free way to drive traffic to the practice website. There is a huge amount of content generated in every veterinary practice and an amazing knowledge base that can be shared. This content can be put into article form (usually 300–600 words) and distributed to free article-hosting sites. Practice articles should be informative, educational and entertaining.

Video marketing

Video marketing is simply publishing the practice message online through video. It can be used to highlight the practice, its products and services – such as a vet or nurse talking, a product demonstration, a promotional campaign or a customer testimonial. These videos do not have to be professionally made; the key is to create a 'buzz' around the video. If it is clever, interesting, relevant or unique in some way it will achieve traffic. Creativity is key. A few simple videos can dramatically increase a business's exposure on the Internet and help drive more traffic to its website.

Once the video has been created it should be uploaded to a commercial video-sharing site; terms and conditions should be checked carefully, as some sites are more restrictive than others on type of content. It is important to include a good description of the video, including the practice's keywords. The video should also be linked back to the practice's website and promoted on the practice's blog, Facebook page, Twitter, etc.

KEY POINT

If the video features a pet or owner, or both, the practice must ensure that it has permission to use it; a simple signed letter should suffice.

List building

Building up a list of leads (potential customers) is an important part of marketing. Whether captured through the website or through social media, leads are what eventually bring in sales. Practices can gather details from clients, e.g. for newsletter sign-ups, via e-mail forms on the website. This can be administratively heavy, and outsourcing may be preferable. An automated process can be set up using a webform. These forms, which usually ask for a visitor's name and e-mail address (Figure 25.14), allow the practice to build up a list of people who have given permission for the practice to market its products and services to them. The information is sensitive and must be kept secure. There are strict guidelines regarding blanket marketing and particularly spamming by e-mail. To comply with the Data Protection Act there should be an 'opt in' opportunity for the recipient to agree beforehand to receive communications such as newsletters by e-mail.

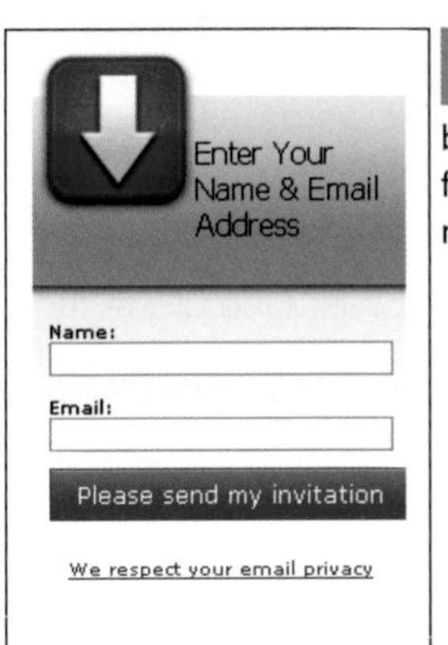
Enter Your Name & Email Address
Name:
Email:
Please send my invitation
We respect your email privacy

25.14 Webforms on the practice website can be used to gather client details for specific purposes, such as newsletter sign-up.

An autoresponder is a computer program that automatically answers e-mail sent to it. For practices that pay a subscription for an autoresponder service, the e-mail distribution list is sent to a third party. It is the responsibility of the list owner (the practice in this case) to make sure that all reasonable steps are taken to ensure the suitability of that third party as a responsible custodian of the data. Reputable autoresponder services will have their own e-mail privacy and anti-spam policies, which are vigorously enforced for the protection of the account holder and subscribers. Using the autoresponder software, messages can be prepared in advance and sent automatically to the practice's subscriber list. This is a great marketing tool.

The webform should ideally be placed 'above the fold' (on the top half of the 'page') on the website, with as little information as possible required from the subscriber. The more information that is requested, the less likely visitors will be to subscribe. The practice should also set out the expectations for its marketing and explain that the practice will respect the user's privacy. The clearer the practice is as to how any information will be used, and who it will be shared or not shared with, then the more willing people tend to be regarding imparting their details. Webforms can be used for newsletter sign-ups, 'recommend a friend' programmes – anything that will help the practice gather information. Webforms need not be confined to the practice website – it is also possible to put one on the practice Facebook business page.

Lead generation incentives

Once a webform is in place, the practice can offer something in exchange for getting that all-important lead. This incentive is something of value that the practice offers its website visitors, but only if they fill out the form, e.g. an e-book on how to care for a pet, or a voucher to spend when they visit the practice or order merchandise online from the practice. Time should be taken to create an offer that is really appealing to potential customers.

E-mail marketing

E-mail marketing is an inexpensive way in which to reach people on the list (customers/potential customers). If done correctly, this type of marketing will take a business to the next level and generate a good return on investment.

- It is important for the practice to have a system in place to ensure that all e-mails are opened and responded to promptly.
- The practice also needs to be able to see the response rate to e-mails that are sent out using an automated system. If the practice is using a reputable autoresponder service then it is possible to track this.
- SPAM-related words such as 'free' and 'special offer' should be avoided.
- The subject line is a big factor in whether the recipient opens the e-mail, so it needs to be appealing and any sensationalism must be avoided.
- All content should be relevant and valuable, educational and/or entertaining.
- It is important to make sure that clients know they can easily 'unsubscribe' at any time.

Care should be taken as to the number of e-mails sent out. A happy medium needs to be found which allows the practice to stay in touch. Regular newsletters and updates on practice events are a great way of fulfilling this. These can be prepared in advance and the whole delivery process can be automated.

Rather than trying to 'sell', the practice can guide its clients through a process which results in their wanting to contact the practice for more information, and this will ultimately lead to more sales. It is usual to have a link back to the website, where clients can contact the practice for more information.

How it all fits together

These days, with sophisticated practice management systems and software, it is possible to automate many of the tasks so that much can run on 'autopilot'. Figure 4.9 (see page 65) shows how new media marketing, including social media, fits together and allows the practice multiple opportunities to 'touch' its clients and prospective clients.

An ideas checklist for marketing

To get down to the practicalities, putting all this to work in a practice can be rather daunting. Some examples of areas to consider for practical marketing initiatives for practices are given in Figure 25.15. This list is not exhaustive, but should be a start to some creative marketing, publicity and service expansion, to spread the word and build the practice's brand.

Reception

- Posters, promotions and offers on products and services
- Practice-branded and educational leaflets
- Merchandise stand
- Pet photo noticeboard
- Staff picture board
- Themed displays
- Trained and knowledgeable reception staff

Nursing staff

- Vaccine clinics
- Senior clinics
- Obesity clinics
- Other clinics
- Puppy classes
- Patient admission and discharges
- Pre- and postoperative checks

Practice open evenings/days

- Preventive healthcare
- Communicate to a selective audience
- Invite bonded clients to bring a friend
- Specific client and complimentary invitations
- Target audience of key opinion-leaders, e.g. groomers, yard managers, breeders
- Obtain company support and sponsorship

Community involvement

- Schools, colleges
- Work experience
- School projects
- Local groups and societies, e.g. WI, riding clubs
- Fêtes, shows, community events

Local advertising

- Village/church magazine
- Sports and community clubs
- Kennels and catteries
- Public posters in shops, feed merchants, saddlers
- Advertise other businesses in your surgery, and your surgery in other businesses

Practice promotions

- Branded free gifts: leads, pens, bags for life
- Bundled products offering compelling discounts
- Special offers, repeated, seasonal
- Discount loyalty schemes
- Encourage and reward endorsements
- Practice literature

25.15 Some areas to consider for practical marketing initiatives.

Acknowledgements

The authors are grateful to the partners at Alfreton Park Veterinary Centre for the use of their image.

Further reading

Fifield P (2007) *Marketing Strategy, 3rd edn.* Butterworth-Heinemann (Elsevier), Oxford

Fifield P (2008) *Marketing Strategy Masterclass.* Butterworth-Heinemann (Elsevier), Oxford

Nicol D (2011) *The Yellow Pages Are Dead – Marketing your Vet Practice in the Digital Age.* Available from www.davenicol.com/ebook; http://www.theyellowpagesaredead.co.uk

Managing service quality to deliver excellence

26

Caroline Jevring-Bäck

Veterinary practice is a service industry committed to serving the needs of clients (pet owners and their pets) through selling veterinary services and products. To be successful, the procedures, policies and protocols that exist within practices should consistently produce satisfied and loyal clients who are willing to continue to buy these services, and this will ultimately improve practice profitability. However, increasing competition means that clients not only have more choice than ever before about where to take their pets, they are also less loyal.

This chapter will highlight some of the key issues behind producing excellence in client service (with a focus on managing and delivering the supporting service), and its relationship to quality, satisfaction and profitability.

When considering giving excellent service to clients, it is useful to include not just the pet owners who use veterinary services and purchase from the practice, but also other companies and businesses that have dealings with the surgery, any departments within the practice, and all members of the practice team. Examples of internal customers are a branch surgery needing to refer an orthopaedic case to the main hospital, and a new employee who will have a customer relationship with the staff who administer the payroll and supply uniforms and locker facilities. The service these internal customers receive may be reflected in the service they, in turn, offer to their external customers. Staff members dealing with customers will learn and reproduce skills that are demonstrated to them by their colleagues and by senior staff in their day-to-day interactions. Poor service levels to staff will therefore translate to poor service levels to customers. The management principles described in this chapter apply to both.

KEY POINTS

In veterinary practice, managing and delivering excellence in client service is made up of two parts:

- Managing veterinary medical and surgical care, to ensure quality and consistency
- Managing the supporting service around this, to ensure client satisfaction.

Client service and the service–profit chain

The lifetime value of a loyal client is enormous, especially when referrals (in this context, recommendations to other potential clients) are added to the economics of client retention and repeat purchase of related services and products. The link between service and profit is captured in the *service–profit chain* (Figure 26.1) which establishes relationships between profitability and client loyalty, and employee satisfaction, loyalty and productivity. The links in the chain are as follows:

- Profit and growth are stimulated primarily by client loyalty
- Loyalty is a near direct result of client satisfaction
- Satisfaction is largely influenced by the value of the services provided to clients
- Value is created by satisfied, loyal and productive practice members
- Practice employee satisfaction results primarily from high-quality support services and policies that enable them to deliver results to clients.

For a detailed description of how the service–profit chain works, the reader is referred to the original paper (Heskett *et al.*, 2008), but the concept forms the backbone to the rest of this chapter. Simply put, what Figure 26.1 shows is that 'happy staff make happy customers'.

In those practices where staff are selected, trained and rewarded for their commitment to client service, results are clearly measurable in terms of increased profitability and client satisfaction. There are three critical aspects to this:

- Recruiting staff that are really interested in people. A detailed description of how to select, develop and reward staff is given in Chapter 19
- A commitment to regular, frequent staff training in the necessary skills to enable *everyone* consistently to deliver the required level of service
- Managing the gap between client expectations about the service provided by the practice and their perceptions of that service (see Chapter 27).

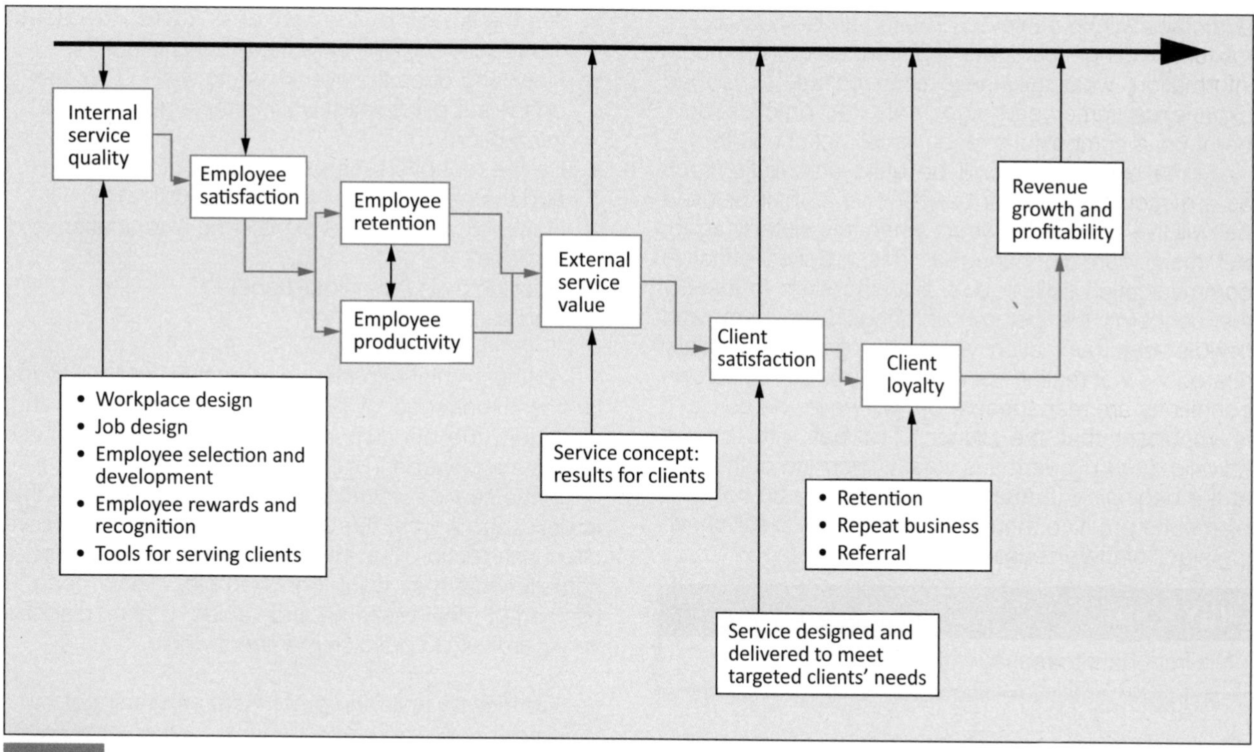

26.1 The links in the service–profit chain. (After Heskett *et al.*, 2008)

Staff recruitment and development

Hiring staff for their attitude and teaching them the necessary skills is the most effective way of rapidly improving the level of service.

KEY POINT

Do not make assumptions about skills or what staff already know. For example, a polite school leaver may be completely overwhelmed by a demanding pet owner; or an experienced locum from another culture may have a very different attitude towards pets and pet ownership, which alienates them from clients.

Excellence in client service is about considerably more than 'educating' staff by 'training' them. In fact, few training programmes in client service are successfully implemented in the daily turmoil of business. This is because providing service excellence is an *attitude* that must underpin all actions. This requires that everyone in the practice pays attention to the many small, individual trivial actions or 'moments of truth', rather than making a few grand gestures.

This does not, of course, mean that staff should *not* receive training – particular skills may need to be learnt or refined, such as how to answer the telephone, soothe an upset client, manage a busy reception area, communicate technical information appropriately, and so on. To be effective, training must be planned, structured and ongoing, and opportunities for improvement should be seized. For example, the weekly staff meeting provides an excellent forum for raising service issues – perhaps to discuss a client complaint, or to review a procedure such as pet handover after hospitalization.

Staff should also be *empowered* to provide a good service. This includes having the tools in place to be able to do a good job. For example: an easy-to-use computer software system; a practice floorplan design that encourages good work flow-through; and clear support from senior staff, such as including client service objectives in annual performance goals for all staff.

KEY POINT

Providing service excellence is an attitude that must underpin all actions.

Managing client expectations and perceptions

Maister's (2003) service experience equation shows how client perceptions and expectations influence satisfaction levels:

Satisfaction = Perception – Expectation

If the client perceives better than expected service then satisfaction is high; if the level of service is lower than expected, the client will not be satisfied. Therefore it is important not only to be interested in managing the client service experience, i.e. their perceptions, but also in helping to *frame* their expectations.

Expectations

When a pet owner visits a practice they bring with them expectations about how their experience will be, how the veterinary surgeon will help them and what outcomes will be achieved. These can be based on a mixture of things: personal experience; word-of-mouth information; what they have seen on the TV; a bad experience some years ago in another practice; and, perhaps, a competitor's recent small act of courtesy.

Some expectations will be quite unrealistic, such as a miraculous cure for cancer or that their beloved pet will live another ten years when it is already aged, but many can be managed. This requires effective communication skills – both listening skills to identify the concerns the pet owner brings with them, and flexible communication styles to gain a mutually shared view of reality. For example, many chronic skin conditions are manageable but will never be cured. It is important that the owner of a pet with, say, a chronic deep pyoderma is clearly informed of this fact at the beginning of treatment so that they do not then blame the practice months later if the pet is still showing signs of the disease.

KEY POINT

It is important to manage client expectations.

The service experience

When a pet owner visits a practice, they are having a *service experience*. This experience is made up of many mini-experiences, all of which contribute to the overall impression of the practice. Identifying and managing these mini-experiences lifts service levels from mediocre to excellent.

Managing mini-experiences is about meticulous attention to detail (these details are definable and teachable) but, most importantly, it is also about taking control over what happens in each client interaction instead of leaving it to chance.

Figure 26.2 illustrates the service experience. If this was for, say, having a pet vaccinated, the service experience might start with receiving a vaccination reminder from the practice. Then the mini-experiences continue:

- Is the phone answered promptly? (the first human interaction)
- How friendly and helpful is the staff member? Could an appointment be booked at a convenient time?
- How easy is it to get to the practice? Are the parking facilities good?
- What does the practice look like from the outside?
- Does anyone greet the client on arrival? (second human interaction)
- How crowded is the waiting room?
- Are the flowers on the front desk fresh? How does the practice smell? How clean does it look?
- How long does the client have to wait? Does the coffee supplied whilst waiting taste good? (third interaction)
- Do the receptionist and vet greet both the owner and the pet by name? (fourth interaction)
- How well does the vet explain the examination and findings?
- How kindly is the animal handled?
- And so on...

All these mini-experiences together add up to the overall experience of having a pet vaccinated and, ultimately, the pet owner's level of satisfaction. These issues are covered in detail in Chapter 27.

In the service–value chain, the service concept that is delivered is what the client experiences. To achieve client satisfaction, it is important that this experience is actually what they want. For example, clients need to be made to feel welcome and valued. Clients respond very positively to practice members who:

- Are friendly and who greet them and their pet by name
- Make the client feel like a friend rather than a number
- Are polite and courteous in their manner
- Look and behave like professionals
- Respect that the client's time is valuable too, by being on time for appointments
- Show interest in and enthusiasm for them, their pets (Figure 26.3) and their children
- Show affection to the pet
- Handle the pet kindly and do not use unnecessary restraint
- Give an accurate estimate of the fees
- Are always willing to help when clients request advice or information.

The most significant of the mini-experiences are the human interactions, whether it is a voice on the phone or a friendly member of staff, but all the other details contribute and can become more weighty if they are either very good or very bad. The most important thing to understand is that the practice owner/manager and every staff member need to manage these myriad mini-experiences *all the time* to ensure consistency resulting in continually satisfied clients. It is not enough just to start the day with a clean fresh-smelling welcoming practice and staff with friendly smiles, everyone must finish the day like this too. This is where the concept of service *quality* comes in, which will be looked at in more detail shortly.

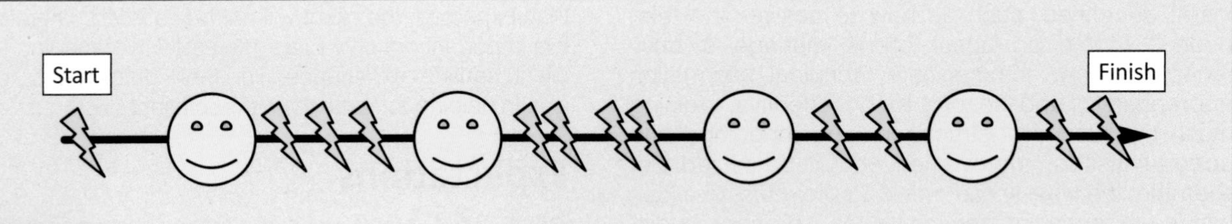

26.2 The service experience: each arrow represents a mini-experience, and each face a human interaction.

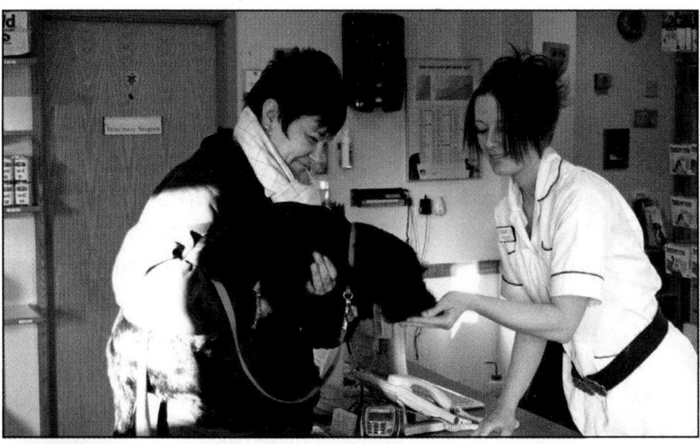

26.3 A consistent friendly welcome to owners and their pets makes all the difference.

Client satisfaction and service quality

In business, quality has a very specific definition that is customer-centred. **A business delivers quality whenever its product or service meets or exceeds customers' needs, requirements and expectations.** The customers pay for the services and products, and it is this money that is the primary revenue for the business.

This means that customer satisfaction and business profitability are closely linked to product and service quality. Higher levels of service quality result in greater customer satisfaction, which often supports higher prices, lower costs due to increased efficiency and, therefore, ultimately greater profitability. A business that satisfies most of its customers' needs most of the time is a quality business and also a successful business. Striving to understand and improve quality should be the top priority of any business.

Defining quality: what do clients want?

One of the simplest definitions of quality is 'providing what clients want'. The only way to find out what clients really want is to ask them. It is equally important to ask and find out what clients are willing to pay for. This does not mean, however, that the practice has to provide everything that the client has requested; the practice can decide at which level it will offer its service and will also work within the existing animal welfare and ethical frameworks.

General surveys from a random selection of clients are a good start to obtaining client viewpoints and identifying areas for improvement. They are also essential for gaining a balanced view from a cross-section of clients.

As the principles of total quality management are adopted (see later), existing services can be improved by using regular and repeated client surveys which are more specific. For example, questionnaires that target users of particular services, and/or at particular times, are helpful in refining and improving services, such as client care throughout the hospitalization process (specific surveys can be given to all owners on discharge of the patient).

Simple questionnaires that focus on certain areas of service provision, which can then be acted upon and outcomes shared with clients, are one of the most powerful ways to gather and use feedback, and show clients that the practice listens to and values their opinions. More on client surveys can be found in Chapter 27.

Judging quality

A challenging concept to grasp is that quality is judged by its user, not announced by its maker. Thus, in a veterinary practice quality is judged by the pet-owning clients who buy the services, not by the veterinary surgeons and their staff who provide those services. At times this can be very frustrating.

Quality is complex, as it is:

- **Situational:** different situations require different standards of 'quality'. For example, diners in a Michelin-starred restaurant want gourmet food, excellent wine and elegant service; customers in a fast-food outlet want predictable food, cheaply, in a hurry. The customer's requirements, and therefore perception of quality, are either fulfilled or not
- **Relative:** what one person perceives as quality may not be as important to another. For example, comparing how parents choose school shoes compared to teenage children: if the latter's canvas trainers suit their needs then the former's choice of sensible leather shoes are not of a quality to interest them
- **Made of symbols:** e.g. a familiar logo, a friendly greeting, a smart uniform, a pet sent home washed and dried after surgery
- **Dynamic:** requiring constant reassessment and change – what was accepted as quality 10 years ago may no longer be valued now.

In relating quality to clinical veterinary work, these definitions still hold. Some owners will expect to have the latest in expensive diagnostic techniques, while others will prefer to pay less for treatment based on clinical examination alone, with perhaps a less certain outcome. Both approaches are consistent with a quality ethical professional service. At the extreme, some owners may opt for euthanasia on cost grounds, whilst others may choose to spend thousands of pounds on treatment. Both will need an ethical and quality service that they feel satisfied with in difficult circumstances. Quality will still be: situational (e.g. charity clinic *versus* referral hospital); relative (e.g. farm cat owner *versus* pedigree cat owner); made of symbols (e.g. what is expected of a particular practice brand); and dynamic (e.g. more owners are expecting their pet's cancer to be treated with chemotherapy nowadays).

Client perceptions of quality may differ from those of the veterinary practice, as illustrated by these examples:

- A surgeon successfully completed a complex piece of spinal surgery on a German Shepherd Dog but was accosted by the owner for doing a poor job when the dog was returned a few days later, as the dog had been shaved asymmetrically over its back
- An angry pet owner complained that a practice was trying to 'rip her off' for selling her a bag of

expensive dog food, even though this was a special diet food that was an important part of the clinical management of that pet
- A pet owner complained because his pet cried out when it was vaccinated.

KEY POINT

Quality is judged by its user, not announced by its maker.

Total quality management and customer satisfaction

To retain and develop customers, a practice must decide at what level it wants to build the relationship – from basic and reactive, to proactive with full partnership. This is the difference between treating the disease problems presented *versus* actively working with established clients to prevent health problems, using tools such as recall systems and client education. Understanding the quality expectations of the customer – and consistently providing them – becomes critical.

Successful practices understand how their customers perceive quality and their customers' expectations regarding quality. They then ensure that they do a better job of meeting these expectations than their competitors. Delivering quality requires full management and employee commitment as well as measurement and reward systems. Total quality management (TQM) is a leading approach to providing customer satisfaction and driving business profitability. Programmes such as Investors in People build on TQM principles and can help practices establish process-driven ways to manage and measure quality systematically.

How TQM works

In the early 1950s, the Japanese started the Total Quality movement, which led to their total market domination with products of superior design and quality. Consumers from around the world flocked to buy high-quality Japanese products, leaving many traditional American and European firms desperately trying to catch up. Today, no business is unaffected by TQM principles and the fundamental aim of the quality movement is 'total customer satisfaction'.

TQM recognizes the following factors.

- **Quality is in the eyes of the customer.** If the customer does not like something, it is a defect. Quality improvements are meaningful only when perceived by the customer. For example, an evaluation of telephone service levels in a vet practice is meaningless to clients if they cannot see noticeable improvements afterwards.
- **Quality must be reflected not just in the business's products, but in every business activity.** This precludes performing advanced orthopaedic surgery in a dirty or cluttered surgical suite: quality is a way of life, and compromises are unacceptable.
- **Quality requires total employee commitment.** Only those practices whose employees commit to quality and who work as a team using training and feedback will consistently deliver it.
- **Quality requires high-quality partners.** Quality businesses need value-chain partners who also deliver quality. For example, suppliers of medical and surgical materials and equipment need to be in tune with the quality needs of their veterinary customers to help them uphold their standards.
- **A quality programme cannot save a poor product.** Promoting a weight management programme to be run by nurses where a substandard dietary product is recommended to save costs will not succeed and will only create dissatisfaction on the part of the pet-owning client.
- **Quality can always improve.** For example, the quality of modern digital radiographs and their speed of production can be compared with the grainy grey images from old X-ray machines where radiographs were then hand-developed in a darkroom. Quality is dynamic – there is no end point.
- **Quality improvement sometimes requires quantum leaps.** Businesses can sometimes obtain small improvements through working harder, but large improvements require fresh solutions and working 'smarter'. For example, however hard a practice tries, the streamlined delivery of quality service will always be limited by a poorly designed clinic.
- **Quality does not necessarily cost more.** Managers have argued that achieving better quality will take both more time and more money. However, improving quality involves learning to do things the right way the first time, i.e. designing in quality rather than inspecting it in.
- **Quality is necessary but may not be sufficient.** Improving quality is necessary to meet the needs of more demanding buyers. However, it may not always be a winning or differentiating advantage, as most businesses increase their service quality by approximately the same amount at the same time. This is frequently seen in the consumer market where a leading brand product – such as a shampoo – develops an attractive 'new and improved' formula, which is quickly matched by competitors, thus giving only a short-term advantage in the marketplace. In veterinary practice this could be equated to how in-house laboratory services have moved from 'best only' practices to becoming standard equipment in most small animal practices.
- **Quality needs long-term commitment.** Quality is not a quick fix but needs to be part of any business's long-term strategy for success. Neglecting this will result in serious consequences for a business.

In providing quality goods or services, a business is entering an (often unspoken) agreement with the customer about what he/she can expect. If this agreement is broken, i.e. the quality is severely substandard, the subsequent loss of trust between supplier and customer can be far-reaching and long term. A clear example of this happened recently in Europe where some human breast implants were found to be made of non-medical grade materials. When trust is lost, it can take a lot of hard work to overcome such setbacks and rebuild faith.

The downside with some users of TQM principles is that too much emphasis may be placed on the power of documentation and the production of quality manuals and Standard Operating Procedures (SOPs). These are important, but it is what actually happens to the individual client at the time that determines whether or not that client is truly satisfied.

Process mapping

Process mapping is an essential tool for delivering service quality. Its purpose is to improve the level of service to the client and to establish a quality standard – 'This is how we all agree to do things here' – by visualizing the provision of services in the practice. Process maps not only streamline procedures but also help solve problems, for example by identifying the reasons behind bottlenecks or communication break downs. This is especially helpful in larger practices where the increased number of staff introduces complexity.

A process can be compared to the flow of a river. Stones and natural bends have shaped and slowed down the flow of this river, so, just as a water engineer might clear the river's path so that it can flow most effectively, a process mapper removes the obstacles and hindrances that reduce the effectiveness of a process in a business (Figure 26.4).

Process mapping results in the production of a workflow diagram that illustrates a clearer, simpler understanding of a service process. The map enables thorough examination of a business process without the 'distraction' of the organizational structure or internal politics. The resulting map is a series of connected steps or actions to achieve an outcome which includes the following characteristics:

- A starting point and an end point – these delineate the scope of the process
- A purpose or aim for the outcome
- An internal or external customer
- Rules governing the standard or quality of inputs throughout the process
- It is usually linked to other processes
- Repeatability.

A process is mapped in three stages:

1. A workflow diagram is drawn of each step of the process 'as is', to identify the current status of the process.
2. Through analysis and review, steps in the process are identified that are the cause of bottlenecks, delays, barriers and errors; and resolutions are found.
3. The finished map describes the re-engineered process and shows the improvements that have been made.

Some examples of process maps are given in Figures 26.5 and 26.6.

- The top line shows the main process delivered by the practice and experienced by the client. Each step includes some further detail. For example, for vaccination (Figure 26.5): How long is an acceptable waiting time? Does the nurse or the vet give the vaccination?
- Further detail is given in the second line. In Figure 26.6 this shows the actions performed by the nurse during triage.
- The third line breaks down one of these steps into even more detail.

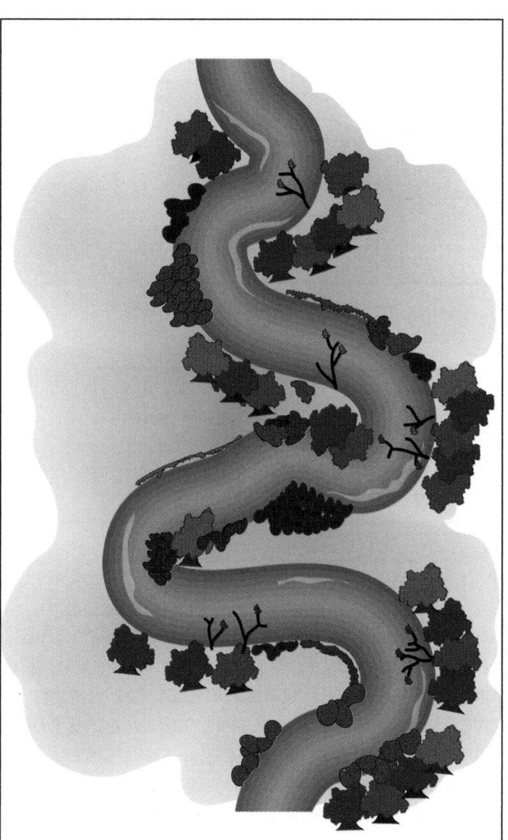

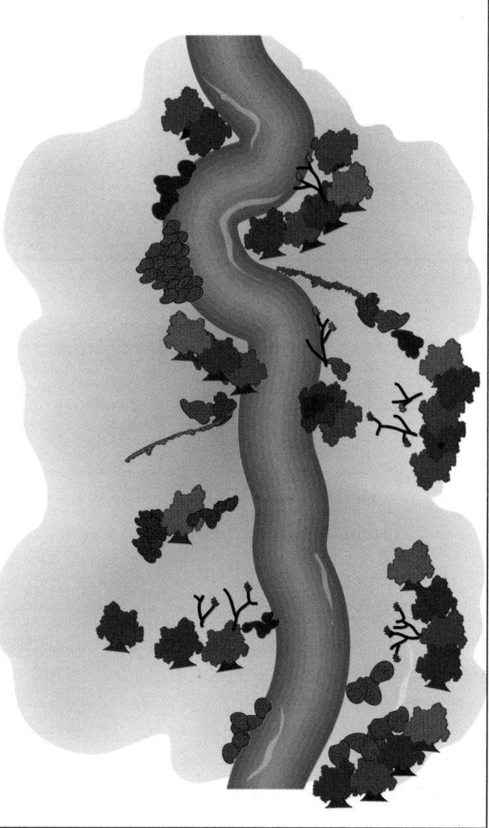

26.4 Clearing obstacles to improve the flow of a river. Process-mapping looks at obstacles and hindrances within the service process so that they can be removed or bypassed.

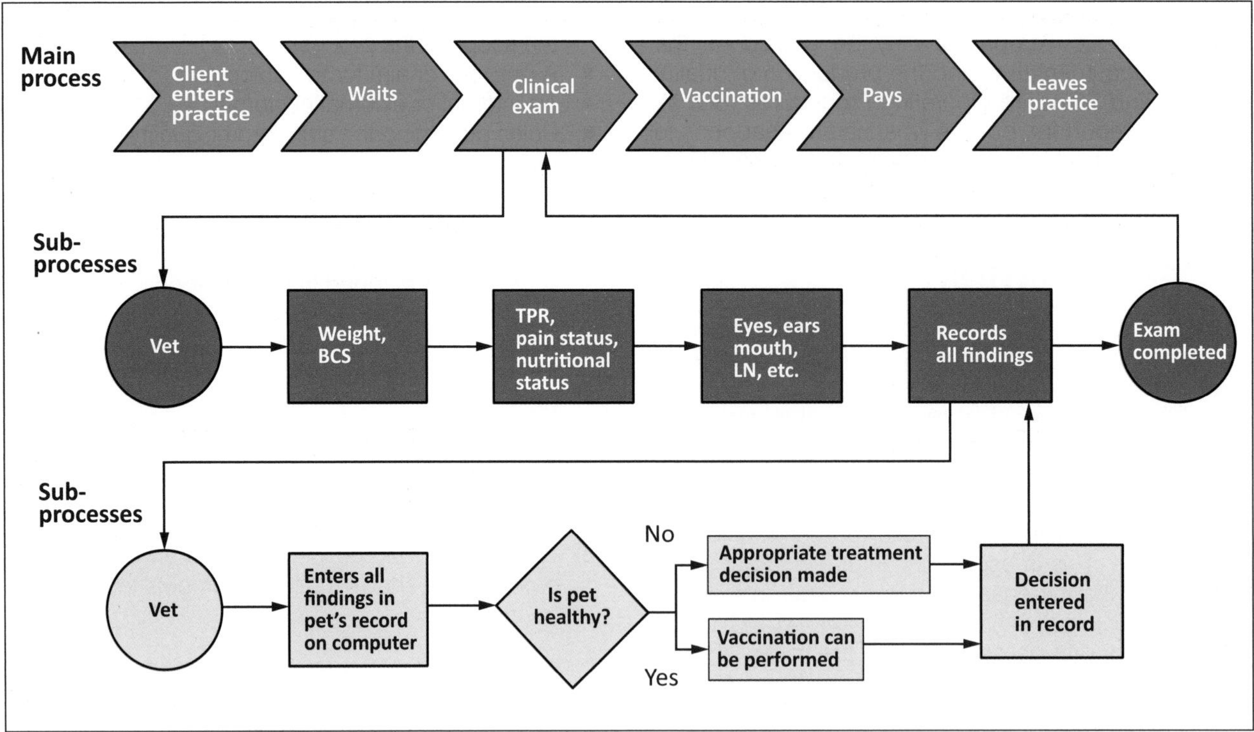

26.5 An example of a process map for a vaccination appointment. BCS, body condition score; TPR, temperature, pulse, respiration; LN, lymph nodes.

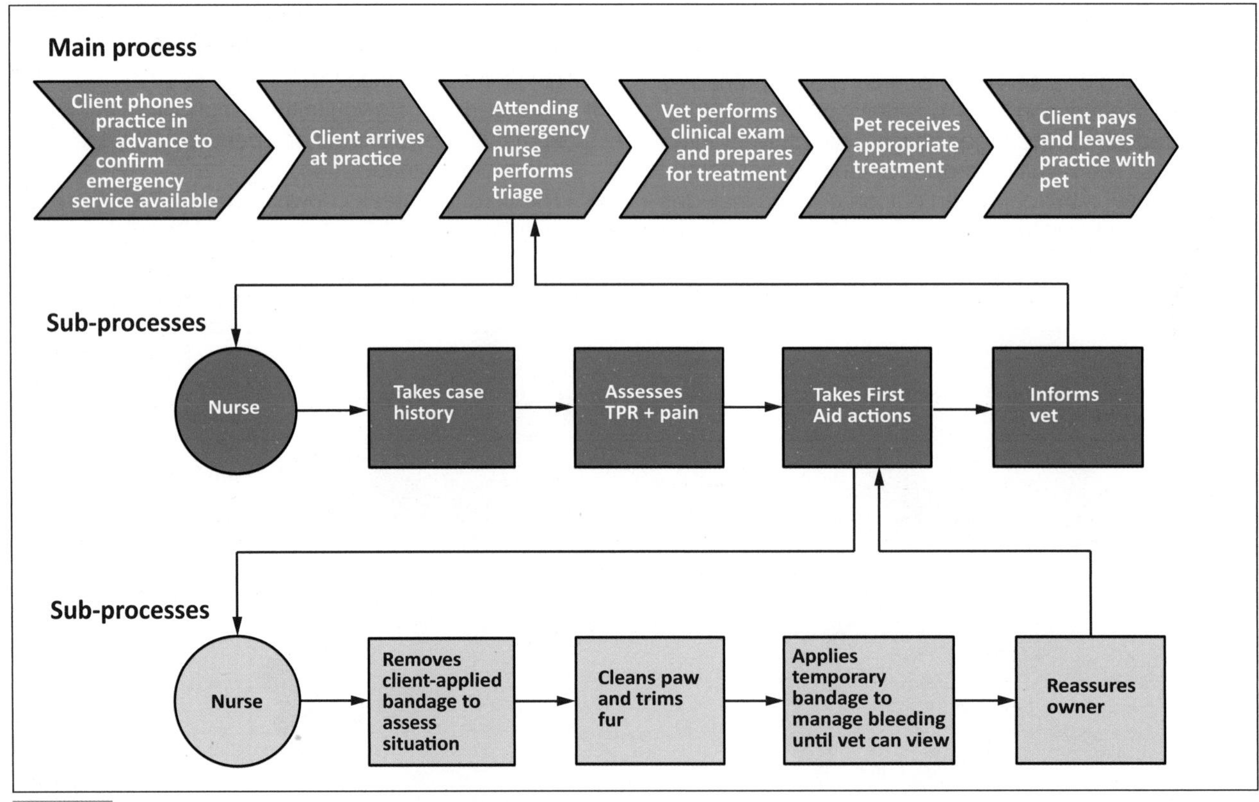

26.6 An example of a process map for dealing with an emergency patient with a cut paw.

Clearly, such a map will vary between practices and could involve several staff members, including the receptionist, nurse and vet who participate in the processes. However, its purpose is to give a clear structure and overview of how a vaccination should progress to create a seamless experience for the client whilst ensuring staff in the practice work most efficiently.

The pet-owning client is not the only 'client' in the process: each internal point of human interaction is also about client service. For example, the quality of the handover from nurse to receptionist when a pet is leaving, from surgeon to nurse for a hospitalized pet, or from day staff to night staff is critical to the overall quality of the care provided and service experienced by the pet owner.

The first process maps take time to produce but they can then be made fairly easily once certain standard procedures are recognized that are common to several services; e.g. how an appointment booking is made; how repeat medications or food are ordered and collected; or how a clinical examination is carried out. In some cases the process maps do not need to be written down because a simple discussion can reveal the obvious improvement. Where practices have chosen to map procedures, not only do they end up with agreed, effective and streamlined routines that help them work more effectively, they have also spent valuable time discussing in detail how procedures *should* happen to provide the consistent quality of service for which the practice is aiming. Most importantly, these discussions give staff a chance to eliminate steps that serve no function and waste time, and to cut down the number of active service steps that have no value to the client.

Figure 26.7 shows how process mapping was used for problem-solving on queues in reception during consulting periods. Process mapping can also be used to streamline internal procedures, such as debt control, requesting holiday, dealing with the drug order or running the payroll.

Breaking down activities into steps in this way is also a useful exercise in developing training manuals or standard operating procedures (SOPs). Indeed, the process of writing down SOPs often reveals some inefficient or unnecessary steps, which can be eliminated or changed in order to streamline procedures.

Factors to be considered in delivering excellence in client service

Client service in a veterinary practice involves managing and delivering these two essential components:

- The veterinary surgical and medical care, to ensure quality and consistency
- The supporting service around this to ensure client satisfaction.

Ensuring medical standards

Clients assume, unless proven otherwise, that the medical care they receive for their pets is of the best level, and in general they are very satisfied with their veterinary surgeon. Standards can vary considerably from practice to practice, however, due to variations in goals and standards set, the facilities available, and the skill levels of individual veterinary surgeons. For example, simply achieving RCVS Hospital status does not necessarily mean that technical service levels are significantly better than at any other good practice, and certainly should not be the only reason for charging higher fees. Conversely, it can be very frustrating for a practice when they are continually undercut by a local 'cheap and cheerful' practice which offers only a fraction of the overall medical service levels of care but is perceived as 'friendly and nice' by pet owners.

The problem

A veterinary hospital had a problem: there were log jams at reception, with clients queuing up waiting to pay. This was causing irritation for, and grumbles from, the clients and was leading to stress for the reception staff, who simply could not manage each individual client more quickly. No amount of customer service training could help the reception nurses, who were already trying to handle the waiting clients as best they could, whilst new clients became increasingly anxious when they could not sign in on time.

The problem-solving process

Discussions at staff team meetings mapped the processes to tease out the reason for the problem: the vets were sending out their clients to pay, and using the few extra minutes then available in the consultation time to write up the case notes and charge up the work without interruption. They felt that by doing this they would save the client having to wait while they wrote up the notes. However, as the reception staff could not access the PMS record until the vets had finished writing, they were powerless to complete the transaction with the client, who tended to stand at the desk waiting. Not only was that client dissatisfied at the delay, but it also held up other incoming clients.
Further discussions, of which there were many, persuaded the vets that they should write up their notes with the client still in the room. It was found that clients liked being part of the case recording process, as they experienced a less rushed appointment. Not only did reception queues get shorter but fee charging was also improved; previously some vets had released the record for reception and then completed the charging later, after the client had paid, occasionally resulting in unexpected charges for the client.
Then came the next stage: vets booked the next visit for the client from the consulting room. They used a quick system accessed from the computerized client records, which enabled the vet to time rechecks around their own availability and avoid interruptions from reception such as 'You said you wanted to see Mrs Jones again in 2 weeks but you are away then – should she come in the following week or should she book with a different vet?' This improved perceived quality of service for clients, as seeing the same vet had also been identified as an important service factor for clients. More effective follow-up also improved compliance.

Lessons learned

Several lessons were learned:

- The vets realized that their perceptions were different from those of the client and the reception staff
- A commitment to excellence in client service meant that all staff focused on what needed to be changed to deliver this level of service, and worked with solutions rather than objections
- Computer software systems can streamline processes and improve effectiveness in managing the client contact, as well as reducing the number of necessary interactions
- By challenging traditional views of who should be making appointments, a more streamlined system was adopted which saved time for vets, reception staff and clients.

26.7 Problem-solving a service issue at reception: an example of the use of process mapping.

The RCVS Practice Standards Scheme in the UK provides a framework for facilities, maintenance, compliance with regulations, staff development and clinical governance, which is used by many practices to improve and maintain their clinical service. The scheme involves regular inspections and spot checks of member practices, but it is the everyday activity of each member of staff that actually produces high medical standards. The growing fields of evidence-based medicine, practice research and clinical governance can all be used to set benchmarks and improve the quality of medical and surgical activity within a practice (see Chapter 28).

Delivering the service to clients

The compliance equation

The important elements in providing quality of care in a veterinary practice are usefully summarized in the 'compliance equation' first described in the American Animal Hospital Association survey of compliance from 2003. This provides a structure around which quality improvement can take place:

$$C = R + A + FT$$

where C = compliance; R= recommendation and reinforcement; A = acceptance; and FT = follow-through.

Compliance

Compliance is achieved when all the other factors are in place. It is about taking the necessary actions to ensure pets receive the treatment and care the veterinary practice has recommended. It can also reflect how well client service is delivered, as compliance and client service are intimately linked.

Recommendation and reinforcement

This is a combination of the veterinary surgeon's recommendation, and the reinforcement of this by the practice team.

Recommendation is the first step in the process. Many vets make the mistake of offering a client too many options without making a clear recommendation about one. This is equivalent to saying 'You could have treatment A, B or C for your pet. Which do you choose?' It is very different from saying, 'There are various treatment options available for your pet – A, B or C. I would recommend A as the best option.'

> **KEY POINT**
>
> Our clients seek us because they want our professional opinion. It is what they pay us for and it is therefore important to give it.

Effective **reinforcement** of that recommendation requires good teamwork with a team of professionals that function well together and support each other. It also requires a commitment to regular staff training about the services and products the practice provides, and how to communicate these effectively to clients.

'R' can also include **routines**. These are the written process maps or practice policies, which describe how each patient should be cared for in the best possible way. Routines start with completing patient records accurately and fully, and finish with ensuring that clients are properly informed, both verbally and in writing, about their pet's health status and what they need to do. Routines mean agreement about what should be included in patient care: for example, is the practice really providing quality service if it does not offer every owner detailed guidance on recognizing pain in their pet, together with appropriate pain relief after every surgical procedure?

Acceptance

Acceptance of the recommendation by the pet owner is vital, as it drives their *actions*. It is not uncommon for pet owners to medicate their pet wrongly, for example, because they have not understood the need to complete a 10-day course of antibiotics, or continue eardrops even though the pet has stopped shaking its head. To achieve acceptance requires solid communication skills (see Chapter 17) to ensure the pet owner truly understands the nature of the problem and the need for the treatment(s) recommended. Acceptance also requires an empathetic understanding of and willingness to look at options to help the pet owner manage the limitations they may experience in trying to follow directions. For example: the elderly owner of a snappy pug may be willing but unable to administer oral medication; or the owner of a large hairy dog may not have the facilities at home for twice-weekly shampoo and soaks to manage a dermatological condition.

> **KEY POINT**
>
> Working together to find solutions that provide the care the pet needs is an essential component of compliance success.

Follow-through

Follow-through is critical to patient care success and really puts the 'icing on the cake' for service delivery. It is also probably the most neglected area of the three components of compliance. Follow-through includes:

- Ensuring no patient leaves the practice without a new appointment booked
- Contacting the client by phone a few days after their visit to ensure they have understood everything and are progressing as they should
- Sending reminders for revisits.

Many clients leave a practice with unanswered questions and concerns, or are willing to follow a treatment but unable to achieve it in their home environment. Contact shortly after their visit would help enormously. Follow-through actions should be part of the practice's processes (routines), to ensure that compliance is being achieved.

Monitoring compliance

For compliance to be achieved and improved, the factors above need to monitored and measured. Recommendations can be measured, for example, by reviewing recorded recommendations in patients' notes and matching these to actual bookings: the vet recommended that a pet have a dental scale and polish – did this result in a booking? Accepted, documented routines and procedures will improve team function and support of recommendations; client questionnaires can assess the quality of communication to deliver messages; the number of actual revisits *versus* the number booked can measure follow-through, and so on.

The 7 Cs of quality

Part of providing excellence in client service is understanding what is important to clients.

Emotional intelligence competencies play an important role in the way staff members and clients evaluate the quality of their experience with the practice. Seven parameters have been identified that are important measures of quality for clients, but they are equally important for employees (Figure 26.8); of these, only the last two are not EQ (emotional quotient) competencies

What is important to clients sometimes differs from the criteria veterinary surgeons *think* are important. For example, one study showed that clients set high value on a prognosis after a consultation, whereas vets focused more on the diagnosis (Manning, 2003). Another example is how many practices, whilst claiming to be service-oriented, actually work mostly to suit their own needs, e.g. by severely restricting the access owners have to their pets whilst they are hospitalized, or by not being open at lunchtimes or after normal working hours when it would be much easier for many clients to come in with their pets.

The key to combining clinical delivery excellence with client service excellence is to monitor the standards of both against a set of measurable parameters and to compare the outcomes against best practice or desired measures. Such parameters include client satisfaction from surveys and specific measures such as waiting time or number of times the phone rings before being answered. Improvements to the level of care are measured by clinical audit and by regular internal staff discussions and surveys and external client surveys to provide feedback (see Chapters 27 and 28).

KEY POINTS

- Commit to understanding and working with excellent client service in all practice activities.
- Hire staff who are genuinely interested in people and develop their skills through regular focused training.
- Define and use measurable quality standards in all areas of the practice (this is TQM in action).
- Work with process mapping to ensure quality service delivery and reduce wasted time and resources.
- Include client service quality measures as part of annual performance evaluation objectives (this is particularly important for senior staff).
- Ask for and act on feedback from your clients – after all, it is they who actually judge the quality of the client service you provide.

Practice competencies	Employee's requirements	Client's requirements
Caring	Feeling I am treated as an individual and not a number; that my employer knows who I am, and something about my background and family situation and is interested in me; that they are committed to helping me to reach my potential	Feeling I am being treated as an individual and not a number; that the practice knows who I and my pet are, and are friendly towards me and interested in me; that staff members show affection towards my pet and show empathy for me, the owner
Compassion	Showing understanding that I am trying to do my best under sometimes challenging circumstances, and being supportive	Feeling that a kindly concern is expressed towards me and my pet and the situation in which I find myself
Commitment	Feeling that the practice is willing to invest in my growth and development both on a personal level but also to be an even better team member	Knowing that the vet and healthcare team are doing all they can to resolve my situation in the best possible way
Communication	Feeling I am part of all activities in the practice and am kept well informed and up to date, both on a general and on a personal level	Creates trust and understanding by taking the necessary time and using the appropriate methods to ensure that I understand what is being said and the options I am being given about my pet's treatment
Courtesy	Being treated with respect and politeness at all times and not shouted at or abused	Being treated with respect; e.g. not being kept waiting unnecessarily; not being left alone in a room to wait for the vet or nurse with no explanation of what is happening and how long it will take
Competence	Colleagues show a good level of effectiveness and efficiency in performing their jobs and help me to achieve the same in mine	I, as a client, assume, until proven otherwise, that you have the medical competence needed to do your job. I will therefore tend to judge competence on what I am familiar with: how quickly you answered the phone; how confident you seem in your manner; how clear you are in your communication to me; how well you handle my pet
Cost	My salary should fairly reflect my contribution to the success of the practice	I can differentiate between levels of service, so I would expect a higher level of service if I have paid a higher price. As a client I would expect to be charged fairly for the treatment my pet has received. If I perceive a gap between what I have paid for and the quality of the service I have received, complaints and dissatisfaction can arise

26.8 The 7 'C's' of quality.

Managing the dissatisfied client: an opportunity to improve quality

Practices deal with a cross-section of the community daily, and it is inevitable that some clients will not be satisfied with the job done. Common sources of irritation to already stressed clients are: being kept waiting; not receiving an accurate estimate of the bill; or insensitive handling of the pet, especially in association with euthanasia. Sometimes there is a genuine error on the part of the practice: a promised phone call to a worried client was not made at the agreed time; or a client was not informed about increased costs before a treatment process. Almost all complaints can be traced back to a miscommunication or misunderstanding.

KEY POINT

Often, what the client complains about may not actually be the problem, as there are unexpressed feelings behind the complaint. For example, a client may complain about the *costs* involved in treating a case, when they are actually upset that the pet has not got better as expected; it is easier to complain about something concrete, such as money, than to talk about very personal things, such as feelings.

In general, only the *highly* dissatisfied clients will actually complain to the practice in such a way that it can respond to, and do something about, their complaint. Dissatisfied clients are less likely to return to the practice and more likely to complain about it to friends, so they are always to be taken seriously. However, studies show that 70% of customers with grievances will stay with a business if efforts are made to remedy their complaint, and 95% will stay if their complaint is rectified on the spot; so, a complaint, although often uncomfortable, may actually be a golden opportunity to improve service and communication levels in the practice, as well as convert an unhappy client to a loyal one.

People express their frustration in different ways and can sometimes be very unpleasant. They may write a scalding letter of complaint to the practice principal, make an official complaint to the veterinary governing bodies, threaten litigation, or phone or visit the practice and offload to the first practice member they meet – usually the receptionist or nurse. This experience is upsetting and unpleasant for all staff members concerned, so it is important that processes are in place in the practice to manage these complaints efficiently and promptly when they arise, including training in effective communication techniques to manage dissatisfied clients. In addition, staff should be empowered to resolve problems, which includes knowing when to pass them on to more senior staff members such as the practice manager. For more on handling complaints see Chapter 17.

References and further reading

American Animal Hospital Association (2003) *The Path to High Quality Care: Practical Tips for Improving Compliance*. AAHA, Colorado

Gray C and Moffett J (2010) *Handbook of Veterinary Communication Skills*. Wiley Blackwell, Oxford

Heppel M (2010) *Five Star Service: How to Deliver Exceptional Customer Service*. Prentice Hall Business, Upper Saddle River, NJ

Heskett JL, James L, Thomas O *et al.* (1994) Putting the Service-Profit Chain to Work. *Harvard Business Review* **72**, 164–70

Irons K (1997) *The Marketing of Services*. McGraw-Hill, Maidenhead

Maister D (2003) *Managing the Professional Service Firm*. Simon and Schuster

Manning PR (2003) *Consultation technique in general veterinary practice*. (MSc Thesis, Middlesex University)

Price B and Jaffe D (2008) *The Best Service is No Service: How to Liberate Your Customers from Customer Service, Keep Them Happy, and Control Costs*. Jossey-Bass, San Francisco

The customer experience

27

Alison Lambert

The concept of the 'customer experience' is not new: it was first explored by Pine and Gilmore in 1998. The idea is a simple one – that a customer, whether existing or potential, forms an impression of a company based on what he/she sees, hears, feels, touches and even smells. The customer interaction is a full-on sensory experience. So, where people used to speak of a business delivering customer service, it is now understood that successful businesses deliver an excellent experience: premises are easy to find and park at, comfortable to wait in, laid out practically, bright and clean, and smell pleasant. This is all before any staff have even interacted with the client, which is undoubtedly the biggest opportunity to influence clients' perception and, ultimately, behaviour.

Points of customer interaction

At a small animal veterinary practice there are some key stages in a pet's life where interaction with the owner is most likely:

- Acquisition: new kittens and puppies are generally vaccinated, wormed, microchipped and then neutered
- Unpredictable accidents, illness and emergencies
- End of life: terminal illness management and euthanasia.

Unless there is good reason to, the majority of pet owners will not attend the practice outside of these three stages. Take up of annual booster vaccination can be low. Pets will hopefully be regularly wormed and treated for fleas, but it is probable that the products used will not be purchased from a veterinary practice. The author's research suggests that almost two-thirds of pet owners purchas e such treatments from non-veterinary sources.

Regardless of *how* customers experience their practice, they will very quickly form a belief about what it *feels* like – reputation, the level of care provided, and so on. This belief is personal to each individual. It may not be in line with the view the practice has of itself nor be one that staff are aware of but, once formed, it can be almost impossible to change.

KEY POINT

Where people used to speak of a business delivering customer *service*, it is now understood that successful businesses deliver an excellent *experience*. Providing a warm and rewarding experience will make the customers *want* to come back.

Client interactions

Clients experience a practice in a number of ways. The following includes some basic points; practices are often aware of the issues raised here, but they also need to address them.

Word of mouth

Prospective clients will *hear* things about a business, e.g. 'it's expensive', 'the lady vet is nice', 'parking is awful', 'they were really kind when Jessie was put to sleep'. Some of these nuggets will have been solicited from friends and acquaintances on the morning dog walk, but many will have been gleaned subconsciously from overheard conversations and half-remembered gossip.

Online

- A survey of 150 vets in 2010 by the author's market research company found that whilst 80.5% of vets had a practice website, only 58.5% were happy with it.
- The Office of National Statistics noted in August 2011 that 77% of the UK population has Internet access.
- According to the Interactive Media in Retail Group (www.imrg.org; January 2012) £68 billion was spent online by UK consumers in 2011; a 16% increase on the previous year.

Animal owners are increasingly using the Internet to research products and services, to buy goods and to access the views of other local owners via forums and blogs. If the practice does not have a website, this should be reviewed. Websites must be informative, professional and easy to read (see Chapter 25). With the burgeoning influence of social media sites such as Twitter and Facebook, the web is a powerful medium that every forward-thinking practice should be using actively. Facebook updates can communicate offers and practice news quickly to clients, friends and pet owners.

Visual first impressions

These include potential customers just passing the premises. A long hard look should be taken at the outside of the practice:

- Is the signage looking a little dated and worn around the edges?
- Does the window have peeling posters of last summer's promotion?
- Is there litter in the car park?

Getting the waiting room and reception area right is vital in creating a good first impression (see Chapter 5).

Telephone calls

A receptionist with a good telephone manner is invaluable. Front-of-house staff will engage callers with the practice, show clients that the practice is caring, friendly and professional, and make money by converting casual enquiries into appointments.

In a survey in 2010 by the author's market research company, telephone calls were made to 150 practices asking the question, 'I've just got a puppy; how much are your vaccines?'. Some of the results were as follows:

- Only 54% of calls were answered by a member of staff who gave their name
- Only 24% of callers felt the receptionist was interested in them and/or their pet
- Crucially, only 13% of practices offered to make an appointment.

The customer experience here is all about what the caller hears and feels. It is therefore important that, whilst on the phone, the receptionist is not distracted by other things and is not eating, drinking or chewing gum. The receptionist's tone should be bright and cheery, giving the impression that the practice is warm, friendly and caring. This can be achieved by making the call more personal, such as the member of staff saying their name when answering the phone, asking open questions to find out more about both the pet and the client's concerns, and using both the pet's name and the client's name during the conversation. If the telephone call is handled professionally, if prices are given at the end of the conversation and if an appointment is always offered (Figure 27.1), the number of speculative callers registering as new clients will be increased.

Effective telephone skills

The key to a successful telephone conversation is to listen to what the caller has to say and to clarify anything that is not clear. If unable to help, the receptionist should be honest with the client and put them through to another member of the team who can, or it should be agreed that the client will be called back with the information that they require. Ideally a time should be allocated, the contact telephone number confirmed and the client informed as to who will call them back. Without the benefit of eye contact, it is even more important to make sure the mouth, brain and ears are all used effectively during telephone conversations.

In order to provide an excellent telephone service the following points are important guidelines.

DO:

- Answer promptly: within 3–4 rings
- Use the hold button if needed to prevent the client from hearing what is going on (ask the client's permission first). This is far more professional than the phone being tucked under the receiver's chin, with the client listening in on what is being said
- Answer with a short but professional greeting: 'Best Practice Vets; this is Angela. How may I help you?'
- Listen: it is easy to be distracted by colleagues or by what is going on around you
- Explain the silence if there is a delay: 'Sorry, the computer is a bit slow this morning'; or 'Just one moment please whilst I go and get the appointment book'
- Have a pen and paper ready to make notes; write the name of the caller as you go to save asking it again later.

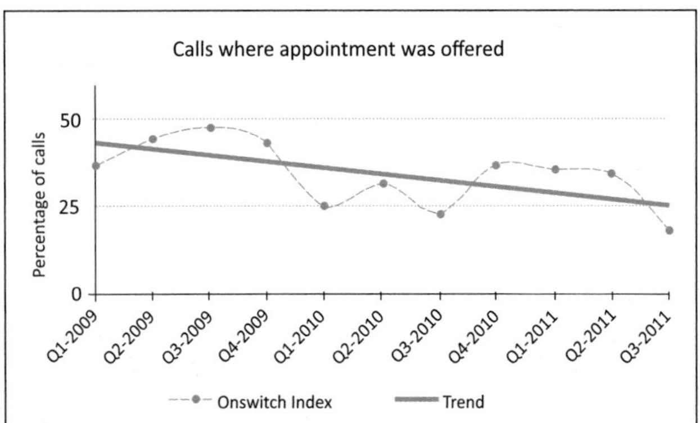

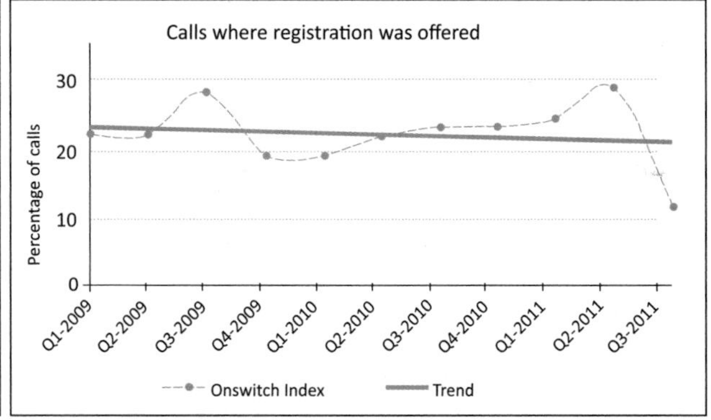

27.1 Mystery shopper results relating to telephone approaches. The Onswitch Index includes data from over 3000 veterinary practices across the UK. An Index practice will receive four calls per month. The reasons for the downward trend shown here have not been identified.

DON'T:

- Put the client on speaker phone whilst you do other things; they will not be able to hear you properly and will feel like you are not paying them your full attention
- Eat or drink whilst speaking on the phone: all the accompanying slurps and chomps will be magnified
- Pause to type without clarifying what you are doing: it can be off-putting if a caller does not think they have your full attention. Reassure them you are typing up their notes
- Cough or sneeze anywhere near the phone, as the caller can still hear.

Although engaging with callers and helping them with their queries is essential good service, the practice is a business, not a free advice shop, so the focus on handling incoming telephone calls should be on caller conversion. Based on the author's research, a successful practice should be aiming to convert 40% of phone enquiries into appointments, without the caller ever feeling pressurized in the process.

There are five key points that should be standard practice when handling telephone calls with clients. Good reception staff should always:

- **Use their own name** when answering the call. This makes the client feel that they are having a conversation with someone who cares, rather than just being given a list of standard information
- **Ask for and use the client's name and the pet's name throughout the conversation –** Doing this shows that the practice cares about the pet, and not just about making money from another faceless patient number. The pet is part of the family, and is the reason the owner is contacting the practice
- **Provide practice information –** directions, opening hours, services, team information, etc. This not only demonstrates competence and care, but also opens up other options for the client to take up additional services. The owner needs validation that this practice is the right choice for them. Welcome packs and information leaflets can be posted out as appropriate and the caller could be referred to the practice website
- **Answer any questions about price at the end of the call –** In this way affiliated services and benefits, such as extra free checks that the client may be entitled to, have already been discussed, thereby justifying the cost. Also, any talk of price can wait until care, love and undivided attention have all been demonstrated
- **Offer an appointment –** Not only make the offer, but do it in a way that is hard to refuse. Avoid closed questions with a yes or no answer such as, 'Would you like to make an appointment?' A better way to ask would be either, 'When would you like to bring Trixie in to see us?' or 'Did you want to bring Trixie in this morning or this afternoon?'. Not only does this demonstrate that staff are keen to help, but it makes the owner feel valued by the practice as well as having the added advantage of converting a free enquiry into practice income.

The veterinary consultation

An owner who has booked an appointment to see a veterinary surgeon will be accessing clinical services, and will often have a serious concern regarding their pet's wellbeing. This means that many owners arriving at the practice may be feeling stressed, worried, embarrassed, upset or guilty. Fear of criticism or of what might be found is also a real emotion that owners may experience, and they may feel very vulnerable. It is important throughout the consultation that the veterinary surgeon understands this mixture of emotions, does not add to the client's negative thoughts, nor criticise, and appreciates that clients are paying for a solution to their problem and for peace of mind. Showing empathy will significantly improve the customer experience and is the basis for trust in the professional relationship. A kind word from the clinical team, for example, reassuring an owner that it is the right time to say goodbye to their beloved pet, will go a long way in helping to minimize the guilt that so many feel at this difficult time. An owner worried about a lump on their pet which initially appears benign will feel a complete relief when the histology results come back 'all clear'. An owner with an elderly pet who is limping badly may purchase anti-inflammatory medication from the practice but they are actually paying for the benefits that this drug gives. The client wants to ensure that their pet continues to be comfortable and have a good quality of life. The consultation process and communication skills are discussed more fully in Chapter 17.

Emergency care provision

In an emergency a client's emotions will be heightened; this can create challenges for the veterinary team as they need to attend to the patient and look after the owner at the same time. Once again it is important to see the situation from the owner's point of view. Whilst the clinical team may quickly ascertain that the injury is not serious and the wound just needs a few stitches, the owner may be under the impression that, due to the amount of blood, a major artery has been hit and their pet may not survive. Whatever the outcome of any situation, particularly one that the owner perceives to be an emergency, it is the little touches and kind considerate gestures that will be remembered for a long time afterwards: the understanding look; the unhurried explanation; the cup of tea and quiet room offered by the nurse; the bereavement card or flowers; and not being asked for credit card details whilst a pet is being euthanased. Unfortunately, the not-so-good things are also remembered, such as receiving a booster reminder when the practice has been informed that their much-loved pet has passed away. All the little things, good and bad, make a big difference to the customer experience.

KEY POINT

All staff need to see things from the customer's emotional point of view – this is called empathy. Showing empathy will significantly improve the customer experience.

Nurse clinics

Where veterinary nurses are given their own consultations there is a huge potential for creating an excellent customer experience, as well as generating extra income for the practice. The nurses will have time to spend with clients in a way that is not always possible in a veterinary consultation, and owners do not always want to 'bother the vet' with what they see as trivial concerns.

All consultations, whether with a vet or a nurse, must be treated in the same manner as any other interaction with clients:

- A professional and caring image must be portrayed
- A proper consultation room must be made available
- Sufficient time must be allocated.

The customer will then leave feeling positive about the practice.

Nurses can also promote special offers, hand out leaflets and carry out small procedures, thereby showing the customer that the practice does that little bit more. It is important to ensure that nurse clinic time is cost-effective for the practice and that it is correctly charged for where appropriate.

The eight-step experience process

There is a recognized continuum through which pet owners progress on their customer experience 'journey':

1. Awareness
2. Information
3. Consideration
4. Selection
5. Experience
6. Repeat experience
7. Recommendation
8. Brand ambassador.

Where and how the customer experience evolves can be assessed in more detail by taking each of these stages in turn.

Awareness

If a practice has a prominent position, there is a high probability that most people in town will know of it, even if they do not have a pet. For the 'average' practice, 85% of their clients live within 3 miles (source: Onswitch 2011), so convenience and location are key considerations for most clients. There may, however, be a number of pet owners in the locality who do not know the practice exists. There are many easy and cost-effective ways to boost local awareness (see Chapter 25). Some of the simplest include:

- Sponsoring or writing pet care features in the local press
- Advertising (not fly posting!) on litter bins, roundabouts, parks, etc.
- Prominent signage (Figure 27.2)
- Open days
- Stalls and dog shows at community events
- Leaflet drops.

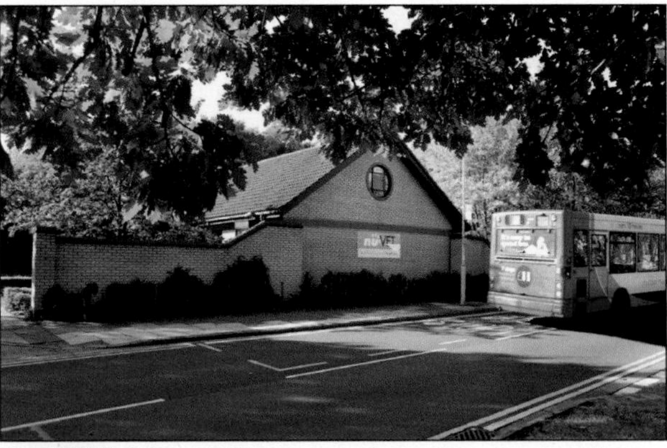

27.2 Clients will be aware of practices prominently situated in a busy position. (Courtesy of Nuvet and *Veterinary Business Journal*. © Veterinary Business Development).

Generally speaking, advertising in a directory such as Yellow Pages or Thomsons's is *not* a cost-effective way to raise awareness. Research by the author's company in 2010 showed that fewer than 5% of all owners ever mentioned using paper or online directories to find their vet, and if they did it was usually due to an emergency need in the middle of the night. The Internet is used more and more for finding local business telephone numbers, so a clear website with good search ratings is now essential.

Information

Having heard about the practice, potential customers will go about gathering information: Do any of their friends and family use it? What do fellow dog-walkers think about it? Is there a website? Is the website interesting, up to date and user-friendly? Is the practice easy to find? Is it convenient for them to get there and to park?

Research in 2010 by the author's company in the UK regarding practice opening times found that few practices were making it easy for busy clients to visit at a time to fit in with their work and home commitments:

- 22% of practices offered routine consultations seven days a week
- 21% of practices consulted after 7 pm
- 4% consulted after 8 pm
- 3% consulted after 9 pm.

If out-of-hours consultations are offered at the practice, it is important to ensure that this benefit is widely advertised.

KEY POINT

It is vital to remember that every request for information is an opportunity for staff to register a new client. This opportunity must be recognized and not missed.

Consideration

Once a potential client is aware that the practice exists, and they have gathered information about the surgery, along with other local practices or regional specialists, a considered choice on which to use can be made. It is important for practices to be aware that for many pet owners this is not a monogamous relationship: customers may use one veterinary practice for emergency care and one for everything else, one for one species of pet (e.g. chickens) and another for a different species (e.g. cat), or they may choose the cheapest practice for routine procedures but be willing to pay more for care somewhere else when their animal is ill.

Selection

Customers may choose to use a practice for a number of reasons, but the decision is usually made along a mixture of pragmatic and emotional lines, with the following factors in order of declining importance:

- Locality and convenience
- Recommendation from a friend or family member
- Recommendation from local key opinion leaders (Figure 27.3).

- Catteries
- Kennels
- Breeders
- Trainers
- Groomers
- Pet shops
- Alternative therapists
- Dog walkers
- Feed merchants
- Rescue centres

27.3 Key opinion leaders. There are numerous businesses in associated pet care professions that may share both the practice catchment area and its clients. These businesses see plenty of pet owners every day and will have their own opinions of a practice – good or bad. They will increasingly also have their own Facebook pages and Twitter accounts, where they can share their thoughts.

The majority of owners will choose their closest practice but in a city there may be several options that are equally close, so then word-of-mouth reputation becomes critical. Selection is far more likely to be swayed by reports of friendly staff, expensive prices, a rude member of the team or a smelly waiting area than by the practice having a state-of-the-art operating theatre, a comprehensive CPD programme or staff with impressive qualifications.

Experience

At last, the customer actually gets to have something to do with the practice – a chance for the practice to shine. The customer has already formed a very firm idea of what their experience is likely to be, and this far along in the process their expectations are high. Every step of the experience needs to meet or exceed these expectations, so the customer must be able to:

- Find the practice and park easily
- Get through the door with a large dog, pet carrier and/or pushchair/wheelchair
- Identify staff members (uniforms and name badges help ensure a professional look)
- Wait without stress (separate areas for cats and dogs, water bowls, recent magazines, toys for children to play with (Figure 27.4), comfortable chairs, drinks machine and toilets are all much appreciated)
- Feel welcome (friendly greetings from staff who smile and use the customer's name and the pet's name)
- Have their queries and concerns addressed
- Have their pet treated quickly and professionally, with treatment regimens and medication costs explained clearly
- Leave the practice on a positive note, with no delays regarding payment or booking any follow-up appointments.

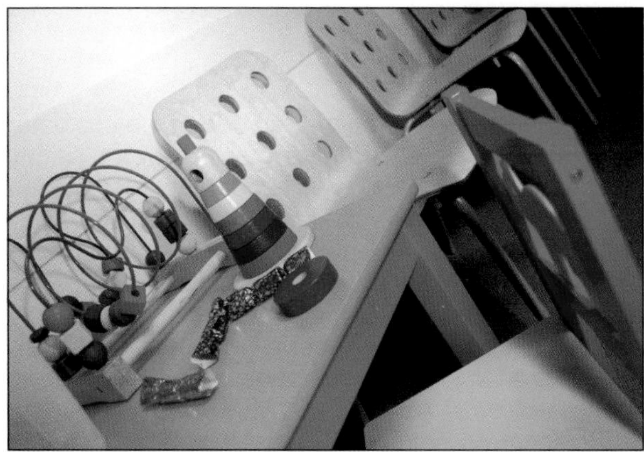

27.4 Providing toys to keep small children occupied in the reception area can greatly improve the experience for parents. (Courtesy of Nuvet and *Veterinary Business Journal*. © Veterinary Business Development).

Very few of these essentials could be classed as uniquely veterinary. Most owners do not care what drug is being dispensed, as long as they know why (i.e. its benefits) and what it costs, and they trust that the practice staff are doing right by their pet.

KEY POINT

Fundamentally, delivering a great customer experience is about making clients feel valued and respected.

Repeat experience

Clients that return to use the services of the practice provide a key indication that it must be doing something right. They have come back, despite the fact that they have other choices. It is therefore essential that their experience is every bit as positive as last time, with a friendly and proactive (but without pressure) service from the whole team.

Recommendation

The Holy Grail of advertising – someone loves the practice so much that they spread the good news to anyone who will listen – free advertising! Powerful advertising too, for when it comes to their pets, owners are far more likely to listen to the opinion of someone they know rather than a clever slogan. When service is great, people will want to talk about it. If there is a practice Facebook page, clients can recommend to friends, 'like' its offers, news and services, and post links on their friends' walls (see Chapter 25). Considering that the 'average' Facebook user has 130 'friends', that is a lot of free recommendation for a practice. Reward schemes such as 'Recommend a friend' help encourage this recommendation, and these are explored later in the chapter.

KEY POINT

Recommending a practice is an accurate indicator that a client's customer service needs have been met or exceeded. In surveys, 'Would you recommend this practice?' is an important question to ask.

Brand ambassador

These clients have got to the very top of the customer experience scale. They have gone beyond simply mentioning the practice when a friend asks for a good vet, to being practically the face of the business. They are able to speak at length about practice facilities and services and will promote special offers to friends and acquaintances. They will potentially be 'tweeting' about the service they receive, and putting photos and links on their Facebook pages, for all their many 'friends' to see.

Personal recommendation is the most powerful call to action to most pet owners, so if there are any brand ambassadors amongst the current client base, it is important to take special care to acknowledge them and maintain the best care and service.

KEY POINT

Losing a brand ambassador will have a significant effect on recommendations.

Why can't the customer experience be just 'good enough'?

In times gone by, when there were not nearly so many veterinary practices, and when customers did not expect so much, practices could just 'do their own thing' and nobody would be any the wiser. If a veterinary surgeon's scientific approach to life or lack of bedside manner rubbed some clients up the wrong way, the client still had to attend the practice. Fortunately for customers, those days are long gone and the market has moved on.

- **Client numbers are not static.** The author's 2010 data suggest that if a business is run without actively attracting new clients, within 5 years there will not be enough clients to make it profitable: around 10% of patients will die each year; and another 10% will move out of the area or switch to another practice.
- **Practice economics have changed.** On average, a small animal practice needs 1000 active households on its database for every full-time-equivalent vet. If clients drift away because they are not happy with their experience, the practice will quickly reach the point where overheads are far bigger than income. Whilst staff may have chosen veterinary practice out of a genuine love for the job, without income-generating clients, the practice's economic position will not be sustainable.
- **Pet owners have much more choice.** In the 10 years between 2000 and 2010 the number of UK practices almost doubled, from 2300 to 4300 (source: Vetfile 2011). Twenty per cent of pet owners use more than one vet (Figure 27.5). In addition, the veterinary practice is increasingly the last port of call for many pet owners. Qualitative research consistently shows that owners will use the Internet, books, paraprofessionals and friends to diagnose issues, find treatments and research behavioural problems.

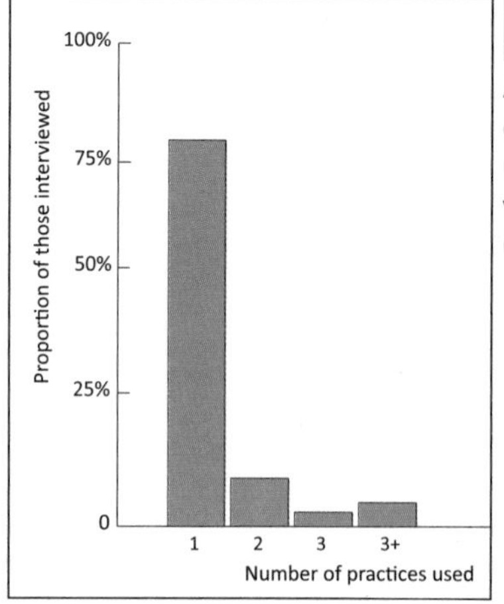

27.5 Approximately 20% of pet owners use more than one veterinary practice. (Onswitch data)

The delivery of a good customer experience must be consistent. This can only be truly achieved if every member of the team as an individual is ensuring that every time they interact with a client they have contributed to making it a positive experience for that client in terms of customer care. This objective is made easier by recruiting staff with the same values and beliefs as the practice. Team training on the practice ethos as well as the practice delivery of client care ensures that everyone has to step up to the mark. The client experience is made up of several mini-experiences ('moments of truth') (see Chapter 26) – it is all the little things that will form the clients' perception of a practice. The team is only as strong as its weakest member and one rude or indifferent member of staff can undo the good work of the rest of the team.

KEY POINT

The delivery of a good customer experience must be consistent. This means that the level of client care must be to the same high standard for every client, every time they visit and at every interaction throughout the process.

Measuring the customer experience

Offering value for money does not have to be about low prices – it is about justifying what is available. If not competing on price, practices need to offer something unique and/or be outstanding in terms of customer care in order for pet owners to believe that they receive good value for money. Looking for information on the Internet does not allow the pet owner to talk to a real person about the best way to worm an awkward cat; signing up for an annual healthcare scheme with the local veterinary practice might prove more cost-effective over the course of a year than the one-off prices on the Internet, particularly if more appropriate care results.

There are three main ways to assess customer experience:

- Mystery shoppers
- Customer feedback surveys, including net promoter score (NPS)
- Team feedback.

KEY POINT

Measuring the customer experience produces real data with which to record and track improvements.

Mystery shoppers

This is a great way to get right to the heart of a practice's customer experience provision. Real pet owners will call or drop in and ask staff a simple question about caring for their pet. They will rate the quality of information provided and, more importantly, the manner in which it was delivered. The practice is given an unbiased and accurate picture of how clients feel about the business and one that is difficult to obtain directly from clients – as people tend not to complain unless they are really unhappy. They will simply go elsewhere, without saying why. Results of research by the author's company using mystery shoppers at approximately 3000 practices across the UK are shown in Figure 27.6.

Customer feedback surveys

Surveys are another good way of gauging the mood of clients. They can both measure the customer experience and give specific feedback to improve client service and processes. It is important to be clear what the survey is aiming to find out, for example:

- Who are the clients, and what are their attitudes and needs?
- What do clients feel about the practice generally?
- How do clients feel about their last or a recent experience at the practice?

Surveys should be kept short and to the point, and questions should be worded to elicit the desired information so the practice can act on it appropriately.

- **General questionnaires** aimed at identifying service gaps can be completed by a random sample of clients during their visit and then posted into a sealed collection box in the waiting room.
- **Questionnaires that target specific areas** can be sent out or taken away to be completed by the appropriate targeted sector of the practice's client base and then returned either to the practice or to a third party to ensure anonymity.

Rather than handing out questionnaires to 'nice' clients, or following routine or easy consultations, it is better to: issue a form to everyone; ask the first five clients each day; or randomly select names from the week's appointments.

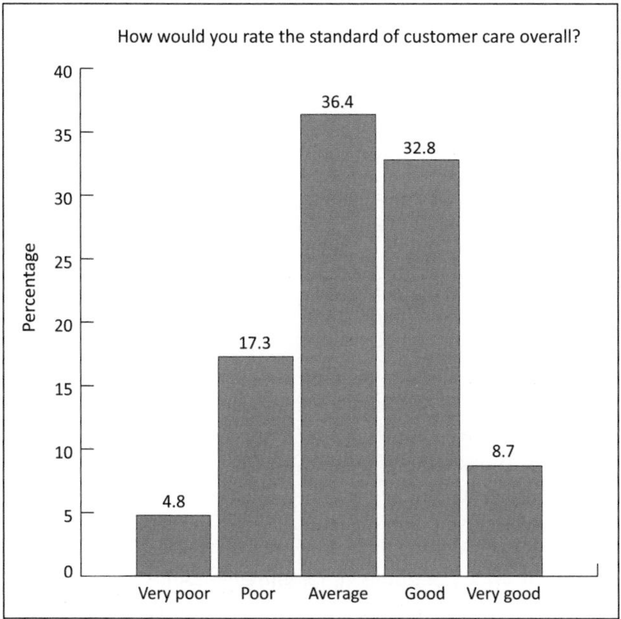

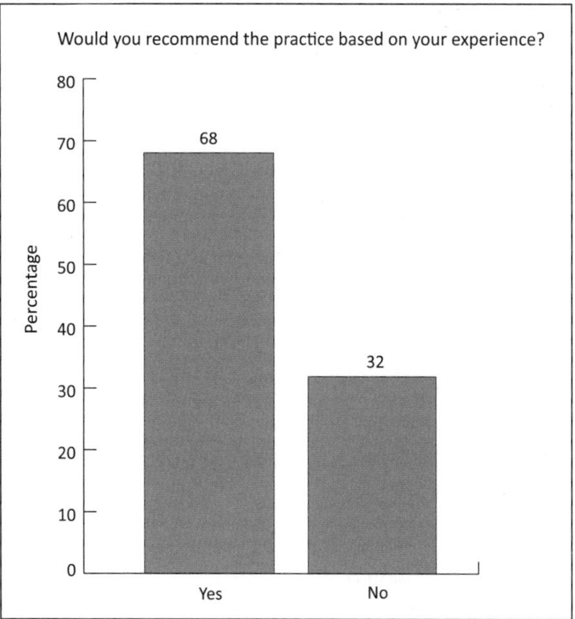

27.6 Mystery shopper results assessing customer experience. Although more than 40% felt they had received good or very good care, fewer than 10% scored it as 'very good'. More than 20% felt that the customer care received was 'worse than average'. The level of customer service experienced was insufficient for 32% to consider recommending the practice. It is important to note that this is not a judgment of the quality of clinical care but purely of customer experience. (Onswitch data 2004 – 2011, from approximately 3000 UK veterinary practices)

It is important that enough forms are completed and returned to allow a balanced picture. A prize draw might be considered to encourage clients to return their questionnaires; a reply-paid or pre-stamped envelope should be supplied if questionnaires are to be returned by post. If targeting particular service areas, return rates can be improved by surveying clients who are likely to revisit the practice; this can double the return rate. For example, a post-operative survey can ask about the admission and discharge processes and the client's experience of their pet having surgery, and can be returned at the follow-up appointment.

A short note about why the process is being undertaken, e.g. to improve the service provided, or investigate whether a new service is needed, should be included. Everyone who agrees to take part should be thanked and asked to answer questions honestly. Clients should be assured that they need not add their name unless they require a specific response.

Questionnaire design

A mix of open (What? Where? Who? How? When? Why?) and closed (can be answered yes or no) questions should be included. Open questions allow clients to articulate their feelings, but do not allow for comparing trends over time. A quantitative score can be used, e.g. 1–6 or 'very satisfied' to 'not very satisfied' (avoiding ranges with a mid-way rating). Alternatively, or in addition, space can be made for freehand comments indicating what went well and what they would have liked to have seen done better.

The actual questions asked will depend on whether the survey is a general one or whether it requires more detailed feedback regarding specific services. The more specific the question, the more useful the responses will be.

A general or feedback survey might include a selection of the following **background questions**:

- Respondent's age and sex – to find out who the practice's clients are, highlight any age or gender-specific issues
- Number and species of animals owned by the respondent
- Does the respondent have pet insurance?
- How far away from the practice does the respondent live?
- Reason for attendance (offer a tick box of options – routine vaccinations, emergency procedure, operation, nurse clinic, etc.)
- Date and time of attendance – to find out whether standards slip towards the weekend or when a particular member of staff is on duty.

Questions can then be asked about the **client experience**, for example:

- On a scale of 1 to 6, where 1 is very poor and 6 is very good, how would you rate:
  - Your overall experience today
  - The level to which the practice appreciates you
  - Contacting the surgery by telephone
  - Greeting on arrival
  - Waiting time
  - The waiting room and reception area
  - How well you were kept informed of delays
  - If your pet was hospitalized, how well you were kept updated of his/her progress
  - Staff:
    - Politeness and courtesy
    - Appearance
    - Identification
    - Friendliness
  - Clarity of information and instructions you were given
  - How well you were informed of costs involved during your pet's treatment
  - How well treatment options were discussed and explained to you
  - Accuracy of price estimates
  - Explanation of the bill and itemized invoices
  - Satisfaction of the level of value for money at the practice
  - Amount of information given by clinical staff.

Space should be allowed after each question for elaboration, if required, and general questions may also be asked, such as:

- What did you particularly like about your visit?
- What could we have done better?

Surveys can also be a useful marketing tool. Questions can be added asking whether respondents would like to join the e-mail newsletter list or to be mailed with regular special offers. Specific questions can highlight practice services; for example:

- Please tick which of the following were important to you in choosing to come to us with your pet:
  - 24-hour emergency service on premises
  - Late appointments on Fridays
  - Sunday opening
  - Wide range of special diet foods
  - Puppy playgroup sessions
  - Fully qualified veterinary nurses always on site.

Many clients will tick services they actually did not know existed until completing the survey!

Results, interpretation and use

One survey can offer some statistical analysis (how many clients were satisfied or very satisfied with an experience; how many clients would recommend the practice?) and also specific pointers to improve current processes and staff behaviour ('It would have been nice if Dan had been groomed before coming home, as happened at our last practice').

Concentrating on scores and yes/no answers will make the data gathered very specific, though usually retrospective. There is no opportunity to gain further insight into what the client's needs and thoughts are or were.

More specific or open questions will often elicit more practical feedback. For example, 'What did we do that was particularly helpful? Was there any other information you would have liked to be given?'. Action can be taken right away where systems or processes can be improved, and individual client needs met as a result of the survey response (e.g. written information can be sent if it was not given at the time, or an appointment can be offered).

All surveys require the information gathered to be collated, interpreted and findings presented in an easy-to-read format. Some practices may prefer to use an independent company to carry out this service.

Findings should be shared with staff and clients alike. Seeing that their comments are being acted upon will encourage future cooperation. Specific reassurances that comments have been taken on board, and acceptance of suggestions can be powerful drivers of loyalty.

Surveys should be an ongoing process: quarterly questionnaires ensure that any issues are picked up early on and allow tracking (and communication) of improvements.

KEY POINT

Surveys should help the practice take positive action to continually improve their service. The implementation of suggestions can be a powerful driver of loyalty.

Net promoter score

Levels of client satisfaction can be illustrated using the net promoter score (NPS). Clients are asked, after a consultation, to rate a practice on a scale of 1 to 10 (where 1 is very unlikely and 10 is very likely) against the statement: 'How likely are you to recommend our practice?' 'Promoters' will score very highly, rating 9s and 10s, whilst 'detractors' will rate between 1 and 6. The net effect for a practice is that active promoters will be offset somewhat by detractors, the effect of which can be calculated as follows. If 86% of clients rate a practice as either 9 or 10, and 10% rate it between 1 and 6, the NPS score would be 86 (promoters) minus 10 (detractors) = 76.

KEY POINT

The net promoter score is a very useful measure of client satisfaction, which can be tracked over time and used as a key performance indicator.

Collated NPS data from practices around the country show that whilst the majority of clients would recommend their practice, a significant minority would not (Figure 27.7). This suggests that there is still some way to go in delivering an excellent customer experience in many practices around the UK. Also, considering that those clients who are very unlikely to recommend are probably actively telling their friends exactly why not, there is every reason for practices to raise their game and deliver improvements to their customer experience.

Team feedback

Staff will all have their own positive and negative experiences, both when dealing with clients and when buying goods or services. A team meeting should be held to brainstorm what everyone thinks of the service provided at the practice, and to suggest areas where this can be improved. The whole team should be included – sometimes the quietest, newest or most junior staff members have the best insight.

KEY POINT

Get the team to discuss their own good and bad experiences as a customer. How can these be related to the customer experience in your own practice? Where are the common areas with your business?

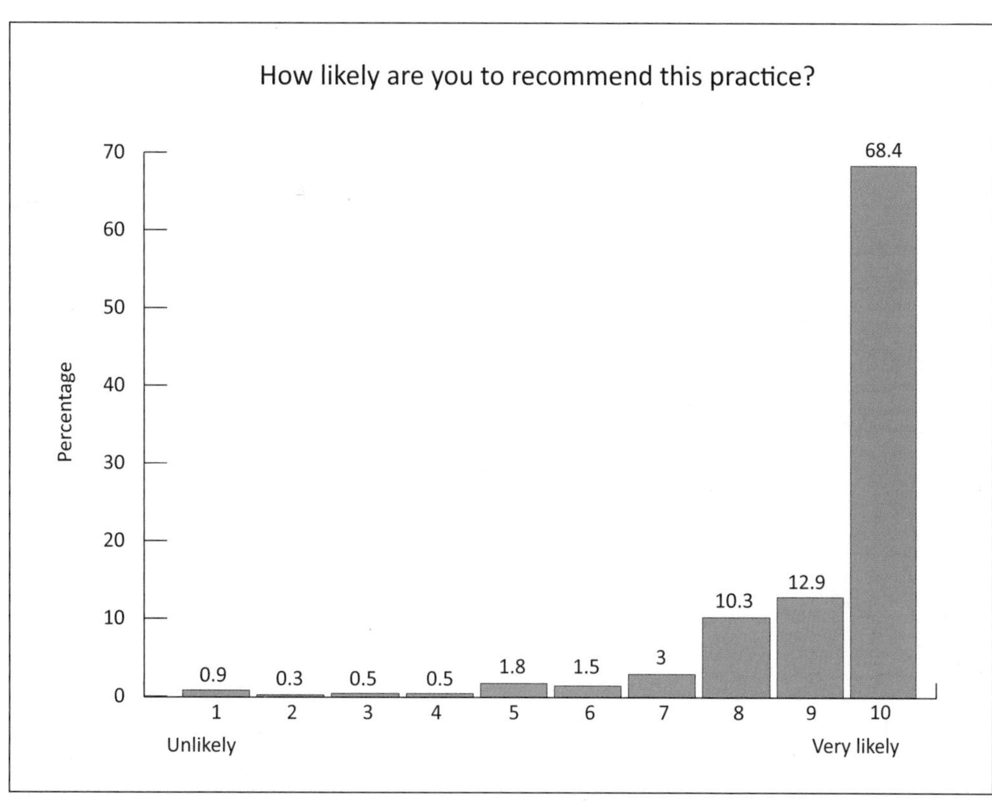

27.7 Client responses to the question 'How likely are you to recommend this practice?'. Calculating the NPS for these data gives a score of 75.8 (81.3 (those rating 9 or 10) minus 5.5 (those rating between 1 and 6)). (Onswitch data)

There are a number of points of client interaction where getting things right is particularly crucial: follow-up phone calls; postoperative calls; customer orders and repeat prescriptions; handling insurance claims; discussing test results; returning ashes. Staff could use role play of these situations, enabling those who are more experienced to impart their wisdom, balanced with the enthusiasm and fresh eyes of the newer team members. It is important to try and distance personal feelings from this process – people need to be comfortable both giving and receiving feedback if improvements are to be made.

Seeking excellence in patient experience

The concept of the excellent customer experience is not unique to the veterinary sector. Manufacturers, banks, service providers, online businesses and retail chains are all building reputations for providing an excellent customer experience. 'Patient experience' is something of a buzz phrase in the human medicine field. It has been a national priority since the publication of Lord Darzi's *Next Stage Review* in June 2008, and measuring and improving the patient experience is now enshrined in the NHS Operating Framework, with a proportion of income conditional on achieving locally agreed customer satisfaction goals.

Recent government initiatives such as 'Choose and book' have given patients a choice of up to five healthcare providers, with plans to extend this much further. Patients can now specify which hospital they visit, and which doctor they want to see. Suddenly it is important to attract patients (customers) with the promise of excellence, so aside from the moral principle of delivering the 'best' care they can, trusts now also have a financial incentive to do so. In order to help patients make their choice, league tables highlighting everything from waiting time to the standard of hospital food and the recovery rate of inpatients can be consulted. Data are collected direct from individual patients via hand-held electronic tablets on which they are asked to assess their recent experience using a wide range of criteria, including 'softer' measures such as:

- Were you involved as much as you wanted to be in decisions about your care and treatment?
- Did you find someone on the hospital staff to talk to about your worries and fears?
- Were you given enough privacy when discussing your condition or treatment?
- Did a member of staff tell you about medication side effects to watch for when you went home?
- Did hospital staff tell you who to contact if you were worried about your condition or treatment after you left hospital?

Pet owners are giving increasing priority to areas such as this when forming their own assessment of the customer experience, and it is in these small but critical details that the route to excellence lies, whether in human medicine or veterinary care.

Using customer experience to build business

The first step to implementing change is to identify where a practice's clients are coming from – are they new or existing? As Figure 27.8 shows, there are a number of means by which to encourage clients to visit the practice more often, and in greater numbers. Branding (see Chapter 25) and recommendation are two of the most powerful ways to attract clients. Recommendation comes either from key opinion leaders (KOLs) or from friends.

Key opinion leaders

If there is a close relationship with some of the most local and influential KOLs (see Figure 27.3), the practice has an opportunity to access a sizeable pool of potential clients. It therefore makes good business sense to find out who the main KOLs are in the area and then implement some or all of the following action plans:

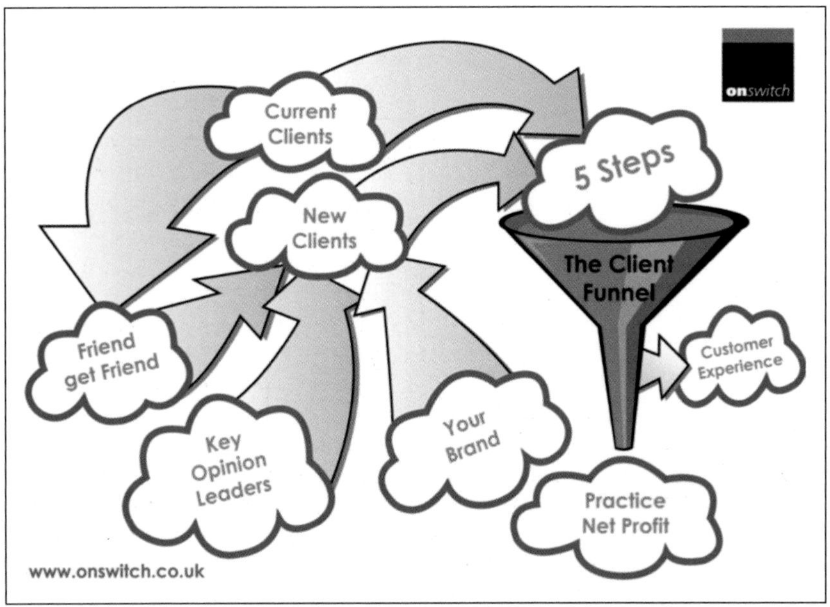

27.8 The 'client funnel' shows the drivers of footfall, which is ultimately the source of practice net profit. Customer experience whilst 'in the funnel' will influence these drivers positively or negatively. © Onswitch.

- Hold a practice open day (Figure 27.9); show KOLs around and answer their questions about what the practice does, and how it does it
- Implement lectures, workshops, client evenings and mutual training sessions, all of which are good ways to build professional and personal relationships and demonstrate why the practice is so good
- Attend events such as local school fêtes, dog shows, etc.
- Hold social evenings, summer BBQs, dog walking fundraisers, etc., as opportunities to understand any local issues or negative perceptions
- Produce newsletters, keeping these KOLs up to date with new services and facilities.

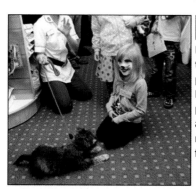

27.9 Demonstrating clicker training during a practice open day. Involving younger people in practice activities builds relationships for the future.

'Recommend a friend' schemes

'Recommend a friend' (Figure 27.10) is a simple process that is used across many industries with impressive results. Most consumers will be aware of the mail order catalogues and mail shots that drop through their letter boxes, and how almost every company is recruiting new customers through such schemes. It works extremely well and, as an added bonus, can be self-funding when used at a practice.

1. A card is given to owners as they leave the building, sent out with booster reminders, handed around at puppy classes, etc. These should be professionally designed and printed.
2. Clients fill in their own details and give it to their friends.
3. When their friend spends £x or more on professional fees this now new client receives £x off and the original client who introduced them also receives a voucher for £x which is redeemable at the practice.

If customers are enjoying their experience, they will often talk about it to others. To be rewarded financially for doing so will be an added bonus; the practice gains more clients and therefore ultimately benefits from an increase in sales. Existing clients receive a lovely warm glow of recognition, and the new client's first impressions are also positive as a result of the introductory offer.

KEY POINT

Make customers feel valued, and they will spend more with the practice as well as recruiting more clients.

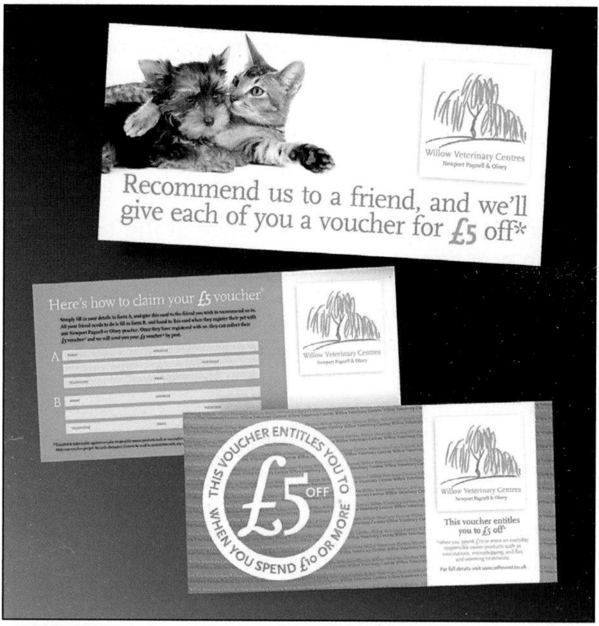

27.10 An example of a 'recommend a friend' scheme.

The importance of the telephone

For customers (both existing and new), the telephone will always be a key interface between a practice and its clients. Without face-to-face contact and body language cues, it is imperative that reception staff members are trained to deliver a consistently excellent telephone service. Regular training reinforcement of the five steps for successful telephone call handling is essential (see earlier). Every time an owner calls a practice, staff should offer an appointment.

All staff who speak to clients on the phone should be fully trained and thus competent and confident when it comes to effective telephone skills. In addition to receptionists and nurses, veterinary surgeons, the practice principal and the management team should all receive training to ensure that there is consistency and that the same high standards are maintained whichever member of the team the client is speaking to.

The long game

Practice reputation is only as good as the last client interaction, so there is no time for complacency. Delivering an excellent customer experience requires an ongoing commitment from the whole team. A team that is engaged, motivated and well trained will achieve this and it is incredibly rewarding to receive glowing feedback from delighted customers.

Increasing numbers of veterinary practices are putting customer care at the very heart of their business: setting objectives to improve further; establishing ongoing training and staff mentoring schemes; and canvassing customers' feedback to monitor changes in satisfaction levels. They are doing this because, as well as maintaining staff morale, and achieving better ongoing patient care, delivering an excellent customer experience is helping them to be more profitable and to grow their client base.

Changing the customer experience is a long-term commitment, not just a chapter to read, a box to tick, and then one more trendy term to forget. If a practice truly believes that the customer experience is key to success, there are some fundamental steps that must be put in place:

- **Place the customer experience at the heart of the practice mission.** Share it with clients and make sure all the team sign up to it
- **Put in place a process to capture client feedback –** either through mystery shoppers or regular surveys. Share the results and communicate what is going to be done differently. Be proud of successes, and do not shy away from highlighting the areas where improvement is needed
- **Hold regular team meetings.** Each member of the team needs to understand the practice approach to customer care and feel that their suggestions count
- **Make everyone accountable for delivery of excellence** in customer care. Each appraisal should require staff to show what they are doing to continue making improvements.

Veterinary medicine is a service industry. Clients demand the best care not only for their pets but also for themselves. If they do not receive it, most will not say so but are more likely to 'vote with their feet' – and then tell their friends.

If the practice gets the basics right, everything else will follow. If commitment to quality and service forms the core of the business, not just an optional extra bolt-on, customers will love the practice (Figure 27.11), be more inclined to seek professional advice, spend more there and tell their friends to do the same. An excellent customer experience motivates staff, attracts customers, provides free advertising and justifies a price premium.

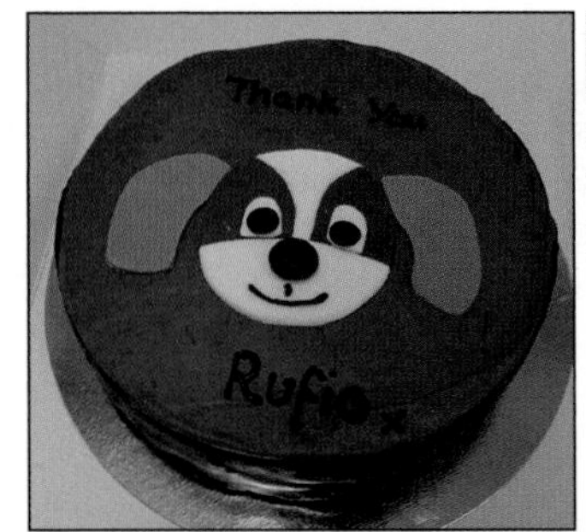

27.11 Gifts from customers should always be acknowledged with a thank you note from the team.

KEY POINT

There are no quick fixes and gimmicks to make the customer experience excellent. The aim to deliver must sit at the heart of the business and be evident in everything it does.

Acknowledgement

The author is grateful to Mill House Veterinary Surgery and Hospital for supplying images for this chapter.

References and further reading

Fornell C (2009) *The Satisfied Customer: Winners and Losers in the Battle for Buyer Preference.* Palgrave Macmillan

Hill N, Roche G and Allen R (2007) *Customer Satisfaction: The Customer Experience through the Customer's Eyes.* Cogent Publishing, London

Hsieh T (2010) *Delivering Happiness: A Path to Profits, Passion and Purpose.* Business Plus

Pine BJ II and Gilmore J (1999) *The Experience Economy: Work Is Theater & Every Business a Stage.* [illustrated edition] Harvard Business School Press, Boston

Shaw C (2007) *The DNA of Customer Experience: How Emotions Drive Value.* Palgrave Macmillan

Smith S and Wheeler J (2002) *Managing the Customer Experience: Turning Customers into Advocates.* Financial Times/Prentice Hall, London

Clinical governance

28

Bradley Viner

The public is increasingly questioning the competence of medical practitioners and demanding evidence of good practice, rather than just relying on professional qualifications as a guarantee, and this is spilling over into veterinary practice. Professional governing bodies in the UK and elsewhere are increasingly calling upon veterinary surgeons to ensure that clinical governance forms part of their professional activities and this requirement is now part of the RCVS Codes of Professional Conduct for Veterinary Surgeons and Veterinary Nurses. The RCVS Practice Standards Scheme (PSS) notes that this should include monitoring and reviewing clinical outcomes, with the aim of improving the care practices provide.

As a basic level of clinical audit, all practices should have a means of monitoring and discussing the clinical outcome of cases and of acting on the results, with some system for monitoring and discussing the clinical outcome of some common procedures. This may vary from clinical audit reports to notes of clinical discussion meetings, but inevitably starts with some form of record-keeping.

Practices that aspire to provide a more advanced level of clinical care, such as veterinary hospitals and referral centres, should have a more sophisticated system in place to audit their results and should strive continually to improve their clinical performance. Regular morbidity and mortality meetings should be held to discuss the outcome of clinical cases, with permanent records of such meetings kept to demonstrate any changes in procedures as a consequence of any resultant action list. Continued monitoring to assess the effectiveness of any changes should be undertaken.

KEY POINT

'Veterinary surgeons must ensure that clinical governance (consideration of animal safety, client experience and effective care) forms part of their professional activities, including monitoring and reviewing clinical outcomes, with the aim of improving the care they provide.' RCVS Code of Professional Conduct for Veterinary Surgeons 2012

It is incumbent upon all individual clinicians to review the quality of their work continually with the aim of improving their quality of care, and for those with management responsibility to ensure that a suitable framework exists to encourage and support an appropriate level of clinical practice. What constitutes appropriate will vary depending upon the circumstances but the concept of continually striving to ensure that the available resources are used in the most effective manner is universally recognized as good business practice. For veterinary practices, quality improvement (see Chapter 26) should be embedded into clinical governance protocols.

Evidence-based veterinary medicine and 'best practice'

Evidence-based veterinary medicine (EBVM) is defined as the conscientious, explicit and judicious use of current best evidence in making decisions about the care of individual patients. This means integrating individual clinical expertise and the best available external clinical evidence from systematic research. The subject is a discipline in its own right, and it is strongly recommended that anyone with an interest in it consults sources such as those listed as further reading at the end of this chapter.

Within human medicine the best available knowledge has become synonymous with evidence largely based on randomized controlled trials (RCTs), meta-analyses and systematic reviews. In veterinary practice, however, as those are in short supply a broader range of evidence needs to be considered (Figure 28.1).

EBVM involves a five-stage process:

1. Convert needs for information into answerable questions, which may be about:
   - The patient or problem being addressed
   - The intervention being considered
   - A comparison intervention (or control)
   - The clinical outcome.
2. Track down, with maximum efficiency, the best evidence with which to answer the questions

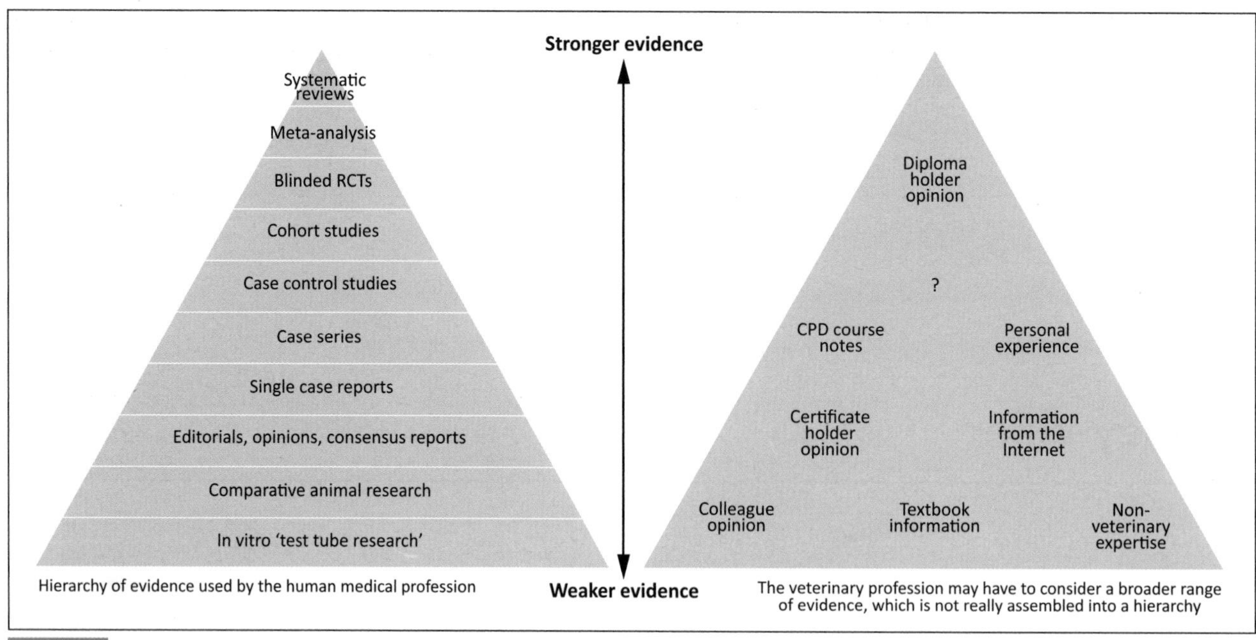

28.1 Hierarchy of evidence. RCTs = randomized clinical trials (Adapted from Cockcroft and Holmes, 2003)

(whether from the clinical examination, the diagnostic laboratory, from research evidence or other sources).

3. Critically appraise the evidence for validity (closeness to the truth) and usefulness (clinical applicability).
4. Apply the results of this appraisal to clinical practice.
5. Evaluate performance.

KEY POINT

The aim of the process is to establish what constitutes 'best practice' for the management of a particular condition under certain circumstances.

'Best practice' can be defined as the most efficient (involving the least amount of effort or expense) and effective (producing the best results) way of accomplishing a task. It is often defined in terms of a local clinical setting where, in addition to any relevant evidence from research, it will take into account the availability of skills and resources as well as individual clinician and client preferences in delivering what is considered optimal for the patient in that context. It may thus vary from one site to another. For example, best practice for the investigation of a chronic cough in a dog may be quite different in a referral *versus* a first-opinion practice.

Elements of clinical governance

The term 'clinical governance' describes the framework (Figure 28.2) and systematic approach through which an organization is accountable for continually improving the quality of its services and safeguarding high standards of care, i.e. quality-assured patient care. It will achieve this by creating an environment in which excellence in clinical care can flourish.

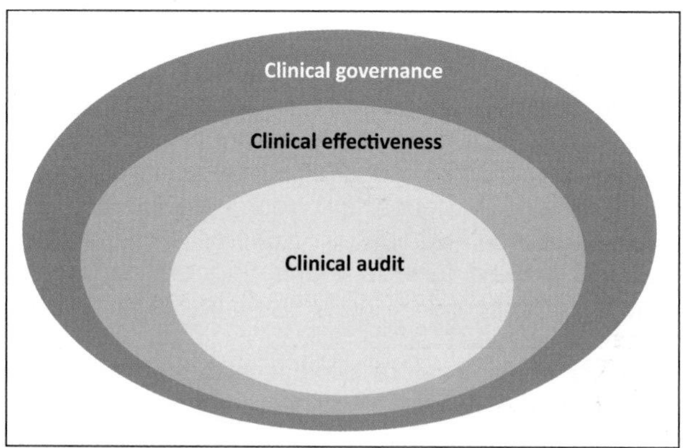

28.2 Clinical effectiveness is an important component of clinical governance and, in turn, incorporates clinical audit as a tool.

Clinical governance can be considered to cover seven broad areas, many of which are covered in previous chapters:

- Risk management (see Chapters 6 to 15 and 22)
- Information management (see Chapters 4, 16 and 24)
- Human resource management and team working (see Chapters 16 to 23)
- Client involvement (see Chapters 5, 17, 21, 25, 26 and 27)
- Continuing professional development (see Chapters 18 and 19)
- Evidence-based veterinary medicine (EBVM)
- Clinical effectiveness (incorporating clinical audit).

Individual responsibility

Continuing professional development

The RCVS has adopted the definition of CPD for vets as 'the systematic maintenance, improvement and broadening of knowledge and skills and the development of personal qualities necessary for the execution of professional and technical duties throughout the member's working life'. Registered veterinary nurses (RVNs) also have a minimum requirement for CPD. There is no restriction on the number of hours of online assessment or mediated distance learning that can be counted towards the requirement.

It is important to realize that what the RCVS considers to be CPD encompasses much more than just attending external courses. Indeed, it could be argued that attending didactic lectures without taking steps to apply the learning in the workplace, and reflect upon its impact, is one of the least effective ways to improve professional performance. The RCVS recognizes that what should count as CPD will vary for each individual, and it is therefore up to each person to decide how best to fulfil his/her own learning needs. CPD planning should be tied in with the strategic objectives of the organization and with the appraisal system. Examples of appropriate activities are given in Figure 28.3.

- Studying towards a qualification
- Shadowing or mentoring in own or another practice
- Participating in 'learning sets' – informal networks of colleagues who learn together, e.g. by comparing and discussing case reports
- In-house sharing of expertise
- Attending organized courses, lectures or seminars
- Participating in webinars and online learning
- Secondments to other practices
- Critical reading of veterinary journals and other relevant publications, combined with keeping a reading diary or notes
- Research, including research in preparation for giving lectures/seminars/presentations/writing articles or books
- Clinical audit activities if combined with an account of how they have contributed to personal learning

28.3 Examples of appropriate activities for continuing professional development (CPD).

KEY POINT

Good governance demands that professional development is inculcated within the culture of the organization, which should have a policy to reflect this (see Chapter 19). Effective CPD not only requires a statement of good intention but also a willingness to allocate the funds and time that is required.

Specific suggestions for encouraging effective CPD within an organization include:

- Incorporating professional development into the appraisal process – many organizations now refer to appraisal sessions as 'developmental reviews' to highlight that emphasis. The process should ensure that team members are clear about the strategic objectives of the business and the role that they should be playing in moving towards achieving them. This should enable them to highlight the most appropriate learning needs that will benefit both themselves and the organization as a whole, and to seek out the most appropriate means of meeting those needs. Structured learning will be far more effective than *ad hoc* CPD undertaken in response to whatever happens to be on offer at a particular time. Progress should be reviewed at least every six months
- Developing a whole practice development plan that integrates development activity across the team
- Considering working within the Investors in People (IiP) framework and extended standards (Figure 28.4), to drive improvement and involvement
- Allocating each team and member of the practice team a realistic CPD budget and giving them the responsibility to plan their own development programme within that budget
- Making best use of the budget allocated to attendance at external meetings and courses, by encouraging attendees to share their key learning points with other members of the team. As well as benefiting the whole group, the act of crystallizing the learning gained from a meeting concisely helps to consolidate it, and feedback from others can often develop it further. The conversion of learning to practice and individual action points is an essential process
- Trying to make learning relevant and enjoyable by organizing clinical clubs or journal clubs, either physical or online, critically discussing cases and clinical papers
- Ensuring that the practice remains open to new thinking as new information is brought into the organization, by discussing it at clinical effectiveness meetings and incorporating that information into new practice guidelines or revising existing ones, where appropriate
- Ensuring clinical staff have access to suitable up-to-date reference material. In multi-site practices certain core texts will need to be kept at each site, but a central reference library can be used to collate other reference books and journals. Consideration could be given to subscribing to online resources that enable easy access to practical and reference material for all of the practice team (e.g. VIN, Vetstream, RCVS library service).

KEY POINT

Structured learning will be far more effective than relying on the *ad hoc* CPD that many practitioners undertake in response to whatever happens to be on offer at a particular time.

Reflective practice

Reflecting upon performance and unexpected critical events is a useful way of learning from outcomes and encouraging veterinary surgeons to make appropriate changes to practice. A reflective learning diary can be a useful tool, as can participating in learning sets and discussing issues with colleagues.

KEY POINT

Reflection should include both clinical and communication performance, within the team and with clients.

Business strategy	Management effectiveness
■ Top managers make sure the practice's strategy is developed through the involvement of managers, people, stakeholders and other sources ■ People can describe how they are involved in developing the practice's strategy ■ People can describe the key performance indicators used by the practice to improve its performance	■ Top managers can describe how they act as role models for inspirational leadership and have an open, honest and trusting management style ■ People can confirm they are able to give constructive feedback to their manager and believe it is well received and acted upon ■ People believe the practice has a culture of openness and trust
Learning and development strategy	**Recognition and reward**
■ Top managers can describe how they have created a culture that encourages continuous learning and promotes the development of skills and knowledge at every level ■ Managers can describe how they involve people in identifying the learning and development needs of their team and the activities planned to meet them ■ People can confirm that their learning and development is planned to build their future capability to contribute to achieving the practice's vision ■ People believe that continuous learning is at the heart of the culture of the practice	■ Top managers can describe how the practice's reward and recognition strategy is linked to its business strategy and externally benchmarked
	Involvement and empowerment
	■ Top managers and managers make sure the practice has effective internal communication systems to encourage knowledge and information to be shared throughout the practice ■ People believe that consultation arrangements are effective and allow them to take part in decision-making ■ People believe they can challenge the way the practice works and can give examples of how they or others have done so
Learning and development	**Performance measurement**
■ People can describe how they are encouraged to try new approaches and learn from their efforts, mistakes and successes ■ People can confirm that they are well supported after learning and development activities and have clear objectives for putting the new skills and knowledge into practice	■ People can give examples of improvements in the performance of the team as a result of people management and development activities
Leadership and management strategy	**Continuous improvement**
■ Managers and top managers can confirm that they are regularly reviewed against the capabilities and receive constructive feedback on their performance	■ People can describe improvements that have been made as a result of their feedback to the way the practice manages and develops people

28.4 Investors in People (IiP) is used by many practices to drive improvements and performance. The extended framework, with opportunity for bronze, silver and gold achievement, has over a hundred evidence requirements across a range of ten management areas, which are all relevant to the topics discussed in this chapter. A flavour of some of these is given here; it is worth taking some time to consider how well your own practice measures up to the standards, and where improvements can be made. The full standards are available at www. investorsinpeople.co.uk. Involvement and trust are crucial to the standard and to a successful 'no blame' culture that encourages continual improvements and clinical excellence. Investors in People assessment is an effective means of benchmarking against an external 'gold standard'.

Peer review

Peer review is an assessment of the quality of care provided by a clinical team with a view to improving clinical care, including interesting or unusual cases. This may be carried out by someone external to the practice, but more commonly will be work colleagues offering constructive criticism (Figure 28.5).

Benchmarking

Comparing one's own level of performance against the level achieved by others is a useful basis for improvement. Performance can also be benchmarked against specific time periods, e.g. looking for improvement year on year. Comparison may be internal (within a practice or group) or external (comparison with similar practices or against an externally set 'gold standard', e.g. Investors in People; see Figure 28.4).

> **KEY POINT**
>
> When benchmarking, care must be taken to ensure that, as far as possible, like is compared with like.

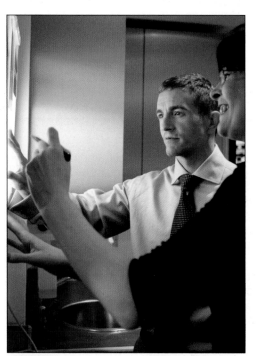

28.5 Work colleagues offering constructive criticism is an important aspect of peer review.

Whilst external benchmarking is common within the NHS, there are currently few areas of veterinary practice where reliable clinical performance data have been accumulated. An exception to this is in the area of postoperative complications of neutering, where data are centrally collated and analysed. This depends upon a reasonably uniform method of grading postoperative complications, which for the purpose of this audit are scored as:

0. Lost to follow-up (when follow-up was expected)
1. No complication reported
2. Complications noted but no treatment required
3. Complications noted but only medical treatment was required
4. Complications noted and surgical treatment was required
5. The animal died.

Information on how to submit practice data for benchmarking and current UK results can be found at www.vetaudit.co.uk.

Team responsibility

Animal safety

Protocols

Clinical protocols (rather than guidelines; see below) are appropriate in some instances, such as when the consequences of not following specific instructions are potentially dire. They are applicable particularly to procedures that are critical to the safety of patients (Figure 28.6). This will be particularly obvious in an area such as the surgical suite, where simple problems such as an interruption in oxygen supply or the administration of an incorrect drug or drug dose can rapidly cause loss of life.

Critical incident review meetings (see below) may be used to review relevant protocols and to consider whether they need to be altered in the light of any problems. However, all protocols should be subject to periodic team review as a matter of course, rather than waiting for a critical event to occur. Involving the practice clinical team in such reviews can also act as a reminder that such protocols exist. It is essential to communicate changes in procedure effectively to the whole practice team and to ensure that internal communication systems are updated accordingly. Recording discussions and changes can be kept very simple, e.g. a desk diary can be used or notes made on the clinical practice management system (PMS) using a 'client' record called, say, 'Clinical governance'.

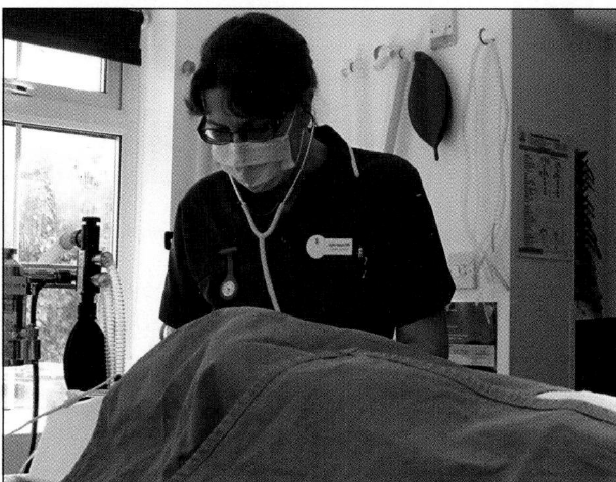

28.6 When a patient is under general anaesthesia, strict monitoring and recording protocols must be followed at all times, with clear lines of responsibility that are understood by the clinical team.

KEY POINTS

- Clear written protocols should be in place to ensure that all staff are familiar with procedures for ensuring patient safety before an incident occurs.
- Management systems should ensure that the protocols:
  - Are embedded into training procedures
  - Are regularly reviewed
  - Are drawn to the attention of all new members of staff and that existing members are reminded of them at regular intervals.

Critical incident review

A formalized peer review is used in specific cases that have caused concern or had an unexpected outcome. Discussion and reflection should enable the team to learn from what has happened, with a view to improvement for future cases. Critical events can include:

- Unexpected medical or surgical complications
- A serious complaint
- An accident
- Unexpected anaesthetic death.

A meeting of all staff involved should be held as soon as possible after the incident, in a no-blame environment where all team members feel free to open up about what took place. All details should be recorded. Creating a 'no-blame' culture can be difficult to achieve, as there are many external pressures that encourage veterinary professionals to behave defensively. The focus should be kept firmly on looking forwards to the improvement of outcomes rather than backwards to attributing blame. Any individual performance issues should be dealt with on an entirely separate basis (see Chapter 19). An example of a detailed critical incident review reporting form is given at the end of this chapter.

KEY POINT

It is essential that critical incident review meetings are used as a positive effort by the clinical team to unravel what went wrong and what could be done differently in future. In order to achieve this it is important that team members feel able to speak freely without fear of censure.

Referrals

Knowing when it is appropriate to offer referral to the client is an essential aspect of professional competence and veterinary surgeons within the organization must be aware of practice policy on this issue. It is entirely appropriate for referrals to be made within a practice or to other general practitioners known to have expertise in a particular area. The referring vet has a responsibility to ensure they are making the referral to a person with an appropriate level of expertise, and that any choice in this area is communicated to the client. Cases that require specialized equipment or expertise should be referred to a referral centre unless external factors make that impossible. In this case, the client should be made aware that the primary care clinician is acting at the limits of his/her expertise and the client must give informed consent to proceed.

KEY POINTS

- Practice policy on case referral should be clear.
- Clinicians should be aware of the specialists to which the practice is confident to direct clients for a particular type of case.

Clinical effectiveness

Clinical effectiveness involves the application of the best available knowledge, derived from research, clinical experience and owner/patient preferences, to achieve optimum processes and outcomes of care for patients.

KEY POINT

Improving clinical effectiveness requires a multifaceted approach to encourage excellence.

Practice meetings

Regular practice meetings (Figure 28.7) should be designed not just to tackle administrative issues but also to deal with clinical matters and staff training. Such meetings could act as a forum for clinical staff to discuss cases that they consider to be interesting or challenging, encouraging their peers to help them reflect upon the clinical decision-making process and what might be considered best practice in a particular situation.

Practice meetings can also be used to update the team about new products that have become available and also to allow staff to debate and have an input into whether new products are to be used and whether others should be discontinued. Sometimes commercial factors will also influence that choice, but those in charge of the financial management of the organization are best placed to make a balanced decision when they have an understanding of how the front line staff feel about the clinical issues involved.

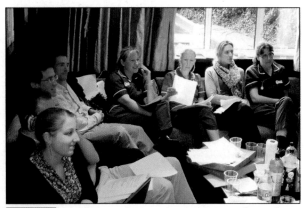

28.7 Regular practice meetings can act as a forum for clinical staff to discuss cases.

Meetings can also be used to refresh and update the clinical team on specific areas of their work, picking up on one or more areas of diagnosis or treatment and either bringing in an outside speaker to talk about the subject or tasking one member with an interest in that area to research the current literature on the topic and put together a presentation.

Good communication is vital at all stages and includes:

- Notifying staff members so that they are kept informed of what is up and coming, and their likely role in the process
- Inviting input to the agenda from clinical staff at all levels to maintain their sense of involvement
- Recording the issues raised during the meeting and any action points that may have been decided during the course of it, and circulating these
- Reviewing any action points at the next meeting to see if they have been acted upon and to reflect upon their effect.

Practices may find it preferable to carry out at least some of this work electronically, such as by organizing online discussion forums to review clinical cases where geography or part-time working make face-to-face meetings difficult. Meeting notes can be made on a specific PMS computer record or in a bound book; full typed minutes are not necessary. For more on communication and meetings see Chapter 17.

Clinical guidelines

These are systematically developed statements designed to assist the practitioner and client in making decisions about appropriate healthcare for patients in specific clinical circumstances; they will enhance clinical effectiveness. The term 'clinical protocol' is used similarly, although it suggests a more rigid set of rules that the clinician is obliged to follow (see earlier).

KEY POINT

Guidelines are much more likely to be embraced by the practice team if they have played a role in their formulation. Individuals can bring their own clinical experience to the discussion, which will help in making the guidelines applicable to the practice situation.

Three key features differentiate guidelines from general clinical advice such as may be given in veterinary texts:

- They involve an explicit attempt systematically to review the literature on the subject in question for the best available evidence. The evidence base for veterinary clinical practice is often very scanty compared to that for human medicine, and evaluating the relative merit of various sources is a skill in its own right

- They represent a consensus in the setting in which they are prepared, rather than the opinion of an individual. This may be a panel of experts if they are nationally developed guidelines, or a team of clinical staff if they are guidelines being written or adapted for local use
- The information is presented in a summarized form, often as a series of bullet points, so as to be readily accessible in a clinical situation.

The use of clinical guidelines can bring several benefits but can also raise concerns (Figure 28.8). However, if applied sensibly, most clinicians find such guidelines supportive rather than restrictive. Within the context of human medical jurisprudence they have not undermined the clinical judgement of doctors and, even where guidelines are laid down as a legal standard, courts still require sensible discretion to be used in applying them. Clinical guidelines are only one source of information available to the clinician, and are not suitable for every clinical decision-making situation.

Advantages
■ Assist the application of evidence-based best practice to individual patients ■ Provide a uniform standard of care ■ Can be used in the education and training of health professionals ■ Help clients to make informed decisions by improving communications and managing expectations ■ Facilitate a cost–benefit analysis of the diagnostic and treatment options
Disadvantages
■ May interfere with the clinical freedom of vets ■ Could be used against the veterinary profession in litigation and therefore increase defensive medicine ■ Could be imposed by insurance companies as a cost-cutting exercise and thus restrict access to potentially useful treatments

28.8 Advantages and disadvantages of clinical guidelines.

Currently few nationally developed clinical guidelines exist within the veterinary profession. In 2007 the Feline Advisory Bureau introduced a series of 23 feline clinical protocols and in 2009 the European Advisory Board on Cat Diseases (ABCD) produced a series of articles providing guidelines on the prevention and management of a whole range of feline infectious diseases that filled one whole issue of the *Journal of Feline Medicine and Surgery.* Nationally produced clinical guidelines are not the only way of communicating the findings of evidence-based veterinary medicine, but they represent a convenient and accessible medium for the busy practitioner and it is likely that their use will become more widespread in the future. Until that time, practitioners wishing to utilize them either independently or as part of the clinical audit process will often need to formulate them locally. In these instances, it falls upon the clinical team to follow the principles of EBVM outlined above.

Internationally, the World Small Animal Veterinary Association (WSAVA) has published International Vaccination Guidelines (Day *et al.*, 2010) and has three groups working on liver, gastrointestinal and renal standardization for histological and clinical diagnosis. In 2010 the International Task Force on Canine Atopic Dermatitis (now International Committee on Allergic Diseases of Animals – ICADA) published peer-reviewed practice guidelines on the treatment of atopic dermatitis in dogs (Olivry *et al.*, 2010); these evidence-based recommendations for general practitioners are endorsed by WSAVA.

Information systems

Effective management of information is essential to the governance of any organization, as it is of no value to have detailed guidelines and protocols in place unless they are communicated adequately to all levels of staff and, where appropriate, clients. This is a two-way process, as nowadays there is a vast flow of information into an organization that needs to be processed and managed appropriately. In a small practice it may be adequate to achieve this through a combination of oral and written communication, but within a larger organization it will inevitably involve computer systems. The intelligent use of e-mails, internal messaging, intranets and other software solutions can bring vast benefits to an organization but can bring problems as well. Information technology is dealt with specifically in Chapter 4, but its relevance to clinical governance includes the following:

- The maintenance of accurate clinical records is fundamental to the effective clinical care of patients and fulfilling professional obligations under the RCVS Code of Professional Conduct. There are many enhancements that can be used to facilitate other governance measures, including the recall of data for the purposes of clinical audit (see later)
- A practice manual, which brings together all the relevant protocols and guidelines for handling and treating patients as well as for managing the practice's interface with the public, can be produced in printed format; but software solutions such as an intranet allow such documents to be readily updated, shared, and information searched for when required
- An internal communication system can be used very effectively to process and handle information that comes into the organization, ensuring that it is passed on to relevant members of staff. Many practice management systems have e-mail servers incorporated, or an external service can be installed across a network
- A staff forum can serve as a more interactive form of communication, helping to involve team members in the decision-making process without having to be physically present at a meeting and to discuss clinical information (see above)
- IT can play an important role in assisting the process of professional development within the organization. This can include the use of an online training forum, the sharing of knowledge acquired by individuals with the practice team (Figure 28.9), and the searching out of information to help determine the evidence base for clinical work.

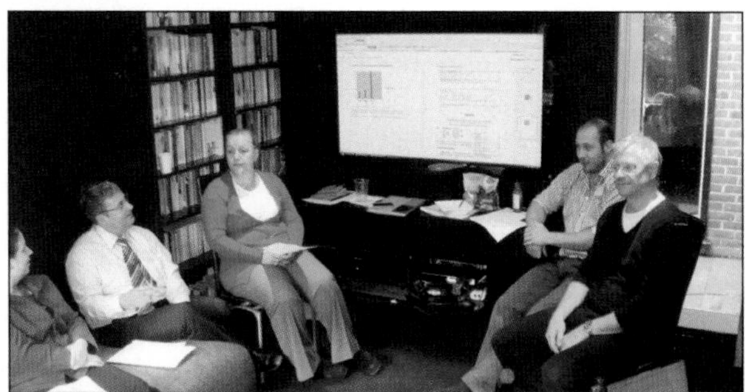

28.9 Sharing knowledge within the practice team is a vital part of clinical governance.

Patient and client experience

Standards of care and continuity

The patient and client experience should be actively considered and the team facilitated to seek ways of continual improvement; nursing staff are often particularly vigilant in this respect. The Feline Advisory Bureau's cat-friendly practice scheme offers wide-ranging advice for feline patients; requirements for other species will be different. Considerations include accommodation and equipment requirements, and day-to-day organizational issues, such as keeping prey and predator species separated and encouraging owners to bring familiar bedding and toys for canine inpatients. Not only will the patients benefit, but their owners are likely to be greatly reassured by the practice's concern about such matters.

Guidelines should be put into place to safeguard pain relief and nursing care for all inpatients. This will involve carefully considering the evidence base for analgesic routines for different species, different procedures and differing circumstances. Veterinary nurses are able to follow clearly laid down guidelines under veterinary direction; but each case should be individually monitored and, if necessary, further veterinary attention sought to gain approval for deviation from standard regimens.

Accurate record-keeping and effective systems will help to ensure continuity of care for patients by facilitating case handovers between clinical staff, but should be augmented by a face-to-face explanation for each patient. Regular monitoring and recording of vital signs and medication administered must be stored in an agreed format for ongoing reference, and kept for retrospective analysis should the need arise (see Chapter 7).

Effective personal communications with owners should also ensure that owners are given accurate and consistent information. A clearly laid down and effective complaints procedure is essential (see Chapter 17). Client feedback should be monitored, taken note of and, where appropriate, acted upon (see Chapter 27).

Clinical audit

Clinical audit has been defined as: a quality improvement process in clinical practice that seeks to establish guidelines for dealing with particular problems, based on documented evidence when it is available, measuring the effectiveness of these guidelines once they have been put into effect, and modifying them as appropriate. It should be an ongoing upward spiral of appraisal and improvement (Figure 28.10).

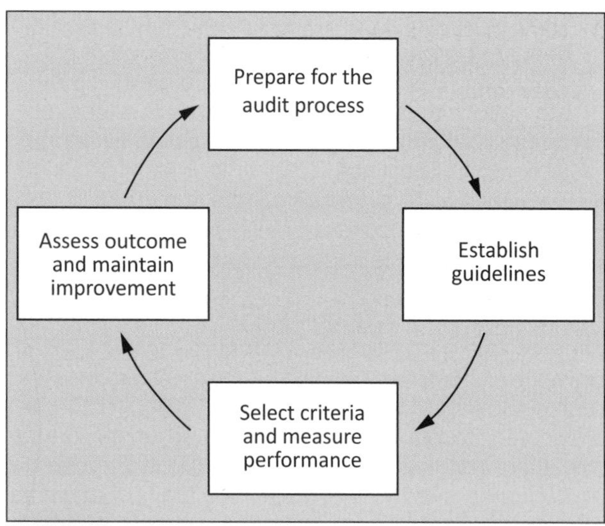

28.10 The clinical audit cycle. The key components can best be visualized schematically as a positive feedback loop.

Clinical audit involves the collection and recording of clinical information with the aim of monitoring the quality of care. As purely a process of measurement it has limited value, although it can play a role in benchmarking the performance of one practice against another for purposes of quality assurance. Auditing can have several important benefits:

- Establishing what is being done, and that what is being done is acceptable
- Serving as a basis to improve clinical effectiveness
- Improving job satisfaction
- Helping to standardize care throughout the practice or practices
- Increasing public confidence in the profession as a whole and in individual practice procedures
- Fulfilling the requirements of the RCVS Practice Standards Scheme
- Assisting in creating a positive culture within the clinical team
- As a management tool it has the potential to increase practice income.

KEY POINT

When used as a positive feedback loop of continual improvement, the clinical audit cycle can be an extremely useful management tool to improve clinical performance.

The clinical audit cycle

1. **Preparation.** This includes:
   - Selecting an area to audit
   - Considering objectives for the audit
   - Making sure that it is possible to record and retrieve information
   - Involving the team in the process, which includes developing a culture in which problems and differences of opinion can be freely discussed.
2. **Establishing guidelines.** Recommendations for the care of patients, using the best available evidence and agreeing best practice in each circumstance.

3. **Selection of criteria.** Criteria are explicit statements that define what is being measured; they represent elements of care that can be measured objectively. Criteria can measure outcomes or processes.
   - Select criteria that:
     - Can be easily understood
     - Can be measured
   - Set targets for each criterion.
4. **Assessing the outcome and maintaining improvement.** This includes:
   - Comparing results with targets
   - Reviewing and discussing how improvements could be made
   - Implementing changes
   - Re-auditing.

Careful thought needs to be given to the choice of area to audit, as it should be:

- Amenable to measurement
- Commonly encountered
- Have room for improvement in performance.

As auditing involves significant costs, it might also be relevant to consider whether the topic is financially significant to the practice and/or animal owner. An example of an audit planning sheet for a small animal practice can be found at the end of this chapter.

Data acquisition

In order to carry out the clinical audit process, in all but the smallest of practices the clinical records will need to be computerized; in the vast majority of small animal practices in the UK they already are. Every practice management system (PMS) will have some system whereby data can be searched under specific criteria and matching records recalled. Some systems are much more sophisticated than others in the manner in which information can be coded when it is entered and then retrieved. This should be considered when a new PMS is being purchased (see Chapter 4) but most of the time it is necessary to manage with the system that is already in place, and often with retrospective data that have already been entered.

KEY POINT

The ability of a PMS to record and handle data for clinical audit purposes should be investigated whenever changing or upgrading a practice computer system.

The clinical audit process will usually involve recalling animals of a particular species (and possibly age) that either have a particular condition (e.g. dogs with chronic nephritis) or have had a specific procedure carried out (e.g. blood pressure measurement). With most PMSs the recall of procedures is straightforward because it is usually possible to search for a procedure or fee that has been associated with them. Searching retrospectively for patients with specific diseases can be more troublesome unless a standardized recording nomenclature or coding system is used to tag them at the time of entry. A veterinary version of the SNOMED medical coding system, called VeNom, has been developed for that purpose (see www.venomcoding.org). The problem with searching for a term entered into a clinical record without such a system is that the same disease may be described in several different ways, or accidentally misspelt. For example, unless a practice has a very disciplined use of terminology, chronic nephritis may also be entered as kidney failure, CIN or renal failure. In such instances it is possible to search for a variety of terms using an 'or' function, or to search for products that are likely to be associated with treating the condition, such as renal diets or ACE inhibitors for chronic nephritis. If the audit is to be prospective, it is usually possible to attach a code or zero-priced product to a case as it is written up to indicate a specific diagnosis; these can usually also be used to print out information for clients or staff that may be of use for reinforcing guidelines or advice.

Data can also be collected by setting specific questions in the PMS to be asked of the clinician for certain procedures. For example, a fixed set of questions could be asked at each postoperative check. The responses on the system could be put into a spreadsheet such as Excel, or into another data file type, such as csv. The data can be interrogated later, giving an instant count of cases seen and a proportion of wound problems of various types, and allow easy linking, for example to different suture patterns and whether protection collars were used, depending on the questions asked. If clinician details and procedure are recorded, a more detailed investigation of anomalies would be possible if necessary. Otherwise, results can be compared with previous years or target benchmarks in real time. In the absence of a computer system, notes could be recorded in writing where this is easier, but analysis of the data will be very time-consuming.

Statistical significance

Figure 28.11 considers the differences between research and clinical audit. Statistical significance is important in a scientific experiment: a control group has to be formed; the numbers involved have to be large enough to be statistically significant; and ideally there will be some form of 'blinding' to minimize bias. Trying to design an audit along these lines, however, will usually result in failure.

This difference is also reflected in the way in which the data generated by an audit should be viewed. If viewed as scientific data and standard tests are applied, it is usually very difficult to measure a statistically significant difference between outcomes before and then after changes were put in place. However, if data are viewed as performance indicators and, where appropriate, investigated qualitatively in more depth, logical actions can be based upon these results. They cannot be 'proven' to be scientifically valid and thus generalizable, but once their effect has been measured with a further review of the audit cycle, they can be used sensibly to guide actions in an informed manner.

Research	Clinical audit
Creates new knowledge	Tests care given against knowledge gained
Generally is based on a hypothesis	Measures against criteria
May involve 'experiments' on animals	Should never involve anything beyond clinical management
May need 'ethical' approval	Abides by an ethical framework but does not usually require ethical approval
May involve random allocation to different treatment groups, including placebo	Never involves random allocation or the use of placebo
Usually carried out on a large scale over a prolonged period of time	Usually carried out on a relatively small number of cases over a short time span
Rigorous methodology; power calculations for sample sizes, statistical tests, etc.	Different methodology from research; less need for large sample sizes and statistical significance
Results are generalizable and hence may be published; aimed at influencing the activities of clinical practice as a whole	Results are only relevant locally, influencing activities of local clinicians and teams. The audit process may be of interest to a wider audience and hence audits should be published

28.11 Differentiating clinical audit from research.

An example of a clinical audit

A veterinary hospital has quite a few diabetic cats on its records. The practice is concerned that once stabilized, many of the patients go 'off the radar' and their progress is not monitored regularly. They discuss this at one of their regular clinical effectiveness meetings and decide they would like to use the clinical audit process to try and improve this. They set up an audit team consisting of one of their vets who has a particular interest in feline medicine, the head nurse, and the head receptionist.

The team considers the issue and agrees that feline diabetes is a suitable area for audit because it is important, common, and the practice has plenty of room to improve its performance. They discuss the various approaches to the issue – such as measuring outcomes in terms of blood fructosamine levels a certain time after diagnosis to see if they are within an acceptable range – but decide that a simple process audit that aims to ensure that all cats diagnosed with diabetes receive at least a 3-monthly check and blood test is sufficient. They agree to go away and examine the evidence base for the frequency of blood testing in diabetic cats and to carry out a retrospective audit of those patients to find out how many are already complying with 3-monthly physical examination and testing.

The team searches the existing database, using the prescribing of insulin as the key to identifying cases, because they do not use oral treatments for diabetes in cats and have no way of coding the diagnoses set up on their system. They pull out the data and find that only 15% of diabetic cats have had a blood test and physical examination within 3 months of the previous one, although 33% have had them after 6 months.

The full clinical effectiveness group meets again to discuss the results and to plan how to take the audit forwards. They agree that although there are no national benchmarks for comparison, the figures leave plenty of room for improvement, so they decide to set a target of 70% of cats to receive a physical examination and blood test within 6 months of the previous one: this is the criterion that they have set, and it is a 'yes' or 'no' criterion. This is a *process audit* as it measures what is being done; an audit that measured, for example, fructosamine levels would be an *outcome audit*.

The group decides that creating a product code on the computer entitled 'diabetes mellitus' would make it easier to track these cases more accurately, and they discuss guidelines that they could put into place to improve concordance. They decide there is a need for increasing the awareness of what needs to be done internally via a series of practice meetings including the front desk staff, who are recognized as having an important role in translating a veterinary recommendation into a booking for a procedure. It is also decided to hand out written advice to owners of all relevant cats, reinforcing the need for regular monitoring and stressing the potentially severe consequences of allowing diabetes to remain improperly controlled.

The meeting after the next 6-month audit period showed an increase in the number of patients that had met the criterion: from 33% to 60%. This was thought to be satisfactory but, in view of the target that had previously been set, it was decided to see if this could be improved further. Awareness of the guidelines was reinforced amongst the whole clinical team every month, and the product on the computer was used to generate a reminder 3 months after the previous visit, that was followed up with a phone call from a veterinary nurse.

At the third audit meeting after another 6 months, the concordance rate had risen to 72%. The extra income from the procedures carried out more than compensated for the time and effort involved, and it was considered that the process had brought significant health benefits to their patients, since many cats had had their insulin regimen adjusted as a result.

Summary

This Manual has covered the framework of skills, structures and procedures that need to be in place to support the clinical activities of the staff working in a practice. A veterinary business cannot function without at least some of them, and to varying degrees each practice will already have many of them in place, but it can be guaranteed that even the best run practice will be able to make significant improvements to its performance. Whilst clinical expertise is undoubtedly important, there is often a tendency for the profession to underestimate the role that all the supporting competencies play in optimizing clinical outcomes, which surely must be the ultimate goal of every veterinary surgeon. This final chapter has drawn together the threads that can be found within this Manual and has looked at practical guidance to assist practitioners to improve their clinical governance procedures and enhance their patient and client outcomes. A sample clinical governance policy is given at the end of the chapter, and more guidance can be found in the supporting guidance to the RCVS Code of Professional Conduct, and for members at www.bsava.com.

References and further reading

American Animal Hospital Association. AAHA guidelines. (available at www.aahanet.org)

Cockcroft P and Holmes M (2003) *Handbook of Evidence-Based Veterinary Medicine*. Blackwell, Oxford

Day MJ, Horzinek MC and Schultz RD (2010) Guidelines for the vaccination of dogs and cats compiled by the Vaccination Guidelines Group (VGG) of the World Small Animal Veterinary Association (WSAVA). *Journal of Small Animal Practice* **51**(6), e1–e32 [editorial]

Feline Advisory Bureau (2009) Clinical protocols. *Journal of Feline Medicine and Surgery,* **11** (also available at www.fabvets.org)

Olivry T, de Boer DJ, Favrot C *et al.* (2010) Treatment of canine atopic dermatitis: 2010 clinical practice guidelines from the International Task Force on Canine Atopic Dermatitis. *Veterinary Dermatology* **21**, 233–248

Viner B (2005) Clinical audit in veterinary practice – the story so far. *In Practice* **27**, 215–218

Viner B (2009) Using audit to improve clinical effectiveness. *In Practice* **31**, 240–243

Viner B (2010) Clinical effectiveness: what does it mean for practitioners – and cats? *Journal of Feline Medicine and Surgery* **12**, 561–568

Viner B (2010) *Success in Veterinary Practice: Maximising Clinical Outcomes and Personal Well-Being*. Wiley-Blackwell, Oxford

Examples of practice policy, clinical audit and critical accident report 

Practice Policy on Clinical Governance

The RCVS Code of Professional Conduct requires that veterinary surgeons must ensure that clinical governance forms part of their professional activities. We support delivery of the best care to our patients.

We will:

- Organize regular clinical discussion meetings for the practice team
- Record minutes of clinical meetings and review any action points at future meetings
- Follow up any clinical issues arising from meetings and case discussions
- Make changes as a result of discussions and monitor these changes to ensure they are effective
- Organize online discussion forums to discuss clinical cases where geography or part-time working make face-to-face meetings difficult
- Have a system in place where all clinical staff can put items on the agenda for clinical meetings
- Have a system whereby ad hoc case discussions between vets can be recorded and so followed up
- Try to include all clinical staff in meetings
- Communicate results of meetings to those staff unable to attend
- In case of any significant event (e.g. unexpected medical or surgical complications, serious complaint, accident or anaesthetic death), hold a no-blame meeting of all staff involved, as soon as possible after the incident, and record all the details
- At the significant event meeting consider what, if anything, could have been done to avoid the incident, and what changes can be made in procedure following the meeting
- Communicate changes in procedure to the whole practice team
- Monitor any changes in procedure
- Organize practice team discussions on guidelines or protocols used in practice
- Organize regular clinical clubs or journal clubs
- Look at the evidence base for common treatment protocols used in the practice and revise these as a result if necessary
- Record the results of common procedures
- Audit the results of clinical procedures of interest to the practice team
- Ensure that individuals feed back interesting information from CPD courses to the rest of the practice team
- Incorporate information learned at CPD courses into practice protocols where appropriate
- Encourage CPD for all vets, nurses and clinical support staff
- Maintain access to suitable up-to-date reference material
- Ensure that information on new veterinary products or new pieces of equipment is communicated to all the clinical team
- Ensure that new members of clinical staff have access to any practice guidelines, protocols or clinical discussion meeting notes, so that they are aware of relevant clinical issues in the practice
- Ensure that any locum veterinary surgeons are aware of practice guidelines and protocols at the earliest opportunity
- Ensure continuity of care for patients by having effective systems of case handovers between vets
- Have effective means of communicating with clients, e.g. newsletters, websites
- Monitor and take note of feedback from clients
- Ensure that the public are aware of the identity of members of staff
- Have protocols known to all relevant staff for dealing with members of the public
- Follow the complaints procedure
- Record all complaints received and the responses to the clients
- Have effective communication systems within the practice and with clients
- Have a performance review system in place for all clinical staff to monitor and plan development

Individual Veterinary Surgeons and Registered Veterinary Nurses will:

- Keep up to date with CPD requirements relevant to the work done
- Communicate information learned at CPD courses to professional colleagues
- Discuss cases with professional colleagues
- Participate in practice clinical meetings
- Give a prompt honest account of any significant events, e.g. unexpected medical or surgical complications, serious complaint, accident or anaesthetic death
- Reflect on results of procedures or clinical cases
- Look at the evidence base for treatment and nursing protocols used
- Make any changes necessary as a result of reflection or searching the evidence base
- Keep up to date with new drugs and equipment used in practice
- Communicate details of any ongoing cases to other vets, nurses and all clinical support staff
- On moving to a new branch, or acting as a locum, ensure awareness of practice guidelines and protocols, and ensure competence in using all necessary equipment, computer systems, etc.
- Communicate honestly and courteously with clients
- Not act outside their own professional competence
- Consult with more experienced or better qualified colleagues when unsure about a case
- Refer cases, or offer referral as an option to the client when appropriate

An example of a clinical governance policy. (Courtesy of Pam Mosedale and Carole Clarke)

PLANNING A CLINICAL AUDIT

This form is to help you to plan your clinical audit project. It is possible that you will not be able to fill in all the details immediately but the aim of the questions is to prompt you to consider all elements that, when put together, make a good quality project.
You will find guidance for completion of this form on the next page.

PROJECT TITLE: (see Note 1)

Project Team: (see Note 2)

Project manager:	
Members of audit team	Role

Background:
What is prompting you to look at this topic?
Why do you think this is a priority area for action?
What benefits for patients do you hope to bring about by doing this audit?
What resources do you need to carry out the audit?
Are you content that these resources will be available to you?

Objectives: (see Note 3)
Will you be introducing new guidelines? If so attach them on a separate sheet.
Criteria: (see Note 3)
Targets: (see Note 3)

Data collection: (see Note 4)
Audit population
How will you identify the relevant population within your practice management system?
What criteria will you use to select your population?
Have you run a data search to identify the numbers involved?
Will you be using your whole data population or a subset? (If the latter, how will you select them?)
What time period will be audited: Start date: End date:
Data collection method (one or more): (see Note 5)
Prospective data collection:
Retrospective search of data on file:
Patient/staff questionnaire:
Further details
or other method:
Do you intend to run a pilot or baseline audit?

Timescale:
Proposed start of data collection:
Proposed date for presentation of results:
To whom?
Proposals for repeat audit:

PTO

An example of a format for planning a clinical audit. (Adapted from an original document courtesy of Carole Clarke.) (continues) ▶

Notes to help you complete your Clinical Audit Plan

1. **Project name**
   A short name for the project that can easily be fitted on to reports and presentations, e.g. 'Screening for hypertension in elderly cats'.

2. **Members of project team**
   To make your project work you should involve:
   - A project manager, who should ideally have a particular interest in the area being audited
   - Representatives of all the staff groups who deliver the aspect of care being audited
   - Key staff who will be involved in implementing any changes identified as necessary to address shortfalls revealed by the audit results.

Ideally include them in the audit team – as a minimum, make sure the senior staff are aware of the project, and willing to cooperate with the action plan.

3. **Objectives, Guidelines, Criteria and Targets**
   - The **Objectives** start with a broad statement or question describing your overall goal (e.g. 'To identify hypertensive cats as early as possible, and before serious sequelae develop by introducing guidelines to encourage better screening of the at-risk population') and should then be broken down into a series of smaller steps.
   - How are you going to bring about an improvement in performance? It will usually involve the introduction of new or revised **Guidelines** to encourage better patient care. Consider how these guidelines will be drawn up and introduced effectively. They will need to be appended to the audit form before you begin your audit.
   - Decide what you will measure to gauge the effect of your intervention. These will be one or more **Criteria** and you need to define them carefully so that they are relevant to your outcome and easily measurable, e.g. 'We will be measuring the proportion of cats diagnosed with renal disease, diabetes mellitus and hyperthyroidism that have their blood pressure measured within one week of diagnosis'.
   - You will need to set some sort of **Target** for your intervention. In human medicine there are many externally set standards against which medical teams can benchmark themselves but except for postoperative complications of neutering (see www.vetaudit.co.uk), very few data exist within the veterinary profession. You may simply estimate what you think a realistic target should be; you may consult with your colleagues to see if they have carried out a similar audit; or you may make a baseline measurement of your current performance and see what improvement you are able to bring about.

4. **Audit sample:**
   - Be careful not to confuse audit with research. Your figures will only be performance indicators so do not need the statistical rigour of a scientific study.
   - As a guide, 20 to 50 cases are usually sufficient to show how well targets are being met.
   - In many veterinary practices finding enough cases may be a problem, but for common conditions or large group practices sampling strategies could include:
     - Taking a random sample of patients seen within your audit timeframe
     - Restricting the timeframe (e.g. all patients seen last month)
     - Choosing (for example) 'the first 20 patients after' or 'the last 30 patients before' a specified date.

5. **Data collection method:**
   - The best method will be dependent on your audit topic and whether the data items you need are already recorded routinely or not.
   - Piloting your data collection method and analysis makes sure your questions are clear and unambiguous and that you can get the information you need. You then have a chance to amend your form as necessary before it is used on the full audit sample.

(continued) An example of a format for planning a clinical audit.

CASE CONTROL QUESTIONNAIRE

Instructions

This form must be completed for ALL perioperative DEATHS (i.e. occurring within 24 hours of termination of a procedure) whether under sedation or anaesthesia by the Veterinary Surgeon performing the procedure.

It should be completed and returned within one week of perioperative fatality.

Section A: Patient's details

1. Owner name: ....

   Patient name: ....

   Address: ....

   ....

2. Please state the patient's species: ❑ Dog ❑ Cat ❑ Exotic (please specify species)
3. What was the patient's BREED? ....
4. Please state the sex of the patient: ❑ Male ❑ Female ❑ Not known

   ❑ Entire ❑ Neutered ❑ Not known
5. What was the patient's age? .... years .... months

   What was the patient's weight? .... kg
6. In your opinion was the patient overweight? ❑ Yes ❑ No
7. What type of case was this? ❑ Primary ❑ Referred
8. Did the patient have any other GENERAL ANAESTHETICS in the last month? ❑ Yes ❑ No

   If YES, please specify the number of GAs: ❑ 1 ❑ 2 ❑ 3 or more
9. Did the patient have any other SEDATION in the last month? ❑ Yes ❑ No ❑ Not known

   If YES, please specify the number of sedations: ❑ 1 ❑ 2 ❑ 3 or more

Section B: Personnel details

10. Name of the Veterinary Surgeon responsible: ....

    How familiar were they with the anaesthetic/sedation used? ❑ Very familiar ❑ Familiar ❑ Unfamiliar

    How familiar were they with the procedure? ❑ Very familiar ❑ Familiar ❑ Unfamiliar
11. Please give the name(s) of the person(s) assisting in monitoring the patient ....

    Is this the same person who undertook the procedure? (**Q10**) ❑ Yes; please go to **Q12** ❑ No

    How familiar were they with the anaesthetic/sedation used? ❑ Very familiar ❑ Familiar ❑ Unfamiliar

    Please state their qualifications: .... Year of qualifying: ....

    Are they: ❑ Vet ❑ Listed or Registered VN ❑ Student VN ❑ Nursing Assistant

    ❑ Other, please specify: ....
12. Were there any OTHER persons involved in the procedure? ❑ Yes ❑ No

    If YES, please state their Name: ....

    Were they a vet or a nurse? ❑ Vet ❑ Listed VN ❑ VN Assistant

    ❑ Other, please specify: ....

    What were they doing? Please specify: ....

Section C: Preoperative evaluation

13. Preoperatively were there any ongoing medical conditions (e.g. heart failure, renal disease, etc.)?

    ❑ Yes ❑ No; please go to **Q14** ❑ Not known

An example of a critical accident report form for a perioperative fatality. (Adapted from original document courtesy of Goddard Veterinary Group) (continues) ▶

If YES, please specify the type of illness and current treatment:

- ❑ Respiratory/cardiac ......
- ❑ Liver/kidney ......
- ❑ Other, please specify: ......

14. In the opinion of the veterinary surgeon, PREoperatively what anaesthetic risk group would you classify the patient as?
    - ❑ Class 1 – fit and healthy, no systemic disease
    - ❑ Class 2 – mild to moderate systemic disease only, e.g. skin tumour, chronic arthritis, fracture without shock
    - ❑ Class 3 – severe systemic disease, showing clinical signs or limiting activity but not incapacitating, e.g. moderate hypovolaemia, anaemia, pyrexia or heart failure
    - ❑ Class 4 – severe systemic disease that is constant threat to life, e.g. severe uraemia, toxaemia, hypovolaemia or heart failure
    - ❑ Class 5 – moribund patient that is not expected to survive 24 hours with or without the procedure, e.g. extreme sepsis/shock

    In light of any information gained from undertaking the procedure, POSToperatively would you give the patient the same anaesthetic risk class?

    ❑ Yes ❑ No, revised anaesthetic risk: ......

15. Was a preoperative clinical examination performed by a veterinary surgeon? ❑ Yes ❑ No

    Please briefly describe any significant clinical findings: ......

    ......

16. Were haematological or biochemical blood tests performed preoperatively? ❑ Yes ❑ No

    If YES, please specify any significant findings: ......

    ......

    ......

17. Were thoracic or abdominal radiographs taken perioperatively? ❑ Yes ❑ No

    If YES, please specify the radiographs taken and any significant findings: ......

    ......

    ......

18. Were any other tests performed preoperatively (e.g. ECG, ultrasound, urine analysis)? ❑ Yes ❑ No

    If YES, please specify the tests performed and any significant results ......

    ......

    ......

19. Was the patient starved prior to the procedure? ❑ Yes ❑ No ❑ Not known

    If YES, for how long? ...... (hours)

20. Was water withheld prior to the procedure? ❑ Yes ❑ No ❑ Not known

    If YES, for how long ...... (hours)

Section D: Procedure details

21. Date of admission ....../....../...... Time of admission (24 hour clock): ...... : ......
22. Date of procedure ....../....../...... Time of admission (24 hour clock): ...... : ......
23. Please classify the procedure type
    - ❑ Emergency – requiring immediate surgery on admission
    - ❑ Urgent – operation required within the next 24 hours
    - ❑ Scheduled/Elective – a procedure not requiring attention within the next 24hrs
24. What procedure was intended? ......

    Was this the procedure performed? ❑ Yes ❑ No

(continued) An example of a critical accident report form for a perioperative fatality. (Adapted from original document courtesy of Goddard Veterinary Group) (continues)

If NO, please briefly describe why the intended procedure was not carried out and what procedure was performed instead (if any).

....

....

25. In the opinion of the surgeon, what was the anticipated risk of death from the procedure?

❑ Minimal risk ❑ Low risk ❑ Moderate risk ❑ High risk

26. In the opinion of the surgeon, how difficult was the procedure that was performed?

❑ Simple ❑ Moderate ❑ Difficult ❑ Very difficult

27. Where did the procedure take place?

❑ Theatre ❑ Prep room ❑ Consulting room ❑ Other ....

28. At which practice premises was the procedure performed?

....

29. What was the patient's main body position during the procedure?

❑ Dorsal recumbency ❑ Left lateral recumbency ❑ Right lateral recumbency ❑ Sternal recumbency

❑ Multiple positions – please describe briefly:..

Section E: Anaesthetic drugs and sedatives administered

30. For the procedure undertaken did the patient receive sedation only or general anaesthesia?

❑ General anaesthesia (defined as complete unconsciousness, allowing ET intubation if required) – please now go to **Q31**

❑ Sedation (defined as chemical restraint without unconsciousness, ET intubation would not be possible) – please now go to **Q32**

31. Was any premedication given prior to anaesthesia? ❑ Yes ❑ No; please go to **Q32**

If YES, what drugs were given?

Drug name	Dose	Concentration	Route given	Time given

What was the effect of premedication?

❑ No effect ❑ Light sedation – patient calm but still alert

❑ Moderate sedation – patient quiet, able to walk, some ataxia

❑ Heavy sedation – patient recumbent, difficult to rouse ❑ Unconsciousness

32. Were any INJECTABLE drugs given for INDUCTION or MAINTENANCE of anaesthesia or sedation (other than premedication recorded in **Q31**)?

❑ Yes ❑ No; please go to **Q33**

If YES, what drugs were given?

Drug name	Dose	Concentration	Route given	Time given

What was the effect of sedation or anaesthesia?

❑ No effect ❑ Light sedation – patient calm but still alert

❑ Moderate sedation – patient quiet, able to walk, some ataxia

❑ Heavy sedation – patient recumbent, difficult to rouse ❑ Unconsciousness

(continued) An example of a critical accident report form for a perioperative fatality. (Adapted from original document courtesy of Goddard Veterinary Group) (continues) ▶

What was the quality of induction of sedation/anaesthesia?

❑ Good – smooth ❑ Moderate ❑ Poor

33. Was an INHALATIONAL anaesthetic used? ❑ Yes ❑ No; please go to **Q34**

If YES, what was used? ❑ Isoflurane ❑ Other, please specify.................................

When was the inhalational agent given? ❑ Induction only ❑ Maintenance only ❑ Both induction and maintenance

34. Was the patient's airway intubated? ❑ Yes ❑ No; please go to **Q35**

If YES, was it a cuffed or uncuffed tube? ❑ Cuffed ❑ Uncuffed ❑ Tube type and size ....

Was local anaesthetic used to desensitize the larynx? ❑ Yes ❑ No ❑ Not known

Was the GA machine checked fully prior to procedure? ❑ Yes ❑ No ❑ Not known

35. Was oxygen supplied during the procedure? ❑ Yes ❑ No

36. Was nitrous oxide supplied during the procedure? ❑ Yes ❑ No

37. Was an anaesthetic circuit used during the procedure? ❑ Yes ❑ No

If YES, what system was used (please specify)?.................................

Was the patient on a heat mat or was a heat source used? ❑ Yes ❑ No ❑ Not known

38. What type of ventilation was mainly used? ❑ Spontaneous breathing ❑ Positive pressure ventilation

39. Were any ANALGESICS or OTHER DRUGS administered PERIoperatively?

❑ Yes ❑ No (excluding those given and recorded during premedication, **Q32**)

If YES, what analgesics or other drugs were given?

Drug name	Dose	Concentration	Route given	Time given

40. Was an intravenous catheter placed PERIoperatively? ❑ Yes ❑ No

41. Were fluids administered PERIoperatively? ❑ Yes ❑ No

If YES, please state the type of fluids:.................... Rate:.................... ml/h

When were they given? (please tick all appropriate) ❑ Preoperatively ❑ During the procedure ❑ Postoperatively

By which route? ❑ Intravenous ❑ Subcutaneous ❑ Other:....................

Section F: Monitoring of anaesthesia and sedation

42. Who monitored the patient?

❑ Operating Vet ❑ Separate Vet ❑ Registered or Listed VN ❑ Student VN ❑ Nursing Assistant

What other duties was this person doing at the time?.................................

43. Is there a written record of the anaesthetic? ❑ Yes; please attach a copy of the anaesthetic record ❑ No

44. What methods of monitoring were used during the procedure?

❑ Body temperature

❑ Finger on pulse: ❑ Peripheral ❑ Central

❑ Pulse oximeter ❑ Capnography ❑ Inhaled gases

❑ Observation of breathing/reservoir bag ❑ Respiratory rate monitor

❑ Oesophageal/standard stethoscope ❑ Electrocardiogram

❑ Arterial blood pressure – direct method

❑ Arterial blood pressure – indirect method (e.g. Doppler, DINAMAP)

❑ Other, please specify:.................................

(continued) An example of a critical accident report form for a perioperative fatality. (Adapted from original document courtesy of Goddard Veterinary Group) (continues) ▶

Section G: Recovery from anaesthesia and sedation

45. Time of termination of the procedure (24 hour clock): .... : ....

46. Duration of anaesthesia or sedation (in minutes): ....

47. Was a reversal agent given at the end of the procedure? ❑ Yes ❑ No

If YES, what drug was given?...Dose: ....mg

48. Please give the approximate time from termination of the procedure until the patient reached the following:

Sternal recumbency: ....Min Standing: ....Min

49. What was the quality of recovery?

❑ Good – smooth ❑ Moderate – minimal excitement ❑ Poor – very violent, fitting etc

50. Where was the patient placed to recover? ❑ Ward kennel/cage ❑ Theatre

❑ Prep room ❑ ICU ❑ Other, please specify:...

51. Was the patient observed during recovery? ❑ Yes ❑ No

If YES, who observed the recovery? ❑ Vet ❑ Listed or Registered VN ❑ Student VN ❑ Nursing Assistant

❑ Other, please specify: ....

How often was the patient checked whilst recovering? ❑ Continuously ❑ Every 5 minutes ❑ Every 10 minute

❑ Other, please specify: ....

52. Was the patient's temperature taken on recovery? ❑ Yes ❑ No If YES what was it? ....°C

53. Were there any NON-FATAL serious perioperative complications (e.g. collapse, hypotension, respiratory obstruction or depression, pulmonary aspiration, fitting, or any problems with ET intubation)?

❑ Yes ❑ No; please go to **Q54**

If YES, when did this occur? ❑ After premedication ❑ During the procedure ❑ On recovery

What type of complication(s) occurred and what were the treatment and outcome (please specify)?

❑ CNS (e.g. fitting): ....

❑ Cardiopulmonary: ....

❑ Other, please specify: ....

Section H: Fatality details Please complete this section for a DEATH/EUTHANASIA only

54. In the opinion of the veterinary surgeon, was the fatility:

❑ Solely as a result of anaesthesia or sedation? ❑ Primarily as a result of anaesthesia or sedation?

❑ Only partly as a result of anaesthesia or sedation? ❑ Not part of GA, e.g. haemorrhage?

55. When did the patient die? Time................ : ....(24 hour clock) Date: ..../.........../.........

Was this: ❑ After premed ❑ During sedation/anaesthesia ❑ On recovery

56. Where did the patient die?

❑ Theatre ❑ Prep room ❑ Ward kennel/cage ❑ Home ❑ Other: ....

57. Did the patient show any abnormal clinical signs, just prior to death? ❑ Yes ❑ No

If yes, please specify: ....

58. Was there an ECG on the patient at the time of death? ❑ Yes ❑ No

If YES, what did the ECG indicate?...

59. Was any procedure being performed around the time of death? ❑ Yes ❑ No

If YES, please specify ....

60. If applicable, what was the vaporizer setting and O_2 just before the complication? ....

61. Was cardiopulmonary resuscitation carried out? ❑ Yes ❑ No

(continued) An example of a critical accident report form for a perioperative fatality. (Adapted from original document courtesy of Goddard Veterinary Group) (continues) ▶

Also what drugs were given?

Drug name	Dose	Concentration	Route given	Time given

Outcome:..

62. If the patient died during the recovery period, did it receive O_2? ☐ Yes ☐ No

    Did the patient receive thermal support? ☐ Yes ☐ No

    What monitoring was carried out during recovery?..

63. What was the cause of death? (please specify)

    ☐ Cardiac complications:..

    ☐ Respiratory complications:..

    ☐ Renal/liver complications:...

    ☐ Other:..

    ☐ Unknown

64. Was a post-mortem examination performed? ☐ Yes ☐ No

    If YES, what were the findings?...

65. On reflection, what would you have done differently?..

    ....

    ....

Section I: Veterinary Surgeon Responsible for Case

Veterinary Surgeon responsible for case:..

Branch:...

Signature:..

Date:...

Thank you very much for completing this questionnaire.

Section J: Any further comments

....

....

....

....

....

....

....

....

....

....

(continued) An example of a critical accident report form for a perioperative fatality. (Adapted from original document courtesy of Goddard Veterinary Group)

Index

Page numbers in *italics* indicate figures

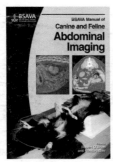

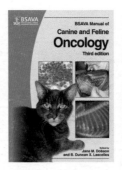

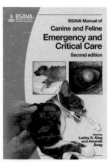

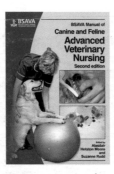

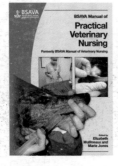

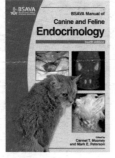

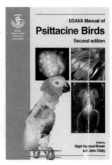

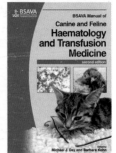

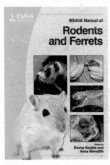

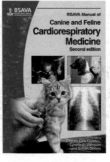

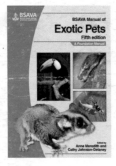

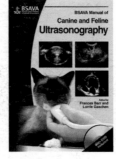

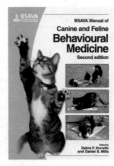

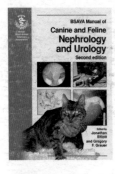

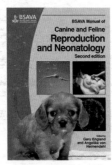

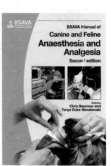

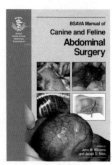

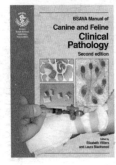

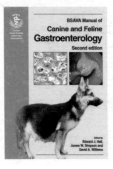

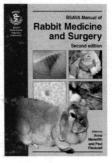

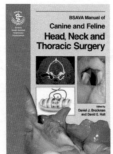

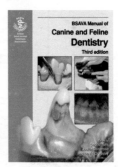

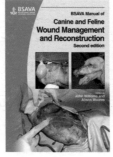

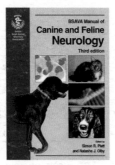

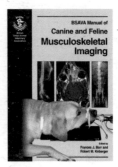